W9-APS-062

(THE NUTRiBASE COMPLETE)

BOOK OF FOOD COUNTS

DR. ART ULENE

Avery Publishing Group
Garden City Park, New York

The information in this book is based upon the latest data made available by government agencies, food manufacturers, and trade associations. It is important to note that all nutrient breakdowns for processed foods are subject to change by manufacturers without notice and may therefore vary from printing to printing.

ISBN 0-89529-667-5

Printed in the United States of America

10   9   8   7   6

CONTENTS

INTRODUCTION

For thousands of years, people have recognized the life-sustaining nature of food. But only during the last four or five decades have we begun to understand the many ways in which our choices of foods can affect the quality of our health and the length of our life. And only during the last four or five years have we really begun to appreciate how profound the effects of those choices can be.

Now we know that some of the so-called "inevitable" diseases like atherosclerosis, osteoporosis, and even cancer are often the consequence of poor nutritional choices. Research has clearly shown the relationship between poor nutritional intake and many of these diseases. The studies prove that high-fat diets can—and often do—contribute to the development of coronary heart disease; that excessive sodium intake can cause hypertension; and that low fiber intake may increase the risk of colon cancer. The list of nutrition-related conditions goes on and on.

But there is also a hopeful side to this story. New studies have clearly demonstrated the positive effects that good nutritional choices can have on our health. Coronary heart disease can be prevented—even reversed—through dietary changes. The incidence of cancer can be reduced with diets that are low in fat and high in fruits and vegetables. Blood pressure can be lowered with sodium restriction. The list of health-promoting nutritional interventions is lengthy, and constantly growing.

THE NEW NUTRITION

Modern research studies are giving rise to a "new" nutrition, one that is both scientifically sound and practical. The new nutrition differs from the old in at least two important ways. First, the old nutrition dealt in generalities, such as the four food groups, and created minimum recommendations designed to prevent deficiency-related disorders. The new nutrition seeks to achieve optimal levels of health, and creates specific recommendations based on individual differences, such as age, sex, lifestyle, and medical factors. Second, the old nutrition left many nutritional decisions up to the health professionals and food marketers, while the new nutrition puts you in control. It empowers you with the information necessary to evaluate confusing and conflicting claims, and enables you to reject foods that do not meet your nutritional needs and goals.

This book is designed to provide you with that empowering information. Use this book to learn more about the foods you should consume—or avoid—so you can meet your particular nutritional needs. Don't be intimidated by the huge number of choices listed or by the impossible-to-memorize nutritional value numbers that accompany the lists. It is not necessary to memorize these numbers. Instead, just try to familiarize yourself with the foods and food categories that are best suited to your needs. Begin by looking up the foods that you eat most often or in the largest quantities. If these foods are not providing you with the nutrients you need, use the book to find better alternatives that are just as tasty. Once you are familiar with the nutritional content of your most common food choices, gradually look up the remainder of the foods in your diet. You'll be surprised by how easy it is to learn about these foods and to make any necessary changes.

As you take more control over the foods you are eating and put more thought into your choices, keep in mind that good nutrition is just one element of a healthy lifestyle. To achieve maximum benefits from the new nutrition, your life should be filled with physical activity and free of cigarette smoke and other toxic substances. In addition, the stress in your life should be under control. Even the best diet can't overcome the problems caused by smoking, immoderate use of alcohol, poorly managed stress, and other health-compromising habits.

Finally, keep in mind that research is constantly adding to our knowledge of nutrition, and, in the process, changing some of our beliefs. As best you can, try to keep up with the new information and, when appropriate, make whatever dietary changes are necessary. But also be skeptical about nutritional news that seems too good to be true. (More often than not, it *isn't* true.) Be wary of nutritional claims made by people who are trying to sell you something. And be cautious—don't make any drastic changes in your nutritional program without first talking to a health professional who is knowledgeable about nutrition and about your particular medical circumstances.

The following section will explain some of the basics of nutrition. After that, you will learn how to locate the information you need to improve your diet.

A QUICK LOOK AT THE BASIC NUTRIENTS

Water, carbohydrates, proteins, and fats are the basic building blocks of a healthy diet. Each works in different ways to fuel the body, to build and repair the cells which make up the body, and to provide the environment in which the cells live.

Water

The human body is two-thirds water by weight. Indeed, water is an essential nutrient that is involved in every function of the body. It helps transport nutrients and waste products in and out of cells. It is necessary for all digestive, absorption, circulatory, and excretory functions, and for the utilization of the water-soluble vitamins. And it is needed to maintain proper body temperature.

Carbohydrates

Carbohydrates provide the body with the energy it needs to function. There are two different types of carbohydrates, generally referred to as "simple" and "complex." Sugars such as glucose, fructose (fruit sugar), and sucrose (table sugar) are examples of simple carbohydrates. Starch, on the other hand, is a complex carbohydrate.

One type of complex carbohydrate you may have heard a good deal about is fiber. Referred to in the past as roughage, fiber is actually the part of plant materials that our body cannot digest. Yet, fiber is known to perform a number of important functions. It promotes feelings of fullness; prevents constipation, hemorrhoids, and other intestinal problems; and may reduce the risk of developing colon cancer. In addition, fiber may help lower blood cholesterol levels, reducing the risk of heart disease. (To learn about the difference between crude fiber and dietary fiber, see page xiii.)

Proteins

Protein is essential for growth and development. It provides the body with energy, and is needed for the manufacture of hormones, antibodies, enzymes, and muscle tissues. It also helps maintain the proper acid-alkali balance.

Fats

Recently, much attention has been focused on the need to reduce dietary fat. Nevertheless, the body does need fats—but only the right fats, and only in appropriate quantities. Specifically, it needs fatty acids, which perform a variety of vital bodily functions. Fatty acids carry the fat-soluble vitamins. They are essential for growth and development, and they provide the body with energy.

Most of us are now aware that there are several kinds of dietary fat—saturated, polyunsaturated, and monounsaturated—and that some are better than others. To understand the difference between these three fats, it is helpful to first learn a little about cholesterol.

Cholesterol is a white, waxy substance found in all foods that come from animal sources. Cholesterol is essential to our well-being, as it helps to build cell membranes, to produce hormones, and to manufacture bile acids. The liver is capable of manufacturing all of the cholesterol needed for good health.

Cholesterol manufactured by the liver is carried through the bloodstream by LDLs (low-density lipoproteins). High levels of LDLs in the bloodstream can result in clogged arteries, causing stroke or heart disease. This is why LDL is referred to as the "bad" cholesterol. Fortunately, in many people, LDL levels can be reduced through proper diet.

HDLs (high-density lipoproteins) carry excess cholesterol from different body tissues to the liver, where it is converted to bile acids and then eliminated through the intestines. High levels of HDLs are linked with a decreased risk of coronary heart disease. This is why HDL is often called the "good" cholesterol. To a limited extent, HDL levels can be raised through regular exercise.

How are the three types of fat related to cholesterol? *Saturated fats*—which come from animal foods like meat, fish, and cheese, as well as from palm, coconut, and palm kernel oil—have been shown to increase total blood cholesterol, especially the undesirable LDL portion. *Polyunsaturated fats*—found mainly in vegetable oils like corn, sunflower, safflower, and soybean—tend to lower levels of both HDL and LDL. *Monounsaturated fats*—found in vegetable and nut oils such as olive and canola—have been shown to reduce total cholesterol without lowering levels of the good cholesterol, HDL. In fact, some monounsaturated fats appear to raise HDL levels.

One other element, *trans-fatty acids*, might also play a role in blood cholesterol levels. Trans-fatty acids occur when polyunsaturated oils are altered through hydrogenation, a process used to harden liquid vegetable oils into solid foods like margarine and shortening. One study found that trans-monounsaturated fatty acids raise LDL cholesterol levels, behaving much like saturated fats. Simultaneously, these trans-fatty acids reduced HDL cholesterol readings. Much more research is necessary about trans-fatty acids, since some studies have not produced clear-cut conclusions about these substances. For now it is clear that when your goal is to lower cholesterol, polyunsaturated and monounsaturated fats are much more desirable than are saturated fats.

A Word About Calories

When we talk about foods, we often mention the number of calories a certain food has. As you have seen, calories are not among the four basic nutrients. What, then, are calories?

A calorie is an energy unit. As already discussed, carbohydrates, protein, and fat provide the body with the energy it needs to function. This energy is measured in calories. There are, for instance, 4 calories in every gram of protein, 4 calories in every gram of carbohydrate, and 9 calories in every gram of fat. It is no wonder, then, that when people try to lose weight, they are often advised to cut down on fatty foods. On a gram-for-gram basis, fat is more than twice as fattening as carbohydrates or protein.

In addition to fat having more calories than protein or carbohydrates, it is important to understand that the way in which the body metabolizes dietary fat is different from the way it metabolizes the other two nutrients. Because dietary fat is similar in chemical composition to body fat, it takes less energy to convert it to body fat. In fact, it takes only 3 percent of the calories in the fat we eat to turn that food into body fat, while it takes at least 25 percent of the carbohydrates and protein calories we eat to convert them into body fat. Remember, though, that if you eat more calories than your body needs, regardless of the nutrient providing these calories, the excess will be stored as body fat.

Being Sodium Wise

Not even a brief look at nutrition would be complete without a word or two about sodium. The mineral sodium is necessary for health. It helps maintain normal fluid levels in the body, is involved in healthy muscle functioning, and supports the blood and lymph systems.

It is important to note, however, that most people get *too much* sodium in their diet. We need less than 500 milligrams of sodium a day to stay healthy. This is enough to accomplish the functions that sodium performs in the body. A quick glance through some randomly selected pages of this book will show you how easy it is to reach the 500-milligram mark. Better yet, read the nutrition labels on some of the foods in your refrigerator and pantry. You'll be surprised by the amount of salt found in the foods you are eating now, and by your typical daily intake.

When trying to reduce your intake of sodium, it is important to be aware of two hidden sources of this mineral. One source includes a number of food ingredients and additives other than salt itself. For instance, both baking powder and baking soda contain sodium, as does the flavor enhancer monosodium glutamate (MSG). In general, by looking for the word *sodium* among ingredient listings, you should be able to identify most sodium sources.

Medications—including over-the-counter cough, antacid, and pain relief preparations—constitute the second hidden source of sodium. Again, any ingredient that contains the word *sodium*—for example, sodium salicylate—should alert you to a possible problem.

THE FOOD GUIDE PYRAMID

Over the years, the United States Department of Agriculture (USDA) has tried to insure adequate nutrition by encouraging Americans to eat a "well-balanced diet"—a concept that has changed dramatically over the years. Most of us still remember the four food groups that the USDA once promoted. These food groups—fruits and vegetables; breads and cereals; meat, poultry, fish, and eggs; and dairy products—were developed to encourage a balanced diet that was rich in meat, poultry, and dairy products. Clearly, we now have a greater understanding of how such a diet affects our health, and the government now recommends a diet high in complex carbohydrates and low in fat. With this in mind, in May 1992, the government abandoned the four food groups in favor of the Food Guide Pyramid, which has dramatically changed the recommended amounts of foods in each group.

At the base of the Food Guide Pyramid is the bread, cereal, rice, and pasta group. Six to eleven servings from this group are recommended daily—more servings than from any other food group. The next level of the pyramid is occupied by the vegetable group, with three to five servings recommended daily, and the fruit group, with two to four servings recommended daily. Moving upward, the next pyramid level is shared by the milk, yogurt, and cheese group—two to three servings—and the meat, poultry, fish, dry beans, eggs, and nuts group—two to three servings. Finally, at the peak of the pyramid are fats, oils, and sweets, a group of foods which is to be eaten only sparingly.

Scaling the Pyramid

To insure that you have adequate servings of healthful foods, it is best to follow the Food Guide Pyramid and, within each group, to choose foods that are high in the nutrients needed for good health. The remainder of this book shows how each food rates in terms of its nutrient values. To make sure that these foods are still high in nutrients when they reach your table, and to help keep your diet low in fat and high in fiber, certain additional guidelines should be followed when selecting foods from each group.

■ When eating foods from the important bread, cereal, rice, and pasta group, always choose whole-grain, high-fiber, low-fat breads and cereals—preferably without added sugar, coloring, or unnecessary preservatives. Choose brown rice over white rice, and whole-wheat or other whole-grain pastas over pastas made from white flour.

■ When eating fruits and vegetables, eat fresh raw produce as often as possible. Water-soluble vitamins, such as vitamin C, may leach out of foods during cooking, be damaged by overprocessing, or be destroyed when foods are overcooked. Even fat-soluble vitamins, which are fairly stable during low-temperature cooking, can be affected by frying. For this reason, it is best to steam or microwave vegetables rather than boiling or frying them. And, unless the produce was grown organically, be sure to peel or thoroughly wash it to eliminate pesticide residues and waxes.

■ When choosing foods from the milk, yogurt, and cheese group, select low-fat and nonfat brands, which provide the most nutrients and the least amount of fat. When eating meat, poultry, and fish, choose the leanest cuts available, trim off any excess fat, and bake and broil the foods instead of frying them.

■ Select as few foods as possible from the fats, oils, and sweets group. When you do use fats and oils, though, choose monounsaturated and polyunsaturated fats instead of saturated fats. Limit your intake of sweets, choosing fresh fruits instead of cakes, cookies, and other high-fat desserts.

The following section should provide you with the details you need to better access and understand the data contained in this volume. I hope that this book will inspire you to learn more about your unique nutritional needs and the foods you are using to meet those needs. You will enjoy the sense of control this knowledge gives you. More important, you will make better food choices and take a major step toward better health. Best wishes for good health always.

Arthur Ulene, MD

HOW TO USE THIS BOOK

This book was designed to provide comprehensive nutritional information on a wide range of foods, both generic and brand name, raw and prepared. The information provided here was gleaned from a number of government agencies, from hundreds of manufacturers, and from food trade associations. This information was compiled and later supplemented through countless hours of follow-up that involved hundreds of additional sources. Because scientific techniques are constantly being improved and nutritional theory continues to advance, this book will be continuously updated to reflect the most current nutritional data available.

FINDING THE LISTING YOU WANT

This easy-to-use guide is an A-to-Z reference to the calories, protein, carbohydrates, sodium, fiber, fat, and cholesterol contents of foods. All of the foods in this reference have been listed alphabetically. For instance, if you were looking for the nutrient values of ground beef, you would turn to the *B*'s and look under *Beef*. For convenience, similar foods have been grouped together in categories such as *Baby Foods, Breads, Candies, Cereals, Cheese, Cookies, Pasta,* and *Sauces*. Therefore, if the food you are looking for is not listed individually by its own name, you should try looking it up under a logical category.

Some foods are known by two or more names. In most cases, the food is listed under just one name, and cross-references have been provided to guide you to the proper listing. For instance, garbanzo beans are also called chick peas and ceci beans. In this book, you will find the nutrient information under *Garbanzo beans*, with cross-references under *Ceci beans* and *Chick peas*.

If you are unable to find a particular food, look for the listing of a similar food. The nutritional data should be close, if not exact, for any product not listed. When doing this, make sure you are comparing weight measure against weight measure and volume measure against volume measure.

After you locate the listing of the food you are interested in, you may find that abbreviations have been used to provide you with the information you need. Refer to page xiv for a complete key to the abbreviations used throughout this book.

UNDERSTANDING FISH, MEAT, AND POULTRY LISTINGS

When examining the nutrient values of cooked fish, meat, poultry, and vegetables, keep in mind that unless otherwise noted, no additional ingredients have been added. Also be aware that unless otherwise noted, the food values for fish, meats, and poultry are for meat only, and do not include skin or bones.

UNDERSTANDING FIBER VALUES

When looking at the fiber values of foods, it is important to understand that as a result of two different methods of analysis, two different types of fiber have been listed in this book. For many years, the acid-based process used to measure the fiber content of foods actually destroyed some of the fiber it was designed to measure. Referred to as "crude fiber," the results of this type of analysis are inaccurate, and almost always show an amount that is lower than the actual amount of fiber present in the food. Later, a more precise enzyme-related process for measuring this nutrient was devised. The fiber analyzed with this system is referred to as "dietary fiber."

In the interest of accuracy, whenever possible, we have provided the most up-to-date, accurate measure of total dietary fiber. You will know that the value reflects *total fiber* when the number is not accompanied by a qualifying symbol. For instance, the amount of fiber found in $1/2$ cup of boiled sliced carrots is listed as *2.6*. This means that according to the most accurate techniques of analysis now available, 2.6 grams of fiber are present in this amount of carrots. Unfortunately, in the case of some foods, only the *crude fiber* value is available at this time. You will know that the value reflects crude fiber when it is preceded by the symbol >—meaning "greater than"—and followed by the letter *c*—meaning "crude." For instance, the amount of fiber found in $1/2$ cup of boiled garbanzo beans is listed as >2.0c. This means that according to crude analysis, at least 2 grams of fiber can be found in this amount of beans. Of course, as techniques of analysis are improved and as additional foods are tested, the listings in this book will be updated.

We hope that you will find *The Nutribase Complete Book of Food Counts* a valuable companion that provides the information you need to take control of your eating habits. Should you have any comments about this book, feel free to write to the following address: Nutribase Comments, c/o Avery Publishing Group, 120 Old Broadway, Garden City Park, NY 11040.

CODES AND ABBREVIATIONS

To provide the most comprehensive nutritional information possible, a number of codes and abbreviations have been used throughout this book. A complete translation is given below.

>	greater than[1]
<	less than
%	percentage
approx	approximately
c	crude fiber[1]
carbs	carbohydrates
chol	cholesterol
diam	diameter
fl	fluid
gm	gram
lb	pound
mcg	microgram(s)
med	medium-sized
mgs	milligrams
(mq)	may contain a measurable quantity[2]

na	not available
pkg	package
prep	prepared according to package directions
prot	protein
raw wt	raw weight
sod	sodium
tbsp	tablespoon
tr	trace
(tr)	may contain a trace amount
tsp	teaspoon
w/	with
w/o	without
wt	weight

[1] The symbols > and c, which are used only in fiber value listings, indicate that the amount shown is the result of crude analysis, and that the actual amount of fiber present most probably is greater than the amount shown. For further explanation, see page xiii.

[2] The food item may contain a quantity ranging from a trace amount to a substantial amount. This quantity depends upon any one of a number of variables—such as soil condition and mineral content of fertilizer used—that may have affected the food item during growing, processing, and/or preparation.

A

Food Name	Serv. Size	Total Cal.	Prot. GMS	Carbs GMS	Sod. MGS	Fiber GMS	Fat GMS	Chol. MGS
ABALONE, MIXED SPECIES, raw	3 oz	89	14.5	5.1	256	0	0.7	72
ACEROLA CHERRY/Barbados cherry								
trimmed	1 cup	31	0.4	7.5	7	1.1	0.3	0
trimmed	1 oz	9	0.1	2.2	2	>.1 c	0.1	0
trimmed	1 fruit	2	0.0	0.4	0	0.1	0.0	0
untrimmed	1 lb	114	1.5	27.9	26	>1.5 c	1.1	0
ACEROLA CHERRY JUICE/Barbados cherry juice								
	1 cup	51	1.0	11.6	7	.7	0.7	0
	1 oz	6	0.1	1.5	1	.1	0.1	0
ACORN								
dried	1 oz	145	2.3	15.2	0	>1.0 c	8.9	0
dried, in shell	1 lb	1432	22.8	150.9	1995	>9.5 c	88.3	0
raw, in shell	1 lb	1037	17.3	114.6	1515	>7.2 c	67.1	0
raw, shelled	1 oz	105	1.8	11.6	0	>.7 c	6.8	0
ACORN FLOUR, full fat	1 oz	142	2.1	15.5	0	>.8 c	8.6	0
ACORN SQUASH. See SQUASH, ACORN.								
ADZUKI BEAN								
boiled, mature seeds	1/2 cup	147	8.6	28.5	9	>2.3 c	0.1	0
raw	1 oz	93	5.6	17.8	1	>1.5 c	0.2	0
raw *(Arrowhead Mills)*	2 oz	190	13.0	35.0	3	14.3	1.0	0
raw, mature seeds	1/2 cup	322	19.5	61.6	5	12.5	0.5	0
yokan, mature seeds, 1/4-inch slice	1 slice	36	0.5	8.5	12	>.2 c	0.0	0
ADZUKI BEAN, CANNED								
mature seeds, sweetened	1/2 cup	351	5.6	81.4	323	>2.3 c	0.0	0
organic, no salt added *(Eden Foods)*	1/2 cup	80	7.0	18.0	10	5.0	<1.0	0
organic, w/liquid *(Eden Foods)*	1/2 cup	100	6.0	17.0	20	4.3	<1.0	0
AGAR								
dried	100 gm	306	6.2	80.9	102	7.7	0.3	0
raw	1 lb	116	2.5	30.6	40	>2.0 c	0.1	0
raw	100 gm	26	0.5	6.8	9	.5	0.0	0
raw	1 oz	7	0.2	1.9	3	>.1 c	tr	0
AHI. See TUNA, YELLOWFIN.								
AKU. See TUNA, SKIPJACK.								
ALBACORE. See TUNA, CANNED; TUNA, FROZEN.								
ALCOHOL-FREE BEVERAGES								
BEER								
(Cutter)	12 oz	76	0.5	19.6	<1	0	0.0	0
(Kaliber)	12 oz	71	1.2	10.6	3	na	0.0	na
(Sharp's)	12 oz	86	1.0	9.5	5	0	0.0	0

Food Name	Serv. Size	Total Cal.	Prot. GMS	Carbs GMS	Sod. MGS	Fiber GMS	Fat GMS	Chol. MGS
MIXED-DRINK MIXERS								
Banana Daiquiri, frozen, diluted w/water								
(Bacardi)	7 oz	150	0.0	35.0	0	na	1.0	na
Bloody Mary								
bottled (Mr. & Mrs. T)	4.5 oz	20	1.0	4.0	670	0	0.0	0
bottled, rich & spicy (Mr. & Mrs. T)	4.5 oz	30	1.0	6.0	500	0	0.0	0
bottled 'Smooth N' Spicy' (Holland House)	1 oz	3	0.0	<1.0	329	(tr)	0.0	0
Daiquiri								
bottled (Holland House)	1 oz	36	0.0	9.0	111	(tr)	0.0	0
instant, dry (Holland House)	.56 oz	65	0.0	16.0	21	(tr)	0.0	0
Grenadine								
syrup (Roses)	1 oz	65	0.0	16.0	27	(tr)	0.0	0
syrup (Roses)	.5 oz	32	1.0	8.0	14	na	<1.0	na
Lime Daiquiri, shelf stable, w/water								
(Bacardi)	7 oz	130	0.0	33.0	10	na	0.0	na
Mai Tai								
bottled (Holland House)	1 oz	32	0.0	8.0	60	(tr)	0.0	0
instant, dry (Holland House)	.56 oz	64	0.0	16.0	4	(tr)	0.0	0
Manhattan, bottled (Holland House)	1 oz	28	0.0	7.0	5	0	0.0	0
Margarita								
bottled (Holland House)	1 oz	27	0.0	6.0	92	(tr)	0.0	0
bottled (Mr. & Mrs. T)	3 oz	80	<1.0	20.0	35	na	<1.0	na
frozen, diluted w/water (Bacardi)	7 oz	90	0.0	24.0	0	na	0.0	na
instant, dry (Holland House)	.5 oz	57	0.0	14.0	4	(tr)	0.0	0
shelf stable, w/water (Bacardi)	7 oz	130	0.0	33.0	10	na	0.0	na
Old Fashioned, bottled (Holland House)	1 oz	33	0.0	8.0	6	0	0.0	0
Peach Daiquiri, frozen, diluted w/water								
(Bacardi)	7 oz	130	0.0	33.0	5	na	0.0	na
Piña Colada								
bottled (Holland House)	1 oz	33	0.0	8.0	4	na	0.0	0
bottled (Mr. & Mrs. T)	4 oz	150	<1.0	39.0	120	na	<1.0	na
frozen, diluted w/water (Bacardi)	7 oz	200	1.0	37.0	25	na	6.0	na
instant, dry (Holland House)	.56 oz	82	0.0	12.0	<1	na	3.0	0
shelf stable, w/water (Bacardi)	7 oz	170	0.0	36.0	20	na	2.0	na
Raspberry Daiquiri, bottled (Holland House)	1 oz	30	0.0	7.0	4	(tr)	0.0	0
Rum Runner, shelf stable, w/water (Bacardi)	7 oz	140	0.0	33.0	15	na	0.0	na
Strawberry Colada, shelf stable, w/water								
(Bacardi)	7 oz	150	0.0	34.0	15	na	1.0	na
Strawberry Daiquiri								
bottled (Holland House)	1 oz	31	0.0	7.0	3	(tr)	0.0	0
frozen, diluted w/water (Bacardi)	7 oz	140	0.0	34.0	0	na	0.0	na
shelf stable, w/water (Bacardi)	7 oz	130	0.0	31.0	15	na	0.0	na

Food Name	Serv. Size	Total Cal.	Prot. GMS	Carbs GMS	Sod. MGS	Fiber GMS	Fat GMS	Chol. MGS
Strawberry Margarita								
bottled (Holland House)	1 oz	31	0.0	7.0	3	na	0.0	0
bottled (Mr. & Mrs. T)	3.5 oz	100	<1.0	24.0	10	na	<1.0	na
instant, dry (Holland House)	.56 oz	66	0.0	16.0	<1	(tr)	0.0	0
Sweet and Sour								
bottled (Mr. & Mrs. T)	3 oz	70	<1.0	17.0	45	na	<1.0	na
liquid (Holland House)	1 oz	34	0.0	8.0	107	na	0.0	0
Tom Collins								
bottled (Holland House)	1 oz	47	0.0	11.0	96	na	0.0	0
instant, dry (Holland House)	.56 oz	65	0.0	16.0	14	na	0.0	0
Whiskey Sour								
bottled (Holland House)	1 oz	37	0.0	9.0	105	na	0.0	0
instant, dry (Holland House)	.56 oz	64	0.0	16.0	16	na	0.0	0
ALCOHOLIC BEVERAGES. See also ALCOHOL-FREE BEVERAGES.								
BEER, ALE, AND MALT LIQUOR								
(Anheuser Marzen)	12 oz	168	2.3	15.2	12	0	0.0	0
(Beck's)	12 oz	148	1.7	10.0	14	0	0.0	0
(Budweiser)	12 oz	144	1.2	11.3	12	0	0.0	0
(Budweiser) 'Bud Light'	12 oz	110	1.1	6.9	12	0	0.0	0
(Busch)	12 oz	144	1.2	11.9	12	0	0.0	0
(Carlsberg)	12 oz	149	1.2	11.9	12	0	0.0	0
(Carlsberg) 'Light'	12 oz	110	1.1	6.5	12	0	0.0	0
(Coors)	12 oz	137	0.6	11.6	<1	0	0.0	0
(Coors) 'Dry'	12 oz	119	0.4	6.0	<1	0	0.0	0
(Coors) 'Dry' 3.2%	12 oz	101	0.6	5.3	<1	0	0.0	0
(Coors) 'Extra Gold'	12 oz	151	1.3	12.5	<1	0	0.0	0
(Coors) 'Extra Gold' 3.2%	12 oz	121	0.6	10.2	<1	0	0.0	0
(Coors) 'Light'	12 oz	103	0.7	4.7	<1	0	0.0	0
(Coors) 'Light' 3.2%	12 oz	98	0.7	4.7	<1	0	0.0	0
(Coors) 3.2%	12 oz	119	0.7	9.7	<1	0	0.0	0
(Coqui)	12 oz	208	1.7	9.8	13	0	0.0	0
(Dribeck's)	12 oz	94	1.0	7.0	14	0	0.0	0
(Elephant)	12 oz	208	1.6	16.9	12	0	0.0	0
(Keystone)	12 oz	121	0.6	6.8	<1	0	0.0	0
(Keystone) 'Dry'	12 oz	121	0.6	6.4	<1	0	0.0	0
(Keystone) 'Light'	12 oz	100	0.6	4.4	<1	0	0.0	0
(Keystone) 'Light' 3.2%	12 oz	99	0.4	5.0	<1	0	0.0	0
(Keystone) 3.2%	12 oz	104	0.5	6.1	<1	0	0.0	0
(Killian's)	12 oz	161	1.0	15.0	<1	0	0.0	0
(Killian's) 3.2%	12 oz	128	1.2	11.4	<1	0	0.0	0
(King Cobra)	12 oz	182	1.4	15.2	12	0	0.0	0
(Knickerbocker)	12 oz	140	0.9	12.3	9	0	0.0	0
(LA) light alcohol	12 oz	114	0.8	16.4	12	0	0.0	0

Food Name	Serv. Size	Total Cal.	Prot. GMS	Carbs GMS	Sod. MGS	Fiber GMS	Fat GMS	Chol. MGS
(Lite) 'Genuine Draft'	12 oz	98	0.8	3.5	6	0	0.0	0
(Lite) 'Lite'	12 oz	96	0.8	2.8	6	0	0.0	0
(Lowenbräu) 'Dark Special'	12 oz	158	1.4	14.3	7	0	0.0	0
(Lowenbräu) 'Special'	12 oz	158	1.4	14.3	7	0	0.0	0
(McSorley's)	12 oz	166	1.7	14.7	6	0	0.0	0
(Meister Brau)	12 oz	141	1.0	12.8	6	0	0.0	0
(Meister Brau) 'Light'	12 oz	98	0.8	3.5	6	0	0.0	0
(Michelob)	12 oz	156	1.5	13.6	12	0	0.0	0
(Michelob) 'Classic Dark'	12 oz	158	1.5	14.4	12	0	0.0	0
(Michelob) 'Dry'	12 oz	133	1.3	7.8	12	0	0.0	0
(Michelob) 'Light'	12 oz	134	1.2	11.9	12	0	0.0	0
(Miller) 'Genuine Draft'	12 oz	147	1.0	13.1	7	0	0.0	0
(Miller) 'High Life'	12 oz	147	1.0	13.1	7	0	0.0	0
(Miller) 'Magnum'	12 oz	162	1.3	10.2	8	0	0.0	0
(Milwaukee) 'Milwaukee's Best'	12 oz	133	0.9	11.4	6	0	0.0	0
(Milwaukee) 'Milwaukee's Best Light'	12 oz	98	0.8	3.5	6	0	0.0	0
(Natural Light)	12 oz	110	1.1	6.6	12	0	0.0	0
(Ortlieb's)	12 oz	140	0.9	12.3	9	0	0.0	0
(Prior) 'Double Dark'	12 oz	171	1.4	15.4	10	0	0.0	0
(Rheingold)	12 oz	148	1.3	12.9	9	0	0.0	0
(Rheingold) 'Light'	12 oz	96	0.7	2.8	7	0	0.0	0
(Rolling Rock) 'Light'	12 oz	104	0.4	8.0	<1	0	0.0	0
(Rolling Rock) 'Premium'	12 oz	145	0.4	10.0	<1	0	0.0	0
(Schmidt's)	12 oz	148	1.0	12.9	9	0	0.0	0
(Schmidt's) 'Classic'	12 oz	144	1.0	12.8	10	0	0.0	0
(Schmidt's) 'Light'	12 oz	96	0.7	2.8	7	0	0.0	0
(Tiger Head)	12 oz	166	1.7	14.7	6	0	0.0	0
(Zima)	12 oz	148	0.2	14.0	2	na	na	na
CHAMPAGNE								
brut *(Jacques Bonet)*	4 oz	92	0.0	2.1	4	0	0.0	0
brut *(Lejon)*	4 oz	92	0.0	3.4	4	0	0.0	0
extra dry *(Jacques Bonet)*	4 oz	97	0.0	3.4	4	0	0.0	0
extra dry *(Lejon)*	4 oz	97	0.0	2.1	4	0	0.0	0
pink *(Jacques Bonet)*	4 oz	98	0.0	3.7	4	0	0.0	0
pink *(Lejon)*	4 oz	98	0.0	3.7	4	0	0.0	0
LIQUOR AND LIQUEUR								
Bourbon								
80 proof, distilled	1 oz	65	0.0	tr	tr	0	0.0	0
86 proof, distilled	1 oz	70	0.0	tr	tr	0	0.0	0
90 proof, distilled	1 oz	74	0.0	tr	tr	0	0.0	0
94 proof, distilled	1 oz	77	0.0	tr	tr	0	0.0	0
100 proof, distilled	1 oz	83	0.0	tr	tr	0	0.0	0

Food Name	Serv. Size	Total Cal.	Prot. GMS	Carbs GMS	Sod. MGS	Fiber GMS	Fat GMS	Chol. MGS
Brandy								
80 proof, distilled	1 oz	65	0.0	tr	tr	0	0.0	0
86 proof, distilled	1 oz	70	0.0	tr	tr	0	0.0	0
90 proof, distilled	1 oz	74	0.0	tr	tr	0	0.0	0
94 proof, distilled	1 oz	77	0.0	tr	tr	0	0.0	0
100 proof, distilled	1 oz	83	0.0	tr	tr	0	0.0	0
Coffee Liqueur								
53 proof	1 oz	117	0.0	16.3	3	0	0.1	0
63 proof	1 oz	107	0.0	11.2	3	0	0.1	0
Creme de Menthe, 72 proof	1 oz	125	0.0	14.0	2	0	0.1	0
Gin								
80 proof, distilled	1 oz	64	0.0	0.0	0	0	0.0	0
86 proof, distilled	1 oz	69	0.0	0.0	0	0	0.0	0
90 proof, distilled	1 oz	73	0.0	0.0	0	0	0.0	0
94 proof, distilled	1 oz	76	0.0	0.0	0	0	0.0	0
100 proof, distilled	1 oz	82	0.0	0.0	0	0	0.0	0
Rum								
80 proof, distilled	1 oz	64	0.0	0.0	0	0	0.0	0
86 proof, distilled	1 oz	69	0.0	0.0	0	0	0.0	0
90 proof, distilled	1 oz	73	0.0	0.0	0	0	0.0	0
94 proof, distilled	1 oz	76	0.0	0.0	0	0	0.0	0
100 proof, distilled	1 oz	82	0.0	0.0	0	0	0.0	0
Rye Whiskey								
80 proof, distilled	1 oz	65	0.0	tr	tr	0	0.0	0
86 proof, distilled	1 oz	70	0.0	tr	tr	0	0.0	0
90 proof, distilled	1 oz	74	0.0	tr	tr	0	0.0	0
94 proof, distilled	1 oz	77	0.0	tr	tr	0	0.0	0
100 proof, distilled	1 oz	83	0.0	tr	tr	0	0.0	0
Scotch								
80 proof, distilled	1 oz	65	0.0	tr	tr	0	0.0	0
86 proof, distilled	1 oz	70	0.0	tr	tr	0	0.0	0
90 proof, distilled	1 oz	74	0.0	tr	tr	0	0.0	0
94 proof, distilled	1 oz	77	0.0	tr	tr	0	0.0	0
100 proof, distilled	1 oz	83	0.0	tr	tr	0	0.0	0
Tequila								
80 proof, distilled	1 oz	65	0.0	tr	tr	0	0.0	0
86 proof, distilled	1 oz	70	0.0	tr	tr	0	0.0	0
90 proof, distilled	1 oz	74	0.0	tr	tr	0	0.0	0
94 proof, distilled	1 oz	77	0.0	tr	tr	0	0.0	0
100 proof, distilled	1 oz	83	0.0	tr	tr	0	0.0	0
Vodka								
80 proof, distilled	1 oz	64	0.0	0.0	0	0	0.0	0
86 proof, distilled	1 oz	69	0.0	0.0	0	0	0.0	0

Food Name	Serv. Size	Total Cal.	Prot. GMS	Carbs GMS	Sod. MGS	Fiber GMS	Fat GMS	Chol. MGS
90 proof, distilled	1 oz	73	0.0	0.0	0	0	0.0	0
94 proof, distilled	1 oz	76	0.0	0.0	0	0	0.0	0
100 proof, distilled	1 oz	82	0.0	0.0	0	0	0.0	0
Whiskey								
80 proof, distilled	1 oz	64	0.0	0.0	0	0	0.0	0
86 proof, distilled	1 oz	69	0.0	0.0	0	0	0.0	0
90 proof, distilled	1 oz	73	0.0	0.0	0	0	0.0	0
94 proof, distilled	1 oz	76	0.0	0.0	0	0	0.0	0
100 proof, distilled	1 oz	82	0.0	0.0	0	0	0.0	0

MIXED DRINKS. See also ALCOHOL-FREE BEVERAGES, MIXED-DRINK MIXERS.

Food Name	Serv. Size	Total Cal.	Prot. GMS	Carbs GMS	Sod. MGS	Fiber GMS	Fat GMS	Chol. MGS
Banana Daiquiri								
frozen, w/1/2-can Rum, diluted as directed								
(Bacardi)	7 oz	210	0.0	35.0	0	na	1.0	na
Bloody Mary, prepared from recipe	5 oz	115	0.7	4.9	332	>.3 c	0.2	na
Bourbon and Soda, prepared from recipe	4 oz	104	0.0	0.0	16	0	0.0	0
Daiquiri								
instant, prepared as directed								
(Bar-Tender's)	3.5 oz	177	0.0	18.0	50	0	0.0	0
prepared from recipe	1 oz	56	0.0	2.0	2	0	0.0	0
Gin and Tonic, prepared from recipe	1 oz	23	0.0	2.1	1	0	0.0	0
Lime Daiquiri, mix, shelf stable, w/1/2-can								
Rum (Bacardi)	7 oz	210	0.0	33.0	10	na	0.0	na
Manhattan, prepared from recipe	1 oz	64	0.0	0.9	1	0	0.0	0
Margarita								
frozen, w/1/2-can Rum, diluted as directed								
(Bacardi)	7 oz	160	0.0	24.0	5	na	0.0	na
shelf stable, w/1/2-can Rum (Bacardi)	7 oz	210	0.0	33.0	10	na	0.0	na
Martini, prepared from recipe	1 oz	63	0.0	0.1	1	0	0.0	0
Peach Daiquiri								
frozen, w/1/2-can Rum, diluted as directed								
(Bacardi)	7 oz	200	0.0	33.0	5	na	0.0	na
Piña Colada								
frozen, w/1/2-can Rum, diluted as directed								
(Bacardi)	7 oz	260	1.0	37.0	25	na	6.0	na
mix, shelf stable, w/1/2-can Rum (Bacardi)	7 oz	240	0.0	36.0	20	na	2.0	na
prepared from recipe	1 oz	58	0.1	8.9	2	>.1 c	0.6	0
Rum Runner, shelf stable, w/1/2-can Rum								
(Bacardi)	7 oz	210	0.0	33.0	15	na	0.0	na
Screwdriver, prepared from recipe	1 oz	25	0.2	2.6	0	0	0.0	0
Strawberry Colada								
mix, shelf stable, w/1/2-can Rum (Bacardi)	7 oz	230	0.0	34.0	15	na	1.0	na

Food Name	Serv. Size	Total Cal.	Prot. GMS	Carbs GMS	Sod. MGS	Fiber GMS	Fat GMS	Chol. MGS
Strawberry Daiquiri								
frozen, w/1/2-can Rum, diluted as directed								
(Bacardi)	7 oz	200	0.0	34.0	0	na	0.0	na
mix, shelf stable, w/1/2-can Rum (Bacardi)	7 oz	200	0.0	31.0	15	na	0.0	na
Tequila Sunrise, prepared from recipe	1 oz	34	0.1	2.7	1	0	0.0	0
Tom Collins, prepared from recipe	1 oz	16	0.0	0.4	5	0	0.0	0
Whiskey Sour								
mix, powder, instant, prepared w/whiskey								
(Bar-Tender's)	3.5 oz	177	0.0	18.0	50	0	0.0	0
prepared from recipe	1 oz	41	0.1	1.7	3	0	0.0	0
WINE. See also WINE, COOKING.								
'Arriba' (Mission Bell)	2 oz	95	0.0	6.8	4	0	0.0	0
'Diamond Red' (Mission Bell)	2 oz	95	0.0	6.8	4	0	0.0	0
'Silver Satin' (Mission Bell)	2 oz	83	0.0	5.4	4	0	0.0	0
'Silver Satin Bitter Lemon' (Mission Bell)	2 oz	83	0.0	5.5	4	0	0.0	0
'Swiss Up' (Mission Bell)	2 oz	84	0.0	5.6	4	0	0.0	0
Barbera, white (Colony)	4 oz	91	0.0	3.5	4	0	0.0	0
Burgundy								
(Bravo)	4 oz	91	0.0	1.7	4	0	0.0	0
(Carlo Rossi)	4 oz	92	0.0	1.6	na	0	0.0	0
(Colony) 'Classic'	4 oz	90	0.0	1.2	4	0	0.0	0
(Gallo)	4 oz	88	0.0	0.8	na	0	0.0	0
(Gallo) 'Hearty'	4 oz	92	0.0	1.6	na	0	0.0	0
(Gambarelli & Davitto) 'Parma'	4 oz	91	0.0	1.7	4	0	0.0	0
(Petri)	4 oz	91	0.0	1.7	4	0	0.0	0
Cabernet Sauvignon								
(Colony)	4 oz	88	0.0	0.7	4	0	0.0	0
(Gallo)	4 oz	88	0.0	0.0	na	0	0.0	0
Carbonated								
(Carlo Rossi) 'Paisano'	4 oz	92	0.0	1.6	na	0	0.0	0
(Jacques Bonet) almond	4 oz	104	0.0	7.7	4	0	0.0	0
(Jacques Bonet) apricot	4 oz	111	0.0	9.5	4	0	0.0	0
(Jacques Bonet) cherry	4 oz	106	0.0	8.3	4	0	0.0	0
(Jacques Bonet) peach	4 oz	111	0.0	9.5	4	0	0.0	0
(Jacques Bonet) raspberry	4 oz	106	0.0	8.3	4	0	0.0	0
Chablis								
(Bravo)	4 oz	86	0.0	1.7	4	0	0.0	0
(Carlo Rossi)	4 oz	84	0.0	2.0	na	0	0.0	0
(Carlo Rossi) pink	4 oz	92	0.0	3.6	na	0	0.0	0
(Colony)	4 oz	98	0.0	4.5	4	0	0.0	0
(Colony) 'Classic'	4 oz	84	0.0	1.8	4	0	0.0	0
(Colony) emerald	4 oz	102	0.0	5.3	4	0	0.0	0
(Colony) gold	4 oz	97	0.0	4.3	4	0	0.0	0

Food Name	Serv. Size	Total Cal.	Prot. GMS	Carbs GMS	Sod. MGS	Fiber GMS	Fat GMS	Chol. MGS
(Colony) ruby	4 oz	104	0.0	5.9	4	0	0.0	0
(Gallo)	4 oz	80	0.0	4.0	na	0	0.0	0
(Gallo) 'Blanc'	4 oz	80	0.0	0.6	na	0	0.0	0
(Gambarelli & Davitto) 'Parma'	4 oz	86	0.0	1.7	4	0	0.0	0
(Petri)	4 oz	98	0.0	4.5	4	0	0.0	0
(Petri) 'Blanc'	4 oz	86	0.0	1.7	4	0	0.0	0
Chardonnay *(Gallo)*	4 oz	88	0.0	na	na	0	0.0	0
Chenin Blanc								
(Colony)	4 oz	86	0.0	2.4	4	0	0.0	0
(Gallo)	4 oz	88	0.0	1.6	na	0	0.0	0
Chianti								
(Carlo Rossi) 'Light'	4 oz	92	0.0	2.4	na	0	0.0	0
(Petri)	4 oz	91	0.0	1.7	4	0	0.0	0
Cold duck								
(Jacques Bonet)	4 oz	108	0.0	5.9	4	0	0.0	0
(Lejon)	4 oz	108	0.0	5.9	4	0	0.0	0
French colombard								
(Colony)	4 oz	84	0.0	1.8	4	0	0.0	0
(Gallo)	4 oz	88	0.0	2.0	na	0	0.0	0
Gewurztraminer *(Gallo)*	4 oz	88	0.0	1.6	na	0	0.0	0
Marsala *(Gambarelli & Davitto)*	4 oz	77	0.0	4.0	4	0	0.0	0
Moselle *(Colony)* 'Rhineskeller'	4 oz	97	0.0	4.3	4	0	0.0	0
Muscatel *(Italian Swiss Colony)*	2 oz	122	0.0	5.9	4	0	0.0	0
Pastoso *(Petri)*	4 oz	92	0.0	1.8	4	0	0.0	0
Port								
(Gallo)	2 oz	64	0.0	2.0	na	0	0.0	0
(Gallo) white	2 oz	86	0.0	5.6	na	0	0.0	0
(Italian Swiss Colony)	2 oz	85	0.0	5.7	4	0	0.0	0
(Italian Swiss Colony) white	2 oz	86	0.0	6.3	4	0	0.0	0
(Livingston Cellars) tawny	2 oz	86	0.0	6.4	na	0	0.0	0
Rhine								
(Bravo)	4 oz	97	0.0	4.3	4	0	0.0	0
(Carlo Rossi)	4 oz	84	0.0	4.4	na	0	0.0	0
(Colony) 'Classic'	4 oz	89	0.0	3.8	4	0	0.0	0
(Gallo)	4 oz	80	0.0	4.0	4	0	0.0	0
(Gambarelli & Davitto) 'Parma'	4 oz	92	0.0	1.2	4	0	0.0	0
(Petri)	4 oz	97	0.0	4.3	4	0	0.0	0
Reisling, *(Gallo)* 'Johannisberg'	4 oz	84	0.0	1.6	na	0	0.0	0
Rosé								
(Bravo)	4 oz	92	0.0	3.1	4	0	0.0	0
(Carlo Rossi) 'Vin Rosé'	4 oz	88	0.0	2.8	na	0	0.0	0
(Colony) 'Classic'	4 oz	89	0.0	3.0	4	0	0.0	0
(Gallo) 'Grenache'	4 oz	88	0.0	2.4	na	0	0.0	0

Food Name	Serv. Size	Total Cal.	Prot. GMS	Carbs GMS	Sod. MGS	Fiber GMS	Fat GMS	Chol. MGS
(Gallo) 'Red Rosé'	4 oz	112	0.0	6.4	na	0	0.0	0
(Gallo) 'Vin Rosé'	4 oz	88	0.0	2.8	na	0	0.0	0
(Gambarelli & Davitto) 'Parma'	4 oz	92	0.0	3.1	4	0	0.0	0
(Petri)	4 oz	92	0.0	3.1	4	0	0.0	0
Sauvignon Blanc, (Gallo)	4 oz	80	0.0	0.8	na	0	0.0	0
Sherry								
(Gallo)	2 oz	64	0.0	2.0	na	0	0.0	0
(Italian Swiss Colony) cream	2 oz	85	0.0	6.8	4	0	0.0	0
(Italian Swiss Colony) dry	2 oz	63	0.0	1.2	4	0	0.0	0
(Livingston Cellars) cream	2 oz	78	0.0	5.6	na	0	0.0	0
(Livingston Cellars) 'Very Dry'	2 oz	60	0.0	1.0	na	0	0.0	0
Tokay (Italian Swiss Colony)	2 oz	82	0.0	5.1	4	0	0.0	0
Vermouth								
(Gallo) dry	2 oz	56	0.0	0.8	na	0	0.0	0
(Gallo) sweet	2 oz	90	0.0	9.4	na	0	0.0	0
(Gambarelli & Davitto) dry	2 oz	64	0.0	1.5	4	0	0.0	0
(Gambarelli & Davitto) sweet	2 oz	77	0.0	8.4	4	0	0.0	0
(Lejon) dry	2 oz	64	0.0	1.5	4	0	0.0	0
(Lejon) sweet	2 oz	77	0.0	8.4	4	0	0.0	0
Zinfandel								
(Colony)	4 oz	91	0.0	0.7	4	0	0.0	0
(Colony) white	4 oz	82	0.0	2.7	4	0	0.0	0
(Gallo)	4 oz	92	0.0	0.0	na	0	0.0	0
WINE COOLERS								
(Bartles & Jaymes) Berry Cooler 'Light'	12 oz	150	0.0	32.0	na	na	0.0	na
(Bartles & Jaymes)								
Black Cherry Cooler 'Light'	12 oz	139	0.0	30.0	na	na	0.0	na
(Bartles & Jaymes) Citrus Cooler 'Light'	6 oz	67	<1.0	12.0	na	na	<1.0	na
(Bartles & Jaymes) Tropical Cooler 'Light'	12 oz	151	0.0	32.0	na	na	0.0	na
ALE. See ALCOHOLIC BEVERAGES.								
ALFALFA SEEDS								
(Arrowhead Mills)	1 cup	40	5.0	4.0	na	(mq)	1.0	0
sprouted, raw	1 lb	132	18.1	17.1	29	10.0	3.1	0
sprouted, raw	1/2 cup	5	0.7	0.6	1	.4	0.1	0
sprouted, raw	1 tbsp	1	0.1	0.1	0	.1	0.0	0
sprouted, raw	1 oz	8	1.1	1.1	2	.6	0.2	0
ALLSPICE								
ground	1 oz	75	1.7	20.4	22	>6.1 c	2.5	0
ground	1 tbsp	16	0.4	4.3	5	1.3	0.5	0
ground	1 tsp	5	0.1	1.4	1	.4	0.2	0
ground (Durkee)	1 tsp	7	0.0	0.0	0	0.0	tr	na
ground (Laurel Leaf)	1 tsp	7	0.0	0.0	0	0.0	tr	na
ground (Spice Islands)	1 tsp	6	0.1	1.3	1	>.4 c	0.1	0

Food Name	Serv. Size	Total Cal.	Prot. GMS	Carbs GMS	Sod. MGS	Fiber GMS	Fat GMS	Chol. MGS
ALMOND								
(Beer Nuts)	1 oz	180	5.0	7.0	51	(mq)	14.4	0
(Dole)	1 oz	170	6.0	12.0	4	(mq)	14.0	0
(Fisher)	1 oz	170	3.0	3.0	0	na	15.0	0
chopped	1 cup	766	25.9	26.5	14	6.1	67.9	0
in shell	1 lb	1069	36.2	37.0	19	>4.9 c	94.7	0
sliced	1 cup	554	18.8	19.2	10	4.4	49.1	0
slivered, tightly packed	1 cup	795	26.9	27.5	15	6.4	70.5	0
whole kernels	1 cup	836	28.3	29.0	16	15.5	74.1	0
whole kernels, approx 24	1 oz	167	5.7	5.8	3	>.8 c	14.8	0
Blanched								
sliced	1 cup	615	21.4	19.5	11	>2.4 c	55.2	0
whole kernels	1 cup	850	29.6	26.9	15	9.7	76.2	0
whole kernels	1 oz	166	5.8	5.3	3	>.7	14.9	0
Dry roasted								
(Planters)	1 oz	170	6.0	6.0	200	(mq)	15.0	0
whole kernels	1 cup	810	22.5	33.4	15	>6.8 c	71.2	0
whole kernels	1 oz	167	4.6	6.9	3	>1.4 c	14.7	0
Honey roasted								
(Planters)	1 oz	170	5.0	9.0	180	na	13.0	0
whole kernels	1 cup	855	26.2	40.2	187	na	71.9	0
whole kernels	1 oz	168	5.2	7.9	37	na	14.1	0
Oil roasted								
whole kernels	1 cup	970	32.0	24.9	16	17.6	90.5	0
whole kernels, approx 22	1 oz	176	5.8	4.5	3	3.2	16.4	0
Oil roasted and blanched								
toasted	1 oz	167	5.8	6.5	3	>1.4 c	14.4	0
toasted	1 cup	870	27.0	25.6	17	15.9	80.3	0
whole kernels, approx 24	1 oz	174	5.4	5.1	3	3.2	16.1	0
Raw								
blanched (Planters)	1 oz	170	6.0	6.0	0	na	15.0	0
sliced (Planters)	1 oz	170	6.0	6.0	0	(mq)	15.0	0
slivered (Planters)	1 oz	170	6.0	6.0	0	(mq)	15.0	0
whole (Planters)	1 oz	170	6.0	6.0	0	na	15.0	0
Toasted								
(Dole)	1 oz	170	6.0	5.0	4	na	14.0	na
unblanched	1 oz	167	5.8	6.5	3	>1.4 c	14.4	0
ALMOND BUTTER								
PLAIN								
	1/2 cup	791	18.9	26.5	14	4.65	73.9	0
	1 oz	179	4.3	6.0	3	>.4 c	16.8	0
blanched, toasted (Hain)	2 tbsp	220	8.0	3.0	10	(mq)	19.0	0
gourmet (Roaster Fresh)	1 oz	184	5.0	6.0	4	na	16.0	na

Food Name	Serv. Size	Total Cal.	Prot. GMS	Carbs GMS	Sod. MGS	Fiber GMS	Fat GMS	Chol. MGS
no salt, crunchy 'Natural' (Westbrae)	2 tbsp	190	7.0	7.0	0	na	17.0	na
no salt, smooth 'Natural' (Westbrae)	2 tbsp	190	7.0	7.0	0	na	17.0	0
raw 'Natural' (Hain)	2 tbsp	190	8.0	3.0	.5	(mq)	18.0	0
raw, organic (Maranatha Natural)	2 tbsp	190	7.0	8.0	5	na	15.0	0
roasted (Maranatha Natural)	2 tbsp	190	7.0	8.0	5	na	15.0	na
salted	1 cup	791	18.9	26.5	563	4.65	73.9	0
salted	1 oz	179	4.3	6.0	128	>.4 c	16.8	0
salted	1 tbsp	101	2.4	3.4	72	>.2 c	9.5	0
HONEY AND CINNAMON								
	1/2 cup	753	19.8	33.7	14	4.65	65.3	0
	1 oz	171	4.5	7.6	3	>.4 c	14.8	0
salted	1/2 cup	753	19.8	33.7	213	4.65	65.3	0
salted	1 oz	171	4.5	7.6	48	>.4 c	14.8	0
ALMOND MEAL								
partially defatted	4 oz	463	44.8	32.8	8	>2.6 c	20.8	0
partially defatted, salted	4 oz	463	44.8	32.8	846	>2.6 c	20.8	0
ALMOND OIL								
	1/2 cup	964	0.0	0.0	0	0	109.0	0
	1 oz	251	0.0	0.0	0	0	28.4	0
	1 tbsp	120	0.0	0.0	0	0	13.6	0
(Hain)	1 tbsp	120	0.0	0.0	0	0	14.0	0
(Spectrum Naturals)	1 tbsp	120	0.0	0.0	0	(tr)	14.0	(tr)
ALMOND PASTE								
	4 oz	506	13.4	49.4	10	16.8	30.8	0
	1 oz	127	3.4	12.4	3	4.2	7.7	0
firmly packed	1 cup	1012	26.9	98.9	20	33.8	61.7	0
ALMOND POWDER								
full-fat	1 oz	168	5.6	6.3	2	>.5 c	14.7	0
full-fat, not packed	1 cup	385	12.9	14.5	4	>1.2 c	33.6	0
partially defatted	1 oz	112	10.6	9.0	3	>.8 c	4.5	0
partially defatted, not packed	1 cup	255	24.4	20.7	7	>1.8 c	10.4	0
ALPINE SPICED CIDER (Krusteaz)	8 oz	80	0.0	21.0	20	na	0.0	0
AMARANTH								
boiled, drained	1/2 cup	14	1.4	2.7	14	>.9 c	0.1	0
raw	1 cup	7	0.7	1.1	6	>.3 c	0.1	0
AMARANTH DINNER, CANNED								
w/garden vegetables 'Fast Menu' fat-free (Health Valley)	7.5 oz	120	8.0	16.0	138	8.3	3.0	0
w/garden vegetables 'Fast Menu' fat-free (Health Valley)	5 oz	70	6.0	11.0	90	5.5	0.0	0
AMARANTH FLOUR (Arrowhead Mills)	2 oz	200	8.0	35.0	<1	3.9	3.0	0
AMARANTH SEED (Arrowhead Mills)	2 oz	200	8.0	35.0	1	3.9	3.0	0

Food Name	Serv. Size	Total Cal.	Prot. GMS	Carbs GMS	Sod. MGS	Fiber GMS	Fat GMS	Chol. MGS
AMBERJACK								
raw	1 lb	386	82.1	0.0	(mq)	0	4.1	(mq)
raw	1 oz	24	5.1	0.0	(mq)	0	0.3	(mq)
AMBROSIA JUICE (Knudsen & Sons)	8 oz	110	<1.0	27.0	na	na	0.0	na
AMBROSIA SALAD (Sunfresh)								
in light syrup	2/3 cup	70	0.0	18.0	30	1.0	0.0	0
ANASAZI BEAN raw (Arrowhead Mills)	2 oz	200	13.0	35.0	3	12.1	1.0	0
ANCHOVY, European, meat only, raw	1 oz	37	5.8	0.0	29	0	1.4	(mq)
ANCHOVY, CANNED								
in olive oil, drained	1 oz	60	8.2	0.0	1040	0	2.8	(mq)
in olive oil, drained, 5 med	.7 oz	42	5.8	0.0	734	0	1.9	(mq)
in olive oil, drained, yield from 2-oz can	1.6 oz	94	13.0	0.0	1651	0	4.4	38
ANGLER FISH. See MONKFISH.								
ANISE SEED								
whole	1 oz	95	5.0	14.2	5	4.1 c	4.5	0
whole	1 tbsp	23	1.2	3.3	1	1.0 c	1.1	0
whole	1 tsp	7	0.4	1.0	0	.3 c	0.3	0
APPLE								
boiled, peeled slices	1/2 cup	60	0.3	15.5	1	2.2	0.4	0
boiled, unpeeled slices	1/2 cup	46	0.2	11.7	1	>.5 c	0.3	0
microwaved, peeled slices	1/2 cup	64	0.3	16.3	1	2.7	0.5	0
microwaved, unpeeled slices	1/2 cup	48	0.2	12.3	1	>.5 c	0.4	0
raw, peeled	1 oz	16	<.1	4.2	tr	.5	0.1	0
raw, peeled slices	1 cup	63	0.2	16.3	0	2.1	0.3	0
raw, peeled whole fruit, approx 3 per lb	1 med	73	0.2	19.0	0	2.4	0.4	0
raw, unpeeled	1 oz	17	0.1	4.3	tr	.6	0.1	0
raw, unpeeled slices	1 cup	65	0.2	16.8	0	3.0	0.4	0
raw, unpeeled whole fruit, approx 3 per lb	1 med	81	0.3	21.0	0	3.7	0.5	0
raw, unpeeled whole fruit	1 lb	244	0.8	63.7	2	11.1	1.5	0
APPLE, CANNED								
Chipped								
(Lucky Leaf)	4 oz	50	0.0	12.0	10	(mq)	0.0	0
(Musselman's)	4 oz	50	0.0	12.0	10	(mq)	0.0	0
(White House) in water	4 oz	50	0.0	12.0	5	(mq)	0.0	0
Diced								
(Lucky Leaf)	4 oz	50	0.0	12.0	10	(mq)	0.0	0
(Musselman's)	4 oz	50	0.0	12.0	10	(mq)	0.0	0
Rings, spiced								
(Lucky Leaf) green	4 oz	100	0.0	24.0	20	(mq)	0.0	0
(Lucky Leaf) red	4 oz	100	0.0	24.0	20	(mq)	0.0	0
(Musselman's) green	4 oz	100	0.0	24.0	20	(mq)	0.0	0
(Musselman's) red	4 oz	100	0.0	24.0	20	(mq)	0.0	0
(White House)	3.5 oz	180	0.0	44.0	25	(mq)	0.0	0

Food Name	Serv. Size	Total Cal.	Prot. GMS	Carbs GMS	Sod. MGS	Fiber GMS	Fat GMS	Chol. MGS
Sliced								
(Lucky Leaf) dessert	4 oz	70	0.0	16.0	25	(mq)	0.0	0
(Lucky Leaf) sweetened, in syrup	4 oz	50	0.0	13.0	35	(mq)	0.0	0
(Lucky Leaf) sweetened, in water	4 oz	50	0.0	12.0	10	(mq)	0.0	0
(Lucky Leaf) sweetened, unpeeled	4 oz	90	0.0	22.0	15	(mq)	0.0	0
(Musselman's) dessert	4 oz	70	0.0	16.0	25	(mq)	0.0	0
(Musselman's) sweetened, in syrup	4 oz	50	0.0	13.0	35	(mq)	0.0	0
(Musselman's) sweetened, in water	4 oz	50	0.0	12.0	10	(mq)	0.0	0
(Musselman's) sweetened, unpeeled	4 oz	90	0.0	22.0	15	(mq)	0.0	0
(White House) sweetened	4 oz	54	0.0	14.0	10	(mq)	0.0	0
(White House) sweetened, in water	4 oz	40	0.0	12.0	5	(mq)	0.0	0
Whole								
(Lucky Leaf) baked	1 apple	110	0.0	28.0	35	(mq)	0.0	0
(Lucky Leaf) sweetened, peeled, cored	1 apple	90	0.0	21.0	10	(mq)	0.0	0
(Musselman's) baked	1 apple	110	0.0	28.0	35	(mq)	0.0	0
(Musselman's) sweetened, peeled, cored	1 apple	90	0.0	21.0	10	(mq)	0.0	0
(White House) baked	3.5 oz	118	0.0	29.0	11	(mq)	0.0	0
APPLE, DEHYDRATED/SULFURED								
chips (Weight Watchers)	.75 oz pkg	70	0.0	19.0	200	4.0	0.0	0
cooked	4 oz	84	0.3	22.6	29	>1.0 c	0.1	0
stewed, low moisture	1/2 cup	72	0.3	19.3	25	>.8 c	0.1	0
uncooked	4 oz	392	1.5	111.7	141	>4.6 c	0.7	0
uncooked, low moisture	1/2 cup	104	0.4	28.1	37	3.7	0.2	0
APPLE, DRIED								
chunks (Sun•Maid)	2 oz	150	1.0	42.0	40	(mq)	0.0	0
chunks (SunSweet)	2 oz	150	1.0	42.0	40	(mq)	0.0	0
sliced, uncooked (Del Monte)	2 oz	140	0.0	37.0	50	(mq)	0.0	0
sulfured, stewed	1/2 cup	73	0.3	19.6	26	2.6	0.1	0
sulfured, uncooked	4 oz	276	1.1	74.7	99	>3.3 c	0.4	0
sulfured, uncooked	1 cup	209	0.8	56.7	75	7.5	0.3	0
sulfured, uncooked, approx 2.3 oz	10 rings	155	0.6	42.2	56	5.6	0.2	0
APPLE, FROZEN								
escalloped (Stouffer's)	4 oz	130	0.0	27.0	15	na	2.0	na
glazed, in raspberry sauce 'Side Dish'								
(Budget Gourmet)	5 oz	110	0.0	22.0	210	(mq)	3.0	10
unsweetened	4 oz	54	0.3	14.0	3	2.3	0.4	0
unsweetened, heated	4 oz	53	0.3	13.6	3	2.2	0.4	0
unsweetened, heated, sliced	1/2 cup	48	0.3	12.4	3	>.6 c	0.3	0
unsweetened, sliced	1/2 cup	41	0.2	10.6	3	1.8	0.3	0
APPLE APRICOT JUICE (Knudsen & Sons)	8 oz	120	<1.0	29.0	na	na	0.0	na
APPLE BANANA JUICE (Knudsen & Sons)	8 oz	85	<1.0	21.0	na	na	0.0	na
APPLE BLACKBERRY JUICE								
(Knudsen & Sons)	8 oz	100	<1.0	24.0	na	na	0.0	na

Food Name	Serv. Size	Total Cal.	Prot. GMS	Carbs GMS	Sod. MGS	Fiber GMS	Fat GMS	Chol. MGS
(Santa Cruz Natural) organic	8 oz	120	<1.0	29.0	na	na	1.0	na
APPLE BOYSENBERRY JUICE								
(Knudsen & Sons)	8 oz	110	<1.0	28.0	na	na	0.0	na
(Santa Cruz Natural) organic	8 oz	120	<1.0	29.0	na	na	1.0	na
APPLE BUTTER								
	1 cup	519	0.3	134.5	0	3.7	0.9	0
	1 tbsp	33	0.0	8.6	0	.2	0.1	0
APPLE CHERRY BERRY DRINK *(Veryfine)*	8 oz	130	0.1	33.0	25	(mq)	0.0	0
APPLE CHERRY CIDER								
(Indian Summer)	6 oz	100	<1.0	25.0	10	(mq)	<1.0	0
(McCain) 100% juice 'Junior'	4.2 oz	50	0.0	13.0	5	na	0.0	na
(Musselman's) 'Breakfast Cocktail'	6 oz	100	1.0	26.0	5	(mq)	0.0	0
(Red Cheek) 'Naturally 100%'	6 oz	113	0.2	28.0	11	(mq)	0.0	0
APPLE CIDER								
(Indian Summer) can or bottle	6 oz	80	<1.0	20.0	10	(mq)	<1.0	0
(Indian Summer) can or bottle, cinnamon	6 oz	90	<1.0	21.0	10	(mq)	<1.0	0
(Lucky Leaf) can or bottle	6 oz	90	0.0	21.0	0	(mq)	0.0	0
(Lucky Leaf) can or bottle, sparkling	6 oz	80	0.0	18.0	45	(mq)	0.0	0
(S. Martinelli) 'Sparkling'	6 oz	100	0.0	25.0	5	na	0.0	0
(Tree Top) canned or frozen, diluted as directed	6 oz	90	0.0	22.0	10	na	0.0	0
APPLE CIDER MIX *(Swiss Miss)*	.776 oz	84	0.0	20.3	58	.9	0.3	0
APPLE CITRUS JUICE *(Tree Top)* canned or frozen	6 oz	90	1.0	22.0	10	(mq)	0.0	0
APPLE CRANBERRY CIDER								
(Indian Summer)	6 oz	100	<1.0	24.0	10	(mq)	<1.0	0
APPLE CRANBERRY DRINK								
(Mott's)	10 oz	176	0.0	44.0	3	(tr)	0.0	0
(Mott's)	9.5 oz	167	0.0	42.0	3	(tr)	0.0	0
(Tropicana)	6 oz	110	<1.0	27.0	15	na	<1.0	na
(Tropicana) 'Single Serve'	10 oz	175	(tr)	43.0	3	(tr)	0.0	0
APPLE CRANBERRY JUICE								
(Apple & Eve)	6 oz	80	0.0	19.0	5	(mq)	0.0	0
(Knudsen & Sons)	8 oz	110	<1.0	28.0	na	na	0.0	na
(Lucky Leaf)	6 oz	130	0.0	32.0	10	(mq)	0.0	0
(Mott's)	9.5 oz	147	0.0	38.0	27	(mq)	0.0	0
(Mott's)	6 oz	83	0.0	24.0	17	(mq)	0.0	0
(Mott's) aseptic box	8.45 oz	136	0.0	34.0	24	(mq)	0.0	0
(Santa Cruz Natural) organic	8 oz	115	<1.0	28.0	na	na	<1.0	na
(Smucker's) 'Naturally 100%'	8 oz	120	0.0	32.0	10	(tr)	0.0	0
(Tree Top) canned	6 oz	100	0.0	25.0	10	(mq)	0.0	0
(Tree Top) frozen	6 oz	100	0.0	25.0	10	(mq)	0.0	0
(Veryfine) cocktail	8 oz	130	0.1	33.0	10	(tr)	0.0	0

Food Name	Serv. Size	Total Cal.	Prot. GMS	Carbs GMS	Sod. MGS	Fiber GMS	Fat GMS	Chol. MGS
APPLE DRINK								
(Hi-C) 'Candy Apple Cooler'	6 oz	94	<.1	23.1	17	(tr)	<.1	0
(Hi-C) 'Candy Apple Cooler'	8.45 oz	132	<.1	32.6	25	(tr)	<.1	0
(Hi-C) 'Jamin' Apple Drink,' aseptic box	6 oz	90	0.0	23.0	20	na	0.0	na
(10-K)	8 oz	60	0.0	15.0	55	na	0.0	na
APPLE DUMPLING frozen								
(Pepperidge Farm)	3 oz	260	2.0	33.0	230	(mq)	13.0	na
APPLE GRAPE CHERRY JUICE								
(Welch's) 'Orchard Cocktail'	6 oz	110	0.0	27.0	20	(tr)	0.0	0
(Welch's) 'Orchard Cocktail-in-a-Box'	8.45 oz	150	0.0	38.0	20	(tr)	0.0	0
(Welch's) 'Orchard Cocktail' frozen	6 oz	90	0.0	22.0	10	(tr)	0.0	0
APPLE GRAPE JUICE								
(Juicy Juice)	6 oz	90	0.0	22.0	10	(mq)	0.0	0
(Juicy Juice) box	8.45 oz	120	1.0	29.0	10	na	0.0	na
(Mott's)	9.5 oz	139	0.0	37.0	27	(mq)	0.0	0
(Mott's)	6 oz	86	0.0	23.0	17	(mq)	0.0	0
(Mott's) aseptic box	8.45 oz	128	0.0	32.0	24	(mq)	0.0	0
(Musselman's) 'Breakfast Cocktail'	6 oz	110	0.0	28.0	5	(tr)	0.0	0
(Red Cheek)	6 oz	109	0.3	27.0	9	(mq)	0.0	0
(Tree Top) canned	6 oz	100	0.0	25.0	10	(mq)	0.0	0
(Tree Top) frozen	6 oz	100	0.0	25.0	10	(mq)	0.0	0
(Welch's) 'Orchard Cocktail'	6 oz	110	0.0	27.0	20	(tr)	0.0	0
(Welch's) 'Orchard Cocktail,' frozen	6 oz	110	0.0	27.0	10	(tr)	0.0	0
(Welch's)'Orchard Cocktail,' frozen, w/raspberry	6 oz	90	0.0	22.0	10	(tr)	0.0	0
(Welch's) 'Orchard Cocktail-in-a Box' w/raspberry	8.45 oz	140	0.0	35.0	20	(tr)	0.0	0
APPLE JUICE								
Can, bottle, or box								
(Heinz) strained, 'Saver Size'	4.2 oz	70	0.0	17.0	15	na	0.0	na
(IGA) 'Unsweetened'	6 oz	74	0.0	18.0	10	(mq)	0.0	0
(Indian Summer)	6 oz	90	<1.0	21.0	10	(mq)	<1.0	0
(J. Hungerford)	9.03 oz	128	0.1	32.2	6	0	0.0	0
(J. Hungerford) 50% juice	9.03 oz	119	0.2	29.9	8	0	0.0	0
(J. Hungerford) 100% juice	9.03 oz	112	0.3	28.0	17	0	0.0	0
(Juicy Juice)	6 oz	90	0.0	21.0	5	(mq)	0.0	0
(Knudsen & Sons) Gravenstein	8 oz	110	<1.0	28.0	na	na	0.0	na
(Knudsen & Sons) 'Natural'	8 oz	85	<1.0	21.0	na	na	0.0	na
(Kraft) 'Pure 100%'	6 oz	80	0.0	20.0	5	(mq)	0.0	0
(Lucky Leaf) 'Individual Portion Control'	3.8 oz	60	0.0	14.0	0	(mq)	0.0	0
(Lucky Leaf) 100% vitamin C enriched	6 oz	90	0.0	21.0	0	(mq)	0.0	0
(Lucky Leaf) regular	6 oz	90	0.0	21.0	0	(mq)	0.0	0
(McCain) 100% juice 'Junior'	4.2 oz	50	0.0	13.0	5	na	0.0	na

Food Name	Serv. Size	Total Cal.	Prot. GMS	Carbs GMS	Sod. MGS	Fiber GMS	Fat GMS	Chol. MGS
(Minute Maid) aseptic box	6 oz	80	0.0	21.0	30	na	0.0	na
(Minute Maid) 'Juices to Go'	6 oz	80	0.0	21.0	30	na	0.0	na
(Mott's)	10 oz	148	0.0	37.0	22	(mq)	0.0	0
(Mott's)	9.5 oz	141	0.0	35.0	20	(mq)	0.0	0
(Mott's)	8.45 oz	124	0.0	31.0	18	(mq)	0.0	0
(Mott's)	6 oz	88	0.0	22.0	13	(mq)	0.0	0
(Mott's) natural style	6 oz	76	0.0	19.0	28	(mq)	0.0	0
(Musselman's) 'Individual Portion Control'	3.8 oz	60	0.0	14.0	0	(mq)	0.0	0
(Musselman's) 100% vitamin C enriched	6 oz	90	0.0	21.0	0	(mq)	0.0	0
(Musselman's) regular	6 oz	90	0.0	21.0	0	(mq)	0.0	0
(Ocean Spray)	6 oz	90	0.0	23.0	15	(mq)	0.0	0
(Red Cheek) 'Natural'	6 oz	97	0.2	24.0	16	(mq)	0.0	0
(Red Cheek) '100% Pure'	6 oz	97	0.2	24.0	7	(mq)	0.0	0
(S&W) '100% Pure Unsweetened'	6 oz	85	0.0	20.0	5	(mq)	0.0	0
(S. Martinelli)	6 oz	100	0.0	25.0	5	na	0.0	0
(S. Martinelli) 'Sparkling'	6 oz	100	0.0	25.0	5	na	0.0	0
(Sippin' Pak) 100% pure, from concentrate	8.45 oz	110	0.0	28.0	25	na	0.0	na
(Snapple) 'Apple Crisp'	8 oz	140	0.0	36.0	30	na	0.0	0
(Tree Top)	6 oz	90	0.0	22.0	10	>.2 c	0.0	0
(TreeSweet)	6 oz	90	0.0	22.0	15	na	0.0	0
(Tropicana) '100% Pure'	8 oz	116	(tr)	28.5	17	(mq)	0.0	0
(Tropicana) '100% Pure'	6 oz	80	<1.0	20.0	15	na	<1.0	na
(Veryfine) '100%'	8 oz	107	0.2	27.0	10	(mq)	0.0	0
(Welch's) sparkling	6 oz	100	0.0	24.0	5	0	0.0	0
(White House)	6 oz	87	0.0	22.0	5	(mq)	0.0	0
Chilled or frozen								
(A&P) diluted as directed	6 oz	90	<1.0	22.0	0	(mq)	<1.0	0
(Knudsen & Sons) clear	8 oz	90	<1.0	22.0	na	na	0.0	na
(Minute Maid) diluted as directed	6 oz	80	0.0	21.0	15	na	0.0	na
(Sunkist) diluted as directed	8 oz	79	0.2	19.4	12	(mq)	0.2	0
(Tree Top) diluted as directed	6 oz	90	0.0	22.0	10	(mq)	0.0	0
(Welch's) 'Orchard Cocktail'	10 oz	170	0.0	42.0	95	0	0.0	0
APPLE ORANGE PINEAPPLE COCKTAIL								
(Welch's) 'Orchard Tropical Cocktails'	6 oz	100	0.0	25.0	20	(tr)	0.0	0
(Welch's) 'Orchard Tropical Cocktails'	8.45 oz	140	0.0	35.0	20	(tr)	0.0	0
APPLE PASTRY								
Fresh								
(Entenmann's) 'Apple Puffs'	1 puff	280	4.0	39.0	320	na	13.0	na
(Tastykake) pocket	3 oz	323	4.3	38.3	222	1.5	17.6	11
Frozen								
(Hormel) 'Apple Dulcita'	4 oz	290	5.0	44.0	350	(mq)	10.0	na
(Mrs. Paul's) 'Apple Fritter'	2 pieces	240	4.0	35.0	500	na	9.0	5

Food Name	Serv. Size	Total Cal.	Prot. GMS	Carbs GMS	Sod. MGS	Fiber GMS	Fat GMS	Chol. MGS
(Pepperidge Farm) 'Apple Dumpling' ..... 3 oz		260	2.0	33.0	230	(mq)	13.0	na
(Pepperidge Farm) apple fruit square ... 1 piece		220	2.0	27.0	170	(mq)	12.0	na
(Pepperidge Farm) 'Berkshire'								
apple crisps .... 1 ramekin		250	2.0	43.0	130	1.0	8.0	4
(Weight Watchers) 'Sweet Celebrations'								
apple crisps .... 3.5 oz		190	1.0	40.0	190	(mq)	5.0	na
APPLE PEACH JUICE (Knudsen & Sons) .. 8 oz		140	<1.0	34.0	na	na	0.0	na
APPLE PEAR JUICE (Tree Top) frozen .... 6 oz		90	0.0	22.0	10	(mq)	0.0	0
APPLE PIE. See PIE.								
APPLE PIE FILLING. See PIE FILLING.								
APPLE PIE SPICE (Tone's) .... 1 tsp		9	0.2	2.4	1	.7	0.2	0
APPLE PUNCH								
(Minute Maid) chilled .... 6 oz		90	0.0	23.0	20	na	0.0	na
(Minute Maid) frozen concentrate .... 6 oz		90	0.0	23.0	0	na	0.0	na
APPLE PUNCH DRINK (Red Cheek) ...... 6 oz		113	0.3	28.0	7	(tr)	0.0	0
APPLE RASPBERRY DRINK								
(Mott's) .... 10 oz		158	0.0	40.0	17	(tr)	0.0	0
(Mott's) .... 9.5 oz		150	0.0	38.0	16	(tr)	0.0	0
APPLE RASPBERRY JUICE								
(Knudsen & Sons) .... 8 oz		110	<1.0	28.0	na	na	0.0	na
(Mott's) .... 9.5 oz		134	0.0	35.0	76	(mq)	0.0	0
(Mott's) .... 6 oz		83	0.0	22.0	48	(mq)	0.0	0
(Mott's) aseptic box .... 8.45 oz		124	0.0	31.0	67	(mq)	0.0	0
(Red Cheek) .... 6 oz		113	0.3	28.0	8	(mq)	0.0	0
(Santa Cruz Natural) organic .... 8 oz		120	<1.0	29.0	na	na	1.0	na
(Tree Top) canned or frozen .... 6 oz		80	0.0	21.0	10	(mq)	0.0	0
(Veryfine) cocktail .... 8 oz		110	0.0	27.0	15	(tr)	0.0	0
APPLE STICKS, frozen, breaded, fried								
(Farm Rich) .... 4 oz		260	2.0	44.0	565	(mq)	8.0	0
APPLE STRAWBERRY JUICE								
(Knudsen & Sons) .... 8 oz		110	<1.0	28.0	na	na	0.0	na
(Santa Cruz Natural) organic .... 8 oz		120	<1.0	29.0	na	na	<1.0	na
APPLE STRAWBERRY NECTAR (Kern's)								
can or bottle .... 6 oz		110	0.0	26.0	0	na	0.0	na
APPLE STRUDEL								
(Aunt Fanny's) individual .... 3 oz		330	4.0	38.0	210	na	18.0	na
(Entenmann's) old fashioned .... 1.5 oz		120	1.0	17.0	110	na	5.0	na
APPLE SYRUP (Knudsen & Sons) .... 1 oz		75	<1.0	15.0	na	na	<1.0	na
APPLE-WHITE GRAPE JUICE								
(Welch's) 'No Sugar Added' frozen cocktail 6 oz		40	0.0	10.0	5	(tr)	0.0	0
APPLESAUCE								
(A&P)								
regular .... 1/2 cup		110	<1.0	25.0	15	(mq)	<1.0	0

Food Name	Serv. Size	Total Cal.	Prot. GMS	Carbs GMS	Sod. MGS	Fiber GMS	Fat GMS	Chol. MGS
unsweetened	1/2 cup	50	<1.0	10.0	0	(mq)	<1.0	0
(Del Monte)								
'Lite'	1/2 cup	50	0.0	13.0	10	(mq)	0.0	0
regular	1/2 cup	90	0.0	24.0	5	(mq)	0.0	0
(Featherweight)	1/2 cup	50	0.0	12.0	3	(mq)	0.0	0
(Finast)								
regular	1/2 cup	105	0.0	25.0	10	(mq)	0.0	0
unsweetened	1/2 cup	56	0.4	15.0	na	(mq)	0.2	0
(Lucky Leaf)								
chunky	4 oz	80	0.0	20.0	20	(mq)	0.0	0
'Juice Pack'	4 oz	50	0.0	12.0	0	(mq)	0.0	0
'Natural' individual portion control	4 oz	50	0.0	13.0	0	(mq)	0.0	0
regular	4 oz	80	0.0	20.0	20	(mq)	0.0	0
'Regular' individual portion control	4 oz	80	0.0	20.0	0	(mq)	0.0	0
unsweetened	4 oz	50	0.0	12.0	0	(mq)	0.0	0
(Mott's)								
chunky	6 oz	86	0.0	21.0	11	(mq)	0.0	0
cinnamon	6 oz	152	0.0	36.0	<1	(mq)	0.0	0
'Natural'	6 oz	80	0.0	20.0	3	(mq)	0.0	0
'Natural Single Serve'	4 oz	53	0.0	13.0	2	(mq)	0.0	0
regular	6 oz	150	0.0	36.0	<1	(mq)	0.0	0
'Single Serve'	4 oz	100	0.0	24.0	<1	(mq)	0.0	0
'Single Serve' cinnamon	4 oz	101	0.0	24.0	<1	(mq)	0.0	0
(Musselman's)								
chunky	4 oz	80	0.0	20.0	20	(mq)	0.0	0
'Juice Pack'	4 oz	50	0.0	12.0	0	(mq)	0.0	0
'Natural' individual portion control	4 oz	50	0.0	13.0	0	(mq)	0.0	0
regular	4 oz	80	0.0	20.0	20	(mq)	0.0	0
'Regular' individual portion control	4 oz	80	0.0	20.0	0	(mq)	0.0	0
unsweetened	4 oz	50	0.0	12.0	0	(mq)	0.0	0
(S&W)								
regular	1/2 cup	90	0.0	24.0	10	(mq)	0.0	0
unsweetened	1/2 cup	55	0.0	14.0	5	(mq)	0.0	0
(S&W Nutradiet)	1/2 cup	55	0.0	14.0	10	(mq)	0.0	0
(Stokely)								
regular	1/2 cup	90	0.0	23.0	30	(mq)	0.0	0
unsweetened	1/2 cup	45	0.0	12.0	5	(mq)	0.0	0
(Tree Top) 'Original'	1/2 cup	80	0.0	21.0	0	(mq)	0.0	0
(White House)								
chunky	4 oz	80	0.0	22.0	5	(mq)	0.0	0
in apple juice	4 oz	50	0.0	13.0	5	(mq)	0.0	0
'Regular'	4 oz	80	0.0	22.0	5	(mq)	0.0	0
unsweetened	4 oz	50	0.0	12.0	5	(mq)	0.0	0

Food Name	Serv. Size	Total Cal.	Prot. GMS	Carbs GMS	Sod. MGS	Fiber GMS	Fat GMS	Chol. MGS
APRICOT								
candied	100 gm	338	0.6	86.5	1	>.6 c	0.2	0
pitted	1 oz	14	0.4	3.2	<1	.4	0.1	0
raw, halves	1 cup	74	2.2	17.2	2	3.7	0.6	0
untrimmed	1 lb	202	5.9	46.9	2	5.6	1.7	0
APRICOT, CANNED								
In extra heavy syrup								
peeled	4 oz	109	0.6	28.2	15	>.4 c	<.1	0
peeled, whole	1/2 cup	118	0.7	30.6	16	>.4 c	0.1	0
In extra light syrup								
unpeeled	4 oz	56	0.7	14.2	2	>.5 c	0.1	0
unpeeled, halves	1/2 cup	61	0.7	15.4	3	>.5 c	0.1	0
In heavy syrup								
peeled	4 oz	94	0.6	24.3	12	>.4 c	0.1	0
peeled, halves	1 cup	214	1.4	55.4	10	>1.0 c	0.2	0
peeled, whole	1/2 cup	107	0.7	27.7	14	>.5 c	0.1	0
peeled, whole (S&W)	1/2 cup	100	0.0	26.0	15	(mq)	0.0	0
unpeeled	4 oz	94	0.6	24.3	5	>.5 c	0.1	0
unpeeled (A&P)	1/2 cup	110	<1.0	28.0	15	(mq)	1.0	0
unpeeled, halves	1/2 cup	107	0.7	27.7	5	1.65	0.1	0
unpeeled, halves (IGA)	1 cup	220	1.0	56.0	15	(mq)	0.0	0
unpeeled, halves (S&W)	1/2 cup	110	0.0	28.0	15	(mq)	0.0	0
In juice								
peeled (Featherweight)	1/2 cup	50	1.0	12.0	10	(mq)	0.0	0
unpeeled	4 oz	54	0.7	14.0	5	.5	<.1	0
unpeeled, halves	1/2 cup	60	0.8	15.3	5	.6	<.1	0
unpeeled, 'Lite' (Libby's)	1/2 cup	60	0.0	17.0	5	(mq)	0.0	0
In light syrup								
unpeeled	4 oz	71	0.6	18.7	5	.5 c	0.1	0
unpeeled, halves	1/2 cup	80	0.7	20.9	5	.5 c	0.1	0
unpeeled, halves 'No Frills' (Pathmark)	1/2 cup	80	0.0	20.0	5	(mq)	0.0	0
In water								
peeled	1/2 cup	25	0.8	6.2	12	>.4 c	<.1	0
peeled, whole (S&W Nutradiet)	1/2 cup	28	0.0	7.0	5	(mq)	0.0	0
unpeeled	4 oz	31	0.8	7.2	3	>.5 c	0.2	0
unpeeled, halves	1/2 cup	33	0.9	7.8	4	1.6	0.2	0
unpeeled, halves (S&W)	1/2 cup	35	0.0	9.0	5	(mq)	0.0	0
unpeeled, halves (S&W Nutradiet)	1/2 cup	35	0.0	9.0	5	(mq)	0.0	0
APRICOT, DEHYDRATED/SULFURED								
cooked	4 oz	143	2.2	37.0	6	>1.8 c	0.3	0
stewed, low-moisture	1/2 cup	156	2.4	40.4	6	>1.9 c	0.3	0
uncooked	4 oz	363	5.6	94.0	15	>4.5 c	0.7	0
uncooked, low-moisture	1/2 cup	192	2.9	49.7	8	>2.4 c	0.4	0

Food Name	Serv. Size	Total Cal.	Prot. GMS	Carbs GMS	Sod. MGS	Fiber GMS	Fat GMS	Chol. MGS
APRICOT, DRIED								
sulfured, cooked	4 oz	96	1.5	24.8	3	>1.2 c	0.2	0
sulfured, stewed, halves	1/2 cup	106	1.6	27.4	4	>1.3 c	0.2	0
sulfured, uncooked	4 oz	270	4.1	70.0	11	8.8	0.5	0
sulfured, uncooked, approx 1.2 oz ...	10 halves	83	1.3	21.6	3	3.2	0.2	0
sulfured, uncooked, halves	1 cup	309	4.7	80.3	13	11.7	0.6	0
(Del Monte)	2 oz	140	2.0	35.0	10	(mq)	0.0	0
(Mariani) California, sun dried, premium	1/4 cup	140	2.0	35.0	10	4.0	0.0	0
(Mariani) Mediterranean, sun dried, premium	1/4 cup	140	2.0	35.0	10	4.0	0.0	0
(SunSweet)	2 oz	140	2.0	35.0	10	(mq)	0.0	0
(Sun•Maid)	2 oz	140	2.0	35.0	10	(mq)	0.0	0
APRICOT, FROZEN								
sweetened	4 oz	111	0.8	28.5	5	>.7 c	0.1	0
sweetened, unthawed	1 cup	237	1.7	60.7	10	4.1	0.2	0
APRICOT KERNEL OIL								
....	1/2 cup	964	0.0	0.0	0	0	109.0	0
....	1 oz	251	0.0	0.0	0	0	28.4	0
....	1 tbsp	120	0.0	0.0	0	0	13.6	0
(Hain)	1 tbsp	120	0.0	0.0	0	0	14.0	0
APRICOT NECTAR								
(Del Monte)	6 oz	100	1.0	26.0	10	(mq)	0.0	0
(Kern's)	6 oz	110	1.0	27.0	0	na	0.0	na
(Knudsen & Sons)	8 oz	105	<1.0	24.0	na	na	0.0	na
(Libby's)	6 oz	110	0.0	26.0	0	(mq)	0.0	0
(S&W)	6 oz	100	0.0	26.0	10	(mq)	0.0	0
APRICOT PIE FILLING. See PIE FILLING.								
APRICOT PINEAPPLE NECTAR								
(Kern's)	6 oz	110	0.0	27.0	5	na	0.0	na
(S&W Nutradiet)	4 oz	35	0.0	12.0	20	(mq)	0.0	0
ARCTIC BONITO. See TUNA, SKIPJACK.								
ARROWHEAD								
boiled, drained	4 oz	88	5.1	18.3	20	>1.7 c	0.1	0
boiled, drained	1 med	9	0.5	1.9	2	>.2 c	0.0	0
raw	1 large	25	1.3	5.1	6	>.2 c	0.1	0
raw	1 med	12	0.6	2.4	3	>.1 c	0.0	0
raw, trimmed	1 oz	28	1.5	5.7	6	>.2 c	0.1	0
raw, untrimmed	1 lb	337	18.2	68.8	75	>2.8 c	1.0	0
ARROWROOT powdered (Tone's)	1 tsp	10	0.0	2.3	1	0	0.0	0
ARROWROOT FLOUR								
....	1 oz	101	0.1	25.0	1	(mq)	<.1	0
....	1/3 cup	154	0.1	37.9	1	(mq)	0.0	0

Food Name	Serv. Size	Total Cal.	Prot. GMS	Carbs GMS	Sod. MGS	Fiber GMS	Fat GMS	Chol. MGS
ARTICHOKE HEARTS								
boiled, drained	4 oz	57	3.9	12.7	108	>1.4 c	0.2	0
boiled, drained	1/2 cup	42	2.9	9.4	80	>1.1 c	0.1	0
canned, marinated *(S&W)*	3.5 oz	225	2.0	6.0	15	(mq)	26.0	0
frozen, boiled, drained	4 oz	51	3.5	10.4	60	>1.0 c	0.6	0
frozen, 'Deluxe' *(Birds Eye)*	3 oz	30	2.0	7.0	140	(mq)	0.0	0
frozen *(Seabrook)*	3 oz	25	3.0	4.0	6	>1.0 c	0.0	0
ARTICHOKES, FRENCH								
boiled, drained	1 med	60	4.2	13.4	114	>1.5 c	0.2	0
boiled, drained, hearts	1/2 cup	42	2.9	9.4	80	4.5	0.1	0
frozen, boiled, drained	3 oz	36	2.5	7.3	42	>.7 c	0.4	0
raw	1 large	76	5.3	17.0	152	8.8	0.2	0
raw	1 med	60	4.2	13.4	120	6.7	0.2	0
ARTICHOKES, GLOBE								
boiled, drained	1 med	60	4.2	13.4	114	>1.5 c	0.2	0
boiled, drained, hearts	1/2 cup	42	2.9	9.4	80	4.54	0.1	0
boiled, drained, trimmed	4 oz	57	3.9	12.7	108	>1.4 c	0.2	0
boiled, drained, untrimmed	4 oz	23	1.6	5.1	43	>.6 c	0.1	0
fresh *(Dole)*	1 large	23	2.0	5.0	65	3.0	0.1	na
frozen, boiled, drained	3 oz	36	2.5	7.3	42	>.7 c	0.4	0
frozen, unprepared	9 oz	97	6.7	19.8	120	9.94	1.1	0
raw	1 large	76	5.3	17.0	152	8.8	0.2	0
raw	1 med	60	4.2	13.4	120	6.9	0.2	0
raw, untrimmed	1 lb	85	5.9	19.1	171	9.4	0.3	0
ARTICHOKES, JERUSALEM								
raw, slices	1/2 cup	57	1.5	13.1	3	1.2	0.0	0
trimmed	1 oz	22	0.6	4.9	na	>.2 c	tr	0
untrimmed	1 lb	238	6.3	54.6	na	>2.5 c	<.1	0
ARUGULA/rocket/roquette/ruculo/rugula								
raw	1 leaf	1	0.1	0.1	1	na	0.0	0
raw	1/2 cup	3	0.3	0.4	3	na	0.1	0
(Frieda's)	1 lb	104	10.0	17.7	68	4.1	1.4	0
(Frieda's)	1 oz	7	0.6	1.1	4	.3	<.1	0
ASPARAGUS								
boiled, drained	1/2 cup	22	2.3	3.8	10	1.9	0.3	0
boiled, drained, cuts and spears	4 oz	28	2.9	5.0	5	>.9 c	0.4	0
fresh *(Dole)*	5 spears	18	2.0	2.0	0	2.0	0.0	na
raw, cuts and spears	1/2 cup	15	2.1	2.5	1	1.41	0.2	0
raw, trimmed	1 oz	6	0.9	1.0	1	.3	0.1	0
raw, untrimmed	1 lb	54	7.3	8.9	5	2.4	0.5	0
ASPARAGUS, CANNED								
Cuts and tips *(Finast)*	1 cup	35	4.0	6.0	720	(mq)	0.0	0
Points, all green *(S&W Nutradiet)*	1/2 cup	17	4.0	3.0	10	(mq)	0.0	0

Food Name	Serv. Size	Total Cal.	Prot. GMS	Carbs GMS	Sod. MGS	Fiber GMS	Fat GMS	Chol. MGS
Spears								
and tips, all green *(Del Monte)*	1/2 cup	20	2.0	3.0	355	(mq)	0.0	0
colossal, all green 'Fancy' *(S&W)*	1/2 cup	20	2.0	4.0	320	(mq)	0.0	0
cut *(Green Giant)*	1/2 cup	18	2.0	3.0	420	1.0	0.0	0
cut, 50% less salt *(Green Giant)*	1/2 cup	18	2.0	3.0	210	1.0	0.0	0
cut, green *(Pathmark)*	1/2 cup	20	3.0	2.0	450	(mq)	0.0	0
cut, green 'No Salt Added' *(Pathmark)*	1/2 cup	20	3.0	2.0	5	(mq)	0.0	0
green *(Stokely)*	1/2 cup	20	2.0	3.0	380	(mq)	0.0	0
green 'Fancy' *(S&W)*	1/2 cup	18	2.0	3.0	320	(mq)	0.0	0
green, w/liquid *(Green Giant)*	1/2 cup	20	2.0	3.0	420	1.0	0.0	0
'No Salt or Sugar Added' *(Stokely)*	1/2 cup	20	2.0	3.0	5	(mq)	0.0	0
white *(Green Giant)*	1/2 cup	16	2.0	3.0	410	1.0	0.0	0
white, w/liquid *(Green Giant)*	1/2 cup	16	2.0	3.0	410	1.0	0.0	0
w/liquid, 50% less salt *(Green Giant)*	1/2 cup	20	2.0	3.0	210	1.0	0.0	0
w/liquid, green, tipped *(Del Monte)*	1/2 cup	20	2.0	3.0	355	(mq)	0.0	0
ASPARAGUS, FROZEN								
boiled, drained	10-oz pkg	82	8.6	14.3	12	>2.5 c	1.2	0
boiled, drained, cuts and spears	4 oz	32	3.3	5.5	5	>1.0 c	0.5	0
cuts *(Birds Eye)*	3.3 oz	25	3.0	4.0	5	(mq)	0.0	0
cuts *(Seabrook)*	3.3 oz	25	3.0	4.0	6	(mq)	0.0	0
cuts 'Harvest Fresh' *(Green Giant)*	1/2 cup	25	3.0	4.0	95	2.0	0.0	0
cuts and spears *(Frosty Acres)*	3.3 oz	25	3.0	4.0	6	(mq)	0.0	0
spears *(Birds Eye)*	3.3 oz	25	3.0	4.0	0	(mq)	0.0	0
spears *(Finast)*	3.3 oz	25	3.0	4.0	5	(mq)	0.0	0
spears *(Frosty Acres)*	3.3 oz	25	3.0	4.0	4	>1.0 c	0.0	0
spears *(Seabrook)*	3.3 oz	25	3.0	4.0	4	>1.0 c	0.0	0
spears *(Southern)*	3.5 oz	27	3.3	4.1	20	(mq)	0.2	0
unprepared	10-oz pkg	68	9.2	11.6	23	6.0	0.7	0
ASPARAGUS BEAN. See YARDLONG BEAN.								
AUBERGINE. See EGGPLANT.								
AU JUS. See GRAVY.								
AVOCADO								
All commercial varieties								
puréed	1/2 cup	185	2.3	8.5	12	>2.4 c	17.6	0
trimmed	1 oz	46	0.6	2.1	3	>.6 c	4.3	0
untrimmed	1 lb	540	6.7	24.8	35	>7.1 c	51.4	0
California								
puréed	1/2 cup	204	2.4	8.0	14	3.1	19.9	0
trimmed	1 oz	50	0.6	2.0	3	.8	4.9	0
untrimmed	1 lb	610	7.3	23.8	42	9.3	59.8	0
Florida								
puréed	1/2 cup	129	1.8	10.3	6	>2.4 c	10.2	0
trimmed	1 oz	32	0.5	2.5	1	>.6 c	2.5	0

Food Name	Serv. Size	Total Cal.	Prot. GMS	Carbs GMS	Sod. MGS	Fiber GMS	Fat GMS	Chol. MGS
untrimmed	1 lb	339	4.8	27.1	14	>6.4 c	26.9	0
AVOCADO OIL								
	1/2 cup	964	0.0	0.0	0	0	109.0	0
	1 oz	251	0.0	0.0	0	0	28.4	0
	1 tbsp	124	0.0	0.0	0	0	1.6	0
(Hain)	1 tbsp	120	0.0	0.0	0	0	14.0	0
AWA/milkfish								
dry-heat cooked	3 oz	161	22.4	0.0	78	0	7.3	57
raw	1 lb	673	93.1	0.0	(mq)	0	30.5	235
raw	1 oz	42	5.8	0.0	(mq)	0	1.9	15

B

Food Name	Serv. Size	Total Cal.	Prot. GMS	Carbs GMS	Sod. MGS	Fiber GMS	Fat GMS	Chol. MGS
BABASSU OIL. See PALM KERNEL OIL.								
BABY FOOD								
CEREAL								
Barley								
dry	1 tbsp	65	2.4	9.0	42	0.2	2.3	81
dry	.5 oz	52	1.6	10.7	7	1.2	0.5	na
instant, dry, '1st Foods' (Gerber)	.5 oz	60	1.0	11.0	na	na	1.0	na
instant, dry, 'Stage 1' (Beech-Nut)	.5 oz	60	1.0	12.0	10	na	0.0	na
instant, .5 oz cereal prepared w/2.4 oz formula, 'Stage 1' (Beech-Nut)	1 serving	120	2.0	18.0	25	na	4.0	na
instant, .5 oz cereal prepared w/2.4 oz whole milk (Gerber)	1 serving	100	3.0	14.0	na	(mq)	4.0	(mq)
instant, .5 oz cereal prepared w/2.4 oz formula	1 serving	110	2.0	16.0	na	na	4.0	na
instant (Heinz)	3.5 oz	370	8.9	78.5	15	na	3.7	na
prepared w/whole milk	3 1/2 oz	111	4.6	16.3	49	>.2 c	3.3	na
Cereal w/applesauce and bananas, '3rd Foods' (Gerber)	7 tbsp	82	1.3	17.9	3	na	0.6	na
Cereal w/egg yolks								
junior	7.5 oz	111	4.1	15.1	70	1.9	3.8	na
junior	1 oz	15	0.5	2.0	9	0.3	0.5	na
strained	1 oz	14	0.5	2.0	9	0	0.5	18
w/bacon, junior	4.5 oz	101	3.2	7.9	61	1.1	6.4	na
w/bacon, junior	1 oz	22	0.7	1.8	14	0.3	1.4	na
w/bacon, strained	7.5 oz	179	5.3	15.1	98	1.9	11.1	na
w/bacon, strained	1 oz	24	0.7	2.0	13	0.3	1.5	na
Cereal w/eggs								
strained	4.5 oz	74	2.8	10.2	49	.1 c	1.9	66

Food Name	Serv. Size	Total Cal.	Prot. GMS	Carbs GMS	Sod. MGS	Fiber GMS	Fat GMS	Chol. MGS
strained	1 oz	16	0.6	2.3	11	0	0.4	15
Corn								
instant, dry, 'Tropical Foods' *(Gerber)*	.5 oz	60	1.0	12.0	na	na	1.0	na
instant, dry, 'Tropical Foods' *(Gerber)*	3.5 oz	390	6.3	80.8	55	na	4.6	na
instant, prepared w/milk, 'Tropical Foods' *(Gerber)*	2.4 oz	110	3.0	15.0	na	na	4.0	na
Grits & egg yolks								
strained	4.5 oz	73	2.3	9.5	45	>.1 c	2.9	na
strained	1 oz	16	0.5	2.1	10	tr	0.7	na
High-protein								
instant, dry	1 tbsp	9	0.9	1.1	1	.2	0.1	na
instant, dry	.5 oz	51	5.1	6.6	7	1.0	0.8	na
instant, 1 oz cereal prepared w/whole milk	1 serving	31	2.5	3.3	14	>.1 c	1.1	na
instant, w/apple and orange, dry	1 tbsp	9	0.6	1.4	3	.2	0.2	na
instant, w/apple and orange, dry	.5 oz	53	3.6	8.2	15	1.0	0.9	na
instant, w/apple and orange, 1 oz cereal prepared w/whole milk	1 serving	32	2.0	3.8	16	>.1 c	1.1	na
Mixed								
dry	1 tbsp	9	0.3	1.8	1	.2	0.1	na
dry	.5 oz	54	1.7	10.4	6	1.1	0.6	na
instant, dry *(Earth's Best)*	.5 oz	60	2.0	11.0	0	(mq)	0.0	0
instant, dry, '2nd Foods' *(Gerber)*	.5 oz	60	1.0	11.0	na	na	1.0	na
instant, dry, 'Stages 2' *(Beech-Nut)*	.5 oz	60	1.0	12.0	10	na	0.0	na
instant, .5 oz cereal prepared w/2.4 oz formula, 'Stages 2' *(Beech-Nut)*	1 serving	120	2.0	17.0	25	na	4.0	na
instant, .5 oz cereal prepared w/2.5 oz formula *(Earth's Best)*	1 serving	110	3.0	16.0	15	(mq)	3.0	na
instant, .5 oz cereal prepared w/2.4 oz whole milk, 'Stages 2' *(Beech-Nut)*	1 serving	100	4.0	14.0	50	(mq)	3.0	(mq)
instant *(Heinz)*	3.5 oz	373	12.8	71.9	12	na	4.9	na
instant, prepared w/apple juice, '2nd Foods' *(Gerber)*	2.4 oz	90	1.0	20.0	na	na	1.0	na
1 oz cereal prepared w/whole milk	1 serving	32	1.4	4.5	13	>.1 c	1.0	na
w/apples and bananas, 'Stages 2' *(Beech-Nut)*	4.5 oz	90	2.0	19.0	0	(mq)	1.0	0
w/apples and bananas, strained *(Heinz)*	3.5 oz	70	1.1	15.7	3	na	0.3	na
w/applesauce and bananas, junior	7.75 oz	183	2.6	40.5	79	2.6	0.9	na
w/applesauce and bananas, junior	1 oz	24	0.3	5.2	10	.3	0.1	na
w/applesauce and bananas, '2nd Foods' *(Gerber)*	4 oz	90	1.0	20.0	na	na	1.0	na
w/applesauce and bananas, '2nd Foods' *(Gerber)*	7 tbsp	81	1.2	17.8	2	na	0.6	na

Food Name	Serv. Size	Total Cal.	Prot. GMS	Carbs GMS	Sod. MGS	Fiber GMS	Fat GMS	Chol. MGS
w/applesauce and bananas, strained ...	4.75 oz	111	1.6	24.2	3	1.6	0.7	na
w/applesauce and bananas, strained	1 oz	23	0.3	5.1	1	.3	0.1	na
w/applesauce and bananas, '3rd Foods' (Gerber)	7 tbsp	82	1.3	18.9	3	na	0.6	na
w/bananas, dry	1 tbsp	9	0.3	1.9	3	.2	0.1	na
w/bananas, dry	.5 oz	56	1.5	10.9	17	1.1	0.7	na
w/bananas, instant, dry, '2nd Foods, (Gerber)	.5 oz	60	1.0	11.0	na	na	1.0	na
w/bananas, 1 oz cereal prepared w/whole milk	1 serving	33	1.3	4.7	17	(mq)	1.0	na
w/fruit and nuts, no sugar added, 1-4 yr., dry (Familia)	1.5 oz	170	4.0	31.0	4	na	3.0	na
w/fruit and nuts, no sugar added, 1-4 yr., 1.5 oz cereal prepared w/whole milk (Familia)	1 serving	270	9.0	38.0	77	na	8.0	na
w/fruit and nuts, 1-4 yr., 1.5 oz cereal prepared w/2/3 cup milk (Familia) ...	1 serving	270	9.0	39.0	74	na	8.0	na
w/fruit and nuts, 100% natural, 1-4 yr., dry (Familia)	1.5 oz	170	4.0	32.0	1	na	3.0	na
w/honey, dry	1 tbsp	9	0.3	1.8	1	(mq)	0.1	na
w/honey, dry	.5 oz	56	2.0	10.4	6	(mq)	0.7	na
w/honey, 1 oz cereal prepared w/whole milk	1 serving	33	1.4	4.5	14	(mq)	1.0	na
Oatmeal								
instant, dry	1 tbsp	10	0.3	1.7	1	.2	0.2	na
instant, dry	.5 oz	57	1.9	9.8	5	.9	1.1	na
prepared w/whole milk	1 oz	33	1.4	4.3	13	>.1 c	1.2	na
w/apples and bananas, 'Stages 2' (Beech-Nut)	4.5 oz	90	2.0	17.0	5	(mq)	1.0	0
w/apples and bananas, strained (Heinz)	3.5 oz	76	1.5	16.1	3	.5	0.6	na
w/apples and cinnamon, instant, '3rd Foods' (Gerber)	1 pkt	90	2.0	16.0	50	na	2.0	na
w/applesauce and bananas, '2nd Foods' (Gerber)	4 oz	90	1.0	20.0	na	(mq)	1.0	0
w/applesauce and bananas, '2nd Foods' (Gerber)	7 tbsp	83	1.4	17.6	2	na	0.8	na
w/applesauce and bananas, '3rd Foods' (Gerber)	7 tbsp	80	1.4	17.0	3	na	0.8	na
w/applesauce and bananas, junior	7.75 oz	165	2.9	34.5	68	1.8	1.5	na
w/applesauce and bananas, junior	1 oz	21	0.4	4.4	9	.2	0.2	na
w/applesauce and bananas, strained ..	4.75 oz	99	1.8	20.8	3	1.1	0.9	na
w/applesauce and bananas, strained	1 oz	21	0.4	4.4	1	.2	0.2	na
w/bananas, dry	1 tbsp	9	0.3	1.8	3	.1	0.1	na

Food Name	Serv. Size	Total Cal.	Prot. GMS	Carbs GMS	Sod. MGS	Fiber GMS	Fat GMS	Chol. MGS
w/bananas, dry	.5 oz	56	1.7	10.4	17	.7	0.9	na
w/bananas, instant, '3rd Foods' (Gerber)	1 pkt	90	2.0	16.0	50	na	2.0	na
w/bananas, prepared w/whole milk	1 oz	33	1.3	4.5	17	>.1 c	1.1	na
w/bananas, prepared w/whole milk	3.5 oz	116	4.7	16.0	61	>.2 c	3.8	na
w/bananas, 100% natural, organic, dry (Healthy Times)	.5 oz	60	2.0	12.0	0	na	0.0	na
w/bananas, organic, .5 oz cereal prepared w/2.4 oz formula (Healthy Times)	.5 oz	100	3.0	17.0	15	na	3.0	na
w/honey, dry	1 tbsp	9	0.3	1.7	1	(mq)	0.2	na
w/honey, dry	1/2 oz	56	1.9	9.8	7	>.1 c	1.0	na
w/honey, prepared w/whole milk	1 oz	33	1.4	4.3	14	(mq)	1.1	na
Rice								
dry	1 tbsp	9	0.2	1.9	1	(mq)	0.1	na
dry	.5 oz	56	1.0	11.0	5	.1 c	0.7	na
dry (Earth's Best)	.5 oz	60	1.0	12.0	0	(mq)	0.0	0
dry (Health Valley)	1 tbsp	60	1.0	10.0	5	.7	1.0	0
dry, .5 oz cereal prepared w/2.5 oz formula (Earth's Best)	3 oz	110	2.0	17.0	15	(mq)	3.0	na
dry, prepared w/whole milk	1 oz	33	1.1	4.7	13	0	1.0	na
instant, dry, '1st Foods' (Gerber)	.5 oz	60	1.0	11.0	na	na	1.0	na
instant, dry, '1st Foods' (Gerber)	3.5 oz	380	8.3	79.3	7	na	3.3	na
instant, dry, 'Stages 1' (Beech-Nut)	.5 oz	60	1.0	12.0	15	(mq)	0.0	0
instant, .5 oz cereal prepared w/2.4 oz formula (Beech-Nut)	.5 oz	120	2.0	18.0	20	na	4.0	na
instant, .5 oz cereal prepared w/2.4 oz whole milk (Beech-Nut)	2.9 oz	110	2.0	17.0	30	(mq)	3.0	na
instant (Heinz)	3.5 oz	376	7.9	78.0	12	na	4.1	na
sprouted (Health Valley)	1 tbsp	60	1.0	10.0	5	2.1	1.0	0
w/apples, instant, dry, 'Stages 2' (Beech-Nut)	.5 oz	60	0.0	13.0	15	(mq)	0.0	0
w/apples, instant, .5 oz cereal prepared w/2.4 oz formula (Beech-Nut)	.5 oz	120	1.0	19.0	20	na	4.0	na
w/apples, instant, .5 oz cereal prepared w/2.4 oz whole milk (Beech-Nut)	2.9 oz	110	3.0	17.0	50	(mq)	3.0	na
w/apples and bananas, 'Stages 2' (Beech-Nut)	4.5 oz	100	2.0	24.0	25	(mq)	0.0	0
w/apples and bananas, strained (Heinz)	3.5 oz	70	0.6	16.2	5	na	0.2	na
w/applesauce and bananas, '2nd Foods' (Gerber)	4 oz	90	1.0	21.0	na	(mq)	0.0	0
w/applesauce and bananas,'2nd Foods' (Gerber)	7 tbsp	79	0.9	18.2	9	na	0.2	na
w/applesauce and bananas, strained	4.75 oz	107	1.6	23.1	38	1.4	0.5	na
w/applesauce and bananas, strained	1 oz	22	0.3	4.8	8	.3	0.1	na

Food Name	Serv. Size	Total Cal.	Prot. GMS	Carbs GMS	Sod. MGS	Fiber GMS	Fat GMS	Chol. MGS
w/bananas, dry	1 tbsp	10	0.2	1.9	2	(mq)	0.1	na
w/bananas, dry	.5 oz	57	1.2	11.4	14	.1	0.6	na
w/bananas, instant, dry, '2nd Foods' (Gerber)	.5 oz	60	1.0	11.0	na	na	1.0	na
w/bananas, instant, dry, 'Stages 2' (Beech-Nut)	.5 oz	60	1.0	13.0	15	(mq)	0.0	0
w/bananas, instant, .5 oz cereal prepared w/2.4 oz formula (Beech-Nut)	.5 oz	120	1.0	19.0	20	na	4.0	na
w/bananas, instant, .5 oz cereal prepared w/2.4 oz whole milk (Beech-Nut)	2.9 oz	100	3.0	17.0	50	(mq)	3.0	(mq)
w/bananas, prepared w/whole milk	1 oz	33	1.2	4.8	16	(mq)	1.0	na
w/formula, instant, '1st Foods' (Gerber)	2.4 oz	110	2.0	16.0	na	na	4.0	na
w/honey, dry	1 tbsp	9	0.2	1.9	1	(mq)	0.1	na
w/honey, dry	.5 oz	56	1.0	11.5	7	(mq)	0.4	na
w/honey, prepared w/whole milk	1 oz	33	1.1	4.8	14	(mq)	0.9	na
w/mango, instant, dry, 'Tropical Foods' (Gerber)	3.5 oz	386	6.4	84.3	20	na	2.6	na
w/mango, instant, prepared w/milk, 'Tropical Foods' (Gerber)	2.4 oz	100	3.0	15.0	na	na	3.0	na
w/mixed fruit, junior	7.75 oz	185	2.2	41.1	24	2.2	0.4	na
w/mixed fruit, junior	1 oz	24	0.3	5.3	3	.3	0.1	na
w/mixed fruit, junior (Gerber)	6 oz	140	1.0	31.0	17	(mq)	1.0	0
w/mixed fruit, '3rd Foods' (Gerber)	7 tbsp	79	0.9	18.3	10	na	0.2	na
DESSERTS AND SNACKS								
Apple betty								
junior	7.75 oz	154	0.9	41.8	20	2.2	0.0	na
junior	1 oz	20	0.1	5.4	3	.3	0.0	na
strained	4.75 oz	97	0.5	26.5	14	1.4	0.0	na
strained	1 oz	20	0.1	5.6	3	.3	0.0	na
Apple Juice Dessert, w/yogurt, 2nd Foods' (Gerber)	4 oz	100	2.0	18.0	na	na	2.0	na
Apple yogurt								
apple yogurt dessert, 'Stages 2' (Beech-Nut)	4.5 oz	120	1.0	25.0	25	na	2.0	na
'Breakfast' (Earth's Best)	4.5 oz	100	3.0	17.0	20	na	2.0	na
Banana yogurt								
'2nd Foods' (Gerber)	7 tbsp	74	1.1	16.4	22	na	0.4	na
'Stages 2' (Beech-Nut)	4.5 oz	120	1.0	26.0	30	na	2.0	na
strained (Heinz)	3.5 oz	83	1.0	18.7	20	na	0.5	na
Banana-apple dessert, 2nd Foods (Gerber)	7 tbsp	68	0.2	16.4	7	na	0.1	na
Banana-pineapple dessert, 'Stages 2' (Beech-Nut)	4.5 oz	110	0.0	27.0	15	na	0.0	na

Food Name	Serv. Size	Total Cal.	Prot. GMS	Carbs GMS	Sod. MGS	Fiber GMS	Fat GMS	Chol. MGS
Banana-vanilla dessert, 'Tropical Foods'								
(Gerber) .... 7 tbsp	7 tbsp	85	0.5	18.7	11	na	0.9	na
Blueberry yogurt, 'Breakfast' (Earth's Best)	4.5 oz	100	3.0	16.0	20	na	2.0	na
Cereal snack								
apple-banana finger snacks, 'Graduates'								
(Gerber) .... 3.2 oz	3.2 oz	405	8.2	82.6	86	na	4.8	na
apple-cinnamon finger snacks,								
'Graduates' (Gerber) .... 3.2 oz	3.2 oz	407	7.9	82.6	84	na	5.0	na
Cherry vanilla dessert								
junior .... 7.75 oz	7.75 oz	152	0.4	40.5	33	.7	0.4	na
junior .... 1 oz	1 oz	20	0.1	5.2	4	.1	0.1	na
strained .... 4.75 oz	4.75 oz	92	0.3	24.0	22	.3 c	0.4	na
strained .... 1 oz	1 oz	19	0.1	5.1	5	.1	0.1	na
Cookies and crackers								
animal-shaped, baked, chunky (Gerber)	3.5 oz	443	6.5	74.8	187	na	13.1	na
apple, organic, 'Hugga Bears'								
(Healthy Times) .... 1 oz	1 oz	120	2.0	17.0	38	na	3.0	0
arrowroot .... 1 oz	1 oz	125	2.2	20.2	105	1.1	4.1	0
arrowroot, baked finger snacks, 'Graduates'								
(Gerber) .... 3.5 oz	3.5 oz	452	8.4	70.3	324	na	15.3	na
arrowroot, w/maple, wheat-free								
(Healthy Times) .... 1 cookie	1 cookie	120	2.0	17.0	38	na	3.0	0
baked, chunky, 'Biter Biscuit' (Gerber)	1 biscuit	50	1.0	9.0	na	na	1.0	na
cinnamon animal crackers, baked,								
'Graduates' (Gerber) .... 3.5 oz	3.5 oz	449	5.9	78.7	369	na	12.3	na
pretzel .... 1 oz	1 oz	113	3.1	23.3	76	.7	0.6	na
pretzel, baked, finger snacks, 'Graduates'								
(Gerber) .... 3.5 oz	3.5 oz	403	10.5	83.0	597	na	3.3	na
strawberry, organic, 'Hugga Bears'								
(Healthy Times) .... 1 oz	1 oz	120	2.0	17.0	38	na	3.0	0
teething biscuit .... 1 biscuit	1 biscuit	43	1.2	8.4	40	.2	0.5	na
teething biscuit .... 1 oz	1 oz	111	3.0	21.7	103	.4	1.2	na
zwieback, baked, chunky (Gerber) ..... 3.5 oz	3.5 oz	432	12.9	69.4	210	na	11.5	na
Cottage cheese w/pineapple								
junior .... 7.75 oz	7.75 oz	172	6.6	35.0	112	>2.2 c	1.5	na
junior .... 1 oz	1 oz	22	0.9	4.5	14	>.3 c	0.2	na
strained .... 4.75 oz	4.75 oz	93	3.9	17.8	70	>1.8 c	1.1	na
strained .... 1 oz	1 oz	20	0.8	3.7	15	>.4 c	0.2	na
'Stages 2' (Beech-Nut) .... 4.5 oz	4.5 oz	130	2.0	26.0	15	(mq)	1.0	(mq)
'Stages 3' (Beech-Nut) .... 6 oz	6 oz	170	3.0	36.0	20	na	2.0	na
Custard/pudding								
banana pudding, 'Stages 2' (Beech-Nut)	4.5 oz	100	0.0	25.0	10	na	0.0	na
banana pudding, strained (Heinz) ...... 3.5 oz	3.5 oz	74	0.7	16.8	9	na	0.5	na

Food Name	Serv. Size	Total Cal.	Prot. GMS	Carbs GMS	Sod. MGS	Fiber GMS	Fat GMS	Chol. MGS
caramel pudding, junior	7.75 oz	168	3.0	36.2	60	>.2 c	1.9	na
caramel pudding, junior	1 oz	22	0.4	4.8	8	(mq)	0.3	na
caramel pudding, strained	4.75 oz	104	1.8	23.2	36	>.1 c	0.9	na
caramel pudding, strained	1 oz	22	0.4	4.9	8	(mq)	0.2	na
cherry vanilla pudding, '2nd Foods' (Gerber)	7 tbsp	69	0.3	16.6	9	na	0.2	na
cherry vanilla pudding, strained (Gerber)	4.5 oz	90	0.0	21.0	12	(mq)	1.0	3
chocolate custard, junior	7.75 oz	196	4.2	38.3	55	1.5	3.5	na
chocolate custard, junior	1 oz	25	0.5	4.9	7	.2	0.5	na
chocolate custard, junior (Heinz)	3.5 oz	75	2.0	14.0	27	na	1.2	na
chocolate custard, strained	4.75 oz	108	2.4	20.6	29	.9	2.2	na
chocolate custard, strained	1 oz	24	0.5	4.6	7	.2	0.5	na
orange pudding, strained	4.75 oz	108	1.5	23.9	27	.8	1.2	na
orange pudding, strained	1 oz	23	0.3	5.0	6	.2	0.3	na
pineapple pudding, junior	7.75 oz	191	3.1	47.5	48	1.8	0.9	na
pineapple pudding, junior	1 oz	25	0.4	6.1	6	.2	0.1	na
pineapple pudding, strained	4.75 oz	104	1.7	26.0	24	.9	0.4	na
pineapple pudding, strained	1 oz	23	0.4	5.8	5	.2	0.1	na
vanilla custard, junior	7.75 oz	196	3.5	35.6	64	>.4 c	5.1	na
vanilla custard, junior	1 oz	25	0.5	4.6	8	>.1 c	0.7	na
vanilla custard, junior (Gerber)	6 oz	150	3.0	31.0	41	na	2.0	23
vanilla custard, '2nd Foods' (Gerber)	7 tbsp	88	1.8	18.2	25	na	0.9	na
vanilla custard, 'Stages 2' (Beech-Nut)	4.5 oz	140	2.0	24.0	60	na	4.0	na
vanilla custard, 'Stages 3' (Beech-Nut)	6 oz	180	3.0	30.0	80	na	5.0	na
vanilla custard, strained	4.75 oz	109	2.0	20.6	36	>.3 c	2.6	na
vanilla custard, strained	1 oz	24	0.5	4.6	8	>.1 c	0.6	na
vanilla custard, strained (Gerber)	4.5 oz	100	2.0	22.0	32	na	1.0	14
vanilla custard, '3rd Foods' (Gerber)	7 tbsp	89	1.7	18.4	24	na	0.9	na
vanilla custard, strained (Heinz)	3.5 oz	75	2.0	14.0	27	na	1.2	na
Dutch apple dessert								
junior	7.75 oz	152	0.0	37.0	35	2.0	2.2	na
junior	1 oz	20	0.0	4.8	5	.3	0.3	na
junior (Heinz)	3.5 oz	69	0.1	16.3	5	na	0.4	na
'2nd Foods' (Gerber)	7 tbsp	79	0.1	17.4	14	na	1.0	na
'Stages 2' (Beech-Nut)	4.5 oz	100	0.0	24.0	15	(mq)	0.0	0
strained	4.75 oz	92	0.0	22.5	22	1.2	1.2	na
strained	1 oz	19	0.0	4.7	5	.3	0.3	na
strained (Heinz)	3.5 oz	69	0.1	16.3	5	na	0.4	na
'3rd Foods' (Gerber)	7 tbsp	77	0.1	16.9	14	na	0.9	na
Fruit dessert								
junior (Gerber)	6 oz	130	0.0	30.0	12	(mq)	1.0	0
junior (Heinz)	3.5 oz	65	0.2	15.7	14	na	0.2	na
'2nd Foods' (Gerber)	7 tbsp	82	0.4	19.7	9	na	0.2	na

Food Name	Serv. Size	Total Cal.	Prot. GMS	Carbs GMS	Sod. MGS	Fiber GMS	Fat GMS	Chol. MGS
'Stages 2' (Beech-Nut)	4.5 oz	80	0.0	20.0	0	(mq)	0.0	0
'Stages 3' (Beech-Nut)	6 oz	120	0.0	28.0	5	(mq)	0.0	0
strained (Gerber)	4.5 oz	100	0.0	24.0	13	(mq)	1.0	0
strained (Heinz)	3.5 oz	66	0.3	15.8	11	na	0.2	na
'3rd Foods' (Gerber)	7 tbsp	73	0.3	17.6	7	na	0.2	na
w/o ascorbic acid, junior	7.75 oz	139	0.7	37.8	29	1.3	0.0	na
w/o ascorbic acid, junior	1 oz	18	0.1	4.9	4	.2	0.0	na
w/o ascorbic acid, strained	4.75 oz	80	0.4	21.6	19	.8	0.0	na
w/o ascorbic acid, strained	1 oz	17	0.1	4.5	4	.2	0.0	na
Guava dessert, w/tapioca, 'Tropical Foods'								
(Gerber)	7 tbsp	69	0.1	16.8	3	na	0.1	na
Hawaiian dessert								
junior (Gerber)	6 oz	150	2.0	33.0	32	(mq)	1.0	3
'2nd Foods' (Gerber)	7 tbsp	86	1.3	19.7	17	na	0.2	na
'3rd Foods' (Gerber)	7 tbsp	87	1.3	20.2	15	na	0.1	na
strained (Gerber)	4.5 oz	120	2.0	25.0	23	(mq)	1.0	2
Mango dessert, w/tapioca 'Tropical Foods'								
(Gerber)	7 tbsp	75	0.2	18.2	2	na	0.2	na
Mango-banana dessert, w/passion fruit,								
'Tropical Foods' (Gerber)	7 tbsp	73	0.2	17.7	9	na	0.1	na
Mixed fruit yogurt, '2nd Foods' (Gerber)	7 tbsp	79	1.0	18.0	15	na	0.3	na
Papaya dessert, w/tapioca, 'Tropical Foods'								
(Gerber)	7 tbsp	62	0.2	15.1	7	na	0.2	na
Papaya-pineapple dessert, 'Tropical Foods'								
(Gerber)	7 tbsp	76	0.2	18.6	8	na	0.0	na
Peach cobbler								
junior	7.75 oz	147	0.7	40.3	20	1.5	0.0	na
junior	1 oz	19	0.1	5.2	3	.2	0.0	na
'2nd Foods' (Gerber)	7 tbsp	77	0.5	18.2	8	na	0.2	na
strained	4.75 oz	88	0.4	24.0	9	.9	0.0	na
strained	1 oz	18	0.1	5.1	2	.2	0.0	na
strained (Heinz)	3.5 oz	72	0.5	16.9	6	.3	0.3	na
'3rd Foods' (Gerber)	7 tbsp	77	0.6	18.4	9	na	0.1	na
Peach melba								
junior	7.75 oz	132	0.7	36.1	20	>.2 c	0.0	na
junior	1 oz	17	0.1	4.7	3	(mq)	0.0	na
strained	4.75 oz	81	0.3	22.3	12	>.3 c	0.0	na
strained	1 oz	17	0.1	4.7	3	>.1 c	0.0	na
Peach yogurt								
'2nd Foods' (Gerber)	7 tbsp	76	1.0	17.2	14	na	0.4	na
'Stages 2' (Beech-Nut)	4.5 oz	120	1.0	25.0	30	na	2.0	na
Peach-mango dessert, 'Tropical Foods'								
(Gerber)	7 tbsp	60	0.3	16.8	7	na	0.2	na

Food Name	Serv. Size	Total Cal.	Prot. GMS	Carbs GMS	Sod. MGS	Fiber GMS	Fat GMS	Chol. MGS
Pear yogurt								
'Stages 2' (Beech-Nut)	4.5 oz	130	1.0	29.0	35	na	2.0	na
strained (Heinz)	3.5 oz	80	0.8	18.1	19	na	0.4	na
Pineapple-banana dessert, 'Tropical Foods'								
(Gerber)	7 tbsp	79	0.3	19.3	9	na	0.1	na
Pineapple-orange dessert								
strained	4.75 oz	90	0.3	24.4	13	.5	0.0	na
strained	1 oz	20	0.1	5.4	3	.1	0.0	na
Tropical fruit dessert								
junior	7.75 oz	132	0.4	36.1	15	>.2 c	0.0	na
junior	1 oz	17	0.1	4.7	2	(mq)	0.0	na
medley, 'Tropical Foods' (Gerber)	7 tbsp	64	0.2	15.4	6	na	0.1	na
w/tapioca, strained	4.5 oz	80	0.0	20.0	6	(mq)	0.0	0
Tropical yogurt, 'Breakfast' (Earth's Best)	4.5 oz	110	3.0	19.0	20	na	2.0	na
Tutti frutti dessert, junior (Heinz)	3.5 oz	67	0.3	15.7	12	.3	0.4	na
DINNERS AND MAIN DISHES								
Apples and chicken dinner, 'Simple Recipe'								
'2nd Foods' (Gerber)	7 tbsp	66	2.4	11.0	13	na	1.4	na
Apples and ham dinner, 'Simple Recipe'								
'2nd Foods' (Gerber)	7 tbsp	67	2.7	12.2	9	na	0.8	na
Apples and turkey dinner								
'Simple Recipe,' '2nd Foods' (Gerber)	4 oz	80	3.0	13.0	20	na	2.0	na
'Simple Recipe,' '2nd Foods' (Gerber)	7 tbsp	67	2.9	11.3	13	na	1.2	na
Beans and rice dinner								
'Tropical Foods' (Gerber)	7 tbsp	52	2.1	7.4	8	na	1.5	na
w/green beans (Earth's Best)	4.5 oz	70	2.0	14.0	0	(mq)	0.0	0
Beef and egg noodle dinner								
'2nd Foods' (Gerber)	7 tbsp	62	2.7	8.3	10	na	2.0	na
'3rd Foods' (Gerber)	7 tbsp	64	2.7	8.9	14	na	1.9	na
strained (Heinz)	3.5 oz	49	2.0	6.3	15	.3 ns	1.8	na
Beef and rice dinner								
toddler	6.25 oz	145	8.9	15.6	632	>.5 c	5.1	na
toddler	1 oz	23	1.4	2.5	101	>.1 c	0.8	na
Beef dinner								
junior (Gerber)	2.5 oz	80	11.0	1.0	38	0	4.0	20
'Stages 1' (Beech-Nut)	2.8 oz	90	10.0	0.0	40	.0	5.0	(mq)
'Stages 3' (Beech-Nut)	6 oz	150	6.0	14.0	45	(mq)	8.0	(mq)
supreme, 'Stages 2' (Beech-Nut)	4.5 oz	120	3.0	13.0	40	na	6.0	(mq)
'3rd Foods' (Gerber)	7 tbsp	103	15.1	0.2	52	na	4.6	na
w/vegetables, lean meat, junior (Gerber)	4.5 oz	100	8.0	10.0	29	(mq)	3.0	12
w/vegetables, lean meat, strained								
(Gerber)	4.5 oz	90	7.0	9.0	32	(mq)	3.0	11

Food Name	Serv. Size	Total Cal.	Prot. GMS	Carbs GMS	Sod. MGS	Fiber GMS	Fat GMS	Chol. MGS
Beef lasagna dinner								
toddler	6.25 oz	136	7.4	17.7	804	>.4 c	3.7	na
toddler	1 oz	22	1.2	2.8	129	>.1 c	0.6	na
Beef noodle dinner								
junior	7.5 oz	121	5.3	15.8	36	2.3	4.1	na
junior	1 oz	16	0.7	2.1	5	.3	0.5	na
strained	4.5 oz	68	2.9	9.0	37	1.4	2.2	na
strained	1 oz	15	0.7	2.0	8	.3	0.5	na
Beef stew								
'Stages Table Time' *(Beech-Nut)*	6 oz	150	10.0	16.0	380	(mq)	6.0	(mq)
toddler	6.25 oz	90	9.0	9.7	611	2.0	2.1	22
toddler	1 oz	14	1.5	1.6	98	.3	0.3	4
Beef vegetable dinner								
high-meat, junior	4.5 oz	109	8.1	6.8	42	1.1	5.9	na
high-meat, junior	1 oz	24	1.8	1.5	9	.3	1.3	na
high-meat, strained	4.5 oz	96	7.3	5.4	46	1.1	5.4	na
high-meat, strained	1 oz	21	1.6	1.2	10	.3	1.2	na
Beef vegetable entrée								
'Stages 2' *(Beech-Nut)*	4.5 oz	90	2.0	10.0	35	(mq)	4.0	(mq)
'Stages 3' *(Beech-Nut)*	6 oz	160	6.0	16.0	70	(mq)	7.0	(mq)
Broccoli-chicken dinner, 'Simple Recipe'								
'2nd Foods' *(Gerber)*	7 tbsp	42	3.7	3.4	20	na	1.5	na
Carrots and beef dinner, 'Simple Recipe'								
'2nd Foods' *(Gerber)*	7 tbsp	59	3.4	5.7	40	na	2.5	na
Chicken dinner								
junior *(Gerber)*	2.5 oz	110	11.0	1.0	28	0	7.0	42
'3rd Foods' *(Gerber)*	7 tbsp	132	15.0	0.2	39	na	7.9	na
vegetable entrée, 'Stages 2' *(Beech-Nut)*	4.5 oz	90	3.0	14.0	65	(mq)	3.0	(mq)
vegetable entrée, 'Stages 3' *(Beech-Nut)*	6 oz	90	7.0	13.0	70	(mq)	2.0	(mq)
w/vegetables, lean meat, junior *(Gerber)*	4.5 oz	90	7.0	10.0	32	(mq)	3.0	19
w/vegetables, lean meat, strained *(Gerber)*	4.5 oz	90	7.0	8.0	31	(mq)	3.0	18
Chicken noodle dinner								
junior	7.5 oz	109	4.1	16.0	36	2.3	3.0	na
junior	1 oz	14	0.5	2.1	5	.3	0.4	na
'2nd Foods' *(Gerber)*	7 tbsp	55	2.5	8.6	14	na	1.2	na
strained	4.5 oz	67	2.7	9.6	20	1.4	1.9	na
strained	1 oz	15	0.6	2.1	5	.3	0.4	na
'3rd Foods' *(Gerber)*	7 tbsp	56	2.5	8.6	14	na	1.3	na
Chicken rice dinner								
'Stages 2' *(Beech-Nut)*	4.5 oz	80	2.0	11.0	40	(mq)	3.0	(mq)
'Tropical Foods' *(Gerber)*	7 tbsp	48	2.3	6.9	14	na	1.3	na
Chicken stew dinner								
toddler	6 oz	133	8.8	10.9	683	1.0	6.3	49

Food Name	Serv. Size	Total Cal.	Prot. GMS	Carbs GMS	Sod. MGS	Fiber GMS	Fat GMS	Chol. MGS
toddler	1 oz	22	1.5	1.8	114	.2	1.0	8
w/noodles, 'Graduates'	3.2 oz	69	4.4	8.5	308	na	2.0	na
Chicken vegetable dinner								
high-meat, junior	4.5 oz	118	9.0	5.4	33	1.1	7.0	na
high-meat, junior	1 oz	26	2.0	1.2	7	.3	1.6	na
high-meat, strained	4.5 oz	100	7.9	7.6	35	1.1	4.6	na
high-meat, strained	1 oz	22	1.8	1.7	8	.3	1.0	na
Green bean dinner, w/turkey, 'Simple Recipe,'								
'2nd Foods' (Gerber)	7 tbsp	55	4.1	6.5	11	na	1.5	na
Ham dinner								
ham and vegetable entrée, 'Stages 2'								
(Beech-Nut)	4.5 oz	80	3.0	12.0	30	(mq)	3.0	(mq)
w/vegetables, lean meat, junior (Gerber)	4.5 oz	110	8.0	11.0	27	(mq)	4.0	11
w/vegetables, lean meat, strained								
(Gerber)	4.5 oz	100	7.0	10.0	26	(mq)	4.0	12
Ham vegetable dinner								
high-meat, junior	4.5 oz	99	8.2	7.8	28	1.1	4.2	23
high-meat, junior	1 oz	22	1.8	1.7	6	.3	0.9	5
high-meat, strained	4.5 oz	97	8.1	7.0	28	1.1	4.5	na
high-meat, strained	1 oz	22	1.8	1.6	6	.3	1.0	na
Lamb and vegetable entrée, 'Stages 2'								
(Beech-Nut)	4.5 oz	90	2.0	13.0	40	(mq)	4.0	(mq)
Lamb noodle dinner								
junior	7.5 oz	138	4.9	18.5	38	>.4 c	4.7	na
junior	1 oz	18	0.7	2.5	5	>.1 c	0.6	na
Macaroni dinner								
tomato beef, '2nd Foods' (Gerber)	7 tbsp	57	2.6	9.1	32	na	1.1	na
tomato beef, '3rd Foods' (Gerber)	7 tbsp	60	2.5	10.2	12	na	0.9	na
tomatoes and beef, junior (Heinz)	3.5 oz	52	2.0	8.2	14	.3	1.2	na
w/bacon, junior	7.5 oz	160	5.3	18.3	166	>.2 c	7.0	na
w/bacon, junior	1 oz	21	0.7	2.4	22	(mq)	0.9	na
w/beef, 'Stages 2' (Beech-Nut)	4.5 oz	90	2.0	13.0	40	(mq)	4.0	(mq)
w/beef, 'Stages 3' (Beech-Nut)	6 oz	160	6.0	17.0	85	(mq)	8.0	(mq)
w/cheese (Earth's Best)	4.5 oz	100	4.0	12.0	10	na	4.0	na
w/cheese, junior	7.5 oz	130	5.5	17.5	162	.6	4.3	na
w/cheese, junior	1 oz	17	0.7	2.3	22	.1	0.6	na
w/cheese, strained	4.5 oz	76	3.3	9.6	93	.4	2.7	na
w/cheese, strained	1 oz	17	0.7	2.1	21	.1	0.6	na
w/cheese, '2nd Foods' (Gerber)	7 tbsp	63	2.8	8.6	88	na	2.0	na
Macaroni main dish								
alphabets w/beef and tomato sauce, chunky								
(Gerber)	7 tbsp	80	4.2	11.4	199	na	2.0	na
w/beef, in sauce, 'Graduates' (Gerber)	3.2 oz	78	4.7	11.1	302	na	1.7	na

Food Name	Serv. Size	Total Cal.	Prot. GMS	Carbs GMS	Sod. MGS	Fiber GMS	Fat GMS	Chol. MGS
w/ham, junior	7.5 oz	128	6.8	18.1	100	>.4 c	3.0	na
w/ham, junior	1 oz	17	0.9	2.4	13	>.1 c	0.4	na
w/tomato and beef, junior	7.5 oz	126	5.3	20.0	36	2.3	2.3	na
w/tomato and beef, junior	1 oz	17	0.7	2.7	5	.3	0.3	na
w/tomato and beef, strained	4.5 oz	70	2.8	11.3	22	1.4	1.4	na
w/tomato and beef, strained	1 oz	16	0.6	2.5	5	.3	0.3	na
Mixed vegetable dinner								
junior	7.5 oz	70	2.1	16.8	19	>.4 c	0.0	na
junior	1 oz	9	0.3	2.2	3	>.1 c	0.0	na
strained	4.5 oz	52	1.5	12.2	10	>.4 c	0.1	na
strained	1 oz	12	0.3	2.7	2	>.1 c	0.0	na
Noodle main dish								
w/beef, chunky, 'Homestyle' (Gerber)	7 tbsp	88	4.4	9.8	216	na	3.5	na
w/chicken, carrots, and peas, chunky (Gerber)	7 tbsp	65	4.1	8.8	207	na	1.5	na
Pasta dinner (Earth's Best)	4.5 oz	90	3.0	13.0	20	na	3.0	na
Potato dinner, w/green beans (Earth's Best)	4.5 oz	100	4.0	13.0	25	na	3.0	na
Ravioli								
beef, w/tomato sauce, 'Graduates' (Gerber)	3.2 oz	97	3.4	16.3	322	na	2.0	na
beef, w/tomato sauce, 'Graduates' micro cup (Gerber)	6 oz	170	6.0	28.0	590	na	4.0	na
cheese, w/tomato sauce, 'Graduates' (Gerber)	3.2 oz	99	3.6	16.3	297	na	2.2	na
cheese, w/tomato sauce, 'Graduates' micro cup (Gerber)	6 oz	170	6.0	28.0	510	na	4.0	na
Rice and lentil dinner, (Earth's Best)	4.5 oz	80	3.0	13.0	25	na	2.0	na
Rice main dish								
saucy, w/chicken, chunky (Gerber)	7 tbsp	67	3.3	10.1	222	na	1.5	na
w/beef and tomato sauce, chunky (Gerber)	7 tbsp	79	3.8	11.7	202	na	1.9	na
Spaghetti								
rings, in meat sauce, 'Stages Table Time' (Beech-Nut)	6 oz	160	7.0	22.0	390	(mq)	4.0	(mq)
w/beef, 'Stages 3' (Beech-Nut)	6 oz	170	6.0	17.0	75	(mq)	8.0	(mq)
w/mini meatballs and sauce,'Graduates' (Gerber)	6 oz	160	7.0	21.0	590	na	5.0	na
w/mini meatballs and sauce, 'Graduates' (Gerber)	3.2 oz	91	4.4	12.0	300	na	2.8	na
w/tomato and meat, junior	7.5 oz	134	5.3	21.5	43	2.3	2.8	na
w/tomato and meat, junior	1 oz	18	0.7	2.9	6	.3	0.4	na
w/tomato and meat, toddler	6.25 oz	133	9.4	19.1	634	>.7 c	1.8	na
w/tomato and meat, toddler	1 oz	21	1.5	3.1	101	>.1 c	0.3	na

Food Name	Serv. Size	Total Cal.	Prot. GMS	Carbs GMS	Sod. MGS	Fiber GMS	Fat GMS	Chol. MGS
w/tomato sauce and beef, chunky								
(Gerber)	7 tbsp	85	4.4	12.5	223	na	1.9	na
w/tomato sauce and beef, junior (Gerber)	6 oz	120	5.0	19.0	41	(mq)	3.0	7
w/tomato sauce and beef, '3rd Foods'								
(Gerber)	7 tbsp	64	2.8	10.6	20	na	1.2	na
w/tomato sauce and meat, junior (Heinz)	3.5 oz	58	2.2	9.6	19	.4	1.3	na
Split pea and ham dinner								
junior	7.5 oz	151	7.0	24.1	30	2.3	2.8	na
junior	1 oz	20	0.9	3.2	4	.3	0.4	na
Sweet potato dinner, w/chicken (Earth's Best)	4.5 oz	90	3.0	13.0	30	na	2.0	na
Turkey dinner								
junior (Gerber)	2.5 oz	100	10.0	1.0	37	0	6.0	38
supreme, 'Stages 2' (Beech-Nut)	4.5 oz	120	4.0	11.0	35	(mq)	6.0	(mq)
Turkey rice dinner								
junior	7.5 oz	104	3.8	15.3	32	2.3	3.0	na
junior	1 oz	14	0.5	2.0	4	.3	0.4	na
junior (Gerber)	6 oz	110	4.0	14.0	34	(mq)	4.0	19
'2nd Foods' (Gerber)	7 tbsp	55	2.7	7.5	15	na	1.5	na
'Stages 2' (Beech-Nut)	4.5 oz	70	2.0	12.0	35	(mq)	2.0	(mq)
'Stages 3' (Beech-Nut)	6 oz	110	6.0	14.0	65	(mq)	4.0	(mq)
strained	4.5 oz	63	2.4	9.3	22	1.4	1.7	13
strained	1 oz	14	0.5	2.1	5	.3	0.4	3
strained (Gerber)	4.5 oz	80	3.0	10.0	20	(mq)	3.0	15
'3rd Foods' (Gerber)	7 tbsp	55	2.7	7.8	17	na	1.4	na
w/vegetables, junior (Heinz)	3.5 oz	42	1.5	7.9	20	.2	0.6	na
w/vegetables, strained (Heinz)	3.5 oz	47	1.2	8.2	21	.6	1.1	na
Turkey stew main dish, w/rice, 'Graduates'								
(Gerber)	3.2 oz	59	4.9	7.6	298	na	1.0	na
Turkey vegetable dinner								
high-meat, junior	4.5 oz	115	7.6	7.6	55	1.1	6.4	na
high-meat, junior	1 oz	26	1.7	1.7	12	.3	1.4	na
high-meat, strained	4.5 oz	111	7.2	7.7	38	1.1	6.1	na
high-meat, strained	1 oz	25	1.6	1.7	9	.3	1.4	na
lean meat, junior (Gerber)	4.5 oz	100	7.0	10.0	31	(mq)	4.0	16
lean meat, strained (Gerber)	4.5 oz	100	7.0	9.0	31	(mq)	4.0	17
Veal vegetable dinner								
high-meat, junior	4.5 oz	93	7.8	7.4	32	1.1	4.0	na
high-meat, junior	1 oz	21	1.7	1.6	7	.3	0.9	na
high-meat, strained	4.5 oz	88	7.6	7.8	31	1.1	3.5	na
high-meat, strained	1 oz	20	1.7	1.7	7	.3	0.8	na
Vegetable bacon dinner								
junior	7.5 oz	151	3.8	16.2	96	2.3	8.3	na
junior	1 oz	20	0.5	2.2	13	.3	1.1	na

Food Name	Serv. Size	Total Cal.	Prot. GMS	Carbs GMS	Sod. MGS	Fiber GMS	Fat GMS	Chol. MGS
'2nd Foods' *(Gerber)*	7 tbsp	73	2.0	8.8	49	na	3.3	na
strained	4.5 oz	88	2.0	11.0	55	1.4	4.2	4
'3rd Foods' *(Gerber)*	7 tbsp	77	2.3	9.3	52	na	3.4	na
Vegetable beef dinner								
(Earth's Best)	4.5 oz	90	3.0	11.0	15	na	3.0	na
junior	7.5 oz	113	5.1	15.8	51	2.3	3.6	na
junior	1 oz	15	0.7	2.1	7	.3	0.5	na
'2nd Foods' *(Gerber)*	7 tbsp	65	2.3	8.5	11	na	2.4	na
strained	4.5 oz	68	2.6	9.0	27	1.4	2.6	na
strained	1 oz	15	0.6	2.0	6	.3	0.6	na
'3rd Foods' *(Gerber)*	7 tbsp	62	2.6	9.2	16	na	1.6	na
Vegetable chicken dinner								
junior	7.5 oz	107	4.1	18.1	19	2.3	2.3	na
junior	1 oz	14	0.5	2.4	3	.3	0.3	na
'2nd Foods' *(Gerber)*	7 tbsp	58	2.3	9.4	10	na	1.4	na
strained	4.5 oz	55	2.4	8.4	14	1.4	1.4	na
strained	1 oz	12	0.5	1.9	3	.3	0.3	na
'3rd Foods' *(Gerber)*	7 tbsp	51	2.1	8.1	17	na	1.1	na
Vegetable dinner, 'Summer' *(Earth's Best)*	4.5 oz	90	3.0	12.0	15	na	3.0	na
Vegetable dumpling dinner								
w/beef, junior	7.5 oz	102	4.5	17.0	111	>.6 c	1.7	na
w/beef, junior	1 oz	14	0.6	2.3	15	>.1 c	0.2	na
w/beef, junior *(Heinz)*	3.5 oz	47	1.9	7.2	16	.4	1.2	na
w/beef, strained	4.5 oz	61	2.6	9.9	63	>.4 c	1.1	na
w/beef, strained	1 oz	14	0.6	2.2	14	>.1 c	0.3	na
w/beef, strained *(Heinz)*	3.5 oz	49	1.9	8.6	15	.4	1.3	na
Vegetable ham dinner								
junior	7.5 oz	111	5.1	14.9	38	2.3	3.6	na
junior	1 oz	15	0.7	2.0	5	.3	0.5	na
'2nd Foods' *(Gerber)*	7 tbsp	59	1.9	8.6	9	na	1.9	na
strained	4.5 oz	61	2.3	8.8	15	1.4	2.2	na
strained	1 oz	14	0.5	2.0	3	.3	0.5	na
'3rd Foods' *(Gerber)*	7 tbsp	61	2.1	9.2	12	na	1.8	na
toddler	6.25 oz	127	7.4	14.0	531	2.0	5.3	14
toddler	1 oz	20	1.2	2.2	85	.3	0.9	2
Vegetable lamb dinner								
junior	7.5 oz	109	4.5	15.1	28	2.3	3.6	na
junior	1 oz	14	0.6	2.0	4	.3	0.5	na
strained	4.5 oz	67	2.6	8.8	26	1.4	2.6	na
strained	1 oz	15	0.6	2.0	6	.3	0.6	na
Vegetable liver dinner								
junior	7.5 oz	94	3.8	17.5	28	2.3	1.3	na
junior	1 oz	12	0.5	2.3	4	.3	0.2	na

Food Name	Serv. Size	Total Cal.	Prot. GMS	Carbs GMS	Sod. MGS	Fiber GMS	Fat GMS	Chol. MGS
strained	4.5 oz	50	2.8	8.8	23	1.4	0.5	na
strained	1 oz	11	0.6	2.0	5	.3	0.1	na
Vegetable main dish								
w/beef, chunky *(Gerber)*	7 tbsp	70	3.8	9.2	201	na	2.0	na
w/chicken, chunky *(Gerber)*	7 tbsp	66	3.8	9.5	202	na	1.4	na
w/ham, chunky *(Gerber)*	7 tbsp	70	3.7	8.7	200	na	2.3	na
w/turkey, chunky *(Gerber)*	7 tbsp	61	3.6	8.4	190	na	4.4	na
Vegetable noodle dinner								
w/chicken, junior	7.5 oz	136	3.6	19.4	55	2.3	4.7	na
w/chicken, junior	1 oz	18	0.5	2.6	7	.3	0.6	na
w/chicken, junior *(Heinz)*	3.5 oz	57	1.6	8.7	21	.3	1.8	na
w/chicken, strained	4.5 oz	81	2.6	10.1	26	1.4	3.2	na
w/chicken, strained	1 oz	18	0.6	2.2	6	.3	0.7	na
w/chicken, strained *(Heinz)*	3.5 oz	54	2.2	7.5	24	.2	1.7	na
w/turkey, junior	7.5 oz	111	3.8	16.2	36	2.3	3.2	na
w/turkey, junior	1 oz	15	0.5	2.2	5	.3	0.4	na
w/turkey, junior *(Heinz)*	3.5 oz	48	1.2	6.4	21	na	2.0	na
w/turkey, strained	4.5 oz	56	1.5	8.7	27	1.4	1.5	na
w/turkey, strained	1 oz	12	0.3	1.9	6	.3	0.3	na
w/turkey, strained *(Heinz)*	3.5 oz	47	1.3	6.7	22	.3	1.6	na
Vegetable stew								
w/beef, 'Graduates' *(Gerber)*	3.2 oz	71	5.8	8.8	290	na	1.4	na
w/beef, 'Graduates' micro cup *(Gerber)*	6 oz	130	10.0	15.0	500	na	3.0	na
w/chicken, 'Stages Table Time' *(Beech-Nut)*	6 oz	190	5.0	23.0	340	(mq)	8.0	(mq)
Vegetable turkey dinner								
(Earth's Best)	4.5 oz	60	3.0	11.0	15	na	1.0	na
junior	7.5 oz	100	3.6	16.4	36	2.3	2.6	na
junior	1 oz	13	0.5	2.2	5	.1 c	0.3	na
'2nd Foods' *(Gerber)*	7 tbsp	49	2.2	7.5	12	na	1.2	na
'3rd Foods' *(Gerber)*	7 tbsp	53	2.2	8.7	13	na	1.0	na
strained	4.5 oz	54	2.2	8.4	17	.3 c	1.5	na
strained	1 oz	12	0.5	1.9	4	.1 c	0.3	na
toddler	6.25 oz	142	8.5	14.2	591	.9 c	6.0	na
toddler	1 oz	23	1.4	2.3	95	.1 c	1.0	na
EGG YOLK								
'2nd Foods' *(Gerber)*	7 tbsp	193	9.5	1.0	42	na	16.8	na
strained	3.3 oz	191	9.4	0.9	37	0	16.3	691
strained	1 oz	58	2.8	0.3	11	0	4.9	208
FRUIT								
Apple *(Earth's Best)*	4.5 oz	60	0.0	14.0	5	(mq)	1.0	0
Apple, peach, and strawberry, 'Stages 2'								
(Beech-Nut)	4.5 oz	100	0.0	24.0	0	(mq)	0.0	0

Food Name	Serv. Size	Total Cal.	Prot. GMS	Carbs GMS	Sod. MGS	Fiber GMS	Fat GMS	Chol. MGS
Apple, pear, and banana, 'Stages 2'								
(Beech-Nut)	4.5 oz	100	0.0	24.0	0	(mq)	0.0	0
Apple and apricot								
(Earth's Best)	4.5 oz	70	0.0	15.0	5	(mq)	1.0	0
strained (Heinz)	3.5 oz	55	0.3	12.9	3	na	0.3	na
Apple and banana								
(Earth's Best)	4.5 oz	80	0.0	18.0	15	(mq)	1.0	0
'2nd Foods' (Gerber)	4 oz	60	0.0	15.0	na	na	0.0	na
Apple and blueberry								
(Earth's Best)	4.5 oz	60	0.0	14.0	na	(mq)	1.0	0
junior	7.75 oz	136	0.4	36.5	29	4.0	0.4	na
junior	1 oz	18	0.1	4.7	4	.5	0.1	na
junior (Gerber)	6 oz	80	0.0	19.0	2	(mq)	1.0	na
'2nd Foods' (Gerber)	7 tbsp	51	0.2	12.1	0	na	0.2	na
strained	4.75 oz	82	0.3	22.0	3	2.4	0.3	na
strained	1 oz	17	0.1	4.6	1	.5	0.1	na
strained (Gerber)	4.5 oz	60	0.0	14.0	1	(mq)	1.0	0
'3rd Foods' (Gerber)	7 tbsp	50	0.2	11.8	1	na	0.2	na
Apple and cranberry, w/tapioca,								
strained (Heinz)	3.5 oz	66	0.1	15.9	6	na	0.3	na
Apple and pear								
(Heinz)	3.5 oz	56	0.2	13.4	2	na	0.2	na
junior	3.5 oz	57	0.2	12.9	1	.6	0.2	na
Apple and plum (Earth's Best)	4.5 oz	70	0.0	16.0	10	(mq)	1.0	0
Apple and raspberry								
w/sugar, junior	7.75 oz	128	0.4	34.1	4	4.6	0.4	na
w/sugar, junior	1 oz	16	0.1	4.4	1	.6	0.1	na
w/sugar, strained	4.75 oz	78	0.3	21.2	3	2.8	0.3	na
w/sugar, strained	1 oz	16	0.1	4.4	1	.6	0.1	na
Applesauce								
'Beginner Foods' (Heinz)	3.5 oz	73	0.1	18.0	1	na	0.1	na
'1st Foods' (Gerber)	2.5 oz	35	0.0	9.0	0	(mq)	0.0	0
'1st Foods' (Gerber)	7 tbsp	56	0.2	13.2	0	na	0.2	na
golden delicious, 'Baby's First'								
(Beech-Nut)	2.5 oz	50	0.0	11.0	0	na	0.0	na
golden delicious, 'Stages 1' (Beech-Nut)	4.5 oz	70	0.0	17.0	0	(mq)	0.0	0
golden delicious, 'Stages 1' (Beech-Nut)	2.8 oz	50	0.0	13.0	0	(mq)	0.0	0
junior	7.5 oz	79	0.0	21.9	4	3.6	0.0	na
junior	1 oz	10	0.0	2.9	1	.5	0.0	na
junior (Gerber)	6 oz	90	0.0	20.0	3	(mq)	1.0	0
junior (Heinz)	3.5 oz	53	0.2	12.4	2	na	0.2	na
'2nd Foods' (Gerber)	7 tbsp	52	0.2	12.3	22	na	0.2	na
'Stages 3' (Beech-Nut)	6 oz	90	0.0	22.0	0	(mq)	0.0	0

Food Name	Serv. Size	Total Cal.	Prot. GMS	Carbs GMS	Sod. MGS	Fiber GMS	Fat GMS	Chol. MGS
strained	4.5 oz	52	0.3	14.0	3	2.2	0.3	na
strained	1 oz	12	0.1	3.1	1	.5	0.1	na
strained (Gerber)	4.5 oz	60	0.0	14.0	3	(mq)	1.0	0
strained (Heinz)	3.5 oz	53	0.2	12.4	2	na	0.2	na
'3rd Foods' (Gerber)	7 tbsp	51	0.2	12.1	1	na	0.2	na
w/apricot, junior	7.75 oz	103	0.4	27.3	7	4.0	0.4	na
w/apricot, junior	1 oz	13	0.1	3.5	1	.5	0.1	na
w/apricot, '2nd Foods' (Gerber)	7 tbsp	53	0.3	12.5	1	na	0.2	na
w/apricot, 'Stages 2' (Beech-Nut)	4.5 oz	80	0.0	19.0	0	(mq)	0.0	0
w/apricot, strained	4.75 oz	61	0.3	15.7	4	2.4	0.3	na
w/apricot, strained	1 oz	13	0.1	3.3	1	.5	0.1	na
w/apricot, strained (Gerber)	4.5 oz	70	0.0	15.0	3	(mq)	1.0	0
w/banana, 'Stages 2' (Beech-Nut)	4.5 oz	80	0.0	18.0	0	(mq)	0.0	0
w/banana, 'Stages 3' (Beech-Nut)	6 oz	100	0.0	25.0	0	(mq)	0.0	0
w/cherry, junior	7.75 oz	106	0.7	29.0	7	3.3	0.0	na
w/cherry, junior	1 oz	14	0.1	3.7	1	.4	0.0	na
w/cherry, 'Stages 2' (Beech-Nut)	4.5 oz	70	0.0	18.0	5	(mq)	0.0	0
w/cherry, 'Stages 3' (Beech-Nut)	6 oz	100	0.0	24.0	0	(mq)	0.0	0
w/cherry, strained	4.75 oz	65	0.4	17.7	3	2.0	0.0	na
w/cherry, strained	1 oz	14	0.1	3.7	1	.4	0.0	na
w/pineapple, junior	7.5 oz	83	0.2	22.4	4	3.2	0.2	na
w/pineapple, junior	1 oz	11	0.0	3.0	1	.4	0.0	na
w/pineapple, strained	4.5 oz	47	0.1	12.9	3	1.9	0.1	na
w/pineapple, strained	1 oz	10	0.0	2.9	1	.4	0.0	na
Apricot								
w/pear, 'Stages 3' (Beech-Nut)	6 oz	120	1.0	27.0	0	(mq)	0.0	0
w/pear and applesauce, 'Stages 2' (Beech-Nut)	4.5 oz	90	0.0	21.0	0	(mq)	0.0	0
w/tapioca, junior	7.75 oz	139	0.7	38.1	13	3.3	0.0	na
w/tapioca, junior	1 oz	18	0.1	4.9	2	.4	0.0	na
w/tapioca, junior (Gerber)	6 oz	130	1.0	29.0	9	(mq)	1.0	0
w/tapioca, junior (Heinz)	3.5 oz	66	0.2	15.9	10	na	0.2	na
w/tapioca, '2nd Foods' (Gerber)	7 tbsp	67	0.3	16.2	6	na	0.2	na
w/tapioca, strained	4.75 oz	81	0.4	22.0	11	2.0	0.0	na
w/tapioca, strained	1 oz	17	0.1	4.6	2	.4	0.0	na
w/tapioca, strained (Gerber)	4.5 oz	90	0.0	20.0	8	(mq)	1.0	0
w/tapioca, strained (Heinz)	3.5 oz	64	0.2	15.3	7	.2	0.2	na
w/tapioca, '3rd Foods' (Gerber)	7 tbsp	71	0.3	17.1	5	na	0.2	na
Banana								
'Beginner Foods' (Heinz)	3.5 oz	107	1.2	25.0	3	na	0.2	na
Chiquita, 'Baby's First' (Beech-Nut)	2.5 oz	70	0.0	16.0	0	na	0.0	na
Chiquita, 'Stages 1' (Beech-Nut)	4.5 oz	110	1.0	26.0	0	(mq)	0.0	0
Chiquita, 'Stages 1' (Beech-Nut)	2.8 oz	70	0.0	16.0	0	(mq)	0.0	0

Food Name	Serv. Size	Total Cal.	Prot. GMS	Carbs GMS	Sod. MGS	Fiber GMS	Fat GMS	Chol. MGS
(Earth's Best)	4.5 oz	100	2.0	22.0	60	(mq)	0.0	0
'1st Foods' *(Gerber)*	2.5 oz	70	1.0	17.0	na	(mq)	0.0	0
'1st Foods' *(Gerber)*	7 tbsp	100	1.2	23.3	3	na	0.3	na
w/pineapple and tapioca, '2nd Foods' *(Gerber)*	7 tbsp	52	0.4	12.3	na	na	0.1	na
w/pineapple and tapioca, '3rd Foods' *(Gerber)*	7 tbsp	52	0.4	12.3	4	na	0.1	na
w/tapioca, junior	7.75 oz	147	0.9	39.2	20	3.5	0.4	na
w/tapioca, junior	1 oz	19	0.1	5.1	3	.5	0.1	na
w/tapioca, junior *(Gerber)*	6 oz	140	1.0	31.0	15	(mq)	1.0	0
w/tapioca, junior *(Heinz)*	3.5 oz	73	0.2	17.6	8	na	0.2	na
w/tapioca, '2nd Foods' *(Gerber)*	7 tbsp	78	0.5	18.5	5	na	0.2	na
w/tapioca, '3rd Foods' *(Gerber)*	7 tbsp	77	0.5	18.4	5	na	0.2	na
w/tapioca, strained	4.75 oz	77	0.5	20.7	12	2.2	0.1	na
w/tapioca, strained	1 oz	16	0.1	4.3	3	.5	0.0	na
w/tapioca, strained *(Gerber)*	4.5 oz	110	1.0	24.0	12	(mq)	1.0	0
w/tapioca, strained *(Heinz)*	3.5 oz	73	0.2	17.6	8	na	0.2	na
Banana and apple, strained *(Gerber)*	4.5 oz	90	0.0	20.0	9	(mq)	1.0	0
Banana and pear, w/applesauce, 'Stages 2' *(Beech-Nut)*	4.5 oz	100	0.0	24.0	0	(mq)	0.0	0
Banana and pineapple 'Stages 2' *(Beech-Nut)*	4.5 oz	110	0.0	27.0	15	(mq)	0.0	0
w/tapioca, junior	4.75 oz	92	0.3	24.8	11	2.2	0.1	na
w/tapioca, junior	1 oz	19	0.1	5.2	2	.5	0.0	na
w/tapioca, junior *(Gerber)*	6 oz	90	1.0	20.0	7	(mq)	1.0	0
w/tapioca, strained	7.75 oz	143	0.4	39.2	13	3.5	0.0	na
w/tapioca, strained	1 oz	18	0.1	5.1	2	.5	0.0	na
w/tapioca, strained *(Gerber)*	4.5 oz	60	1.0	15.0	5	(mq)	0.0	0
w/tapioca, strained *(Heinz)*	3.5 oz	64	0.2	15.3	8	.1	0.2	na
Guava w/tapioca, strained	4.5 oz	86	0.4	23.4	3	2.3	0.0	na
w/tapioca, strained	1 oz	19	0.1	5.2	1	.5	0.0	na
w/tapioca, strained *(Gerber)*	4.5 oz	90	0.0	20.0	3	(mq)	1.0	0
w/tapioca, strained, 'Stages 2' *(Beech-Nut)*	4.5 oz	100	0.0	24.0	10	(mq)	0.0	0
Guava and papaya w/tapioca, strained	4.5 oz	81	0.3	21.8	5	>.6 c	0.1	na
w/tapioca, strained	1 oz	18	0.1	4.8	1	>.1 c	0.0	na
Mango tropical fruit dessert, 'Stages 2' *(Beech-Nut)*	4.5 oz	100	0.0	25.0	15	(mq)	0.0	0
w/tapioca, strained	4.75 oz	108	0.4	29.2	5	1.4	0.3	na
w/tapioca, strained	1 oz	23	0.1	6.1	1	.3	0.1	na

Food Name	Serv. Size	Total Cal.	Prot. GMS	Carbs GMS	Sod. MGS	Fiber GMS	Fat GMS	Chol. MGS
w/tapioca, strained *(Gerber)*	4.5 oz	90	0.0	21.0	4	(mq)	1.0	0
Mango and banana, w/passion fruit and								
tapioca, strained *(Gerber)*	4.5 oz	100	0.0	25.0	12	(mq)	0.0	0
Papaya								
'Stages 2' *(Beech-Nut)*	4.5 oz	100	0.0	24.0	15	(mq)	0.0	0
w/tapioca, strained *(Gerber)*	4.5 oz	80	0.0	19.0	9	(mq)	1.0	0
Papaya and applesauce								
w/tapioca, strained	4.5 oz	90	0.3	24.2	6	1.8	0.1	na
w/tapioca, strained	1 oz	20	0.1	5.4	1	.4	0.0	na
Peach								
'Beginner Foods' *(Heinz)*	3.5 oz	80	1.2	18.3	2	na	0.2	na
'1st Foods' *(Gerber)*	2.5 oz	30	0.0	7.0	na	(mq)	0.0	0
'1st Foods' *(Gerber)*	7 tbsp	43	0.7	9.6	1	na	0.2	na
junior *(Gerber)*	6 oz	110	1.0	25.0	5	(mq)	1.0	0
junior *(Heinz)*	3.5 oz	68	0.9	15.4	7	.7	0.3	na
'2nd Foods' *(Gerber)*	7 tbsp	66	0.7	15.3	3	na	0.2	na
'Stages 3' *(Beech-Nut)*	6 oz	90	1.0	22.0	0	(mq)	0.0	0
strained *(Gerber)*	4.5 oz	90	1.0	19.0	4	(mq)	1.0	0
strained *(Heinz)*	3.5 oz	68	0.9	15.4	7	.7	0.3	na
'3rd Foods' *(Gerber)*	7 tbsp	65	0.7	15.1	2	na	0.2	na
w/mango and tapioca, strained *(Gerber)*	4.5 oz	100	0.0	24.0	9	(mq)	1.0	0
w/oatmeal and banana *(Earth's Best)*	4.5 oz	70	2.0	15.0	5	(mq)	1.0	0
w/sugar, junior	7.75 oz	156	1.1	41.6	11	3.3	0.4	na
w/sugar, junior	1 oz	20	0.1	5.4	1	.4	0.1	na
w/sugar, strained	4.75 oz	96	0.7	25.5	8	2.0	0.3	na
w/sugar, strained	1 oz	20	0.1	5.4	2	.4	0.1	na
w/yogurt, 'Stages 2' *(Beech-Nut)*	4.5 oz	120	1.0	25.0	30	(mq)	2.0	(mq)
yellow cling, 'Baby's First' *(Beech-Nut)*	2.5 oz	45	0.0	10.0	0	na	0.0	na
yellow cling, 'Stages 1' *(Beech-Nut)*	4.5 oz	70	0.0	15.0	0	(mq)	0.0	0
yellow cling, 'Stages 1' *(Beech-Nut)*	2.8 oz	50	0.0	12.0	0	(mq)	0.0	0
Pear								
Bartlett, 'Baby's First' *(Beech-Nut)*	2.5 oz	50	0.0	12.0	0	na	0.0	0
Bartlett, 'Stages 1' *(Beech-Nut)*	4.5 oz	70	0.0	18.0	0	(mq)	0.0	0
Bartlett, 'Stages 1' *(Beech-Nut)*	2.8 oz	50	0.0	13.0	0	(mq)	0.0	0
Bartlett, 'Stages 3' *(Beech-Nut)*	6 oz	100	0.0	24.0	5	(mq)	0.0	0
Bartlett, w/applesauce, 'Stages 2'								
(Beech-Nut)	4.5 oz	80	0.0	20.0	0	(mq)	0.0	0
Bartlett, w/pineapple, 'Stages 2'								
(Beech-Nut)	4.5 oz	90	0.0	21.0	0	(mq)	0.0	0
'Beginner Foods' *(Heinz)*	3.5 oz	76	0.5	18.0	3	na	0.2	na
(Earth's Best)	4.5 oz	60	0.0	14.0	11	(mq)	0.0	0
'1st Foods' *(Gerber)*	2.5 oz	40	0.0	11.0	2	(mq)	0.0	0
'1st Foods' *(Gerber)*	7 tbsp	57	0.4	13.2	1	na	0.3	na

Food Name	Serv. Size	Total Cal.	Prot. GMS	Carbs GMS	Sod. MGS	Fiber GMS	Fat GMS	Chol. MGS
junior	7.5 oz	92	0.6	24.7	4	7.7	0.2	na
junior	1 oz	12	0.1	3.3	1	1.0	0.0	na
junior (Gerber)	6 oz	100	1.0	21.0	2	(mq)	1.0	0
junior (Heinz)	3.5 oz	60	0.4	14.1	3	na	0.2	na
'2nd Foods' (Gerber)	7 tbsp	55	0.4	12.9	0	na	0.2	na
strained	4.5 oz	52	0.4	13.8	3	4.6	0.3	na
strained	1 oz	12	0.1	3.1	1	1.0	0.1	na
strained (Gerber)	4.5 oz	80	1.0	16.0	3	(mq)	1.0	0
strained (Heinz)	3.5 oz	60	0.4	14.1	3	na	0.2	na
'3rd Foods' (Gerber)	7 tbsp	55	0.4	12.9	2	na	0.2	na
Pear and pineapple								
junior	7.5 oz	94	0.6	24.3	2	5.5	0.4	na
junior	1 oz	12	0.1	3.2	0	.7	0.1	na
junior (Gerber)	6 oz	100	1.0	21.0	3	(mq)	1.0	0
'2nd Foods' (Gerber)	7 tbsp	55	0.4	12.8	1	na	0.2	na
strained	4.5 oz	52	0.4	14.0	5	3.3	0.1	na
strained	1 oz	12	0.1	3.1	1	.7	0.0	na
strained (Gerber)	4.5 oz	80	1.0	16.0	3	(mq)	1.0	0
'3rd Foods' (Gerber)	7 tbsp	54	0.4	12.7	2	na	0.2	na
Pears and raspberries, (Earth's Best)	4.5 oz	60	0.0	15.0	0	na	0.0	na
Plum								
w/banana and rice (Earth's Best)	4.5 oz	90	2.0	19.0	15	(mq)	0.0	0
w/rice, 'Stages 2' (Beech-Nut)	4.5 oz	150	1.0	34.0	0	(mq)	0.0	0
w/tapioca, junior (Gerber)	6 oz	130	1.0	30.0	3	(mq)	1.0	0
w/tapioca, '2nd Foods' (Gerber)	7 tbsp	74	0.3	17.7	3	na	0.2	na
w/tapioca, strained (Gerber)	4.5 oz	90	0.0	22.0	5	(mq)	0.0	na
w/tapioca, strained (Heinz)	3.5 oz	67	0.2	16.2	9	na	0.2	na
w/tapioca, '3rd Foods' (Gerber)	7 tbsp	75	0.3	18.1	2	na	0.2	na
w/tapioca, w/o ascorbic acid, junior	7.75 oz	163	0.2	44.9	18	2.6	0.0	na
w/tapioca, w/o ascorbic acid, junior	1 oz	21	0.0	5.8	2	.3	0.0	na
w/tapioca, w/o ascorbic acid, strained	4.75 oz	96	0.1	26.6	8	1.6	0.0	na
w/tapioca, w/o ascorbic acid, strained	1 oz	20	0.0	5.6	2	.3	0.0	na
Prune								
'1st Foods' (Gerber)	2.5 oz	70	1.0	17.0	na	(mq)	0.0	0
'1st Foods' (Gerber)	7 tbsp	101	1.0	23.8	6	na	0.2	na
w/oatmeal (Earth's Best)	4.5 oz	100	1.0	24.0	20	(mq)	0.0	0
w/pear, 'Stages 2' (Beech-Nut)	4.5 oz	90	0.0	22.0	0	(mq)	0.0	0
w/tapioca, '2nd Foods' (Gerber)	7 tbsp	77	0.7	18.1	4	na	0.2	na
w/tapioca, strained (Gerber)	4.5 oz	100	1.0	22.0	5	(mq)	1.0	0
w/tapioca, strained (Heinz)	3.5 oz	90	0.5	21.5	8	na	0.2	na
w/tapioca, w/o ascorbic acid, junior	7.75 oz	154	1.3	41.1	4	5.9	0.2	na
w/tapioca, w/o ascorbic acid, junior	1 oz	20	0.2	5.3	1	.8	0.0	na
w/tapioca, w/o ascorbic acid, strained	4.75 oz	94	0.8	25.0	7	3.7	0.1	na

Food Name	Serv. Size	Total Cal.	Prot. GMS	Carbs GMS	Sod. MGS	Fiber GMS	Fat GMS	Chol. MGS
w/tapioca, w/o ascorbic acid, strained	1 oz	20	0.2	5.2	1	.8	0.0	na
INFANT FORMULA								
Mix								
liquid, iron-fortified, prepared, 'Follow-Up' (Carnation)	5 oz	100	2.6	13.2	39	na	4.1	na
liquid, iron-fortified, prepared, 'Good Start' (Carnation)	5 oz	100	2.4	11.0	24	na	5.1	na
liquid, low-iron, prepared (Enfamil)	5 oz	100	2.2	10.3	27	na	5.6	na
liquid, low-iron, prepared (Gerber)	5 oz	100	3.0	10.0	47	na	5.3	na
liquid, low-iron, prepared (Similac)	5 oz	100	2.1	10.7	27	na	5.4	na
liquid, soy, iron-fortified, milk-free (Nursoy)	.5 oz	100	2.7	10.2	30	na	5.3	na
liquid, soy, iron-fortified, milk-free, prepared (Gerber)	5 oz	100	3.0	10.0	47	na	5.3	na
liquid, soy, iron-fortified, milk-free, prepared (ProSobee)	5 oz	100	3.0	10.0	36	na	5.3	na
liquid, soy, w/iron, milk-free, prepared (Isomil)	5 oz	100	2.5	10.3	44	na	5.4	na
liquid, w/iron, prepared (Enfamil)	5 oz	100	2.2	10.3	27	na	5.6	na
liquid, w/iron, prepared (Gerber)	5 oz	100	2.2	10.7	33	na	5.4	na
liquid, w/iron, prepared (Similac)	5 oz	100	2.1	10.7	27	na	5.4	na
powder, iron-fortified, prepared, 'Follow-Up' (Carnation)	5 oz	100	2.6	13.2	39	na	4.1	na
powder, iron-fortified, prepared, 'Good Start' (Carnation)	5 oz	100	2.4	11.0	24	na	5.1	na
powder, low-iron, prepared (Enfamil)	5 oz	100	2.2	10.3	27	na	5.6	na
powder, low-iron, prepared (Gerber)	5 oz	100	3.0	10.0	47	na	5.3	na
powder, low-iron, prepared (Similac)	5 oz	100	2.1	10.7	27	na	5.4	na
powder, soy, iron-fortified, milk-free, prepared (Gerber)	5 oz	100	3.0	10.0	47	na	5.3	na
powder, soy, iron-fortified, milk-free, prepared (ProSobee)	5 oz	100	3.0	10.0	36	na	5.3	na
powder, soy, w/iron, milk-free, prepared (Isomil)	5 oz	100	2.5	10.3	44	na	5.5	na
powder, w/iron, prepared (Enfamil)	5 oz	100	2.2	10.3	27	na	5.6	na
powder, w/iron, prepared (Gerber)	5 oz	100	2.2	10.7	33	na	5.4	na
powder, w/iron, prepared (Similac)	5 oz	100	2.1	10.7	27	na	5.4	na
Ready to use								
iron-fortified, 'Follow-Up' (Carnation)	5 oz	100	2.6	13.2	39	na	4.1	na
iron-fortified, 'Good Start' (Carnation)	5 oz	100	2.4	11.0	24	na	5.1	na
low-iron (Enfamil)	5 oz	100	2.2	10.3	27	na	5.6	na
low-iron (Gerber)	5 oz	100	3.0	10.0	47	na	5.3	na
low-iron (Similac)	5 oz	100	2.1	10.7	27	na	5.4	na
soy, iron-fortified, milk-free (Gerber)	5 oz	100	3.0	10.0	47	na	5.3	na

Food Name	Serv. Size	Total Cal.	Prot. GMS	Carbs GMS	Sod. MGS	Fiber GMS	Fat GMS	Chol. MGS
soy, iron-fortified, milk-free *(ProSobee)* ...	5 oz	100	3.0	10.0	36	na	5.3	na
soy, w/iron, milk-free *(Isomil)*	5 oz	100	2.5	10.3	44	na	5.4	na
w/iron *(Enfamil)*	5 oz	100	2.2	10.3	27	na	5.6	na
w/iron *(Gerber)*	5 oz	100	2.2	10.7	33	na	5.4	na
w/iron *(Similac)*	5 oz	100	2.1	10.7	27	na	5.4	na
JUICE								
Apple								
....	4.2 oz	61	0.0	15.2	4	.1	0.1	na
....	1 oz	15	0.0	3.6	1	tr	0.0	na
(Earth's Best)	4.2 oz	60	0.0	14.0	20	(mq)	0.0	0
'Graduates' *(Gerber)*	6 oz	80	0.0	21.0	0	na	0.0	na
'Graduates' *(Gerber)*	3.2 oz	48	0.1	11.7	2	na	0.1	na
100% juice, 'Junior' *(McCain)*	4.2 oz	50	0.0	13.0	5	na	0.0	na
'Stages 1' *(Beech-Nut)*	4.2 oz	60	0.0	14.0	5	(mq)	0.0	0
strained, '1st Foods' *(Gerber)*	4 oz	60	0.0	14.0	2	(mq)	0.0	0
strained, '1st Foods' *(Gerber)*	3.2 oz	46	0.1	11.0	1	na	0.1	na
strained *(Heinz)*	3.5 oz	48	0.1	11.7	5	.1	0.2	na
strained, 'Saver Size' *(Heinz)*	4.2 oz	70	0.0	17.0	15	na	0.0	na
w/yogurt, 2nd Foods' *(Gerber)*	3.2 oz	73	2.0	14.2	32	na	0.9	na
Apple-apricot, strained *(Heinz)*	3.5 oz	47	0.2	11.2	8	.2	0.2	na
Apple-banana								
(Earth's Best)	4.2 oz	60	0.0	14.0	2	(mq)	0.0	0
'Graduates' *(Gerber)*	6 oz	90	0.0	23.0	10	na	0.0	na
'Graduates' *(Gerber)*	3.2 oz	51	0.1	12.5	2	na	0.1	na
'2nd Foods' *(Gerber)*	3.2 oz	51	0.2	12.3	2	na	0.1	na
strained *(Heinz)*	3.5 oz	52	0.1	12.5	6	na	0.2	na
Apple-carrot								
'3rd Foods' *(Gerber)*	4 oz	50	0.0	12.0	15	na	0.0	na
'3rd Foods' *(Gerber)*	3.2 oz	42	0.1	10.0	10	na	0.1	na
Apple-cherry								
....	4.2 oz	53	0.1	12.9	4	.1	0.3	na
....	1 oz	13	0.0	3.1	1	tr	0.1	na
'Graduates' *(Gerber)*	6 oz	80	0.0	21.0	25	na	0.0	na
'Graduates' *(Gerber)*	3.2 oz	51	0.1	12.4	3	na	0.1	na
100% juice, 'Junior' *(McCain)*	4.2 oz	50	0.0	13.0	5	na	0.0	na
'2nd Foods' *(Gerber)*	4 oz	60	0.0	14.0	na	na	0.0	na
'2nd Foods' *(Gerber)*	3.2 oz	48	0.2	11.5	5	na	0.1	na
'Stages 2' *(Beech-Nut)*	4 oz	60	0.0	14.0	5	(mq)	0.0	0
strained *(Heinz)*	3.5 oz	45	0.1	10.7	7	.1	0.2	na
Apple-cranberry								
'Stages 2' *(Beech-Nut)*	4 oz	60	0.0	14.0	5	(mq)	0.0	0
strained *(Heinz)*	3.5 oz	48	0.1	11.5	7	na	0.2	na

Food Name	Serv. Size	Total Cal.	Prot. GMS	Carbs GMS	Sod. MGS	Fiber GMS	Fat GMS	Chol. MGS
Apple-grape								
....	4.2 oz	60	0.1	14.8	4	.1	0.3	na
....	1 oz	14	0.0	3.5	1	tr	0.1	na
(Earth's Best)	4.2 oz	60	0.0	14.0	15	(mq)	0.0	0
'Graduates' (Gerber)	6 oz	90	0.0	22.0	40	na	0.0	na
'Graduates' (Gerber)	3.2 oz	51	0.0	12.4	3	na	0.1	na
'2nd Foods' (Gerber)	4 oz	60	0.0	15.0	na	na	0.0	na
'2nd Foods' (Gerber)	3.2 oz	48	0.1	11.7	7	na	0.1	na
'Stages 2' (Beech-Nut)	4 oz	70	0.0	16.0	15	(mq)	0.0	0
strained (Heinz)	3.5 oz	47	0.1	11.3	7	na	0.2	na
Apple-peach								
....	4.2 oz	55	0.3	13.6	1	.1	0.1	na
....	1 oz	13	0.1	3.3	0	tr	0.0	na
'2nd Foods' (Gerber)	3.2 oz	47	0.2	11.3	5	na	0.1	na
'2nd Foods' (Gerber)	4 oz	60	0.0	14.0	na	na	0.0	na
strained (Heinz)	3.5 oz	44	0.2	10.4	7	.2	0.2	na
Apple-pineapple, strained (Heinz)	3.5 oz	47	0.2	11.1	6	na	0.2	na
Apple-plum								
....	4.2 oz	64	0.1	16.0	1	.1	0.0	na
....	1 oz	15	0.0	3.8	0	tr	0.0	na
'2nd Foods' (Gerber)	4 oz	60	0.0	15.0	na	na	0.0	na
'2nd Foods' (Gerber)	3.2 oz	48	0.2	11.7	8	na	0.1	na
Apple-prune								
....	4.2 oz	95	.0.3	23.4	7	.1	0.1	na
....	1 oz	23	0.1	5.6	2	tr	0.0	na
'2nd Foods' (Gerber)	4 oz	60	0.0	16.0	na	na	0.0	na
'2nd Foods' (Gerber)	3.2 oz	53	0.2	12.8	4	na	0.1	na
strained (Heinz)	3.5 oz	50	0.2	11.9	7	na	0.2	na
Apple-sweet potato, '3rd Foods' (Gerber) ..	3.2 oz	48	0.3	11.4	5	na	0.1	na
Banana								
w/yogurt, '2nd Foods' (Gerber)	4 oz	110	3.0	21.0	na	na	2.0	na
w/yogurt, '2nd Foods' (Gerber)	3.2 oz	84	2.2	16.5	37	na	1.0	na
Grape								
'Juice Plus,' 'Stages 2' (Beech-Nut)	4 oz	90	0.0	22.0	10	(mq)	0.0	0
red, '1st Foods' (Gerber)	4 oz	80	0.0	20.0	na	na	0.0	na
red, '1st Foods' (Gerber)	3.2 oz	65	0.4	15.4	5	na	0.1	na
white, '1st Foods' (Gerber)	4 oz	80	0.0	19.0	na	na	0.0	na
white, '1st Foods' (Gerber)	3.2 oz	65	0.4	15.6	6	na	0.1	na
white, 'Stages 1' (Beech-Nut)	4.2 oz	80	0.0	20.0	10	(mq)	0.0	0
white, strained (Heinz)	3.5 oz	58	0.4	13.8	6	.2	0.2	na
Guava, w/mixed fruit, 'Tropical Foods'								
(Gerber)	3.2 oz	58	0.3	13.8	6	na	0.1	na

Food Name	Serv. Size	Total Cal.	Prot. GMS	Carbs GMS	Sod. MGS	Fiber GMS	Fat GMS	Chol. MGS
Mango, w/mixed fruit, 'Tropical Foods'								
(Gerber)	3.2 oz	59	0.2	14.2	5	na	0.1	na
Mango nectar, w/grape and pear juice								
'Stages 2' (Beech-Nut)	4 oz	80	0.0	19.0	5	na	0.0	na
Mixed fruit								
	4.2 oz	61	0.1	15.1	5	.1	0.1	na
	1 oz	15	0.0	3.6	1	tr	0.0	na
100% juice, 'Junior' (McCain)	4.2 oz	60	0.0	15.0	5	na	0.0	na
'2nd Foods' (Gerber)	4 oz	60	0.0	14.0	na	na	0.0	na
'2nd Foods' (Gerber)	3.2 oz	49	0.3	11.8	4	na	0.1	na
'Stages 2' (Beech-Nut)	4 oz	70	0.0	16.0	10	(mq)	0.0	0
strained (Heinz)	3.5 oz	50	0.3	11.7	6	na	0.2	na
w/yogurt, '2nd Foods' (Gerber)	4 oz	100	3.0	18.0	na	na	2.0	na
w/yogurt, '2nd Foods' (Gerber)	3.2 oz	75	2.2	14.4	36	na	0.9	na
Orange								
	4.2 oz	57	0.8	13.3	1	.1	0.4	na
	1 oz	14	0.2	3.2	0	tr	0.1	na
'2nd Foods' (Gerber)	4 oz	60	1.0	13.0	na	na	0.0	na
'2nd Foods' (Gerber)	3.2 oz	46	0.7	10.3	2	na	0.3	na
'Stages 3' (Beech-Nut)	4 oz	60	0.0	14.0	0	(mq)	0.0	0
strained (Heinz)	3.5 oz	48	0.7	10.7	5	na	0.3	na
Orange-apple								
	4.2 oz	56	0.5	13.1	4	.1	0.3	na
	1 oz	13	0.1	3.1	1	tr	0.1	na
strained (Heinz)	3.5 oz	50	0.4	11.4	8	na	0.3	na
w/banana	4.2 oz	61	0.5	14.9	5	.1	0.1	na
w/banana	1 oz	15	0.1	3.6	1	tr	0.0	na
Orange-apricot								
	4.2 oz	60	1.0	14.2	8	.1	0.1	na
	1 oz	14	0.3	3.4	2	tr	0.0	na
Orange-banana								
	4.2 oz	65	0.9	15.5	4	.1	0.1	na
	1 oz	15	0.2	3.7	1	tr	0.0	na
Orange-carrot, '3rd Foods' (Gerber)	3.2 oz	43	0.5	9.9	10	na	0.1	na
Orange-pineapple								
	4.2 oz	62	0.7	15.2	3	.1	0.1	na
	1 oz	15	0.2	3.6	1	tr	0.0	na
Papaya, w/mixed fruit, 'Tropical Foods'								
(Gerber)	3.2 oz	57	0.3	13.5	5	na	0.2	na
Papaya nectar, w/pear and grape juice,								
'Stages 2' (Beech-Nut)	4 oz	70	0.0	17.0	10	na	0.0	na
Peach nectar, w/pear and grape juice,								
'Stages 2' (Beech-Nut)	4 oz	70	0.0	17.0	10	na	0.0	na

Food Name	Serv. Size	Total Cal.	Prot. GMS	Carbs GMS	Sod. MGS	Fiber GMS	Fat GMS	Chol. MGS
Pear								
(Earth's Best)	4.2 oz	60	0.0	15.0	0	(mq)	0.0	0
'Stages 1' (Beech-Nut)	4 oz	60	0.0	15.0	5	(mq)	0.0	0
strained (Heinz)	3.5 oz	49	0.2	11.7	9	na	0.2	na
strained, '1st Foods' (Gerber)	4 oz	60	0.0	14.0	6	(mq)	0.0	0
strained, '1st Foods' (Gerber)	3.2 oz	46	0.1	11.1	1	na	0.1	na
strained, 'Saver Size' (Heinz)	4.2 oz	70	0.0	15.0	25	na	1.0	na
Pear-grape, strained (Heinz)	3.5 oz	43	0.1	10.5	4	na	0.1	na
Pear-peach								
w/yogurt, '2nd Foods' (Gerber)	4 oz	90	3.0	18.0	na	na	1.0	na
w/yogurt, '2nd Foods' (Gerber)	3.2 oz	72	2.2	14.0	34	na	0.9	na
Pineapple-carrot								
'3rd Foods' (Gerber)	4 oz	60	1.0	13.0	15	na	0.0	na
'3rd Foods' (Gerber)	3.2 oz	47	0.4	11.0	10	na	0.1	na
Prune-orange								
	4.2 oz	91	0.8	21.8	3	.1	0.4	na
	1 oz	22	0.2	5.2	1	tr	0.1	na
Tropical blend, 'Stages 2' (Beech-Nut)	4 oz	70	0.0	17.0	5	(mq)	0.0	0
Tropical blend nectar, 'Stages 2' (Beech-Nut)	4 oz	90	0.0	21.0	10	na	0.0	na
MEAT								
Beef								
junior	3.5 oz	105	14.4	0.0	65	0	4.8	na
junior	1 oz	30	4.1	0.0	19	0	1.4	na
'2nd Foods' (Gerber)	7 tbsp	100	14.4	0.1	52	na	4.7	na
strained	3.5 oz	106	13.5	0.0	80	0	5.3	na
strained	1 oz	30	3.9	0.0	23	0	1.5	na
'3rd Foods' (Gerber)	7 tbsp	103	15.1	0.2	52	na	4.6	na
w/beef heart, strained	3.5 oz	93	12.6	0.0	62	0	4.4	na
w/beef heart, strained	1 oz	27	3.6	0.0	18	0	1.3	na
w/broth, junior (Heinz)	3.5 oz	123	14.6	0.3	53	.4	7.2	na
w/broth, 'Stages 1' (Beech-Nut)	2.5 oz	80	9.0	0.0	40	na	5.0	na
w/broth, strained (Heinz)	3.5 oz	123	14.6	0.3	53	.4	7.2	na
w/egg yolks, strained (Gerber)	2.5 oz	80	10.0	0.0	38	0	4.0	21
Chicken								
junior	3.5 oz	148	14.5	0.0	50	0	9.5	na
junior	1 oz	42	4.2	0.0	14	0	2.7	na
'2nd Foods' (Gerber)	7 tbsp	128	14.1	0.0	40	na	7.9	na
'Stages 1' (Beech-Nut)	2.8 oz	80	10.0	0.0	55	0	4.0	(mq)
strained	3.5 oz	129	13.6	0.1	47	0	7.8	na
strained	1 oz	37	3.9	0.0	13	0	2.2	na
'3rd Foods' (Gerber)	7 tbsp	132	15.0	0.2	39	na	7.9	na
w/broth, junior (Heinz)	3.5 oz	143	13.5	0.7	59	.1	9.7	na

Food Name	Serv. Size	Total Cal.	Prot. GMS	Carbs GMS	Sod. MGS	Fiber GMS	Fat GMS	Chol. MGS
w/broth, 'Stages 1' *(Beech-Nut)*	2.5 oz	70	9.0	0.0	55	na	4.0	na
w/broth, strained *(Heinz)*	3.5 oz	143	13.5	0.7	59	.1	9.7	na
Chicken sticks								
finger snacks, 'Graduates' *(Gerber)*	10 sticks	143	15.4	1.6	445	na	8.3	na
junior	1 stick	19	1.5	0.1	48	0	1.4	na
Ham								
junior	3.5 oz	124	14.9	0.0	66	0	6.6	na
junior	1 oz	35	4.3	0.0	19	0	1.9	na
junior *(Gerber)*	2.5 oz	90	11.0	0.0	30	0	5.0	21
'2nd Foods' *(Gerber)*	7 tbsp	120	13.7	0.2	42	na	7.1	na
strained	3.5 oz	110	13.8	0.0	41	0	5.7	na
strained	1 oz	31	3.9	0.0	12	0	1.6	na
'3rd Foods' *(Gerber)*	7 tbsp	123	14.5	0.1	42	na	7.2	na
w/egg yolks, strained *(Gerber)*	2.5 oz	90	10.0	1.0	30	0	5.0	17
Lamb								
junior	3.5 oz	111	15.1	0.0	72	0	5.2	na
junior	1 oz	32	4.3	0.0	21	0	1.5	na
'2nd Foods' *(Gerber)*	7 tbsp	104	15.1	0.0	51	na	4.8	na
'Stages 1' *(Beech-Nut)*	2.8 oz	70	9.0	0.0	50	0	3.0	(mq)
strained	3.5 oz	102	14.0	0.1	61	0	4.7	na
strained	1 oz	29	4.0	0.0	18	0	1.3	na
w/broth, 'Stages 1' *(Beech-Nut)*	2.5 oz	60	9.0	0.0	50	na	3.0	na
w/broth, strained *(Heinz)*	3.5 oz	129	15.3	0.2	59	.2	7.6	na
w/egg yolks, strained *(Gerber)*	2.5 oz	70	10.0	1.0	36	0	3.0	27
Liver								
strained	3.5 oz	100	14.2	1.4	73	0	3.8	182
strained	1 oz	29	4.1	0.4	21	0	1.1	52
w/liver broth, strained *(Heinz)*	3.5 oz	100	14.3	3.6	49	.1	3.2	na
Meat sticks								
finger snacks, 'Graduates' *(Gerber)*	10 sticks	150	14.5	1.5	451	na	9.6	na
junior	1 stick	18	1.3	0.1	55	0	1.5	na
Pork								
strained	3.5 oz	123	13.9	0.0	42	0	7.0	na
strained	1 oz	35	4.0	0.0	12	0	2.0	na
Turkey								
junior	3.5 oz	128	15.2	0.0	71	0	7.0	na
junior	1 oz	37	4.4	0.0	20	0	2.0	na
'2nd Foods' *(Gerber)*	7 tbsp	109	13.7	0.2	54	na	5.9	na
'Stages 1' *(Beech-Nut)*	2.8 oz	100	9.0	0.0	50	0	6.0	(mq)
strained	3.5 oz	113	14.2	0.1	54	0	5.7	na
strained	1 oz	32	4.1	0.0	16	0	1.6	na
'3rd Foods' *(Gerber)*	7 tbsp	115	14.8	0.1	52	na	6.1	na
w/broth, 'Stages 1' *(Beech-Nut)*	2.5 oz	90	8.0	0.0	40	na	6.0	na

Food Name	Serv. Size	Total Cal.	Prot. GMS	Carbs GMS	Sod. MGS	Fiber GMS	Fat GMS	Chol. MGS
w/broth, strained *(Heinz)*	3.5 oz	137	14.9	0.4	49	.8	8.6	na
w/egg yolks, strained *(Gerber)*	2.5 oz	100	10.0	1.0	38	0	6.0	42
Turkey sticks								
finger snacks, 'Graduates' *(Gerber)* ...	10 sticks	141	14.5	1.5	425	na	8.5	na
junior	1 stick	18	1.4	0.1	48	.1	1.4	na
Veal								
junior	3.5 oz	109	15.1	0.0	68	0	4.9	na
junior	1 oz	31	4.3	0.0	20	0	1.4	na
junior *(Gerber)*	2.5 oz	80	11.0	0.0	39	0	4.0	19
'2nd Foods' *(Gerber)*	7 tbsp	102	14.1	0.1	55	na	5.1	na
'Stages 1' *(Beech-Nut)*	2.8 oz	60	10.0	0.0	50	0	2.0	(mq)
strained	3.5 oz	100	13.4	0.0	63	0	4.8	na
strained	1 oz	29	3.8	0.0	18	0	1.4	na
'3rd Foods' *(Gerber)*	7 tbsp	108	15.5	0.0	56	na	5.0	na
w/broth, 'Stages 1' *(Beech-Nut)*	2.5 oz	70	10.0	0.0	50	na	3.0	na
w/broth, strained *(Heinz)*	3.5 oz	130	15.1	0.2	57	.5	7.9	na
w/egg yolks, strained *(Gerber)*	2.5 oz	80	10.0	1.0	38	0	4.0	18
Veal and beef								
junior *(Gerber)*	6 oz	110	4.0	16.0	31	(mq)	3.0	7
strained *(Gerber)*	4.5 oz	90	3.0	11.0	17	(mq)	4.0	5
Veal and ham								
junior *(Gerber)*	6 oz	120	3.0	17.0	24	(mq)	4.0	7
strained *(Gerber)*	4.5 oz	80	2.0	11.0	14	(mq)	3.0	4
Veal and turkey								
junior *(Gerber)*	6 oz	100	3.0	15.0	24	(mq)	3.0	19
strained *(Gerber)*	4.5 oz	70	2.0	10.0	17	(mq)	2.0	12
SOUP								
Chicken								
hearty, w/stars, 'Stages Table Time'								
(Beech-Nut)	6 oz	180	4.0	20.0	350	(mq)	9.0	(mq)
strained	4.5 oz	64	2.0	9.2	20	1.4	2.2	na
strained	1 oz	14	0.5	2.0	5	.3	0.5	na
strained *(Heinz)*	3.5 oz	49	1.5	7.2	20	.3	1.7	na
Cream of broccoli, '3rd Foods' *(Gerber)* ...	3.2 oz	26	1.4	2.7	83	na	1.1	na
Cream of chicken								
strained	4.5 oz	74	3.2	10.8	24	0	2.0	na
strained	1 oz	16	0.7	2.4	5	0	0.5	na
Cream of potato, '3rd Foods' *(Gerber)*	3.2 oz	33	1.2	5.2	69	na	0.8	na
Cream of tomato, '3rd Foods' *(Gerber)*	3.2 oz	41	1.4	7.3	73	na	0.7	na
Cream of vegetable, '3rd Foods'								
(Gerber)	3.2 oz	29	1.2	4.4	48	na	0.8	na

Food Name	Serv. Size	Total Cal.	Prot. GMS	Carbs GMS	Sod. MGS	Fiber GMS	Fat GMS	Chol. MGS
VEGETABLES								
Beet								
'2nd Foods' (Gerber)	7 tbsp	39	1.2	8.1	91	na	0.2	na
strained	4.5 oz	44	1.7	9.9	106	2.4	0.1	na
strained	1 oz	10	0.4	2.2	24	.5	0.0	na
strained (Gerber)	4.5 oz	60	1.0	11.0	115	(mq)	1.0	0
strained (Heinz)	3.5 oz	40	1.1	8.3	34	na	0.2	na
Broccoli, carrot, and cheese, '3rd Foods'								
(Gerber)	7 tbsp	44	1.6	7.2	46	na	1.0	na
Carrot								
(Earth's Best)	4.5 oz	40	1.0	7.0	70	(mq)	1.0	0
'Beginner Foods' (Heinz)	3.5 oz	30	0.8	6.1	32	na	0.3	na
buttered, junior	7.5 oz	70	1.7	14.3	34	>.9 c	1.3	na
buttered, junior	1 oz	9	0.2	1.9	5	>.1 c	0.2	na
buttered, strained	4.5 oz	46	1.0	9.5	23	>.4 c	0.8	na
buttered, strained	1 oz	10	0.2	2.1	5	>.1 c	0.2	na
diced, 'Graduates' (Gerber)	3.2 oz	22	0.5	4.7	26	na	0.1	na
'1st Foods' (Gerber)	2.5 oz	25	1.0	5.0	na	(mq)	0.0	0
'1st Foods' (Gerber)	7 tbsp	34	0.9	6.9	78	na	0.3	na
junior	7.5 oz	68	1.7	15.3	104	3.6	0.4	na
junior	1 oz	9	0.2	2.0	14	.5	0.1	na
junior (Gerber)	6 oz	80	3.0	16.0	83	(mq)	1.0	0
junior (Heinz)	3.5 oz	23	0.5	4.9	44	na	0.2	na
'Regal Imperial, 'Baby's First'								
(Beech-Nut)	2.5 oz	25	0.0	6.0	80	na	0.0	0
'Regal Imperial,' 'Stages 1' (Beech-Nut)	4.5 oz	40	1.0	9.0	130	(mq)	0.0	0
'Regal Imperial,' 'Stages 1' (Beech-Nut)	2.8 oz	30	0.0	7.0	80	(mq)	0.0	0
'2nd Foods' (Gerber)	7 tbsp	30	0.8	6.1	40	na	0.2	na
'Stages 3' (Beech-Nut)	6 oz	60	1.0	13.0	170	(mq)	0.0	0
strained	4.5 oz	35	1.0	7.7	47	2.2	0.1	na
strained	1 oz	8	0.2	1.7	10	.5	0.0	na
strained (Gerber)	4.5 oz	35	1.0	8.0	46	(mq)	0.0	0
strained (Heinz)	3.5 oz	23	0.5	4.9	44	na	0.2	na
'3rd Foods' (Gerber)	7 tbsp	29	0.8	6.0	49	na	0.2	na
Carrot and parsnip (Earth's Best)	4.5 oz	60	0.0	14.0	30	na	0.0	na
Corn, creamed								
junior	7.5 oz	138	3.0	34.7	111	4.5	0.9	na
junior	1 oz	18	0.4	4.6	15	.6	0.1	na
junior (Heinz)	3.5 oz	65	0.9	14.1	14	.4	0.5	na
'2nd Foods' (Gerber)	7 tbsp	62	1.8	12.7	8	na	0.5	na
'Stages 2' (Beech-Nut)	4.5 oz	100	2.0	20.0	25	(mq)	1.0	na
strained	4.5 oz	73	1.8	18.0	55	2.7	0.5	na
strained	1 oz	16	0.4	4.0	12	.6	0.1	na

Food Name	Serv. Size	Total Cal.	Prot. GMS	Carbs GMS	Sod. MGS	Fiber GMS	Fat GMS	Chol. MGS
strained *(Gerber)*	4.5 oz	80	2.0	16.0	12	(mq)	1.0	na
strained *(Heinz)*	3.5 oz	63	0.8	14.0	16	.3	0.4	na
Garden vegetable								
(Earth's Best)	4.5 oz	70	1.0	15.0	15	na	0.0	na
'2nd Foods' *(Gerber)*	7 tbsp	39	2.3	6.4	20	na	0.4	na
'Stages 2' *(Beech-Nut)*	4.5 oz	60	2.0	11.0	35	(mq)	0.0	0
strained	4.5 oz	47	2.9	8.7	45	1.9	0.3	na
strained	1 oz	10	0.7	1.9	10	.4	0.1	na
strained *(Gerber)*	4.5 oz	50	3.0	8.0	26	(mq)	1.0	0
Green bean								
'Beginner Foods' *(Heinz)*	3.5 oz	30	1.2	5.9	3	na	0.3	na
buttered, junior	7.25 oz	66	2.7	12.6	4	>.8 c	1.9	na
buttered, junior	1 oz	9	0.4	1.7	1	>.1 c	0.3	na
buttered, strained	4.5 oz	42	1.5	8.4	4	>.4 c	1.0	na
buttered, strained	1 oz	9	0.3	1.9	1	>.1 c	0.2	na
creamed, junior	7.5 oz	68	2.1	15.3	26	3.4	0.9	na
creamed, junior	1 oz	9	0.3	2.0	3	.5	0.1	na
creamed, junior *(Gerber)*	6 oz	80	3.0	16.0	14	(mq)	1.0	na
creamed, junior *(Heinz)*	3.5 oz	41	1.4	6.6	13	na	1.0	na
creamed, '3rd Foods' *(Gerber)*	7 tbsp	45	1.6	9.1	8	>.5 c	0.2	na
diced, 'Graduates' *(Gerber)*	3.2 oz	21	0.8	4.2	23	na	0.1	na
'1st Foods' *(Gerber)*	2.5 oz	25	1.0	5.0	na	(mq)	0.0	0
'1st Foods' *(Gerber)*	7 tbsp	32	1.3	6.2	1	na	0.2	na
junior	7.25 oz	52	2.5	11.7	4	3.9	0.2	na
junior	1 oz	7	0.3	1.6	1	.5	0.0	na
'2nd Foods' *(Gerber)*	7 tbsp	30	1.3	5.8	1	na	0.2	na
'Stages 3' *(Beech-Nut)*	6 oz	45	2.0	10.0	80	(mq)	0.0	0
'Stages 1' *(Beech-Nut)*	4.5 oz	35	1.0	8.0	0	(mq)	0.0	0
strained	4.5 oz	32	1.7	7.6	3	2.4	0.1	na
strained	1 oz	7	0.4	1.7	1	.5	0.0	na
strained *(Heinz)*	3.5 oz	25	1.0	4.9	2	.7	0.2	na
Mixed								
junior	7.5 oz	87	3.0	17.5	77	3.2	0.9	na
junior	1 oz	12	0.4	2.3	10	.4	0.1	na
junior *(Gerber)*	6 oz	70	2.0	14.0	32	(mq)	1.0	0
'2nd Foods' *(Gerber)*	7 tbsp	42	1.2	8.4	17	na	0.4	na
'Stages 2' *(Beech-Nut)*	4.5 oz	50	1.0	12.0	30	(mq)	0.0	0
strained	4.5 oz	52	1.5	10.2	17	1.9	0.6	na
strained	1 oz	12	0.3	2.3	4	.4	0.1	na
strained *(Gerber)*	4.5 oz	60	1.0	11.0	15	(mq)	1.0	0
strained *(Heinz)*	3.5 oz	44	1.4	8.8	21	na	0.4	na
'3rd Foods' *(Gerber)*	7 tbsp	39	1.3	8.0	14	na	0.2	na

Food Name	Serv. Size	Total Cal.	Prot. GMS	Carbs GMS	Sod. MGS	Fiber GMS	Fat GMS	Chol. MGS
Peas								
'Beginner Foods' (Heinz)	3.5 oz	55	3.6	9.5	13	1.4	0.5	na
buttered, junior	7.25 oz	124	7.2	23.3	10	>2.3 c	2.7	na
buttered, junior	1 oz	17	1.0	3.2	1	>.3 c	0.4	na
buttered, strained	4.5 oz	72	4.7	13.6	10	>.9 c	1.4	na
buttered, strained	1 oz	16	1.0	3.0	2	>.2 c	0.3	na
buttered, tender, sweet, 'Stages 1' (Beech-Nut)	4.5 oz	60	4.0	10.0	0	(mq)	0.0	0
buttered, tender, sweet, 'Stages 1' (Beech-Nut)	2.8 oz	40	2.0	6.0	0	(mq)	0.0	0
creamed, strained	4.5 oz	68	2.8	11.4	18	2.4	2.4	na
creamed, strained	1 oz	15	0.6	2.5	4	.5	0.5	na
creamed, strained (Heinz)	3.5 oz	52	2.0	7.6	11	na	1.5	na
diced, 'Graduates' (Gerber)	3.2 oz	44	2.7	8.4	9	na	0.1	na
'1st Foods' (Gerber)	2.5 oz	30	2.0	6.0	na	(mq)	0.0	0
'1st Foods' (Gerber)	7 tbsp	47	3.0	7.7	6	na	0.4	na
junior (Gerber)	6 oz	90	5.0	16.0	5	(mq)	1.0	0
'2nd Foods' (Gerber)	7 tbsp	47	3.0	7.7	5	na	0.5	na
strained	4.5 oz	51	4.5	10.4	5	2.7	0.4	na
strained	1 oz	11	1.0	2.3	1	.6	0.1	na
strained (Gerber)	4.5 oz	60	4.0	10.0	6	(mq)	1.0	0
tender, sweet, 'Baby's First' (Beech-Nut)	2.5 oz	40	2.0	7.0	0	na	0.0	na
'3rd Foods' (Gerber)	7 tbsp	47	3.0	7.8	6	na	0.4	na
Peas and brown rice (Earth's Best)	4.5 oz	80	5.0	16.0	10	na	0.0	na
Peas and carrots, 'Stages 2' (Beech-Nut)	4.5 oz	60	2.0	11.0	35	(mq)	0.0	0
Potato, diced, 'Graduates' (Gerber)	3.2 oz	38	1.0	8.5	6	na	0.1	na
Spinach, creamed								
junior	7.5 oz	89	6.4	13.6	117	3.8	3.0	na
junior	1 oz	12	0.9	1.8	16	.5	0.4	na
'2nd Foods' (Gerber)	7 tbsp	47	3.1	7.3	57	na	0.6	na
strained	4.5 oz	47	3.2	7.3	63	2.3	1.7	na
strained	1 oz	10	0.7	1.6	14	.5	0.4	na
strained (Gerber)	4.5 oz	60	4.0	9.0	73	(mq)	1.0	0
Spinach and potato (Earth's Best)	4.5 oz	60	2.0	8.0	25	na	2.0	na
Squash								
'Beginner Foods' (Heinz)	3.5 oz	36	1.2	7.3	5	na	0.2	na
buttered, junior	7.5 oz	64	1.5	13.6	4	>.4 c	1.3	na
buttered, junior	1 oz	9	0.2	1.8	1	>.1 c	0.2	na
buttered, strained	4.5 oz	37	0.8	8.8	3	>.3 c	0.4	na
buttered, strained	1 oz	8	0.2	2.0	1	>.1 c	0.1	na
butternut, and corn (Earth's Best)	4.5oz	90	2.0	15.0	0	na	2.0	na
butternut, 'Baby's First' (Beech-Nut)	2.5 oz	30	0.0	7.0	0	na	0.0	na
butternut, 'Stages 1' (Beech-Nut)	4.5 oz	50	1.0	11.0	0	(mq)	0.0	0

Food Name	Serv. Size	Total Cal.	Prot. GMS	Carbs GMS	Sod. MGS	Fiber GMS	Fat GMS	Chol. MGS
butternut, 'Stages 1' (Beech-Nut)	2.8 oz	30	0.0	7.0	0	(mq)	0.0	0
'1st Foods' (Gerber)	2.5 oz	25	1.0	5.0	na	(mq)	0.0	0
'1st Foods' (Gerber)	7 tbsp	33	0.8	7.0	1	na	0.3	na
junior	7.5 oz	51	1.7	11.9	2	4.5	0.4	na
junior	1 oz	7	0.2	1.6	0	.6	0.1	na
junior (Gerber)	6 oz	60	1.0	11.0	3	(mq)	1.0	0
'2nd Foods' (Gerber)	7 tbsp	32	0.8	6.8	1	na	0.2	na
strained	4.5 oz	31	1.0	7.2	3	2.7	0.3	na
strained	1 oz	7	0.2	1.6	1	.6	0.1	na
strained (Gerber)	4.5 oz	35	1.0	8.0	3	(mq)	0.0	0
strained (Heinz)	3.5 oz	32	0.9	6.6	2	.8	0.3	na
'3rd Foods' (Gerber)	7 tbsp	33	0.9	6.8	1	na	0.2	na
winter (Earth's Best)	4.5 oz	50	1.0	12.0	10	(mq)	0.0	0
Sweet potato								
(Earth's Best)	4.5 oz	60	1.0	12.0	15	(mq)	1.0	0
'Baby's First' (Beech-Nut)	2.5 oz	50	1.0	11.0	10	na	0.0	na
'Beginner Foods' (Heinz)	3.5 oz	69	1.0	15.7	14	na	0.2	na
buttered, junior	7.75 oz	125	1.8	26.8	18	>.4 c	1.5	na
buttered, junior	1 oz	16	0.2	3.5	2	>.1 c	0.2	na
buttered, strained	4.75 oz	76	1.2	15.9	11	>.1 c	0.9	na
buttered, strained	1 oz	16	0.3	3.3	2	(mq)	0.2	na
'1st Foods' (Gerber)	2.5 oz	45	1.0	10.0	na	(mq)	0.0	0
'1st Foods' (Gerber)	7 tbsp	67	1.2	15.0	15	na	0.2	na
junior	7.75 oz	132	2.4	30.6	48	3.3	0.2	na
junior	1 oz	17	0.3	3.9	6	.4	0.0	na
junior (Gerber)	6 oz	110	1.0	24.0	39	(mq)	1.0	0
junior (Heinz)	3.5 oz	69	1.0	15.6	11	na	0.3	na
'2nd Foods' (Gerber)	7 tbsp	62	1.0	14.1	17	na	0.2	na
'Stages 1' (Beech-Nut)	2.8 oz	60	0.0	14.0	10	(mq)	0.0	0
'Stages 1' (Beech-Nut)	4.5 oz	90	1.0	20.0	80	(mq)	0.0	0
'Stages 3' (Beech-Nut)	6 oz	110	1.0	26.0	80	(mq)	0.0	0
strained	4.75 oz	77	1.5	17.8	27	2.0	0.1	na
strained	1 oz	16	0.3	3.7	6	.4	0.0	na
strained (Gerber)	4.5 oz	80	1.0	18.0	22	(mq)	1.0	0
strained (Heinz)	3.5 oz	69	1.0	15.6	11	na	0.3	na
'3rd Foods' (Gerber)	7 tbsp	63	1.1	14.2	23	na	0.2	na
WATER, w/fluoride, sodium-free								
(Beech-Nut)	4 oz	0	0.0	0.0	0	na	0.0	na
BACON								
cooked, yield from 1 lb raw	4.5 oz	732	38.7	0.8	2026	0	62.5	107
cured, approx 20 slices per lb, cooked	3 slices	109	5.8	0.1	303	0	9.4	16
cured, breakfast strips, cooked	3 slices	156	9.8	0.4	714	0	12.5	36
cured, broiled	4.5 oz	732	38.7	0.8	2027	0	62.5	108

Food Name	Serv. Size	Total Cal.	Prot. GMS	Carbs GMS	Sod. MGS	Fiber GMS	Fat GMS	Chol. MGS
cured, broiled	3 med slices	109	5.8	0.1	303	0	9.4	16
cured, canned	100 gm	685	8.5	1.0	680	0	71.5	89
cured, pan-fried	4.5 oz	732	38.7	0.8	2027	0	62.5	108
cured, pan-fried	3 med slices	109	5.8	0.1	303	0	9.4	3.3
cured, roasted	4.5 oz	732	38.7	0.8	2027	0	62.5	108
cured, roasted	3 med slices	109	5.8	0.1	303	0	9.4	16
cured, strips, cooked	6 oz	780	49.2	1.8	3568	0	62.4	178
cured, 12 slices per lb, raw	1 slice	211	3.3	0.0	277	0	21.9	25
cured, strips, 15 slices per 12 oz, raw ..	3 slices	264	8.0	0.5	671	0	25.3	47
raw	1 oz	158	2.5	<.1	194	0	16.3	19
(Hormel)								
'Black Label' cooked	1 oz	142	3.0	2.0	192	na	14.0	18
'Black Label' low salt, cooked	1.76 oz	250	5.0	2.0	260	na	25.0	32
'Black Label' sliced, cooked	2 slices	60	4.0	0.0	298	0	5.0	(mq)
'Range' thick sliced, cooked	1 oz	152	2.0	2.0	199	na	16.0	17
(JM)								
cooked	2 slices	100	4.0	1.0	370	0	9.0	12
'Lower Sodium' cooked	2 slices	100	4.0	1.0	260	0	9.0	(mq)
'Lower Sodium' raw	2 slices	290	5.0	1.0	250	0	30.0	((mq)
raw	2 slices	280	4.0	1.0	530	0	29.0	38.
(Jones Dairy Farm), raw	1 slice	165	2.3	tr	187	0	17.0	25
(Kahn's), 'American Beauty,' cooked	2 slices	100	5.0	na	(mq)	0	9.0	(mq)
(Oscar Mayer)								
'Center Cut' cooked, approx .2-oz slices	1 slice	25	2.0	0.1	113	0	1.8	6
'Center Cut' cooked, yield from 1 lb raw ..	6 oz	852	68.8	3.5	3813	0	62.5	189
cooked, approx .2-oz slices	1 slice	33	2.0	0.1	138	0	2.8	5
cooked, yield from 16-oz pkg raw	5 oz	784	47.1	3.0	3236	0	64.9	127
'Lower Salt' cooked, approx .2-oz slices	1 slice	33	2.2	0.1	104	0	2.6	6
'Lower Salt,' cooked, yield from 1 lb raw	5.6 oz	870	57.2	2.3	2768	0	70.3	170
thick sliced, cooked, approx .4-oz slices	1 slice	58	3.6	0.1	259	0	4.8	9
thick sliced, cooked, yield from 1 lb raw ...	5 oz	811	50.6	1.1	3656	0	67.1	123
(Range Brand) 'Sliced,' cooked	2 slices	110	6.0	0.0	392	0	9.0	(mq)
(Red Label) cooked	3 slices	110	6.0	0.0	(mq)	0	10.0	(mq)

BACON, ALTERNATIVE

BEEF

Food Name	Serv. Size	Total Cal.	Prot. GMS	Carbs GMS	Sod. MGS	Fiber GMS	Fat GMS	Chol. MGS
heated *(JM)*	2 slices	100	7.0	1.0	320	0	7.0	20
heated *(Sizzlean)*	2 strips	70	6.0	0.0	480	0	5.0	(mq)
heated, yield from 12-oz pkg	6 oz	764	53.2	2.4	700	0	58.5	202
raw	1 oz	115	2.8	0.2	271	0	11.0	23
raw *(JM)*	2 slices	200	9.0	1.0	430	0	18.0	53.
unheated	1 oz	115	2.8	0.2	271	0	11.0	23

PORK

Food Name	Serv. Size	Total Cal.	Prot. GMS	Carbs GMS	Sod. MGS	Fiber GMS	Fat GMS	Chol. MGS
80% fat-free *(Louis Rich)* ....,	1 slice	35	2.0	<1.0	185	na	2.0	10

Food Name	Serv. Size	Total Cal.	Prot. GMS	Carbs GMS	Sod. MGS	Fiber GMS	Fat GMS	Chol. MGS
heated *(Sizzlean)*	2 strips	90	6.0	0.0	530	0	8.0	(mq)
heated, brown sugar cured *(Sizzlean)*	2 strips	110	6.0	2.0	490	0	9.0	(mq)
heated, yield from 12-oz pkg	6 oz	780	49.2	1.8	3568	0	62.4	179
raw	1 oz	110	3.3	0.2	280	0	10.5	20
TURKEY, heated *(Louis Rich)*	1 slice	32	2.4	0.3	186	0	2.4	10
VEGETARIAN								
	1 cup	446	15.4	9.1	2110	3.7	42.5	0
	1 oz	88	3.0	1.8	415	.2	8.4	0
(Morningstar Farms) 'Breakfast Strips'								
frozen	3 strips	80	3.0	4.0	350	na	6.0	0
(White Wave SoyFood) 'Healthy'	1 oz	27	4.0	4.0	310	3.3	1.0	0
(Worthington) 'Stripples' frozen	4 strips	120	4.0	6.0	460	na	9.0	0
Canadian style								
(Heartline)	2 oz	176	19.0	9.0	260	na	7.0	0
(Heartline) 'Canadian Bacon Style' lite	.5 oz	22	5.0	1.0	135	3.0	0.0	0
BACON, CANADIAN-STYLE								
cured, grilled	2 slices	86	11.3	0.6	719	0	3.9	27
cured, grilled, yield from 6 oz raw	4.9 oz	257	33.7	1.9	2149	0	11.7	81
cured, packed 6 slices per 6 oz,								
unheated	2 slices	89	11.7	1.0	799	0	4.0	28
cured, unheated	6 oz	267	35.1	2.9	2395	0	11.9	85
unheated	1 oz	45	5.9	0.5	399	0	2.0	14
(Hormel) 'Sliced'	1 oz	45	6.0	0.5	315	0	2.0	(mq)
(Jones Dairy Farm) unheated	1 slice	25	3.2	tr	144	0	1.0	7
(Light & Lean)	2 slices	35	6.0	0.0	(mq)	0	1.0	(mq)
(Oscar Mayer)	.8 oz	28	4.7	0.1	305	0	1.0	11
BACON BITS								
(Hormel)	1 oz	117	12.0	1.0	1008	na	7.0	16
(Hormel)	1 tbsp	30	3.0	0.0	313	0	2.0	na
(Libby's) 'Bacon Crumbles'	1 tbsp	25	2.0	2.0	(mq)	0	1.0	na
(Oscar Mayer)	3 oz	248	31.6	2.5	2224	0	12.4	67
(Oscar Mayer)	1 tbsp	20	2.6	0.2	183	0	1.0	6
BACON BITS, ALTERNATIVE								
(Bac•Os)	2 tsp	25	2.0	2.0	90	na	1.0	na
(McCormick) 'Bac'N Pieces'								
no cholesterol	1 1/2tbsp	30	3.0	2.0	240	na	1.0	0
(Schilling) 'Bac'N Pieces'	1 tsp	26	2.0	2.0	51	na	0.4	na
BACON PIECES *(Hormel)*	1 oz	94	12.0	2.0	654	na	5.0	26
BAGEL								
BLUEBERRY								
(Earth Grains) 3 oz	1 bagel	245	9.0	48.0	210	na	0.0	0
(Western Bagel)	1 bagel	240	8.0	43.0	410	2.0	4.0	0

Food Name	Serv. Size	Total Cal.	Prot. GMS	Carbs GMS	Sod. MGS	Fiber GMS	Fat GMS	Chol. MGS
CINNAMON-RAISIN								
(Dunkin' Donuts)	1 bagel	250	8.0	49.0	370	na	2.0	0
(Earth Grains) 3 oz	1 bagel	245	9.0	48.0	210	na	0.0	0
(Thomas') 'Deli Style'	1 bagel	170	6.0	33.0	230	2.0	2.0	0
(Western Bagel)	1 bagel	230	8.0	40.0	410	4.0	4.0	0
EGG								
	1 oz	79	3.0	15.0	143	na	0.6	7
(Dunkin' Donuts)	1 bagel	250	9.0	47.0	380	na	2.0	15
(Lender's) 'Bagel Shop'	1 bagel	230	9.0	41.0	460	2.0	2.5	15
(Lender's) 'Bakery Style'	1 bagel	210	9.0	41.0	450	2.0	2.0	5
HONEY WHEAT (Earth Grains) 3 oz	1 bagel	240	9.0	45.0	210	na	0.0	0
ONION								
enriched, 3.5 inch diam	1 bagel	195	7.5	37.9	379	1.5	1.1	0
enriched, w/calcium proprianate, 3.5 inch diam	1 bagel	195	7.5	37.9	379	1.5	1.1	0
enriched, w/calcium proprianate, toasted	1 oz	84	3.2	16.3	163	na	0.5	0
unenriched, 3.5 inch diam	1 bagel	195	7.5	37.9	379	1.5	1.1	0
unenriched, w/calcium proprianate, 3.5 inch diam	1 bagel	195	7.5	37.9	379	1.5	1.1	0
(Dunkin' Donuts)	1 bagel	230	9.0	46.0	480	na	1.0	0
(Earth Grains) 3 oz	1 bagel	240	9.0	45.0	210	na	0.0	0
(Lender's) 'Bagel Shop'	1 bagel	220	9.0	40.0	460	2.0	2.0	0
(Western Bagel)	1 bagel	220	8.0	39.0	430	4.0	4.0	0
PLAIN								
enriched, 3.5 inch diam	1 bagel	195	7.5	37.9	379	1.5	1.1	0
enriched, w/calcium proprianate, 3.5 inch diam	1 bagel	195	7.5	37.9	379	1.5	1.1	0
unenriched, 3.5 inch diam	1 bagel	195	7.5	37.9	379	1.5	1.1	0
unenriched, w/calcium proprianate, 3.5 inch diam	1 bagel	195	7.5	37.9	379	1.5	1.1	0
(Dunkin' Donuts)	1 bagel	240	9.0	47.0	450	na	1.0	0
(Earth Grains) 3 oz	1 bagel	240	9.0	45.0	210	na	0.0	0
(Lender's) 'Bagel Shop'	1 bagel	210	10.0	40.0	350	1.0	1.5	0
(Lender's) 'Bakery Style'	1 bagel	210	8.0	42.0	450	2.0	2.0	0
POPPY SEED								
enriched, 3.5 inch diam	1 bagel	195	7.5	37.9	379	1.5	1.1	0
enriched, w/calcium proprianate, 3.5 inch diam	1 bagel	195	7.5	37.9	379	1.5	1.1	0
enriched, w/calcium proprianate, toasted	1 oz	84	3.2	16.3	163	na	0.5	0
unenriched, 3.5 inch diam	1 bagel	195	7.5	37.9	379	1.5	1.1	0

Food Name	Serv. Size	Total Cal.	Prot. GMS	Carbs GMS	Sod. MGS	Fiber GMS	Fat GMS	Chol. MGS
unenriched, w/calcium proprianate,								
3.5 inch diam	1 bagel	195	7.5	37.9	379	1.5	1.1	0
RAISIN								
(Lender's) 'Bagel Shop'	1 bagel	240	8.0	44.0	350	2.0	3.0	0
(Lender's) 'Bakery Style'	1 bagel	220	8.0	44.0	380	2.0	2.0	na
RAISIN-HONEY CINNAMON								
(Finast) 2.5 oz	1 bagel	200	8.0	40.0	305	(mq)	1.0	0
SESAME								
enriched, 3.5 inch diam	1 bagel	195	7.5	37.9	379	1.5	1.1	0
enriched, w/calcium proprianate,								
3.5 inch diam	1 bagel	195	7.5	37.9	379	1.5	1.1	0
enriched, w/calcium proprianate,								
toasted	1 oz	84	3.2	16.3	163	na	0.5	0
unenriched, 3.5 inch diam	1 bagel	195	7.5	37.9	379	1.5	1.1	0
unenriched, w/calcium proprianate,								
3.5 inch diam	1 bagel	195	7.5	37.9	379	1.5	1.1	0
WATER *(Western Bagel)*	1 bagel	230	8.0	41.0	420	2.0	4.0	0
BAGEL, FROZEN								
BLUEBERRY *(Lender's)* 2.5 oz	1 bagel	190	7.0	38.0	250	(mq)	1.0	0
CINNAMON-RAISIN								
(Lender's) 'Big'n Crusty' 3 1/8 oz	1 bagel	250	8.0	49.0	370	(mq)	2.0	0
(Sara Lee) 3.1 oz	1 bagel	240	8.0	48.0	280	(mq)	2.0	0
(Sara Lee) 2.5 oz	1 bagel	200	7.0	39.0	230	(mq)	2.0	0
EGG								
(Lender's) 2 oz	1 bagel	150	7.0	29.0	360	(mq)	1.0	5
(Lender's) 'Big'n Crusty' 3 1/8 oz	1 bagel	250	9.0	47.0	380	(mq)	2.0	15
(Sara Lee) 3.1 oz	1 bagel	250	9.0	48.0	450	(mq)	2.0	20
(Sara Lee) 2.5 oz	1 bagel	200	8.0	38.0	360	(mq)	2.0	15
GARLIC								
(Lender's) 2 oz	1 bagel	160	6.0	32.0	340	(mq)	1.0	0
(Lender's) 'Big'n Crusty' 3 1/8 oz	1 bagel	250	9.0	50.0	530	(mq)	1.0	0
OAT BRAN								
(Lender's) 2.5 oz	1 bagel	170	7.0	36.0	290	3.0	2.0	0
(Sara Lee) 3 oz	1 bagel	220	9.0	47.0	450	(mq)	1.0	0
(Sara Lee) 2.5 oz	1 bagel	180	8.0	38.0	360	(mq)	1.0	0
ONION								
(Lender's) 2 oz	1 bagel	160	7.0	31.0	290	(mq)	1.0	0
(Lender's) 'Bagelettes' .9 oz	1 bagel	70	3.0	14.0	135	<.1 c	<1.0	0
(Lender's) 'Big'n Crusty' 3 1/8 oz	1 bagel	230	9.0	46.0	480	(mq)	1.0	0
(Sara Lee) 3.1 oz	1 bagel	230	9.0	45.0	560	(mq)	1.0	0
(Sara Lee) 2.5 oz	1 bagel	190	7.0	37.0	450	(mq)	1.0	0
PLAIN								
(Lender's) 2 oz	1 bagel	150	6.0	30.0	320	(mq)	1.0	0

Food Name	Serv. Size	Total Cal.	Prot. GMS	Carbs GMS	Sod. MGS	Fiber GMS	Fat GMS	Chol. MGS
(Lender's) 'Bagelettes' .9 oz	1 bagel	70	3.0	13.0	170	(mq)	<1.0	
(Lender's) 'Big'n Crusty'	1 bagel	240	9.0	47.0	450	(mq)	1.0	
(Lender's) soft, 2.5 oz	1 bagel	210	7.0	36.0	350	(mq)	3.0	1
(Sara Lee) 3.1 oz	1 bagel	230	9.0	46.0	580	(mq)	1.0	
(Sara Lee) 2.5 oz	1 bagel	190	8.0	38.0	460	(mq)	1.0	
POPPY SEED								
(Lender's) 2 oz	1 bagel	160	7.0	29.0	370	(mq)	1.0	
(Sara Lee) 3.1 oz	1 bagel	230	9.0	46.0	560	(mq)	1.0	n.
(Sara Lee) 2.5 oz	1 bagel	190	8.0	37.0	450	(mq)	1.0	
PUMPERNICKEL (Lender's) 2 oz	1 bagel	160	6.0	31.0	330	(mq)	1.0	
RAISIN (Lender's) 'Bagelettes' .9 oz	1 bagel	70	2.0	14.0	110	(mq)	<1.0	
RAISIN-HONEY (Lender's) 2.5 oz	1 bagel	200	8.0	40.0	310	(mq)	1.0	
RYE (Lender's) 2 oz	1 bagel	150	6.0	30.0	310	(mq)	1.0	
SESAME								
(Lender's) 2 oz	1 bagel	160	7.0	31.0	320	(mq)	1.0	
(Sara Lee) 3.1 oz	1 bagel	240	9.0	46.0	550	(mq)	2.0	
(Sara Lee) 2.5 oz	1 bagel	190	8.0	37.0	440	(mq)	1.0	
WHEAT-RAISIN (Lender's) 2.5 oz	1 bagel	190	6.0	39.0	310	(mq)	1.0	
BAGEL CHIP								
(Burns & Ricker) cinnamon raisin								
'Original Bagel Crisps'	1 oz	130	4.0	20.0	170	1.0	4.0	
(Burns & Ricker) garlic 'Original Bagel								
Crisps'	1 oz	130	4	20.0	190	1.0	4.0	
BAKED BEANS, CANNED. See also BEANS, CANNED.								
(Allens)	1/2 cup	170	6.0	21.0	330	(mq)	6.0	n.
(Grandma Brown's)	1 cup	301	14.6	53.9	655	15.5	3.0	<
(Green Giant)	1/2 cup	150	5.0	28.0	670	na	2.0	n
(Open Range)	4.656 oz	152	6.6	30.5	425	6.7	2.3	
(Van Camp's)	1 cup	260	11.0	52.0	1020	(mq)	2.0	n
bacon and brown sugar, 'Premium'								
(Van Camp's)	6 oz	170	8.0	36.0	790	8.3	2.0	n
barbecue (B&M)	8 oz	260	15.0	48.0	1000	11.0	6.0	
barbecue (Campbell's)	7 7/8 oz	210	10.0	43.0	900	(mq)	4.0	n.
Boston (Health Valley)	4 oz	213	11.0	43.0	74	22.3	1.0	
Boston, 'No Salt Added' (Health Valley)	4 oz	213	11.0	43.0	25	22.3	1.0	
Boston, w/ham 'Homestyle' (Hunt's)	9.03 oz	248	15.9	41.8	740	9.8	1.9	
'Brick Oven' (S&W)	1/2 cup	160	7.0	28.0	560	(mq)	2.0	n.
brown sugar (Van Camp's)	1 cup	290	11.6	51.0	640	>3.2 c	5.1	n.
'Deluxe' (Van Camp's)	1 cup	320	13.0	57.0	970	(mq)	4.0	n.
'Dry Beans in Sauce' (Green Giant)	1/2 cup	130	6.0	30.0	570	6.0	1.0	
'Dry Beans in Sauce' (Joan of Arc)	1/2 cup	130	6.0	30.0	570	6.0	1.0	
'Home Style' (Campbell's)	8 oz	220	11.0	48.0	820	(mq)	4.0	n.
honey (B&M)	8 oz	240	15.0	50.0	940	11.0	2.0	

Food Name	Serv. Size	Total Cal.	Prot. GMS	Carbs GMS	Sod. MGS	Fiber GMS	Fat GMS	Chol. MGS
hot 'n spicy (B&M)	8 oz	240	14.0	50.0	990	12.0	3.0	3
in homestyle sauce (Bush's Best)	4 oz	110	5.0	25.0	350	6.0	1.0	na
in molasses, brown sugar, 'Old Fashioned' (Campbell's)	8 oz	230	11.0	49.0	730	(mq)	3.0	na
in tomato sauce (B&M)	8 oz	230	12.0	48.0	1010	10.0	3.0	1
in tomato sauce (Campbell's)	8 oz	200	10.0	43.0	770	(mq)	3.0	na
in tomato sauce (Pathmark)	1/2 cup	150	7.0	23.0	440	(mq)	2.0	na
in tomato sauce, 40-oz can (Finast)	1/2 cup	120	7.0	21.0	930	(mq)	1.0	na
in tomato sauce, 'No Frills' (Pathmark)	1/2 cup	160	7.0	28.0	390	(mq)	2.0	na
in tomato sauce, 16-oz can (Finast)	1 cup	270	13.0	50.0	1180	(mq)	3.0	na
maple (B&M)	8 oz	240	14.0	52.0	890	11.0	2.0	5
maple (Friends)	8 oz	240	14.0	52.0	890	11.0	2.0	5
no salt added, fat-free (Health Valley)	7.5 oz	190	8.0	41.0	20	5.0	0.0	0
pea beans (B&M)	8 oz	270	14.0	50.0	750	11.0	6.0	5
pea, small (Friends)	8 oz	360	17.0	62.0	1040	15.0	4.0	6
pea, small, w/pork (Friends)	8 oz	260	14.0	53.0	890	11.0	5.0	5
pork and beans, 'Deluxe' (Bush's Best)	4 oz	110	5.0	25.0	350	6.0	1.0	na
pork and beans, 'Showboat' (Bush's Best)	4 oz	80	6.0	19.0	470	na	<1.0	na
regular, fat-free (Health Valley)	7.5 oz	190	8.0	41.0	290	5.0	0.0	0
'Saucepan' (Grandma Brown's)	1 cup	307	13.7	52.3	592	14.8	4.8	<1
vegetarian	1/2 cup	118	6.1	26.0	504	9.8	0.6	0
vegetarian (A&P)	1/2 cup	130	7.0	25.0	420	(mq)	<1.0	0
vegetarian (Allens)	1/2 cup	110	6.0	19.0	380	(mq)	1.0	0
vegetarian (B&M)	8 oz	230	14.0	50.0	370	11.0	3.0	0
vegetarian (Campbell's)	7.75 oz	170	11.0	40.0	780	(mq)	1.0	0
vegetarian 'Vegetarian Style' (Van Camp's)	1 cup	206	10.0	42.0	950	(mq)	0.6	0
vegetarian, w/miso 'Vegetarian' (Health Valley)	4 oz	90	6.0	19.0	134	6.5	1.0	0
w/beef	1/2 cup	161	8.5	22.5	632	>1.4 c	4.6	29
w/franks	1/2 cup	182	8.6	19.7	550	8.8	8.4	8
w/franks, 'Beanee Weenee' (Van Camp's)	1 cup	326	15.2	31.7	990	7.0	15.4	15
w/onions, approx 1/2 cup (Bush's Best)	4 oz	110	6.0	27.0	550	7.0	1.0	na
w/pork	1/2 cup	134	6.5	25.2	522	6.9	2.0	9
w/pork (A&P)	1/2 cup	150	7.0	25.0	440	(mq)	2.0	(mq)
w/pork (Hunt's)	4 oz	140	6.0	26.0	400	(mq)	1.0	(mq)
w/pork (S&W)	1/2 cup	130	5.0	22.0	135	(mq)	2.0	(mq)
w/pork (Van Camp's)	1 cup	216	10.9	41.0	1000	9.9	1.9	(mq)
w/pork 'Extra Fancy' (Allens)	1/2 cup	125	5.0	24.0	540	(mq)	1.0	(mq)
w/pork, 'Extra Standard' (Allens)	1/2 cup	90	5.0	15.0	350	(mq)	1.0	(mq)
w/pork, 'Fancy' (Allens)	1/2 cup	110	6.0	18.0	430	(mq)	1.0	((mq)

Food Name	Serv. Size	Total Cal.	Prot. GMS	Carbs GMS	Sod. MGS	Fiber GMS	Fat GMS	Chol. MGS
w/pork, 'Micro-Cup' *(Hormel)*	7.5 oz	254	11.0	41.0	650	(mq)	5.0	30
w/pork and sweet sauce	1/2 cup	140	6.7	26.5	423	6.9	1.8	9
w/pork and tomato sauce	1/2 cup	123	6.5	24.4	554	6.9	1.3	9
w/pork and tomato sauce *(Green Giant)*	1/2 cup	90	5.0	21.0	420	5.0	1.0	0
w/pork and tomato sauce *(Joan of Arc)*	1/2 cup	90	5.0	21.0	420	5.0	1.0	0
BAKING POWDER								
....	1 tbsp	11	0.0	2.6	1050	0	0.0	0
....	1 tsp	3	0.0	0.7	290	0	0.0	0
commercial	3 1/2 oz	109	0.1	26.5	16804	0	0.0	0
commercial *(Calumet)*	1/4 tsp	0	0.0	0.0	100	0	0.0	0
cream of tartar, w/tartaric acid	1 tbsp	7	0.0	1.8	694	0	0.0	0
double-acting, sodium aluminum sulfate	1 tsp	2	0.0	1.3	488	na	0.0	0
double-acting, straight phosphate	1 tsp	2	0.0	1.1	363	na	0.0	0
'Low Salt' *(Featherweight)*	1 tsp	8	0.0	2.0	2	0	0.0	0
low-sodium	1 tsp	5	0.0	2.3	5	0	0.0	0
low-sodium, commercial	1 tbsp	23	0.0	5.6	1	0	0.0	0
low-sodium, commercial	1 tsp	7	0.0	1.8	0	0	0.0	0
low-sodium, non-commercial	1 tsp	2	0.0	0.6	0	0	0.0	0
w/monohydrate	1 tbsp	14	0.0	3.4	1205	0	0.0	0
w/monohydrate	1 tsp	4	0.0	0.9	329	0	0.0	0
w/straight phosphate	1 tbsp	15	0.0	3.7	1028	0	0.0	0
w/straight phosphate	1 tsp	5	0.0	1.1	312	0	0.0	0
BAKING SODA								
....	1 tsp	0	0.0	0.0	1259	na	0.0	0
(Arm & Hammer)	1/2 tsp	0	0.0	0.0	476	0	0.0	0
BALSAM PEAR/bitter melon								
Leafy tips								
boiled, drained	4 oz	40	4.1	7.7	15	2.1	0.2	0
boiled, drained	1/2 cup	10	1.0	2.0	4	.6	0.1	0
raw	1/2 cup	7	1.3	0.8	3	>.6 c	0.2	0
raw, trimmed	1 oz	9	1.5	0.9	3	>.6 c	0.2	0
raw, untrimmed	1 lb	52	9.1	5.7	18	>3.9 c	1.2	0
Pods								
boiled, drained	4 oz	22	1.0	4.9	7	2.5	0.2	0
boiled, drained, 1/2-inch pieces	1/2 cup	12	0.5	2.7	4	1.2	0.1	0
raw	1 pear	21	1.2	4.6	6	3.5	0.2	0
raw, approx 9 3/8 inch x 1 1/2 inch, 5.3 oz each	1 pod	21	1.2	4.6	6	3.5	0.2	0
raw, 1/2-inch pieces	1 cup	16	0.9	3.4	5	2.6	0.2	0
raw, trimmed	1 oz	5	0.3	1.1	1	>.4 c	0.1	0
raw, untrimmed	1 lb	64	3.8	13.9	20	>5.3 c	0.6	0
BAMBOO SHOOTS								
boiled, drained	4 oz	14	1.7	2.2	5	>.7 c	0.2	0
boiled, drained, 1/2-inch slices	1 cup	14	1.8	2.3	5	>.8 c	0.3	0

Food Name	Serv. Size	Total Cal.	Prot. GMS	Carbs GMS	Sod. MGS	Fiber GMS	Fat GMS	Chol. MGS
canned *(LaChoy)*	1.5 oz	8	0.7	1.4	3	(mq)	0.2	0
canned *(LaChoy)*	2 tbsp	3	0.2	0.7	0	>.4 c	0.1	0
canned, drained solids, 1/8-inch slices	1 cup	25	2.3	4.2	9	3.9	0.5	0
raw, 1/2-inch slices	1 cup	41	3.9	7.8	6	3.3	0.5	0
raw, trimmed	1 oz	8	0.7	1.5	1	.7	0.1	0
raw, w/sheath	1 lb	36	3.4	6.8	6	3.4	0.4	0
BANANA								
fresh *(Dole)*	1 fruit	120	1.0	28.0	na	3.0	1.0	0
mashed	1/2 cup	104	1.2	26.4	1	1.8	0.5	0
peeled	1 oz	26	0.3	6.6	<1	.5	0.1	0
powdered	1 oz	98	1.1	25.0	1	>.5 c	0.5	0
powdered	1/4 cup	87	1.0	22.1	1	>.5 c	0.5	0
powdered	1 tbsp	21	0.2	5.5	tr	>.1 c	0.1	0
raw, w/o skin and seeds	1 fruit	105	1.2	26.7	1	1.8	0.6	0
unpeeled	1 lb	271	3.1	69.1	3	4.7	1.4	0
BANANA, COOKING. See PLANTAIN.								
BANANA, DEHYDRATED								
	1 oz	98	1.1	25.0	1	1.8	0.5	0
	1/4 cup	87	1.0	22.1	1	1.8	0.5	0
BANANA, RED								
raw	100 gm	90	1.2	23.4	1	>.4 c	0.2	0
raw, approx 7.25 inch x 1.5 inch	1 med	118	1.6	30.7	1	(mq)	0.3	0
raw, sliced	1/2 cup	68	0.9	17.6	1	(mq)	0.2	0
BANANA BERRY DRINK								
'Stompin' Banana Berry Drink' *(Hi-C)*	6 oz	90	0.0	22.0	25	na	0.0	na
BANANA BREAD. See BREAD, QUICK.								
BANANA CHIPS								
	1 oz	147	0.7	16.6	2	>.7 c	9.5	0
freeze-dried *(Mountain House)*	1/2 cup	248	2.0	15.0	na	(mq)	8.0	0
premium *(Mariani)*	1 oz	150	1.0	17.0	<10	na	9.0	0
BANANA NECTAR *(Libby's)*	6 oz	110	0.0	26.0	15	na	0.0	na
BANANA PEPPER. See PEPPER, BANANA.								
BANANA PINEAPPLE NECTAR *(Kern's)*	6 oz	110	1.0	27.0	0	na	0.0	na
BANANA SQUASH. See SQUASH, BANANA.								
BANNER BEAN SEED, whole, dried	1 oz	95	6.3	17.4	na	>2.2 c	0.3	0
BARBADOS CHERRY. See ACEROLA CHERRY.								
BARBADOS CHERRY JUICE. See ACEROLA CHERRY JUICE.								
BARBECUE SAUCE								
(Bull's Eye)	.5 oz	22	0.0	5.0	47	na	0.0	0
(Cattleman's) mild	1 tbsp	25	0.0	5.0	260	na	0.0	0
(Enrico's) 'Original'	1 tbsp	18	1.0	3.0	4	na	1.0	0
(Healthy Choice) original	1.1 oz	25	0.3	5.7	229	.5	0.2	0
(Heinz) 'Old Fashioned'	1 tbsp	18	0.2	4.1	180	tr	0.1	0

Food Name	Serv. Size	Total Cal.	Prot. GMS	Carbs GMS	Sod. MGS	Fiber GMS	Fat GMS	Chol. MGS
(Heinz) 'Select'	1 oz	40	0.0	9.0	275	na	0.0	0
(Heinz) 'Thick and Rich' old fashioned	1 oz	35	0.0	8.0	350	na	0.0	0
(Heinz) 'Thick and Rich' original	1 oz	35	0.0	8.0	390	na	0.0	0
(Hunt's) 'Bold' original	1.2 oz	46	0.3	10.8	315	.5	0.3	0
(Hunt's) 'Light' original	1.1 oz	26	0.5	6.1	223	.6	0.1	0
(Hunt's) original	1.2 oz	40	0.5	9.4	410	1.0	0.3	0
(Kraft)	2 tbsp	45	0.0	10.0	460	na	1.0	0
(Kraft) 'Thick 'n Spicy' original	2 tbsp	50	0.0	12.0	430	na	1.0	0
(Open Range) original	1.2 oz	38	0.6	9.0	333	.9	0.2	0
(Ott's)	1 tbsp	14	0.2	3.2	147	.1	0.1	<1
(Skipper's)	1 tbsp	25	0.0	5.0	226	na	1.0	0
CAJUN STYLE								
(Golden Dipt)	1 oz	90	0.0	5.0	360	na	8.0	0
(Heinz)	1 tbsp	15	0.3	3.4	108	>.1 c	0.1	na
(Heinz) 'Thick and Rich'	1 oz	35	0.0	8.0	360	na	0.0	0
CHUNKY								
(Heinz) 'Thick and Rich'	1 oz	30	1.0	6.0	380	na	0.0	0
(Kraft) 'Thick 'n Spicy'	2 tbsp	60	0.0	13.0	420	na	1.0	0
COUNTRY STYLE								
(Hunt's)	1.2 oz	39	0.4	8.8	399	.3	0.3	0
(Hunt's)	1 tbsp	20	<1.0	5.0	140	<1.0	<1.0	0
DIJON AND HONEY								
(Estee)	1 tbsp	18	<1.0	3.0	5	na	<1.0	0
(Lawry's)	1/2 cup	203	4.7	27.0	1768	>.4 c	1.2	na
GARLIC *(Kraft)*	2 tbsp	40	0.0	9.0	420	na	0.0	0
HAWAIIAN STYLE								
(Heinz)	1 tbsp	19	0.2	4.4	108	>.1 c	0.1	na
(Heinz) 'Thick and Rich'	1 oz	40	0.0	10.0	210	na	0.0	0
HICKORY								
(Healthy Choice)	1.1 oz	26	0.4	5.6	229	.5	0.2	0
(Heinz) 'Select'	1 oz	35	0.0	8.0	260	na	0.0	0
(Hunt's)	1 tbsp	20	<1.0	5.0	160	<1.0	<1.0	0
(Hunt's) bold	1.2 oz	46	0.4	10.6	283	.6	0.4	0
(Hunt's) 'Light'	1.1 oz	27	0.5	6.2	245	.7	0.2	0
(Open Range)	1.2 oz	37	0.5	8.6	423	1.0	0.2	0
HICKORY SMOKE								
(Heinz)	1 tbsp	19	0.3	4.4	56	>.1 c	0.1	na
(Heinz) 'Thick and Rich'	1 oz	35	0.0	8.0	380	na	0.0	0
(Heinz) 'Thick and Rich'	1 tbsp	20	0.0	5.0	220	na	0.0	0
(Kraft)	2 tbsp	45	0.0	10.0	440	na	1.0	0
(Kraft) 'Thick 'n Spicy'	2 tbsp	50	0.0	12.0	430	na	1.0	0
(Kraft) w/onion bits	2 tbsp	50	0.0	11.0	340	na	1.0	0
HOMESTYLE *(Hunt's)*	1.2 oz	41	0.5	9.8	381	.5	0.1	0

Food Name	Serv. Size	Total Cal.	Prot. GMS	Carbs GMS	Sod. MGS	Fiber GMS	Fat GMS	Chol. MGS
HONEY								
(Hain)	1 tbsp	14	0.0	1.0	120	na	1.0	0
(Kraft) 'Thick 'n Spicy'	2 tbsp	60	0.0	13.0	340	na	1.0	0
HONEY MUSTARD (Hunt's)	1.2 oz	48	0.4	11.5	450	.6	0.2	0
HOT								
(Healthy Choice) and spicy	1.1 oz	25	0.3	5.7	229	.5	0.2	0
(Heinz) 'Thick and Rich'	1 tbsp	20	0.0	5.0	220	na	0.0	0
(Hunt's) and spicy	1.2 oz	48	0.4	11.5	450	.6	0.2	0
(Kraft)	2 tbsp	45	0.0	9.0	520	na	1.0	0
(Kraft) hickory smoke	2 tbsp	45	0.0	9.0	360	na	1.0	0
ITALIAN SEASONING (Kraft)	2 tbsp	50	0.0	10.0	280	na	1.0	0
KANSAS CITY STYLE								
(Hunt's)	1.2 oz	43	0.4	10.0	220	.6	0.2	0
(Kraft)	2 tbsp	50	0.0	11.0	270	na	1.0	0
(Kraft) 'Thick 'n Spicy'	2 tbsp	60	0.0	13.0	270	na	1.0	0
MESQUITE SMOKE								
(Enrico's)	1 tbsp	18	1.0	3.0	4	na	1.0	0
(Heinz) 'Thick and Rich'	1 oz	30	0.0	7.0	380	na	0.0	0
(Hunt's)	2 tbsp	40	<1.0	9.0	360	<1.0	0.0	0
(Kraft)	2 tbsp	45	0.0	10.0	410	na	1.0	0
(Kraft) 'Thick 'n Spicy'	2 tbsp	50	0.0	12.0	430	na	1.0	0
MUSHROOM								
(Heinz)	1 tbsp	14	0.3	3.2	219	>.1 c	0.1	na
(Heinz) 'Thick and Rich'	1 oz	30	1.0	6.0	460	na	0.0	0
NEW ORLEANS STYLE (Hunt's)	1.2 oz	41	0.5	9.4	383	.7	0.2	0
ONION								
(Heinz)	1 tbsp	15	0.3	3.4	255	>.1 c	0.1	na
(Heinz) 'Thick and Rich'	1 oz	30	0.0	7.0	420	na	0.0	0
(Kraft) w/onion bits	2 tbsp	50	0.0	11.0	340	na	1.0	0
ORANGE JUICE, 'California Grill' (Lawry's)	1/4 cup	34	3.8	3.4	3846	>.1 c	0.7	na
ORIENTAL (LaChoy)	1 tbsp	16	0.7	3.8	304	<1.0	<.1	0
SALSA STYLE (Kraft)	2 tbsp	45	0.0	9.0	420	0	0.0	0
SLOPPY JOE, w/beef (Libby's)	1/3 cup	110	5.0	7.0	190	na	7.0	(mq)
SMOKY								
(Cattleman's)	1 tbsp	25	0.0	5.0	300	na	0.0	0
(Maull's)	1 tbsp	20	<1.0	4.0	139	>.7 c	<1.0	<1
(Ott's)	1 tbsp	14	0.2	3.3	149	.1	0.1	<1
SOUTHERN STYLE (Hunt's)	1 tbsp	20	<1.0	5.0	170	<1.0	<1.0	0
TEXAS STYLE								
(Heinz) hot 'Thick and Rich'	1 oz	30	0.0	7.0	390	na	0.0	0
(Hunt's)	1 tbsp	25	<1.0	6.0	150	<1.0	<1.0	0
WESTERN STYLE (Hunt's)	1 tbsp	20	<1.0	5.0	170	<1.0	<1.0	0
BARBECUE SPICE (Tone's)	1 tsp	9	0.3	1.4	713	.3	0.4	0

Food Name	Serv. Size	Total Cal.	Prot. GMS	Carbs GMS	Sod. MGS	Fiber GMS	Fat GMS	Chol. MGS
BARLEY								
....	1 cup	651	23.0	135.2	22	31.8	4.2	0
flakes (Arrowhead Mills)	2 oz	200	5.0	45.0	1	7.2	1.0	0
pearled, cooked	1 cup	193	3.5	44.3	5	6.0	0.7	0
pearled, cooked	4 oz	139	2.6	32.0	1	4.5	0.5	0
pearled, raw	1 cup	704	19.8	155.4	18	31.2	2.3	0
pearled, raw	1 oz	100	2.8	22.0	3	4.4	0.3	0
pearled, raw (Arrowhead Mills)	2 oz	200	5.0	45.0	1	7.2	1.0	0
pearled, raw, medium 'Scotch Brand' 1.7 oz (Quaker)	1/4 cup	172	5.0	36.3	0	5.0	0.5	0
pearled, raw, quick 'Scotch Brand' (Quaker)	1/3 cup	172	5.5	36.3	0	5.0	0.5	0
raw	1 oz	100	3.5	20.8	3	4.9	0.7	0
BARLEY FLOUR (Arrowhead Mills)	2 oz	200	7.0	35.0	1	7.2	1.0	0
BARRACUDA, PACIFIC								
raw	1 lb	426	89.4	0.0	(mq)	0	5.0	(mq)
raw	100 gm	113	21.0	0.0	40	0	2.6	55
raw	1 oz	27	5.6	0.0	(mq)	0	0.3	(mq)
BASELLA. See VINE SPINACH.								
BASIL								
dried (Golden Dipt)	2 grams	8	0.0	1.0	36	na	0.0	0
dried, crumbled	1 oz	71	4.1	17.3	10	>5.0 c	1.1	0
dried, crumbled	1 tbsp	11	0.7	2.7	2	.8	0.2	0
dried, crumbled (Spice Islands)	1 tsp	3	0.1	0.7	<1	>.2 c	<.1	0
dried, ground (Durkee)	1 tsp	5	0.0	0.0	0	0	tr	na
dried, ground (Laurel Leaf)	1 tsp	5	0.0	0.0	0	0	tr	na
fresh	2 tbsp	1	0.1	0.2	0	na	0.0	0
fresh	5 leaves	1	0.1	0.1	0	na	0.0	0
BASS, FRESHWATER, MIXED SPECIES								
dry-heat cooked	3 oz	124	20.6	0.0	77	0	4.0	74
raw	1 lb	516	85.5	0.0	317	0	16.7	308
raw	3 oz	97	16.0	0.0	59	0	3.1	58
raw	1 oz	32	5.3	0.0	20	0	1.0	19
BASS, SEA, MIXED SPECIES								
baked	4 oz	141	26.8	0.0	99	0	2.9	60
broiled	4 oz	141	26.8	0.0	99	0	2.9	60
dry-heat cooked	3 oz	105	20.1	0.0	74	0	2.2	45
microwaved	4 oz	141	26.8	0.0	99	0	2.9	60
raw	1 lb	439	83.6	0.0	308	0	9.1	186
raw	3 oz	82	15.7	0.0	58	0	1.7	35
raw	1 oz	27	5.2	0.0	19	0	0.6	12
BASS, STRIPED								
dry-heat cooked	3 oz	105	19.3	0.0	75	0	2.5	88

Food Name	Serv. Size	Total Cal.	Prot. GMS	Carbs GMS	Sod. MGS	Fiber GMS	Fat GMS	Chol. MGS
raw	1 lb	439	80.4	0.0	313	0	10.6	363
raw	3 oz	82	15.1	0.0	59	0	2.0	68
raw	1 oz	27	5.0	0.0	23	0	0.7	23
BATTER MIX								
beer, dry mix *(Golden Dipt)*	1 oz	100	2.0	22.0	650	na	0.0	0
corn dog, dry mix *(Golden Dipt)*	1 oz	100	3.0	22.0	490	(mq)	0.0	0
fish and chips, dry mix *(Golden Dipt)*	1.25 oz	120	2.0	27.0	910	(mq)	0.0	0
onion ring, dry mix *(Golden Dipt)*	1 oz	100	2.0	22.0	570	(mq)	0.0	0
original, dry mix *(Golden Dipt)*	1 oz	100	3.0	21.0	740	(mq)	0.0	0
tempura, dry mix *(Golden Dipt)*	1 oz	100	3.0	22.0	130	(mq)	0.0	0
BAY LEAF								
dried, crumbled	1 oz	89	2.2	21.3	7	>7.4 c	2.4	0
dried, crumbled	1 tbsp	6	0.1	1.4	0	.5	0.2	0
dried, crumbled	1 tsp	2	0.1	0.5	0	.2	0.1	0
dried, crumbled *(Durkee)*	1 tsp	2	0.0	0.0	0	0	tr	na
dried, crumbled *(Laurel Leaf)*	1 tsp	2	0.0	0.0	0	0	tr	na
dried, crumbled *(Spice Islands)*	1 tsp	5	0.1	0.3	<1	>.3 c	0.1	0
BEAN. See individual listings.								
BEAN DINNER, W/FRANKFURTERS, FROZEN								
(Banquet)	10 oz	520	17.0	57.0	1230	(mq)	25.0	35
(Morton)	10 oz	350	11.0	46.0	1490	(mq)	13.0	30
(Swanson)	10.5 oz	440	14.0	53.0	900	(mq)	19.0	(mq)
BEAN ENTRÉE, MICROWAVE								
w/frankfurters, in sauce, 'Diner' micro cup								
(Libby's)	7.75 oz	330	15.0	38.0	930	4.3	15.0	55
w/wieners, microwave cup								
(Kid's Kitchen)	7.5 oz	310	13.0	36.0	750	na	13.0	45
BEAN MIX								
Cajun, w/sauce, dry *(Lipton)*	1/4 pkg	130	5.0	28.0	400	(mq)	<1.0	na
Cajun, w/sauce, prepared *(Lipton)*	1/2 cup	160	5.0	28.0	440	(mq)	3.0	(mq)
chicken and sauce, dry *(Lipton)*	1/4 pkg	120	6.0	26.0	470	(mq)	1.0	na
chicken and sauce, prepared *(Lipton)*	1/2 cup	150	6.0	26.0	500	(mq)	4.0	(mq)
'Kettle Creations' bean medley with pasta, dry *(Lipton)*	1/4 cup	130	6.0	23.0	690	4.0	1.5	0
BEAN SALAD, CANNED								
four-bean *(Joan of Arc)*	1/2 cup	100	3.0	23.0	660	3.3	1.0	0
four-bean *(Read)*	1/2 cup	100	3.0	23.0	660	3.3	1.0	0
green bean, German-style *(Joan of Arc)*	1 cup	180	3.0	27.0	920	3.6	7.0	na
green bean, German-style *(Read)*	1 cup	180	3.0	27.0	920	3.6	7.0	na
three-bean *(Joan of Arc)*	1/2 cup	90	2.0	22.0	710	3.0	0.0	0
three-bean *(Read)*	1/2 cup	90	2.0	22.0	710	3.0	0.0	0
'Three Bean Salad' *(Green Giant)*	1/2 cup	70	2.0	18.0	470	3.0	<1.0	0

Food Name	Serv. Size	Total Cal.	Prot. GMS	Carbs GMS	Sod. MGS	Fiber GMS	Fat GMS	Chol. MGS
BEAN SPROUTS, CANNED								
(LaChoy)	2 oz	6	0.7	1.4	17	.7	0.1	0
(LaChoy)	2.928 oz	12	1.1	2.2	20	1.1	0.1	0
BEANS, BAKED. See BAKED BEANS, CANNED.								
BEANS, CANNED. See also BAKED BEANS, CANNED; BEAN SPROUTS, CANNED;								
BEAN SALAD, CANNED; and individual listings.								
barbecue (Open Range)	4.75 oz	185	7.1	36.4	687	7.9	3.3	1
'Beans 'N Fixins' (Big John's)	4.7 oz	127	7.1	22.6	590	6.0	3.5	3
'Big John's Beans 'n Fixin's' (Hunt's)	4 oz	170	5.0	26.0	490	6.0	6.0	6
'Mexe-Beans' (Old El Paso)	1/2 cup	163	10.0	31.0	627	13.0	1.0	0
'Mix and Serve' (Hunt's)	4.75 oz	125	1.8	30.3	575	7.8	2.8	1
mixed (Bush's Best)	1/2 cup	70	6.0	17.0	410	6.0	0.0	na
'Pork and Beans' (Hunt's)	4.5 oz	130	6.2	27.5	516	4.3	1.2	0
'Pork and Beans' (Open Range)	4.6 oz	157	6.1	26.8	621	7.4	4.8	2
ranch (Open Ranch)	4.7 oz	124	6.2	22.7	628	8.3	3.2	1
spiced (Gebhardt)	4.5 oz	100	7.2	19.3	654	7.6	1.6	0
vegetarian, 'Deluxe' (Bush's Best)	4 oz	110	5.0	25.0	350	6.0	0.0	na
'Vegetarian Style' (Van Camp's)	1 cup	206	10.9	42.0	950	na	0.6	na
w/beef, 'Homestyle' (Hunt's)	9 oz	246	16.1	30.6	944	11.9	6.5	16
w/franks, 'Homestyle' (Hunt's)	9 oz	319	16.5	41.0	735	12.5	9.9	23
w/sausage, 'Homestyle' (Hunt's)	9 oz	306	18.7	35.7	567	11.6	9.8	18
BEARNAISE. See SAUCE.								
BEECHNUT, DRIED								
in shell	1 lb	1595	17.2	92.7	(mq)	>10.2 c	138.4	0
shelled	1 oz	164	1.8	9.5	11	>1.0 c	14.2	0
BEEF								
(NOTE: TRIMMED = Lean; separable fat removed after cooking. UNTRIMMED =								
Separable fat not removed.)								
BRAIN								
pan-fried	3 oz	167	10.7	0.0	134	0	13.5	1696
raw	4 oz	142	11.1	0.0	116	0	10.5	1889
simmered	4 oz	181	12.6	0.0	136	0	14.2	2329
BRISKET, FLAT HALF								
Trimmed								
all grades, 0-inch fat, braised	4 oz	217	35.7	0.0	71	0	7.0	108
all grades, 0-inch fat, braised	3 oz	162	26.8	0.0	54	0	5.3	81
all grades, 1/4-inch fat, braised	3 oz	189	26.8	0.0	54	0	8.2	81
all grades, 1/2-inch fat, braised	3 oz	180	26.8	0.0	54	0	7.3	81
Untrimmed								
all grades, 0-inch fat, braised	4 oz	244	34.6	0.0	70	0	10.7	108
all grades, 1/4-inch fat, braised	11.5 oz	1189	81.2	0.0	183	0	93.1	310
all grades, 1/4-inch fat, braised	3 oz	309	21.3	0.0	48	0	24.2	81
all grades, 1/4-inch fat, raw	4 oz	328	20.2	0.0	70	0	26.7	79

Food Name	Serv. Size	Total Cal.	Prot. GMS	Carbs GMS	Sod. MGS	Fiber GMS	Fat GMS	Chol. MGS
all grades, 1/2-inch fat, braised	3 oz	311	21.0	0.0	48	0	24.6	81
all grades, 1/2-inch fat, raw	1 lb	1338	79.5	0.0	277	0	110.7	322
all grades, 1/2-inch fat, raw	1 oz	84	5.0	0.0	17	0	6.9	20

BRISKET, POINT HALF
Trimmed

Food Name	Serv. Size	Total Cal.	Prot. GMS	Carbs GMS	Sod. MGS	Fiber GMS	Fat GMS	Chol. MGS
all grades, 0-inch fat, braised	4 oz	277	31.8	0.0	87	0	15.6	103
all grades, 0-inch fat, braised	3 oz	207	23.8	0.0	65	0	11.7	77
all grades, 1/4-inch fat, braised	3 oz	222	23.8	0.0	65	0	13.3	77
all grades, 1/2-inch fat, braised	3 oz	224	23.8	0.0	65	0	13.5	77
all grades, 1-inch fat, braised	4 oz	296	31.8	0.0	87	0	17.8	103

Untrimmed

Food Name	Serv. Size	Total Cal.	Prot. GMS	Carbs GMS	Sod. MGS	Fiber GMS	Fat GMS	Chol. MGS
all grades, 0-inch fat, braised	3 oz	304	20.0	0.0	58	0	24.2	78
all grades, 1/4-inch fat, braised	3 oz	343	18.8	0.0	55	0	29.1	78
all grades, 1/4-inch fat, raw	1 lb	1501	73.1	0.0	295	0	131.9	345
all grades, 1/4-inch fat, raw	1 oz	94	4.6	0.0	18	0	8.3	22
all grades, 1/2-inch fat, braised	3 oz	347	18.7	0.0	55	0	29.6	78
all grades, 1/2-inch fat, raw	1 lb	1601	71.5	0.0	290	0	143.5	345
all grades, 1/2-inch fat, raw	1 oz	100	4.5	0.0	18	0	9.0	22

BRISKET, WHOLE
Trimmed

Food Name	Serv. Size	Total Cal.	Prot. GMS	Carbs GMS	Sod. MGS	Fiber GMS	Fat GMS	Chol. MGS
all grades, 0-inch fat, braised	4 oz	247	33.7	0.0	79	0	11.4	105
all grades, 0-inch fat, braised	3 oz	185	25.3	0.0	59	0	8.6	79
all grades, 1/4-inch fat, braised	4 oz	274	33.7	0.0	79	0	14.5	105
all grades, 1/4-inch fat, braised	3 oz	206	25.3	0.0	59	0	10.9	79
all grades, 1/2-inch fat, braised	3 oz	205	25.0	0.0	61	0	10.9	79

Untrimmed

Food Name	Serv. Size	Total Cal.	Prot. GMS	Carbs GMS	Sod. MGS	Fiber GMS	Fat GMS	Chol. MGS
all grades, 0-inch fat, braised	3 oz	247	22.8	0.0	55	0	16.6	79
all grades, 1/4-inch fat, braised	3 oz	327	20.0	0.0	52	0	26.8	80
all grades, 1/4-inch fat, raw	1 lb	1415	76.8	0.0	290	0	120.4	331
all grades, 1/4-inch fat, raw	1 oz	88	4.8	0.0	18	0	7.5	21
all grades, 1/2-inch fat, braised	3 oz	332	19.5	0.0	52	0	27.6	79
all grades, 1/2-inch fat, raw	1 lb	1474	75.4	0.0	281	0	127.7	336
all grades, 1/2-inch fat, raw	1 oz	92	4.7	0.0	18	0	8.0	21

CHUCK, ARM POT ROAST
Trimmed

Food Name	Serv. Size	Total Cal.	Prot. GMS	Carbs GMS	Sod. MGS	Fiber GMS	Fat GMS	Chol. MGS
all grades, 0-inch fat, braised	3 oz	178	28.1	0.0	56	0	6.5	86
all grades, 1/4-inch fat, braised	3 oz	184	28.1	0.0	56	0	7.1	86
all grades, 1/2-inch fat, braised	3 oz	196	28.1	0.0	56	0	8.5	86
choice, 0-inch fat, braised	3 oz	186	28.1	0.0	56	0	7.4	86
choice, 1/4-inch fat, braised	3 oz	191	28.1	0.0	56	0	7.9	86
choice, 1/2-inch fat, braised	3 oz	199	28.1	0.0	56	0	8.8	86
prime, 1/2-inch fat, braised	3 oz	222	28.1	0.0	56	0	11.4	86
prime, 1/2-inch fat, raw	1 lb	699	96.4	0.0	304	0	31.6	272

Food Name	Serv. Size	Total Cal.	Prot. GMS	Carbs GMS	Sod. MGS	Fiber GMS	Fat GMS	Chol. MGS
prime, 1/2-inch fat, raw	1 oz	44	6.0	0.0	19	0	2.0	17
select, 0-inch fat, braised	3 oz	168	28.1	0.0	56	0	5.3	86
select, 1/4-inch fat, braised	3 oz	175	28.1	0.0	56	0	6.1	86
select, 1/2-inch fat, braised	3 oz	189	28.1	0.0	56	0	7.6	86
Untrimmed								
all grades, 0-inch fat, braised	3 oz	238	25.2	0.0	53	0	14.5	85
all grades, 1/4-inch fat, braised	3 oz	282	23.3	0.0	51	0	20.2	84
all grades, 1/4-inch fat, raw	1 lb	1111	84.0	0.0	268	0	83.3	308
all grades, 1/4-inch fat, raw	1 oz	69	5.3	0.0	17	0	5.2	19
all grades, 1/2-inch fat, braised	3 oz	297	23.0	0.0	51	0	22.1	84
all grades, 1/2-inch fat, raw	1 lb	1166	83.1	0.0	268	0	89.8	313
all grades, 1/2-inch fat, raw	1 oz	73	5.2	0.0	17	0	5.6	20
choice, 0-inch fat, braised	3 oz	249	25.0	0.0	53	0	15.8	85
choice, 1/4-inch fat, braised	3 oz	296	22.9	0.0	50	0	21.9	84
choice, 1/4-inch fat, raw	1 lb	1157	83.4	0.0	268	0	88.8	313
choice, 1/4-inch fat, raw	1 oz	72	5.2	0.0	17	0	5.6	20
choice, 1/2-inch fat, braised	3 oz	301	22.9	0.0	50	0	22.5	84
choice, 1/2-inch fat, raw	1 lb	1188	82.6	0.0	263	0	92.9	313
choice, 1/2-inch fat, raw	1 oz	74	5.2	0.0	16	0	5.8	20
prime, 1/2-inch fat, braised	3 oz	332	22.2	0.0	49	0	26.3	84
prime, 1/2-inch fat, raw	1 lb	1334	80.5	0.0	259	0	109.6	318
prime, 1/2-inch fat, raw	1 oz	83	5.0	0.0	16	0	6.8	20
select, 0-inch fat, braised	3 oz	221	25.6	0.0	54	0	12.4	85
select, 1/4-inch fat, braised	3 oz	268	23.7	0.0	51	0	18.5	85
select, 1/4-inch fat, raw	1 lb	1061	84.6	0.0	268	0	77.4	308
select, 1/4-inch fat, raw	1 oz	66	5.3	0.0	17	0	4.8	19
select, 1/2-inch fat, braised	3 oz	286	23.3	0.0	51	0	20.8	84
select, 1/2-inch fat, raw	1 lb	1075	84.8	0.0	272	0	79.2	308
select, 1/2-inch fat, raw	1 oz	67	5.3	0.0	17	0	4.9	19
CHUCK, BLADE ROAST								
Trimmed								
all grades, 0-inch fat, braised	3 oz	215	26.4	0.0	60	0	11.3	90
all grades, 1/4-inch fat, braised	3 oz	213	26.4	0.0	60	0	11.1	90
all grades, 1/2-inch fat, braised	3 oz	229	26.4	0.0	60	0	13.0	90
choice, 0-inch fat, braised	3 oz	225	26.4	0.0	60	0	12.5	90
choice, 1/4-inch fat, braised	3 oz	224	26.4	0.0	60	0	12.2	90
choice, 1/2-inch fat, braised	3 oz	234	26.4	0.0	60	0	13.4	90
prime, 1/2-inch fat, braised	3 oz	270	26.4	0.0	60	0	17.5	90
prime, 1/2-inch fat, raw	1 lb	921	87.3	0.0	349	0	60.8	295
prime, 1/2-inch fat, raw	1 oz	58	5.5	0.0	22	0	3.8	18
select, 0-inch fat, braised	3 oz	202	26.4	0.0	60	0	9.9	90
select, 1/4-inch fat, braised	3 oz	201	26.4	0.0	60	0	9.9	90
select, 1/2-inch fat, braised	3 oz	218	26.4	0.0	60	0	11.6	90

Food Name	Serv. Size	Total Cal.	Prot. GMS	Carbs GMS	Sod. MGS	Fiber GMS	Fat GMS	Chol. MGS
Untrimmed								
all grades, 0-inch fat, braised	3 oz	284	23.1	0.0	55	0	20.5	88
all grades, 1/4-inch fat, braised	3 oz	293	22.6	0.0	54	0	21.8	88
all grades, 1/4-inch fat, raw	1 lb	1152	77.3	0.0	304	0	91.2	327
all grades, 1/4-inch fat, raw	1 oz	72	4.8	0.0	19	0	5.7	20
all grades, 1/2-inch fat, braised	3 oz	326	21.6	0.0	54	0	25.8	88
all grades, 1/2-inch fat, raw	1 lb	1288	75.6	0.0	299	0	107.0	331
all grades, 1/2-inch fat, raw	1 oz	81	4.7	0.0	19	0	6.7	21
choice, 0-inch fat, braised	3 oz	296	22.9	0.0	55	0	22.0	88
choice, 1/4-inch fat, braised	3 oz	309	22.2	0.0	54	0	23.6	88
choice, 1/4-inch fat, raw	1 lb	1234	76.3	0.0	299	0	100.8	327
choice, 1/4-inch fat, raw	1 oz	77	4.8	0.0	19	0	6.3	20
choice, 1/2-inch fat, braised	3 oz	330	21.6	0.0	54	0	26.4	88
choice, 1/2-inch fat, raw	1 lb	1320	75.2	0.0	295	0	110.7	331
choice, 1/2-inch fat, raw	1 oz	83	4.7	0.0	18	0	6.9	21
prime, 1/2-inch fat, braised	3 oz	354	21.7	0.0	54	0	29.0	88
prime, 1/2-inch fat, raw	1 lb	1488	74.1	0.0	290	0	129.6	336
prime, 1/2-inch fat, raw	1 oz	93	4.6	0.0	18	0	8.1	21
select, 0-inch fat, braised	3 oz	266	23.5	0.0	56	0	18.4	88
select, 1/4-inch fat, braised	3 oz	277	22.9	0.0	55	0	19.9	88
select, 1/4-inch fat, raw	1 lb	1066	78.3	0.0	308	0	81.3	322
select, 1/4-inch fat, raw	1 oz	67	4.9	0.0	19	0	5.1	20
select, 1/2-inch fat, braised	3 oz	311	21.9	0.0	54	0	24.1	88
select, 1/2-inch fat, raw	1 lb	1179	76.9	0.0	304	0	94.4	327
select, 1/2-inch fat, raw	1 oz	74	4.8	0.0	19	0	5.9	20
FLANK								
Trimmed								
choice, 0-inch fat, braised	3 oz	201	23.8	0.0	61	0	11.0	60
choice, 0-inch fat, broiled	3 oz	176	23.0	0.0	71	0	8.6	57
Untrimmed								
choice, 0-inch fat, braised	3 oz	224	22.9	0.0	59	0	14.0	61
choice, 0-inch fat, broiled	3 oz	192	22.5	0.0	69	0	10.6	58
choice, 0-inch fat, raw	1 oz	51	5.6	0.0	20	0	3.0	15
choice, 0-inch fat, raw	4 oz	203	22.3	0.0	80	0	12.0	59
HEART								
raw	4 oz	132	19.3	2.9	71	0	4.3	158
simmered	3 oz	149	24.5	0.4	54	0	4.8	164
KIDNEY								
raw	4 oz	121	18.8	2.5	202	0	3.5	322
simmered	3 oz	122	21.7	0.8	114	0	2.9	329
LEAN CUTS								
bottom round steak, 'Lite' *(Heritage Lifestyle)*								
uncooked	3 oz	108	19.0	0.0	40	na	4.0	50

Food Name	Serv. Size	Total Cal.	Prot. GMS	Carbs GMS	Sod. MGS	Fiber GMS	Fat GMS	Chol. MGS
(Brae Beef) raw	4 oz	120	26.0	0.0	60	0	2.0	57
brisket 'Lite' (Heritage Lifestyle) uncooked	3 oz	98	18.0	0.0	40	na	3.0	48
burger (Lean and Free) raw	4 oz	174	22.5	0.0	64	0	9.3	77
chuck, arm pot roast, 'Lite' (Heritage Lifestyle) uncooked	3 oz	101	18.0	0.0	40	na	3.0	52
chuck blade roast, 'Lite' (Heritage Lifestyle) uncooked	3 oz	128	17.0	0.0	45	na	7.0	52
cube steak (Lean and Free) raw	4 oz	109	23.8	0.0	(mq)	0	1.0	61
eye round steak, 'Lite' (Heritage Lifestyle) uncooked	3 oz	111	19.0	0.0	38	na	4.0	41
ground, lean, 'Lite' (Heritage Lifestyle) uncooked	3 oz	118	18.0	0.0	45	na	5.0	54
lean cuts, raw (Lean and Free)	4 oz	161	21.5	0.0	(mq)	0	7.5	67
rib eye (Lean and Free) raw	4 oz	121	24.7	0.0	59	0	2.6	71
rib roast, large end, 'Lite' (Heritage Lifestyle) uncooked	3 oz	142	18.0	0.0	40	na	8.0	50
rib steak, small end, 'Lite' (Heritage Lifestyle) uncooked	3 oz	118	19.0	0.0	35	na	5.0	43
rolled (Lean and Free) raw	4 oz	125	25.4	0.0	60	0	2.8	(mq)
round steak (Lean and Free) raw	4 oz	111	25.7	0.0	60	0	1.1	(mq)
round tip roast, 'Lite' (Heritage Lifestyle) uncooked	3 oz	91	18.0	0.0	43	na	1.5	49
sirloin steak (Lean and Free) raw	4 oz	111	24.2	0.0	67	0	1.8	66
sirloin steak, 'Lite' (Heritage Lifestyle) uncooked	3 oz	103	18.0	0.0	45	na	3.0	49
sirloin tip (Lean and Free) raw	4 oz	110	23.2	0.0	62	0	1.2	66
strip loin steak (Lean and Free) raw	4 oz	113	25.2	0.0	61	0	1.8	67
T-bone (Lean and Free) raw	4 oz	125	25.5	0.0	54	0	2.7	(mq)
tenderloin fillet steak (Lean and Free) raw	4 oz	116	23.6	0.0	68	0	2.4	61
tenderloin steak, 'Lite' (Heritage Lifestyle) uncooked	3 oz	109	18.0	0.0	40	na	4.0	53
top loin steak, 'Lite' (Heritage Lifestyle) uncooked	3 oz	114	19.0	0.0	40	na	4.0	44
top round (Lean and Free) raw	4 oz	134	24.6	0.0	49	0	4.5	(mq)
top round steak, 'Lite' (Heritage Lifestyle) uncooked	3 oz	100	19.0	0.0	40	na	3.0	48
LIVER								
braised	3 oz	137	20.7	2.9	59	0	4.2	331
pan-fried	3 oz	184	22.7	6.7	90	0	6.8	410
pan-fried in vegetable oil	4 oz	246	30.3	8.9	120	0	9.1	547
raw	4 oz	162	22.6	6.6	82	0	4.3	400
LUNG								
braised	3 oz	102	17.3	0.0	86	0	3.2	235

Food Name	Serv. Size	Total Cal.	Prot. GMS	Carbs GMS	Sod. MGS	Fiber GMS	Fat GMS	Chol. MGS
raw	4 oz	104	18.3	0.0	224	0	2.8	273
PANCREAS								
braised	3 oz	230	23.0	0.0	51	0	14.6	223
raw	4 oz	266	17.7	0.0	76	0	21.0	232
PORTERHOUSE								
Trimmed								
choice, 1/4-inch fat, broiled	3 oz	185	23.9	0.0	56	0	9.2	68
choice, 1/2-inch fat, broiled	3 oz	185	23.9	0.0	56	0	9.2	68
Untrimmed								
choice, 1/4-inch fat, broiled	3 oz	259	21.1	0.0	52	0	18.8	71
choice, 1/4-inch fat, raw	1 lb	1229	80.2	0.0	222	0	98.4	313
choice, 1/4-inch fat, raw	1 oz	77	5.0	0.0	14	0	6.2	20
choice, 1/2-inch fat, broiled	3 oz	254	21.3	0.0	52	0	18.0	71
choice, 1/2-inch fat, raw	1 lb	1288	78.8	0.0	222	0	105.6	318
choice, 1/2-inch fat, raw	1 oz	81	4.9	0.0	14	0	6.6	20
RIB, LARGE END								
Trimmed								
all grades, ribs 6-9, 0-inch fat, roasted	3 oz	202	23.4	0.0	62	0	11.4	69
all grades, ribs 6-9, 1/4-inch fat, broiled	3 oz	190	21.4	0.0	61	0	11.0	65
all grades, ribs 6-9, 1/4-inch fat, roasted	3 oz	201	23.4	0.0	62	0	11.2	69
all grades, ribs 6-9, 1/2-inch fat, broiled	3 oz	198	20.9	0.0	59	0	12.1	70
all grades, ribs 6-9, 1/2-inch fat, roasted	3 oz	207	23.4	0.0	62	0	11.9	69
choice, ribs 6-9, 0-inch fat, roasted	3 oz	215	23.4	0.0	62	0	12.7	69
choice, ribs 6-9, 1/4-inch fat, broiled	3 oz	204	21.4	0.0	61	0	12.4	65
choice, ribs 6-9, 1/4-inch fat, roasted	3 oz	213	23.4	0.0	62	0	12.5	69
choice, ribs 6-9, 1/2-inch fat, broiled	3 oz	203	20.9	0.0	59	0	12.6	70
choice, ribs 6-9, 1/2-inch fat, roasted	3 oz	211	23.4	0.0	62	0	12.3	69
prime, ribs 6-9, 1/4-inch fat, broiled	3 oz	250	20.9	0.0	59	0	17.7	70
prime, ribs 6-9, 1/4-inch fat, roasted	3 oz	241	23.4	0.0	62	0	15.6	69
prime, ribs 6-9, 1/2-inch fat, broiled	3 oz	250	20.9	0.0	59	0	17.7	70
prime, ribs 6-9, 1/2-inch fat, roasted	3 oz	241	23.4	0.0	62	0	15.6	69
select, ribs 6-9, 0-inch fat, roasted	3 oz	187	23.4	0.0	62	0	9.7	69
select, ribs 6-9, 1/4-inch fat, broiled	3 oz	175	21.4	0.0	61	0	9.3	65
select, ribs 6-9, 1/4-inch fat, roasted	3 oz	187	23.4	0.0	62	0	9.7	69
select, ribs 6-9, 1/2-inch fat, broiled	3 oz	183	20.9	0.0	59	0	10.4	70
select, ribs 6-9, 1/2-inch fat, roasted	3 oz	197	23.4	0.0	62	0	10.8	69
Untrimmed								
all grades, ribs 6-9, 0-inch fat, roasted	3 oz	300	19.7	0.0	55	0	24.0	72
all grades, ribs 6-9, 1/4-inch fat, broiled	3 oz	295	18.1	0.0	54	0	24.2	69
all grades, ribs 6-9, 1/4-inch fat, raw	1 lb	1465	73.0	0.0	249	0	127.9	322
all grades, ribs 6-9, 1/4-inch fat, raw	1 oz	92	4.6	0.0	16	0	8.0	20
all grades, ribs 6-9, 1/4-inch fat, roasted	3 oz	310	19.2	0.0	54	0	25.3	72
all grades, ribs 6-9, 1/2-inch fat, broiled	3 oz	321	17.1	0.0	51	0	27.5	74

Food Name	Serv. Size	Total Cal.	Prot. GMS	Carbs GMS	Sod. MGS	Fiber GMS	Fat GMS	Chol. MGS
all grades, ribs 6-9, 1/2-inch fat, raw	1 lb	1588	70.6	0.0	240	0	142.3	331
all grades, ribs 6-9, 1/2-inch fat, raw	1 oz	99	4.4	0.0	15	0	8.9	21
all grades, ribs 6-9, 1/2-inch fat, roasted	3 oz	313	19.3	0.0	54	0	25.5	72
choice, ribs 6-9, 0-inch fat, roasted	10.2 oz	1080	66.1	0.0	186	0	88.4	246
choice, ribs 6-9, 0-inch fat, roasted	3 oz	316	19.4	0.0	54	0	25.9	72
choice, ribs 6-9, 1/4-inch fat, broiled	3 oz	312	17.8	0.0	54	0	26.2	69
choice, ribs 6-9, 1/4-inch fat, raw	1 lb	1565	71.4	0.0	240	0	139.8	331
choice, ribs 6-9, 1/4-inch fat, raw	1 oz	98	4.5	0.0	15	0	8.7	21
choice, ribs 6-9, 1/4-inch fat, roasted	3 oz	326	19.0	0.0	54	0	27.2	72
choice, ribs 6-9, 1/2-inch fat, broiled	3 oz	326	17.0	0.0	51	0	28.1	74
choice, ribs 6-9, 1/2-inch fat, raw	1 lb	1615	70.2	0.0	240	0	145.6	336
choice, ribs 6-9, 1/2-inch fat, raw	1 oz	101	4.4	0.0	15	0	9.1	21
choice, ribs 6-9, 1/2-inch fat, roasted	3 oz	316	19.3	0.0	54	0	25.9	72
prime, ribs 6-9, 1/4-inch fat, broiled	3 oz	351	17.3	0.0	52	0	30.8	73
prime, ribs 6-9, 1/4-inch fat, raw	1 lb	1710	70.4	0.0	240	0	156.5	331
prime, ribs 6-9, 1/4-inch fat, raw	1 oz	107	4.4	0.0	15	0	9.8	21
prime, ribs 6-9, 1/4-inch fat, roasted	3 oz	342	19.1	0.0	54	0	28.9	72
prime, ribs 6-9, 1/2-inch fat, broiled	3 oz	361	16.9	0.0	51	0	32.1	74
prime, ribs 6-9, 1/2-inch fat, raw	1 lb	1737	69.8	0.0	236	0	159.6	336
prime, ribs 6-9, 1/2-inch fat, raw	1 oz	109	4.4	0.0	15	0	10.0	21
prime, ribs 6-9, 1/2-inch fat, roasted	3 oz	346	18.9	0.0	54	0	29.4	72
select, ribs 6-9, 0-inch fat, roasted	3 oz	281	20.0	0.0	55	0	21.7	71
select, ribs 6-9, 1/4-inch fat, broiled	3 oz	275	18.3	0.0	54	0	21.9	68
select, ribs 6-9, 1/4-inch fat, raw	1 lb	1379	74.0	0.0	249	0	117.7	322
select, ribs 6-9, 1/4-inch fat, raw	1 oz	86	4.6	0.0	16	0	7.4	20
select, ribs 6-9, 1/4-inch fat, roasted	3 oz	289	19.7	0.0	55	0	22.7	72
select, ribs 6-9, 1/2-inch fat, broiled	3 oz	301	17.4	0.0	52	0	25.1	73
select, ribs 6-9, 1/2-inch fat, raw	1 lb	1488	72.0	0.0	245	0	130.7	327
select, ribs 6-9, 1/2-inch fat, raw	1 oz	93	4.5	0.0	15	0	8.2	20
select, ribs 6-9, 1/2-inch fat, roasted	3 oz	303	19.4	0.0	54	0	24.5	72

RIB, SHORTRIB

Trimmed, choice, braised .... 3 oz 251 26.1 0.0 49 0 15.4 79

Untrimmed

choice, braised	3 oz	400	18.3	0.0	43	0	35.7	80
choice, raw	1 lb	1760	65.3	0.0	222	0	164.3	345
choice, raw	1 oz	110	4.1	0.0	14	0	10.3	22

RIB, SMALL END

Trimmed

all grades, ribs 10-12, 0-inch fat, broiled	3 oz	181	23.8	0.0	59	0	8.8	68
all grades, ribs 10-12, 1/4-inch fat, roasted	3 oz	185	22.8	0.0	60	0	9.8	67
all grades, ribs 10-12, 1/2-inch fat, broiled	3 oz	188	23.8	0.0	59	0	9.5	68
all grades, ribs 10-12, 1/2-inch fat, roasted	3 oz	201	22.7	0.0	64	0	11.5	68
all grades, ribs 10-12, 1/4-inch fat, broiled	3 oz	188	23.8	0.0	59	0	9.5	68

Food Name	Serv. Size	Total Cal.	Prot. GMS	Carbs GMS	Sod. MGS	Fiber GMS	Fat GMS	Chol. MGS
choice, ribs 10-12, 0-inch fat, broiled	3 oz	191	23.8	0.0	59	0	9.9	68
choice, ribs 10-12, 1/4-inch fat, broiled	3 oz	198	23.8	0.0	59	0	10.7	68
choice, ribs 10-12, 1/4-inch fat, roasted	3 oz	197	22.8	0.0	60	0	11.1	67
choice, ribs 10-12, 1/2-inch fat, broiled	3 oz	191	23.8	0.0	59	0	9.9	68
choice, ribs 10-12, 1/2-inch fat, roasted	3 oz	207	22.7	0.0	64	0	12.1	68
prime, ribs 10-12, 1/4-inch fat, broiled	3 oz	221	23.8	0.0	59	0	13.2	68
prime, ribs 10-12, 1/4-inch fat, roasted	3 oz	258	22.7	0.0	64	0	17.9	68
prime, ribs 10-12, 1/2-inch fat, broiled	3 oz	221	23.8	0.0	59	0	13.2	68
prime, ribs 10-12, 1/2-inch fat, roasted	3 oz	258	22.7	0.0	64	0	17.9	68
select, ribs 10-12, 0-inch fat, broiled	3 oz	168	23.8	0.0	59	0	7.4	68
select, ribs 10-12, 1/4-inch fat, broiled	3 oz	176	23.8	0.0	59	0	8.2	68
select, ribs 10-12, 1/4-inch fat, roasted	3 oz	173	22.8	0.0	60	0	8.3	67
select, ribs 10-12, 1/2-inch fat, broiled	3 oz	178	23.8	0.0	59	0	8.4	68
select, ribs 10-12, 1/2-inch fat, roasted	3 oz	184	22.7	0.0	64	0	9.6	68
Untrimmed								
all grades, ribs 10-12, 0-inch fat, broiled	3 oz	252	21.2	0.0	54	0	17.9	71
all grades, ribs 10-12, 1/4-inch fat, broiled	3 oz	286	20.1	0.0	53	0	22.1	71
all grades, ribs 10-12, 1/4-inch fat, raw	1 lb	1352	76.2	0.0	240	0	113.9	318
all grades, ribs 10-12, 1/4-inch fat, raw	1 oz	84	4.8	0.0	15	0	7.1	20
all grades, ribs 10-12, 1/4-inch fat, roasted	3 oz	295	19.0	0.0	54	0	23.8	71
all grades, ribs 10-12, 1/2-inch fat, broiled	3 oz	277	20.4	0.0	53	0	21.1	71
all grades, ribs 10-12, 1/2-inch fat, raw	1 lb	1388	75.9	0.0	245	0	117.8	318
all grades, ribs 10-12, 1/2-inch fat, raw	1 oz	87	4.7	0.0	15	0	7.4	20
all grades, ribs 10-12, 1/2-inch fat, roasted	3 oz	305	18.9	0.0	55	0	24.9	72
choice, ribs 10-12, 0-inch fat, broiled	3 oz	265	21.0	0.0	54	0	19.4	71
choice, ribs 10-12, 1/4-inch fat, broiled	3 oz	297	20.0	0.0	53	0	23.5	71
choice, ribs 10-12, 1/4-inch fat, raw	1 lb	1429	75.1	0.0	240	0	122.8	322
choice, ribs 10-12, 1/4-inch fat, raw	1 oz	89	4.7	0.0	15	0	7.7	20
choice, ribs 10-12, 1/4-inch fat, roasted	3 oz	312	18.7	0.0	53	0	25.7	71
choice, ribs 10-12, 1/2-inch fat, broiled	3 oz	282	20.4	0.0	53	0	21.6	71
choice, ribs 10-12, 1/2-inch fat, raw	1 lb	1415	75.5	0.0	240	0	121.2	318
choice, ribs 10-12, 1/2-inch fat, raw	1 oz	88	4.7	0.0	15	0	7.6	20
choice, ribs 10-12, 1/2-inch fat, roasted	3 oz	312	18.8	0.0	55	0	25.7	72
prime, ribs 10-12, 1/4-inch fat, broiled	3 oz	307	20.3	0.0	53	0	24.4	71
prime, ribs 10-12, 1/4-inch fat, raw	1 lb	1551	75.1	0.0	240	0	136.4	322
prime, ribs 10-12, 1/4-inch fat, raw	1 oz	97	4.7	0.0	15	0	8.5	20
prime, ribs 10-12, 1/4-inch fat, roasted	3 oz	354	18.6	0.0	55	0	30.5	71
prime, ribs 10-12, 1/2-inch fat, broiled	3 oz	309	20.2	0.0	53	0	24.7	71
prime, ribs 10-12, 1/2-inch fat, raw	1 lb	1583	74.3	0.0	240	0	140.2	322
prime, ribs 10-12, 1/2-inch fat, raw	1 oz	99	4.7	0.0	15	0	8.8	20
prime, ribs 10-12, 1/2-inch fat, roasted	3 oz	357	18.5	0.0	54	0	30.8	72
select, ribs 10-12, 0-inch fat, broiled	3 oz	242	21.2	0.0	54	0	16.8	71
select, ribs 10-12, 1/4-inch fat, broiled	3 oz	273	20.3	0.0	53	0	20.6	71

Food Name	Serv. Size	Total Cal.	Prot. GMS	Carbs GMS	Sod. MGS	Fiber GMS	Fat GMS	Chol. MGS
select, ribs 10-12, 1/4-inch fat, raw	1 lb	1297	76.7	0.0	245	0	107.4	318
select, ribs 10-12, 1/4-inch fat, raw	1 oz	81	4.8	0.0	15	0	6.7	20
select, ribs 10-12, 1/4-inch fat, roasted	3 oz	281	19.1	0.0	54	0	22.2	71
select, ribs 10-12, 1/2-inch fat, broiled	3 oz	263	20.7	0.0	54	0	19.4	71
select, ribs 10-12, 1/2-inch fat, raw	1 lb	1288	77.2	0.0	245	0	106.4	313
select, ribs 10-12, 1/2-inch fat, raw	1 oz	81	4.8	0.0	15	0	6.7	20
select, ribs 10-12, 1/2-inch fat, roasted	3 oz	283	19.2	0.0	56	0	22.3	71

RIB, WHOLE
Trimmed

Food Name	Serv. Size	Total Cal.	Prot. GMS	Carbs GMS	Sod. MGS	Fiber GMS	Fat GMS	Chol. MGS
all grades, ribs 6-12, 1/4-inch fat, broiled	3 oz	190	22.4	0.0	60	0	10.4	65
all grades, ribs 6-12, 1/4-inch fat, roasted	3 oz	195	23.2	0.0	61	0	10.6	68
all grades, ribs 6-12, 1/2-inch fat, broiled	3 oz	194	22.1	0.0	59	0	11.0	70
all grades, ribs 6-12, 1/2-inch fat, roasted	3 oz	204	23.1	0.0	63	0	11.7	69
choice, ribs 6-12, 1/4-inch fat, broiled	3 oz	201	22.4	0.0	60	0	11.7	65
choice, ribs 6-12, 1/4-inch fat, roasted	3 oz	207	23.2	0.0	61	0	11.9	68
choice, ribs 6-12, 1/2-inch fat, broiled	3 oz	198	22.1	0.0	59	0	11.5	70
choice, ribs 6-12, 1/2-inch fat, roasted	3 oz	209	23.1	0.0	63	0	12.2	69
prime, ribs 6-12, 1/4-inch fat, broiled	3 oz	238	22.1	0.0	59	0	15.9	69
prime, ribs 6-12, 1/4-inch fat, roasted	3 oz	248	23.1	0.0	63	0	16.5	69
prime, ribs 6-12, 1/2-inch fat, broiled	3 oz	238	22.1	0.0	59	0	15.9	70
prime, ribs 6-12, 1/2-inch fat, roasted	3 oz	248	23.1	0.0	63	0	16.5	69
select, ribs 6-12, 1/4-inch fat, broiled	3 oz	175	22.4	0.0	60	0	8.9	65
select, ribs 6-12, 1/4-inch fat, roasted	3 oz	181	23.2	0.0	61	0	9.1	68
select, ribs 6-12, 1/2-inch fat, broiled	3 oz	181	22.1	0.0	59	0	9.6	70
select, ribs 6-12, 1/2-inch fat, roasted	3 oz	191	23.1	0.0	63	0	10.3	69

Untrimmed

Food Name	Serv. Size	Total Cal.	Prot. GMS	Carbs GMS	Sod. MGS	Fiber GMS	Fat GMS	Chol. MGS
all grades, ribs 6-12, 1/4-inch fat, broiled	3 oz	291	18.9	0.0	54	0	23.3	70
all grades, ribs 6-12, 1/4-inch fat, raw	1 lb	1420	74.3	0.0	245	0	122.4	322
all grades, ribs 6-12, 1/4-inch fat, raw	1 oz	89	4.6	0.0	15	0	7.7	20
all grades, ribs 6-12, 1/4-inch fat, roasted	3 oz	304	19.1	0.0	54	0	24.7	71
all grades, ribs 6-12, 1/2-inch fat, broiled	3 oz	308	18.3	0.0	52	0	25.5	73
all grades, ribs 6-12, 1/2-inch fat, raw	1 lb	1501	72.8	0.0	240	0	132.2	327
all grades, ribs 6-12, 1/2-inch fat, raw	1 oz	94	4.6	0.0	15	0	8.3	20
all grades, ribs 6-12, 1/2-inch fat, roasted	3 oz	324	18.6	0.0	54	0	27.0	72
choice, ribs 6-12, 1/4-inch fat, broiled	3 oz	306	18.7	0.0	53	0	25.1	70
choice, ribs 6-12, 1/4-inch fat, raw	1 lb	1510	72.9	0.0	240	0	133.2	327
choice, ribs 6-12, 1/4-inch fat, raw	1 oz	94	4.6	0.0	15	0	8.3	20
choice, ribs 6-12, 1/4-inch fat, roasted	3 oz	320	18.8	0.0	54	0	26.5	72
choice, ribs 6-12, 1/2-inch fat, broiled	3 oz	313	18.2	0.0	52	0	26.1	73
choice, ribs 6-12, 1/2-inch fat, raw	1 lb	1533	72.4	0.0	240	0	135.5	327
choice, ribs 6-12, 1/2-inch fat, raw	1 oz	96	4.5	0.0	15	0	8.5	20
choice, ribs 6-12, 1/2-inch fat, roasted	3 oz	328	18.6	0.0	54	0	27.6	72
prime, ribs 6-12, 1/4-inch fat, broiled	3 oz	333	18.5	0.0	53	0	28.2	72

Food Name	Serv. Size	Total Cal.	Prot. GMS	Carbs GMS	Sod. MGS	Fiber GMS	Fat GMS	Chol. MGS
prime, ribs 6-12, 1/4-inch fat, raw	1 lb	1651	72.2	0.0	240	0	149.0	331
prime, ribs 6-12, 1/4-inch fat, raw	1 oz	103	4.5	0.0	15	0	9.3	21
prime, ribs 6-12, 1/4-inch fat, roasted	3 oz	348	18.9	0.0	54	0	29.6	72
prime, ribs 6-12, 1/2-inch fat, broiled	3 oz	347	17.9	0.0	51	0	29.9	73
prime, ribs 6-12, 1/2-inch fat, raw	1 lb	1678	71.4	0.0	236	0	152.4	331
prime, ribs 6-12, 1/2-inch fat, raw	1 oz	105	4.5	0.0	15	0	9.5	21
prime, ribs 6-12, 1/2-inch fat, roasted	3 oz	361	18.3	0.0	54	0	31.4	73
select, ribs 6-12, 1/4-inch fat, broiled	3 oz	275	19.1	0.0	54	0	21.4	70
select, ribs 6-12, 1/4-inch fat, raw	1 lb	1347	75.1	0.0	249	0	113.7	318
select, ribs 6-12, 1/4-inch fat, raw	1 oz	84	4.7	0.0	16	0	7.1	20
select, ribs 6-12, 1/4-inch fat, roasted	3 oz	286	19.4	0.0	54	0	22.5	71
select, ribs 6-12, 1/2-inch fat, broiled	3 oz	289	18.6	0.0	52	0	23.3	72
select, ribs 6-12, 1/2-inch fat, raw	1 lb	1411	74.0	0.0	245	0	121.2	322
select, ribs 6-12, 1/2-inch fat, raw	1 oz	88	4.6	0.0	15	0	7.6	20
select, ribs 6-12, 1/2-inch fat, roasted	3 oz	306	19.0	0.0	54	0	24.9	72

RIB EYE, SMALL END
Trimmed

Food Name	Serv. Size	Total Cal.	Prot. GMS	Carbs GMS	Sod. MGS	Fiber GMS	Fat GMS	Chol. MGS
choice, ribs 10-12, 0-inch fat, broiled	3 oz	191	23.8	0.0	59	0	9.9	68
choice, ribs 10-12, 1/4-inch fat, broiled	4 oz	255	31.8	0.0	78	0	13.3	91

Untrimmed

Food Name	Serv. Size	Total Cal.	Prot. GMS	Carbs GMS	Sod. MGS	Fiber GMS	Fat GMS	Chol. MGS
choice, ribs 10-12, 0-inch fat, broiled	3 oz	261	21.2	0.0	54	0	18.9	71
choice, ribs 10-12, 0-inch fat, raw	1 lb	1243	79.4	0.0	254	0	100.1	308
choice, ribs 10-12, 0-inch fat, raw	1 oz	78	5.0	0.0	16	0	6.3	19

ROUND, BOTTOM
Trimmed

Food Name	Serv. Size	Total Cal.	Prot. GMS	Carbs GMS	Sod. MGS	Fiber GMS	Fat GMS	Chol. MGS
all grades, 0-inch fat, braised	3 oz	173	26.9	0.0	43	0	6.5	82
all grades, 0-inch fat, roasted	3 oz	156	24.4	0.0	56	0	5.7	66
all grades, 1/4-inch fat, braised	3 oz	178	26.9	0.0	43	0	7.0	82
all grades, 1/4-inch fat, roasted	3 oz	161	24.4	0.0	56	0	6.3	66
all grades, 1/2-inch fat, braised	3 oz	189	26.9	0.0	43	0	8.2	82
choice, 0-inch fat, braised	3 oz	181	26.9	0.0	43	0	7.4	82
choice, 0-inch fat, roasted	3 oz	164	24.4	0.0	56	0	6.6	66
choice, 1/4-inch fat, braised	3 oz	187	26.9	0.0	43	0	8.0	82
choice, 1/4-inch fat, roasted	3 oz	168	24.4	0.0	56	0	7.1	66
choice, 1/2-inch fat, braised	3 oz	191	26.9	0.0	43	0	8.5	82
prime, 1/2-inch fat, braised	3 oz	212	26.9	0.0	43	0	10.8	82
prime, 1/2-inch fat, raw	1 lb	721	99.2	0.0	268	0	33.1	268
prime, 1/2-inch fat, raw	1 oz	45	6.2	0.0	17	0	2.1	17
select, 0-inch fat, braised	3 oz	163	26.9	0.0	43	0	5.3	82
select, 0-inch fat, roasted	3 oz	145	24.4	0.0	56	0	4.6	66
select, 1/4-inch fat, braised	3 oz	167	26.9	0.0	43	0	5.8	82
select, 1/4-inch fat, roasted	10.5 oz	534	86.0	0.0	197	0	18.5	232
select, 1/4-inch fat, roasted	3 oz	152	24.4	0.0	56	0	5.3	66

Food Name	Serv. Size	Total Cal.	Prot. GMS	Carbs GMS	Sod. MGS	Fiber GMS	Fat GMS	Chol. MGS
select, 1/2-inch fat, braised	3 oz	182	26.9	0.0	43	0	7.4	82
Untrimmed								
all grades, 0-inch fat, braised	3 oz	181	26.5	0.0	43	0	7.5	82
all grades, 0-inch fat, roasted	3 oz	160	24.3	0.0	56	0	6.3	66
all grades, 1/4-inch fat, braised	3 oz	234	24.4	0.0	43	0	14.4	82
all grades, 1/4-inch fat, raw	1 lb	943	91.8	0.0	249	0	60.9	290
all grades, 1/4-inch fat, raw	1 oz	59	5.7	0.0	16	0	3.8	18
all grades, 1/4-inch fat, roasted	3 oz	211	22.6	0.0	54	0	12.7	68
all grades, 1/2-inch fat, braised	3 oz	222	25.3	0.0	43	0	12.6	82
all grades, 1/2-inch fat, raw	1 lb	1021	90.2	0.0	249	0	70.5	295
all grades, 1/2-inch fat, raw	1 oz	64	5.6	0.0	16	0	4.4	18
choice, 0-inch fat, braised	3 oz	193	26.3	0.0	43	0	9.0	82
choice, 0-inch fat, roasted	3 oz	173	24.2	0.0	55	0	7.7	66
choice, 1/4-inch fat, braised	3 oz	241	24.4	0.0	43	0	15.2	82
choice, 1/4-inch fat, raw	1 lb	989	91.1	0.0	249	0	66.7	290
choice, 1/4-inch fat, raw	1 oz	62	5.7	0.0	16	0	4.2	18
choice, 1/4-inch fat, roasted	3 oz	221	22.5	0.0	54	0	13.9	68
choice, 1/2-inch fat, braised	3 oz	224	25.3	0.0	43	0	12.9	82
choice, 1/2-inch fat, raw	1 lb	1030	90.1	0.0	249	0	71.5	295
choice, 1/2-inch fat, raw	1 oz	64	5.6	0.0	16	0	4.5	18
prime, 1/2-inch fat, braised	3 oz	252	24.9	0.0	43	0	16.2	82
prime, 1/2-inch fat, raw	1 lb	1021	91.3	0.0	249	0	69.8	290
prime, 1/2-inch fat, raw	1 oz	64	5.7	0.0	16	0	4.4	18
select, 0-inch fat, braised	3 oz	171	26.5	0.0	43	0	6.4	82
select, 0-inch fat, roasted	3 oz	150	24.3	0.0	56	0	5.1	66
select, 1/4-inch fat, braised	3 oz	220	24.5	0.0	43	0	12.8	82
select, 1/4-inch fat, raw	1 lb	885	92.4	0.0	254	0	54.3	286
select, 1/4-inch fat, raw	1 oz	55	5.8	0.0	16	0	3.4	18
select, 1/4-inch fat, roasted	3 oz	199	22.8	0.0	54	0	11.3	68
select, 1/2-inch fat, braised	3 oz	215	25.4	0.0	43	0	11.8	82
select, 1/2-inch fat, raw	1 lb	984	90.9	0.0	249	0	66.0	290
select, 1/2-inch fat, raw	1 oz	62	5.7	0.0	16	0	4.1	18
ROUND, EYE OF								
Trimmed								
all grades, 0-inch fat, roasted	3 oz	141	24.6	0.0	53	0	4.0	59
all grades, 1/4-inch fat, roasted	3 oz	143	24.6	0.0	53	0	4.2	59
all grades, 1/2-inch fat, roasted	3 oz	156	24.6	0.0	53	0	5.5	59
choice, 0-inch fat, roasted	3 oz	149	24.6	0.0	53	0	4.8	59
choice, 1/4-inch fat, roasted	3 oz	149	24.6	0.0	53	0	4.8	59
choice, 1/2-inch fat, roasted	3 oz	156	24.6	0.0	53	0	5.7	59
prime, 1/2-inch fat, roasted	3 oz	213	23.0	0.0	50	0	12.7	61
prime, 1/2-inch fat, raw	1 lb	676	98.7	0.0	240	0	28.4	245
prime, 1/2-inch fat, raw	1 oz	42	6.2	0.0	15	0	1.8	15

Food Name	Serv. Size	Total Cal.	Prot. GMS	Carbs GMS	Sod. MGS	Fiber GMS	Fat GMS	Chol. MGS
prime, 1/2-inch fat, roasted	3 oz	168	24.6	0.0	53	0	7.0	59
select, 0-inch fat, roasted	3 oz	132	24.6	0.0	53	0	3.0	59
select, 0-inch fat, roasted	10.4 oz	460	85.8	0.0	184	0	10.4	204
select, 1/4-inch fat, roasted	3 oz	136	24.6	0.0	53	0	3.4	59
select, 1/2-inch fat, roasted	3 oz	151	24.6	0.0	53	0	5.1	59
Untrimmed								
all grades, 0-inch fat, roasted	3 oz	145	24.5	0.0	53	0	4.6	59
all grades, 1/4-inch fat, raw	1 lb	966	89.4	0.0	222	0	64.8	277
all grades, 1/4-inch fat, raw	1 oz	60	5.6	0.0	14	0	4.1	17
all grades, 1/4-inch fat, roasted	3 oz	195	22.8	0.0	50	0	10.8	61
all grades, 1/2-inch fat, raw	1 lb	903	91.0	0.0	227	0	57.1	272
all grades, 1/2-inch fat, raw	1 oz	56	5.7	0.0	14	0	3.6	17
all grades, 1/2-inch fat, roasted	3 oz	207	22.8	0.0	50	0	12.1	62
choice, 0-inch fat, braised	3 oz	176	30.7	0.0	38	0	4.9	77
choice, 0-inch fat, roasted	3 oz	153	24.5	0.0	53	0	5.4	59
choice, 1/4-inch fat, raw	1 lb	989	89.4	0.0	222	0	67.1	277
choice, 1/4-inch fat, raw	1 oz	62	5.6	0.0	14	0	4.2	17
choice, 1/4-inch fat, roasted	3 oz	205	22.6	0.0	50	0	12.0	61
choice, 1/2-inch fat, raw	1 lb	916	90.8	0.0	227	0	58.8	272
choice, 1/2-inch fat, raw	1 oz	57	5.7	0.0	14	0	3.7	17
choice, 1/2-inch fat, roasted	3 oz	207	22.8	0.0	50	0	12.2	62
prime, 1/2-inch fat, raw	1 lb	1002	90.3	0.0	227	0	68.3	272
prime, 1/2-inch fat, raw	1 oz	63	5.6	0.0	14	0	4.3	17
select, 0-inch fat, roasted	3 oz	137	24.5	0.0	53	0	3.5	59
select, 1/4-inch fat, raw	1 lb	916	90.0	0.0	227	0	59.1	272
select, 1/4-inch fat, raw	1 oz	57	5.6	0.0	14	0	3.7	17
select, 1/4-inch fat, roasted	1 oz	184	22.9	0.0	51	0	9.6	61
select, 1/4-inch fat, roasted	4 oz	246	30.6	0.0	68	0	12.8	82
select, 1/2-inch fat, raw	1 lb	853	91.6	0.0	227	0	51.4	268
select, 1/2-inch fat, raw	1 oz	53	5.7	0.0	14	0	3.2	17
select, 1/2-inch fat, roasted	3 oz	201	22.8	0.0	50	0	11.5	61
ROUND, FULL CUT								
Trimmed								
choice, 1/4-inch fat, broiled	3 oz	162	24.8	0.0	54	0	6.2	66
select, 1/4-inch fat, broiled	3 oz	146	24.9	0.0	54	0	4.4	66
select, 1/2-inch fat, broiled	3 oz	156	24.2	0.0	54	0	5.9	70
Untrimmed								
choice, 1/4-inch fat, broiled	3 oz	204	23.3	0.0	52	0	11.6	68
choice, 1/4-inch fat, raw	1 lb	921	92.4	0.0	240	0	58.1	286
choice, 1/4-inch fat, raw	1 oz	58	5.8	0.0	15	0	3.6	18
choice, 1/2-inch fat, broiled	3 oz	233	21.7	0.0	51	0	15.5	71
choice, 1/2-inch fat, raw	1 lb	1093	87.9	0.0	231	0	79.6	299
choice, 1/2-inch fat, raw	1 oz	68	5.5	0.0	14	0	5.0	19

Food Name	Serv. Size	Total Cal.	Prot. GMS	Carbs GMS	Sod. MGS	Fiber GMS	Fat GMS	Chol. MGS
select, 1/4-inch fat, broiled	3 oz	190	23.3	0.0	53	0	10.0	47
select, 1/4-inch fat, raw	1 lb	866	92.4	0.0	240	0	52.6	286
select, 1/4-inch fat, raw	1 oz	54	5.8	0.0	15	0	3.3	18
select, 1/2-inch fat, broiled	3 oz	223	21.8	0.0	51	0	14.3	71
select, 1/2-inch fat, raw	1 lb	1048	88.5	0.0	231	0	74.1	295
select, 1/2-inch fat, raw	1 oz	65	5.5	0.0	14	0	4.6	18
ROUND, TIP								
Trimmed								
all grades, 0-inch fat, roasted	3 oz	150	24.4	0.0	55	0	5.0	69
all grades, 1/4-inch fat, roasted	3 oz	157	24.4	0.0	55	0	5.9	69
all grades, 1/2-inch fat, roasted	3 oz	161	24.4	0.0	55	0	6.4	69
choice, 0-inch fat, roasted	3 oz	153	24.4	0.0	55	0	5.4	69
choice, 1/4-inch fat, roasted	3 oz	160	24.4	0.0	55	0	6.2	69
choice, 1/2-inch fat, roasted	3 oz	164	24.4	0.0	55	0	6.6	69
prime, 1/4-inch fat, roasted	3 oz	181	24.4	0.0	55	0	8.6	69
prime, 1/2-inch fat, roasted	3 oz	181	24.4	0.0	55	0	8.6	69
select, 0-inch fat, roasted	3 oz	144	24.4	0.0	55	0	4.5	69
select, 1/4-inch fat, roasted	3 oz	153	24.4	0.0	55	0	5.4	69
select, 1/2-inch fat, roasted	3 oz	156	24.4	0.0	55	0	5.7	69
Untrimmed								
all grades, 0-inch fat, roasted	3 oz	162	23.9	0.0	54	0	6.7	69
all grades, 1/4-inch fat, raw	1 lb	912	87.6	0.0	259	0	59.8	295
all grades, 1/4-inch fat, raw	1 oz	57	5.5	0.0	16	0	3.7	18
all grades, 1/4-inch fat, roasted	3 oz	199	22.9	0.0	54	0	11.3	70
all grades, 1/2-inch fat, raw	1 lb	934	87.5	0.0	259	0	62.4	295
all grades, 1/2-inch fat, raw	1 oz	58	5.5	0.0	16	0	3.9	18
all grades, 1/2-inch fat, roasted	3 oz	213	22.5	0.0	53	0	13.0	71
choice, 0-inch fat, roasted	3 oz	170	23.8	0.0	54	0	7.6	70
choice, 1/4-inch fat, raw	1 lb	962	87.0	0.0	259	0	65.2	299
choice, 1/4-inch fat, raw	1 oz	60	5.4	0.0	16	0	4.1	19
choice, 1/4-inch fat, roasted	3 oz	210	22.6	0.0	53	0	12.6	71
choice, 1/2-inch fat, raw	1 lb	948	87.3	0.0	259	0	64.0	295
choice, 1/2-inch fat, raw	1 oz	59	5.5	0.0	16	0	4.0	18
choice, 1/2-inch fat, roasted	3 oz	216	22.5	0.0	53	0	13.3	71
prime, 1/4-inch fat, raw	1 lb	971	88.2	0.0	263	0	66.1	295
prime, 1/4-inch fat, raw	1 oz	61	5.5	0.0	16	0	4.1	18
prime, 1/4-inch fat, roasted	3 oz	233	22.4	0.0	53	0	15.2	71
prime, 1/2-inch fat, raw	1 lb	1012	86.8	0.0	259	0	72.9	299
prime, 1/2-inch fat, raw	1 oz	63	5.4	0.0	16	0	4.6	19
prime, 1/2-inch fat, roasted	3 oz	241	22.1	0.0	52	0	16.3	71
select, 0-inch fat, roasted	3 oz	158	23.9	0.0	54	0	6.2	69
select, 1/4-inch fat, raw	1 lb	848	89.6	0.0	256	0	51.2	288
select, 1/4-inch fat, raw	1 oz	53	5.6	0.0	16	0	3.2	18

Food Name	Serv. Size	Total Cal.	Prot. GMS	Carbs GMS	Sod. MGS	Fiber GMS	Fat GMS	Chol. MGS
select, 1/4-inch fat, roasted	3 oz	191	23.0	0.0	54	0	10.3	70
select, 1/2-inch fat, raw	1 lb	875	88.4	0.0	263	0	55.7	295
select, 1/2-inch fat, raw	1 oz	55	5.5	0.0	16	0	3.5	18
select, 1/2-inch fat, roasted	3 oz	205	22.6	0.0	53	0	12.0	71
ROUND, TOP								
Trimmed								
all grades, 0-inch fat, braised	3 oz	169	30.7	0.0	38	0	4.3	77
all grades, 1/4-inch fat, braised	3 oz	174	30.7	0.0	38	0	4.8	77
all grades, 1/4-inch fat, broiled	3 oz	153	26.9	0.0	52	0	4.2	71
all grades, 1/2-inch fat, broiled	3 oz	162	26.9	0.0	52	0	5.3	71
choice, 1/4-inch fat, braised	3 oz	181	30.7	0.0	38	0	5.5	77
choice, 1/4-inch fat, broiled	3 oz	161	26.9	0.0	52	0	5.0	71
choice, 1/4-inch fat, pan-fried	3 oz	193	29.8	0.0	60	0	7.3	82
choice, 1/4-inch fat, pan-fried in vegetable oil	4 oz	257	39.8	0.0	81	0	9.7	110
choice, 1/2-inch fat, broiled	3 oz	165	26.9	0.0	52	0	5.5	71
choice, 1/2-inch fat, pan-fried	3 oz	193	29.8	0.0	60	0	7.3	82
prime, 1/4-inch fat, broiled	3 lb	183	26.9	0.0	52	0	7.5	71
prime, 1/2-inch fat, broiled	3 oz	183	26.9	0.0	52	0	7.5	71
select, 0-inch fat, braised	3 oz	161	30.7	0.0	38	0	3.4	77
select, 1/4-inch fat, braised	3 oz	167	30.7	0.0	38	0	3.9	77
select, 1/4-inch fat, broiled	3 oz	144	26.9	0.0	52	0	3.2	71
select, 1/2-inch fat, broiled	3 oz	156	26.9	0.0	52	0	4.6	71
Untrimmed								
all grades, 0-inch fat, braised	3 oz	178	30.3	0.0	38	0	5.4	77
all grades, 1/4-inch fat, braised	3 oz	211	28.8	0.0	38	0	9.7	77
all grades, 1/4-inch fat, broiled	3 oz	184	25.6	0.0	51	0	8.2	72
all grades, 1/4-inch fat, raw	1 lb	798	97.4	0.0	227	0	42.5	277
all grades, 1/4-inch fat, raw	1 oz	50	6.1	0.0	14	0	2.7	17
all grades, 1/2-inch fat, broiled	3 oz	179	26.2	0.0	51	0	7.5	72
all grades, 1/2-inch fat, raw	1 lb	780	98.7	0.0	227	0	39.7	272
all grades, 1/2-inch fat, raw	1 oz	49	6.2	0.0	14	0	2.5	17
choice, 0-inch fat, braised	3 oz	184	30.3	0.0	38	0	6.0	77
choice, 1/4-inch fat, broiled	3 oz	190	25.6	0.0	51	0	9.0	72
choice, 1/4-inch fat, pan-fried	3 oz	235	27.5	0.0	58	0	13.1	82
choice, 1/4-inch fat, pan-fried in vegetable oil	4 oz	314	36.7	0.0	77	0	17.4	110
choice, 1/4-inch fat, raw	1 lb	821	97.4	0.0	227	0	45.0	277
choice, 1/4-inch fat, raw	1 oz	51	6.1	0.0	14	0	2.8	17
choice, 1/2-inch fat, braised	3 oz	221	28.5	0.0	38	0	10.9	77
choice, 1/2-inch fat, broiled	3 oz	181	26.2	0.0	51	0	7.7	72
choice, 1/2-inch fat, pan-fried	3 oz	247	26.9	0.0	57	0	14.5	82
choice, 1/2-inch fat, raw	1 lb	789	98.7	0.0	227	0	40.7	272

Food Name	Serv. Size	Total Cal.	Prot. GMS	Carbs GMS	Sod. MGS	Fiber GMS	Fat GMS	Chol. MGS
choice, 1/2-inch fat, raw	1 oz	49	6.2	0.0	14	0	2.5	17
prime, 1/4-inch fat, broiled	3 oz	195	26.4	0.0	51	0	9.1	71
prime, 1/4-inch fat, raw	1 lb	816	100.1	0.0	231	0	42.9	268
prime, 1/4-inch fat, raw	1 oz	51	6.3	0.0	14	0	2.7	17
prime, 1/2-inch fat, broiled	3 oz	201	26.1	0.0	51	0	9.9	72
prime, 1/2-inch fat, raw	1 lb	853	98.9	0.0	227	0	47.9	272
prime, 1/2-inch fat, raw	1 oz	53	6.2	0.0	14	0	3.0	17
select, 0-inch fat, braised	3 oz	170	30.3	0.0	38	0	4.5	77
select, 1/4-inch fat, braised	3 oz	199	29.0	0.0	38	0	8.4	77
select, 1/4-inch fat, broiled	3 oz	175	25.6	0.0	51	0	7.2	72
select, 1/4-inch fat, raw	1 lb	744	98.1	0.0	227	0	36.2	272
select, 1/4-inch fat, raw	1 oz	46	6.1	0.0	14	0	2.3	17
select, 1/2-inch fat, broiled	3 oz	176	26.1	0.0	51	0	7.1	72
select, 1/2-inch fat, raw	1 lb	748	98.8	0.0	227	0	36.3	272
select, 1/2-inch fat, raw	1 oz	47	6.2	0.0	14	0	2.3	17
SIRLOIN, TOP								
Trimmed								
all grades, 0-inch fat, broiled	3 oz	162	25.8	0.0	56	0	5.8	76
all grades, 1/4-inch fat, broiled	3 oz	166	25.8	0.0	56	0	6.1	76
all grades, 1/2-inch fat, broiled	3 oz	177	25.8	0.0	56	0	7.4	76
choice, 0-inch fat, broiled	4 oz	227	34.4	0.0	75	0	8.8	101
choice, 0-inch fat, broiled	3 oz	170	25.8	0.0	56	0	6.6	76
choice, 1/4-inch fat, broiled	4 oz	229	34.4	0.0	75	0	9.1	101
choice, 1/4-inch fat, broiled	3 oz	172	25.8	0.0	56	0	6.8	76
choice, 1/4-inch fat, pan-fried	3 oz	202	27.6	0.0	65	0	9.3	84
choice, 1/4-inch fat, pan-fried in vegetable oil	4 oz	270	36.8	0.0	87	0	12.4	112
choice, 1/2-inch fat, broiled	3 oz	179	25.8	0.0	56	0	7.7	76
choice, 1/2-inch fat, pan-fried	3 oz	202	27.6	0.0	65	0	9.3	84
prime, 1/2-inch fat, broiled	3 oz	201	25.8	0.0	56	0	10.1	76
prime, 1/2-inch fat, raw	1 lb	703	96.3	0.0	263	0	32.1	277
prime, 1/2-inch fat, raw	1 oz	44	6.0	0.0	16	0	2.0	17
select, 0-inch fat, broiled	3 oz	153	25.8	0.0	56	0	4.8	76
select, 1/4-inch fat, broiled	3 oz	158	25.8	0.0	56	0	5.3	76
select, 1/2-inch fat, broiled	3 oz	170	25.8	0.0	56	0	6.6	76
Untrimmed								
all grades, 0-inch fat, broiled	3 oz	183	25.0	0.0	55	0	8.5	76
all grades, 1/4-inch fat, broiled	3 oz	219	23.6	0.0	54	0	13.1	77
all grades, 1/4-inch fat, raw	1 lb	984	86.9	0.0	240	0	68.2	304
all grades, 1/4-inch fat, raw	1 oz	62	5.4	0.0	15	0	4.3	19
all grades, 1/2-inch fat, broiled	3 oz	238	23.3	0.0	54	0	15.3	77
all grades, 1/2-inch fat, raw	1 lb	1179	82.7	0.0	236	0	91.5	313
all grades, 1/2-inch fat, raw	1 oz	74	5.2	0.0	15	0	5.7	20

Food Name	Serv. Size	Total Cal.	Prot. GMS	Carbs GMS	Sod. MGS	Fiber GMS	Fat GMS	Chol. MGS
choice, 0-inch fat, broiled	3 oz	195	24.8	0.0	54	0	9.8	76
choice, 1/4-inch fat, broiled	3 oz	229	23.5	0.0	53	0	14.2	77
choice, 1/4-inch fat, pan-fried	3 oz	277	23.9	0.0	59	0	19.4	83
choice, 1/4-inch fat, pan-fried in								
vegetable oil	4 oz	370	31.9	0.0	79	0	25.9	111
choice, 1/4-inch fat, raw	1 lb	1030	86.3	0.0	240	0	73.5	304
choice, 1/4-inch fat, raw	1 oz	64	5.4	0.0	15	0	4.6	19
choice, 1/2-inch fat, broiled	3 oz	241	23.3	0.0	53	0	15.7	77
choice, 1/2-inch fat, pan-fried	3 oz	288	23.3	0.0	58	0	20.9	83
choice, 1/2-inch fat, raw	1 lb	1198	82.5	0.0	231	0	93.8	318
choice, 1/2-inch fat, raw	1 oz	75	5.2	0.0	14	0	5.9	20
prime, 1/2-inch fat, broiled	3 oz	271	22.7	0.0	53	0	19.4	77
prime, 1/2-inch fat, raw	1 lb	1320	80.8	0.0	231	0	108.0	322
prime, 1/2-inch fat, raw	1 oz	83	5.1	0.0	14	0	6.8	20
select, 0-inch fat, broiled	3 oz	166	25.2	0.0	55	0	6.4	76
select, 1/4-inch fat, broiled	3 oz	208	23.8	0.0	54	0	11.8	77
select, 1/4-inch fat, raw	1 lb	939	87.4	0.0	245	0	62.5	304
select, 1/4-inch fat, raw	1 oz	59	5.5	0.0	15	0	3.9	19
select, 1/2-inch fat, broiled	3 oz	232	23.3	0.0	53	0	14.8	77
select, 1/2-inch fat, raw	1 lb	1116	83.8	0.0	236	0	84.0	313
select, 1/2-inch fat, raw	1 oz	70	5.2	0.0	15	0	5.3	20
SHANK CROSSCUTS								
Trimmed								
choice, 1/4-inch fat, simmered	4 oz	228	38.2	0.0	73	0	7.2	88
choice, 1/4-inch fat, simmered	3 oz	171	28.6	0.0	54	0	5.4	66
choice, 1/2-inch fat, simmered	3 oz	171	28.6	0.0	54	0	5.4	66
Untrimmed								
choice, 1/4-inch fat, raw	1 oz	50	5.8	0.0	17	0	2.8	12
choice, 1/4-inch fat, raw	3 oz	150	17.5	0.0	51	0	8.4	37
choice, 1/4-inch fat, simmered	3 oz	224	26.1	0.0	52	0	12.5	68
choice, 1/2-inch fat, raw	1 lb	721	95.1	0.0	277	0	35.1	195
choice, 1/2-inch fat, raw	1 oz	45	5.9	0.0	17	0	2.2	12
choice, 1/2-inch fat, simmered	3 oz	207	26.9	0.0	53	0	10.3	67
SPLEEN								
braised	3 oz	123	21.3	0.0	48	0	3.6	295
calf, raw	100 gm	104	18.3	0.0	86	0	3.0	250
raw	4 oz	119	20.7	0.0	96	0	3.4	297
T-BONE								
Trimmed								
choice, 1/4-inch fat, broiled	3 oz	182	23.9	0.0	56	0	8.8	68
choice, 1/2-inch fat, broiled	3 oz	182	23.9	0.0	56	0	8.8	68
Untrimmed								
choice, 1/4-inch fat, broiled	3 oz	253	21.2	0.0	52	0	18.0	71

Food Name	Serv. Size	Total Cal.	Prot. GMS	Carbs GMS	Sod. MGS	Fiber GMS	Fat GMS	Chol. MGS
choice, 1/4-inch fat, raw	1 lb	1234	79.8	0.0	222	0	99.2	313
choice, 1/4-inch fat, raw	1 oz	77	5.0	0.0	14	0	6.2	20
choice, 1/2-inch fat, broiled	3 oz	275	20.4	0.0	51	0	20.9	71
choice, 1/2-inch fat, raw	1 lb	1393	76.1	0.0	218	0	118.5	322
choice, 1/2-inch fat, raw	1 oz	87	4.8	0.0	14	0	7.4	20
TENDERLOIN								
Trimmed								
all grades, 0-inch fat, broiled	3 oz	175	24.0	0.0	54	0	8.1	71
all grades, 1/4-inch fat, broiled	3 oz	179	24.0	0.0	54	0	8.5	71
all grades, 1/4-inch fat, roasted	3 oz	189	23.5	0.0	52	0	9.8	71
all grades, 1/2-inch fat, broiled	3 oz	173	24.0	0.0	54	0	7.9	71
all grades, 1/2-inch fat, roasted	3 oz	186	23.4	0.0	50	0	9.6	73
choice, 0-inch fat, broiled	3 oz	180	24.0	0.0	54	0	8.6	71
choice, 1/4-inch fat, broiled	3 oz	189	24.0	0.0	54	0	9.5	71
choice, 1/4-inch fat, roasted	4 oz	262	31.4	0.0	82	0	14.2	94
choice, 1/4-inch fat, roasted	3 oz	196	23.5	0.0	61	0	10.6	71
choice, 1/2-inch fat, broiled	3 oz	176	24.0	0.0	54	0	8.1	71
choice, 1/2-inch fat, roasted	3 oz	190	23.4	0.0	50	0	9.9	73
prime, 1/4-inch fat, broiled	3 oz	197	24.0	0.0	54	0	10.5	71
prime, 1/4-inch fat, roasted	3 oz	217	23.4	0.0	50	0	13.0	73
prime, 1/2-inch fat, broiled	3 oz	197	24.0	0.0	54	0	10.5	71
prime, 1/2-inch fat, roasted	3 oz	217	23.4	0.0	50	0	13.0	73
select, 0-inch fat, broiled	3 oz	170	24.0	0.0	54	0	7.5	71
select, 1/4-inch fat, broiled	3 oz	169	24.0	0.0	54	0	7.4	71
select, 1/4-inch fat, roasted	3 oz	179	23.5	0.0	52	0	8.8	71
select, 1/2-inch fat, broiled	3 oz	167	24.0	0.0	54	0	7.1	71
select, 1/2-inch fat, roasted	3 oz	177	23.4	0.0	50	0	8.6	73
Untrimmed								
all grades, 0-inch fat, broiled	3 oz	200	23.1	0.0	53	0	11.2	72
all grades, 1/4-inch fat, broiled	3 oz	247	21.5	0.0	50	0	17.2	73
all grades, 1/4-inch fat, raw	1 lb	1284	80.6	0.0	218	0	104.4	322
all grades, 1/4-inch fat, raw	1 oz	80	5.0	0.0	14	0	6.5	20
all grades, 1/4-inch fat, roasted	3 oz	282	20.1	0.0	48	0	21.8	73
all grades, 1/2-inch fat, broiled	3 oz	226	22.1	0.0	52	0	14.6	72
all grades, 1/2-inch fat, raw	1 lb	1093	84.1	0.0	222	0	81.6	313
all grades, 1/2-inch fat, roasted	3 oz	258	20.8	0.0	48	0	18.7	74
choice, 0-inch fat, broiled	3 oz	207	23.0	0.0	52	0	12.2	72
choice, 1/4-inch fat, broiled	4 oz	356	29.4	0.0	69	0	25.6	101
choice, 1/4-inch fat, broiled	3 oz	258	21.3	0.0	50	0	18.6	73
choice, 1/4-inch fat, raw	1 lb	1306	80.6	0.0	218	0	106.8	322
choice, 1/4-inch fat, raw	1 oz	82	5.0	0.0	14	0	6.7	20
choice, 1/4-inch fat, roasted	3 oz	288	20.1	0.0	55	0	22.4	73
choice, 1/2-inch fat, broiled	3 oz	230	22.0	0.0	51	0	15.1	73

Food Name	Serv. Size	Total Cal.	Prot. GMS	Carbs GMS	Sod. MGS	Fiber GMS	Fat GMS	Chol. MGS
choice, 1/2-inch fat, raw	1 lb	1116	83.8	0.0	222	0	83.9	313
choice, 1/2-inch fat, roasted	3 oz	262	20.7	0.0	48	0	19.2	74
prime, 1/4-inch fat, broiled	3 oz	269	21.2	0.0	50	0	19.9	73
prime, 1/4-inch fat, raw	1 lb	1288	81.2	0.0	218	0	104.6	318
prime, 1/4-inch fat, raw	1 oz	81	5.1	0.0	14	0	6.5	20
prime, 1/4-inch fat, roasted	3 oz	300	20.1	0.0	47	0	23.7	75
prime, 1/2-inch fat, broiled	3 oz	270	21.2	0.0	50	0	19.9	73
prime, 1/2-inch fat, raw	1 lb	1306	80.7	0.0	218	0	106.8	322
prime, 1/2-inch fat, roasted	3 oz	304	19.9	0.0	47	0	24.4	75
select, 0-inch fat, broiled	3 oz	195	23.1	0.0	53	0	10.6	72
select, 1/4-inch fat, broiled	3 oz	230	21.8	0.0	51	0	15.2	73
select, 1/4-inch fat, raw	1 lb	1261	80.6	0.0	218	0	101.6	322
select, 1/4-inch fat, raw	1 oz	79	5.0	0.0	14	0	6.3	20
select, 1/4-inch fat, roasted	3 oz	275	20.1	0.0	48	0	21.0	73
select, 1/2-inch fat, broiled	3 oz	216	22.2	0.0	52	0	13.4	73
select, 1/2-inch fat, raw	1 lb	1043	84.7	0.0	222	0	75.7	313
select, 1/2-inch fat, roasted	3 oz	245	21.0	0.0	48	0	17.3	74
THYMUS								
braised	3 oz	271	18.6	0.0	99	0	21.2	250
raw	4 oz	267	13.8	0.0	108	0	23.0	252
TONGUE								
potted or deviled	100 gm	290	18.6	0.7	1430	0	23.0	110
raw	4 oz	253	16.8	4.2	78	0	18.2	98
simmered	3 oz	241	18.8	0.3	51	0	17.6	91
smoked	100 gm	328	17.2	0.9	73	0	28.8	68
whole, canned or pickled	100 gm	267	19.3	0.3	1021	0	20.3	90
TOP LOIN								
Trimmed								
all grades, 0-inch fat, broiled	3 oz	168	24.3	0.0	58	0	7.1	65
all grades, 1/4-inch fat, broiled	3 oz	176	24.3	0.0	58	0	8.0	65
all grades, 1/2-inch fat, broiled	3 oz	173	24.3	0.0	58	0	7.6	65
choice, 0-inch fat, broiled	4 oz	237	32.5	0.0	77	0	10.9	86
choice, 0-inch fat, broiled	3 oz	178	24.3	0.0	58	0	8.2	65
choice, 1/4-inch fat, broiled	4 oz	243	32.5	0.0	77	0	11.5	86
choice, 1/4-inch fat, broiled	3 oz	182	24.3	0.0	58	0	8.6	65
choice, 1/2-inch fat, broiled	3 oz	176	24.3	0.0	58	0	8.0	65
prime, 1/4-inch fat, broiled	3 oz	208	24.3	0.0	58	0	11.6	65
prime, 1/2-inch fat, broiled	3 oz	208	24.3	0.0	58	0	11.6	65
select, 0-inch fat, broiled	3 oz	156	24.3	0.0	58	0	5.9	65
select, 1/4-inch fat, broiled	3 oz	164	24.3	0.0	58	0	6.6	65
select, 1/2-inch fat, broiled	3 oz	161	24.3	0.0	58	0	6.4	65
Untrimmed								
all grades, 0-inch fat, broiled	3 oz	180	23.9	0.0	57	0	8.7	65

Food Name	Serv. Size	Total Cal.	Prot. GMS	Carbs GMS	Sod. MGS	Fiber GMS	Fat GMS	Chol. MGS
all grades, 1/4-inch fat, broiled	3 oz	244	21.7	0.0	54	0	16.8	67
all grades, 1/4-inch fat, raw	1 lb	1102	86.2	0.0	240	0	81.3	304
all grades, 1/2-inch fat, broiled	3 oz	238	21.9	0.0	54	0	16.0	67
all grades, 1/2-inch fat, raw	1 lb	1284	82.3	0.0	236	0	103.6	313
choice, 0-inch fat, broiled	3 oz	194	23.7	0.0	57	0	10.2	65
choice, 1/4-inch fat, broiled	3 oz	253	21.6	0.0	54	0	17.8	67
choice, 1/4-inch fat, raw	1 lb	1179	85.0	0.0	240	0	90.4	304
choice, 1/2-inch fat, broiled	3 oz	243	21.8	0.0	54	0	16.6	67
choice, 1/2-inch fat, raw	1 lb	1311	82.0	0.0	231	0	106.7	313
prime, 1/4-inch fat, broiled	3 oz	275	21.6	0.0	54	0	20.3	67
prime, 1/4-inch fat, raw	1 lb	1383	83.1	0.0	236	0	114.2	313
prime, 1/2-inch fat, broiled	3 oz	288	21.0	0.0	53	0	22.0	68
prime, 1/2-inch fat, raw	1 lb	1461	81.1	0.0	231	0	123.7	318
select, 0-inch fat, broiled	3 oz	169	23.9	0.0	57	0	7.5	65
select, 1/4-inch fat, broiled	3 oz	226	22.0	0.0	54	0	14.6	67
select, 1/4-inch fat, raw	1 lb	1043	86.8	0.0	245	0	74.6	299
select, 1/2-inch fat, broiled	3 oz	223	22.1	0.0	54	0	14.2	67
select, 1/2-inch fat, raw	1 lb	1198	83.6	0.0	236	0	93.0	308
TRIPE								
canned *(Armour)*	6 oz	180	33.0	1.0	230	na	4.0	na
pickled	100 gm	62	11.8	0.0	46	0	1.3	68
raw	4 oz	111	16.5	0.0	52	0	4.5	107
BEEF, ALTERNATIVE								
(Heartline) 'Beef Fillet Style'	2 oz	176	19.0	9.0	480	na	7.0	0
(Heartline) 'Beef Fillet Style' lite	.5 oz	22	5.0	1.0	135	3.0	0.0	0
(Heartline) 'Ground Beef Style'	2 oz	176	19.0	9.0	480	na	7.0	0
(Heartline) 'Ground Beef Style' lite	.5 oz	22	2.0	1.0	135	3.0	0.0	0
(Heartline) 'Teriyaki Beef Style'	2 oz	176	19.0	9.0	450	na	7.0	0
Canned								
(Worthington) 'Prime Stakes'	3.25-oz piece	160	10.0	7.0	410	(mq)	10.0	0
(Worthington) 'Savory Slices'								
2-oz slices	2 slices	100	8.0	4.0	340	(mq)	6.0	0
(Worthington) 'Vegetable Steaks'								
approx 1.28-oz pieces	3.2 oz	110	17.0	5.0	400	(mq)	2.0	0
Frozen								
(Worthington) roll, approx 1.25-oz								
slices	2 slices	130	12.0	7.0	750	(mq)	6.0	0
(Worthington) roll, smoked, frozen, approx								
2/3-oz slices	3 slices	120	10.0	7.0	790	(mq)	6.0	0
(Worthington) 'Stakelets'	2.5 oz	150	13.0	7.0	460	(mq)	8.0	0
BEEF, CANNED, chopped *(Armour)*	3 oz	280	11.0	3.0	1290	na	24.0	na
BEEF, CORNED								
(Healthy Deli)	1 oz	35	5.7	0.7	210	0	1.0	11

Food Name	Serv. Size	Total Cal.	Prot. GMS	Carbs GMS	Sod. MGS	Fiber GMS	Fat GMS	Chol. MGS
(Hillshire Farm)	1 oz	31	6.0	<1.0	230	0	0.4	(mq)
(Oscar Mayer)	.6 oz	17	3.4	0.1	204	0	0.3	8
brisket, cured, cooked	3 oz	213	15.4	0.4	964	0	16.1	83
brisket, cured, raw	1 lb	898	66.6	0.6	553	0	67.6	245
brisket, cured, raw	1 oz	56	4.2	0.0	35	0	4.2	15
canned (Dinty Moore)	2 oz	130	15.0	0.0	(mq)	0	8.0	(mq)
canned, cured	1 oz	71	7.7	0.0	285	0	4.2	24
canned, '7 oz can' (Libby's)	2.3 oz	160	17.0	2.0	720	0	9.0	(mq)
canned, '12 oz can' (Libby's)	2.4 oz	160	17.0	2.0	750	0	9.0	(mq)
'St. Paddy's' (Healthy Deli)	1 oz	24	3.9	1.1	290	0	0.4	7
'Slender Sliced' (Eckrich)	1 oz	40	6.0	1.0	270	0	1.0	(mq)
BEEF, CORNED, ALTERNATIVE								
roll, frozen (Worthington)	2.5 oz	150	12.0	9.0	660	(mq)	7.0	0
roll, frozen (Worthington) approx								
.5-oz slices	4 slices	120	9.0	8.0	740	(mq)	6.0	0
BEEF, CORNED, HASH								
canned (Armour)	7.5 oz	390	18.0	18.0	900	na	27.0	na
canned, '15 oz can' (Libby's)	7 1/2 oz	400	18.0	20.0	1260	(mq)	27.0	(mq)
canned, '15 oz can' (Mary Kitchen)	7 1/2 oz	360	20.0	19.0	1386	(mq)	24.0	(mq)
canned (Mary Kitchen)	1 oz	47	3.0	2.0	111	na	3.0	9
canned (Nalley's)	8 oz	420	17.0	27.0	940	(mq)	27.0	(mq)
canned, 'No Frills' (Pathmark)	7 1/2 oz	410	16.0	27.0	1250	(mq)	26.0	(mq)
canned, '25 oz can' (Mary Kitchen)	8 1/3 oz	400	22.0	19.0	1429	(mq)	27.0	(mq)
canned, '24 oz can' (Libby's)	8 oz	420	19.0	21.0	1330	(mq)	28.0	(mq)
canned, w/potato	1 cup	398	19.4	23.5	1188	>1.1 c	24.9	73
microwave cup (Dinty Moore)	7.5 oz	350	19.0	19.0	850	na	22.0	65
25% less salt, 'Premium' (Armour)	7.5 oz	350	19.0	21.0	790	na	21.0	na
BEEF, CORNED, SPREAD, canned								
(Hormel)	.5 oz	35	2.0	0.0	(mq)	(tr)	3.0	(mq)
BEEF, DRIED								
chipped, cooked, creamed	1 cup	377	20.1	17.4	1754	0	25.2	98
cured	1 oz	47	8.3	0.4	984	0	1.1	12
sliced (Armour)	1.1 oz	60	8.0	2.0	na	na	2.0	na
BEEF, GROUND								
Extra lean								
baked, medium-cooked	3 oz	213	20.8	0.0	42	0	13.7	70
baked, well-done	3 oz	233	25.8	0.0	54	0	13.6	91
broiled, medium-cooked	3 oz	218	21.6	0.0	59	0	13.9	71
broiled, well-done	3 oz	225	24.3	0.0	70	0	13.4	84
pan-fried, medium-cooked	3 oz	217	21.2	0.0	59	0	14.0	69
pan-fried, well-done	3 oz	224	23.8	0.0	69	0	13.6	79
raw	1 oz	66	5.3	0.0	19	0	4.8	20
raw	4 oz	264	21.1	0.0	75	0	19.3	78

Food Name	Serv. Size	Total Cal.	Prot. GMS	Carbs GMS	Sod. MGS	Fiber GMS	Fat GMS	Chol. MGS
Lean								
baked, medium-cooked	3 oz	228	20.3	0.0	48	0	15.6	66
baked, well-done	3 oz	248	25.2	0.0	60	0	15.6	84
broiled, medium-cooked	3 oz	231	21.0	0.0	65	0	15.7	74
broiled, well-done	3 oz	238	24.0	0.0	76	0	15.0	86
pan-fried, medium-cooked	3 oz	234	20.6	0.0	65	0	16.2	71
pan-fried, well-done	3 oz	235	23.4	0.0	74	0	15.0	81
raw	1 oz	75	5.0	0.0	20	0	5.9	21
raw	4 oz	298	20.0	0.0	78	0	23.4	85
Regular								
baked, medium-cooked	3 oz	244	19.6	0.0	51	0	17.8	74
baked, well-done	3 oz	269	24.5	0.0	64	0	18.3	92
broiled, frozen patty, medium-cooked	3 oz	240	20.8	0.0	65	0	16.7	80
broiled, medium-cooked	3 oz	246	20.5	0.0	71	0	17.6	77
broiled, well-done	3 oz	248	23.1	0.0	79	0	16.5	86
pan-fried, medium-cooked	3 oz	260	20.3	0.0	71	0	19.2	76
pan-fried, well-done	3 oz	243	23.0	0.0	79	0	16.1	83
raw	1 oz	88	4.7	0.0	19	0	7.5	24
raw	4 oz	350	18.8	0.0	77	0	30.0	96
raw, frozen patty	3 oz	240	14.5	0.0	58	0	19.7	67
BEEF DINNER, FROZEN. See also BEEF ENTRÉE, FROZEN.								
and gravy *(Swanson)*	11.25 oz	310	26.0	38.0	770	(mq)	6.0	(mq)
chopped *(Banquet)*	11 oz	420	21.0	14.0	600	(mq)	32.0	80
chopped steak, 'Hungry Man'								
(Swanson)	16.75 oz	640	35.0	41.0	1600	(mq)	37.0	(mq)
'Extra Helping' *(Banquet)*	16 oz	870	34.0	50.0	810	(mq)	61.0	120
in barbecue sauce *(Swanson)*	11 oz	460	30.0	51.0	860	(mq)	17.0	(mq)
Mexicana *(Budget Gourmet)*	12.8 oz	560	33.0	56.0	1290	(mq)	23.0	50
patty, charbroiled *(Freezer Queen)*	10 oz	300	17.0	20.0	1260	(mq)	17.0	(mq)
Salisbury steak *(Banquet)*	11 oz	500	23.0	26.0	600	(mq)	34.0	80
Salisbury steak *(Freezer Queen)*	10 oz	380	18.0	28.0	1260	(mq)	22.0	(mq)
Salisbury steak *(Healthy Choice)*	11.5 oz	300	19.0	41.0	480	na	7.0	50
Salisbury steak *(Le Menu)*	10.5 oz	370	20.0	28.0	880	(mq)	20.0	(mq)
Salisbury steak *(Morton)*	10 oz	300	12.0	23.0	1420	(mq)	17.0	40
Salisbury steak *(Swanson)*	10.75 oz	400	18.0	43.0	880	(mq)	17.0	(mq)
Salisbury steak, charbroiled flavor								
'Healthy Balance' *(Banquet)*	10.5 oz	270	14.0	34.0	800	na	8.0	35
Salisbury steak 'Classics' *(Armour)*	11.25 oz	350	22.0	26.0	1430	(mq)	17.0	55
Salisbury steak 'Classics Lite' *(Armour)*	11.5 oz	300	21.0	29.0	1020	(mq)	2.0	35
Salisbury steak 'Extra Helping' *(Banquet)*	18 oz	910	50.0	49.0	740	(mq)	60.0	175
Salisbury steak 'Hungry Man' *(Swanson)*	16.5 oz	680	41.0	37.0	1730	(mq)	41.0	(mq)
Salisbury steak 'Lightstyle' *(Le Menu)*	10 oz	280	18.0	31.0	400	(mq)	9.0	(mq)

Food Name	Serv. Size	Total Cal.	Prot. GMS	Carbs GMS	Sod. MGS	Fiber GMS	Fat GMS	Chol. MGS
Salisbury steak, parmigiana 'Classics' (Armour)	11.5 oz	410	22.0	32.0	1120	(mq)	21.0	60
Salisbury steak, sirloin (Budget Gourmet)	11.5 oz	410	26.0	28.0	890	(mq)	22.0	105
Salisbury steak, w/mushroom gravy 'Extra Helping' (Banquet)	18 oz	890	51.0	48.0	685	(mq)	58.0	169
sirloin, chopped (Le Menu)	12.25 oz	430	25.0	28.0	1010	(mq)	24.0	(mq)
sirloin, chopped (Swanson)	10.75 oz	340	20.0	28.0	790	(mq)	16.0	(mq)
sirloin, roast, 'Classics' (Armour)	10.45 oz	190	19.0	21.0	970	(mq)	4.0	55
sirloin, w/barbecue sauce (Healthy Choice)	11 oz	280	17.0	44.0	240	na	4.0	25
sirloin tips (Healthy Choice)	11.25 oz	270	22.0	29.0	360	na	7.0	65
sliced (Morton)	10 oz	220	24.0	20.0	950	(mq)	5.0	65
sliced, 'Hungry Man' (Swanson)	15.25 oz	450	37.0	49.0	1060	(mq)	12.0	(mq)
sliced, w/gravy (Freezer Queen)	10 oz	210	18.0	18.0	1010	(mq)	7.0	(mq)
steak Diane, 'Classics Lite' (Armour)	10 oz	290	27.0	25.0	440	(mq)	9.0	80
tips (Le Menu)	11.5 oz	400	30.0	29.0	760	(mq)	18.0	(mq)
tips 'Classics' (Armour)	10.25 oz	230	22.0	20.0	820	(mq)	7.0	70
tips, in Burgundy sauce (Budget Gourmet)	11 oz	310	24.0	28.0	720	(mq)	11.0	65
BEEF ENTRÉE, ALTERNATIVE								
'Country Stew' (Worthington)	9.5 oz	220	10.0	23.0	760	(mq)	10.0	0
pie, frozen (Worthington)	8 oz	360	9.0	44.0	1940	(mq)	16.0	0
BEEF ENTRÉE, CANNED								
chow mein (LaChoy)	3/4 cup	40	5.0	5.0	960	2.0	2.0	16
chow mein, 'Bi-Pack' (LaChoy)	8.748 oz	83	9.3	11.1	998	3.5	0.9	12
chow mein, 'Bi-Pack' (LaChoy)	3/4 cup	70	7.0	8.0	840	1.0	1.0	20
Oriental, w/noodles, 'Bi-Pack' (LaChoy)	9 oz	148	11.7	24.3	1101	3.4	1.2	13
pepper, 'Bi-Pack' (LaChoy)	3/4 cup	80	7.0	10.0	950	2.0	2.0	17
pepper Oriental, 'Bi-Pack' (LaChoy)	8.783 oz	101	10.1	12.7	1219	3.7	2.0	12
pepper Oriental, 'Bi-Pack' (LaChoy)	3/4 cup	80	7.0	10.0	950	1.0	2.0	18
stew (Armour)	8 oz	210	11.0	16.0	1200	na	11.0	na
stew (Dinty Moore)	8 oz	220	11.0	16.0	870	na	13.0	30
stew (Estee)	7.5 oz	210	14.0	15.0	65	(mq)	11.0	30
stew (Featherweight)	7.5 oz	160	17.0	17.0	400	(mq)	3.0	35
stew (Wolf Brand)	1 cup	179	9.6	18.3	1043	>.6 c	7.5	(mq)
stew, 'Big Chunk' (Nalley's)	7.5 oz	200	10.0	24.0	790	(mq)	7.0	(mq)
stew, '15-oz can' (Dinty Moore)	7.5 oz	200	10.0	15.0	810	na	12.0	30
stew, '15-oz pkg' (Libby's)	7.5 oz	160	12.0	18.0	870	(mq)	5.0	(mq)
stew, 'Homestyle' (Nalley's)	8 oz	180	11.0	22.0	810	(mq)	5.0	(mq)
stew, '40-oz can' (Dinty Moore)	8 oz	210	13.0	16.0	971	(mq)	11.0	(mq)
stew, 'No Frills' (Pathmark)	8 oz	190	10.0	25.0	625	(mq)	4.0	(mq)
stew, '24-oz can' (Dinty Moore)	8 oz	220	12.0	15.0	980	(mq)	12.0	(mq)

Food Name	Serv. Size	Total Cal.	Prot. GMS	Carbs GMS	Sod. MGS	Fiber GMS	Fat GMS	Chol. MGS
stew, '24-oz pkg' *(Libby's)*	8 oz	170	12.0	19.0	930	(mq)	6.0	(mq)
pepper Oriental *(LaChoy)*	3/4 cup	100	7.0	12.0	1340	2.0	4.0	9
BEEF ENTRÉE, FREEZE-DRIED								
beef and rice w/onions, prepared								
(Mountain House)	1 cup	330	11.0	42.0	265	(mq)	12.0	(mq)
stew, prepared *(Mountain House)*	1 cup	260	16.0	26.0	75	(mq)	9.0	(mq)
BEEF ENTRÉE, FROZEN. See also BEEF DINNER, FROZEN.								
and broccoli, w/rice, 'Fresh & Lite'								
(LaChoy)	11 oz	260	17.0	42.0	1299	5.2	5.0	51
Cantonese, w/rice, 'Stir Fry'								
(Weight Watchers)	9 oz	200	14.0	27.0	530	na	4.0	15
casserole, 'Microwave Classic' *(Pillsbury)*	1 pkg	430	16.0	34.0	1100	(mq)	25.0	(mq)
champignon, 'Gourmet Selection'								
(Tyson)	10.5 oz	370	27.0	31.0	830	(mq)	15.0	(mq)
creamed, chipped *(Myers)*	3.5 oz	136	9.0	7.0	863	na	8.0	(mq)
creamed, chipped *(Stouffer's)*	5.5 oz	230	9.0	9.0	850	na	17.0	na
creamed, chipped, 'Cookin' Bag'								
(Banquet)	4 oz	100	7.0	9.0	(mq)	na	4.0	(mq)
creamed, chipped, 'Cook-In-Pouch'								
(Freezer Queen)	5 oz	80	5.0	11.0	500	(mq)	2.0	(mq)
Dijon, w/pasta and vegetables								
(Right Course)	9.5 oz	290	20.0	31.0	580	(mq)	9.0	40
fiesta, w/corn pasta *(Right Course)*	8 7/8 oz	270	18.0	33.0	590	(mq)	7.0	30
homestyle, w/noodles, gravy, and								
vegetable *(Stouffer's)*	8 3/8 oz	230	16.0	26.0	720	na	7.0	na
Jade garden, 'Stir Fry' *(Weight Watchers)*	9 oz	150	13.0	17.0	490	na	3.0	20
London broil *(Ultimate 200)*	7.5 oz	110	17.0	4.0	320	na	3.0	25
London broil, in mushroom sauce								
(Weight Watchers)	7.37 oz	140	18.0	9.0	510	na	3.0	40
Oriental, w/vegetables and rice								
(Lean Cuisine)	8 5/8 oz	290	20.0	31.0	590	na	9.0	40
patty, charbroiled, w/mushroom and								
onion gravy *(Banquet)*	8 oz	300	12.0	14.0	(mq)	na	21.0	(mq)
patty, charbroiled, w/ mushroom and								
onion gravy *(Freezer Queen)*	7 oz	200	13.0	10.0	960	na	12.0	(mq)
patty, charbroiled, w/mushroom gravy								
(Banquet)	8 oz	290	13.0	13.0	(mq)	na	21.0	(mq)
patty, charbroiled, w/mushroom gravy								
(Banquet)	5 oz	210	9.0	8.0	(mq)	na	15.0	(mq)
patty, charbroiled, w/ mushroom gravy								
(Freezer Queen)	7 oz	180	12.0	9.0	1050	na	11.0	(mq)
patty, charbroiled, w/ mushroom gravy								
(Freezer Queen)	5 oz	90	10.0	7.0	900	na	3.0	(mq)

Food Name	Serv. Size	Total Cal.	Prot. GMS	Carbs GMS	Sod. MGS	Fiber GMS	Fat GMS	Chol. MGS
pepper, Oriental (Chun King)	13 oz	310	17.0	53.0	1300	(mq)	3.0	(mq)
pie (Banquet)	7 oz	510	12.0	39.0	870	(mq)	33.0	25
pie (Myers)	3.5 oz	123	7.0	10.0	343	(mq)	6.0	(mq)
pie (Stouffer's)	10 oz	460	18.0	37.0	1130	na	27.0	na
pie, 'Supreme Microwave' (Banquet)	7 oz	440	14.0	30.0	730	(mq)	29.0	35
'Platters' (Banquet)	10 oz	460	22.0	20.0	630	(mq)	34.0	75
pot pie (Swanson)	7 oz	370	12.0	36.0	730	(mq)	19.0	(mq)
pot pie, 'Hungry Man' (Swanson)	16 oz	610	24.0	58.0	1360	(mq)	31.0	(mq)
ragoût, w/rice pilaf (Right Course)	10 oz	300	19.0	38.0	550	(mq)	8.0	50
rib, boneless, seasoned, w/barbecue sauce (Healthy Choice)	11 oz	330	28.0	40.0	530	na	6.0	70
Romanoff supreme, w/pasta and vegetables (Weight Watchers)	9 oz	230	12.0	29.0	540	na	7.0	20
Salisbury steak (Dining Lite)	9 oz	200	18.0	14.0	1000	na	8.0	55
Salisbury steak, charbroiled, w/vegetable medley 'Single Serve' (Freezer Queen)	9 oz	330	22.0	14.0	990	(mq)	22.0	(mq)
Salisbury steak, homestyle, w/gravy, macaroni and cheese (Stouffer's)	9 5/8 oz	350	25.0	23.0	1130	na	17.0	na
Salisbury steak, 'Homestyle Recipe' (Swanson)	10 oz	320	21.0	22.0	980	(mq)	16.0	(mq)
Salisbury steak, supreme 'Gourmet Selection' (Tyson)	10 oz	430	16.0	34.0	810	(mq)	26.0	(mq)
Salisbury steak, w/gravy 'Cook-In-Pouch' (Freezer Queen)	5 oz	160	9.0	7.0	850	na	11.0	(mq)
Salisbury steak, w/gravy 'Cookin' Bags' (Banquet)	5 oz	190	9.0	8.0	(mq)	na	14.0	(mq)
Salisbury steak, w/gravy 'Family Entrées' (Banquet)	8 oz	300	13.0	12.0	(mq)	na	22.0	(mq)
Salisbury steak, w/gravy 'Family Suppers' (Freezer Queen)	7 oz	200	13.0	9.0	1110	na	13.0	(mq)
Salisbury steak, w/gravy and scalloped potatoes (Lean Cuisine)	9.5 oz	240	23.0	22.0	580	na	7.0	45
Salisbury steak, w/mushroom gravy 'Classics' (Healthy Choice)	11 oz	280	21.0	35.0	500	na	6.0	55
sirloin roast (Budget Gourmet)	9.5 oz	330	13.0	36.0	700	(mq)	14.0	85
sirloin tips (Ultimate 200)	7.5 oz	200	20.0	20.0	560	na	6.0	30
sirloin tips, w/Burgundy sauce, Homestyle Recipe (Swanson)	7 oz	160	12.0	16.0	550	(mq)	5.0	(mq)
sirloin tips, w/country-style vegetables (Budget Gourmet)	10 oz	310	16.0	21.0	570	na	18.0	40
sliced beef, w/barbecue sauce, 'Cookin' Bag' (Banquet)	4 oz	100	9.0	11.0	(mq)	na	2.0	(mq)

Food Name	Serv. Size	Total Cal.	Prot. GMS	Carbs GMS	Sod. MGS	Fiber GMS	Fat GMS	Chol. MGS
sliced beef, w/gravy, 'Cookin' Bag' (Banquet)	4 oz	100	8.0	5.0	(mq)	na	5.0	(mq)
sliced beef, w/gravy, 'Cook-In-Pouch' (Freezer Queen)	4 oz	60	9.0	4.0	500	na	1.0	(mq)
sliced beef, w/gravy, 'Deluxe Family Suppers' (Freezer Queen)	7 oz	130	15.0	10.0	870	na	3.0	(mq)
sliced beef, w/gravy, 'Family Entrées' (Banquet)	8 oz	160	20.0	8.0	(mq)	(mq)	5.0	(mq)
steak, breaded (Hormel)	4 oz	370	14.0	13.0	(mq)	(mq)	30.0	(mq)
steak and mushroom hand-held pie, 'Aussie Pie' (Mrs. Paterson's)	5.5 oz	410	14.0	43.0	820	na	20.0	80
Szechuan (Chun King)	13 oz	340	20.0	57.0	1810	(mq)	3.0	(mq)
teriyaki (Chun King)	13 oz	380	22.0	68.0	2200	(mq)	2.0	(mq)
teriyaki (Dining Lite)	9 oz	270	20.0	36.0	850	(mq)	5.0	45
teriyaki, w/rice and vegetables, 'Fresh & Lite' (LaChoy)	10 oz	240	17.0	39.9	1198	2.0	5.0	57
stew, 'Family Entrées' (Banquet)	7 oz	140	6.0	18.0	(mq)	(mq)	5.0	(mq)
stew, 'Family Suppers' (Freezer Queen)	7 oz	150	9.0	15.0	820	(mq)	6.0	(mq)
BEEF ENTRÉE, MICROWAVE								
beef and mushrooms, 'Health Selections' micro cup (Hormel)	7 oz	210	21.0	25.0	390	na	3.0	45
ribs, boneless, microwave bowl (Top Shelf)	1 serving	440	28.0	29.0	550	(mq)	24.0	90
roast, tender, microwave bowl (Top Shelf)	1 serving	240	27.0	18.0	980	(mq)	7.0	65
roast beef, w/gravy and potatoes, 'American Classics' (Dinty Moore)	10 oz	260	26.0	26.0	910	na	6.0	45
Salisbury steak, w/potatoes, microwave bowl (Top Shelf)	1 serving	254	29.0	22.0	1211	(mq)	6.0	88
stew (Armour)	7.5 oz	150	10.0	15.0	870	na	5.0	na
stew, chunky, microwave cup (Weight Watchers)	7.5 oz	120	14.0	14.0	450	na	2.0	20
stew, 'Diner' microwave cup (Libby's)	7.75 oz	240	12.0	22.0	790	0	12.0	40
stew, hearty, 'Microeasy,' 1/4 pkg prepared w/1.5 lbs beef (Lipton)	1 serving	370	31.0	14.0	800	(mq)	20.0	(mq)
stew, hearty, microwave cup (Lunch Bucket)	7.5 oz	180	8.0	13.0	870	na	11.0	40
stew, micro cup (Hormel)	7.5 oz	230	13.0	11.0	1140	na	15.0	45
stew, microwave bowl (Dinty Moore)	10 oz	260	15.0	19.0	1180	na	14.0	45
stew, microwave cup (Dinty Moore)	7.5 oz	180	11.0	15.0	830	na	9.0	30
sukiyaki, microwave bowl (Top Shelf)	1 serving	330	24.0	36.0	1700	(mq)	10.0	45
w/macaroni, 'Diner' microwave cup (Libby's)	7.75 oz	230	10.0	34.0	670	2.5	6.0	20

Food Name	Serv. Size	Total Cal.	Prot. GMS	Carbs GMS	Sod. MGS	Fiber GMS	Fat GMS	Chol. MGS
BEEF ENTRÉE, PACKAGED								
Salisbury steak *(Top Shelf)* . . . . 10 oz		320	25.0	22.0	910	na	15.0	70
Salisbury steak, w/mushroom gravy								
(Ultra Slim Fast) . . . . 10.5 oz		290	19.0	44.0	830	na	5.0	35
BEEF JERKY								
'Arrowhead' *(Pemmican)* . . . . .7-oz piece		70	8.0	2.0	580	0	3.0	(mq)
'Big Jerk' *(Slim Jim)* . . . . .25-oz piece		25	3.0	1.0	220	0	1.0	(mq)
'Giant Jerk' *(Slim Jim)* . . . . .63-oz piece		60	7.0	2.0	510	0	2.0	(mq)
jalapeño *(Pemmican)* . . . . 1.3-oz piece		110	16.0	5.0	1150	0	3.0	(mq)
jalapeño *(Pemmican)* . . . . 1.1 oz		90	13.0	4.0	960	0	2.0	(mq)
jalapeño flavored steak *(Pemmican)* . . . . .25 oz		25	3.0	1.0	220	0	1.0	(mq)
'Lumberjack' *(Hormel)* . . . . 1 oz		101	5.0	0.0	304	0	9.0	(mq)
natural *(Pemmican)* . . . . 1.3-oz piece		110	16.0	5.0	1150	0	3.0	(mq)
natural *(Pemmican)* . . . . 1.1 oz		90	13.0	4.0	960	0	2.0	(mq)
natural *(Pemmican)* . . . . 1 oz		80	12.0	4.0	880	0	2.0	(mq)
natural flavored steak *(Pemmican)* . . . . . .25 oz		25	3.0	1.0	220	0	1.0	(mq)
peppered *(Pemmican)* . . . . 1.3-oz piece		110	16.0	5.0	1150	0	3.0	(mq)
peppered *(Pemmican)* . . . . 1.1 oz		90	13.0	4.0	960	0	2.0	(mq)
peppered steak *(Pemmican)* . . . . .25 oz		25	3.0	1.0	220	0	1.0	(mq)
regular *(Frito-Lay's)* . . . . .21 oz		25	3.0	1.0	200	0	1.0	10
regular *(Hickory Farms)* . . . . 1 oz		100	16.0	4.0	1360	0	3.0	73
regular *(Slim Jim)* . . . . .14-oz piece		20	2.0	1.0	120	0	1.0	(mq)
regular 'Super Jerk' approx .31 oz								
(Slim Jim) . . . . 1 piece		30	4.0	1.0	250	0	1.0	(mq)
'Steakers' *(Pemmican)* . . . . 1.1-oz pouch		80	14.0	4.0	470	0	1.0	(mq)
'Steakers' *(Pemmican)* . . . . 1 strip		40	5.0	2.0	160	0	1.0	(mq)
Tabasco *(Pemmican)* . . . . 1.3-oz piece		110	16.0	5.0	1150	0	3.0	(mq)
Tabasco *(Pemmican)* . . . . 1.1 oz		90	13.0	4.0	960	0	2.0	(mq)
Tabasco flavored steak *(Pemmican)* . . . . .25 oz		25	3.0	1.0	220	0	1.0	(mq)
Tabasco 'Super Jerk' *(Slim Jim)* . . .31-oz piece		30	4.0	1.0	250	0	1.0	(mq)
'Tender' *(Frito-Lay's)* . . . . .7 oz		120	5.0	2.0	370	0	10.0	25
'Tender Brave' *(Pemmican)* . . . . 1 oz		80	14.0	2.0	830	0	2.0	(mq)
'Tender Chief' *(Pemmican)* . . . . 1 oz		80	14.0	2.0	830	0	2.0	(mq)
'Tender Tomahawk' *(Pemmican)* . . .25-oz piece		20	3.0	1.0	210	0	1.0	(mq)
'Tender Trail' *(Pemmican)* . . . . 1 oz		80	14.0	2.0	830	0	2.0	(mq)
'Tender Tribe' *(Pemmican)* . . . . 1 oz		80	14.0	2.0	830	0	2.0	(mq)
teriyaki, natural style *(Pemmican)* . . . . 1 oz		80	12.0	4.0	800	0	2.0	(mq)
teriyaki, natural style *(Pemmican)* . . .25-oz piece		20	3.0	1.0	200	0	1.0	(mq)
teriyaki, natural style, slab *(Pemmican)* . . 1.3 oz		100	15.0	5.0	1030	0	2.0	(mq)
BEEF JERKY, ALTERNATIVE								
'Jerquee' vegetable protein product *(Stonewall's)* .5 oz		50	5.0	2.0	125	1.0	2.0	0
'Spicy Italian Style' *(Cajun Jerky)* . . . . .5 oz		50	5.0	2.0	125	1.0	2.0	0

BEEF POT PIE. See BEEF ENTRÉE, FROZEN.

Food Name	Serv. Size	Total Cal.	Prot. GMS	Carbs GMS	Sod. MGS	Fiber GMS	Fat GMS	Chol. MGS
BEEF SEASONING MIX								
(French's) dry ground, w/onions	1/4 pkg	25	1.0	6.0	440	na	0.0	0
(Lawry's) marinade	1 pkg	49	1.2	10.7	7284	>.1 c	0.2	0
(Schilling) Stroganoff	1/4 pkg	32	1.0	6.0	1078	na	0.3	na
BEEF STEW. See BEEF ENTRÉE, CANNED; BEEF ENTRÉE, DRIED; BEEF ENTRÉE, FROZEN; BEEF ENTRÉE, MICROWAVE.								
BEEF STEW MIX, hearty, 'Microeasy'								
(Lipton) dry	1/4 pkg	70	2.0	14.0	730	(mq)	<1.0	na
BEEF STEW SEASONING MIX								
(French's) dry mix	1/6 pkg	25	0.0	5.0	770	na	0.0	0
(Lawry's) 'Seasoning Blends'	1 pkg	131	5.4	25.7	3181	>1.2 c	0.7	0
(Schilling)	1/2 pkg	33	1.3	6.0	806	na	0.3	na
(Schilling) 'Bag'n Season'	1 pkg	87	7.5	11.0	4320	na	1.0	1
BEEF SUET, raw	1 oz	242	0.4	0.0	2	0	26.7	19
BEEF TALLOW								
	1 cup	1849	0.0	0.0	0	0	205.0	223
	1 oz	256	0.0	0.0	0	0	28.4	31
	1 tbsp	115	0.0	0.0	0	0	12.8	14
BEEFALO								
composite of cuts, diced, roasted	1 cup	263	42.9	0.0	115	0	8.8	81
composite of cuts, roasted	4 oz	213	34.8	0.0	93	0	7.2	66
raw	1 lb	649	105.7	0.0	354	na	21.8	200
raw	1 oz	40	6.5	0.0	22	na	1.3	12
roasted	3 oz	160	26.1	0.0	70	na	5.4	49
BEER. See ALCOHOLIC BEVERAGES.								
BEER, NONALCOHOLIC. See ALCOHOL-FREE BEVERAGES.								
BEER SALAMI. See LUNCHEON MEAT.								
BEERWURST								
beef	1 oz	92	3.5	0.5	264	0	8.3	16
beef, 4-inch diam	1/8-inch slice	76	2.8	0.4	236	0	6.9	14
beef, 2.75-inch diam	1/16-inch slice	20	0.7	0.1	62	0	1.8	4
pork	1 oz	67	4.0	0.6	352	0	5.3	17
pork, 4-inch diam	1/8-inch slice	55	3.3	0.5	285	0	4.3	14
pork, 2.75-inch diam	1/16-inch slice	14	0.9	0.1	74	0	1.1	4
pork, cured, 4-inch diam	1/8-inch slice	55	3.3	0.5	285	0	4.3	14
pork, cured, 2.75-inch diam	1/16-inch slice	14	0.9	0.1	74	0	1.1	4
BEET								
boiled, drained	4 oz	35	1.2	7.6	56	>1.0 c	0.1	0
boiled, drained, sliced	1/2 cup	37	1.4	8.5	65	1.4	0.2	0
raw, sliced	1/2 cup	29	1.1	6.5	53	1.9	0.1	0
raw, trimmed	1 oz	12	0.4	2.8	20	.3	<.1	0
raw, untrimmed	1 lb	133	4.5	30.4	220	3.0	0.4	0

Food Name	Serv. Size	Total Cal.	Prot. GMS	Carbs GMS	Sod. MGS	Fiber GMS	Fat GMS	Chol. MGS
BEET, CANNED								
cut *(Stokely)*	1/2 cup	40	1.0	8.0	300	(mq)	0.0	0
diced *(S&W)*	1/2 cup	40	1.0	9.0	270	(mq)	0.0	0
diced *(Stokely)*	1/2 cup	35	1.0	7.0	300	(mq)	0.0	0
Harvard *(Stokely)*	1/2 cup	70	1.0	18.0	135	(mq)	0.0	0
Harvard, sliced, w/liquid	1/2 cup	90	1.0	22.4	199	>.8 c	0.1	0
julienne *(S&W)*	1/2 cup	40	1.0	9.0	270	(mq)	0.0	0
'No Salt or Sugar Added' *(Stokely)*	1/2 cup	40	1.0	8.0	40	(mq)	0.0	0
pickled *(Freshlike)*	1/2 cup	40	1.0	9.0	650	na	0.0	na
pickled *(Stokely)*	1/2 cup	100	1.0	25.0	400	(mq)	0.0	0
pickled *(Veg·All)*	1/2 cup	100	1.0	25.0	650	na	0.0	na
pickled, crinkle sliced, w/liquid								
(Del Monte)	1/2 cup	80	1.0	19.0	375	(mq)	0.0	0
pickled 'Jars' *(Stokely)*	1/2 cup	90	1.0	22.0	280	(mq)	0.0	0
pickled, sliced, w/liquid	1/2 cup	74	0.9	18.6	301	>.7 c	0.1	0
pickled, sliced, w/red wine vinegar 'Party'								
(S&W)	1/2 cup	70	1.0	16.0	215	(mq)	0.0	0
pickled, sliced, w/red wine vinegar								
'Regular' *(S&W)*	1/2 cup	70	1.0	16.0	215	0.0	0.0	0
pickled, whole, extra small *(S&W)*	1/2 cup	70	1.0	16.0	215	(mq)	0.0	0
regular pack, w/liquid	1/2 cup	36	1.0	8.3	323	1.4	0.1	0
sliced *(A&P)*	1/2 cup	40	1.0	9.0	300	(mq)	<1.0	0
sliced *(Featherweight)*	1/2 cup	45	1.0	10.0	55	(mq)	0.0	0
sliced *(Finast)*	1/2 cup	40	1.0	9.0	390	(mq)	0.0	0
sliced *(Pathmark)*	1/2 cup	45	1.0	10.0	330	(mq)	0.0	0
sliced *(S&W Nutradiet)*	1/2 cup	35	1.0	9.0	40	(mq)	0.0	0
sliced *(Stokely)*	1/2 cup	40	1.0	8.0	300	(mq)	0.0	0
sliced, drained	1/2 cup	26	0.8	6.1	233	1.5	0.1	0
sliced, 'No Salt Added' *(A&P)*	1/2 cup	35	1.0	8.0	50	(mq)	<1.0	0
sliced, 'No Salt Added' *(Finast)*	1/2 cup	40	1.0	9.0	40	(mq)	0.0	0
sliced, 'No Salt Added' *(Pathmark)*	1/2 cup	35	1.0	7.0	35	(mq)	0.0	0
sliced, water packed, w/o salt								
(Freshlike)	1/2 cup	40	1.0	9.0	50	na	0.0	na
sliced, water packed, w/o sugar or salt								
(Freshlike)	1/2 cup	40	1.0	9.0	50	na	0.0	na
sliced, w/liquid, 'No Salt Added'								
(Del Monte)	1/2 cup	35	1.0	8.0	100	(mq)	0.0	0
small, sliced *(Freshlike)*	1/2 cup	40	1.0	9.0	260	na	0.0	na
small, sliced, 'Premium' *(S&W)*	1/2 cup	40	1.0	9.0	270	(mq)	0.0	0
small, whole *(Freshlike)*	1/2 cup	40	1.0	9.0	260	na	0.0	na
small, whole *(S&W)*	1/2 cup	40	1.0	9.0	270	(mq)	0.0	0
special dietary pack, w/liquid	1/2 cup	36	1.0	8.3	57	1.4	0.1	0
tiny, whole, w/liquid *(Del Monte)*	1/2 cup	35	1.0	8.0	290	(mq)	0.0	0

Food Name	Serv. Size	Total Cal.	Prot. GMS	Carbs GMS	Sod. MGS	Fiber GMS	Fat GMS	Chol. MGS
whole *(A&P)*	1/2 cup	40	1.0	9.0	300	(mq)	<1.0	0
whole *(IGA)*	1/2 cup	40	1.0	9.0	275	(mq)	0.0	0
whole *(Stokely)*	1/2 cup	40	1.0	8.0	300	(mq)	0.0	0
whole, sliced, w/liquid *(Del Monte)*	1/2 cup	35	1.0	8.0	290	(mq)	0.0	0
BEET GREENS								
boiled, drained	4 oz	31	2.9	6.2	273	>1.2 c	0.2	0
boiled, drained, 1-inch pieces	1/2 cup	19	1.9	3.9	174	2.1	0.1	0
raw, approx 2 oz	1 leaf	6	0.6	1.3	64	1.2	<.1	0
raw, 1-inch pieces	1/2 cup	4	0.4	0.8	38	.7	0.0	0
raw, untrimmed	1 lb	49	4.6	10.1	510	>3.3 c	0.2	0
raw, untrimmed	1 oz	5	0.5	1.1	57	>.4 c	<.1	0
BEET ROOT JUICE, bottled *(Biotta)*	6 oz	75	1.8	15.9	128	(mq)	0.1	0
BELLYFISH. See MONKFISH.								
BERLINER								
beef and pork	1 oz	65	4.3	0.7	368	0	4.9	13
beef and pork, 2.5 inch diam	1/4-inch slice	53	3.5	0.6	298	0	4.0	11
BERRY DRINK								
'Berries & Berries' *(Tropicana)*	6 oz	90	<1.0	23.0	20	na	<1.0	na
'Berries & Berries' juice *(Tropicana)*	10 oz	156	(tr)	39.0	3	(tr)	0.0	0
'Berry B. Wild' *(Squeezit)*	6.75 oz	120	0.0	29.0	5	na	0.0	na
berry blend juice, 'Fruit Box' *(Tang)*	8.45 oz	140	0.0	36.0	10	na	0.0	0
berry citrus drink, frozen, prepared								
(Five Alive)	6 oz	90	0.0	22.0	5	na	0.0	na
berry juice, bottled *(Juicy Juice)*	6 oz	90	1.0	22.0	10	na	0.0	na
berry juice, boxed *(Juicy Juice)*	8.45 oz	130	1.0	30.0	15	na	0.0	na
berry juice, canned *(Juicy Juice)*	6 oz	90	0.0	22.0	10	(mq)	0.0	0
berry nectar, organic *(Santa Cruz Natural)*	8 oz	90	<1.0	22.0	na	na	<1.0	na
berry punch, aseptic box or chilled								
(Minute Maid)	6 oz	90	0.0	23.0	20	na	0.0	na
berry punch, frozen concentrate								
(Minute Maid)	6 oz	90	0.0	23.0	0	na	0.0	na
'Bopin' Berry' *(Hi-C)*	6 oz	90	0.0	23.0	25	na	0.0	na
'Great Bluedini' *(Kool-Aid)* 'Kool Bursts'	6.75 oz	110	0.0	28.0	10	na	0.0	0
'Great Bluedini' *(Kool-Aid)* 'Koolers'	8.45 oz	110	0.0	29.0	10	na	0.0	0
Mountain Berry Punch *(Kool-Aid)*								
'Koolers'	8.45 oz	140	0.0	37.0	10	na	0.0	0
'Very Berry' *(Hawaiian Punch)*	6 oz	90	0.0	22.0	30	(tr)	0.0	0
BERRY DRINK MIX								
berry blend, sugar-free w/NutraSweet, prepared								
(Crystal Light)	8 oz	4	0.0	0.0	0	na	0.0	0
'Berry Blue' sugar-free w/NutraSweet, prepared								
(Kool-Aid)	8 oz	4	0.0	0.0	5	na	0.0	0

Food Name	Serv. Size	Total Cal.	Prot. GMS	Carbs GMS	Sod. MGS	Fiber GMS	Fat GMS	Chol. MGS
'Berry Blue' sugar-sweetened, prepared (Kool-Aid)	8 oz	80	0.0	21.0	5	na	0.0	0
'Berry Blue' unsweetened, prepared w/sugar (Kool-Aid)	8 oz	100	0.0	25.0	0	na	0.0	0
'Berry Blue' unsweetened, prepared w/o sugar (Kool-Aid)	8 oz	2	0.0	0.0	0	na	0.0	0
'Great Bluedini' sugar-free w/NutraSweet, prepared (Kool-Aid)	8 oz	4	0.0	0.0	0	na	0.0	0
'Great Bluedini' sugar-sweetened, prepared (Kool-Aid)	8 oz	70	0.0	18.0	0	na	0.0	0
'Great Bluedini' unsweetened, prepared w/sugar (Kool-Aid)	8 oz	100	0.0	25.0	0	na	0.0	0
'Great Bluedini' unsweetened, prepared w/o sugar (Kool-Aid)	8 oz	2	0.0	0.0	0	na	0.0	0
Mountain Berry Punch, sugar-free w/NutraSweet, prepared (Kool-Aid)	8 oz	4	0.0	0.0	35	na	0.0	0
Mountain Berry Punch, sugar-sweetened, prepared (Kool-Aid)	8 oz	80	0.0	20.0	15	na	0.0	0
Mountain Berry Punch, unsweetened, prepared w/sugar (Kool-Aid)	8 oz	100	0.0	25.0	15	na	0.0	0
Mountain Berry Punch, unsweetened, prepared w/o sugar (Kool-Aid)	8 oz	2	0.0	0.0	15	na	0.0	0
'Surfin' Berry' sugar-free w/NutraSweet, prepared (Kool-Aid)	8 oz	4	0.0	0.0	10	na	0.0	0
'Surfin' Berry' unsweetened, prepared w/sugar (Kool-Aid)	8 oz	100	0.0	25.0	25	na		
'Surfin' Berry' unsweetened, prepared w/o sugar (Kool-Aid)	8 oz	2	0.0	0.0	25	na	0.0	0

BEVERAGES. See ALCOHOL-FREE BEVERAGES; ALCOHOLIC BEVERAGES; COFFEE; DIET DR MILK; SOFT DRINKS AND MIXERS; SPORTS DRINK; TEA; WATER; and individual listings.

BIBB LETTUCE. See LETTUCE.

BISCUIT

Food Name	Serv. Size	Total Cal.	Prot. GMS	Carbs GMS	Sod. MGS	Fiber GMS	Fat GMS	Chol. MGS
buttermilk, commercially baked	1 oz	103	1.8	13.8	298	na	4.7	0
mixed grain, dough, baked	1 oz	86	2.0	15.6	221	na	1.8	0
plain, commercially baked	1 oz	103	1.8	13.8	298	na	4.7	0
(Awrey's) country	3-inch biscuit	160	4.0	23.0	530	1.0	5.0	0
(Awrey's) round	1 oz	80	2.0	12.0	260	0	3.0	0
(Awrey's) sliced	2 oz	160	4.0	23.0	520	1.0	5.0	0
(Awrey's) square	1 oz	80	2.0	12.0	260	0	3.0	0
(Awrey's) unsliced	2 oz	160	4.0	23.0	520	1.0	5.0	0
(Mrs. Winner's)	1 biscuit	245	4.0	45.0	503	na	5.0	na
(Weight Watchers) buttermilk	1.8 oz	100	3.0	23.0	410	na	1.0	na
(Wonder)	1 biscuit	80	2.0	14.0	140	.6	1.0	na

Food Name	Serv. Size	Total Cal.	Prot. GMS	Carbs GMS	Sod. MGS	Fiber GMS	Fat GMS	Chol. MGS
BISCUIT, FROZEN (Bridgford)	2 oz	180	4.0	28.0	632	(mq)	6.0	1
BISCUIT, REFRIGERATED								
(Ballard) buttermilk, extra lights, 'Ovenready'	1 biscuit	50	1.0	10.0	180	na	0.0	0
(Ballard) buttermilk, 'Ovenready'	1 biscuit	50	1.0	10.0	180	(mq)	1.0	na
(Ballard) extra lights, 'Ovenready'	1 biscuit	50	1.0	10.0	180	na	0.0	0
(Ballard) 'Ovenready'	1 biscuit	50	1.0	10.0	180	(mq)	1.0	0
(Big Country) 'Butter Tastin'	1 biscuit	100	2.0	14.0	320	(mq)	4.0	0
(Big Country) buttermilk	1 biscuit	100	2.0	14.0	320	(mq)	4.0	0
(Big Country) Southern style	1 biscuit	100	2.0	14.0	320	(mq)	4.0	0
(1869 Brand) baking powder	1 biscuit	100	2.0	12.0	310	(mq)	5.0	0
(1869 Brand) 'Butter Tastin'	1 biscuit	100	2.0	12.0	300	(mq)	5.0	0
(1869 Brand) buttermilk	1 biscuit	100	2.0	12.0	310	(mq)	5.0	0
(Good 'N Buttery) fluffy	1 biscuit	90	1.0	11.0	270	(mq)	5.0	0
(Grands Inch) 'Butter Tastin'	1 biscuit	190	4.0	22.0	560	na	9.0	0
(Grands Inch) cinnamon raisin	1 biscuit	190	3.0	27.0	540	na	7.0	0
(Grands Inch) flaky	1 biscuit	190	4.0	23.0	530	na	8.0	0
(Hungry Jack) buttermilk, 'Extra Rich'	1 biscuit	50	1.0	9.0	180	(mq)	1.0	0
(Hungry Jack) buttermilk, flaky	1 biscuit	90	2.0	12.0	300	(mq)	4.0	0
(Hungry Jack) buttermilk, fluffy	1 biscuit	90	2.0	12.0	280	(mq)	4.0	0
(Hungry Jack) flaky, 'Butter Tastin'	1 biscuit	90	2.0	11.0	280	(mq)	4.0	0
(Hungry Jack) flaky	1 biscuit	80	2.0	12.0	300	(mq)	4.0	0
(Hungry Jack) honey, flaky, 'Honey Tastin'	1 biscuit	90	2.0	13.0	290	(mq)	4.0	0
(Hungry Jack) Southern style, flaky	1 biscuit	80	2.0	12.0	300	na	4.0	0
(Pillsbury) 'Big Premium Heat 'n Eat'	2 biscuits	280	5.0	32.0	610	(mq)	15.0	0
(Pillsbury) butter	1 biscuit	50	1.0	10.0	180	(mq)	1.0	0
(Pillsbury) buttermilk, 'Heat 'n Eat'	2 biscuits	170	4.0	27.0	530	(mq)	5.0	0
(Pillsbury) buttermilk	1 biscuit	50	1.0	10.0	180	(mq)	1.0	0
(Pillsbury) buttermilk, 'Tender Layer'	1 biscuit	50	1.0	9.0	170	(mq)	1.0	0
(Pillsbury) 'Country'	1 biscuit	50	1.0	10.0	180	(mq)	1.0	0
(Roman Meal) oat bran, honey nut	1 biscuit	131	2.4	19.7	278	.9	4.7	0
(Roman Meal) white	2 biscuits	180	4.2	32.2	456	1.4	3.8	0
(Roman Meal) white, 'Premium'	1 biscuit	127	2.4	18.8	308	(mq)	4.7	0
BISCUIT, TOASTER								
(Oroweat) 'Australian'	1 biscuit	180	6.0	30.0	440	1.0	5.0	0
(Oroweat) cinnamon raisin	1 biscuit	200	5.0	34.0	410	1.0	5.0	0
(Oroweat) cornbread	1 biscuit	200	5.0	39.0	230	1.0	3.0	5
BISCUIT MIX								
(Arrowhead Mills)	2 oz	100	4.0	19.0	96	(mq)	1.0	0
(Bisquick)	1/2 cup	240	4.0	37.0	700	(mq)	8.0	0
(Gold Medal) 'Pouch Mix,' prepared w/skim milk	1/8 recipe	90	2.0	14.0	270	(mq)	3.0	0

Food Name	Serv. Size	Total Cal.	Prot. GMS	Carbs GMS	Sod. MGS	Fiber GMS	Fat GMS	Chol. MGS
(Health Valley) buttermilk, 'Biscuit & Pancake'	1 oz	100	4.0	20.0	170	3.3	1.0	0
(Krusteaz) cinnamon raisin, w/glaze, prepared from mix	3-inch biscuit	200	2.0	39.0	150	1.0	4.0	0
(Krusteaz) prepared from mix	2-inch biscuit	90	2.0	14.0	260	na	3.0	1
(Martha White) prepared from mix, 'BixMix,' made w/2% milk, rolled	2-inch biscuit	90	2.0	15.0	240	na	2.0	2
(Robin Hood) 'Pouch Mix,' prepared w/skim milk	1/8 recipe	90	2.0	14.0	270	(mq)	3.0	0
BLACK BEAN								
boiled	4 oz	150	10.0	26.9	1	4.8	0.6	0
boiled	1/2 cup	114	7.6	20.4	1	7.5	0.5	0
raw	1/2 cup	331	21.0	60.5	5	14.7	1.4	0
raw	1 oz	97	6.1	17.7	1	3.7	0.4	0
raw *(Arrowhead Mills)*	2 oz	190	13.0	35.0	9	11.3	1.0	0
BLACK BEAN, CANNED								
(Eden Foods) organic, very low sodium, no salt added	1/2 cup	70	7.0	17.0	15	6.0	<1.0	0
(Green Giant)	1/2 cup	90	7.0	21.0	580	6.0	0.0	0
(Joan of Arc)	1/2 cup	90	7.0	21.0	580	6.0	0.0	0
(Progresso)	1/2 cup	90	9.0	19.0	350	6.5	1.0	0
BLACK BEAN DINNER, CANNED								
Western, w/garden vegetables, 'Fast Menu' *(Health Valley)*	7.5 oz	120	13.0	14.0	170	14.5	1.0	0
BLACK BEAN MIX, INSTANT								
prepared w/o added ingredients *(Fantastic Foods)*	1/2 cup	157	10.0	28.0	400	(mq)	2.0	na
prepared w/2 tbsp salted butter *(Fantastic Foods)*	1/2 cup	207	10.0	28.0	469	(mq)	8.0	(mq)
BLACK CHERRY DRINK MIX								
unsweetened, prepared w/sugar *(Kool-Aid)*	8 oz	100	0.0	25.0	0	na	0.0	0
unsweetened, prepared w/o sugar *(Kool-Aid)*	8 oz	2	0.0	0.0	0	na	0.0	0
BLACK CHERRY JUICE								
(Knudsen & Sons)	8 oz	150	2.0	38.0	na	na	0.0	na
(Smucker's) 'Naturally 100%'	8 oz	130	0.0	31.0	10	(mq)	0.0	0
BLACK PUDDING. See BLOOD SAUSAGE.								
BLACK TURTLE BEAN								
boiled	1/2 cup	120	7.5	22.4	3	4.9	0.3	0
canned	1/2 cup	109	7.2	19.9	461	>1.4 c	0.4	0
raw	1/2 cup	312	19.5	58.2	8	22.9	0.8	0
BLACK WALNUT FLAVOR DRINK								
canned, liquid nutrition *(Ensure)*	8 oz	250	8.8	34.3	na	na	8.8	na

Food Name	Serv. Size	Total Cal.	Prot. GMS	Carbs GMS	Sod. MGS	Fiber GMS	Fat GMS	Chol. MGS
BLACKBERRY								
raw	1/2 cup	37	0.5	9.2	0	3.6	0.3	0
trimmed	1 oz	15	0.2	3.6	tr	1.3	0.1	0
untrimmed	1 lb	225	3.1	56.0	1	19.7	1.7	0
BLACKBERRY, CANNED								
in heavy syrup	4 oz	104	1.5	26.2	3	>2.9 c	0.2	0
in heavy syrup, w/liquid	1/2 cup	118	1.7	29.6	4	4.3	0.2	0
in water (Allens)	1/2 cup	25	1.0	4.0	15	(mq)	<1.0	0
BLACKBERRY, FROZEN								
unsweetened	18-oz pkg	326	6.0	79.9	5	25.5	2.2	0
unsweetened	1 cup	97	1.8	23.7	2	7.6	0.7	0
unsweetened	1/2 cup	49	0.9	11.8	1	>2.0 c	0.3	0
BLACKBERRY SYRUP (Knott's Berry Farm)	1 oz	120	0.0	30.0	0	na	0.0	na
BLACK-EYED PEAS/cowpeas/yellow-eyed peas								
boiled, drained	1/2 cup	79	2.6	16.7	3	4.1	0.3	0
boiled, drained	4 oz	110	3.6	23.1	5	5.7	0.4	0
leafy tips, boiled, drained	4 oz	25	5.3	3.2	7	>3.0 c	0.1	0
leafy tips, raw, chopped	1/2 cup	5	0.7	0.9	1	>.2 c	<.1	0
leafy tips, raw, trimmed	1 oz	8	1.2	1.4	2	>.4 c	0.1	0
leafy tips, raw, untrimmed	1 lb	68	9.7	11.4	16	>3.1 c	0.6	0
raw, in pods	1 lb	208	6.8	43.7	9	>4.2 c	0.8	0
raw, trimmed	1 oz	26	0.8	5.4	1	>.5 c	0.1	0
raw, trimmed	1/2 cup	65	2.1	13.6	3	>1.3 c	0.3	0
young pods w/seeds, raw, approx 11 7/8 inches x 5/16 inch	1 pod	5	0.4	1.1	tr	>.2 c	<.1	0
young pods, w/seeds, raw, trimmed	1 oz	12	0.9	2.7	1	>.5 c	0.1	0
young pods, w/seeds, raw, trimmed	1/2 cup	21	1.6	4.5	2	>.8 c	0.1	0
young pods, w/seeds, raw, untrimmed	1 lb	182	13.6	39.2	17	>7.0 c	1.2	0
BLACK-EYED PEAS, CANNED								
(A&P) mature	7.5 oz	120	7.0	20.0	410	(mq)	1.0	(mq)
(Allens)	1/2 cup	100	7.0	18.0	370	(mq)	<1.0	0
(Allens) mature	1/2 cup	105	5.0	18.0	300	(mq)	1.0	(mq)
(Allens) w/snaps	1/2 cup	100	5.0	20.0	370	(mq)	<1.0	0
(Bush's Best) packed from fresh shelled	1/2 cup	70	5.0	16.0	350	3.0	0.0	na
(Bush's Best) packed from soaked dry	1/2 cup	70	5.0	16.0	350	3.0	0.0	na
(Bush's Best) seasoned w/bacon	1/2 cup	90	7.0	16.0	420	3.0	1.0	na
(Green Giant) mature	1/2 cup	90	7.0	18.0	300	4.0	1.0	0
(Joan of Arc) mature	1/2 cup	90	7.0	18.0	300	4.0	1.0	0
(Luck's) mature, w/pork	1/2 cup	200	11.0	25.0	760	7.0	6.0	(mq)
BLACK-EYED PEAS, DRIED								
mature, boiled	1/2 cup	100	6.7	17.9	3	8.3	0.5	0
mature, boiled	4 oz	132	8.8	23.6	5	10.9	0.6	0
mature, boiled (A&P)	1 cup	230	15.0	41.0	15	(mq)	1.0	0

Food Name	Serv. Size	Total Cal.	Prot. GMS	Carbs GMS	Sod. MGS	Fiber GMS	Fat GMS	Chol. MGS
mature, raw	1 oz	95	6.7	17.0	5	7.7	0.4	0
mature, raw	1/2 cup	283	19.8	50.4	14	22.7	1.1	0
BLACK-EYED PEAS, FROZEN								
	10-oz pkg	396	25.5	71.4	17	>4.6 c	2.0	0
boiled, drained	1/2 cup	112	7.2	20.2	5	>1.3 c	0.6	0
boiled, drained	4 oz	150	9.6	26.9	6	>1.7 c	0.7	0
(Freshlike)	3.3 oz	130	9.0	23.0	5	na	1.0	na
(Frosty Acres)	3.3 oz	130	9.0	23.0	6	>1.0 c	1.0	0
(Seabrook)	3.3 oz	130	9.0	23.0	6	>1.0 c	1.0	0
(Southern)	3.5 oz	136	8.9	24.2	20	(mq)	0.7	0
(Veg•All)	3.3 oz	130	9.0	23.0	5	na	1.0	na
BLINTZ								
(Golden) blueberry	1 blintz	90	2.0	18.0	150	na	1.0	10
(Golden) cheese, low fat	1 blintz	80	6.0	13.0	135	na	2.0	13
(Golden) cherry	1 blintz	95	3.0	18.0	145	na	1.0	5
(King Kold) frozen	2.5 oz	113	6.0	18.9	272	(mq)	1.6	(mq)
(King Kold) frozen 'No Salt Added'	1.5 oz	96	6.4	18.6	78	(mq)	0.5	(mq)
BLOOD PUDDING. See BLOOD SAUSAGE.								
BLOOD SAUSAGE/black pudding/blood pudding								
	1 oz	107	4.1	0.4	193	0	9.8	34
approx 5 inches x 4 5/8 inches .. 1/16-inch slice		94	3.7	0.3	170	0	8.6	30
BLOODY MARY. See ALCOHOLIC BEVERAGES.								
BLOODY MARY MIX. See ALCOHOL-FREE BEVERAGES.								
BLUEBERRY								
trimmed	1 pint	225	2.7	56.8	24	9.3	1.5	0
trimmed	1 cup	81	1.0	20.5	9	3.3	0.6	0
trimmed	1/2 cup	41	0.5	10.2	5	1.7	0.3	0
trimmed	1 oz	16	0.2	4.0	2	.7	0.1	0
untrimmed	1 lb	250	3.0	62.8	27	10.2	1.7	0
untrimmed	1 pint	226	2.7	56.8	24	9.2	1.5	0
BLUEBERRY, CANNED								
in heavy syrup	4 oz	100	0.7	25.0	3	1.7	0.4	0
in heavy syrup (A&P)	1/2 cup	110	<1.0	28.0	25	(mq)	<1.0	0
in heavy syrup (S&W)	1/2 cup	111	0.0	30.0	10	(mq)	0.0	0
in heavy syrup, w/liquid	1/2 cup	113	0.8	28.2	4	1.9	0.4	0
in water (Lucky Leaf)	4 oz	40	0.0	9.0	0	(mq)	0.0	0
in water (Musselman's)	4 oz	40	0.0	9.0	0	(mq)	0.0	0
BLUEBERRY, FROZEN								
sweetened	10-oz pkg	230	1.1	62.3	3	6.0	0.4	0
sweetened	1/2 cup	94	0.5	25.2	2	2.5	0.2	0
unsweetened	20-oz pkg	289	2.4	69.0	6	15.3	3.6	0
unsweetened	1 cup	79	0.7	18.9	2	4.2	1.0	0
unsweetened	1/2 cup	39	0.3	9.4	1	2.5	0.5	0

Food Name	Serv. Size	Total Cal.	Prot. GMS	Carbs GMS	Sod. MGS	Fiber GMS	Fat GMS	Chol. MGS
BLUEBERRY NECTAR (Knudsen & Sons) ..	8 oz	135	<1.0	34.0	na	na	0.0	na
BLUEBERRY SYRUP								
(Estee) 'Breakfast'	1 tbsp	12	0.0	3.0	10	na	0.0	0
(Featherweight)	1 tbsp	16	0.0	4.0	35	(tr)	0.0	0
(Knott's Berry Farm)	1 oz	120	0.0	30.0	0	na	0.0	na
(Knott's Berry Farm) 'Light'	1 oz	50	0.0	12.0	0	na	0.0	na
(Knudsen & Sons)	1 oz	75	<1.0	19.0	na	na	<1.0	na
BLUEFISH								
dry-heat cooked	3 oz	135	21.8	0.0	65	0	4.6	65
raw	1 lb	562	90.9	0.0	272	0	19.2	266
raw	3 oz	105	17.0	0.0	51	0	3.6	50
raw	1 oz	35	5.7	0.0	17	0	1.2	17
BLUEGILL								
raw	1 lb	404	88.0	0.0	368	0	3.2	304
raw	1.7-oz fillet	43	9.3	0.0	38	0	0.3	32
raw	1 oz	25	5.5	0.0	23	0	0.2	19
BOBWHITE. See QUAIL.								
BOCKWURST								
	1 oz	87	3.8	0.1	313	0	7.8	17
7 links per lb	1 link	200	8.7	0.3	718	0	17.9	38
BOK CHOY								
boiled, drained	4 oz	14	1.8	2.0	39	1.8	0.2	0
boiled, drained, shredded	1/2 cup	10	1.3	1.5	29	1.4	0.1	0
raw, shredded	1 cup	9	1.0	1.5	46	.7	0.1	0
raw, shredded	1/2 cup	5	0.5	0.8	23	.4	0.1	0
raw, shredded (Dole)	1/2 cup	5	1.0	1.0	23	na	0.1	na
raw, trimmed	1 oz	4	0.4	0.6	19	.3	0.1	0
raw, untrimmed	1 lb	52	6.0	8.7	257	4.0	0.8	0
BOLOGNA. See LUNCHEON MEAT.								
BONITO. See also TUNA, SKIPJACK.								
Caribbean, raw	1 lb	626	106.6	0.0	(mq)	0	19.1	(mq)
Caribbean, raw	1 oz	39	6.7	0.0	(mq)	0	1.2	(mq)
Japanese, raw	1 lb	585	117.0	1.8	200	0	9.1	(mq)
Japanese, raw	1 oz	37	7.3	0.1	12	0	0.6	(mq)
BORAGE								
boiled, drained	4 oz	28	2.4	4.0	98	>1.2 c	0.9	0
boiled, drained	3.5 oz	25	2.1	3.5	88	>1.1 c	0.8	0
raw, 1-inch pieces	1/2 cup	9	0.8	1.4	35	>.4 c	0.3	0
raw, trimmed	1 oz	6	0.5	0.9	23	>.3 c	0.2	0
raw, untrimmed	1 lb	76	6.5	11.1	290	>3.3 c	2.5	0
BORECOLE. See KALE.								
BORLOTTI BEAN. See CRANBERRY BEAN.								
BOSTON CREAM PIE. See CAKE.								

Food Name	Serv. Size	Total Cal.	Prot. GMS	Carbs GMS	Sod. MGS	Fiber GMS	Fat GMS	Chol. MGS
BOTTLE GOURD. See GOURD, BOTTLE.								
BOUILLON. See SOUP.								
BOURBON. See ALCOHOLIC BEVERAGES.								
BOYSENBERRY, CANNED, in heavy								
syrup	1/2 cup	113	1.3	28.6	4	3.3	0.2	0
BOYSENBERRY, FROZEN								
unsweetened, unthawed	10-oz pkg	142	3.1	34.6	3	11.1	0.7	0
unsweetened, unthawed	1 cup	66	1.5	16.1	1	5.2	0.3	0
BOYSENBERRY DRINK								
boysenberry juice, 'Naturally 100%'								
(Smucker's)	8 oz	120	0.0	30.0	10	(mq)	0.0	0
boysenberry nectar (Knudsen & Sons)	8 oz	110	<1.0	33.0	na	na	0.0	na
BOYSENBERRY SYRUP								
(Knott's Berry Farm)	1 oz	120	0.0	30.0	0	na	0.0	na
(Knott's Berry Farm) 'Light'	1 oz	50	0.0	12.0	0	na	0.0	na
BRAMBLE. See RASPBERRY.								
BRANDY. See ALCOHOLIC BEVERAGES.								
BRATWURST								
(Eckrich)	1 link	310	11.0	1.0	820	0	30.0	(mq)
(Hickory Farms) 'Brotwurst'	1 oz	90	4.0	1.0	277	0	8.0	8
(Hickory Farms) cheddar, 'Cheddy Brots'	1 oz	98	4.0	1.0	259	0	9.0	7
(Hillshire Farm) fresh	2 oz	190	7.0	1.0	410	0	17.0	(mq)
(Hillshire Farm) 'Fully Cooked'	2 oz	170	7.0	1.0	380	0	16.0	(mq)
(Hickory Farms) hot, 'Hot Brots'	1 oz	96	4.0	1.0	269	0	9.0	8
(Hillshire Farm) smoked	2 oz	190	8.0	1.0	540	0	17.0	(mq)
(Hillshire Farm) spicy	2 oz	180	8.0	1.0	(mq)	0	17.0	(mq)
(Kahn's)	1 link	190	7.0	2.0	490	0	17.0	(mq)
BRAUNSCHWEIGER								
(Hormel)	1 oz	80	4.0	0.0	322	0	7.0	(mq)
(JM)	1 oz	80	3.0	2.0	260	0	6.0	(mq)
(Oscar Mayer) 'German Brand'	1 oz	96	4.0	0.5	329	0	8.7	45
(Oscar Mayer) liver sausage	1 oz	100	4.0	<1.0	230	na	9.0	50
(Oscar Mayer) 'Slices'	1 oz	96	3.9	0.6	327	0	8.7	50
(Oscar Mayer) 'Tube'	1 oz	97	3.9	0.7	301	0	8.7	47
BRAZIL NUT/butternut/cream nut/paranut								
in shell, unblanched	1 lb	1428	31.2	27.9	3	>5.0 c	144.2	0
shelled, unblanched, approx 6–8 kernels	1 oz	186	4.1	3.6	tr	>.7 c	18.8	0
shelled, unblanched, approx 32 kernels	1 cup	919	20.1	17.9	2	8.0	92.7	0
BREAD. See also BAGEL; BISCUIT; BUN; CROISSANT; ENGLISH MUFFIN; ROLL; MUFFIN/PASTRY, TOASTER.								
APPLE-WALNUT (Arnold)	1 slice	64	2.1	12.6	103	1.3	1.3	1
BARBECUE, 'BBQ Loaf' (Colombo Brand)	2 oz	139	7.9	23.5	318	(mq)	1.6	na

Food Name	Serv. Size	Total Cal.	Prot. GMS	Carbs GMS	Sod. MGS	Fiber GMS	Fat GMS	Chol. MGS
BRAN								
and oat, 'Light' (Oatmeal Goodness)	1 slice	40	2.0	6.0	90	(mq)	<1.0	0
'Bran'nola' (Brownberry)	1 slice	85	3.9	17.5	137	2.9	1.4	tr
'Bran'nola Original' (Arnold)	1 slice	85	3.9	17.5	137	2.9	1.4	tr
'Gold'N Bran' (Earth Grains)	1 oz	70	3.0	12.0	150	na	1.0	0
honey bran, '1.5-lb loaf' (Pepperidge Farm)	1 slice	90	3.0	18.0	160	1.0	1.0	0
original, natural 'Bran'nola' (Oroweat)	1 slice	100	4.0	19.0	160	2.0	1.0	0
raisin (Brownberry)	1 slice	61	2.2	12.4	108	1.8	1.3	0
BROWN								
Boston, w/white corn meal, 3.25 inch diam	1/2-inch slice	95	2.5	20.5	113	>.3 c	0.6	0
Boston, w/yellow corn meal, 3.25 inch diam	1/2-inch slice	95	2.5	20.5	113	>.3 c	0.6	0
canned (B&M)	1.6 oz	94	2.0	22.0	320	2.0	0.0	0
canned (Friends)	1.6 oz	94	2.0	22.0	320	2.0	0.0	0
canned, Boston	1 oz	55	1.5	12.3	179	1.3	0.4	0
canned, 'New England' (S&W)	2 slices	76	2.0	17.0	172	(mq)	0.0	0
canned, raisin (B&M)	1.6 oz	92	2.0	21.0	345	2.0	0.0	0
canned, raisin (Friends)	1.6 oz	92	2.0	21.0	345	2.0	0.0	0
plain (B&M)	1/2-inch slice	92	2.0	21.0	345	2.0	0.0	0
plain (Friends)	1/2-inch slice	92	2.0	21.0	345	2.0	0.0	0
raisin (B&M)	1/2-inch slice	94	2.0	22.0	320	2.0	0.0	0
raisin (Friends)	1/2-inch slice	94	2.0	22.0	320	2.0	0.0	0
BUTTERMILK								
(Grant's Farm)	1-oz slice	70	3.0	12.0	190	na	1.0	0
(Oroweat)	1 slice	100	4.0	20.0	210	1.0	1.0	0
CRESCENT (Pillsbury)	1 serving	100	2.0	11.0	230	na	6.0	0
CRISP, hard crispbread or toast	4 oz	473	15.6	80.2	278	>.2 c	9.8	10
EGG	1 oz	81	2.7	13.5	139	na	1.7	14
FRENCH								
enriched	1 oz	78	2.5	14.7	173	.8	0.9	0
enriched, 5 inches x 2.5 inches	1 slice	101	3.2	19.4	203	>.1 c	1.0	1
extra sour (Colombo Brand)	2 oz	150	7.7	26.9	311	(mq)	1.3	0
extra sour, sliced (Colombo Brand)	2 oz	153	7.6	27.2	310	(mq)	1.6	0
'Hearth' (Pepperidge Farm)	1 oz	75	2.5	14.0	160	.5	1.0	0
'Parisian' (DiCarlo)	1 slice	70	3.0	13.0	180	.7	1.0	na
sweet, 'French Stick' (Colombo Brand)	2 oz	154	7.2	27.1	331	(mq)	1.9	na
twin (Farm Hearth)	1 oz	80	3.0	15.0	160	0	1.0	0
unenriched, 5 inches x 2.5 inches	1 slice	101	3.2	19.4	203	>.1 c	1.0	1
GARLIC (Colombo Brand)	2 oz	185	6.2	17.3	331	(mq)	10.1	na
GRAIN								
'Bran'nola' (Arnold)	1 slice	85	3.9	17.4	144	3.0	1.6	tr

Food Name	Serv. Size	Total Cal.	Prot. GMS	Carbs GMS	Sod. MGS	Fiber GMS	Fat GMS	Chol. MGS
'Bran'nola Nutty Grains' (Brownberry) ...	1 slice	85	3.9	17.4	144	3.0	1.6	tr
honey grain (Grant's Farm)	1-oz slice	70	3.0	13.0	170	na	1.0	0
honey grain, 'Family Recipe' (Colonial)	1-oz slice	70	3.0	14.0	180	na	1.0	0
honey grain, 'Family Recipe' (Kilpatrick's)	1-oz slice	70	3.0	14.0	180	na	1.0	0
honey grain, 'Family Recipe' (Rainbo)	1-oz slice	70	3.0	14.0	180	na	1.0	0
5-grain, organic (BreadMill Bakery)	1 slice	122	6.0	23.0	298	na	1.0	0
mixed grain, 'Round Top' (Roman Meal)	1 slice	67	2.9	13.2	140	1.2	0.8	0
mixed grain, 'Thin Sliced Sandwich' (Roman Meal)	1 slice	55	2.4	10.7	114	1.0	0.7	0
mixed grain, toasted	1 oz	77	3.1	14.3	150	na	1.2	0
mixed grain, whole grain	1 oz	71	2.8	13.1	138	2.0	1.1	0
multi-grain (Hearty Grains)	1 slice	80	2.0	15.0	230	1.0	2.0	0
multi-grain (Weight Watchers)	1 slice	40	2.0	9.0	100	(mq)	<1.0	0
9-grain, 'Light' (Oroweat)	1 slice	40	2.0	10.0	135	2.0	0.0	0
7-grain (Aunt Hattie's)	1 slice	100	4.0	17.0	200	na	2.0	0
7-grain (Grant's Farm)	1-oz slice	60	3.0	13.0	140	na	1.0	0
7-grain, 'Hearty Slice' (Pepperidge Farm)	2 slices	180	5.0	36.0	340	2.0	2.0	0
7-grain, 'Light' (Grant's Farm)	.75-oz slice	40	2.0	9.0	115	na	<1.0	0
'Sun Grain' (Roman Meal)	1 slice	68	3.2	12.3	140	1.7	1.4	0
12-grain (Earth Grains)	1 oz	70	3.0	13.0	140	na	1.0	0
12-grain (Oroweat)	1 slice	110	5.0	20.0	210	1.0	2.0	0
GRANOLA, oat and honey (Pepperidge Farm)	1 slice	60	2.0	12.0	105	2.0	2.0	0
HAWAIIAN (King's Hawaiian Bread)	2 oz	180	6.0	30.0	160	2.0	4.0	20
HEALTH NUT								
(Brownberry)	1 slice	71	2.3	12.4	158	2.5	2.6	0
(Oroweat)	1 slice	110	4.0	20.0	200	2.0	2.0	0
HIGH-CALCIUM								
dark	1 oz	69	2.8	13.9	161	na	0.7	0
light	1 oz	64	2.4	12.5	196	1.4	0.6	0
HOLLYWOOD								
'Dark' (Hollywood)	1 slice	70	3.0	13.0	160	.8	1.0	na
'Light' (Hollywood)	1 slice	70	3.0	13.0	150	.7	1.0	na
HONEY NUT, and oat bran (Aunt Hattie's)	1 slice	100	5.0	16.0	180	1.0	na	0
HONEY OAT NUT (Earth Grains)	1 oz	80	3.0	14.0	85	na	2.0	0
HONEY WHEAT BRAN (Grant's Farm)	1-oz slice	70	3.0	14.0	120	na	1.0	0
HONEY WHEATBERRY								
(Earth Grains)	1 oz	70	3.0	12.0	160	na	1.0	0
(Oroweat)	1 slice	90	3.0	17.0	180	2.0	1.0	0
INDIAN FRY, Navajo, 5 inch diam	1 slice	296	6.4	48.0	626	gna	8.6	0

Food Name	Serv. Size	Total Cal.	Prot. GMS	Carbs GMS	Sod. MGS	Fiber GMS	Fat GMS	Chol. MGS
ITALIAN								
'Family' (Wonder)	1 slice	70	2.0	13.0	160	.7	1.0	na
'Francisco International' (Arnold)	1-oz slice	72	2.9	14.1	190	.8	1.1	0
'Hearth' (Pepperidge Farm)	1 oz	80	2.0	14.0	150	0	1.0	0
'Hi-Fibre' (Monk's)	1 slice	70	3.0	13.0	80	1.4	1.0	0
light, 'Bakery' (Arnold)	1 slice	45	2.4	9.9	90	2.0	0.5	tr
'Light' (Brownberry)	1 slice	44	2.3	9.9	89	2.0	0.5	tr
thick sliced, 'Francisco International' (Arnold)	1 slice	66	2.3	13.7	111	.9	0.8	0
OAT								
'Bran'nola Country' (Arnold)	1 slice	90	3.7	17.8	166	2.8	2.0	tr
'Bran'nola Country' (Brownberry)	1 slice	90	3.7	17.8	166	2.8	2.0	tr
country oat, 'Light' (Oroweat)	1 slice	40	2.0	10.0	135	2.0	0.0	0
crunchy (Pepperidge Farm)	2 slices	190	8.0	34.0	290	3.0	4.0	0
split top, 'Family Recipe' (Colonial)	1-oz slice	70	3.0	13.0	140	na	1.0	0
split top, 'Family Recipe' (Kilpatrick's)	1-oz slice	70	3.0	13.0	140	na	1.0	0
split top, 'Family Recipe' (Rainbo)	1-oz slice	70	3.0	13.0	140	na	1.0	0
OAT BRAN								
country oat, natural, 'Bran'nola' (Oroweat)	2 slices	230	8.0	39.0	390	3.0	4.0	0
honey (Roman Meal)	1 slice	71	3.2	12.7	130	.9	1.2	0
honey (Earth Grains)	1 oz	80	3.0	13.0	105	na	1.0	0
honey, w/whole wheat, organic (BreadMill Bakery)	1 slice	121	5.0	23.0	315	na	1.0	0
honey nut (Roman Meal)	1 slice	72	3.3	12.1	130	1.0	1.6	0
organic, 'Light' (BreadMill Bakery)	1 slice	113	4.0	22.0	229	na	1.0	0
plain (Awrey's)	1 slice	50	2.0	10.0	130	1.0	0.0	0
plain (Grant's Farm)	1-oz slice	70	3.0	14.0	140	na	1.0	0
plain (Weight Watchers)	1 slice	40	1.0	10.0	100	(mq)	<1.0	0
'Split-Top' (Roman Meal)	1 slice	68	2.9	13.2	140	1.1	0.9	0
OATMEAL								
cinnamon (Oatmeal Goodness)	1 slice	90	4.0	15.0	140	1.0	2.0	0
country twists (Hearty Grains)	1 slice	80	2.0	15.0	120	1.0	2.0	0
light, 'Bakery' (Arnold)	1 slice	44	2.3	9.6	98	1.9	0.6	tr
light, 'Light Style' (Pepperidge Farm)	1 slice	45	2.0	9.0	95	1.0	0.0	0
'1.5 lb loaf' (Pepperidge Farm)	1 slice	90	3.0	17.0	200	1.0	1.0	0
plain (Pepperidge Farm)	1 slice	70	2.0	12.0	160	1.0	1.0	0
raisin, 'Hearty Grain' (Pillsbury)	1 slice	90	2.0	16.0	210	1.0	2.0	0
toasted almond (Grant's Farm)	1-oz slice	80	3.0	14.0	135	na	1.0	0
'Very Thin' (Pepperidge Farm)	1 slice	40	1.0	8.0	80	0	1.0	0
w/bran (Oatmeal Goodness)	1 slice	90	4.0	15.0	140	1.0	2.0	0
w/sunflower seed (Oatmeal Goodness)	1 slice	90	4.0	15.0	140	1.0	2.0	0
OATNUT (Orowheat)	1 slice	100	3.0	18.0	200	1.0	2.0	0

Food Name	Serv. Size	Total Cal.	Prot. GMS	Carbs GMS	Sod. MGS	Fiber GMS	Fat GMS	Chol. MGS
PITA								
oat bran *(Sahara)*	1/2 pita	66	2.4	15.3	163	1.8	0.3	0
onion, no fats, no oils, pre-sliced, 1.2 oz								
(Kangaroo)	1 pocket	75	4.0	15.0	160	na	0.0	0
white *(Sahara)*	1/2 pita	79	2.9	15.6	147	(mq)	0.5	0
white, enriched	1 oz	78	2.6	15.8	152	.5	0.3	0
white, enriched	1 pita	165	5.5	33.4	322	1.0	0.7	0
white, mini *(Sahara)*	1 pita	79	2.9	15.6	147	(mq)	0.5	0
white, unenriched	1 oz	78	2.6	15.8	152	.5	0.3	0
white, unenriched	1 pita	165	5.5	33.4	322	1.0	0.7	0
whole-wheat	1 oz	75	2.8	15.6	151	2.1	0.7	0
whole-wheat	1 pita	170	6.3	35.2	340	4.8	1.7	0
whole-wheat, approx 2 oz *(Sahara)*	1 pita	150	6.0	28.0	320	>.7 c	2.0	0
PROTEIN, includes gluten	1 oz	69	3.4	12.4	155	na	0.6	0
PUMPERNICKEL								
	1 oz	71	2.5	13.5	190	1.7	0.9	0
'Family' *(Pepperidge Farm)*	1 slice	80	3.0	15.0	230	2.0	1.0	0
plain *(Arnold)*	1 slice	70	2.7	14.7	198	1.3	0.9	0
small, 'Party' *(Pepperidge Farm)*	4 slices	60	2.0	12.0	160	1.0	1.0	0
RAISIN								
cinnamon *(Arnold)*	1 slice	67	2.1	12.9	86	.8	1.4	2
cinnamon *(Brownberry)*	1 slice	66	2.2	12.8	107	.9	1.3	tr
cinnamon *(Monk's)*	1 slice	70	3.0	10.0	85	(mq)	2.0	0
cinnamon *(Pepperidge Farm)*	1 slice	90	2.0	16.0	100	2.0	2.0	0
cinnamon swirl *(Pepperidge Farm)*	1 slice	90	2.0	16.0	100	1.0	2.0	0
orange *(Brownberry)*	1 slice	67	2.3	13.0	83	.8	1.2	tr
unenriched	1 oz	84	2.4	16.1	120	na	1.4	0
walnut *(Brownberry)*	1 slice	68	2.2	11.4	96	2.3	2.7	tr
walnut, royal *(Northridge)*	1 slice	90	2.0	16.0	90	na	2.0	na
whole wheat, organic *(BreadMill Bakery)*	1 slice	120	5.0	24.0	327	na	1.0	0
RICE BRAN								
golden *(Monk's)*	1 slice	70	3.0	14.0	80	1.6	1.0	0
honey nut *(Roman Meal)*	1 slice	71	2.6	12.8	127	1.3	1.6	0
plain *(Roman Meal)*	1 slice	70	2.8	12.4	132	1.3	1.5	0
RYE								
caraway, 'Natural' *(Brownberry)*	1 slice	73	2.8	15.4	185	1.2	0.8	0
Dijon *(Pepperidge Farm)*	1 slice	50	2.0	9.0	170	1.0	1.0	0
Dijon, 'Hearty' *(Pepperidge Farm)*	1 slice	70	3.0	15.0	260	2.0	1.0	0
dill *(Arnold)*	1 slice	71	2.8	14.4	187	1.3	1.0	0
'Hearty' *(Beefsteak)*	1 slice	70	3.0	13.0	180	.7	1.0	na
hearty rye, 'Light' *(Oroweat)*	1 slice	40	2.0	10.0	135	2.0	0.0	0
honey cracked *(Grant's Farm)*	1-oz slice	70	3.0	13.0	190	na	1.0	0
Jewish, seeded *(Levy's)*	1 slice	76	2.8	15.9	181	1.4	0.9	0

Food Name	Serv. Size	Total Cal.	Prot. GMS	Carbs GMS	Sod. MGS	Fiber GMS	Fat GMS	Chol. MGS
Jewish, seedless *(Levy's)*	1 slice	75	2.8	16.0	178	1.3	0.8	0
'Mild' *(Beefsteak)*	1 slice	70	3.0	13.0	180	.7	1.0	na
'Old Allegheny' *(Braun's)*	1 slice	70	3.0	13.0	160	.7	1.0	0
onion *(Beefsteak)*	1 slice	70	3.0	12.0	170	1.0	1.0	0
plain *(Weight Watchers)*	1 slice	40	2.0	10.0	100	(mq)	<1.0	0
seeded, 'Family' *(Pepperidge Farm)*	1 slice	80	3.0	16.0	220	2.0	1.0	0
seedless, 'Family' *(Pepperidge Farm)*	1 slice	80	3.0	16.0	210	2.0	1.0	0
seedless, 'Natural Thin Sliced' *(Brownberry)*	1 slice	45	1.7	9.8	118	.8	0.6	0
small, 'Party' *(Pepperidge Farm)*	4 slices	60	2.0	12.0	250	1.0	1.0	0
'Soft' *(Beefsteak)*	1 slice	70	3.0	13.0	170	.9	1.0	0
very thin, light *(Earth Grains)*	1 oz	70	3.0	14.0	230	na	1.0	0
wheatberry *(Beefsteak)*	1 slice	70	3.0	13.0	160	1.0	1.0	0
SOURDOUGH								
French *(Boudin)*, approx 2-oz slices	2 slices	130	5.0	27.0	297	(mq)	1.0	0
'Light' *(Earth Grains)*	.75 oz	40	2.0	9.0	115	na	1.0	0
'Light' *(Rainbo)*	.75-oz slice	40	2.0	9.0	110	2.0	<1.0	0
plain *(DiCarlo)*	1 slice	70	3.0	12.0	140	.7	1.0	0
SUNFLOWER								
and bran *(Monk's)*	1 slice	70	3.0	12.0	80	1.6	1.0	0
'Texas Toast' *(Golden Corral)*	1 serving	170	5.0	26.0	230	na	6.0	0
whole wheat, organic *(BreadMill Bakery)*	1 slice	129	6.0	21.0	287	na	2.0	0
VIENNA								
light, 'Light Style' *(Pepperidge Farm)*	1 slice	45	2.0	10.0	100	1.0	0.0	0
thick sliced, 'Hearth' *(Pepperidge Farm)*	1 slice	70	2.0	13.0	125	0	1.0	0
WHEAT								
	1 oz	74	2.6	13.4	150	1.2	1.2	0
apple honey *(Brownberry)*	1 slice	69	2.3	11.4	148	1.5	1.9	0
'Brick Oven' *(Arnold)*	1 slice	57	2.4	10.6	104	1.7	1.5	tr
'Butter Top' *(Home Pride)*	1 slice	70	3.0	13.0	140	.8	1.0	na
buttertop *(Aunt Hattie's)*	1 slice	70	3.0	13.0	140	na	1.0	<5
cracked	1 oz	74	2.5	14.0	153	1.5	1.1	0
cracked *(Earth Grains)*	1 oz	70	2.0	12.0	180	na	1.0	0
cracked *(Pepperidge Farm)*	1 slice	70	2.0	13.0	140	1.0	1.0	0
cracked *(Wonder)*	1 slice	70	3.0	13.0	180	.8	1.0	na
cracked wheat and honey twists *(Hearty Grains)*	1 serving	80	2.0	14.0	120	1.0	2.0	0
dark, 'Bran'nola' *(Arnold)*	1 slice	83	4.1	17.6	166	2.8	1.0	tr
'Family Recipe' *(Colonial)*	1-oz slice	70	3.0	14.0	150	na	1.0	0
'Family Recipe' *(Kilpatrick's)*	1-oz slice	70	3.0	14.0	150	na	1.0	0
'Family Recipe' *(Rainbo)*	1-oz slice	70	3.0	14.0	150	na	1.0	0
'Family', 2-lb loaf *(Pepperidge Farm)*	1 slice	70	2.0	13.0	130	2.0	1.0	0
fat-free, 'Light' *(Wonder)*	1 slice	40	3.0	7.0	120	na	<1.0	0

Food Name	Serv. Size	Total Cal.	Prot. GMS	Carbs GMS	Sod. MGS	Fiber GMS	Fat GMS	Chol. MGS
'Hearth' (Brownberry)	1 oz	70	3.1	13.6	150	2.0	1.4	0
'Hearty' (Beefsteak)	1 slice	70	3.0	11.0	160	1.4	1.0	0
hearty, 'Bran'nola' (Arnold)	1 slice	88	3.8	17.1	197	2.7	1.9	tr
hearty, 'Bran'nola' (Brownberry)	1 slice	88	3.8	17.1	197	2.7	1.9	tr
honey buttered, split top, 'Family Recipe' (Colonial)	1-oz slice	70	3.0	14.0	140	na	1.0	0
honey buttered, split top, 'Family Recipe' (Kilpatrick's)	1-oz slice	70	3.0	14.0	140	na	1.0	0
honey buttered, split top, 'Family Recipe' (Rainbo)	1-oz slice	70	3.0	14.0	140	na	1.0	0
honey wheatberry (Arnold)	1 slice	77	3.1	16.5	143	2.4	1.2	tr
'Light' (Grant's Farm)	.75-oz slice	40	2.0	9.0	115	na	<1.0	0
'Light' (Rainbo)	.75-oz slice	40	2.0	9.0	100	2.0	<1.0	0
light, golden, 'Bakery' (Arnold)	1 slice	44	2.3	9.5	86	2.0	0.5	tr
'Light Style' (Pepperidge Farm)	1 slice	45	2.0	9.0	90	1.0	0.0	0
'Light 35' (Earth Grains)	1 oz	35	2.0	8.0	100	na	<1.0	0
loaf (Pipin' Hot)	1-inch slice	70	2.0	12.0	170	na	2.0	0
multi-grain (Beefsteak)	1 slice	70	3.0	11.0	130	1.6	1.0	0
'Natural' (Brownberry)	1 slice	80	3.0	17.0	183	2.3	1.3	0
oatmeal (Oatmeal Goodness)	1 slice	90	4.0	15.0	140	1.0	2.0	0
oatmeal, 'Light' (Oatmeal Goodness)	1 slice	40	2.0	6.0	90	(mq)	<1.0	0
1.5-lb loaf (Pepperidge Farm)	1 slice	90	3.0	18.0	190	2.0	2.0	0
plain (Country Grain)	1 slice	70	3.0	12.0	160	1.3	1.0	na
plain (Fresh & Natural)	1 slice	70	3.0	13.0	140	1.8	1.0	0
plain (Weight Watchers)	1 slice	40	2.0	9.0	100	(mq)	<1.0	0
sesame, 'Hearty' (Pepperidge Farm)	2 slices	190	7.0	36.0	340	3.0	3.0	0
'7-Grain' (Home Pride)	1 slice	70	3.0	12.0	140	.8	1.0	na
'Soft' (Beefsteak)	1 slice	70	3.0	12.0	160	1.6	1.0	0
soft (Brownberry)	1 slice	74	2.8	13.1	127	1.0	1.8	tr
soft, made w/buttermilk (Aunt Hattie's)	1 slice	70	3.0	12.0	130	na	1.0	na
sprouted (Pepperidge Farm)	1 slice	70	3.0	11.0	100	2.0	2.0	0
stone ground (Grant's Farm)	1-oz slice	60	3.0	12.0	150	na	1.0	0
stone ground, 'Family Recipe' (Colonial)	1-oz slice	70	3.0	14.0	150	na	1.0	0
stone ground, 'Family Recipe' (Kilpatrick's)	1-oz slice	70	3.0	14.0	150	na	1.0	0
stone ground, 'Family Recipe' (Rainbo)	1-oz slice	70	3.0	14.0	150	na	1.0	0
'Stoneground' (Home Pride)	1 slice	70	3.0	12.0	140	1.9	1.0	0
very thin (Earth Grains)	1 oz	70	2.0	13.0	150	na	1.0	0
WHEAT GERM	1 oz	74	2.7	13.7	157	na	0.8	0
WHEATBERRY (Grant's Farm)	1-oz slice	70	3.0	13.0	150	na	1.0	0

Food Name	Serv. Size	Total Cal.	Prot. GMS	Carbs GMS	Sod. MGS	Fiber GMS	Fat GMS	Chol. MGS
WHITE								
....	1 oz	76	2.3	14.0	153	.7	1.0	0
'Brick Oven' (Arnold)	1 slice	61	2.2	11.3	134	.8	1.2	tr
'Butter Top' (Home Pride)	1 slice	70	3.0	13.0	140	.7	1.0	na
buttermilk (Wonder)	1 slice	70	2.0	13.0	160	.7	1.0	na
buttertop, 'Homestyle' (Aunt Hattie's) ...	1 slice	70	3.0	13.0	140	na	1.0	0
'Country White' (Arnold)	1 slice	98	3.4	18.6	204	1.0	1.8	tr
enriched, 'Country Style' (Holsum)	1 slice	70	2.0	14.0	135	na	1.0	0
extra fiber, 'Brick Oven' (Arnold)	1 slice	55	2.2	12.1	93	2.1	0.8	tr
'Hearty Country' (Pepperidge Farm) ...	2 slices	190	7.0	38.0	340	2.0	2.0	0
'High Fiber' (Wonder)	1 slice	40	2.0	6.0	80	2.9	0.0	0
honey buttered, split-top, 'Family Recipe' (Colonial)	1-oz slice	80	3.0	14.0	140	na	1.0	0
honey buttered, split-top, 'Family Recipe' (Kilpatrick's)	1-oz slice	80	3.0	14.0	140	na	1.0	0
honey buttered, split-top, 'Family Recipe' (Rainbo)	1-oz slice	80	3.0	14.0	140	na	1.0	0
'Large Family,' 2-lb loaf (Pepperidge Farm)	1 slice	70	2.0	13.0	150	0	1.0	0
'Light' (Grant's Farm)	.75-oz slice	40	2.0	9.0	115	na	<1.0	0
'Light' (Rainbo)	.75-oz slice	40	2.0	9.0	100	2.0	<1.0	na
'Light' (Wonder)	1 slice	40	3.0	7.0	110	2.0	0.0	0
'Light Premium' (Arnold)	1 slice	42	2.3	9.6	89	2.2	0.5	tr
'Light Premium' (Brownberry)	1 slice	42	2.3	9.6	89	2.2	0.5	tr
'Light 35' (Earth Grains)	1 oz	35	2.0	8.0	105	na	<1.0	0
'Natural' (Brownberry)	1 slice	59	2.2	11.1	136	.6	1.1	tr
old fashioned (Northridge)	1 slice	70	2.0	13.0	125	na	1.0	na
plain (Monk's)	1 slice	60	3.0	10.0	95	(mq)	1.0	0
plain (Weight Watchers)	1 slice	40	2.0	10.0	100	(mq)	<1.0	0
plain (Wonder)	1 slice	70	3.0	13.0	140	.7	1.0	na
'Robust' (Beefsteak)	1 slice	70	3.0	13.0	140	.7	1.0	na
sandwich (Pepperidge Farm)	2 slices	130	4.0	24.0	260	0	2.0	0
special recipe, 'Iron Kids' (Rainbo)	1 slice	60	3.0	13.0	140	2.0	1.0	0
thin (Holsum)	1 slice	70	2.0	14.0	160	na	1.0	0
'Thin Sliced' (Wonder)	1 slice	50	2.0	10.0	120	.5	1.0	0
'Thin Sliced,' 1-lb size (Pepperidge Farm)	1 slice	80	2.0	14.0	130	0	2.0	0
toasting (Pepperidge Farm)	1 slice	90	3.0	17.0	200	1.0	1.0	0
very thin (Earth Grains)	1 oz	80	2.0	14.0	160	na	1.0	0
'Very Thin' (Pepperidge Farm)	1 slice	40	1.0	8.0	80	0	0.0	0
white loaf (Pipin' Hot)	1-inch slice	70	2.0	12.0	170	na	2.0	0
w/buttermilk, 'Homestyle' (Aunt Hattie's)	1 slice	80	3.0	13.0	140	na	1.0	na
WHOLE BRAN, 'Natural' (Brownberry) ...	1 slice	58	2.3	11.7	167	2.1	1.4	0

Food Name	Serv. Size	Total Cal.	Prot. GMS	Carbs GMS	Sod. MGS	Fiber GMS	Fat GMS	Chol. MGS
WHOLE WHEAT								
....	1 oz	70	2.8	13.1	149	2.0	1.2	0
'Family' *(Wonder)*	1 slice	70	3.0	13.0	140	.8	1.0	na
'High Fiber' *(Wonder)*	1 slice	40	2.0	6.0	80	2.9	0.0	0
'Light' *(Wonder)*	1 slice	40	3.0	7.0	120	2.0	0.0	0
100% *(Northridge)*	1 slice	60	3.0	11.0	120	2.0	1.0	0
'100% Stone Ground' *(Monk's)*	1 slice	70	3.0	13.0	110	(mq)	1.0	0
100% whole wheat *(Earth Grains)*	1 oz	70	3.0	11.0	150	na	1.0	0
'100%' *(Wonder)*	1 slice	70	3.0	12.0	160	1.8	1.0	na
plain *(Aunt Hattie's)*	1 slice	90	4.0	14.0	170	na	2.0	0
plain *(Daily)*	2-oz slice	140	6.0	26.0	0	(mq)	0.0	0
'Soft 100%' *(Wonder)*	1 slice	70	4.0	10.0	140	1.8	1.0	0
'Stoneground 100%' *(Arnold)*	1 slice	48	2.4	9.9	97	1.6	0.7	tr
stoneground, 100% *(Oroweat)*	1 slice	60	3.0	11.0	125	2.0	1.0	0
'Thin Sliced', 1-lb loaf *(Pepperidge Farm)*	1 slice	60	2.0	12.0	110	2.0	1.0	0
'Very Thin' *(Pepperidge Farm)*	1 slice	35	2.0	7.0	75	0	0.0	0
BREAD, BROWN AND SERVE								
'Austrian' *(Du Jour)*	1 oz	70	3.0	13.0	140	.6	1.0	0
'French' *(Du Jour)*	1 oz	70	3.0	13.0	140	.6	1.0	0
'Italian' *(Pepperidge Farm)*	1 oz	80	2.0	14.0	150	0	1.0	0
BREAD, QUICK, MIX								
APPLE CINNAMON								
(Pillsbury) mix only, dry	1/12 pkg	140	2.0	30.0	160	na	1.0	0
(Pillsbury) prepared as directed	1/12 loaf	170	3.0	27.0	200	(mq)	6.0	na
(Pillsbury) prepared w/1/4 cup oil, 1/4 cup egg substitute	1/12 loaf	190	2.0	31.0	170	na	6.0	0
(Pillsbury) prepared w/water, 1/4 cup oil, 1 egg	1/12 loaf	180	2.0	31.0	170	na	6.0	20
(Pillsbury) prepared w/water, 1/4 cup oil, 1/4 cup egg substitute	1/12 loaf	190	2.0	31.0	170	na	6.0	0
BANANA								
(Pillsbury) mix only, dry	1/12 pkg	120	2.0	27.0	190	na	1.0	0
(Pillsbury) prepared w/water, 3 tbsp oil, 1/2 cup egg substitute	1/12 loaf	170	2.0	27.0	210	na	6.0	0
(Pillsbury) prepared w/water, 3 tbsp oil, and 2 eggs	1/12 loaf	170	3.0	27.0	200	na	5.0	35
BANANA NUT *(Krusteaz)* prepared as directed	3/4-inch slice	190	3.0	33.0	300	2.0	6.0	3
BLUEBERRY NUT								
(Pillsbury) mix only, dry	1/12 pkg	130	2.0	29.0	160	na	1.0	0
(Pillsbury) prepared as directed	1/12 loaf	150	2.0	26.0	150	(mq)	4.0	na
(Pillsbury) prepared w/1/4 cup oil, 1/4 cup egg substitute	1/12 loaf	180	2.0	30.0	170	na	6.0	0

Food Name	Serv. Size	Total Cal.	Prot. GMS	Carbs GMS	Sod. MGS	Fiber GMS	Fat GMS	Chol. MGS
(Pillsbury) prepared w/water, 1/4 cup oil, 1 egg	1/12 loaf	180	2.0	30.0	160	na	6.0	20
(Pillsbury) prepared w/water, 1/4 cup oil, 1/4 cup egg substitute	1/12 loaf	180	2.0	30.0	170	na	6.0	0
CHERRY NUT *(Pillsbury)* prepared as directed	1/12 loaf	180	3.0	29.0	150	(mq)	5.0	na
CORNBREAD								
(Aunt Jemima) 'Easy,' prepared as directed	1 piece	196	3.5	32.7	679	1.4	6.3	13
(Ballard) mix only, dry	1/16 pkg	120	2.0	24.0	560	na	2.0	0
(Ballard) prepared as directed	1/8 pan	140	3.0	25.0	570	(mq)	3.0	na
(Ballard) prepared w/1 cup milk, 1 egg	1/16 pan	150	4.0	25.0	580	na	3.0	30
(Dromedary) mix only, dry	3 tbsp	100	2.0	19.0	280	(mq)	2.0	na
(Dromedary) prepared as directed	2-inch square	130	3.0	20.0	480	(mq)	3.0	na
(Gold Medal) white, 'Pouch Mix, prepared w/egg and whole milk	1/6 pan	150	4.0	22.0	490	(mq)	5.0	(mq)
(Gold Medal) yellow, 'Pouch Mix,' prepared w/egg and whole milk	1/6 pan	150	4.0	23.0	500	(mq)	5.0	(mq)
(Krusteaz) honey, prepared as directed	1/16 pan	120	2.0	21.0	230	na	3.0	17
(Krusteaz) Southern, prepared as directed	2-inch square	140	3.0	27.0	450	na	3.0	8
(Martha White) buttermilk, prepared w/water	1/6 pan	110	2.0	21.0	360	na	2.0	0
(Martha White) 'Cotton Pickin' prepared as directed	1/4 pan	170	3.0	31.0	540	(mq)	3.0	2
(Martha White) 'Cotton Pickin' prepared w/water	1/6 pan	110	2.0	21.0	360	na	2.0	0
(Martha White) Mexican, prepared w/2% milk	1/6 pan	140	2.0	24.0	410	na	4.0	25
(Martha White) yellow, 'Light Crust,' prepared as directed	2 oz	140	4.0	21.0	400	(mq)	4.0	26
(Robin Hood) white, 'Pouch Mix,' prepared w/egg and whole milk	1/6 pan	150	4.0	22.0	490	(mq)	5.0	(mq)
CRANBERRY								
(Pillsbury) mix only, dry	1/12 pkg	140	2.0	30.0	150	na	1.0	0
(Pillsbury) prepared as directed	1/12 loaf	160	2.0	30.0	160	(mq)	4.0	na
(Pillsbury) prepared w/water, 2 tbsp oil, 1 egg	1/12 loaf	160	2.0	30.0	150	na	4.0	20
(Pillsbury) prepared w/water, 2 tbsp oil, 1/4 cup egg substitute	1/12 loaf	170	3.0	30.0	160	na	4.0	0
DATE								
(Pillsbury) prepared w/water, 1 tbsp oil, 1 egg	1/12 pkg	160	2.0	32.0	150	na	3.0	0

Food Name	Serv. Size	Total Cal.	Prot. GMS	Carbs GMS	Sod. MGS	Fiber GMS	Fat GMS	Chol. MGS
(Pillsbury) prepared w/water, 1 tbsp oil,								
1/4 cup egg substitute	1/12 loaf	160	2.0	32.0	150	na	3.0	0
DATE NUT								
(Dromedary) mix only, dry	1/12 pkg	166	2.0	26.0	242	(mq)	7.0	na
(Dromedary) prepared as directed	1/12 loaf	183	2.0	26.0	248	(mq)	8.0	na
GINGERBREAD								
(Betty Crocker) 'Classic' mix only, dry	1/9 pkg	200	2.0	35.0	320	na	6.0	0
(Betty Crocker) 'Classic,' prepared								
w/cholesterol-free egg product	1/9 pan	210	3.0	35.0	330	(mq)	6.0	0
(Betty Crocker) 'Classic,' prepared								
w/egg	1/9 pan	220	3.0	35.0	330	(mq)	7.0	30
(Dromedary) mix only, dry	3 tbsp	100	1.0	19.0	190	(mq)	2.0	na
(Pillsbury) mix only, dry	1/9 pkg	180	2.0	32.0	300	na	5.0	0
(Pillsbury) prepared as directed	3-inch square	190	2.0	36.0	310	(mq)	4.0	na
NUT								
(Pillsbury) mix only, dry	1/12 pkg	150	3.0	27.0	180	na	3.0	0
(Pillsbury) prepared w/water, 2 tbsp oil,								
1 egg	1/12 loaf	170	3.0	27.0	190	na	6.0	20
(Pillsbury) prepared w/water, 2 tbsp oil,								
1/4 cup egg substitute	1/12 loaf	170	3.0	28.0	190	na	6.0	0
OATMEAL RAISIN								
(Pillsbury) mix only, dry	1/12 pkg	140	3.0	30.0	170	na	2.0	0
(Pillsbury) prepared w/water, 1/4 cup oil,								
1 egg	1/12 loaf	190	3.0	30.0	180	na	7.0	20
(Pillsbury) prepared w/water, 1/4 cup oil,								
1/4 cup egg substitute	1/12 loaf	190	3.0	30.0	180	na	7.0	0
BREAD CRUMBS								
Italian style *(Devonsheer)*	1 oz	104	3.6	21.1	408	.9	1.3	0
Italian style *(Progresso)*	2 tbsp	60	2.0	11.0	240	(mq)	<1.0	0
Italian style, whole-wheat *(Jaclyn's)*	.5 oz	28	4.0	13.0	5	(mq)	1.0	0
plain	1 cup	427	13.5	78.3	931	4.5	5.8	0
plain	1 oz	112	3.5	20.6	244	1.2	1.5	0
plain *(Devonsheer)*	1 oz	108	3.9	21.6	272	.9	1.4	0
plain *(Progresso)*	2 tbsp	60	2.0	11.0	110	(mq)	<1.0	0
seasoned	1 cup	440	17.0	84.5	3180	na	3.1	2
seasoned	1 oz	104	4.0	20.0	751	na	0.7	1
seasoned *(Contadina)*	1 cup	426	16.5	81.5	2970	.7	3.6	na
seasoned *(Contadina)*	1 tbsp	35	1.0	7.0	250	.1	<1.0	na
BREAD DOUGH								
cornbread twists, refrigerated *(Pillsbury)*	1 twist	70	1.0	8.0	150	(mq)	4.0	0
French, crusty, refrigerated *(Pillsbury)*	1-inch slice	60	2.0	11.0	120	(mq)	<1.0	0
honey walnut, frozen *(Bridgford)*	1 oz	76	3.0	13.8	152	(mq)	0.9	0
refrigerated *(Roman Meal)*	1 oz	85	2.3	12.6	199	.6	2.8	0

Food Name	Serv. Size	Total Cal.	Prot. GMS	Carbs GMS	Sod. MGS	Fiber GMS	Fat GMS	Chol. MGS
wheat, refrigerated *(Pipin' Hot)*	1-inch slice	70	0.0	12.0	170	(mq)	2.0	0
white, frozen *(Bridgford)*	1 oz	76	2.5	13.8	156	(mq)	1.2	0
white, frozen *(Rich's)*	2 slices	120	4.0	23.0	300	(mq)	1.0	0
white, refrigerated *(Pipin' Hot)*	1-inch slice	70	3.0	12.0	170	(mq)	2.0	0
BREADFRUIT								
raw	1 cup	227	2.3	59.7	4	10.8	0.5	0
raw	1/4 small	99	1.0	26.0	2	4.7	0.2	0
trimmed	1/2 cup	114	1.2	29.8	2	5.4	0.3	0
trimmed	1 oz	29	0.3	7.7	1	1.4	0.1	0
untrimmed	1 lb	365	3.8	96.0	6	>5.2 c	0.8	0
BREADFRUIT SEEDS								
boiled	1 oz	48	1.5	9.1	7	>.5 c	0.7	0
Pacific, in soft shell, boiled	1 lb	274	8.7	52.3	na	>2.9 c	3.8	0
Pacific, shelled, boiled	1 oz	48	1.5	9.1	na	>.5 c	0.7	0
raw	1 oz	54	2.1	8.3	7	>.5 c	1.6	0
roasted	1 oz	59	1.8	11.4	8	>.6 c	0.8	0
shelled, raw	1 oz	54	2.1	8.3	na	>.5 c	1.6	0
South American, in shell, raw	1 lb	590	22.8	90.2	na	>5.2 c	17.2	0
South American, shelled, roasted	1 oz	59	1.8	11.4	na	>.6 c	0.8	0
BREADNUT TREE SEEDS/Jamaican breadnut								
dried	1 oz	104	2.5	22.5	15	4.2	0.5	0
raw	1 oz	62	1.7	13.1	9	>.7 c	0.3	0
BREADSTICK								
garlic, Italian style *(Barbara's Bakery)*	1 oz	120	4.0	18.0	170	na	3.0	0
onion *(Stella D'oro)*	1 stick	40	1.2	6.1	(mq)	(mq)	1.3	na
pizza *(Fattorie & Pandea)*	3 sticks	59	2.0	10.0	100	(mq)	1.0	0
pizza *(Stella D'oro)*	1 stick	43	1.3	6.9	(mq)	(mq)	1.2	na
plain *(Stella D'oro)*	1 stick	41	1.0	6.5	(mq)	(mq)	1.2	na
plain, dietetic *(Stella D'oro)*	1 stick	46	1.3	7.3	10	(mq)	1.4	na
regular *(Barbara's Bakery)*	1 oz	120	4.0	18.0	170	na	3.0	0
sesame *(Fattorie & Pandea)*	3 sticks	65	2.0	10.0	100	(mq)	2.0	0
sesame *(Stella D'oro)*	1 stick	51	1.4	6.3	(mq)	(mq)	2.2	na
sesame, dietetic *(Stella D'oro)*	1 stick	49	1.3	6.1	10	(mq)	2.1	na
sesame, Italian style *(Barbara's Bakery)*	1 oz	120	4.0	18.0	170	na	3.0	0
soft, refrigerated *(Pillsbury)*	1 stick	100	3.0	17.0	230	(mq)	2.0	0
soft, refrigerated *(Roman Meal)*	1 stick	117	3.1	17.4	274	.8	3.9	0
wheat *(Stella D'oro)*	1 stick	42	1.3	6.1	(mq)	(mq)	1.4	na
whole wheat *(Fattorie & Pandea)*	3 sticks	57	2.0	10.0	100	(mq)	1.0	0
BREAKFAST BAR. See SNACK BAR.								
BREAKFAST DRINK MIX, INSTANT								
CHOCOLATE FLAVOR								
(Carnation) 'Instant Breakfast' dry mix	1 pouch	130	6.0	24.0	160	.2	2.0	3

Food Name	Serv. Size	Total Cal.	Prot. GMS	Carbs GMS	Sod. MGS	Fiber GMS	Fat GMS	Chol. MGS
(Carnation) 'Instant Breakfast' dry mix,								
no sugar added . . . . 1 pouch		70	4.0	12.0	90	1.0	1.0	<5
(Pillsbury) 'Instant Breakfast' from variety								
pack, dry mix . . . . 1/10 pkg		130	6.0	25.0	135	na	0.0	0
(Pillsbury) 'Instant Breakfast' from variety								
pack, prepared w/8 oz 2% milk . . . . 1 cup		250	14.0	37.0	250	na	5.0	20
(Pillsbury) 'Instant Breakfast' from variety								
pack, prepared w/8 oz whole milk . . . . . 1 cup		290	14.0	38.0	310	(mq)	9.0	(mq)
CHOCOLATE MALT FLAVOR								
(Carnation) 'Instant Breakfast' dry mix . . 1 pouch		130	6.0	24.0	160	.2	2.0	3
(Carnation) 'Instant Breakfast' dry mix,								
no sugar added . . . . 1 pouch		70	6.0	8.0	135	.2	2.0	2
(Pillsbury) 'Instant Breakfast' dry mix . . 1 pouch		130	6.0	26.0	190	na	0.0	0
COFFEE FLAVOR								
(Carnation) 'Instant Breakfast' dry mix . . 1 pouch		130	6.0	25.0	150	.1	0.2	3
VANILLA FLAVOR								
(Carnation) 'Instant Breakfast' dry mix . . 1 pouch		130	6.0	25.0	135	.1	0.2	3
(Carnation) 'Instant Breakfast' dry mix,								
no sugar added . . . . 1 pouch		70	6.0	10.0	120	.5	0.0	3
(Pillsbury) 'Instant Breakfast' dry mix . . 1 pouch		140	6.0	29.0	210	(mq)	0.0	na
(Pillsbury) 'Instant Breakfast' prepared								
w/whole milk . . . . 1 cup		300	14.0	41.0	330	na	9.0	(mq)
(Pillsbury) 'Instant Breakfast' from variety								
pack, dry mix . . . . 1/10 pkg		130	6.0	28.0	100	na	0.0	0
(Pillsbury) 'Instant Breakfast' from variety								
pack, prepared w/8 oz 2% milk . . . . 1 cup		260	14.0	40.0	220	na	5.0	20
BREAKFAST JUICE. See also individual listings.								
(Health Valley) . . . . 1/2 cup		26	3.0	5.0	24	3.2	0.0	0
(Knudsen & Sons) 'Natural' . . . . 8 oz		90	2.0	21.0	na	na	0.0	na
(Smucker's) orange banana,								
'Naturally 100%' . . . . 8 oz		120	0.0	30.0	10	(mq)	0.0	0
BREAKFAST STRIPS. See also BACON; BACON, ALTERNATIVE.								
beef, cured, cooked . . . . 6 oz		763	53.2	2.4	3830	0	58.5	202
beef, cured, cooked . . . . 3 slices		153	10.6	0.5	766	0	11.7	40
beef, cured, raw . . . . 3 slices		276	8.5	0.5	649	0	26.4	56
beef, cured, unheated . . . . 3 slices		276	8.5	0.5	649	0	26.4	56
BREATH MINT. See CANDY, HARD.								
BROAD BEAN								
boiled, drained . . . . 4 oz		64	5.4	11.5	47	3.1	0.6	0
immature, boiled, drained . . . . 100 gm		56	4.8	10.1	41	>1.9 c	0.5	0
immature, raw . . . . 1 cup		78	6.1	12.7	54	4.6	0.7	0
mature, boiled . . . . 1/2 cup		94	6.5	16.7	4	4.6	0.3	0
mature, raw . . . . 1/2 cup		256	19.6	43.7	10	18.8	1.1	0

Food Name	Serv. Size	Total Cal.	Prot. GMS	Carbs GMS	Sod. MGS	Fiber GMS	Fat GMS	Chol. MGS
raw, trimmed	1 oz	20	1.6	3.3	14	1.5	0.2	0
raw, untrimmed	1 lb	317	24.6	51.5	220	24.0	2.6	0
BROAD BEAN, DRIED								
mature, boiled	1/2 cup	93	6.5	16.7	4	4.3	0.3	0
mature, boiled	4 oz	125	8.6	22.3	6	5.8	0.5	0
mature, raw	1/2 cup	256	19.6	43.7	9	10.9	1.2	0
mature, raw	1 oz	97	7.4	16.5	4	4.1	0.4	0
BROCCOLI								
boiled, drained	4 oz	32	3.4	5.7	29	2.9	0.4	0
boiled, drained, chopped	1/2 cup	22	2.3	4.0	20	2.0	0.3	0
florets, raw, chopped	1/2 cup	12	1.3	2.3	12	>.5 c	0.2	0
fresh *(Dole)*	1 med spear	40	5.0	4.0	75	5.0	1.0	na
leaves, raw, chopped	1/2 cup	12	1.3	2.3	12	>.5 c	0.2	0
raw, chopped	1/2 cup	12	1.3	2.3	12	1.2	0.2	0
raw, trimmed	1 oz	8	0.8	1.5	8	.8	0.1	0
raw, untrimmed	1 lb	77	8.3	14.5	73	7.7	1.0	0
BROCCOLI, FROZEN. See also BROCCOLI DISHES, FROZEN; BROCCOLI ENTRÉE, FROZEN.								
chopped *(A&P)*	3.3 oz	25	3.0	5.0	25	(mq)	<1.0	0
chopped *(Birds Eye)*	3.3 oz	25	3.0	5.0	15	3.0	0.0	0
chopped *(Finast)*	3.3 oz	25	3.0	5.0	20	(mq)	0.0	0
chopped *(Frosty Acres)*	3.3 oz	25	3.0	5.0	18	>1.0 c	0.0	0
chopped *(Seabrook)*	3.3 oz	25	3.0	5.0	18	>1.0 c	0.0	0
chopped *(Southern)*	3.5 oz	28	2.9	4.4	25	(mq)	0.3	0
chopped, boiled, drained	4 oz	32	3.5	6.1	27	2.5	0.1	0
chopped, boiled, drained	1/2 cup	26	2.8	4.9	22	2.8	0.1	0
chopped, unprepared	10-oz pkg	74	8.0	13.6	68	8.5	0.8	0
cuts *(A&P)*	3.3 oz	25	3.0	5.0	25	(mq)	<1.0	0
cuts *(Birds Eye)*	3.2 oz	25	3.0	5.0	25	3.0	0.0	0
cuts *(Frosty Acres)*	3.3 oz	25	3.0	5.0	50	>1.0 c	0.0	0
cuts *(Seabrook)*	3.3 oz	25	3.0	5.0	50	>1.0 c	0.0	0
cuts, 'Harvest Fresh' *(Green Giant)*	1/2 cup	16	2.0	3.0	95	2.0	0.0	0
cuts, 'Plain Polybag' *(Green Giant)*	1/2 cup	18	2.0	5.0	25	4.0	0.0	0
cuts, 'Portion Pack' *(Birds Eye)*	3 oz	20	3.0	4.0	20	2.0	0.0	0
cuts, 'Singles' *(Stokely)*	3 oz	25	3.0	5.0	15	(mq)	1.0	0
florets *(Frosty Acres)*	3.3 oz	30	3.0	5.0	14	>1.0 c	0.0	0
florets, 'Deluxe' *(Birds Eye)*	3.3 oz	25	3.0	5.0	20	3.0	0.0	0
spears *(A&P)*	3.3 oz	25	3.0	5.0	20	(mq)	<1.0	0
spears *(Birds Eye)*	3.3 oz	25	3.0	5.0	20	3.0	0.0	0
spears *(Frosty Acres)*	3.3 oz	25	3.0	5.0	20	>1.0 c	0.0	0
spears *(Seabrook)*	3.3 oz	25	3.0	5.0	20	>1.0 c	0.0	0
spears *(Southern)*	3.5 oz	30	3.0	4.8	30	(mq)	0.2	0
spears, baby *(Seabrook)*	3.3 oz	30	3.0	5.0	14	>1.0 c	0.0	0
spears, baby, 'Deluxe' *(Birds Eye)*	3.3 oz	30	3.0	5.0	15	3.0	0.0	0

Food Name	Serv. Size	Total Cal.	Prot. GMS	Carbs GMS	Sod. MGS	Fiber GMS	Fat GMS	Chol. MGS
spears, boiled, drained	4 oz	32	3.5	6.1	27	2.5	0.1	0
spears, boiled, drained	10-oz pkg	70	7.8	13.4	60	7.5	0.3	0
spears, boiled, drained	1/2 cup	26	2.8	4.9	22	2.7	0.1	0
spears, 'Harvest Fresh' (Green Giant)	1/2 cup	20	2.0	4.0	115	2.0	0.0	0
spears, mini, 2 1/2 inch x 1/4 inch, approx .6 oz (Green Giant)	1/5 pkg	18	2.0	5.0	25	3.0	0.0	0
spears, unprepared	10-oz pkg	82	8.7	15.2	48	8.5	1.0	0
spears, whole, 'Farm Fresh' (Birds Eye)	4 oz	30	4.0	6.0	25	3.0	0.0	0
spears and florets, 'Deluxe' (Birds Eye)	3.3 oz	25	3.0	5.0	20	3.0	0.0	0
BROCCOLI DISHES, FROZEN								
cuts, in butter sauce, 'One Serving' (Green Giant)	4.5 oz	45	3.0	7.0	420	3.0	2.0	5
cuts, in cheese sauce, (Finast)	3.3 oz	45	3.0	6.0	310	(mq)	0.0	0
cuts, in cheese sauce, 'One Serving' (Green Giant)	5 oz	80	4.0	13.0	700	2.0	2.0	5
cuts, in cheese sauce, 'Singles' (Stokely)	4 oz	80	5.0	7.0	200	(mq)	4.0	15
fanfare, 'Valley Combinations' (Green Giant)	1/2 cup	80	3.0	14.0	340	3.0	2.0	0
in cheese flavored sauce (Green Giant)	1/2 cup	60	3.0	9.0	530	2.0	2.0	2
in cheese sauce, 'Family Side Dishes' (Freezer Queen)	4.5 oz	48	2.0	8.0	280	(mq)	1.0	na
spears, 'Butter Sauce' (Green Giant)	1/2 cup	40	2.0	6.0	350	2.0	2.0	5
spears, 'Butter Sauce Combinations' (Birds Eye)	3.3 oz	45	2.0	5.0	320	2.0	2.0	5
w/baby carrots and water chestnuts, 'Farm Fresh' (Birds Eye)	4 oz	45	2.0	10.0	35	3.0	0.0	0
w/cauliflower (A&P)	3.2 oz	25	2.0	4.0	20	(mq)	<1.0	0
w/cauliflower, 'Valley Combinations' medley (Green Giant)	1/2 cup	30	2.0	10.0	80	3.0	1.0	0
w/cauliflower, 'Singles' (Stokely)	3 oz	20	2.0	4.0	15	(mq)	1.0	0
w/cauliflower, 'Swiss Mix' (Frosty Acres)	3 oz	25	2.0	5.0	36	>1.0 c	0.0	0
w/red peppers, 'Select' (Green Giant)	1/2 cup	25	2.0	4.0	15	2.0	0.0	0
w/whole baby carrots and chestnuts, 'Singles' (Stokely)	3 oz	30	2.0	6.0	22	(mq)	1.0	0
BROCCOLI ENTRÉE, FROZEN								
and baked potato wedges w/cheese sauce, 9.5-oz pkg (Healthy Choice)	1 serving	240	8.0	41.0	510	na	5.0	15
au gratin w/rice, 'For One' (Birds Eye)	5.75 oz	180	6.0	27.0	430	1.0	6.0	5
in pastry, w/cheese (Pepperidge Farm)	1 pastry	230	5.0	18.0	380	(mq)	16.0	(mq)
pot pie w/cheddar cheese, organic (Amy's Kitchen)	8 oz	390	10.0	46.0	500	3.0	18.0	na

BROTH. See SOUP.

BROWN BREAD. See BREAD.

Food Name	Serv. Size	Total Cal.	Prot. GMS	Carbs GMS	Sod. MGS	Fiber GMS	Fat GMS	Chol. MGS
BRUSSELS SPROUTS								
boiled, drained	4 oz	44	2.9	9.8	24	4.9	0.6	0
boiled, drained	1/2 cup	30	2.0	6.8	16	3.3	0.4	0
boiled, drained	1 sprout	8	0.5	1.8	4	.9	0.1	0
fresh *(Dole)*	1/2 cup	19	1.0	4.0	11	2.0	0.1	na
'Plain Polybag' *(Green Giant)*	1/2 cup	25	2.0	6.0	10	2.0	0.0	0
raw	1/2 cup	19	1.5	3.9	11	1.9	0.1	0
raw	1 sprout	8	0.6	1.7	5	.8	0.1	0
raw, trimmed	1 oz	12	1.0	2.5	7	>.4 c	0.1	0
raw, untrimmed	1 lb	174	13.8	36.6	101	>6.2 c	1.2	0
BRUSSELS SPROUTS, FROZEN								
boiled, drained	4 oz	48	4.1	9.4	26	2.0	0.4	0
boiled, drained	1/2 cup	33	2.8	6.5	18	>1.1 c	0.3	0
(A&P)	3.3 oz	35	3.0	7.0	15	(mq)	<1.0	0
(Birds Eye)	3.3 oz	35	3.0	7.0	15	3.0	0.0	0
(Birds Eye) baby, 'Cheese Sauce Combinations'	4.5 oz	130	6.0	12.0	500	2.0	7.0	5
(Frosty Acres)	3.3 oz	35	3.0	7.0	12	>1.0 c	0.0	0
(Green Giant) in butter sauce	1/2 cup	40	3.0	8.0	280	4.0	1.0	5
(Seabrook)	3.3 oz	35	3.0	7.0	12	>1.0 c	0.0	0
(Seabrook) baby	3.3 oz	40	4.0	7.0	5	>1.0 c	0.0	0
(Southern)	3.5 oz	37	3.2	7.5	20	(mq)	0.0	0
(Stokely) in butter sauce, 'Singles'	4 oz	50	4.0	10.0	325	(mq)	1.0	5
(Stokely) 'Singles'	3 oz	35	4.0	7.0	10	(mq)	0.0	0
BUBBLE GUM. See CANDY.								
BUCKWHEAT								
whole-grain	1/2 cup	292	11.3	60.8	1	8.5	2.9	0
whole-grain	1 oz	97	3.8	20.3	<1	(mq)	1.0	0
BUCKWHEAT FLOUR								
whole-grain	1 cup	402	15.1	84.7	na	(mq)	3.7	0
whole-grain	1 oz	95	3.6	20.0	na	(mq)	0.9	0
whole-grain *(Arrowhead Mills)*	2 oz	190	7.0	41.0	0	7.1	1.0	0
whole-groat	1/2 cup	201	7.6	42.4	7	6.0	1.9	0
BUCKWHEAT GROATS/kasha								
brown *(Arrowhead Mills)*	2 oz	190	7.0	41.0	1	7.1	1.0	0
roasted, cooked	1/2 cup	91	3.3	19.7	4	>.5 c	0.6	0
roasted, cooked	4 oz	104	3.8	22.6	5	>.6 c	0.7	0
roasted, dry	1/2 cup	284	9.6	61.5	9	>1.4 c	2.2	0
roasted, dry	1 oz	98	3.3	21.2	3	>.5 c	0.8	0
white *(Arrowhead Mills)*	2 oz	190	7.0	41.0	1	7.1	1.0	0
BULGUR. See also TABBOULEH MIX.								
cooked	4 oz	94	3.5	21.1	6	5.1	0.3	0
cooked	1/2 cup	76	2.8	16.9	5	4.1	0.2	0

Food Name	Serv. Size	Total Cal.	Prot. GMS	Carbs GMS	Sod. MGS	Fiber GMS	Fat GMS	Chol. MGS
dry	1/2 cup	239	8.6	53.1	12	12.8	0.9	0
dry	1 oz	97	3.5	21.5	5	5.2	0.4	0

BULLOCK'S HEART. See CUSTARD APPLE.

BUN. See also BISCUIT; CROISSANT; ENGLISH MUFFIN; ROLL.

Food Name	Serv. Size	Total Cal.	Prot. GMS	Carbs GMS	Sod. MGS	Fiber GMS	Fat GMS	Chol. MGS
brown and serve, partially baked	2.5-inch roll	85	2.3	14.2	146	>.1 c	2.0	2
brown and serve, partially baked, unbrowned	2.5-inch roll	78	2.0	13.2	133	>.1 c	1.8	2
enriched, browned	2.5-inch roll	85	2.3	14.2	146	>.1 c	2.0	2
enriched, unbrowned	2.5-inch roll	84	2.2	14.2	144	>.1 c	1.9	2
hard, enriched, ready to cook	3.75-inch roll	156	4.9	29.7	313	>.1 c	1.6	2
hard, enriched, ready to cook	2.5-inch roll	78	2.5	14.9	156	>.1 c	0.8	1
Kaiser, 'Big' (Holsum)	1 bun	200	5.0	38.0	320	na	3.0	0
sesame seed, 'Big BBQ Buns' (Holsum)	1 bun	200	5.0	38.0	320	na	3.0	0
'Sof-Buns' (Holsum)	1 bun	120	3.0	23.0	190	na	2.0	0

BUN, FRANKFURTER

Food Name	Serv. Size	Total Cal.	Prot. GMS	Carbs GMS	Sod. MGS	Fiber GMS	Fat GMS	Chol. MGS
Dijon (Pepperidge Farm)	1 bun	160	5.0	23.0	230	2.0	5.0	0
'Light' (Wonder)	1 bun	80	5.0	13.0	210	4.0	1.0	na
mixed grain	1 bun	113	4.1	19.2	197	1.9	2.6	0
'New England Style' (Arnold)	1 bun	108	3.7	20.9	178	1.4	2.0	0
oat bran (Awrey's)	1 bun	110	4.0	20.0	210	1.0	2.0	0
'Original' (Roman Meal)	1 bun	104	4.3	19.5	210	1.8	1.9	0
plain	1 bun	123	3.7	21.6	241	na	2.2	0
plain (Arnold)	1 bun	100	3.2	19.6	162	1.2	1.8	0
plain (Country Grain)	1 bun	100	4.0	18.0	230	.9	1.0	na
plain (Pepperidge Farm)	1 bun	140	5.0	24.0	270	.5	3.0	0
plain (Wonder)	1 bun	80	2.0	14.0	150	.6	1.0	na
potato (Aunt Hattie's)	1 bun	150	5.0	23.0	260	na	4.0	0
reduced calorie	1 bun	84	3.6	18.1	190	2.7	0.9	0
reduced calorie	1 oz	56	2.3	11.9	125	1.8	0.6	0
whole grain (Roman Meal)	1 bun	120	4.0	19.0	210	na	3.0	0

BUN, HAMBURGER

Food Name	Serv. Size	Total Cal.	Prot. GMS	Carbs GMS	Sod. MGS	Fiber GMS	Fat GMS	Chol. MGS
'Light' (Wonder)	1 bun	80	5.0	13.0	210	4.0	1.0	na
mixed grain	1 bun	113	4.1	19.2	197	1.9	2.6	0
mixed grain	1 oz	75	2.7	12.6	130	1.2	1.7	0
'Original' (Roman Meal)	1 bun	113	4.7	21.1	228	2.0	1.9	0
plain	1 bun	123	3.7	21.6	241	na	2.2	0
plain	1 oz	81	2.4	14.3	159	na	1.5	0
plain (Arnold)	1 bun	115	4.3	22.0	223	1.8	2.2	0
plain (Pepperidge Farm)	1 bun	130	5.0	22.0	240	.5	2.0	0
plain (Wonder)	1 bun	120	4.0	21.0	230	.9	2.0	na
potato (Aunt Hattie's)	1 bun	150	5.0	23.0	260	na	4.0	0
reduced calorie	1 bun	84	3.6	18.1	190	2.7	0.9	0
reduced calorie	1 oz	56	2.3	11.9	125	1.8	0.6	0

Food Name	Serv. Size	Total Cal.	Prot. GMS	Carbs GMS	Sod. MGS	Fiber GMS	Fat GMS	Chol. MGS
whole grain *(Roman Meal)* .... 1 bun		130	4.0	20.0	230	na	3.0	0
BUN, SWEET								
apple honey, multi pak, 1.5 oz								
(Break Cake) .... 1 bun		170	2.0	20.0	90	na	10.0	0
cheese-topped *(Entenmann's)* .... 1 bun		240	5.0	29.0	240	na	12.0	na
cinnamon *(Entenmann's)* .... 1 bun		230	4.0	31.0	200	na	10.0	na
cinnamon, frozen 'Ever Fresh' 2.5 oz								
(Rich's) .... 1 bun		293	4.0	38.0	(mq)	(mq)	14.6	na
cinnamon, frozen '2/pkg'								
(Pepperidge Farm) .... 1 bun		280	4.0	34.0	190	(mq)	14.0	na
cinnamon, homestyle *(Awrey's)* .... 1 bun		240	4.0	40.0	200	1.0	7.0	5
cinnamon, iced, refrigerated								
(Hungry Jack) .... 2 buns		290	3.0	37.0	570	(mq)	14.0	na
cinnamon swirl 'Grande' *(Awrey's)* ...... 1 bun		340	4.0	46.0	370	1.0	16.0	10
honey *(Aunt Fanny's)* .... 3 oz		360	4.0	42.0	150	na	30.0	10
honey *(Break Cake)* 3 oz .... 1 bun		420	4.0	38.0	160	na	28.0	0
honey, apple bear *(Aunt Fanny's)* .... 4 oz		460	6.0	50.0	220	na	26.0	5
honey, birdie, jelly-filled *(Aunt Fanny's)* .... 4 oz		450	6.0	53.0	210	na	24.0	5
honey, bogie, creme-filled *(Aunt Fanny's)* .. 4 oz		460	6.0	49.0	200	na	27.0	10
honey, frozen, mini, 'Ever Fresh', 1.36 oz								
(Rich's) .... 1 bun		133	1.8	17.5	(mq)	(mq)	6.6	na
honey, lemon bear *(Aunt Fanny's)* .... 4 oz		440	5.0	52.0	200	na	23.0	5
honey, multi pak *(Break Cake)* .... 1 bun		380	3.0	34.0	150	na	24.0	0
honey, snow bear *(Aunt Fanny's)* .... 4 oz		480	6.0	60.0	220	na	24.0	5
honey glazed *(Tastykake)* .... 3.25 oz		362	5.9	42.3	219	3.6	20.4	2
honey glazed *(Hostess)* .... 1 bun		360	5.0	38.0	230	.8	21.0	15
honey iced *(Tastykake)* .... 3.25 oz		348	5.0	50.0	254	1.5	14.9	2
honey iced *(Hostess)* .... 1 bun		430	5.0	55.0	240	1.7	22.0	20
pecan-caramel swirl *(Hostess)* .... 1 bun		240	3.0	23.0	160	1.8	15.0	10
BURBOT								
dry-heat cooked .... 3 oz		98	21.0	0.0	105	0	0.9	65
raw .... 1 lb		407	87.6	0.0	438	0	3.7	270
raw .... 1 oz		26	5.5	0.0	27	0	0.2	17
raw .... 3 oz		77	16.4	0.0	82	0	0.7	51
BURDOCK ROOT/gobo								
boiled, drained .... 4 oz		100	2.4	24.0	5	2.1	0.2	0
boiled, drained .... 1 root		146	3.5	35.1	7	3.0	0.2	0
boiled, drained .... 1 cup		110	2.6	26.4	5	2.3	0.2	0
raw .... 1 root		112	2.4	27.1	8	5.2	0.2	0
raw, 1-inch pieces .... 1 cup		85	1.8	20.5	6	3.9	0.2	0
raw, trimmed .... 1 oz		20	0.4	4.9	1	.9	<.1	0
raw, untrimmed .... 1 lb		245	5.2	59.0	17	>6.6 c	0.5	0

Food Name	Serv. Size	Total Cal.	Prot. GMS	Carbs GMS	Sod. MGS	Fiber GMS	Fat GMS	Chol. MGS
BURGER, VEGETARIAN								
canned 'Vegetarian Burger'								
(Worthington)	1/2 cup	150	19.0	9.0	780	(mq)	4.0	0
canned 'Vegetarian Burger No Salt Added'								
(Worthington)	1/2 cup	160	17.0	9.0	500	(mq)	6.0	0
frozen 'FriPats' (Worthington)	2.25-oz piece	180	13.0	5.0	350	(mq)	12.0	0
frozen 'Grillers'								
(Morningstar Farms)	2.25-oz patty	180	13.0	5.0	350	(mq)	12.0	0
frozen 'Harvest Burger' original flavor								
(Green Giant)	1 burger	140	18.0	8.0	380	5.0	4.0	0
frozen 'Harvest Burger' southwest style								
(Green Giant)	1 burger	140	16.0	9.0	370	5.0	4.0	0
frozen, organic (Amy's Kitchen)	2.5 oz	173	6.0	22.0	181	1.0	4.0	0
BURGER MIX, VEGETARIAN								
(Fantastic Foods) w/tofu, prep,								
excluding cooking fat	3.4-oz burger	133	11.0	14.0	320	(mq)	5.0	na
(Love Natural Foods) 'Loveburger'								
prepared	4-oz burger	245	17.0	20.0	224	8.0	11.0	0
(Nature's Burger) barbecue,								
prepared, excluding cooking fat	3-oz burger	117	4.0	24.0	423	(mq)	0.8	0
(Nature's Burger) 'Original' prepared,								
excluding cooking fat	3-oz burger	152	7.0	21.0	228	(mq)	4.0	0
(Nature's Burger) pizza, prep,								
excluding cooking fat	3-oz burger	121	5.0	24.0	406	(mq)	1.0	0
(Worthington) 'Granburger' prepared,								
excluding cooking fat	1 burger	110	19.9	7.0	700	(mq)	1.0	0
BURRITO, FROZEN								
(Amy's Kitchen) bean and rice	6 oz	251	8.0	44.0	364	6.0	5.0	0
(Don Miguel) cheese, no beans	1 burrito	410	18.0	52.0	950	3.0	14.0	45
(Don Miguel) cheese and green chili	1 burrito	390	20.0	53.0	910	3.0	11.0	40
(Las Campanas) bean and cheese,								
no lard	1 burrito	272	10.0	42.0	480	6.0	7.0	3
(Las Campanas) beef and bean, no lard	1 burrito	304	10.0	39.0	504	5.0	12.0	12
(Maria's) jalapeño bean and cheese	1 burrito	360	12.0	54.0	620	8.0	11.0	10
(Marquez) beef, green chili, and cheese,								
'Primera'	1 burrito	330	14.0	43.0	950	2.0	11.0	30
(Old El Paso) bean and cheese	1 burrito	330	14.0	45.0	740	(mq)	11.0	(mq)
(Swanson) hot and spicy 'Great Starts'	1 burrito	220	9.0	30.0	490	3.0	7.0	55
(Swanson) original, w/cheese and chili								
peppers 'Great Starts'	1 burrito	200	8.0	25.0	510	2.0	8.0	60
(Swanson) w/egg, bacon, cheese								
'Great Starts'	1 burrito	250	10.0	27.0	540	na	11.0	90

Food Name	Serv. Size	Total Cal.	Prot. GMS	Carbs GMS	Sod. MGS	Fiber GMS	Fat GMS	Chol. MGS
(Swanson) w/egg, ham, cheese 'Great Starts'	1 burrito	210	9.0	29.0	350	na	6.0	60
(Swanson) w/egg, pizza sauce, cheese, pepperoni 'Great Starts'	1 burrito	240	9.0	28.0	410	na	9.0	60
BURRITO DINNER MIX								
(Amy's Kitchen) beans, rice, and cheese, organic	6 oz	279	10.0	43.0	370	6.0	8.0	9
(Hormel) beef	1 burrito	205	9.0	31.0	780	(mq)	8.0	(mq)
(Old El Paso) prepared, w/filling	1 burrito	299	11.0	36.0	430	4.0	13.0	23
(Patio)	12 oz	517	18.0	74.0	1643	(mq)	16.0	(mq)
(Tio Sancho) 'Dinner Kit'	1 burrito	125	3.3	24.0	569	>.1 c	1.9	na
BURRITO DINNER, FROZEN								
beef and bean *(Patio)*	5 oz	370	11.0	43.0	830	(mq)	16.0	(mq)
beef and bean 'Britos' *(Patio)*	3.63 oz	250	6.0	33.0	340	(mq)	10.0	15
beef and bean 'Festive Dinners' *(Old El Paso)*	11 oz	470	23.0	72.0	1180	(mq)	9.0	(mq)
beef and bean, green chili *(Patio)*	5 oz	330	12.0	43.0	770	(mq)	12.0	(mq)
beef and bean, hot *(Old El Paso)*	1 burrito	310	12.0	41.0	710	(mq)	11.0	(mq)
beef and bean, medium *(Old El Paso)*	1 burrito	330	13.0	41.0	630	(mq)	13.0	29
beef and bean, mild *(Old El Paso)*	1 burrito	320	13.0	42.0	500	(mq)	11.0	(mq)
beef and bean, nacho 'Britos' *(Patio)*	3.63 oz	270	9.0	30.0	420	(mq)	13.0	25
beef and bean 'Quick Meals' 1 serving *(Healthy Choice)*	5.2 oz	270	12.0	42.0	520	na	7.0	15
beef and bean, red chili *(Patio)*	5 oz	340	11.0	44.0	810	(mq)	13.0	(mq)
beef steak fajita, 'Supreme' 5-oz pkg *(Ruiz)*	1 burrito	290	11.0	42.0	240	1.0	9.0	5
cheese *(Hormel)*	1 burrito	210	9.0	32.0	792	(mq)	5.0	(mq)
cheese, nacho, 'Britos' *(Patio)*	3.63 oz	250	7.0	32.0	330	(mq)	10.0	20
chicken, spicy, 'Britos' *(Patio)*	3.63 oz	250	6.0	33.0	330	(mq)	10.0	25
chicken and rice *(Hormel)*	1 burrito	200	9.0	32.0	594	(mq)	4.0	(mq)
chicken con queso 'Quick Meals' *(Healthy Choice)*	5.4 oz	280	15.0	40.0	500	na	8.0	20
chicken fajita, 'Supreme,' 5-oz pkg *(Ruiz)*	1 burrito	260	12.0	50.0	500	10.0	1.0	5
chili, hot *(Hormel)*	1 burrito	240	9.0	33.0	619	(mq)	8.0	(mq)
green chili 'Britos' *(Patio)*	3.63 oz	250	6.0	33.0	420	(mq)	10.0	15
red chili 'Britos' *(Patio)*	3.63 oz	240	6.0	31.0	370	(mq)	10.0	15
red hot *(Patio)*	5 oz	360	12.0	43.0	800	(mq)	15.0	(mq)
BURRITO FILLING FIX, beans *(Del Monte)*	1/2 cup	110	6.0	20.0	900	na	1.0	na
BURRITO SEASONING MIX								
(Lawry's) 'Seasoning Blends' dry mix	1 pkg	132	6.0	23.3	2516	>.9 c	1.7	0
(Old El Paso)	1/8 pkg	17	1.0	3.0	275	1.0	0.0	0
(Tio Sancho) 'Dinner Kit'	3.25 oz	265	12.3	49.3	5031	>5.5 c	2.1	na

Food Name	Serv. Size	Total Cal.	Prot. GMS	Carbs GMS	Sod. MGS	Fiber GMS	Fat GMS	Chol. MGS
BUSH NUT. See MACADAMIA NUT.								
BUTTER, CLARIFIED. See GHEE.								
BUTTER, REGULAR								
lightly salted (Breakstone's)	1 tbsp	100	0.0	0.0	90	na	11.0	35
lightly salted (Darigold)	1 tsp	25	0.0	0.0	25	0	3.0	7
lightly salted (Hotel Bar)	1 tsp	35	0.0	0.0	35	0	4.0	(mq)
lightly salted (Kellers)	1 tsp	35	0.0	0.0	35	na	4.0	na
lightly salted (Land O'Lakes)	1 tbsp	35	0.0	0.0	40	na	4.0	10
salted	4-oz stick	813	1.0	0.0	937	0	92.0	248
salted	1 tbsp	100	0.0	0.0	115	0	11.4	31
salted	1 tsp	34	<.1	0.0	39	0	3.8	10
salted (Challenge)	1 tbsp	100	0.0	0.0	90	na	11.0	30
salted (Darigold)	1 tsp	35	0.0	0.0	40	0	4.0	11
salted (Hotel Bar)	1 tsp	35	0.0	0.0	35	0	4.0	(mq)
salted (Kellers)	1 tsp	35	0.0	0.0	35	0	4.0	(mq)
salted (Land O'Lakes)	1 tsp	35	0.0	0.0	40	0	4.0	10
salted (Seal of Arizona)	1 tbsp	100	0.0	0.0	90	na	11.0	30
salted, packed 90 pats per 1 lb	1 pat	36	<.1	0.0	41	0	4.1	11
unsalted	4-oz stick	813	1.0	0.1	12	0	92.0	248
unsalted	1 tbsp	100	0.1	0.0	1	0	11.4	31
unsalted	1 pat	36	0.0	0.0	1	0	4.1	11
unsalted	1 tsp	34	<.1	0.0	<1	0	3.8	10
unsalted (Breakstone's)	1 tbsp	100	0.0	0.0	0	na	11.0	35
unsalted (Challenge)	1 tbsp	100	0.0	0.0	2	na	11.0	30
unsalted (Land O'Lakes)	1 tbsp	35	0.0	0.0	0	na	4.0	10
BUTTER, WHIPPED								
lightly salted (Breakstone's)	1 tbsp	70	0.0	0.0	65	na	7.0	20
lightly salted (Land O'Lakes)	1 tsp	25	0.0	0.0	25	na	3.0	5
salted	1 tbsp	67	0.1	tr	78	0	7.6	20
salted	1 tsp	23	tr	tr	26	0	2.6	7
salted (Land O'Lakes)	1 tsp	25	0.0	0.0	25	0	3.0	5
salted, packed 120 pats per 1 lb	1 pat	27	<.1	tr	31	0	3.1	8
unsalted	1 tbsp	67	0.1	tr	1	0	7.6	20
unsalted	1 tsp	23	tr	tr	<1	0	2.6	7
unsalted (Breakstone's)	1 tbsp	70	0.0	0.0	0	na	7.0	20
unsalted (Darigold)	1 tsp	25	0.0	0.0	2	0	3.0	7
unsalted (Land O'Lakes)	1 tsp	25	0.0	0.0	0	0	3.0	5
BUTTER FLAVORED OIL (Wesson)	1 tbsp	122	0.0	0.0	0	0	13.6	0
BUTTER FLAVORED TOPPING								
(Molly McButter)	1/2 tsp	4.0	0.0	1.0	60	na	0.0	0
BUTTER OIL								
	1 oz	248	0.1	0.0	na	0	28.2	73
anhydrous	1 cup	1796	0.6	0.0	3	0	204.0	525

Food Name	Serv. Size	Total Cal.	Prot. GMS	Carbs GMS	Sod. MGS	Fiber GMS	Fat GMS	Chol. MGS
anhydrous	1 tbsp	112	0.0	0.0	0	0	12.7	33

BUTTERBEAN. See LIMA BEAN.

BUTTERBUR/Fuki

boiled, drained	4 oz	9	0.3	2.4	5	>.9 c	<.1	0
raw	1 cup	13	0.4	3.4	7	>1.2 c	0.0	0
raw, approx .2 oz	1 stalk	1	<.1	0.2	tr	>.1 c	tr	0
raw, trimmed	1/2 cup	7	0.2	1.7	4	>.6 c	<.1	0
raw, trimmed	1 oz	4	0.1	1.0	2	>.4 c	<.1	0
raw, untrimmed	1 lb	57	1.6	14.4	28	>5.2 c	0.2	0

BUTTERBUR, CANNED

	4 oz	12	0.1	0.4	5	>1.2 c	0.1	0
chopped	1 cup	4	0.1	0.5	5	>1.1 c	0.2	0
stalks	3 stalks	1	0.1	0.2	2	>.4 c	0.1	0

BUTTERFISH

dry-heat cooked	3 oz	159	18.8	0.0	97	0	8.7	71
raw	1 lb	663	78.4	0.0	401	0	36.4	295
raw	3 oz	124	14.7	0.0	76	0	6.8	55
raw	1 oz	41	4.9	0.0	25	0	2.3	18

BUTTERHEAD LETTUCE. See LETTUCE.

BUTTERMILK

blend, cultured, dry (Saco Foods)	3.5 tbsp	79	7.5	10.7	168	na	0.7	0
cultured	1 cup	99	8.1	11.7	257	0	2.2	9
cultured	1 oz	11	0.9	1.4	30	0	0.2	1
cultured (A&P)	1 cup	90	8.0	12.0	260	0	1.0	(mq)
cultured (Crowley)	1 cup	110	9.0	12.0	390	0	4.0	15
cultured, 1.5% 'Golden Churn' (Borden)	1 cup	120	8.0	11.0	250	0	4.0	(mq)
cultured, 1.5% 'Unsalted' (Friendship)	1 cup	120	9.0	12.0	125	0	4.0	14
cultured, 2% (Knudsen)	1 cup	120	8.0	12.0	140	0	5.0	(mq)
cultured, 'Unsalted' (Crowley)	1 cup	110	9.0	12.0	130	0	4.0	15
sweet cream, dry	1 cup	464	41.2	58.8	621	0	6.9	83
sweet cream, dry	1 oz	110	9.7	13.9	147	0	1.6	20
sweet cream, dry	1 tbsp	25	2.2	3.2	34	0	0.4	5

BUTTERNUT. See BRAZIL NUT.

BUTTERNUT SQUASH. See SQUASH, BUTTERNUT

BUTTERSCOTCH TOPPING

	2 tbsp	103	0.6	27.0	143	0	0.0	0
(Kraft)	1 tbsp	60	0.0	13.0	70	(tr)	1.0	0
(Mrs. Richardson's) caramel	2 tbsp	130	<1.0	28.0	90	na	2.0	5
(Mrs. Richardson's) caramel fudge, microwavable	2 tbsp	130	<1.0	28.0	90	na	2.0	5
(Smucker's)	2 tbsp	140	0.0	33.0	75	(tr)	1.0	0
(Smucker's) caramel flavor 'Special Recipe'	2 tbsp	160	1.0	33.0	40	(tr)	3.0	na

C

Food Name	Serv. Size	Total Cal.	Prot. GMS	Carbs GMS	Sod. MGS	Fiber GMS	Fat GMS	Chol. MGS
CABBAGE								
boiled, drained	1 head	278	12.9	56.3	101	35.34	5.4	0
boiled, drained	4 oz	24	1.1	5.4	22	>.7 c	0.3	0
boiled, drained, shredded	1/2 cup	16	0.8	3.3	6	2.1	0.3	0
raw, approx 2.5 lbs	1 head	227	13.1	49.3	163	20.9	2.5	0
raw, medium size (Dole)	1/12 head	18	1.0	3.0	30	2.0	0.0	na
raw, shredded	1/2 cup	9	0.5	1.9	6	.8	0.1	0
raw, trimmed	1 oz	7	0.3	1.5	5	.3	0.1	0
raw, untrimmed	1 lb	86	4.4	19.5	65	4.0 d	0.7	0
CABBAGE, DANISH								
fresh	1 head	218	11.0	48.8	163	>7.3 c	1.6	0
fresh, shredded	1/2 cup	8	0.4	1.9	6	>.3 c	0.1	0
CABBAGE, NAPA/Chinese cabbage								
boiled, drained	1 leaf	2	0.2	0.3	1	>.1 c	0.0	0
boiled, drained, shredded	1/2 cup	10	1.3	1.5	29	>.5 c	0.1	0
bok-choy, boiled, drained	4 oz	14	1.8	2.0	39	1.8	0.2	0
bok-choy, boiled, drained, shredded	1/2 cup	10	1.3	1.5	29	1.4	0.1	0
bok-choy, raw, shredded	1/2 cup	5	0.5	0.8	23	.4	0.1	0
bok-choy, raw, trimmed	1 oz	4	0.4	0.6	19	.3	0.1	0
bok-choy, raw, untrimmed	1 lb	52	6.0	8.7	257	4.0	0.8	0
pe-tsai, boiled, drained	4 oz	16	1.7	2.7	10	1.8	0.2	0
pe-tsai, boiled, drained, shredded	1/2 cup	8	0.9	1.4	6	1.0	0.1	0
pe-tsai, raw, trimmed	1 oz	5	0.3	0.9	3	.3	0.1	0
pe-tsai, raw, untrimmed	1 lb	68	5.1	13.6	38	4.2	0.8	0
raw, shredded	1/2 cup	5	0.5	0.8	23	.4	0.1	0
CABBAGE, RED								
boiled, drained	4 oz	24	1.2	5.3	9	2.7	0.2	0
boiled, drained, shredded	1/2 cup	16	0.8	3.5	6	1.8	0.2	0
raw, shredded	1/2 cup	9	0.5	2.1	4	.7	0.1	0
raw, trimmed	1 oz	8	0.4	1.7	3	.6	0.1	0
CABBAGE, SAVOY								
boiled, drained	4 oz	27	2.0	6.1	27	>.8 c	0.1	0
boiled, drained, shredded	1/2 cup	18	1.3	4.0	18	>.5 c	0.1	0
raw, shredded	1/2 cup	9	0.7	2.1	10	1.0	0.0	0
raw, trimmed	1 oz	8	0.6	1.7	8	>.2 c	<.1	0
raw, untrimmed	1 lb	100	7.3	22.1	102	>2.9 c	0.4	0
CABBAGE, SKUNK/swamp cabbage/water convolvulus								
boiled, drained	4 oz	23	2.4	4.2	138	>1.0 c	0.3	0
boiled, drained, chopped	1/2 cup	10	1.0	1.8	60	.9	0.1	0
raw	1 shoot	2	0.3	0.4	15	.3	0.0	0

Food Name	Serv. Size	Total Cal.	Prot. GMS	Carbs GMS	Sod. MGS	Fiber GMS	Fat GMS	Chol. MGS
raw, chopped	1/2 cup	10	1.0	1.8	60	1.2	0.1	0
raw, trimmed, chopped	1/2 cup	6	0.7	0.9	32	.6	0.1	0
raw, untrimmed	1 lb	67	9.1	11.0	395	>3.8 c	0.7	0
CABBAGE ENTRÉE, FROZEN								
w/meat, and tomato sauce (Lean Cuisine)	9.5 oz	210	13.0	26.0	560	na	6.0	30
CABBAGE TURNIP. See KOHLRABI.								
CAESAR SALAD, 'Easy Caesar Kit' (Saco)	.75 oz	98	2.0	7.0	246	na	7.0	4
CAIMIT/star apple								
ripe, trimmed	1 oz	19	0.2	4.1	(mq)	>.3 c	0.5	0
CAJUN SEASONING (Tone's)	1 tsp	9	0.4	2.1	215	.5	0.2	0
CAJUN STYLE MARINADE, barbecue sauce								
(Golden Dipt)	1 oz	90	0.0	5.0	360	na	8.0	0
CAKE. See also BREAD, QUICK.								
'Best Wishes' 6 inch (Awrey's)	1/4 cake	150	1.0	18.0	170	0	9.0	25
'Four-in-One Occasion' (Awrey's)	1.3 oz	150	1.0	18.0	170	0	8.0	25
Banana								
loaf (Entenmann's)	1.3 oz	90	2.0	20.0	125	na	0.0	0
single-layer, iced, frozen (Sara Lee)	1/8 cake	170	1.0	28.0	160	(mq)	6.0	na
Black forest								
torte (Awrey's)	1/14 cake	350	3.0	38.0	330	1.0	21.0	50
two-layer, frozen (Sara Lee)	1/8 cake	190	2.0	28.0	100	(mq)	8.0	na
Blueberry crunch (Entenmann's)	1 oz	70	1.0	16.0	85	(mq)	0.0	0
Boston cream 'Supreme' frozen								
(Pepperidge Farm)	2.875 oz	290	3.0	39.0	190	(mq)	14.0	50
Carrot								
cream cheese icing 'Old Fashioned' frozen								
(Pepperidge Farm)	1.5 oz	150	1.0	19.0	160	(mq)	9.0	15
frozen (Weight Watchers)	3 oz	170	4.0	27.0	280	(mq)	5.0	5
single-layer, iced, frozen (Sara Lee)	1/8 cake	250	3.0	30.0	240	(mq)	13.0	25
supreme, iced (Awrey's)	1 piece	210	3.0	23.0	170	0	12.0	25
three-layer, cream cheese icing (Awrey's)	1/12 cake	390	5.0	44.0	310	1.0	23.0	45
Cheesecake								
brownie 'Sweet Celebrations' frozen								
(Weight Watchers)	3.5 oz	200	9.0	34.0	260	(mq)	5.0	10
cream cheese, cherry, frozen (Sara Lee)	1/6 cake	243	4.0	35.0	184	(mq)	8.0	(mq)
cream cheese, frozen (Sara Lee)	1/6 cake	230	5.0	27.0	153	(mq)	11.0	(mq)
cream cheese, strawberry, frozen								
(Sara Lee)	1/6 cake	222	4.0	34.0	171	(mq)	8.0	(mq)
French 'Classics' frozen (Sara Lee)	1/8 cake	250	4.0	23.0	120	(mq)	16.0	20
frozen (Weight Watchers)	3.9 oz	210	10.0	29.0	230	(mq)	7.0	20
nondairy 'Better Than Cheesecake'								
frozen (Tofutti)	1/10 cake	160	2.0	16.0	110	(mq)	10.0	0

Food Name	Serv. Size	Total Cal.	Prot. GMS	Carbs GMS	Sod. MGS	Fiber GMS	Fat GMS	Chol. MGS
strawberry, French 'Classics' frozen								
(Sara Lee)	1/8 cake	240	3.0	28.0	125	(mq)	13.0	20
strawberry 'Sweet Celebrations' frozen								
(Weight Watchers)	3.9 oz	180	7.0	28.0	210	(mq)	4.0	20
triple chocolate 'Sweet Celebrations'								
frozen (Weight Watchers)	1 cake	190	8.0	30.0	220	na	4.0	5
Cherry, and cream, frozen								
(Weight Watchers)	3 oz	190	3.0	32.0	200	(mq)	6.0	5
Chocolate								
(Awrey's)	.8 oz	70	1.0	11.0	110	0	3.0	15
devil's food, fudge icing (Entenmann's)	1.2 oz	130	2.0	19.0	120	na	5.0	na
devil's food, layer, frozen								
(Pepperidge Farm)	1 5/8 oz	180	1.0	24.0	135	(mq)	9.0	20
devil's food, white icing (Awrey's)	1 piece	150	1.0	17.0	160	1.0	8.0	25
double, iced (Awrey's)	1 piece	130	2.0	21.0	150	1.0	6.0	15
double, three-layer (Awrey's)	1/12 cake	310	3.0	48.0	290	2.0	14.0	35
double, three-layer, frozen (Sara Lee)	1/8 cake	220	3.0	26.0	130	(mq)	11.0	20
double, torte (Awrey's)	1/14 cake	340	3.0	51.0	300	2.0	15.0	35
double, two-layer (Awrey's)	1/12 cake	250	3.0	38.0	260	1.0	11.0	35
double, fudge, frozen								
(Weight Watchers)	2.75 oz	200	4.0	34.0	190	(mq)	5.0	5
'Free & Light' frozen (Sara Lee)	1/8 cake	110	2.0	26.0	140	(mq)	0.0	0
frozen (Weight Watchers)	2.5 oz	180	5.0	31.0	250	(mq)	5.0	5
fudge, layer, frozen (Pepperidge Farm)	1 5/8 oz	180	1.0	23.0	140	(mq)	10.0	20
fudge stripe, layer, frozen								
(Pepperidge Farm)	1 5/8 oz	170	2.0	20.0	140	(mq)	9.0	20
German, frozen (Weight Watchers)	2.5 oz	200	4.0	31.0	220	(mq)	7.0	5
German, iced (Awrey's)	2-inch sq.	160	2.0	19.0	150	0	9.0	20
German, single-layer, frozen								
(Pepperidge Farm)	1 5/8 oz	180	1.0	22.0	170	(mq)	10.0	20
German, three-layer (Awrey's)	1/12 cake	350	3.0	46.0	300	1.0	18.0	40
'Happy Birthday' (Awrey's)	1.4 oz	150	1.0	18.0	150	1.0	8.0	25
milk, and yellow, two-layer (Awrey's)	1/12 cake	290	3.0	33.0	320	0	17.0	50
mousse 'Classics' frozen (Sara Lee)	1/8 cake	260	3.0	23.0	100	(mq)	17.0	20
'Supreme' frozen (Pepperidge Farm)	2 7/8 oz	300	3.0	37.0	140	(mq)	16.0	25
two-layer, white icing (Awrey's)	1/12 cake	270	3.0	34.0	290	1.0	15.0	40
Cinnamon swirl, refrigerated (Pillsbury)	1/8 cake	180	2.0	22.0	170	(mq)	9.0	0
Coconut								
butter cream (Awrey's)	1 piece	160	1.0	19.0	180	0	9.0	25
layer, frozen (Pepperidge Farm)	1 5/8 oz	180	1.0	24.0	120	(mq)	8.0	20
and yellow, three-layer (Awrey's)	1/12 cake	350	3.0	40.0	340	0	21.0	50
Coffeecake								
all butter, cheese, frozen (Sara Lee)	1/8 cake	210	4.0	25.0	220	(mq)	11.0	(mq)

Food Name	Serv. Size	Total Cal.	Prot. GMS	Carbs GMS	Sod. MGS	Fiber GMS	Fat GMS	Chol. MGS
all butter, pecan, frozen *(Sara Lee)*	1/8 cake	160	3.0	19.0	180	(mq)	8.0	(mq)
all butter, streusel, frozen *(Sara Lee)*	1/8 cake	160	3.0	20.0	160	(mq)	7.0	(mq)
caramel nut *(Awrey's)*	1/12 cake	140	2.0	15.0	150	0	8.0	5
cheese *(Entenmann's)*	1.6 oz	150	3.0	20.0	140	na	7.0	na
cinnamon swirl, iced *(Pillsbury)*	1 piece	230	3.0	29.0	240	na	11.0	0
crumb *(Entenmann's)*	1.3 oz	160	3.0	21.0	160	na	7.0	na
crumb, cheese-filled *(Entenmann's)*	1.4 oz	130	3.0	18.0	140	na	6.0	na
'Long John' *(Awrey's)*	1/12 cake	160	2.0	19.0	130	0	8.0	10
pecan crumb, iced *(Pillsbury)*	1 piece	230	3.0	29.0	240	na	12.0	0
French crumb, all butter *(Entenmann's)*	1.6 oz	180	2.0	26.0	220	na	8.0	na
Golden								
layer, frozen *(Pepperidge Farm)*	1 5/8 oz	180	1.0	24.0	110	(mq)	9.0	20
thick fudge icing *(Entenmann's)*	1.2 oz	130	2.0	20.0	120	na	6.0	na
Lemon								
coconut 'Supreme' frozen								
(Pepperidge Farm)	3 oz	280	3.0	38.0	220	(mq)	13.0	30
cream 'Supreme' frozen								
(Pepperidge Farm)	1 5/8 oz	170	2.0	21.0	120	(mq)	9.0	20
three-layer *(Awrey's)*	1/12 cake	320	2.0	38.0	310	0	19.0	45
yellow, two-layer *(Awrey's)*	1/12 cake	290	2.0	33.0	310	0	17.0	45
Louisiana crunch *(Entenmann's)*	1.7 oz	180	2.0	27.0	180	na	8.0	na
Neapolitan torte *(Awrey's)*	1/14 cake	380	3.0	43.0	370	0	22.0	55
Orange								
frosty, iced *(Awrey's)*	1 piece	150	1.0	19.0	170	0	8.0	20
three-layer *(Awrey's)*	1/12 cake	320	2.0	40.0	320	0	17.0	35
Peanut butter torte *(Awrey's)*	1/14 cake	380	7.0	44.0	340	1.0	22.0	40
Pecan streusel, refrigerated *(Pillsbury)*	1/8 cake	180	2.0	21.0	170	(mq)	9.0	0
Pineapple								
cream 'Supreme' frozen *(Pepperidge Farm)*	2 oz	190	1.0	28.0	130	(mq)	7.0	20
crunch *(Entenmann's)*	1 oz	70	1.0	16.0	85	(mq)	0.0	0
Pistachio torte *(Awrey's)*	1/12 cake	370	3.0	41.0	370	1.0	22.0	35
Pound								
(Drake's)	1/10 cake	110	2.0	16.0	70	(mq)	5.0	25
all butter 'Family Size Original' frozen								
(Sara Lee)	1/15 cake	130	2.0	14.0	85	(mq)	7.0	(mq)
all butter, loaf *(Entenmann's)*	1 oz	110	2.0	15.0	150	na	5.0	na
all butter 'Original' frozen *(Sara Lee)*	1/10 cake	130	2.0	14.0	85	(mq)	7.0	(mq)
'Free & Light' frozen *(Sara Lee)*	1/10 cake	70	1.0	17.0	105	(mq)	0.0	0
golden *(Awrey's)*	1/14 loaf	130	2.0	19.0	150	0	5.0	20
'Old Fashioned Cholesterol Free' frozen								
(Pepperidge Farm)	1 oz	110	1.0	13.0	85	(mq)	6.0	0
sour cream, loaf *(Entenmann's)*	1 oz	120	1.0	14.0	90	na	7.0	na
Raisin spice, iced *(Awrey's)*	1 piece	160	1.0	21.0	120	0	8.0	20

Food Name	Serv. Size	Total Cal.	Prot. GMS	Carbs GMS	Sod. MGS	Fiber GMS	Fat GMS	Chol. MGS
Raspberry nut (Awrey's) .... 1/16 cake		310	3.0	39.0	220	0	16.0	30
Shortcake								
strawberry 'Dessert Lights' frozen, 3 oz								
(Pepperidge Farm) .... 1 piece		170	2.0	30.0	50	1.0	5.0	70
strawberry, frozen (Sara Lee) .... 1/8 cake		190	2.0	26.0	90	(mq)	8.0	na
Sponge (Awrey's) .... 2-inch sq.		80	1.0	11.0	125	0	3.0	15
Strawberry								
cream 'Supreme' frozen (Pepperidge Farm) 2 oz		190	1.0	30.0	120	(mq)	7.0	20
stripe, layer, frozen (Pepperidge Farm) .. 1.5 oz		160	1.0	21.0	120	(mq)	8.0	20
supreme, torte (Awrey's) .... 1/14 cake		270	3.0	38.0	310	1.0	12.0	45
Vanilla, layer, frozen (Pepperidge Farm) 1 5/8 oz		190	1.0	25.0	120	(mq)	8.0	20
Walnut torte (Awrey's) .... 1/14 cake		320	2.0	38.0	290	0	19.0	30
Yellow								
(Awrey's) .... .9 oz		80	1.0	12.0	135	0	3.0	20
white icing (Awrey's) .... 2-inch sq.		150	1.0	18.0	180	0	9.0	25
CUPCAKE								
Creme, 'Kreme Kup' (Tastykake) .... 1 cupcake		86	1.3	14.6	113	.6	2.8	4
White (Break Cake) .... 1 cupcake		130	1.0	24.0	115	na	3.0	0
SNACK CAKE								
bar (Sunbelt) .... 1.31 oz		130	1.0	28.0	130	(mq)	2.0	<1
'Be My Valentine' (Little Debbie) .... 2.5 oz		330	2.0	44.0	125	(mq)	17.0	<1
'Best Wishes, Miniature' (Awrey's) .... 3 oz		320	5.0	33.0	280	0	22.0	0
'Caravella' (Little Debbie) .:........ 1.2 oz		200	2.0	26.0	95	(mq)	9.0	<1
'Christmas Tree' (Little Debbie) .... 1.6 oz		220	1.0	28.0	80	(mq)	11.0	<1
coconut covered 'Sno Balls' (Hostess) 1 piece		150	1.0	26.0	160	1.0	4.0	2
dessert cup (Hostess) .... 1 piece		90	2.0	18.0	170	.4	2.0	15
dessert cup (Little Debbie) .... .79 oz		80	1.0	4.0	170	(mq)	1.0	<1
'Doodle Dandies' (Little Debbie) .... 2.5 oz		320	2.0	44.0	140	(mq)	16.0	<1
'Easter Bunny' (Little Debbie) .... 2.5 oz		320	2.0	45.0	135	(mq)	15.0	<1
fancy (Little Debbie) .... 2.6 oz		340	2.0	46.0	150	(mq)	16.0	<1
filled twins, 3 oz (Break Cake) .... 2 pieces		310	2.0	53.0	260	na	10.0	15
filled twins, multi pak, 1.5 oz								
(Break Cake) .... 1 piece		150	1.0	26.0	130	na	5.0	5
'Funny Bones' (Drake's) .... 1.25 oz		150	3.0	18.0	110	(mq)	8.0	0
'Lil' Angels' (Hostess) .... 1 piece		90	1.0	14.0	95	(mq)	2.0	2
'Poppets' (Erewhon) .... 1 oz		110	2.0	24.0	10	1.0	1.0	na
'Star Crunch' (Little Debbie) .... 1.08 oz		150	1.0	22.0	95	(mq)	6.0	<1
Swiss roll (Little Debbie) .... 2.25 oz		280	2.0	40.0	135	(mq)	12.0	<1
'Tasty Twist' (Tastykake) .... 1 piece		18	0.3	2.7	(mq)	(mq)	0.6	na
'Tiger Tail' (Hostess) .... 1 piece		240	4.0	38.0	290	1.3	8.0	25
'Zoinks' (Drake's) .... 1.25 oz		130	1.0	20.0	130	(mq)	5.0	10
Apple streusel (Awrey's) .... 1 piece		160	2.0	18.0	120	0	9.0	15
Banana, iced (Awrey's) .... 1 piece		140	1.0	17.0	120	0	8.0	20

Food Name	Serv. Size	Total Cal.	Prot. GMS	Carbs GMS	Sod. MGS	Fiber GMS	Fat GMS	Chol. MGS
Brownie								
À la mode 'Sweet Celebrations' frozen								
(Weight Watchers)	1 serving	180	5.0	35.0	150	0	4.0	5
chocolate 'Sweet Celebrations' frozen								
(Weight Watchers)	1/3 pkg	100	3.0	16.0	150	(mq)	3.0	5
chocolate chip 'Toll House Ready to								
Bake' frozen *(Nestlé)*	1.4 oz	150	2.0	19.0	60	(mq)	7.0	na
chocolate nut, mini *(Break Cake)*	.5 oz	70	1.0	9.0	60	na	4.0	0
Dutch chocolate 'Cake' *(Awrey's)*	1/16 cake	340	3.0	40.0	260	1.0	20.0	35
fudge *(Break Cake)*	2.8 oz	370	4.0	47.0	260	na	18.0	35
fudge *(Little Debbie)*	3 oz	350	4.0	57.0	180	(mq)	12.0	<1
fudge *(Little Debbie)*	2 oz	240	3.0	39.0	140	(mq)	8.0	<1
fudge nut *(Frito-Lay's)*	3 oz	360	3.0	56.0	225	na	14.0	8
fudge nut, iced 'Sheet Cake' *(Awrey's)* . .	2.5 oz	300	3.0	36.0	210	1.0	17.0	40
fudge nut 'Sheet Cake' *(Awrey's)*	1.25 oz	150	2.0	16.0	115	1.0	9.0	25
fudge walnut *(Tastykake)*	3 oz	335	3.9	53.4	222	5.4	14.2	22
hot fudge 'Newport' frozen								
(Pepperidge Farm)	1 ramekin	400	4.0	50.0	160	(mq)	20.0	80
low-fat, fudge, chocolate icing 'Lights'								
(Hostess)	1 brownie	140	2.0	29.0	95	1.0	2.6	10
mint frosting 'Sweet Celebrations'								
frozen *(Weight Watchers)*	1.23 oz	100	2.0	18.0	130	na	2.0	5
peanut butter fudge 'Sweet Celebrations'								
frozen *(Weight Watchers)*	1.23 oz	100	2.0	18.0	140	na	3.0	5
Swiss mocha fudge 'Sweet Celebrations'								
frozen *(Weight Watchers)*	1.23 oz	90	2.0	18.0	140	na	2.0	5
Caramel								
fudge, À la mode, frozen								
(Weight Watchers)	1 serving	180	4.0	35.0	170	na	3.0	5
peanut filled, chocolate coated								
(Little Debbie)	1 piece	230	3.0	28.0	120	(mq)	12.0	<1
Carrot								
(Break Cake)	2 pieces	370	3.0	64.0	380	na	12.0	20
'Classic' frozen, 2.5 oz								
(Pepperidge Farm)	1 piece	260	2.0	32.0	280	(mq)	16.0	50
'Deluxe' frozen, 1.8 oz *(Sara Lee)*	1 piece	180	3.0	26.0	200	(mq)	7.0	na
'Lights' frozen, 2.5 oz *(Sara Lee)*	1 piece	170	4.0	30.0	75	(mq)	4.0	5
multi pak, 1.2 oz *(Break Cake)*	1 piece	120	1.0	20.0	115	na	4.0	5
Cheesecake								
brownie 'Sweet Celebrations' frozen								
(Weight Watchers)	3.5 oz	200	9.0	34.0	260	na	5.0	10
classic, frozen, 2 oz *(Sara Lee)*	1 piece	200	4.0	16.0	150	(mq)	14.0	na
French 'Lights' frozen, 3.2 oz *(Sara Lee)*	1 piece	150	5.0	24.0	90	(mq)	4.0	15

Food Name	Serv. Size	Total Cal.	Prot. GMS	Carbs GMS	Sod. MGS	Fiber GMS	Fat GMS	Chol. MGS
French, strawberry 'Lights' frozen, 3.5 oz								
(Sara Lee) .... 1 piece	1 piece	150	3.0	29.0	65	(mq)	2.0	5
strawberry 'Manhattan' frozen								
(Pepperidge Farm) .... 1 piece	1 piece	300	6.0	49.0	250	(mq)	9.0	150
strawberry 'Sweet Celebrations' frozen								
(Weight Watchers) .... 3.9 oz	3.9 oz	180	7.0	28.0	210	na	4.0	20
Cinnamon, twirl (Aunt Fanny's) .... 1 oz	1 oz	110	2.0	16.0	85	na	4.0	0
Coffeecake								
(Little Debbie) .... 2.1 oz	2.1 oz	250	3.0	39.0	210	(mq)	9.0	<1
apple cinnamon, individually wrapped,								
frozen (Sara Lee) .... 1 piece	1 piece	290	4.0	40.0	270	(mq)	13.0	na
butter streusel, individually wrapped,								
frozen (Sara Lee) .... 1 piece	1 piece	230	4.0	27.0	270	(mq)	12.0	(mq)
cinnamon crumb (Drake's) .... 1.33 oz	1.33 oz	150	2.0	22.0	110	(mq)	6.0	10
cinnamon streusel 'Microwave' frozen								
(Weight Watchers) .... 1 piece	1 piece	190	3.0	28.0	250	(mq)	7.0	5
cream filled 'Koffee Kake' (Tastykake) .... 1 oz	1 oz	110	1.4	17.5	81	.4	4.0	16
crumb (Hostess) .... 1 piece	1 piece	120	1.0	19.0	80	.7	5.0	10
crumb 'Light' (Hostess) .... 1 piece	1 piece	80	1.0	19.0	95	.4	1.0	0
'Jr.' (Drake's) .... 1.1 oz	1.1 oz	140	2.0	18.0	90	(mq)	6.0	10
'Koffee Kake Juniors' (Tastykake) ...... 2.5 oz	2.5 oz	261	3.4	43.8	212	.9	8.5	410
pecan, individually wrapped, frozen								
(Sara Lee) .... 1 piece	1 piece	280	5.0	30.0	270	(mq)	16.0	na
'Small' (Drake's) .... 2 oz	2 oz	220	3.0	33.0	160	(mq)	9.0	15
Oatmeal, creme pie, individually wrapped								
(Little Debbie) .... 1.35 oz	1.35 oz	170	2.0	29.0	140	na	8.0	0
Shortcake								
strawberry, À la mode, frozen								
(Weight Watchers) .... 1 piece	1 piece	170	3.0	33.0	150	na	2.0	5
strawberry 'Dessert Lights' frozen								
(Pepperidge Farm) ...., 1 piece	1 piece	170	2.0	30.0	50	1.0	5.0	70
CAKE, MICROWAVE								
apple streusel, prepared (MicroRave) 1/12 cake	1/12 cake	240	2.0	33.0	190	(mq)	11.0	45
banana, w/vanilla frosting 'Snack'								
prepared (Pillsbury) .... 1/9 cake	1/9 cake	170	1.0	26.0	160	na	7.0	10
carrot, w/cream cheese frosting 'Snack'								
prepared (Pillsbury) .... 1/9 cake	1/9 cake	170	1.0	25.0	200	na	7.0	10
cinnamon pecan, prepared (MicroRave) 1/6 cake	1/6 cake	290	3.0	39.0	210	(mq)	13.0	45
cinnamon streusel, prepared								
(Streusel Swirl) .... 1/8 cake	1/8 cake	240	2.0	33.0	180	(mq)	11.0	na
chocolate, prepared (Pillsbury) ...... 1/8 cake	1/8 cake	210	2.0	23.0	260	(mq)	13.0	na
chocolate, w/chocolate frosting, prepared								
(Pillsbury) .... 1/8 cake	1/8 cake	300	2.0	35.0	310	(mq)	17.0	na

Food Name	Serv. Size	Total Cal.	Prot. GMS	Carbs GMS	Sod. MGS	Fiber GMS	Fat GMS	Chol. MGS
chocolate, w/vanilla frosting, prepared								
(Pillsbury) .... 1/8 cake	300	2.0	36.0	300	(mq)	17.0	na
chocolate supreme, double, prepared								
(Pillsbury) .... 1/8 cake	330	3.0	39.0	340	(mq)	19.0	na
devil's food, w/chocolate frosting, dry mix								
(MicroRave) .... 1/6 pkg	210	2.0	35.0	240	na	7.0	0
German chocolate, w/coconut pecan								
frosting, dry mix (MicroRave) .... 1/6 pkg	230	2.0	37.0	240	na	8.0	0
lemon, prepared (Pillsbury) .... 1/8 cake	220	2.0	23.0	180	(mq)	13.0	na
lemon, w/lemon frosting, prepared								
(MicroRave) .... 1/6 cake	300	2.0	37.0	250	(mq)	16.0	45
lemon, w/lemon frosting, prepared								
(Pillsbury) .... 1/8 cake	300	2.0	37.0	220	(mq)	17.0	na
lemon supreme, double, prepared								
(Pillsbury) .... 1/8 cake	300	2.0	40.0	210	(mq)	15.0	na
yellow, w/chocolate frosting, prepared								
(Pillsbury) .... 1/8 cake	300	2.0	36.0	220	(mq)	17.0	na
yellow, w/chocolate frosting 'Singles' dry mix								
(MicroRave) .... 1/6 pkg	210	1.0	36.0	210	na	7.0	0
SNACK CAKE								
Brownie								
caramel 'Supreme' prepared								
(Betty Crocker) .... 1 brownie	110	1.0	21.0	110	na	2.0	0
caramel 'Supreme' prepared								
(General Mills) .... 1 brownie	110	1.0	21.0	110	na	2.0	0
caramel fudge chunk, prepared								
(Pillsbury) .... 1 brownie	170	2.0	25.0	105	(mq)	7.0	na
carrot, dry mix (Pillsbury) .... 1/9 pkg	110	1.0	17.0	170	na	5.0	10
chocolate chip 'Supreme' prepared								
(Betty Crocker) .... 1 brownie	110	1.0	20.0	85	na	3.0	0
chocolate chip 'Supreme' prepared								
(General Mills) .... 1 brownie	110	1.0	20.0	85	na	3.0	0
double chocolate, prepared								
(Great Additions) .... 1 brownie	140	1.0	19.0	75	na	6.0	10
double fudge 'Brownies Plus' prepared								
(Duncan Hines) .... 1 brownie	150	2.0	22.0	105	na	6.0	na
double fudge, prepared (Pillsbury) ... 1 brownie	160	2.0	24.0	105	(mq)	6.0	na
frosted, prepared (MicroRave) .... 1 brownie	180	2.0	27.0	130	na	7.0	0
frosted 'Supreme' prepared								
(Betty Crocker) .... 1 brownie	140	1.0	26.0	100	na	3.0	0
frosted 'Supreme' prepared								
(General Mills) .... 1 brownie	140	1.0	26.0	100	na	3.0	0
fudge, mix only (Duncan Hines) ..... 1 brownie	100	1.0	18.0	85	na	18.0	na

Food Name	Serv. Size	Total Cal.	Prot. GMS	Carbs GMS	Sod. MGS	Fiber GMS	Fat GMS	Chol. MGS
fudge, 21.5-oz pkg, dry mix *(Pillsbury)*	1/24 pkg	100	1.0	20.0	85	na	2.0	0
fudge, 15-oz pkg, dry mix *(Pillsbury)*	1/16 pkg	110	1.0	21.0	90	na	2.0	0
fudge 'Family Size' prepared *(General Mills)*	1 brownie	110	1.0	22.0	95	na	2.0	0
fudge 'Light' prepared *(General Mills)*	1 brownie	100	1.0	21.0	90	na	1.0	0
fudge, prepared *(Pillsbury)*	1 brownie	190	2.0	25.0	105	(mq)	9.0	na
fudge, prepared *(Duncan Hines)*	1 brownie	130	1.0	18.0	90	na	5.0	na
fudge, prepared *(Krusteaz)*	1 brownie	190	1.0	28.0	135	na	8.0	19
fudge, prepared *(Lovin' Lites)*	1/24 pkg	100	1.0	19.0	80	na	2.0	10
fudge 'Pouch Mix' dry mix *(Gold Medal)*	1/16 pkg	100	1.0	16.0	85	(mq)	4.0	na
fudge 'Pouch Mix' dry mix *(Robin Hood)*	1/16 pkg	100	1.0	16.0	85	(mq)	4.0	na
fudge 'Regular Size' prepared *(General Mills)*	1 brownie	110	1.0	23.0	100	na	2.0	0
fudge 'Ultra Moist' dry mix *(Finast)*	1/16 pkg	130	2.0	20.0	120	(mq)	5.0	na
fudge, w/fudge frosting, prepared *(Pillsbury)*	1/9 pkg	240	2.0	32.0	140	na	11.0	0
fudge deluxe 'Family Size' prepared *(Pillsbury)*	1 brownie	150	1.0	20.0	95	(mq)	7.0	na
fudge deluxe, prepared *(Pillsbury)*	1 brownie	150	2.0	21.0	100	(mq)	6.0	na
fudge deluxe, w/walnuts, prepared *(Pillsbury)*	1 brownie	150	2.0	19.0	90	(mq)	8.0	na
'Funfetti Frosted' prepared *(Great Additions)*	1 brownie	160	1.0	23.0	100	na	7.0	10
German chocolate 'Supreme' prepared *(Betty Crocker)*	1 brownie	130	1.0	24.0	105	na	3.0	0
German chocolate 'Supreme' prepared *(General Mills)*	1 brownie	130	1.0	24.0	105	na	3.0	0
'Gourmet Turtle' prepared *(Duncan Hines)*	1 brownie	200	2.0	27.0	125	na	9.0	na
milk chocolate 'Brownies Plus' prepared *(Duncan Hines)*	1 brownie	160	1.0	20.0	95	na	8.0	na
original 'Supreme' prepared *(Betty Crocker)*	1 brownie	120	1.0	22.0	90	na	3.0	0
original 'Supreme' prepared *(General Mills)*	1 brownie	120	1.0	22.0	90	na	3.0	0
party 'Supreme' prepared *(Betty Crocker)*	1 brownie	140	1.0	26.0	100	na	3.0	0
party 'Supreme' prepared *(General Mills)*	1 brownie	140	1.0	26.0	100	na	3.0	0
peanut butter 'Brownies Plus' prepared *(Duncan Hines)*	1 brownie	150	3.0	16.0	105	na	8.0	na

Food Name	Serv. Size	Total Cal.	Prot. GMS	Carbs GMS	Sod. MGS	Fiber GMS	Fat GMS	Chol. MGS
peanut butter candies 'Supreme'								
prepared *(Betty Crocker)*	1 brownie	140	2.0	21.0	85	na	5.0	na
prepared *(Estee)*	1 brownie	50	<1.0	11.0	0	na	2.0	0
rocky road, fudge *(Pillsbury)*	1 brownie	170	2.0	24.0	95	(mq)	8.0	na
'Singles' prepared *(MicroRave)*	1 brownie	250	4.0	39.0	230	na	9.0	0
triple fudge, chunky *(Pillsbury)*	1 brownie	170	2.0	25.0	105	(mq)	7.0	na
walnut 'Brownies Plus' prepared								
(Duncan Hines)	1 brownie	150	1.0	19.0	90	na	7.0	na
walnut, prepared *(MicroRave)*	1 brownie	160	2.0	21.0	95	(mq)	7.0	0
walnut, prepared *(Great Additions)*	1 brownie	140	2.0	16.0	70	na	8.0	10
walnut 'Supreme' prepared								
(Betty Crocker)	1 brownie	110	1.0	18.0	85	na	4.0	0
walnut 'Supreme' prepared								
(General Mills)	1 brownie	110	1.0	18.0	85	na	4.0	0
walnut 'Ultra Moist' prepared *(Finast)*	1 brownie	130	1.0	19.0	110	(mq)	6.0	na
w/hot fudge topping 'Singles' prepared								
(MicroRave)	1 brownie	340	5.0	54.0	270	na	12.0	0
CAKE MIX								
Angel food								
chocolate, dry mix *(General Mills)*	1/12 pkg	150	3.0	34.0	300	(mq)	0.0	0
confetti, dry mix *(General Mills)*	1/12 pkg	150	3.0	34.0	300	(mq)	0.0	0
dry mix *(Duncan Hines)*	1/12 pkg	140	3.0	30.0	130	na	0.0	na
dry mix *(Lovin' Loaf)*	1/8 pkg	90	2.0	20.0	210	na	0.0	0
lemon custard, dry mix *(General Mills)*	1/12 pkg	150	3.0	34.0	300	na	0.0	0
lemon pudding, dry mix *(General Mills)*	1/12 pkg	150	3.0	34.0	300	(mq)	0.0	0
strawberry, dry mix *(General Mills)*	1/12 pkg	150	3.0	35.0	260	(mq)	0.0	0
'Traditional' dry mix *(Betty Crocker)*	1/12 pkg	130	3.0	30.0	170	(mq)	0.0	0
white, one-step, dry mix *(General Mills)*	1/12 pkg	150	3.0	34.0	300	na	0.0	0
Apple cinnamon, prepared *(SuperMoist)*	1/12 cake	250	3.0	36.0	280	(mq)	10.0	55
Banana								
dry mix *(Duncan Hines)*	1/12 pkg	190	2.0	36.0	280	na	4.0	0
dry mix *(Pillsbury Plus)*	1/12 pkg	180	2.0	34.0	270	na	4.0	0
Black forest								
cherry 'Bundt Ring Cake' dry mix								
(Pillsbury)	1/16 pkg	200	2.0	40.0	310	na	4.0	0
mousse 'Tiarra' prepared								
(Duncan Hines)	1/12 cake	260	3.0	33.0	270	(mq)	13.0	na
Blueberry streusel, dry mix								
(Streusel Swirl)	1/16 pkg	210	2.0	39.0	190	na	5.0	0
Boston cream, chocolate Eclair 'Bundt								
Ring Cake' dry mix *(Pillsbury)*	1/16 pkg	210	1.0	42.0	280	na	4.0	0
Butter brickle, prepared *(SuperMoist)*	1/12 cake	250	3.0	38.0	280	(mq)	10.0	55
Butter pecan, dry mix *(SuperMoist)*	1/12 pkg	180	1.0	35.0	300	na	4.0	0

Food Name	Serv. Size	Total Cal.	Prot. GMS	Carbs GMS	Sod. MGS	Fiber GMS	Fat GMS	Chol. MGS
Butter recipe								
chocolate, dry mix *(Pillsbury Plus)*	1/12 pkg	170	2.0	32.0	330	na	4.0	0
chocolate, dry mix *(SuperMoist)*	1/12 pkg	190	2.0	35.0	300	na	5.0	0
dry mix *(Pillsbury Plus)*	1/12 pkg	170	2.0	35.0	270	na	3.0	0
fudge, dry mix *(Duncan Hines)*	1/12 pkg	190	2.0	34.0	240	na	4.0	0
golden, dry mix *(Duncan Hines)*	1/12 pkg	190	2.0	36.0	160	na	4.0	0
yellow, dry mix *(SuperMoist)*	1/12 pkg	170	1.0	37.0	250	na	2.0	0
Carrot								
dry mix *(SuperMoist)*	1/12 pkg	180	1.0	36.0	280	na	3.0	0
'n' spice, dry mix *(Pillsbury Plus)*	1/12 pkg	180	2.0	33.0	280	na	5.0	0
prepared *(Dromedary)*	1/12 cake	232	3.0	23.0	292	(mq)	15.0	na
prepared *(Estee)*	1/10 cake	100	1.0	18.0	65	(mq)	2.0	0
Cheesecake								
lemon 'No Bake' dry mix *(Jell-O)*	1 pkg	170	4.0	31.0	300	na	3.0	0
lite 'No-Bake' prepared *(Royal)*	1/8 cake	210	5.0	23.0	380	(mq)	10.0	na
New York style 'No Bake' dry mix *(Jell-O)*	1 pkg	180	4.0	33.0	320	na	3.0	0
'No Bake' dry mix *(Jell-O)*	1 pkg	160	3.0	30.0	250	na	4.0	0
real 'No-Bake' prepared *(Royal)*	1/8 cake	280	5.0	31.0	370	(mq)	9.0	na
Cherry, and cream 'Tiarra' prepared								
(Duncan Hines)	1/12 cake	250	4.0	34.0	265	(mq)	11.0	na
Cherry chip, dry mix *(SuperMoist)*	1/12 pkg	180	2.0	37.0	250	na	3.0	0
Chocolate								
caramel 'Bundt Ring Cake' dry mix								
(Pillsbury)	1/16 pkg	220	2.0	43.0	350	na	5.0	5
chocolate chip, dry mix *(SuperMoist)* ..	1/12 pkg	190	2.0	34.0	380	na	5.0	0
dark, dry mix *(Pillsbury Plus)*	1/12 pkg	170	2.0	32.0	330	na	5.0	0
devil's food, dry mix *(Duncan Hines)* ..	1/12 pkg	190	2.0	33.0	360	na	5.0	0
devil's food, dry mix *(Lovin' Lites)*	1/12 pkg	160	3.0	32.0	370	na	2.0	0
devil's food, dry mix *(Pillsbury Plus)* ..	1/12 pkg	170	2.0	32.0	330	na	4.0	0
devil's food, dry mix *(SuperMoist)*	1/12 pkg	190	2.0	35.0	410	na	5.0	0
devil's food 'Light' dry mix *(SuperMoist)*	1/12 pkg	180	2.0	36.0	330	na	3.0	0
devil's food, prepared *(Krusteaz)*	1/12 cake	190	4.0	37.0	330	na	2.0	25
devil's food 'Ultra Moist' prepared								
(Finast)	1/12 cake	250	3.0	33.0	360	(mq)	11.0	na
Dutch fudge, dark, dry mix								
(Duncan Hines)	1/12 pkg	190	2.0	33.0	455	na	5.0	0
fudge, dry mix *(SuperMoist)*	1/12 pkg	180	2.0	35.0	430	na	4.0	0
fudge 'Tunnel of Fudge' dry mix								
(Pillsbury)	1/16 pkg	210	2.0	42.0	330	na	4.0	0
fudge marble, dry mix *(Duncan Hines)*	1/12 pkg	190	2.0	36.0	280	na	4.0	0
fudge marble, dry mix *(SuperMoist)* ...	1/12 pkg	180	1.0	36.0	270	na	4.0	0
fudge swirl, dry mix *(Pillsbury Plus)* ...	1/12 pkg	190	2.0	36.0	280	na	5.0	0
German, dry mix *(Pillsbury Plus)*	1/12 pkg	170	2.0	33.0	270	na	4.0	0

Food Name	Serv. Size	Total Cal.	Prot. GMS	Carbs GMS	Sod. MGS	Fiber GMS	Fat GMS	Chol. MGS
German, dry mix *(SuperMoist)*	1/12 pkg	180	2.0	35.0	400	na	4.0	0
macaroon 'Bundt Ring Cake' dry mix								
(Pillsbury)	1/16 pkg	210	2.0	37.0	330	na	7.0	0
milk, dry mix *(SuperMoist)*	1/12 pkg	190	2.0	34.0	320	na	5.0	0
mousse, amaretto 'Tiarra' prepared								
(Duncan Hines)	1/12 cake	270	3.0	29.0	230	(mq)	16.0	na
mousse 'Bundt Ring Cake' dry mix								
(Pillsbury)	1/16 pkg	180	2.0	37.0	300	na	4.0	0
mousse 'Tiarra' prepared								
(Duncan Hines)	1/12 cake	270	3.0	29.0	235	(mq)	16.0	na
prepared *(Estee)*	1/10 cake	100	1.0	18.0	100	(mq)	2.0	0
pudding 'Classic Dessert' dry mix								
(Betty Crocker)	1/6 pkg	220	2.0	44.0	240	na	4.0	0
Swiss, dry mix *(Duncan Hines)*	1/12 pkg	190	2.0	33.0	360	na	5.0	0
Chocolate chip								
dry mix *(Pillsbury Plus)*	1/12 pkg	180	2.0	34.0	270	na	5.0	0
dry mix *(SuperMoist)*	1/12 pkg	180	2.0	35.0	280	na	4.0	0
Cinnamon streusel, dry mix								
(Streusel Swirl)	1/16 pkg	200	2.0	38.0	190	na	5.0	0
Coffeecake								
apple cinnamon, prepared *(Pillsbury)*	1/8 cake	240	3.0	40.0	150	(mq)	7.0	na
'Flako' prepared *(Quaker)*	1 piece	156	2.1	27.1	279	.7	4.4	1
prepared *(Aunt Jemima)*	1 piece	156	2.1	27.1	279	.7	4.4	1
Lemon								
'Bundt Tunnel of Lemon' dry mix								
(Pillsbury)	1/16 pkg	210	1.0	44.0	270	na	4.0	0
chiffon 'Classic Dessert' dry mix								
(Betty Crocker)	1/12 pkg	190	3.0	36.0	190	na	4.0	0
dry mix *(Pillsbury Plus)*	1/12 pkg	170	2.0	34.0	260	na	3.0	0
dry mix *(SuperMoist)*	1/12 pkg	180	1.0	36.0	260	na	4.0	0
prepared *(Estee)*	1/10 cake	100	1.0	18.0	68	(mq)	2.0	0
pudding 'Classic Dessert' dry mix								
(Betty Crocker)	1/6 pkg	220	1.0	45.0	260	na	4.0	0
supreme, dry mix *(Duncan Hines)*	1/12 pkg	190	2.0	36.0	280	na	4.0	0
supreme, dry mix *(Streusel Swirl)*	1/16 pkg	200	2.0	37.0	290	na	6.0	0
Orange, supreme, dry mix								
(Duncan Hines)	1/12 pkg	190	2.0	36.0	280	na	4.0	0
Pineapple								
creme 'Bundt Ring Cake' dry mix								
(Pillsbury)	1/16 pkg	200	1.0	42.0	270	na	3.0	0
supreme, dry mix *(Duncan Hines)*	1/12 pkg	190	2.0	36.0	280	na	4.0	0
upside down 'Classic Dessert' dry mix								
(Betty Crocker)	1/9 pkg	240	1.0	43.0	200	na	7.0	0

Food Name	Serv. Size	Total Cal.	Prot. GMS	Carbs GMS	Sod. MGS	Fiber GMS	Fat GMS	Chol. MGS
Pound								
dry mix *(Dromedary)*	5 tbsp	130	1.0	20.0	140	(mq)	5.0	na
golden 'Classic Dessert' dry mix								
(Betty Crocker)	1/12 pkg	190	1.0	28.0	150	na	8.0	0
prepared *(Estee)*	1/8 cake	120	<1.5	23.0	85	na	2.5	0
prepared *(Martha White)*	1/10 cake	120	2.0	19.0	110	(mq)	4.0	8
Rainbow chip, party cake, dry mix								
(SuperMoist)	1/12 pkg	180	2.0	35.0	300	na	4.0	0
Sour cream								
chocolate, dry mix *(SuperMoist)*	1/12 pkg	180	2.0	35.0	410	na	4.0	0
white, dry mix *(SuperMoist)*	1/12 pkg	180	2.0	36.0	280	na	3.0	0
Spice								
dry mix *(Duncan Hines)*	1/12 pkg	190	2.0	36.0	280	na	4.0	0
dry mix *(SuperMoist)*	1/12 pkg	180	1.0	36.0	300	na	4.0	0
prepared *(Estee)*	1/8 cake	120	<1.0	23.0	80	na	3.0	0
Strawberry								
dry mix *(Pillsbury Plus)*	1/12 pkg	180	2.0	35.0	290	na	4.0	0
supreme, dry mix *(Duncan Hines)*	1/12 pkg	190	2.0	36.0	280	na	4.0	0
Swirl, party cake, prepared *(SuperMoist)*	1/12 cake	260	3.0	36.0	280	na	11.0	55
Vanilla								
French, dry mix *(Duncan Hines)*	1/12 pkg	190	2.0	36.0	280	na	4.0	0
golden, dry mix *(SuperMoist)*	1/12 pkg	180	1.0	36.0	250	na	4.0	0
golden, prepared *(MicroRave)*	1/6 cake	320	2.0	40.0	230	(mq)	17.0	35
sunshine, dry mix *(Pillsbury Plus)*	1/12 pkg	180	2.0	34.0	280	na	5.0	0
White								
dry mix *(Duncan Hines)*	1/12 pkg	190	2.0	36.0	250	na	4.0	0
dry mix *(Lovin' Lites)*	1/12 pkg	170	2.0	35.0	300	na	2.0	0
dry mix *(Lovin' Loaf)*	1/12 pkg	170	2.0	35.0	300	na	2.0	0
dry mix *(Pillsbury Plus)*	1/12 pkg	180	2.0	34.0	280	na	4.0	0
dry mix *(SuperMoist)*	1/12 pkg	180	2.0	34.0	300	na	4.0	0
'Funfetti' dry mix *(Pillsbury Plus)*	1/12 pkg	180	2.0	35.0	280	na	4.0	0
'Light' dry mix *(SuperMoist)*	1/12 pkg	180	1.0	37.0	320	na	3.0	0
'n fudge swirl, dry mix *(Pillsbury Plus)*	1/12 pkg	190	2.0	36.0	280	na	4.0	0
prepared *(Estee)*	1/10 cake	100	1.0	18.0	68	(mq)	2.0	0
prepared *(Krusteaz)*	1/12 cake	190	3.0	37.0	280	na	3.0	2
Yellow								
dry mix *(Duncan Hines)*	1/12 pkg	190	2.0	36.0	280	na	4.0	0
dry mix *(Pillsbury Plus)*	1/12 pkg	180	2.0	34.0	280	na	5.0	0
dry mix *(SuperMoist)*	1/12 pkg	180	1.0	36.0	280	na	4.0	0
'Light' dry mix *(SuperMoist)*	1/12 pkg	180	1.0	37.0	290	na	3.0	0
prepared *(Krusteaz)*	1/12 cake	200	3.0	36.0	330	.5	5.0	0
prepared *(Lovin' Loaf)*	1/12 cake	180	3.0	35.0	300	na	3.0	35
'Ultra Moist' prepared *(Finast)*	1/12 cake	240	3.0	34.0	280	(mq)	10.0	na

Food Name	Serv. Size	Total Cal.	Prot. GMS	Carbs GMS	Sod. MGS	Fiber GMS	Fat GMS	Chol. MGS
CALAMANSI PUNCH, 'Rain Forest'								
(Knudsen & Sons)	8 oz	115	<1.0	27.0	na	na	0.0	na
CALAMARI. See SQUID, MIXED SPECIES.								
CALICO BASS. See SUNFISH.								
CALIFORNIA SHEEPSHEAD. See SHEEPSHEAD.								
CANADIAN BACON. See BACON, CANADIAN-STYLE.								
CANDLEFISH/eulachon								
dry-heat cooked	4 oz	141	25.6	0.0	87	0	3.5	102
raw	1 lb	440	80.0	0.0	272	0	11.0	318
raw	1 oz	27	5.0	0.0	17	0	0.7	20
CANDY								
'Bridge Mix' (Brach's)	1 oz	140	2.0	17.0	30	na	7.0	na
'Estee-ets' (Estee)	5 pieces	35	1.0	4.0	10	na	2.0	<1
'Home Fashioned Favorites'								
(Russell Stover)	1.4 oz	170	1.0	27.0	60	1.0	7.0	5
'Smoothie' 1.6 oz (Boyer)	2 pieces	250	5.0	24.0	na	na	15.0	na
'Smoothie' .5 oz (Boyer)	1 piece	75	2.5	12.5	na	na	7.5	na
'Smoothie' .275 oz (Boyer)	1 piece	38	1.3	6.3	na	na	3.8	na
ALMOND								
'Almond Delights' (Russell Stover)	1.4 oz	210	3.0	22.0	55	1.0	12.0	10
chocolate covered (Estee)	2 squares	60	1.0	4.5	10	(mq)	4.5	2
chocolate covered (Featherweight)	1 section	90	1.0	6.0	20	(mq)	7.0	na
'Golden Almond Solitaires' chocolate								
covered (Hershey's)	1.5 oz	240	6.0	19.0	25	na	16.0	5
'Golden Almond Solitaires' chocolate								
covered (Hershey's)	3 oz	455	9.9	40.0	46	>4.1 c	31.5	10
'Jordan Almonds' candy coated (Brach's)	1 oz	120	2.0	23.0	0	(mq)	2.0	na
'Kisses w/Almonds' chocolate								
w/almonds, 1 oz (Hershey's)	6 pieces	160	3.0	14.0	25	na	10.0	na
'M&M's' candy coated almonds								
(M&M/Mars)	1 oz	150	2.0	17.0	30	na	8.0	na
'Solitaires' chocolate covered, 1.6 oz								
(Hershey's)	1/2 bar	260	6.0	20.0	25	(mq)	17.0	5
AMARETTO CHOCOLATE, 'Buffalo Ball'								
confection (Great Cakes)	1 ball	105	3.0	27.0	15	6.0	3.5	0
BAR								
'Aero' milk chocolate, dark chocolate								
(Nestlé)	1 bar	210	0.0	20.0	20	na	12.0	na
'Aero' milk chocolate, dark chocolate,								
bite size (Nestlé)	2 bars	85	0.0	10.0	10	na	5.0	na
'Almond Crunch' date sweetened, carob								
(Carafection)	1 oz	139	2.0	17.0	26	na	7.0	na
'Almond Joy' 1.76 oz (Hershey's)	1 bar	232	2.3	29.2	67	>.6 c	13.9	1

Food Name	Serv. Size	Total Cal.	Prot. GMS	Carbs GMS	Sod. MGS	Fiber GMS	Fat GMS	Chol. MGS
'Almond Joy' miniatures (Hershey's) ... 2 pieces		120	1.0	14.0	35	na	7.0	na
'Almond Joy' snack size (Hershey's) .... 1 bar		93	0.9	11.7	27	>.2 c	5.5	0
'Alpine White' white chocolate w/almonds (Nestlé) .... 1 bar		197	3.5	17.6	4	na	12.9	26
'Alpine White' white chocolate w/almonds, 2.2 oz (Nestlé) .... 1 bar		350	6.2	31.3	7	na	22.9	45
'A-Ok' fruit juice sweetened (Natures Warehouse) .... 1 oz		130	3.2	16.5	32	na	6.2	na
'Baby Ruth' chocolate w/peanuts (Nestlé) 1 bar		277	5.6	37.2	14	>2.0 c	13.3	133
'Baby Ruth' chocolate w/peanuts, fun size (Nestlé) .... 1 bar		110	2.0	15.0	55	na	5.0	0
'Bar None' 1.5 oz (Bar None) .... 1 bar		224	3.5	22.5	45	1.4	14.6	7
'Bounty' dark chocolate (M&M/Mars) ..... 1 oz		140	1.0	17.0	20	na	8.0	na
'Bounty' milk chocolate (M&M/Mars) ...... 1 oz		140	1.0	17.0	30	na	7.0	na
'Brazil Nut Crunch' (Yogafection) .... 1 oz		180	2.0	17.0	70	0	10.0	5
'Butterfinger' 2.16 oz (Nestlé) .... 1 bar		267	4.7	40.5	83	>.8 c	11.3	1
'Butterfinger' snack size (Nestlé) .... 1 bar		92	1.6	13.9	29	>.3 c	3.9	0
'Caramello' 5 oz (Cadbury) .... 1 bar		694	8.7	93.7	175	>2.1 c	35.9	34
'Caramello' 1.6 oz (Cadbury) .... 1 bar		220	2.7	29.7	55	>.7 c	11.4	11
carob (Caroby) .... 4 sections		150	4.0	13.0	55	(mq)	9.0	na
carob candy, plain, date sweetened (Carafection) .... 1 oz		139	2.0	17.0	26	na	7.0	na
carob coated (Tiger's Milk) .... 1 bar		160	6.0	22.0	100	na	6.0	na
carob coated 'Light' (Tiger's Milk) .... 1 bar		110	3.0	24.0	na	na	3.0	na
'Cashew Coconut Crunch' carob candy (Carafection) .... 1 oz		139	2.0	17.0	26	na	7.0	na
'Cashew Nut Crunch' (Yogafection) ...... 1 oz		180	2.0	17.0	70	0	10.0	5
'Chew!' nougat, chocolate coated, all flavors (Charleston) .... 1 oz		120	1.0	22.0	40	(mq)	3.0	na
chocolate tofu truffle w/pralines (Barat) .... 1 oz		170	4.0	12.0	10	(mq)	11.0	0
chocolate tofu w/almonds (Barat) .... 1 oz		170	3.0	13.0	10	(mq)	11.0	0
chocolate tofu w/almonds and raisins (Barat) .... 1 oz		160	3.0	14.0	10	(mq)	11.0	0
chocolate w/almonds, w/o sugar, extra thick (Fifty 50) .... 1 section		90	2.0	6.0	20	na	6.0	na
chocolate w/coconut (Estee) .... 2 squares		60	1.0	5.0	15	na	4.0	5
chocolate w/crisps and honey (Cadbury) .. 1 oz		150	2.0	18.0	40	(mq)	7.0	na
chocolate w/fruit and nuts (Cadbury) ..... 1 oz		150	2.0	17.0	40	(mq)	8.0	na
chocolate w/fruit and nuts (Estee) ... 2 squares		60	1.0	4.5	10	(mq)	4.5	2
chocolate w/fruit and nuts, w/o sugar, extra thick (Fifty 50) .... 1 section		80	1.0	6.0	20	na	5.0	na
chocolate w/roasted almonds (Cadbury) ... 1 oz		150	3.0	15.0	40	(mq)	9.0	na
'Chunky' 1.4 oz (Nestlé) .... 1 bar		198	3.6	22.8	21	>1.7 c	11.7	4

Food Name	Serv. Size	Total Cal.	Prot. GMS	Carbs GMS	Sod. MGS	Fiber GMS	Fat GMS	Chol. MGS
'Chunky' 1.25 oz (Nestlé)	1 bar	173	3.2	20.0	19	>1.5 c	10.2	4
'Chunky' w/raisins, peanuts and cashews (Nestlé)	1.4 oz	170	4.0	21.0	20	na	12.0	na
'Cookies 'N' Mint' mint chocolate, cookie pieces Hershey's)	1 bar	220	3.0	26.0	75	na	12.0	na
'Crispy Crunch' carob candy, date sweetened (Carafection)	1 oz	139	2.0	17.0	26	na	7.0	na
crunch (Estee)	2 squares	45	1.0	4.0	10	(mq)	3.0	2
crunch, chocolate, w/o sugar, extra thick (Fifty 50)	1 section	70	1.0	6.0	20	na	5.0	na
'Crunch' milk chocolate w/crisp rice, 1.4 oz (Nestlé)	1 bar	210	3.0	26.0	35	(mq)	10.0	na
'Crunch' milk chocolate w/crisp rice, fun size (Nestlé)	2 bars	100	1.0	13.0	15	na	5.0	na
'Crunch' milk chocolate w/crisp rice, snack size(Nestlé)	1 bar	49	0.6	6.4	15	0	2.6	2
'Dairy Milk' milk chocolate (Cadbury)	1 oz	150	2.0	17.0	45	(mq)	8.0	(mq)
dark chocolate, deluxe (Estee)	2 squares	50	<1.0	6.0	0	na	3.0	0
'Dove' dark chocolate, miniatures (M&M/Mars)	4 pieces	130	1.0	14.0	0	na	8.0	na
'Dove' milk chocolate, miniatures (M&M/Mars)	4 pieces	130	1.0	14.0	20	na	8.0	na
'5th Avenue' 4.2 oz (Hershey's)	1 pkg	555	9.4	80.9	221	>1.1 c	25.2	5
'5th Avenue' 2.1 oz (Hershey's)	1 bar	280	4.7	40.8	112	>.5 c	12.7	2
French chocolate (Russell Stover)	1 bar	200	3.0	20.0	30	1.0	13.0	10
French chocolate mint (Russell Stover)	1 bar	230	3.0	20.0	25	2.0	15.5	10
'Golden Almond' chocolate w/almonds, 3 oz (Hershey's)	1 bar	466	8.9	41.3	54	>2.0 c	32.1	10
'Golden III' 3.2 oz (Hershey's)	1 bar	471	5.9	50.8	79	>4.9 c	30.0	17
'Halvah' (Fantastic Foods)	1.5 oz	232	8.0	17.0	0	(mq)	10.0	0
'Hershey's Milk Chocolate Bar' (Hershey's)	1.55 oz	240	4.0	25.0	40	na	14.0	10
'Hershey's Milk Chocolate Bar w/Almonds' (Hershey's)	1.45 oz	230	5.0	20.0	55	na	14.0	10
'Kit Kat' chocolate covered wafer, 3.375 oz (Hershey's)	1 bar	490	6.4	59.4	97	.9	27.4	24
'Kit Kat' chocolate covered wafer, 1.625 oz (Hershey's)	1 bar	235	3.1	28.5	46	.4	13.1	11
'Kit Kat' chocolate covered wafer, snack size (Hershey's)	1.12 oz	170	2.0	20.0	40	na	9.0	na
'Krackel' chocolate w/rice crisps, 2.6 oz (Hershey's)	1 bar	371	4.6	45.8	101	>.3 c	20.6	14

Food Name	Serv. Size	Total Cal.	Prot. GMS	Carbs GMS	Sod. MGS	Fiber GMS	Fat GMS	Chol. MGS
'Krackel' chocolate w/rice crisps, 1.65 oz (Hershey's)	1 bar	236	2.9	29.1	64	>.2 c	13.1	9
'Mars Almond, 1.76 oz (M&M/Mars)	1 bar	233	4.1	31.4	85	1.0	11.5	5
milk chocolate (Estee)	2 squares	60	1.0	5.0	15	na	4.0	5
milk chocolate, mini (Fifty 50)	4 pieces	90	2.0	6.0	20	na	6.0	na
milk chocolate w/o sugar, extra thick (Fifty 50)	1 section	80	1.0	6.0	25	na	6.0	na
'Milky Way' dark chocolate (M&M/Mars)	1.76 oz	220	1.0	36.0	115	na	8.0	na
'Milky Way' milk chocolate, 2.1 oz (M&M/Mars)	1 bar	251	2.7	43.5	144	1.0	9.1	12
'Milky Way' milk chocolate, minis (M&M/Mars)	1 piece	40	0.0	6.0	15	na	1.0	na
'Milky Way' milk chocolate, snack size (M&M/Mars)	1 bar	75	0.8	13.1	43	.3	2.7	4
mint (Estee)	2 squares	50	<1.0	6.0	0	na	3.0	0
'Mint' date sweetened, carob candy (Carafection)	1 oz	139	2.0	17.0	26	na	7.0	na
'Mint Honey Graham' carob coated (Carafection)	1 oz	139	2.0	17.0	26	na	7.0	na
'Mounds' chocolate covered coconut, 1.9 oz (Hershey's)	1 pkg	195	1.9	31.3	68	1.7	11.7	0
'Mounds' chocolate covered coconut, minis (Hershey's)	2 pieces	110	1.0	13.0	30	na	6.0	na
'Mounds' chocolate covered coconut, snack size (Hershey's)	1 bar	72	0.7	11.6	25	.6	4.3	0
'Mr. GoodBar' milk chocolate w/peanuts, 2.8 oz (Hershey's)	1 bar	406	9.9	40.5	27	3.4	25.5	16
'Mr. GoodBar' milk chocolate w/peanuts, 1.75 oz (Hershey's)	1 bar	257	6.3	25.6	17	2.2	16.1	10
'Munch' (M&M/Mars)	1.42 oz	220	6.0	19.0	110	na	14.0	na
'My O My' fruit juice sweetened (Natures Warehouse)	1 oz	103	2.2	20.5	42	na	1.4	na
'No How' peanut butter, fruit juice sweetened (Natures Warehouse)	1 oz	140	6.0	11.0	48	na	10.0	na
'Non Stop' fruit juice sweetened (Natures Warehouse)	1 oz	122	2.0	18.2	48	na	5.0	na
'Nut Wit' carob, caramel, and peanuts (Natures Warehouse)	1 oz	135	3.2	16.5	32	na	6.3	na
'Oh Henry!' chocolate covered caramel w/peanuts, 2 oz (Nestlé)	1 bar	246	6.2	36.9	5	>1.5 c	9.6	135
'100 Grand' 1.5 oz (Nestlé)	1 bar	195	1.5	30.9	4	>.1 c	8.5	80
'Original' (Cocofection)	1 oz	155	2.0	15.0	23	na	10.0	na

Food Name	Serv. Size	Total Cal.	Prot. GMS	Carbs GMS	Sod. MGS	Fiber GMS	Fat GMS	Chol. MGS
'Original Honey Graham' carob coated								
(Carafection)	1 oz	139	2.0	17.0	26	na	7.0	na
'Pay Day' (Pay Day)	1.85 oz	250	9.0	28.0	200	na	12.0	na
peanut butter (Russell Stover)	1 bar	290	7.0	22.0	130	3.0	19.0	5
peanut butter, carob coated (Tiger's Milk)	1 bar	160	6.0	20.0	105	na	7.0	na
peanut butter, carob coated 'Light'								
(Tiger's Milk)	1 bar	110	3.0	24.0	25	4.0	3.0	na
peanut butter and honey, carob coated								
(Tiger's Milk)	1 bar	160	6.0	23.0	90	na	5.0	na
'Peanut Crunch' carob candy, date								
sweetened (Carafection)	1 oz	139	2.0	17.0	26	na	7.0	na
'Protein Blast' high-energy, chocolate								
(Weider)	1 bar	270	18.0	40.0	110	4.0	6.0	na
'Skor' toffee, 1.4 oz (Hershey's)	1 bar	211	1.8	22.0	92	>.1 c	13.8	24
'Sky Bar' (Necco)	1.5 oz	196	1.9	31.5	57	0	7.1	na
'Snickers' 2.16 oz (M&M/Mars)	1 bar	278	5.9	36.8	163	1.8	13.6	7
'Snickers,' minis (M&M/Mars)	1 piece	45	1.0	5.0	25	na	2.0	na
'Snickers' snack size (M&M/Mars)	1 bar	68	1.4	9.0	40	.5	3.3	2
'Soft'n Crunchy Bar' 1 3/16 oz (Heath)	2 pieces	190	1.0	19.0	85	na	12.0	na
'Special Dark' sweet chocolate bar,								
2.8 oz (Hershey's)	1 bar	376	3.7	48.7	8	4.3	23.9	0
'Special Dark' sweet chocolate bar,								
1.45 oz (Hershey's)	1 bar	195	1.9	25.3	4	2.3	12.4	0
'Symphony' milk chocolate, 2.4 oz								
(Hershey's)	1 bar	355	5.3	38.6	58	>.3 c	22.0	19
'Symphony' milk chocolate, 1.4 oz								
(Hershey's)	1 bar	209	3.1	22.7	34	>.2 c	13.0	11
'Symphony' milk chocolate w/almonds								
and toffee chips (Hershey's)	1.4 oz	220	4.0	20.0	40	na	14.0	na
'3 Musketeers' 2.13 oz (M&M/Mars)	1 bar	250	1.9	46.1	116	1.0	7.7	7
'3 Musketeers' snack size (M&M/Mars)	1 bar	75	0.6	13.8	35	.3	2.3	2
'Twix' caramel, 2.0 oz (M&M/Mars)	1 pkg	272	3.1	37.5	115	1.0	13.4	5
'Twix' cookies-n-creme (M&M/Mars)	1 bar	120	2.0	13.0	50	na	7.0	na
'Twix' peanut butter, 1.77 oz (M&M/Mars)	1 pkg	253	5.4	28.5	148	1.6	14.5	6
'Whatchamacallit' 1.8 oz (Hershey's)	1 bar	257	4.7	30.0	116	1.5	13.2	11
BUBBLE GUM								
(Beechies) candy coated	1 piece	6	0.0	2.0	0	0	0.0	0
(Bubble Yum)								
all flavors	1 piece	25	0.0	7.0	0	na	0.0	na
sugarless, all flavors	1 piece	20	0.0	5.0	0	na	0.0	na
(Bubblicious)								
	1 piece	25	tr	6.2	0	0	tr	tr
'Sugarless'	1 piece	5	tr	1.3	0	0	tr	tr

Food Name	Serv. Size	Total Cal.	Prot. GMS	Carbs GMS	Sod. MGS	Fiber GMS	Fat GMS	Chol. MGS
(Care Free) sugarless, all flavors	1 piece	10	0.0	2.0	0	na	0.0	na
(Chiclets)								
candy coated	1 piece	6	tr	1.5	0	0	tr	tr
'Tiny' candy coated	1 pkg	8	tr	<.1	0	0	tr	tr
(Clorets) candy coated	1 piece	6	tr	1.5	0	0	tr	tr
(Extra)								
classic	1 piece	6	(mq)	(mq)	0	na	(mq)	(mq)
original	1 piece	7	(mq)	(mq)	0	na	(mq)	(mq)
(Fruit Stripe) all flavors	1 piece	8	0.0	2.0	0	na	0.0	na
fruit	1 piece	8	0.0	2.0	0	na	0.0	na
grape	1 piece	8	0.0	2.0	0	na	0.0	na
lemon	1 piece	8	0.0	2.0	0	na	0.0	na
(Hubba Bubba)								
regular, all flavors except cola	1 piece	23	0.0	5.8	0	0	0.0	0
regular, cola	1 piece	23	0.0	5.3	0	0	0.0	0
'Sugar-free' grape	1 piece	13	0.0	(mq)	0	0	0.0	0
sugar-free, original	1 piece	14	0.0	(mq)	0	0	0.0	0
BUTTERSCOTCH, squares *(Russell Stover)*	1.4 oz	180	1.0	29.0	65	1.0	6.5	5
CARAMEL								
(Allen Wertz)	1 piece	37	0.0	6.0	2	na	2.0	1
(Featherweight)	1 piece	30	0.0	5.0	10	(tr)	1.0	0
(Kraft)	1 piece	30	0.0	6.0	25	(tr)	1.0	0
butter cream, squares *(Russell Stover)*	1.4 oz	170	1.0	26.0	95	1.0	7.5	10
chocolate *(Estee)*	1 piece	20	<1.0	3.0	10	(tr)	1.0	0
chocolate coated *(Pom Poms)*	1 oz	100	1.0	15.0	70	(mq)	3.0	na
marshmallow, milk chocolate, squares *(Russell Stover)*	1.4 oz	190	2.0	25.0	85	5.0	10.0	4
milk chocolate coated, approx 1.93 oz *(Rolo)*	8 pieces	270	3.0	37.0	110	(tr)	12.0	15
'Milk Maid' *(Brach's)*	1 oz	110	1.0	22.0	70	(tr)	2.0	na
'Milk Maid' chocolate *(Brach's)*	1 oz	110	1.0	20.0	55	(tr)	3.0	na
'Nip' *(Pearson)*	1 oz	120	1.0	23.0	70	na	3.0	na
nougat swirl *(Allen Wertz)*	1 piece	32	0.0	6.0	2	na	1.0	1
pop *(Sugar Daddy)*	1 3/8 oz	150	1.0	33.0	85	(tr)	1.0	na
'Regular' 1 5/8 oz *(Sugar Babies)*	1 pkg	180	1.0	40.0	85	(tr)	2.0	na
'Rolos' milk chocolate covered *(Hershey's)*	1.93 oz	270	3.0	37.0	110	na	12.0	15
'Tidbits' 1 5/8 oz *(Sugar Babies)*	1 pkg	180	1.0	40.0	85	(tr)	2.0	na
vanilla *(Estee)*	1 piece	20	<1.0	3.0	10	(tr)	1.0	0
CHERRY								
'Cherry Cordials' *(Russell Stover)*	1.4 oz	170	1.0	25.0	25	2.0	7.5	5
chocolate cream *(Brach's)*	1 oz	110	1.0	21.0	20	(mq)	2.0	na
dark chocolate coated *(Brach's)*	1 oz	110	1.0	22.0	20	(mq)	2.0	na

Food Name	Serv. Size	Total Cal.	Prot. GMS	Carbs GMS	Sod. MGS	Fiber GMS	Fat GMS	Chol. MGS
'Nibs' *(Y&S)*	1 oz	106	0.8	26.2	67	0	0.7	0
squares *(Russell Stover)*	1.4 oz	160	1.0	28.0	40	1.0	5.5	na
'Villa' milk chocolate covered *(Brach's)*	1 oz	110	1.0	22.0	20	na	2.0	na
CHEWING GUM								
(Beech-Nut) all flavors	1 piece	10	0.0	2.0	0	na	0.0	na
(Brach's) 'Gumdinger' balls, all flavors	1 oz	110	0.0	24.0	5	0	2.0	0
(Care Free) sugarless, all flavors	1 piece	8	0.0	2.0	0	na	0.0	na
(Chewels) all flavors	1 piece	8	tr	2.0	0	0	tr	tr
(Clorets) stick, all flavors	1 piece	9	tr	2.3	0	0	tr	tr
(Dentyne)								
all flavors	1 piece	6	tr	1.5	0	0	tr	tr
'Sugarless' all flavors	1 piece	5	tr	1.1	0	0	tr	tr
(Estee) gumdrops	4 pieces	25	0.0	6.0	0	na	0.0	0
(Extra) all flavors	1 stick	8	(mq)	(mq)	0	na	(mq)	(mq)
(Freedent) all flavors	1 stick	10	(mq)	2.0	0	na	(mq)	(mq)
(Freshen-Up) all flavors	1 piece	13	tr	3.1	0	0	tr	tr
(Fruit Stripe) all flavors	1 piece	10	0.0	2.0	0	na	0.0	na
(Sticklets) all flavors	1 piece	7	tr	1.9	0	0	tr	tr
(Wrigley's)								
'Big Red'	1 piece	10	0.0	2.3	0	0	0.0	0
'Doublemint'	1 piece	10	0.0	2.3	0	0	0.0	0
'Juicy Fruit'	1 piece	10	0.0	2.3	0	0	0.0	0
'Spearmint'	1 piece	10	0.0	2.3	0	0	0.0	0
CHOCOLATE								
assorted, wrapped, 1-lb bag *(Brach's)*	1 oz	110	0.0	23.0	25	(mq)	2.0	na
'Bits' tofu pastilles *(Barat)*	.75 oz	120	2.0	11.0	10	(mq)	8.0	0
chewy roll *(Tootsie Roll)*	1 oz	112	0.3	22.8	6	(tr)	2.5	tr
'Choc'Oh's' *(Saco Foods)*	1.5 oz	111	1.1	13.8	14	na	6.6	0
chunks *(Saco Foods)*	3.5 oz	466	4.4	66.8	26	na	26.4	0
coated, creme center *(Spangler)*	1 piece	80	<1.0	15.0	40	(mq)	2.0	0
coated, creme center caramel, w/nuts *(Spangler)*	1 piece	100	2.0	11.0	30	(mq)	6.0	0
coated, creme center cherry, w/nuts *(Spangler)*	1 piece	110	2.0	12.0	20	(mq)	5.0	0
coated, creme center fudge, w/nuts *(Spangler)*	1 piece	140	2.0	17.0	25	(mq)	6.0	0
coated, creme center fudge, w/pecans *(Spangler)*	1 piece	140	1.0	18.0	40	(mq)	7.0	0
coated, creme center maple, w/nuts *(Spangler)*	1 piece	110	2.0	12.0	15	(mq)	5.0	0
coated, creme center vanilla, w/nuts *(Spangler)*	1 piece	110	2.0	13.0	20	(mq)	5.0	0
cream *(Callard & Bowser)*	1 oz	120	0.3	22.3	na	(mq)	3.7	na

Food Name	Serv. Size	Total Cal.	Prot. GMS	Carbs GMS	Sod. MGS	Fiber GMS	Fat GMS	Chol. MGS
creamy milk, w/almonds and toffee chips								
(Hershey's) .... .75 oz		280	5.0	26.0	50	(mq)	17.0	(mq)
crunch (Featherweight) .... 1 section		80	1.0	7.0	20	(mq)	6.0	na
'Gift Box' dark and milk mix								
(Russell Stover) .... 1.4 oz		180	2.0	26.0	45	na	8.5	5
'Gourmet' assortment (Allen Wertz) 11.9 grams		55	1.0	9.0	13	na	2.0	1
'Jots' (Brach's) .... 1 oz		130	1.0	21.0	30	(mq)	5.0	na
'Kisses' (Hershey's) .... 6 pieces		150	2.0	16.0	25	na	9.0	5
'M&M's' plain (M&M/Mars) ...... 10 pieces		33	0.4	4.8	7	.2	1.5	1
'M&M's' plain, 1.69 oz (M&M/Mars) ..... 1 pkg		228	3.0	32.7	49	1.5	10.7	7
'Malted Milk Balls' milk coated (Brach's) .. 1 oz		130	1.0	21.0	40	(mq)	5.0	(mq)
malted milk balls, milk coated (Whoppers) 1 oz		136	<1.0	20.0	na	na	6.0	na
milk (Featherweight) .... 1 section		80	1.0	7.0	20	(mq)	6.0	na
milk, assortment (Russell Stover) ...... 1.4 oz		190	2.0	27.0	50	na	8.5	5
'Passionettes' tofu (Barat) .... 1 piece		70	1.0	6.0	5	(mq)	5.0	0
'Stars' (Brach's) .... 1 oz		150	2.0	17.0	30	(mq)	8.0	na
'Stars' approx 13 pieces (Nabisco) ...... 1 oz		160	2.0	19.0	35	(mq)	8.0	na
trail mix, premium (Cocofection) .... 1 oz		130	4.0	13.0	14	na	9.0	na
COCONUT								
'Macaroo' chocolate coated (Sunbelt) .... 2 oz		288	3.0	33.0	75	(mq)	16.0	<1
Neapolitan (Brach's) .... 1 oz		120	1.0	24.0	40	(mq)	2.0	na
COFFEE								
(Brach's) .... 1 oz		120	0.0	25.0	35	0	2.0	na
'Coffee Time' (Allen Wertz) .... 1 piece		20	0.0	4.0	2	na	1.0	1
'Coffee Time' assorted (Allen Wertz) ... 1 piece		28	0.0	5.0	2	na	1.0	1
'Coffee Time' decaffeinated (Allen Wertz) 1 piece		20	0.0	4.0	2	na	1.0	1
'Nip' (Pearson) .... 1 oz		120	1.0	23.0	70	na	3.0	na
FONDANT, candy corn .... 1 cup		728	0.2	179.2	424	0	4.0	0
FRUIT								
(Bonkers!) chews, all flavors .... 1 piece		20	0.0	5.0	0	0	0.0	0
(Brach's)								
orange sticks, chocolate coated .... 1 oz		110	1.0	23.0	25	(mq)	2.0	na
'Orangettes' .... 1 oz		100	0.0	24.0	20	0	0.0	0
(Featherweight)								
berry patch .... 1 piece		12	0.0	3.0	0	0	0.0	0
drops, all flavors .... .33 oz		30	0.0	8.0	15	0	0.0	0
orchard .... 1 piece		12	0.0	3.0	0	0	0.0	0
tropical blend .... 1 piece		12	0.0	3.0	0	0	0.0	0
(Glenny's) 'Drops'								
black cherry .... 1 drop		6	<1.0	1.0	<1	na	<1.0	na
Mandarin orange .... 1 drop		6	<1.0	1.0	<1	na	<1.0	na
mixed fruit .... 1 drop		6	<1.0	1.0	<1	na	<1.0	na
twist of lemon .... 1 drop		6	<1.0	1.0	<1	na	<1.0	na

Food Name	Serv. Size	Total Cal.	Prot. GMS	Carbs GMS	Sod. MGS	Fiber GMS	Fat GMS	Chol. MGS
(Jujyfruits)	11 pieces	100	<1.0	25.0	0	0	<1.0	0
(Rascals) chews, all flavors	1 piece	4	tr	1.0	0	0	tr	tr
(Russell Stover) lemon squares	1.4 oz	160	1.0	27.0	35	2.0	5.5	na
'Skittles' *(M&M/Mars)*								
candy coated, bite size	1 oz	120	0.0	26.0	15	na	1.0	na
candy coated, bite size, 2.3 oz	1 pkg	255	0.2	62.4	30	0	2.0	0
'Starburst' *(M&M/Mars)*								
original fruit chews	2 oz	240	0.0	48.0	30	na	5.0	na
tropical fruit chews	2 oz	240	0.0	48.0	30	na	5.0	na
(Soda-Licious) all flavors	1 pouch	100	<1.0	22.0	20	na	1.0	na
(SweeTARTS) chewy	1 oz	113	0.0	25.0	na	na	1.0	na
'Twizzlers' *(Y&S)*								
strawberry sticks, 5 oz	1 pkg	525	4.7	131.6	393	>.1 c	2.3	0
strawberry sticks, 2.5 oz	1 pkg	263	2.3	65.8	197	>.1 c	1.1	0
FUDGE								
chocolate, w/walnuts *(Woodys)*	1 oz	120	2.0	18.0	25	(mq)	4.0	5
'Fudgies' *(Kraft)*	1 piece	35	0.0	6.0	25	(mq)	1.0	0
maple walnut *(Woodys)*	1 oz	120	1.0	19.0	25	(mq)	4.0	5
mint, w/walnuts *(Woodys)*	1 oz	120	2.0	18.0	25	(mq)	4.0	5
w/walnuts *(Woodys)*	1 oz	120	2.0	18.0	25	(mq)	4.0	5
HARD CANDY								
(Brach's)								
'Cut Rock'	1 oz	110	0.0	27.0	10	0	0.0	0
'Disks' butterscotch	1 oz	110	0.0	27.0	220	(tr)	0.0	na
'Disks' cinnamon	1 oz	110	0.0	27.0	15	0	0.0	0
filled, assorted	1 oz	110	0.0	27.0	15	tr	0.0	0
'Imperials' cinnamon	1 oz	110	0.0	27.0	5	0	0.0	0
lemon drops	1 oz	110	0.0	27.0	5	0	0.0	0
raspberry filled	1 oz	110	0.0	27.0	15	(tr)	0.0	0
ribbon, crimp	1 oz	110	0.0	27.0	15	0	0.0	0
'Royals'	1 oz	100	1.0	20.0	60	(mq)	2.0	na
sour balls	1 oz	110	0.0	27.0	15	0	0.0	0
'Spicettes'	1 oz	100	0.0	26.0	15	0	0.0	0
(Breath Savers)								
cores, mint-cinnamon	1 piece	2	0.0	<1.0	0	na	0.0	0
cores, peppermint	1 piece	2	0.0	<1.0	0	na	0.0	0
cores, spearmint	1 piece	2	0.0	<1.0	0	na	0.0	0
cores, wintergreen	1 piece	2	0.0	<1.0	0	na	0.0	0
mint-cinnamon	1 piece	8	0.0	2.0	0	na	0.0	0
peppermint	1 piece	8	0.0	2.0	0	na	0.0	0
spearmint	1 piece	8	0.0	2.0	0	na	0.0	0
wintergreen	1 piece	8	0.0	2.0	0	na	0.0	0
(Callard & Bowser) butterscotch	1 oz	115	0.0	25.2	na	(tr)	1.9	na

Food Name	Serv. Size	Total Cal.	Prot. GMS	Carbs GMS	Sod. MGS	Fiber GMS	Fat GMS	Chol. MGS
(Ce De) 'Smarties'	1 roll	25	0.0	6.0	0	na	0.0	na
(Certs)								
sugar-free, mini	1 piece	1	tr	0.4	tr	0	tr	0
sugar-free, mints	1 piece	6	tr	1.6	0	0	tr	tr
(Clorets)								
clear mint	1 piece	8	tr	2.1	0	0	tr	tr
pressed mints	1 piece	6	tr	1.6	0	0	tr	tr
(Estee)	2 pieces	25	0.0	6.0	0	na	0.0	0
(Featherweight)								
butterscotch	1 piece	25	0.0	6.0	25	tr	0.0	0
'Sweet Pretenders' tropical blend	1 piece	12	0.0	3.0	0	na	0.0	na
(Fruit Juicers)								
citrus fruits	1 piece	8	0.0	2.0	0	na	0.0	0
fruit punch	1 piece	8	0.0	2.0	0	na	0.0	0
grape	1 piece	8	0.0	2.0	0	na	0.0	0
mixed berries	1 piece	8	0.0	2.0	0	na	0.0	0
strawberry	1 piece	8	0.0	2.0	0	na	0.0	0
(Glenny's)								
fruit	1 piece	19	<1.0	4.0	<1	na	<1.0	na
peppermint	1 piece	19	<1.0	4.0	<1	na	<1.0	na
(Jolly Joes)	1 piece	9	<.1	2.1	1	0	tr	0
(Jolly Rancher)								
apple	1 piece	23	na	6.0	5	na	0.0	na
butterscotch	1 piece	25	na	6.0	37	na	<1.0	na
cherry	1 piece	23	na	6.0	3	na	0.0	na
fire cinnamon	1 piece	23	na	6.0	5	na	0.0	na
fruit punch	1 piece	23	na	6.0	5	na	0.0	na
grape	1 piece	23	na	6.0	5	na	0.0	na
lemon	1 piece	23	na	6.0	5	na	0.0	na
orange	1 piece	23	na	6.0	4	na	0.0	na
peach	1 piece	23	na	6.0	3	na	0.0	na
peppermint	1 piece	23	na	6.0	3	na	0.0	na
pink lemonade	1 piece	23	na	6.0	5	na	0.0	na
raspberry	1 piece	23	na	6.0	5	na	0.0	na
strawberry	1 piece	23	na	6.0	3	na	0.0	na
watermelon	1 piece	23	na	6.0	5	na	0.0	na
(Jurassic Park)								
'Raptor Bites' wild cherry	13 pieces	60	0.0	15.0	0	na	0.0	na
'Spitters' tropical flavors	13 pieces	60	0.0	15.0	0	na	0.0	na
(Life Savers)								
butter creme mint	1 piece	8	0.0	2.0	5	0	0.0	0
butter rum	1 piece	8	0.0	2.0	10	0	0.0	0
butterscotch	1 piece	8	0.0	2.0	10	0	0.0	0

Food Name	Serv. Size	Total Cal.	Prot. GMS	Carbs GMS	Sod. MGS	Fiber GMS	Fat GMS	Chol. MGS
candy coated, bite size .... 10 pieces		43	0.0	10.6	5	0	0.3	na
'Cin-O-Mon' .... 1 piece		8	0.0	2.0	0	0	0.0	0
'Cryst-O-Mint' .... 1 piece		8	0.0	2.0	0	na	0.0	0
fancy fruits .... 1 piece		8	0.0	2.0	0	na	0.0	0
five flavor .... 1 piece		8	0.0	2.0	0	na	0.0	0
holes, butter rum .... 1 piece		2	0.0	<1.0	0	na	0.0	na
holes, five flavor .... 1 piece		2	0.0	<1.0	0	na	0.0	na
holes, 'Pep-O-Mint' .... 1 piece		2	0.0	<1.0	0	na	0.0	na
holes, sunshine fruits .... 1 piece		2	0.0	<1.0	0	na	0.0	na
holes, tangerine .... 1 piece		2	0.0	<1.0	0	na	0.0	na
holes, 'Wint-O-Green' .... 1 piece		2	0.0	<1.0	0	na	0.0	na
'Pep-O-Mint' .... 1 piece		8	0.0	2.0	0	na	0.0	0
root beer .... 1 piece		8	0.0	2.0	0	0	0.0	0
'Spear-O-Mint' .... 1 piece		8	0.0	2.0	0	na	0.0	0
sunshine fruits .... 1 piece		8	0.0	2.0	0	na	0.0	0
tropical fruits .... 1 piece		8	0.0	2.0	0	na	0.0	0
wild cherry .... 1 piece		8	0.0	2.0	0	na	0.0	0
'Wint-O-Green' .... 1 piece		8	0.0	2.0	0	na	0.0	0
(Mike & Ike) .... 1 piece		9	<.1	2.1	1	0	tr	0
(Pearson) 'Nip' butter rum .... 1 oz		120	1.0	24.0	70	na	3.0	na
(Russell Stover) sugar-free, mix ...... 3 pieces		70	0.0	18.0	5	na	0.0	na
(Spree) fruit .... 1 oz		110	0.0	26.0	na	na	0.0	na
(SweeTARTS) fruit .... 1 oz		110	0.0	26.0	na	na	0.0	na
HOLIDAY								
assorted, chocolate (Brach's) .... 1 oz		110	0.0	23.0	25	(mq)	2.0	na
autumn leaves (Brach's) .... 1 oz		100	0.0	26.0	15	0	0.0	0
bell, chocolate, in foil (Brach's) .... 1 oz		150	2.0	17.0	25	(mq)	8.0	na
holiday mints (Brach's) .... 1 oz		110	0.0	26.0	0	0	1.0	0
holiday mix (Brach's) .... 1 oz		110	0.0	27.0	10	0	0.0	0
Christmas								
candy cane (Brach's) .... 1 oz		110	0.0	27.0	10	0	0.0	0
candy cane (Spangler) .... 1 piece		60	<1.0	14.0	0	0	<1.0	0
jellies (Brach's) .... 1 oz		100	0.0	24.0	10	0	0.0	0
jellies, snowbase (Brach's) .... 1 oz		100	0.0	24.0	5	0	0.0	0
'Jots' (Brach's) .... 1 oz		130	1.0	21.0	30	na	5.0	0
nougat (Brach's) .... 1 oz		110	0.0	24.0	20	(mq)	2.0	0
ornaments (Brach's) .... 1 oz		150	2.0	17.0	50	na	8.0	0
'Pearls' mint (Brach's) .... 1 oz		110	0.0	25.0	5	0	1.0	0
'Perkys' (Brach's) .... 1 oz		90	0.0	23.0	20	0	0.0	0
Santa, chocolate, in foil (Brach's) .... 1 oz		140	2.0	18.0	40	(mq)	7.0	na
Santa, marshmallow (Brach's) .... 1 oz		120	1.0	23.0	35	0	3.0	na
snowmen, marshmallow, large pieces								
(Just Born) .... 1 piece		111	0.7	26.8	8	0	0.1	na

Food Name	Serv. Size	Total Cal.	Prot. GMS	Carbs GMS	Sod. MGS	Fiber GMS	Fat GMS	Chol. MGS
snowmen, marshmallow, small pieces								
(Just Born) .... 1 piece		37	0.2	8.9	3	0	<.1	na
'Starlight' mint (Brach's) .... 1 oz		110	0.0	27.0	15	0	0.0	0
trees, marshmallow, large pieces								
(Just Born) .... 1 piece		111	0.7	26.8	8	0	0.1	na
trees, marshmallow, small pieces								
(Just Born) .... 1 piece		37	0.2	8.9	3	0	<.1	na
Easter								
'Chicks & Rabbits' assorted (Brach's) .... 1 oz		100	0.0	26.0	10	0	0.0	0
corn (Brach's) .... 1 oz		100	0.0	26.0	66	0	0.0	0
'Easter Fun' assorted (Brach's) .... 1 oz		100	0.0	26.0	10	0	0.0	0
eggs, chocolate, in foil (Brach's) .... 1 oz		150	2.0	17.0	25	(mq)	8.0	na
eggs, chocolate malted milk (Brach's) .... 1 oz		130	1.0	21.0	40	(mq)	5.0	na
eggs, creme (Cadbury) .... 1.37 oz		190	2.0	26.0	0	na	8.0	na
eggs, creme, chocolate coated buttercream								
(Brach's) .... 1 oz		120	1.0	22.0	50	(mq)	3.0	na
eggs, creme, chocolate coated cherry								
(Brach's) .... 1 oz		110	1.0	23.0	20	(mq)	2.0	na
eggs, creme, chocolate coated coconut								
(Brach's) .... 1 oz		110	0.0	22.0	40	(mq)	3.0	na
eggs, creme, chocolate coated fruit and nut								
(Brach's) .... 1 oz		110	0.0	23.0	35	2.0	na	
eggs, creme, chocolate coated maple								
(Brach's) .... 1 oz		110	0.0	23.0	30	(mq)	2.0	na
eggs, creme, chocolate coated vanilla								
(Brach's) .... 1 oz		110	0.0	23.0	25	(mq)	2.0	na
eggs, creme, mini (Cadbury) .... 1 oz		140	2.0	20.0	na	na	7.0	na
eggs, 'Fiesta' pastel (Brach's) .... 1 oz		120	1.0	23.0	25	0	3.0	na
eggs 'Hide'n Seek' (Brach's) .... 1 oz		110	0.0	27.0	5	0	0.0	0
eggs, jelly (Brach's) .... 1 oz		100	0.0	24.0	15	0	0.0	0
eggs, jelly, speckled (Brach's) .... 1 oz		110	0.0	27.0	40	0	0.0	0
eggs, jelly, spiced (Brach's) .... 1 oz		90	0.0	22.0	10	0	0.0	0
eggs, jelly 'Tiny' (Brach's) .... 1 oz		100	0.0	26.0	10	0	0.0	0
eggs, marshmallow (Brach's) .... 1 oz		100	0.0	25.0	5	0	0.0	0
eggs, 'Robin's Eggs' (Brach's) .... 1 oz		140	1.0	20.0	30	0	6.0	na
nougats (Brach's) .... 1 oz		100	0.0	24.0	25	(mq)	1.0	0
peeps, marshmallow (Just Born) .... 1 piece		27	0.2	6.6	2	0	<.1	0
rabbits, 'Jube' (Brach's) .... 1 oz		100	0.0	24.0	15	0	0.0	0
rabbits, marshmallow (Brach's) .... 1 oz		120	1.0	22.0	55	0	3.0	0
'Starlight' mint (Brach's) .... 1 oz		110	0.0	27.0	15	0	0.0	0
Halloween								
cats, marshmallow (Just Born) .... 1 piece		28	0.2	6.7	2	0	<.1	0
cats 'Scary Cats' (Brach's) .... 1 oz		100	0.0	26.0	85	0	0.0	0

Food Name	Serv. Size	Total Cal.	Prot. GMS	Carbs GMS	Sod. MGS	Fiber GMS	Fat GMS	Chol. MGS
corn, Indian (Brach's)	1 oz	100	0.0	26.0	75	0	0.0	0
corn, three color (Brach's)	1 oz	100	0.0	26.0	95	0	0.0	0
jelly beans (Brach's)	1 oz	100	0.0	26.0	15	0	0.0	0
lollipops 'Picture Pops' (Brach's)	1 oz	110	0.0	27.0	10	0	0.0	0
'Mellowcremes' (Brach's)	1 oz	100	0.0	26.0	40	0	0.0	0
pumpkin heads, crazy (Brach's)	1 oz	100	0.0	24.0	15	0	1.0	0
pumpkins (Brach's)	1 oz	100	0.0	26.0	65	0	0.0	0
pumpkins, marshmallow, large pieces (Just Born)	1 piece	111	0.7	26.8	8	0	0.1	0
pumpkins, marshmallow, small pieces (Just Born)	1 piece	14	0.1	3.4	1	0	<.1	0
'Trick or Treat Party Pack' (Brach's)	1 oz	110	0.0	27.0	20	0	0.0	0
witches' teeth (Brach's)	1 oz	100	0.0	26.0	75	0	0.0	0
Valentine's Day								
'Heart Box, 1-lb' (Brach's)	1 oz	110	1.0	23.0	30	na	2.0	na
'Heart Box, 1/2-lb' (Brach's)	1 oz	110	1.0	23.0	35	na	2.0	na
'Heart Box, 1/3-lb' (Brach's)	1 oz	110	1.0	23.0	25	na	2.0	na
hearts 'Conversation' large (Brach's)	1 oz	110	0.0	27.0	5	0	0.0	0
hearts 'Conversation' small (Brach's)	1 oz	110	0.0	27.0	0	0	0.0	0
hearts, fruity (Brach's)	1 oz	100	0.0	24.0	5	0	0.0	0
hearts 'Imperial' cinnamon (Brach's)	1 oz	110	0.0	27.0	5	0	0.0	0
hearts, 'Jube' cherry (Brach's)	1 oz	100	0.0	26.0	20	0	0.0	0
hearts, red jelly (Brach's)	1 oz	100	0.0	24.0	10	0	0.0	0
hearts 'Sassy Hearts' (Brach's)	1 oz	100	0.0	25.0	0	0	0.0	0
'I Luv U' chocolate (Brach's)	1 oz	150	2.0	17.0	25	na	8.0	na
kisses, nougat (Brach's)	1 oz	110	0.0	24.0	15	na	2.0	na
lollipop, pastels (Life Savers)	1 lollipop	40	0.0	10.0	0	na	0.0	na
'Love' (Brach's)	1 oz	150	2.0	17.0	25	na	8.0	na
'Mellowcremes' (Brach's)	1 oz	100	0.0	26.0	75	0	0.0	0
JELLIED AND GUMMED								
cinnamon bears (Brach's)	1 oz	80	0.0	21.0	10	0	0.0	0
eggs (Rodda)	1 piece	7	<.1	1.7	1	0	tr	0
'Fruit Bunch' (Brach's)	1 oz	100	0.0	24.0	10	na	0.0	na
gummi bears (Brach's)	1 oz	100	2.0	22.0	15	na	0.0	na
gummi dinosaurs, tropical (Jurassic Park)	15 pieces	140	3.0	31.0	na	0	0.0	na
gummi savers (Life Savers)	1 piece	12	0.0	3.0	0	na	0.0	na
gummi worms (Brach's)	1 oz	100	2.0	22.0	15	na	0.0	na
gummy bears (Estee)	4 pieces	20	1.0	4.0	0	0	0.0	0
gummy bears 'Amazin Fruit' approx 12 pieces (Hershey's)	1 oz	90	2.0	21.0	20	na	<1.0	na
gummy bears, tropical 'Amazin Fruit' (Hershey's)	1 oz	90	2.0	21.0	20	na	<1.0	na

Food Name	Serv. Size	Total Cal.	Prot. GMS	Carbs GMS	Sod. MGS	Fiber GMS	Fat GMS	Chol. MGS
hot cinnamon (Hot Tamales)	1 piece	9	<.1	2.1	1	0	tr	0
jelly beans (Brach's)	1 oz	100	0.0	26.0	5	na	0.0	na
jelly nougat (Brach's)	1 oz	100	0.0	24.0	35	(mq)	1.0	0
'Jels' sour cherry (Brach's)	1 oz	100	0.0	26.0	10	0	0.0	0
'Jube Jels' (Brach's)	1 oz	100	0.0	24.0	10	na	0.0	na
juicy (Callard & Bowser)	1 oz	90	0.0	22.9	0	0	0.0	na
mint, assorted (Brach's)	1 oz	100	0.0	26.0	0	0	0.0	0
'Petite' eggs (Just Born)	1 piece	4	tr	1.1	<1	0	tr	0
'Rainbow Bears' (Brach's)	1 oz	100	0.0	24.0	10	0	0.0	0
'Spearmint Leaves' (Brach's)	1 oz	100	0.0	24.0	5	na	0.0	na
spicettes (Brach's)	1 oz	100	0.0	26.0	15	na	0.0	na
'Teenee Beanee Gourmet' (Just Born)	1 piece	4	tr	1.1	<1	0	tr	0
LICORICE								
candy coated (Good & Fruity)	1 oz	106	0.6	25.7	8	0	0.1	0
candy coated (Good & Plenty)	1 oz	106	1.0	25.9	52	0	<.1	0
'Cherry Nibs' (Y&S)	1 oz	100	1.0	23.0	80	na	<1.0	0
'Nip' (Pearson)	1 oz	120	1.0	23.0	70	0	3.0	0
'Red Laces' (Brach's)	1 oz	100	2.0	22.0	10	0	0.0	0
'Twin Twists' (Brach's)	1 oz	100	2.0	22.0	10	0	0.0	0
'Twists' (Brach's)	1 oz	100	2.0	22.0	50	0	1.0	0
'Twizzlers Bites' cherry (Y&S)	1 oz	100	1.0	23.0	85	na	<1.0	0
'Twizzlers' strawberry (Y&S)	1 oz	100	1.0	23.0	95	0	1.0	0
LOLLIPOP								
all flavors (Estee)	1 lollipop	30	0.0	7.0	0	na	0.0	0
all flavors (Life Savers)	1 lollipop	45	0.0	11.0	10	na	0.0	na
all flavors bubble gum center (Spangler)	1 lollipop	57	<1.0	14.0	5	0	<1.0	0
all flavors 'Dum Dums' (Spangler)	1 lollipop	25	<1.0	6.0	0	0	<1.0	0
all flavors except chocolate (Tootsie Pop)	1 oz	111	0.1	26.4	1	(tr)	0.6	tr
all fruit flavors (Sorbee)	1 lollipop	22	0.0	5.0	0	na	0.0	na
all flavors 'Pops' (Brach's)	1 oz	110	0.0	27.0	10	0	0.0	0
all flavors 'Saf-T-Pops' (Spangler)	1 lollipop	45	<1.0	11.0	0	0	<1.0	0
black raspberry (Fruit Juicers)	1 lollipop	40	0.0	10.0	0	na	0.0	na
chocolate (Tootsie Pop)	1 oz	110	0.1	26.2	2	(tr)	0.6	tr
fruit (Glenny's)	1 lollipop	21	<1.0	5.0	<1	na	<1.0	na
fruit punch (Fruit Juicers)	1 lollipop	40	0.0	10.0	0	na	0.0	na
pineapple (Fruit Juicers)	1 lollipop	40	0.0	10.0	0	na	0.0	na
strawberry (Fruit Juicers)	1 lollipop	40	0.0	10.0	0	na	0.0	na
swirled (Life Savers)	1 lollipop	45	0.0	11.0	10	na	0.0	na
vitamin 'C' (Glenny's)	1 lollipop	35	<1.0	8.0	<1	na	<1.0	na
MARSHMALLOW								
'Circus Peanuts' approx 1 oz (Spangler)	4 pieces	110	<1.0	26.0	5	0	<1.0	0

Food Name	Serv. Size	Total Cal.	Prot. GMS	Carbs GMS	Sod. MGS	Fiber GMS	Fat GMS	Chol. MGS
'Mallow Cup' 1.6 oz *(Boyer)*	2 pieces	224	2.0	30.0	na	0	11.0	na
'Mallow Cup' .5 oz *(Boyer)*	1 piece	71	1.0	15.0	na	0	5.0	na
'Mallow Cup' .275 oz *(Boyer)*	1 piece	36	0.5	7.5	na	0	2.5	na
'Perkys Circus Peanuts' *(Brach's)*	1 oz	100	0.0	26.0	10	0	0.0	0
toasted coconut *(Just Born)*	1 piece	30	0.3	6.1	6	.7	0.6	0
MINT								
'After Dinner' tofu, chocolate *(Barat)*	1 piece	40	1.0	4.0	0	(mq)	2.0	0
'After Eight' dark chocolate *(Rowntree)*	1 mint	35	0.0	6.0	0	na	1.0	na
all flavors except cocoamint *(Velamints)*	1 mint	7	0.0	1.7	0	na	0.0	0
'Bits' tofu, chocolate *(Barat)*	.75 oz	120	2.0	11.0	15	(mq)	8.0	0
butter *(Kraft)*	1 piece	8	0.0	2.0	0	0	0.0	0
cocoamint *(Velamints)*	1 mint	7	4.7	1.5	0	na	0.3	0
'Cool Blue' *(Featherweight)*	1 piece	25	0.0	6.0	0	0	0.0	0
'Coolers/Starlight' *(Brach's)*	1 oz	110	0.0	27.0	15	0	0.0	0
creme, chocolate covered, regular *(Brach's)*	1 oz	110	0.0	24.0	10	na	2.0	na
'Creme de Menthe' *(Brach's)*	1 oz	150	2.0	16.0	20	0	9.0	na
'Creme de Menthe' chocolate *(Andes)*	6 pieces	150	2.0	16.0	20	na	9.0	na
dark chocolate coated *(Spangler)*	1 piece	80	<1.0	14.0	25	(mq)	2.0	0
'Dessert Mints' assorted *(Brach's)*	1 oz	110	0.0	27.0	0	0	0.0	na
'Drops' *(Glenny's)*	1 drop	6	<1.0	1.0	<1	na	<1.0	0
filled straws *(Brach's)*	1 oz	110	0.0	26.0	10	0	1.0	0
'Jots/Pearls' *(Brach's)*	1 oz	120	0.0	25.0	10	0	2.0	0
'Junior Mints' chocolate covered, 1 oz	12 pieces	120	1.0	24.0	10	na	3.0	na
'Kentucky Mints' *(Brach's)*	1 oz	110	0.0	27.0	0	0	0.0	na
'Meltaway' .33 oz *(Mint)*	1 piece	50	0.0	5.0	0	0	3.0	na
'Nip' chocolate *(Pearson)*	1 oz	120	1.0	23.0	70	na	3.0	na
'Mint Oh's' *(Saco Foods)*	1.5 oz	111	1.0	13.8	14	na	6.6	0
parfait *(Brach's)*	1 oz	150	2.0	16.0	35	(tr)	9.0	na
party *(Kraft)*	1 piece	8	0.0	2.0	0	0	0.0	0
peppermint kisses *(Brach's)*	1 oz	100	0.0	24.0	25	na	1.0	na
'Peppermint Pattie' large patties *(York)*	1 piece	149	1.3	33.6	17	>.2 c	3.9	0
'Peppermint Pattie' small patties *(York)*	1 piece	38	0.3	8.6	4	>.1 c	1.0	0
peppermint swirls *(Featherweight)*	1 piece	20	0.0	5.0	0	0	0.0	0
squares *(Russell Stover)*	1.4 oz	160	1.0	28.0	35	1.0	5.0	na
thin, chocolate covered, regular *(Brach's)*	1 oz	110	0.0	24.0	10	na	2.0	na
NONPAREILS								
dark chocolate *(Brach's)*	1 oz	140	1.0	20.0	20	(mq)	6.0	na
'Sno-Caps' *(Nestlé)*	1 oz	140	1.0	21.0	0	(mq)	6.0	na
PEANUT								
'Bits' chocolate tofu, dipped *(Barat)*	1 oz	120	4.0	8.0	15	(mq)	8.0	0
candy coated *(Estee)*	10 pieces	70	2.0	8.0	10	na	4.0	0
caramel cluster *(Brach's)*	1 oz	150	4.0	15.0	50	(mq)	8.0	na
chocolate coated *(Cocofection)*	1 oz	140	5.0	10.0	12	na	12.0	na

Food Name	Serv. Size	Total Cal.	Prot. GMS	Carbs GMS	Sod. MGS	Fiber GMS	Fat GMS	Chol. MGS
chocolate coated *(Estee)* .... 2 squares		60	1.0	4.5	10	(mq)	4.5	2
chocolate coated, approx 14 pieces								
(Nabisco) .... 1 oz		160	4.0	14.0	15	(mq)	9.0	na
chocolate coated 'Small' *(Brach's)* .... 1 oz		140	4.0	15.0	40	(mq)	7.0	na
filled *(Brach's)* .... 1 oz		110	1.0	25.0	20	(mq)	1.0	na
French, burnt *(Brach's)* .... 1 oz		130	4.0	18.0	5	(mq)	5.0	0
'Goobers' chocolate covered *(Nestlé)* 10 pieces		51	1.4	4.9	4	>.2 c	3.3	1
'Goobers' chocolate covered, 1 3/8 oz								
(Nestlé) .... 1 pkg		200	6.0	16.0	15	na	13.0	na
'Jots' *(Brach's)* .... 1 oz		140	3.0	18.0	25	(mq)	6.0	na
'M&M's' candy coated chocolate								
peanuts *(M&M/Mars)* .... 10 pieces		99	2.1	11.8	19	>.3 c	5.4	3
'M&M's' candy coated chocolate peanuts,								
fun size *(M&M/Mars)* .... 1 pkg		110	2.0	13.0	20	na	5.0	na
milk chocolate coated *(Brach's)* .... 1 oz		150	3.0	15.0	30	(mq)	9.0	(mq)
'Nut Goodies' *(Brach's)* .... 1 oz		130	2.0	21.0	10	(mq)	4.0	na
parfait *(Brach's)* .... 1 oz		160	3.0	14.0	60	(mq)	10.0	na
'Peanut Clusters' *(Brach's)* .... 1 oz		150	3.0	15.0	25	(mq)	9.0	na
'Peanut Delights' *(Russell Stover)* ...... 1.4 oz		210	4.0	22.0	130	1.0	12.0	10
PEANUT BRITTLE								
(Estee) .... .5 oz		60	<1.0	10.0	20	na	2.0	0
(Estee) .... .25 oz		35	<1.0	5.0	30	(mq)	1.0	0
(Kraft) .... 1 oz		130	3.0	20.0	135	(mq)	5.0	0
(Sophie Mae) .... 1.4 oz		170	4.0	30.0	130	1.0	5.0	0
PEANUT BUTTER								
'Bar None' *(Hershey's)* .... 1.5 oz		240	4.0	23.0	50	na	14.0	10
cup *(Estee)* .... 1 cup		40	1.0	3.0	20	(mq)	3.0	<1
cup, 1.6 oz *(Boyer)* .... 2 pieces		250	5.0	23.0	na	(mq)	15.0	na
cup, .5 oz *(Boyer)* .... 1 piece		75	2.5	12.0	na	(mq)	7.5	na
cup, .275 oz *(Boyer)* .... 1 piece		38	1.3	6.0	na	(mq)	3.8	na
kisses *(Brach's)* .... 1 oz		110	1.0	22.0	135	(mq)	2.0	na
'Kudos' chocolate covered *(M&M/Mars)* .. 1.3 oz		200	4.0	19.0	80	na	12.0	na
'M&M's' candy coated *(M&M/Mars)* .... 1.63 oz		240	5.0	28.0	60	na	12.0	na
'M&M's' candy coated *(M&M/Mars)* ...... 1 oz		150	3.0	17.0	60	na	7.0	na
'PB Max' chocolate covered cookie								
(M&M/Mars) .... 1 piece		240	5.0	20.0	150	na	15.0	na
'Reese's Crunchy Peanut Butter Cups'								
(Hershey's) .... 1.8 oz		280	7.0	24.0	130	na	18.0	5
'Reese's Peanut Butter Cups' *(Hershey's)* 1.6 oz		250	6.0	23.0	160	na	15.0	5
'Reese's Peanut Butter Cups' *(Hershey's)* 1.8 oz		247	5.6	24.4	148	2.1	15.9	8
'Reese's Peanut Butter Cups' miniatures								
(Hershey's) .... 6 cups		204	4.6	20.1	122	1.8	13.1	6

Food Name	Serv. Size	Total Cal.	Prot. GMS	Carbs GMS	Sod. MGS	Fiber GMS	Fat GMS	Chol. MGS
'Reese's Peanut Butter Cups' snack size								
(Hershey's) .... 1 cup	100	2.0	9.0	60	na	6.0	na
'Reese's Pieces' candy coated								
(Hershey's) .... 1.63 oz	230	7.0	28.0	80	na	10.0	0
'Reese's Pieces' candy coated								
(Hershey's) .... 10 pieces	38	1.0	5.0	12	.3	1.7	0
'Reese's Pieces' candy coated, 1.95 oz								
(Hershey's) .... 1 pkg	258	7.2	34.2	83	2.3	11.4	2
toffee (Flavor House) .... 1 oz	150	4.0	17.0	90	(mq)	7.0	na
PECAN								
'Demet's Turtles' milk chocolate, pecans,								
caramel (Demet's) .... 1 piece	82	1.1	9.9	16	>.4 c	4.7	4
'Pecan Crowns' (Russell Stover) ..... 1.4 oz	200	2.0	19.0	60	1.0	13.0	5
'Pecan Delights' (Russell Stover) .... 1.4 oz	220	2.0	19.0	55	1.0	14.5	5
POWDER CANDY								
(Lik-m-aid Fun Dip) .... 1 oz	110	0.0	26.0	na	na	0.0	na
(Pixy Stix) .... 1 oz	100	0.0	26.0	na	na	0.0	na
RAISIN								
'Bits' chocolate tofu covered (Barat) ..... 1 oz	120	1.0	14.0	10	(mq)	7.0	0
chocolate coated (Brach's) .... 1 oz	130	1.0	20.0	30	(mq)	5.0	na
chocolate coated (Cocofection) .... 1 oz	120	1.0	20.0	14	na	5.0	na
chocolate coated (Estee) .... 8 pieces	30	<1.0	5.0	5	na	1.0	0
chocolate coated, approx 29 pieces								
(Nabisco) .... 1 oz	130	1.0	21.0	15	(mq)	5.0	<1
'Raisinets' chocolate covered (Nestlé) .. 1 3/8 oz	180	2.0	28.0	10	na	6.0	na
'Raisinets' chocolate covered (Nestlé) 10 pieces	41	0.5	7.1	4	>.1 c	1.6	0
'Raisinets' chocolate covered (Nestlé) .. 1.58 oz	185	2.1	32.0	16	>.3 c	7.2	2
TAFFY								
all flavors 'Salt Water Taffy' (Brach's) ..... 1 oz	100	0.0	24.0	30	0	1.0	0
apple flavor 'Laffy Taffy' 1 oz (Beich's) 2 pieces	110	0.0	26.0	55	0	1.0	0
banana flavor 'Laffy Taffy' 1 oz (Beich's) 2 pieces	120	0.0	26.0	55	0	1.0	0
cherry flavor 'Laffy Taffy' 1 oz (Beich's) 2 pieces	110	0.0	26.0	55	0	1.0	0
grape flavor 'Laffy Taffy' 1 oz (Beich's) 2 pieces	110	0.0	26.0	60	0	1.0	0
honey flavor (Bit-O-Honey) .... 1.7 oz	200	1.0	39.0	125	na	4.0	na
passion punch flavor 'Laffy Taffy' 1 oz								
(Beich's) .... 2 pieces	120	0.0	26.0	50	0	1.0	0
strawberry flavor 'Laffy Taffy' 1 oz								
(Beich's) .... 2 pieces	110	0.0	26.0	55	0	1.0	0
tangy flavor (Tangy Taffy) .... 1 oz	120	0.0	23.0	na	0	2.5	na
watermelon flavor 'Laffy Taffy' 1 oz								
(Beich's) .... 2 pieces	110	0.0	26.0	55	0	1.0	0
TOFFEE								
(Brach's) .... 1 oz	110	1.0	23.0	80	0	2.0	0

Food Name	Serv. Size	Total Cal.	Prot. GMS	Carbs GMS	Sod. MGS	Fiber GMS	Fat GMS	Chol. MGS
(Callard & Bowser)	1 oz	135	0.5	19.2	0	0	6.5	na
'Bits'O Brickle' *(Heath)*	3 oz	448	1.0	50.0	472	na	28.0	na
English *(Bits'O Heath)*	3.5 oz	520	3.0	62.0	390	na	31.0	na
English, 'Heath Bar' 1 3/16 oz *(Heath)*	2 pieces	180	1.0	20.0	130	(mq)	11.0	na
CANDY APPLE. See APPLE KIT.								
CANE SYRUP								
table blends	1/2 cup	397	0.0	102.4	6	0	0.0	0
table blends	1 tbsp	50	0.0	12.8	tr	0	0.0	0
CANNELLINI BEAN, canned, white								
(Pathmark)	1/2 cup	100	6.0	18.0	390	(mq)	0.0	0
CANNELLONI, CANNED, mini								
(Chef Boyardee)	7.5 oz	230	9.0	33.0	1050	(mq)	7.0	(mq)
CANNELLONI ENTRÉE, frozen								
beef, w/tomato sauce *(Lean Cuisine)*	9 5/8 oz	200	14.0	28.0	490	na	3.0	25
cheese *(Dining Lite)*	9 oz	310	19.0	38.0	650	(mq)	9.0	70
cheese, w/tomato sauce *(Lean Cuisine)*	9 1/8 oz	270	23.0	27.0	590	na	8.0	25
Florentine *(Celentano)*	12 oz	350	21.0	48.0	620	(mq)	8.0	na
CANOLA AND VEGETABLE OIL,								
'Best Blend' *(Wesson)*	1 tbsp	120	0.0	0.0	0	na	14.0	0
CANOLA OIL								
	1/2 cup	964	0.0	0.0	0	0	109.0	0
	1 oz	251	0.0	0.0	0	0	28.4	0
	1 tbsp	124	0.0	0.0	0	0	14.0	na
(Country Pure)	1 tbsp	120	0.0	0.0	0	na	14.0	0
(Hain)	1 tbsp	120	0.0	0.0	0	0	14.0	0
(Kroger)	1 tbsp	122	0.0	0.0	0	0	13.6	0
(Nucoa) 'Heart Beat'	1 tbsp	120	0.0	0.0	0	0	14.0	0
(Spectrum Naturals)	1 tbsp	120	0.0	0.0	0	(tr)	14.0	(tr)
(Spectrum Naturals) organic	1 tbsp	120	0.0	0.0	0	(tr)	14.0	(tr)
(Wesson)	1 tbsp	120	0.0	0.0	0	0	14.0	0
(Wesson) 'Food Service'	1 tbsp	122	0.0	0.0	0	0	13.6	0
CANOLA OIL SPRAY. See COOKING SPRAY.								
CANTALOUPE /muskmelon								
approx 5 inch diam	1/2 fruit	93	2.3	22.3	24	2.1	0.8	0
cubed	1/2 cup	29	0.7	6.7	7	.6	0.2	0
pulp	1 oz	10	0.2	2.4	3	.3	0.1	0
untrimmed	1 lb	82	2.0	19.3	20	1.9	0.6	0
untrimmed *(Dole)*	1/4 fruit	50	1.0	11.0	35	0	0.0	na
CAPE GOOSEBERRY /ground cherry /poha								
in husk	1 lb	226	8.1	47.8	(mq)	>11.9 c	3.0	0
raw	1/2 cup	37	1.3	7.8	na	>2.0 c	0.5	0
trimmed	1/2 cup	37	1.3	7.8	(mq)	>2.0 c	0.5	0
trimmed	1 oz	15	0.5	3.2	(mq)	>.8 c	0.2	0

Food Name	Serv. Size	Total Cal.	Prot. GMS	Carbs GMS	Sod. MGS	Fiber GMS	Fat GMS	Chol. MGS
CAPOCOLLA. See LUNCHEON MEAT.								
CAPPUCCINO. See COFFEE, FLAVORED.								
CARAMBOLA. See STAR FRUIT.								
CARAMEL TOPPING								
(Kraft)	1 tbsp	60	1.0	13.0	45	0	0.0	0
(Mrs. Richardson's) fat-free	2 tbsp	130	1.0	31.0	55	na	0.0	0
(Smucker's) hot	2 tbsp	150	1.0	28.0	75	0	4.0	0
CARAWAY SEED								
whole	1 oz	94	5.6	14.1	5	>3.6 c	4.1	0
whole	1 tbsp	22	1.3	3.3	1	2.5	1.0	0
whole	1 tsp	7	0.4	1.0	0	.8	0.3	0
whole (Durkee)	1 tsp	9	0.0	0.0	0	0	<0.1	na
whole (Laurel Leaf)	1 tsp	9	0.0	0.0	0	0	<0.1	na
whole (Spice Islands)	1 tsp	8	0.4	0.8	<1	>.2 c	0.4	0
CARDAMOM								
ground	1 oz	88	3.1	19.4	5	>3.2 c	1.9	0
ground	1 tbsp	18	0.6	4.0	1	>.7 c	0.4	0
ground	1 tsp	6	0.2	1.4	0	>.2 c	0.1	0
ground (Durkee)	1 tsp	7	0.0	0.0	0	0	tr	na
ground (Laurel Leaf)	1 tsp	7	0.0	0.0	0	0	tr	na
CARDAMOM SEED (Spice Islands)	1 tsp	6	0.2	1.3	tr	>.2 c	0.1	0
CARDONI. See CARDOON.								
CARDOON/cardoni								
boiled, drained	4 oz	25	0.9	6.0	200	(mq)	0.1	0
raw, shredded	1 cup	36	1.3	8.7	303	2.9	0.2	0
raw, shredded	1/2 cup	18	0.6	4.3	151	1.4	0.1	0
raw, trimmed	1 oz	6	0.2	1.4	48	(mq)	<.1	0
raw, untrimmed	1 lb	44	1.6	10.9	378	(mq)	0.2	0
CARISSA/natal plum								
raw, approx .8 oz	1 med	12	0.1	2.7	1	.2	0.3	0
raw, sliced	1 cup	93	0.8	20.4	5	>1.4 c	2.0	0
raw, w/o skin and seeds, approx .8 oz	1 fruit	12	0.1	2.7	1	>.2 c	0.3	0
trimmed	1 oz	18	0.1	3.9	1	>.3 c	0.4	0
untrimmed	1 lb	240	2.0	53.2	11	>3.5 c	5.1	0
CAROB FLAVOR DRINK								
mix, powder	1 oz	105	0.5	26.5	29	>.5 c	0.1	0
mix, powder	3 tsp	45	0.2	11.2	12	>.2 c	0.0	0
mix, prepared w/1 cup whole milk	1 cup	195	8.2	22.6	132	>.3 c	8.2	33
mix, prepared w/1 cup 2% milk	1 cup	166	8.3	22.9	134	>.2 c	4.7	18
mix, prepared w/1 cup 1% milk	1 cup	147	8.2	22.9	135	>.2 c	2.6	10
mix, prepared w/1 cup skim milk	1 cup	131	8.6	23.1	138	>.2 c	0.4	4
CAROB FLOUR								
	1 cup	394	4.8	91.5	36	41.0	0.7	0

Food Name	Serv. Size	Total Cal.	Prot. GMS	Carbs GMS	Sod. MGS	Fiber GMS	Fat GMS	Chol. MGS
....	1 oz	51	1.3	25.2	10	3.0	0.2	0
....	1 tbsp	31	0.4	7.1	3	3.2	0.1	0
CARP								
dry-heat cooked	3 oz	138	19.4	0.0	54	0	6.1	71
dry-heat cooked, approx 7.7 oz raw wt ..	1 fillet	275	38.9	0.0	107	0	12.2	143
raw	1 lb	574	80.9	0.0	223	0	25.4	298
raw	3 oz	108	15.2	0.0	42	0	4.8	56
raw	1 oz	36	5.1	0.0	14	0	1.6	19
raw, approx 7.7 oz	1 fillet	277	38.9	0.0	107	0	12.2	144
CARROT								
baby, raw	1 large	6	0.1	1.2	5	na	0.1	0
baby, raw	1 med	4	0.1	0.8	4	na	0.1	0
boiled, drained	4 oz	51	1.2	11.9	75	2.2	0.2	0
boiled, drained	1 med	21	0.5	4.8	30	1.6	0.1	0
boiled, drained, sliced	1/2 cup	35	0.9	8.2	51	2.6	0.1	0
raw	1 med	31	0.7	7.3	25	2.3	0.1	0
raw *(Dole)*	1 med	40	1.0	8.0	40	1.0	1.0	na
raw, shredded	1/2 cup	24	0.6	5.6	19	1.7	0.1	0
raw, trimmed	1 oz	12	0.3	2.9	10	.9	0.1	0
raw, untrimmed	1 lb	174	4.1	41.0	139	12.9	0.8	0
CARROT, CANNED								
Crinkle sliced								
(A&P)	1/2 cup	30	1.0	6.0	300	(mq)	<1.0	0
(Freshlike)	1/2 cup	30	1.0	6.0	300	na	0.0	na
(Veg•All)	1/2 cup	30	1.0	6.0	300	na	0.0	na
Diced								
(Allens)	1/2 cup	30	1.0	5.0	190	(mq)	<1.0	0
'Fancy' *(S&W)*	1/2 cup	30	1.0	7.0	240	(mq)	0.0	0
julienne 'Fancy' *(S&W)*	1/2 cup	30	1.0	7.0	240	(mq)	0.0	0
'No Salt Added' *(A&P)*	1/2 cup	25	<1.0	6.0	40	(mq)	<1.0	0
'No Salt or Sugar Added'*(Stokely)*	1/2 cup	35	1.0	7.0	35	(mq)	0.0	0
w/liquid *(Del Monte)*	1/2 cup	30	0.0	7.0	265	(mq)	0.0	0
Sliced								
(Featherweight)	1/2 cup	30	1.0	6.0	30	(mq)	0.0	0
(Finast)	1/2 cup	35	1.0	8.0	370	(mq)	0.0	0
(IGA)	1/2 cup	30	1.0	6.0	300	(mq)	0.0	0
(Pathmark)	1/2 cup	35	1.0	7.0	310	(mq)	0.0	0
(S&W Nutradiet)	1/2 cup	30	0.0	7.0	50	(mq)	0.0	0
(Stokely)	1/2 cup	35	1.0	7.0	300	(mq)	0.0	0
'Fancy' *(S&W)*	1/2 cup	30	1.0	7.0	240	(mq)	0.0	0
large *(Allens)*	1/2 cup	30	1.0	7.0	250	(mq)	<1.0	0
medium *(Allens)*	1/2 cup	30	1.0	7.0	250	(mq)	<1.0	0
'No Salt Added' *(Finast)*	1/2 cup	35	1.0	8.0	30	(mq)	0.0	0

Food Name	Serv. Size	Total Cal.	Prot. GMS	Carbs GMS	Sod. MGS	Fiber GMS	Fat GMS	Chol. MGS
'No Salt Added' (Pathmark)	1/2 cup	35	1.0	8.0	35	(mq)	0.0	0
regular pack, drained	1/2 cup	17	0.5	4.0	176	1.1	0.1	0
regular pack, w/liquid	1/2 cup	28	0.8	6.2	297	1.4	0.2	0
regular pack, w/liquid, low-sodium	1/2 cup	28	0.8	6.2	48	1.4	0.2	0
small (Allens)	1/2 cup	30	1.0	7.0	250	(mq)	<1.0	0
special dietary pack, drained	1/2 cup	17	0.5	4.0	31	>.6 c	0.1	0
special dietary pack, w/liquid	1/2 cup	28	0.8	6.2	48	>.9 c	0.2	0
water-packed, w/o salt (Freshlike)	1/2 cup	30	1.0	6.0	40	na	0.0	na
water-packed, w/o sugar or salt (Freshlike)	1/2 cup	30	1.0	6.0	40	na	0.0	na
w/liquid (Del Monte)	1/2 cup	30	0.0	7.0	265	(mq)	0.0	0
Whole								
baby (Allens)	1/2 cup	30	1.0	6.0	240	(mq)	<1.0	0
tiny 'Fancy' (S&W)	1/2 cup	30	1.0	7.0	240	(mq)	0.0	0
w/liquid	1/2 cup	26	0.7	5.7	273	1.2	0.2	0
CARROT, FROZEN								
	10 oz	112	3.1	25.5	167	4.0	0.6	0
(A&P)	3.3 oz	40	1.0	9.0	45	(mq)	<1.0	0
(Seabrook)	3.3 oz	40	1.0	9.0	44	>1.0 c	0.0	0
baby, whole 'Deluxe' (Bird's Eye)	3.3 oz	40	1.0	9.0	45	2.0	0.0	0
baby whole, 'Harvest Fresh' (Green Giant)	1/2 cup	18	1.0	5.0	75	2.0	0.0	0
baby, whole 'Select' (Green Giant)	1/2 cup	20	1.0	7.0	35	2.0	0.0	0
baby whole, 'Singles' (Stokely)	3 oz	35	1.0	8.0	50	(mq)	0.0	0
boiled, drained	4 oz	41	1.3	9.4	67	2.0	0.1	0
Parisienne 'Deluxe' (Deluxe)	2.6 oz	30	1.0	7.0	35	2.0	0.0	0
sliced (Birds Eye)	3.2 oz	35	1.0	8.0	40	1.0	0.0	0
sliced (Frosty Acres)	3.3 oz	40	1.0	9.0	44	>1.0 c	0.0	0
sliced, boiled, drained	1/2 cup	26	0.9	6.0	43	>.9 c	0.1	0
sliced, unprepared	1/2 cup	25	0.7	5.8	38	2.1	0.1	0
whole (Southern)	3.5 oz	42	1.2	8.7	60	(mq)	0.2	0
w/sweet peas, pearl onions 'Deluxe' (Birds Eye)	3.3 oz	50	2.0	10.0	60	2.0	0.0	0
CARROT JUICE								
canned	6 oz	74	1.8	17.1	53	1.5	0.3	0
canned	1/2 cup	49	1.2	11.4	36	1.0	0.2	0
canned (Biotta)	6 oz	51	1.5	11.3	158	(mq)	0.1	0
canned (Hain)	6 oz	80	1.0	17.0	170	(mq)	0.0	0
canned (Hollywood)	6 oz	80	1.0	17.0	170	2.0	0.0	0
CASABA MELON								
cubed	1 cup	44	1.5	10.5	20	1.4	0.2	0
1/10 of 7.75-inch melon	2-in. slice	43	1.5	10.2	20	1.3	0.2	0
pulp	1 oz	7	0.3	1.8	3	>.1 c	<.1	0

Food Name	Serv. Size	Total Cal.	Prot. GMS	Carbs GMS	Sod. MGS	Fiber GMS	Fat GMS	Chol. MGS
untrimmed	1 lb	71	2.5	16.9	33	>1.4 c	0.3	0
CASHEW/heart nut								
(Beer Nuts)	1 oz	170	5.0	8.0	65	(mq)	13.0	0
Dry roasted								
halves (Fisher)	1 oz	160	5.0	8.0	na	na	13.0	0
lightly salted (Planters)	1 oz	160	5.0	9.0	115	na	13.0	0
salted	1 oz	163	4.3	9.3	182	.9	13.2	0
salted (Pathmark)	1 oz	170	4.0	9.0	150	(mq)	13.0	0
salted (Planters)	1 oz	160	5.0	9.0	230	(mq)	13.0	0
salted, 'No Frills' (Pathmark)	1 oz	170	5.0	8.0	220	(mq)	13.0	0
salted, wholes and halves	1 cup	787	21.0	44.8	877	7.8	63.5	0
unsalted	1 oz	163	4.3	9.3	5	.9	13.2	0
'Unsalted' (Planters)	1 oz	160	5.0	9.0	0	(mq)	13.0	0
unsalted, approx 14 large or 26 small kernels	1 oz	163	4.4	9.3	4	1.7	13.2	0
unsalted, wholes and halves	1 cup	787	21.0	44.8	21	7.8	63.5	0
wholes (Fisher)	1 oz	160	5.0	8.0	100	na	13.0	0
Honey roasted								
(Frito-Lays)	1 oz	170	4.0	9.0	115	na	14.0	0
(Planters)	1 oz	170	4.0	11.0	170	(mq)	12.0	0
halves (Fisher)	1 oz	150	4.0	7.0	na	na	13.0	0
wholes (Fisher)	1 oz	150	4.0	7.0	90	na	13.0	0
w/peanuts (Planters)	1 oz	170	5.0	9.0	170	(mq)	12.0	0
Oil roasted								
halves (Fisher)	1 oz	170	5.0	8.0	155	na	14.0	0
lightly salted (Planters)	1 oz	160	5.0	8.0	80	na	14.0	0
pieces (Fisher)	1 oz	170	5.0	8.0	135	na	14.0	0
salted	1 oz	164	4.6	8.1	178	1.1	13.7	0
salted (Flavor House)	1 oz	180	7.0	3.0	125	(mq)	16.0	0
salted (Pathmark)	1 oz	170	5.0	8.0	150	(mq)	14.0	0
salted, approx 14 large or 18 medium kernels	1 oz	163	4.6	8.1	177	1.1	13.7	0
salted, 'Fancy' (Planters)	1 oz	170	5.0	8.0	135	(mq)	14.0	0
salted, halves (Planters)	1 oz	170	5.0	8.0	135	(mq)	14.0	0
salted, 'No Frills' (Pathmark)	1 oz	170	5.0	8.0	150	(mq)	14.0	0
salted, wholes (Guy's)	1 oz	170	5.0	5.0	140	(mq)	14.0	0
salted, wholes and halves	1 cup	749	21.0	37.1	814	7.8	62.7	0
unsalted	1 oz	164	4.6	8.1	5	1.1	13.7	0
unsalted, approx 14 large or 18 medium kernels	1 oz	163	4.6	8.1	5	1.1	13.7	0
unsalted, 'Fancy' (Planters)	1 oz	170	5.0	8.0	0	na	14.0	0
unsalted, halves	1 cup	749	21.0	37.1	22	7.8	62.7	0
'Unsalted' halves (Planters)	1 oz	170	5.0	8.0	0	(mq)	14.0	0

Food Name	Serv. Size	Total Cal.	Prot. GMS	Carbs GMS	Sod. MGS	Fiber GMS	Fat GMS	Chol. MGS
wholes *(Fisher)*	1 oz	170	5.0	8.0	110	na	14.0	0
w/almonds *(Fisher)*	1 oz	170	5.0	6.0	95	na	15.0	0
CASHEW BUTTER								
gourmet *(Roaster Fresh)*	1 oz	165	4.0	9.0	4	na	14.0	na
peanut date *(Maranatha Natural)*	2 tbsp	190	8.0	8.0	8	na	14.0	na
peanut date 'Natural' *(Westbrae)*	2 tbsp	200	6.0	8.0	2	na	15.0	na
plain	1 oz	167	5.0	7.8	4	.6	14.0	0
plain	1 tbsp	94	2.8	4.4	2	.3	7.9	0
raw *(Hain)*	2 tbsp	190	6.0	8.0	(mq)	(mq)	15.0	0
raw 'Natural' *(Westbrae)*	2 tbsp	300	6.0	8.0	0	na	28.0	0
raw, unsalted *(Hain)*	2 tbsp	210	5.0	8.0	10	(mq)	19.0	0
roasted *(Maranatha Natural)*	2 tbsp	190	6.0	10.0	5	na	14.0	na
roasted 'Natural' *(Westbrae)*	2 tbsp	190	6.0	8.0	0	na	17.0	na
toasted *(Hain)*	2 tbsp	210	7.0	7.0	15	(mq)	17.0	0
CASSAVA/manioc/yuca								
trimmed	1 lb	544	14.1	122.1	36	>11.3 c	1.8	0
trimmed	1 oz	34	0.9	7.6	2	>.7 c	0.1	0
raw	100 gm	120	3.1	26.9	8	1.6	0.4	0
CATFISH, CHANNEL								
Farmed								
dry-heat cooked	3 oz	129	15.9	0.0	68	0	6.8	54
frozen, fillets *(Delta Pride)*	4 oz	132	18.0	4.8	<1	0	4.9	62
raw	3 oz	115	13.2	0.0	45	0	6.4	40
raw	1 oz	33	5.2	0.0	18	0	1.2	16
Wild								
dry-heat cooked	3 oz	89	15.7	0.0	43	0	2.4	61
raw	3 oz	81	13.9	0.0	37	0	2.4	49
CATFISH, OCEAN. See WOLF FISH.								
CATSUP/ketchup	1 oz	29	0.4	7.7	336	.5	0.1	0
	1 tbsp	16	0.2	4.1	178	.2	0.1	0
	.2-oz pkt	6	0.1	1.6	71	.1	0.0	0
(Del Monte)	1/4 cup	60	1.0	16.0	675	(mq)	0.0	0
(Estee)	1 tbsp	6	0.0	0.0	20	(mq)	0.0	0
(Featherweight)	1 tbsp	6	0.0	1.0	5	(mq)	0.0	0
(Healthy Choice)	.5 oz	9	0.3	2.0	97	.3	0.1	0
(Heinz)	1 tbsp	16	0.2	3.8	213	>.2 c	0.0	0
(Hunt's)	1 tbsp	16	0.3	3.7	158	.3	0.1	0
(Smucker's)	1 tsp	8	0.0	2.0	45	(mq)	0.0	0
(Snider's)	1 tbsp	16	0.3	3.7	158	.3	0.1	0
(Stokely)	1 tbsp	20	0.0	5.0	190	(mq)	0.0	0
(Weight Watchers)	2 tsp	8	0.0	2.0	110	(mq)	0.0	0
'All Natural' *(Life)*	1 tbsp	17	0.0	4.0	10	(mq)	0.0	0
'Food Service' *(Hunt's)*	1 tbsp	15	0.3	3.6	158	.2	0.1	0

Food Name	Serv. Size	Total Cal.	Prot. GMS	Carbs GMS	Sod. MGS	Fiber GMS	Fat GMS	Chol. MGS
fruit-sweetened (Westbrae)	1 tbsp	12	0.0	2.0	110	na	0.0	0
fruit-sweetened, no salt (Westbrae)	1 tbsp	12	0.0	2.0	10	na	0.0	0
hot (Heinz)	1 tbsp	16	0.3	3.7	195	>.1 c	0.0	0
'Lite' (Heinz)	1 tbsp	8	0.4	1.7	115	>.2 c	0.0	0
low-sodium	1 oz	29	0.4	7.7	6	.5	0.1	0
low-sodium	1 tbsp	16	0.2	4.1	3	>.2 c	0.1	0
low-sodium	.2-oz pkt	6	0.1	1.6	1	>.1 c	0.0	0
'Natural' (Hain)	1 tbsp	16	0.0	4.0	155	(mq)	0.0	0
'Natural No Salt Added' (Hain)	1 tbsp	16	0.0	4.0	5	(mq)	0.0	0
'No Salt Added' (Del Monte)	1/4 cup	60	1.0	16.0	25	(mq)	0.0	0
'No Salt Added' (Hunt's)	1 tbsp	20	0.0	5.0	0	(mq)	0.0	0
organic (Millina's Finest)	1 oz	17	0.5	4.0	143	na	0.1	na
portion pack (Hunt's)	.3175 oz	10	0.2	2.2	75	.2	0.1	0
w/onions (Heinz)	1 tbsp	19	4.5	0.1	289	>.2 c	(tr)	0
CAULIFLOWER								
boiled, drained	4 oz	27	2.1	5.2	7	2.5	0.2	0
boiled, drained, approx 1.9 oz	3 flowerets	12	1.0	2.2	8	1.5	0.2	0
boiled, drained, 1-inch pieces	1/2 cup	14	1.1	2.5	9	1.7	0.3	0
fresh, medium size (Dole)	1/6 head	18	2.0	3.0	45	2.0	0.0	na
green, fresh (Dole)	1/5 head	35	3.0	7.0	30	2.0	0.0	na
raw, approx 5 oz	3 flowerets	14	1.1	2.9	17	1.4	0.1	0
raw, 1-inch pieces	1/2 cup	13	1.0	2.6	15	1.3	0.1	0
raw, trimmed	1 oz	7	0.6	1.4	4	.7	0.1	0
raw, untrimmed	1 lb	42	3.5	8.7	26	4.2	0.3	0
Frozen								
	10 oz	68	5.7	13.3	68	6.5	0.8	0
(A&P)	3.3 oz	25	2.0	5.0	20	(mq)	<1.0	0
(Birds Eye)	3.3 oz	25	2.0	5.0	20	2.0	0.0	0
(Finast)	3.3 oz	25	2.0	5.0	15	(mq)	0.0	0
(Frosty Acres)	3.3 oz	25	2.0	5.0	16	>1.0 c	0.0	0
(Kohl's)	3 oz	20	2.0	4.0	15	(mq)	<1.0	0
(Seabrook)	3.3 oz	25	2.0	5.0	16	>1.0 c	0.0	0
(Southern)	3.5 oz	26	2.0	4.8	30	(mq)	0.2	0
boiled, drained	4 oz	22	1.8	4.3	20	>.9 c	0.2	0
boiled, drained, 1-inch pieces	1/2 cup	17	1.5	3.4	16	>.7 c	0.2	0
cuts (Green Giant)	1/2 cup	12	1.0	3.0	25	1.0	0.0	0
florets 'Plain Polybag' (Green Giant)	1/2 cup	12	1.0	3.0	25	2.0	0.0	0
in cheddar cheese sauce 'Side Dish'								
(Budget Gourmet)	5 oz	110	6.0	10.0	300	(mq)	5.0	25
in cheese flavored sauce (Green Giant)	1/2 cup	60	2.0	10.0	500	2.4	2.0	na
in cheese sauce (Finast)	3.3 oz	40	2.0	5.0	240	(mq)	0.0	0
in cheese sauce 'One Serving' (Green Giant)	5.5 oz	80	3.0	14.0	690	2.0	2.0	5
in cheese sauce 'Singles' (Stokely)	4 oz	70	4.0	7.0	170	(mq)	3.0	15

Food Name	Serv. Size	Total Cal.	Prot. GMS	Carbs GMS	Sod. MGS	Fiber GMS	Fat GMS	Chol. MGS
'Singles' (Stokely)	3 oz	20	2.0	4.0	20	(mq)	0.0	0
unprepared, 1-inch pieces	1/2 cup	16	1.3	3.1	16	1.5	0.2	0
Pickled								
'Hot & Spicy' (Vlasic)	1 oz	4	0.0	1.0	435	(mq)	0.0	0
sweet (Vlasic)	1 oz	35	0.0	9.0	225	(mq)	0.0	0
CAVIAR								
black, granular	1 oz	71	6.9	1.1	420	0	5.0	165
black, granular	1 tbsp	40	3.9	0.6	240	0	2.9	94
red, granular	1 oz	71	6.9	1.1	420	0	5.0	165
red, granular	1 tbsp	40	3.9	0.6	240	0	2.9	94
CAYENNE PEPPER								
ground	1 oz	90	3.4	16.1	9	>7.1 c	4.9	0
ground	1 tbsp	17	0.6	3.0	2	>1.3 c	0.9	0
ground	1 tsp	6	0.2	1.0	1	>.5 c	0.3	0
ground (Spice Islands)	1 tsp	9	0.3	1.1	<1	>.5 c	0.3	0
CECI. See GARBANZO BEAN.								
CELERIAC/celery root								
boiled, drained	4 oz	28	1.1	6.7	69	>.9 c	0.2	0
boiled, drained	100 gm	25	1.0	5.9	61	>.8 c	0.2	0
raw	1/2 cup	30	1.2	7.2	78	1.4	0.2	0
raw (Frieda's)	3.5 oz	40	1.8	8.5	100	(mq)	0.3	0
raw, trimmed	1 oz	11	0.4	2.6	28	>.4 c	0.1	0
raw, untrimmed	1 lb	154	5.9	35.9	390	>5.1 c	1.2	0
CELERY								
boiled, drained	4 oz	20	0.9	4.5	103	>1.0 c	0.1	0
boiled, drained, diced	1/2 cup	14	0.6	3.0	68	1.2	0.1	0
fresh, medium size (Dole)	2 stalks	20	1.0	4.0	140	1.4	0.0	na
raw, diced	1/2 cup	10	0.5	2.2	52	1.0	0.1	0
raw, trimmed	1 oz	5	0.2	1.0	25	.5	<.1	0
raw, untrimmed	1 lb	65	3.0	14.7	352	6.5	0.6	0
CELERY FLAKES (Tone's)	1 tsp	9	0.4	0.9	4	.3	0.5	0
CELERY ROOT. See CELERIAC.								
CELERY ROOT JUICE, bottled (Biotta)	6 oz	67	2.7	13.1	195	(mq)	0.2	0
CELERY SALT (Tone's)	1 tsp	6	0.3	0.6	1584	.2	0.4	0
CELERY SEED								
whole	1 oz	111	5.1	11.7	45	>3.4 c	7.2	0
whole	1 tbsp	25	1.2	2.7	10	.8	1.6	0
whole	1 tsp	8	0.4	0.8	3	.2	0.5	0
whole (Durkee)	1 tsp	9	0.0	0.0	0	0	<0.1	na
whole (Laurel Leaf)	1 tsp	9	0.0	0.0	0	0	<0.1	na
whole (Spice Islands)	1 tsp	11	0.4	1.1	4	>.3 c	0.5	0
CELLOPHANE NOODLES. See NOODLE, CHINESE.								

Food Name	Serv. Size	Total Cal.	Prot. GMS	Carbs GMS	Sod. MGS	Fiber GMS	Fat GMS	Chol. MGS
CELTUCE								
raw, approx .4 oz	1 leaf	2	0.1	0.3	1	(mq)	0.0	0
trimmed	1 oz	6	0.2	1.0	3	>.1 c	0.1	0
untrimmed	1 lb	76	2.9	12.4	36	>1.4 c	1.0	0
CEREAL, HOT								
(NOTE: All of the following hot cereals are dry unless otherwise noted.)								
BARLEY *(Erewhon)* organic plus	1 oz	110	3.0	22.0	0	1.0	1.0	0
BRAN *(H-O Brand)* 'Super Bran'	1/3 cup	110	4.0	18.0	0	8.0	2.0	0
BULGUR WHEAT								
(Arrowhead Mills)	2 oz	200	6.0	43.0	0	5.4	1.0	0
(Krusteaz) 'Ala'	1/4 cup	150	4.0	33.0	0	7.0	0.0	0
CORN GRITS. See GRITS.								
FARINA								
(H-O Brand) cream	3 tbsp	120	3.0	26.0	0	3.0	0.0	0
(H-O Brand) instant	1 pkt	110	3.0	22.0	235	3.0	0.0	0
(Krusteaz)	1 oz	100	3.0	22.0	1	1.0	0.0	0
(Malt•O•Meal) 'Maple Brown Sugar' 30% formulation	1 oz	100	3.0	22.0	0	1.0	0.0	0
GRAIN, MIXED								
(Arrowhead Mills) four grain	1 oz	94	4.0	18.0	1	7.4	1.0	0
(Arrowhead Mills) seven grain	1 oz	100	4.0	17.0	<1	4.0	1.0	0
(Breadshop) 'Triple Bran'	1 oz	100	6.0	15.0	5	6.0	2.0	0
(Maltex) wheat and barley	1 oz	105	3.0	21.0	0	3.0	1.0	0
(Malt•O•Meal) wheat and barley, chocolate flavor	1 tbsp	38	1.1	8.0	1	>.1 c	0.1	0
(Malt•O•Meal) wheat and barley, plain . . .	1 tbsp	38	1.1	8.0	1	>.1 c	0.1	0
(Pritikin) hearty multi-grain, microwave instant	1 pkt	150	5.0	32.0	0	na	na	0
(Quaker) multi-grain	1/2 cup	130	5.0	24.0	0	5.0	1.5	0
(Roman Meal) multi-grain, apple, and cinnamon	2/3 cup	112	3.7	23.8	14	5.7	2.8	<1
(Roman Meal) oat, wheat, dates, raisins, and almonds	1.3 oz	140	4.0	26.0	0	3.0	3.0	0
(Roman Meal) oat, wheat, honey, coconut, and almonds	1.3 oz	150	5.0	21.0	5	3.1	6.0	0
(Roman Meal) oat and wheat, rye, bran, and flax	1.2 oz	116	5.0	25.0	5	5.0	1.7	0
OAT BRAN								
(Arrowhead Mills)	1 oz	110	6.0	17.0	1	5.1 d	1.0	0
(Breadshop) 'Oat Bran Müesli'	1 oz	100	4.0	20.0	5	3.0	2.0	0
(Breadshop) 'Oat Bran' 100% pure	1 oz	100	6.0	17.0	5	4.0	2.0	0
(Erewhon) toasted wheat germ	1 oz	115	5.0	18.0	15	3.0	2.0	0

Food Name	Serv. Size	Total Cal.	Prot. GMS	Carbs GMS	Sod. MGS	Fiber GMS	Fat GMS	Chol. MGS
(Health Valley) 'Natural' apple and cinnamon	1 oz	100	3.0	19.0	10	3.8	1.0	0
(Health Valley) 'Natural' raisins and spice	1 oz	110	3.0	19.0	10	3.8	1.0	0
(Malt•O•Meal) 'Plus 40% Oat Bran'	1.3 oz	130	6.0	25.0	0	3.0	2.0	0
(Mother's)	1/3 cup	92	5.7	16.6	1	4.2	2.1	0
(Quaker)	1 oz	92	5.7	16.6	1	4.2	2.1	0
(3-Minute Brand) instant	1 oz	90	6.0	17.0	0	4.1	2.0	0
(3-Minute Brand) 'Regular'	1 oz	90	6.0	17.0	0	4.1	2.0	0
(Wholesome 'N Hearty)	1 oz	100	4.0	18.0	0	5.0	2.0	0
(Wholesome 'N Hearty) instant, apple cinnamon	1 3/8 oz	130	3.0	30.0	160	5.0	2.0	0
(Wholesome 'N Hearty) instant, honey	1.25 oz	110	3.0	26.0	160	5.0	2.0	0
OATMEAL AND OATS								
(Arrowhead Mills) instant	1 oz	100	5.8	18.0	0	4.3	2.0	0
(Arrowhead Mills) instant, apple, date, and almond	1 oz	130	5.0	23.0	3	3.7	3.0	0
(Arrowhead Mills) instant, apple spice	1 oz	130	5.0	23.0	1	3.4	2.0	0
(Arrowhead Mills) instant, cinnamon, raisin, and almond	1 oz	140	6.0	23.0	3	4.3	3.0	0
(Erewhon) instant, apple and cinnamon	1.25 oz	145	4.0	25.0	100	na	3.0	na
(Erewhon) instant, apple and raisin	1.3 oz	150	4.0	27.0	100	na	3.0	na
(Erewhon) instant, maple spice	1.2 oz	140	4.0	24.0	100	na	3.0	na
(Erewhon) instant, oat bran	1.25 oz	125	6.0	23.0	0	4.0	3.0	na
(Erewhon) instant, raisins, dates, and walnuts	1.2 oz	130	3.0	24.0	60	3.0	3.0	na
(General Mills) instant, apple and cinnamon	1.5 oz	150	4.0	32.0	105	3.0	2.0	0
(General Mills) instant, cinnamon raisin	1.8 oz	170	4.0	38.0	130	3.0	2.0	0
(General Mills) 'Oatmeal Swirlers' instant, apple and cinnamon	1.7 oz	160	3.0	34.0	120	2.0	2.0	0
(General Mills) 'Oatmeal Swirlers' instant, cherry	1.7 oz	150	3.0	33.0	130	2.0	2.0	0
(General Mills) 'Oatmeal Swirlers' instant, cinnamon and spice	1.6 oz	160	3.0	35.0	100	2.0	2.0	0
(General Mills) 'Oatmeal Swirlers' instant, maple and brown sugar	1.6 oz	160	3.0	35.0	100	2.0	2.0	0
(General Mills) 'Oatmeal Swirlers' instant, milk chocolate	1.7 oz	170	3.0	37.0	100	2.0	2.0	0
(General Mills) 'Oatmeal Swirlers' instant, strawberry	1.6 oz	150	3.0	32.0	120	2.0	2.0	0
(H-O Brand) 'Gourmet'	1/3 cup	100	5.0	18.0	0	3.0	2.0	0
(H-O Brand) instant	1 pkt	110	4.0	18.0	230	3.0	2.0	0
(H-O Brand) instant, apple and cinnamon	1 pkt	130	3.0	26.0	220	3.0	2.0	0

Food Name	Serv. Size	Total Cal.	Prot. GMS	Carbs GMS	Sod. MGS	Fiber GMS	Fat GMS	Chol. MGS
(H-O Brand) instant, box	1/2 cup	130	5.0	22.0	5	3.0	2.0	0
(H-O Brand) instant, maple and brown sugar	1 pkt	160	4.0	32.0	285	3.0	2.0	0
(H-O Brand) instant, raisins and spice	1 pkt	150	4.0	32.0	240	3.0	2.0	0
(H-O Brand) instant, sweet 'n mellow	1 pkt	150	5.0	30.0	270	3.0	2.0	0
(H-O Brand) 'Quick'	1/2 cup	130	5.0	23.0	5	3.0	2.0	0
(H-O Brand) w/fiber, instant	1 pkt	110	5.0	18.0	140	3.0	2.0	0
(H-O Brand) w/fiber, instant, apple and bran	1 pkt	130	3.0	26.0	140	3.0	2.0	0
(H-O Brand) w/fiber, instant, box	1/3 cup	100	5.0	15.0	5	3.0	2.0	0
(H-O Brand) w/fiber, instant, raisin, and bran	1 pkt	150	4.0	32.0	140	3.0	2.0	0
(Maypo)	1 cup	362	12.4	67.7	18	10.1	5.0	0
(Maypo) '30 Second' quick	1 oz	100	4.0	19.0	0	2.0	1.0	0
(Maypo) 'Vermont Style' maple flavor	1 oz	105	4.0	20.0	0	2.0	1.0	0
(Mother's) instant	1 oz	110	5.0	18.0	0	.3	2.0	0
(Quaker)	1/3 cup	99	4.4	18.6	1	2.7	2.0	0
(Quaker) 'Extra'	1 pkt	95	4.4	17.6	219	2.9	2.0	0
(Quaker) 'Extra' apples and spice	1 pkt	133	4.3	26.7	191	3.0	1.9	0
(Quaker) 'Extra' raisins and cinnamon	1 pkt	129	4.1	26.6	119	2.7	1.9	0
(Quaker) instant	1 pkt	94	3.8	18.0	270	2.8	2.0	0
(Quaker) instant, apple and cinnamon	1 pkt	118	3.3	26.0	128	3.0	1.5	0
(Quaker) instant, cinnamon and spice	1 pkt	164	4.5	34.9	322	3.1	2.1	0
(Quaker) instant, maple and brown sugar	1 pkt	152	4.5	31.6	320	2.8	2.1	0
(Quaker) instant, peaches and cream	1 pkt	129	3.4	26.3	179	2.3	2.2	0
(Quaker) instant, raisins and spice	1 pkt	149	4.1	31.5	266	2.8	2.0	0
(Quaker) instant, raisins, dates, and walnuts	1 pkt	141	4.0	25.1	216	2.4	3.8	0
(Quaker) instant, strawberries and cream	1 pkt	129	3.4	26.6	204	2.2	2.0	0
(Quaker) 'Kids' Choice' instant, cinnamon graham cookie	1 pkt	140	4.0	29.0	170	2.6	2.0	0
(Quaker) 'Kids' Choice' instant, maple and brown sugar	1 pkt	140	4.0	31.0	240	2.9	2.0	0
(Quaker) 'Kids' Choice' instant, radical raspberry	1 pkt	150	4.0	28.0	170	2.9	3.0	0
(Quaker) 'Kids' Choice' instant, strawberries and stuff	1 pkt	140	4.0	30.0	170	2.6	2.0	0
(Quaker) 'Old Fashioned'	1 oz	99	4.4	18.6	1	2.7	2.0	0
(Quaker) plus fiber	1/2 cup	130	6.0	21.0	0	6.0	2.5	0
(Quaker) plus fiber, oatmeal raisin bran	1 pkt	150	4.0	28.0	65	6.0	2.0	0
(Quaker) 'Quick'	1 oz	99	4.4	18.6	1	2.7	2.0	0
(Ralston)	1 cup	402	16.6	85.1	13	>2.5 c	2.5	0
(Roman Meal)	1 cup	340	14.5	68.5	20	>2.3 c	4.0	0

Food Name	Serv. Size	Total Cal.	Prot. GMS	Carbs GMS	Sod. MGS	Fiber GMS	Fat GMS	Chol. MGS
(3-Minute Brand) oat bran and raisins	1 oz	100	4.0	18.0	0	3.0	2.0	0
(3-Minute Brand) 'Old Fashioned'	1 oz	100	5.0	18.0	0	3.0	2.0	0
(3-Minute Brand) 'Quick'	1 oz	100	5.0	18.0	0	3.0	2.0	0
(3-Minute Brand) 'Quick' oat bran	1 oz	100	5.0	18.0	0	3.3	2.0	0
(3-Minute Brand) raisins	1 oz	100	5.0	18.0	0	3.0	2.0	0
(Total) instant	1.2 oz	110	4.0	22.0	220	3.0	2.0	0
(Total) instant, maple and brown sugar	1.6 oz	160	4.0	34.0	150	3.0	2.0	0
(Total) 'Quick'	1 oz	90	4.0	18.0	0	2.5	2.0	0
QUINOA (Ancient Harvest) steam-rolled flakes	1/3 cup	105	2.6	23.0	5	2.8	1.0	0
RICE								
(Cream of Rice)	1 tbsp	38	0.6	8.4	1	0	0.1	0
(Lundberg Family) 'Hot'n Creamy' cooked	1 oz	110	3.0	23.0	20	na	1.0	na
(Lundberg Family) 'Hot'n Creamy' almonds and dates, cooked	1 oz	110	2.0	24.0	25	na	1.0	na
RICE, BROWN								
(Arrowhead Mills) 'Rise & Shine'	1.5 oz	160	3.0	35.0	<1	1.6	1.0	0
(Erewhon) cream of brown rice	1 oz	110	3.0	23.0	20	na	1.0	na
RYE								
(Breadshop) 'Rye Date Müesli'	1 oz	100	3.0	19.0	5	4.0	2.0	na
(Roman Meal) cream of rye	1.3 oz	110	4.0	27.0	0	5.4	<1.0	0
WHEAT								
(Arrowhead Mills) 'Bear Mush'	1 oz	100	3.0	21.0	<1	1.3	0.0	0
(Arrowhead Mills) cracked wheat	2 oz	180	7.0	40.0	1	2.3	1.0	0
(Cream of Wheat)	1 tbsp	39	1.1	8.1	1	0	0.2	0
(Cream of Wheat) instant	1 oz	100	3.0	22.0	0	1.0	<1.0	5
(Cream of Wheat) instant	1 tbsp	42	1.2	8.7	2	0	0.2	0
(Cream of Wheat) 'Mix'n Eat' instant	1 oz	100	3.0	21.0	170	1.0	0.0	0
(Cream of Wheat) 'Mix'n Eat' instant, apple and cinnamon	1 oz	130	2.0	29.0	250	1.0	0.0	0
(Cream of Wheat) 'Mix'n Eat' instant, apple, banana, and maple	1 pkt	132	2.4	28.9	241	0	0.4	0
(Cream of Wheat) 'Mix'n Eat' instant, brown sugar and cinnamon	1 oz	130	2.0	29.0	230	1.0	0.0	0
(Cream of Wheat) 'Mix'n Eat' instant, maple and brown sugar	1 oz	130	2.0	29.0	180	1.0	0.0	0
(Cream of Wheat) 'Quick'	1 tbsp	38	1.1	7.9	41	0	0.1	0
(General Mills) 'Wheat Hearts'	1 oz	110	4.0	20.0	0	1.0	1.0	0
(Krusteaz) 'Zoom'	1/3 cup	120	5.0	24.0	0	4.0	0.0	0
(Maltex)	1 cup	532	16.9	116.7	26	6.3	3.2	0
(Mother's)	1/3 cup	92	2.9	20.9	1	2.2	0.6	0
(Quaker)	1/3 cup	92	2.9	20.9	1	2.2	0.6	0
(Wheatena)	1 oz	100	3.0	21.0	0	4.0	1.0	0

Food Name	Serv. Size	Total Cal.	Prot. GMS	Carbs GMS	Sod. MGS	Fiber GMS	Fat GMS	Chol. MGS
CEREAL, READY-TO-SERVE								
(NOTE: All of the following ready-to-serve cereals are in their dry form.)								
'Addam's Family' *(Ralston)*	1 oz	110	1.0	25.0	65	na	1.0	0
'All Bran' extra fiber *(Kellogg's)*	1 oz	50	4.0	22.0	140	14.0	0.0	0
'All Bran' wheat bran *(Kellogg's)*	1 oz	71	4.1	21.1	320	10.1	0.5	0
'Almond Flavor O's' fat-free *(Health Valley)*	1 oz	90	3.0	19.0	5	5.0	0.0	0
'Almond Raisin' low fat *(Golden Temple)*	1 oz	110	2.0	22.0	57	2.0	1.5	0
'Almond Raisin' nectarsweet premium *(Breadshop)*	1 oz	120	3.5	18.0	2	2.5	4.0	0
'Alpha Bits' oat and other grains *(Post)*	1 oz	111	2.2	24.6	180	1.2	0.7	0
'Alpha Bits' super swirl marshmallows *(Post)*	1 oz	150	6.0	31.0	220	1.0	1.0	0
'Apple Almond Müesli' *(Ralston)*	1.45 oz	150	4.0	31.0	140	3.0	2.0	0
'Apple & Cinnamon Toasted Oat' *(Malt•O•Meal)*	1 oz	110	2.0	22.0	180	1.0	2.0	0
'Apple Cinnamon Cheerios' *(General Mills)*	1 oz	110	2.0	22.0	180	1.5	2.0	0
'Apple Cinnamon Corn Flakes' *(Wonder)*	1 oz	110	2.0	25.0	200	na	0.0	0
'Apple Cinnamon' low fat *(Golden Temple)*	1 oz	110	2.0	22.0	59	2.0	1.5	0
'Apple Cinnamon O's' fat-free *(Health Valley)*	1 oz	90	3.0	19.0	5	5.0	0.0	0
'Apple Cinnamon Squares' *(Kellogg's)*	1 oz	90	2.0	23.0	5	2.0	0.0	0
'Apple Jacks' corn and other grains *(Kellogg's)*	1 oz	110	1.5	25.8	125	.5	0.1	0
'Apple Raisin Crisp' *(Kellogg's)*	1 oz	130	2.0	32.0	230	3.0	0.0	0
'Aztec' *(Erewhon)*	1 oz	100	2.0	24.0	85	1.0	0.0	0
'Banana Nut Crunch' *(Post)*	1 oz	120	3.0	20.0	95	2.0	3.0	0
'Banana O's' *(Erewhon)*	1 oz	110	2.0	24.0	15	na	0.0	na
'Banana Walnut Müesli' *(Ralston)*	1.45 oz	150	4.0	30.0	150	3.0	3.0	0
'Basic 4' *(General Mills)*	3/4 cup	130	3.0	28.0	210	2.0	2.0	0
'Batman Returns' *(Ralston)*	1 oz	110	1.0	26.0	190	na	0.0	0
'Berry Berry Kix' *(General Mills)*	1 oz	110	1.0	25.0	170	na	1.0	0
'Blueberry 'N Cream' nectarsweet gourmet *(Breadshop)*	1 oz	115	3.7	18.7	2	2.5	3.0	0
'Blueberry Squares' *(Kellogg's)*	1 oz	90	2.0	23.0	5	3.0	0.0	0
'Body Buddies Natural Fruit' *(General Mills)*	1 oz	110	2.0	24.0	280	na	1.0	0
'Booberry' *(General Mills)*	1 oz	110	1.0	24.0	210	na	1.0	0
'Bran Buds' wheat bran *(Kellogg's)*	1 oz	73	4.0	21.6	174	10.6	0.7	0
'Bran Chex' wheat bran and corn *(Kellogg's)*	1 oz	91	2.9	22.6	264	4.6	0.8	0
'Bran Flakes' *(Arrowhead Mills)*	1 oz	100	5.0	21.0	100	4.0	1.0	0
'Bran Flakes' *(Kellogg's)*	1 oz	90	3.0	22.0	220	5.0	0.0	0
'Bran Flakes' *(Malt•O•Meal)*	1 oz	90	3.0	23.0	210	5.0	1.0	0
'Bran Flakes' *(Post)*	1 oz	90	3.0	23.0	210	5.0	0.0	0

Food Name	Serv. Size	Total Cal.	Prot. GMS	Carbs GMS	Sod. MGS	Fiber GMS	Fat GMS	Chol. MGS
'Breakfast O's' (Barbara's Bakery)	1 oz	120	4.0	21.0	90	na	2.0	0
Brown rice, crisp (Erewhon)	1 oz	110	2.0	24.0	185	4.0	1.0	na
Brown rice, crisp, low sodium (Erewhon)	1 oz	110	2.0	24.0	5	4.0	1.0	na
'Brown Rice Crisps' (Barbara's Bakery)	1 oz	120	2.0	26.0	105	na	1.0	0
'Buñuelitos' (General Mills)	1 oz	120	1.0	25.0	120	na	2.0	0
'C.W. Post Hearty Granola Cereal' (Post)	1 oz	130	2.0	21.0	80	(tr)	4.0	0
'C.W. Post' oats and other grains (Post)	1 oz	126	2.6	20.3	49	2.1	4.4	0
'C.W. Post' oats and other grains, raisins (Post)	1 oz	123	2.4	20.4	44	3.8	4.1	0
'California Orange Crunch' honeysweet premium (Breadshop)	1 oz	130	3.5	18.0	1	2.4	5.0	0
'Captain Crunch' corn and other grains (Quaker)	1 oz	120	1.5	23.0	213	.5	2.6	0
'Captain Crunch Crunchberries' corn and oat (Quaker)	1 oz	118	1.5	23.1	198	.5	2.4	0
'Captain Crunch Peanut Butter' corn (Quaker)	1 oz	125	2.0	21.5	217	.4	3.7	0
'Cashew Almond Granola' (Golden Temple)	1 oz	129	4.0	19.0	3	3.5	3.5	0
'Cheerios' oat and wheat (General Mills)	1 oz	111	4.3	19.6	308	2.0	1.8	0
'Cinnamon & Raisin' 100%natural (Nature Valley)	1 oz	120	2.0	20.0	50	1.0	4.0	0
'Cinnamon & Spice Crunch' psyllium and chia seed (Golden Temple)	1 oz	132	3.0	20.0	26	2.0	4.5	0
'Cinnamon Apple Raisin Granola' (Golden Temple)	1 oz	125	3.0	20.0	3	2.0	3.5	0
'Cinnamon Mini Buns' (Kellogg's)	1 oz	110	2.0	25.0	220	1.0	1.0	0
'Cinnamon Toast Crunch' (General Mills)	1 oz	120	1.0	22.0	210	1.0	3.0	0
'Cinnamon Toast Crunch' breakfast pack (General Mills)	1 oz	140	1.0	26.0	240	1.0	4.0	0
'Cinnapple Spice' honeysweet premium (Breadshop)	1 oz	125	3.4	18.5	2	2.0	4.5	0
'Clusters' (General Mills)	1 oz	110	3.0	22.0	140	2.0	2.0	0
'Cocoa Krispies' rice (Kellogg's)	1 oz	110	1.5	25.2	217	.2	0.4	0
'Cocoa Pebbles' rice (Post)	1 oz	116	1.3	24.4	136	.5	1.5	0
'Cocoa Puffs' (General Mills)	1 oz	110	1.0	25.0	180	na	1.0	0
'Coconut Almond Granola' (Golden Temple)	1 oz	145	4.0	18.0	26	3.0	7.0	0
'Common Sense Oat Bran' (Kellogg's)	1 oz	100	4.0	22.0	250	3.0	1.0	0
'Common Sense Oat Bran' raisins (Kellogg's)	3/4 cup	130	4.0	29.0	250	3.0	1.0	0
'Complete' bran flakes, beta carotene (Kellogg's)	1 oz	90	3.0	23.0	220	5.0	<1.0	0
'Cookie-Crisp' chocolate chip and vanilla (Ralston)	1 oz	114	1.5	24.9	196	>.1 c	1.0	0

Food Name	Serv. Size	Total Cal.	Prot. GMS	Carbs GMS	Sod. MGS	Fiber GMS	Fat GMS	Chol. MGS
'Corn Bran' corn bran and other grains								
(Ralston)	1 oz	98	1.9	23.9	244	>1.1 c	1.0	0
'Corn Chex' *(Ralston)*	1 oz	111	2.0	24.9	272	>.1 c	0.1	0
'Corn Flakes' *(Arrowhead Mills)*	1 oz	100	2.0	25.0	100	2.0	0.0	0
'Corn Flakes' *(Barbara's Bakery)*	1 oz	110	2.0	24.0	70	na	0.0	0
'Corn Flakes' *(Kellogg's)*	1 oz	110	2.3	24.4	291	.7	0.1	0
'Corn Flakes' *(Krusteaz)*	1 oz	110	2.0	24.0	280	1.0	1.0	0
'Corn Flakes' *(Malt•O•Meal)*	1 oz	110	2.0	25.0	290	1.0	0.0	0
'Corn Flakes' *(Ralston)*	1 oz	111	2.2	24.6	272	>.1 c	0.1	0
'Corn Flakes' sugar frosted *(Kellogg's)*	1 oz	108	1.4	25.7	230	.5	0.1	0
'Corn Flakes' sugar frosted *(Ralston)*	1 oz	111	1.5	25.6	184	>.1 c	0.4	0
'Corn Pops' *(Kellogg's)*	1 oz	110	1.0	26.0	90	1.0	0.0	0
'Count Chocula' *(General Mills)*	1 oz	110	1.0	25.0	180	na	1.0	0
'Country Corn Flakes' *(General Mills)*	1 oz	110	2.0	25.0	270	na	1.0	0
'Cracklin' Bran' wheat bran and other grains								
(Kellogg's)	1 oz	108	2.6	19.5	230	4.7	4.2	0
'Cracklin' Oat Bran' *(Kellogg's)*	1 oz	110	3.0	21.0	140	4.0	3.0	0
'Cranberry Walnut Müesli' *(Ralston)*	1.45 oz	150	4.0	30.0	95	3.0	3.0	0
'Crisp N' Crackling Rice' *(Malt•O•Meal)*	1 oz	110	2.0	25.0	240	0	0.0	0
'Crisp Rice' *(Krusteaz)*	1 oz	110	2.0	25.0	270	1.0	0.0	0
'Crispix' *(Kellogg's)*	1 oz	110	2.0	25.0	220	0	0.0	0
'Crispy Wheats 'N Raisins' wheat								
(General Mills)	1 oz	99	2.0	23.2	135	1.9	0.5	0
'Crunch Graham Oat Rings' *(Wonder)*	1 oz	110	2.0	24.0	125	na	1.0	0
'Crunchies' brown rice *(Lundberg Family)*	1 cup	171	3.0	38.0	7	na	0.8	na
'Crunchy Oat Bran' nectarsweet gourmet								
(Breadshop)	1 oz	120	3.0	18.0	2	2.5	5.0	na
'Date Almond Müesli' *(Ralston)*	1.45 oz	140	4.0	32.0	95	3.0	2.0	0
'Dino Pebbles' *(Post)*	1 oz	110	1.0	25.0	150	tr	1.0	0
'Double Chex' *(Ralston)*	1 oz	100	1.0	25.0	260	0	0.0	0
'Double Dip Crunch' *(Kellogg's)*	1 oz	120	2.0	23.0	160	0	2.0	0
'Fiber One' aspartame *(General Mills)*	1 oz	60	2.0	23.0	140	13.0	1.0	0
'Fiberwise' *(Kellogg's)*	1 oz	90	3.0	23.0	140	5.0	1.0	0
'Fingos' cinnamon *(General Mills)*	1 oz	110	1.0	22.0	170	2.0	3.0	0
'Fingos' honey toasted oat *(General Mills)*	1 oz	110	2.0	21.0	210	1.5	3.0	0
'40% Bran Flakes' wheat bran *(Kellogg's)*	1 oz	93	3.6	22.2	220	4.0	0.5	0
'40% Bran Flakes' wheat bran *(Post)*	1 oz	92	3.2	22.5	260	5.5	0.5	0
'40% Bran Flakes' wheat bran *(Ralston)*	1 oz	92	3.3	22.7	264	>1.2 c	0.4	0
'Frankenberry' *(General Mills)*	1 oz	110	1.0	24.0	210	na	1.0	0
'Froot Loops' corn and other grains								
(Kellogg's)	1 oz	111	1.7	25.1	145	.6	0.5	0
'Frosted Chex Juniors' *(Ralston)*	1 oz	110	2.0	25.0	200	na	0.0	0
'Frosted Flakes' *(Kellogg's)*	1 oz	110	1.0	26.0	200	1.0	0.0	0

Food Name	Serv. Size	Total Cal.	Prot. GMS	Carbs GMS	Sod. MGS	Fiber GMS	Fat GMS	Chol. MGS
'Frosted Funnies' (Barbara's Bakery) .... 1 cup		110	2.0	27.0	100	na	0.0 .	0
'Frosted Krispies' (Kellogg's) .... 1 oz		110	1.0	26.0	220	0	0.0	0
'Frosted Mini Wheats' (Kellogg's) .... 1 oz		100	3.0	24.0	0	3.0	0.0	0
'Frosted Mini Wheats' bite size (Kellogg's) 1 oz		100	3.0	24.0	0	3.0	0.0	0
'Frosted Mini Wheats' brown sugar and								
cinnamon (Kellogg's) .... 1 oz		102	2.9	23.4	8	2.2	0.3	0
'Frosted Rice Krinkles' rice .... 1 oz		109	1.4	25.9	179	.2	0.1	0
'Frosted Rice Krispies' rice (Kellogg's) .... 1 oz		109	1.4	25.7	240	.2	0.1	0
'Fruit & Fibre' oat, dates, raisins, and								
walnuts (Post) .... 1.25 oz		120	3.0	27.0	170	5.0	2.0	0
'Fruit & Fibre' oat, peaches, raisins, and								
almonds (Post) .... 1.25 oz		120	3.0	26.0	170	5.0	2.0	0
'Fruit & Fibre' oat, pineapple, banana,								
and coconut (Post) .... 1.25 oz		120	3.0	27.0	170	5.0	3.0	0
'Fruit & Fibre' oat, tropical fruit (Post) ... 1.25 oz		120	3.0	27.0	170	5.0	3.0	0
'Fruit & Frosted O's' mixed grain								
(Malt•O•Meal) .... 1 oz		110	2.0	25.0	120	1.0	1.0	0
'Fruit & Nut' 100%natural (Nature Valley) .. 1 oz		130	2.0	19.0	45	1.0	5.0	0
'Fruit 'N Nut Granola' (Golden Temple) .... 1 oz		129	3.0	19.0	26	2.0	4.5	0
'Fruit 'n Wheat' (Erewhon) .... 1 oz		100	2.0	21.0	75	3.0	1.0	0
'Fruit Wheats' apple (Nabisco) .... 1 oz		90	2.0	23.0	15	3.0	0.0	0
'Fruit Whirls' (Krusteaz) .... 1 oz		110	1.0	25.0	120	1.0	1.0	0
'Fruitful Bran' fruit (Kellogg's) .... 1 oz		120	3.0	31.0	240	5.0	0.0	0
'Fruity Marshmallow Krispies' (Kellogg's) 1 1/4 cups		140	2.0	32.0	210	0	0.0	0
'Fruity Pebbles' rice (Post) .... 1 oz		115	1.1	24.4	158	.4	1.5	0
'Golden Crisp' (Post) .... 1 oz		110	2.0	26.0	45	(tr)	0.0	0
'Golden Grahams' corn and wheat								
(General Mills) .... 1 oz		109	1.6	24.2	281	1.0	1.1	0
'Golden Granola' (Golden Temple) .... 1 oz		138	4.0	19.0	25	2.0	6.0	0
'Golden Maple Nut' honeysweet premium								
(Breadshop) .... 1 oz		130	3.5	17.0	2	2.0	5.0	na
'Gone Nuts!' nectarsweet premium								
(Breadshop) .... 1 oz		125	3.5	17.0	2	2.5	5.0	na
'Graham Chex' (Ralston) .... 1 oz		110	2.0	24.0	220	1.0	1.0	0
'Graham Crackos' wheat .... 1 oz		103	2.1	24.5	185	1.7	0.2	0
Granola, banana almond (Sunbelt) ...... 1 oz		130	3.0	20.0	25	na	4.0	2
Granola, date and almond, fat-free								
(Health Valley) .... 1 oz		90	2.0	21.0	20	2.5	0.0	0
Granola, fruit and nut (Sunbelt) .... 1 oz		120	3.0	19.0	20	na	5.0	na
Granola, raisin cinnamon, fat-free								
(Health Valley) .... 1 oz		90	2.0	21.0	20	2.5	0.0	0
Granola, tropical fruit, fat-free								
(Health Valley) ...:............. 1 oz		90	2.0	21.0	20	2.5	0.0	0

Food Name	Serv. Size	Total Cal.	Prot. GMS	Carbs GMS	Sod. MGS	Fiber GMS	Fat GMS	Chol. MGS
'Granola' toasted oat mix (Nature Valley)	1 oz	126	2.9	19.0	58	1.5	4.9	0
'Grape-Nuts' wheat and barley (Post)	1 oz	101	3.3	23.3	197	2.8	0.1	0
'Grape-Nuts Flakes' wheat and barley (Post)	1 oz	102	3.0	23.2	160	2.8	0.3	0
'Great Grains' double pecan (Post)	1 oz	120	3.0	20.0	60	3.0	3.0	0
'Great Grains' raisins, dates, and pecans (Post)	1.25 oz	140	3.0	27.0	70	3.0	3.0	0
'Hawaiian Granola' (Golden Temple)	1 oz	126	4.0	19.0	3	2.0	4.0	0
'Hazelnut Boysenberry' organic oats (Golden Temple)	1 oz	135	4.0	19.0	2	3.0	5.5	0
'Heritage O's' (Natures Path)	1 cup	165	5.0	34.0	140	4.5	<1.0	0
'High Fiber O's' fat-free (Health Valley)	1 oz	90	3.0	19.0	5	5.0	0.0	0
'High 5' (Barbara's Bakery)	3/4 cup	100	3.0	23.0	180	na	0.5	0
'High Protein Granola' (Golden Temple)	1 oz	124	4.0	19.0	6	2.0	3.5	0
'Honey Almond Delight' (Ralston)	1 oz	110	2.0	23.0	200	1.0	2.0	0
'Honey Almond Granola' (Golden Temple)	1 oz	130	4.0	20.0	25	3.0	3.5	0
'Honey & Nut Toasted Oat' (Malt•O•Meal)	1 oz	110	3.0	23.0	190	2.0	1.0	0
'Honey Apple Blueberry' honeysweet premium(Breadshop)	1 oz	125	3.5	18.0	1	2.5	5.0	na
'Honey Blueberry Apple Granola' (Golden Temple)	1 oz	128	4.0	20.0	2	2.0	3.5	0
'Honey Bunches of Oats' almonds (Post)	1 oz	120	2.0	22.0	160	1.0	3.0	0
'Honey Bunches of Oats' honey roasted (Post)	1 oz	110	2.0	24.0	180	1.0	2.0	0
'Honey Gone Nuts!' honeysweet premium (Breadshop)	1 oz	130	3.5	17.5	2	2.5	5.5	na
'Honey Nut' toasted oatmeal (Quaker)	1 oz	120	3.0	20.0	110	2.0	3.0	0
'Honey Nut Cheerios' oat and wheat (General Mills)	1 oz	107	3.1	22.8	257	1.3	0.7	0
'Honey Nut Cheerios' oat and wheat, breakfast pack(General Mills)	4/5 cup	100	2.0	21.0	230	1.0	1.0	0
'Honey Nut Crispy Rice' (Wonder)	1 oz	110	2.0	25.0	205	na	1.0	0
'Honey Nut O's' (Krusteaz)	1 oz	110	3.0	23.0	190	2.0	1.0	0
'HoneyComb' corn and oats (Post)	1 oz	111	1.6	25.3	160	.8	0.5	0
'Just Right' fiber nuggets (Kellogg's)	1 oz	100	2.0	24.0	200	2.0	1.0	0
'Just Right' raisins, dates, and nuts (Kellogg's)	3/4 cup	140	3.0	30.0	190	2.0	1.0	0
'Kaboom' (General Mills)	1 oz	110	2.0	23.0	270	na	1.0	0
'Kamut Flakes' (Erewhon)	1 oz	90	4.0	18.0	60	4.0	0.0	na
'Kenmei Rice Bran' (Kellogg's)	1 oz	110	2.0	24.0	230	1.0	1.0	0
'King Vitaman' corn and other grains	1 oz	115	1.5	24.1	218	.4	1.6	0
'Kix' corn and other grains (General Mills)	1 oz	110	2.6	23.5	291	.5	0.7	0
'Life' oat and other grains (Quaker)	1 oz	105	5.2	20.3	148	1.7	0.5	0

Food Name	Serv. Size	Total Cal.	Prot. GMS	Carbs GMS	Sod. MGS	Fiber GMS	Fat GMS	Chol. MGS
'Life' oat and other grains, cinnamon (Quaker)	1 oz	105	5.2	20.3	148	>.4 c	0.5	0
'Lite Müesli' (Golden Temple)	1 oz	102	3.0	20.0	60	2.0	1.0	0
'Lite 'N Crunchy Granola' (Golden Temple)	1 oz	129	4.0	19.0	9	2.0	4.5	0
'Lucky Charms' oat and other grains (General Mills)	1 oz	111	2.6	23.2	202	1.2	1.1	0
'Lucky Charms' oat and other grains, breakfast pack (General Mills)	7/8 oz	110	2.0	24.0	180	na	1.0	0
'Maple Almond Granola' (Golden Temple)	1 oz	129	4.0	20.0	25	2.0	3.5	0
'Maple Corns' (Arrowhead Mills)	1 oz	100	3.0	23.0	75	3.0	1.0	na
'Maple Frosted Corn' mini puffs (Glenny's)	1 oz	109	4.0	20.0	50	na	<.5	na
'Marshmallow Alpha Bits' (Post)	1 oz	110	2.0	25.0	150	1.0	1.0	0
'Most' wheat bran and wheat	1 oz	96	4.0	21.6	151	4.0	0.3	0
'Müeslix Crispy Blend' (Kellogg's)	2/3 cup	150	3.0	32.0	150	3.0	2.0	0
'Müeslix Golden Crunch' (Kellogg's)	1/2 cup	120	3.0	25.0	170	3.0	2.0	0
'Multi Grain Cheerios' (General Mills)	1 oz	100	2.0	23.0	220	2.0	1.0	0
'Multi-Bran Chex' (Ralston)	1 oz	90	2.0	23.0	200	4.0	1.0	0
'Natural Blueberry Granola' (Golden Temple)	1 oz	132	4.0	19.0	3	2.0	5.0	0
'Natural Blueberry Granola' coconut-free (Golden Temple)	1 oz	131	4.0	19.0	3	2.0	4.5	0
'Natural Bran Flakes' (Post)	1 oz	90	3.0	23.0	240	5.0	0.0	0
'Natural Delite Granola' (Golden Temple)	1 oz	128	3.0	20.0	26	2.0	3.5	0
'Natural Foods Apple Cinnamon' low fat (Golden Temple)	1 oz	110	3.0	22.0	3	2.0	1.0	0
'Natural Foods Raisin Almond' low fat (Golden Temple)	1 oz	110	3.0	22.0	3	2.0	1.0	0
'Natural Foods Strawberry/Raspberry' low fat (Golden Temple)	1 oz	111	3.0	22.0	3	2.0	1.0	0
'Natural' oat and wheat germ (Heartland)	1 oz	123	2.9	19.4	72	1.7	4.4	0
'Natural' oat and wheat germ, coconut (Heartland)	1 oz	125	3.0	19.3	58	2.0	4.6	0
'Natural' oat and wheat germ, raisins (Heartland)	1 oz	121	2.8	19.6	58	1.6	4.0	0
'Natural Raisin Bran' (Post)	1.4 oz	120	3.0	31.0	200	6.0	1.0	0
'Nut & Honey Crunch' (Kellogg's)	1 oz	110	2.0	24.0	200	0	1.0	0
'Nut & Honey Crunch O's' (Kellogg's)	1 oz	110	2.0	22.0	190	1.0	2.0	0
'Nutri-Grain' barley (Kellogg's)	1 oz	106	3.1	23.5	192	1.6	0.2	0
'Nutri-Grain' corn (Kellogg's)	1 oz	108	2.3	24.0	187	1.8	0.7	0
'Nutri-Grain' rye (Kellogg's)	1 oz	102	2.5	24.0	193	1.8	0.2	0
'Nutri-Grain' wheat (Kellogg's)	1 oz	102	2.5	24.0	193	1.8	0.3	0
'Nutri-Grain Almond Raisin' (Kellogg's)	2/3 cup	140	3.0	31.0	220	3.0	2.0	0
'Nutri-Grain Raisin Bran' (Kellogg's)	1 cup	130	4.0	31.0	200	5.0	1.0	0

Food Name	Serv. Size	Total Cal.	Prot. GMS	Carbs GMS	Sod. MGS	Fiber GMS	Fat GMS	Chol. MGS
'Oat Bran Almond' *(Golden Temple)*	1 oz	120	4.0	20.0	3	3.0	3.5	0
'Oat Bran Apple' *(Golden Temple)*	1 oz	112	4.0	19.0	3	3.0	3.5	0
'Oat Bran Flakes' *(Arrowhead Mills)*	1 oz	100	5.0	19.0	100	3.0	2.0	0
'Oat Bran Granola' berries *(Golden Temple)*	1 oz	120	4.0	20.0	3	3.0	3.5	0
'Oat Bran Granola' raisins and almonds *(Golden Temple)*	1 oz	119	3.0	19.0	3	3.0	3.5	0
'Oat Bran Müesli' dates and almonds *(Golden Temple)*	1 oz	108	3.0	21.0	79	2.0	1.5	0
'Oat Bran Müesli' raisins and hazelnuts *(Golden Temple)*	1 oz	102	3.0	20.0	59	3.0	1.5	0
'Oat Bran Oregonberry' *(Golden Temple)*	1 oz	116	4.0	20.0	3	3.0	3.5	0
'Oat Flakes' *(Arrowhead Mills)*	2 oz	220	10.0	39.0	1	8.1	4.0	0
'Oat Flakes' *(Post)*	1 oz	110	4.0	21.0	130	2.0	1.0	0
'Oat Mini Puffs' *(Glenny's)*	1 oz	108	4.5	22.0	30	na	<.5	na
'Oat Mini Puffs' w/o salt, w/o sugar *(Glenny's)*	1 oz	108	4.5	22.0	7	na	<.5	na
'Oatbake Honey Bran' *(Kellogg's)*	1 oz	110	2.0	21.0	190	3.0	3.0	0
'Oatbake Raisin Nut' *(Kellogg's)*	1 oz	110	2.0	21.0	190	3.0	3.0	0
'Oatmeal Crisp' *(General Mills)*	1 oz	110	3.0	21.0	180	1.0	2.0	0
'Oatmeal Crisp With Apples' *(General Mills)*	1 oz	110	2.0	23.0	180	1.0	1.0	na
'Oatmeal Raisin Crisp' *(General Mills)*	1/2 cup	130	3.0	25.0	170	1.5	2.0	0
'100% Bran' wheat bran and barley *(Nabisco)*	1 oz	76	3.5	20.7	197	>2.1 c	1.4	0
'100% Natural Almond' *(Golden Temple)*	1 oz	123	3.0	18.0	15	2.0	4.0	0
'100% Natural Apple/Cinnamon' *(Golden Temple)*	1 oz	120	3.0	18.0	14	2.0	4.0	0
'100% Natural' mixed grain *(Quaker)*	1 oz	127	3.3	18.0	14	2.0	5.5	0
'100% Natural' mixed grain, raisins, low fat *(Quaker)*	1 oz	110	3.0	21.0	15	2.1	2.0	0
'100% Natural Oat Bran' *(Golden Temple)*	1 oz	70	5.0	19.0	1	5.0	2.5	0
'100% Natural' oats and wheat *(Quaker)*	1 oz	133	3.3	17.8	12	2.4	6.1	0
'100% Natural' oats and wheat, apple and cinnamon *(Quaker)*	1 oz	130	2.9	13.1	14	1.9	5.3	0
'100% Natural' oats and wheat, raisins, low fat *(Quaker)*	1 oz	150	7.0	27.0	80	2.0	2.0	0
'100% Natural' oats and wheat, raisins and dates *(Quaker)*	1 oz	128	2.9	18.7	12	1.9	5.3	0
'100% Natural Raisin/Almond' *(Golden Temple)*	1 oz	120	3.0	19.0	7	2.0	4.0	0
'100% Organic Blue Corn Flakes' *(Health Valley)*	1 oz	90	3.0	19.0	10	2.8	<1.0	0
'Orange Almond' nectarsweet premium *(Breadshop)*	1 oz	120	3.5	18.0	2	2.5	4.0	na

Food Name	Serv. Size	Total Cal.	Prot. GMS	Carbs GMS	Sod. MGS	Fiber GMS	Fat GMS	Chol. MGS
'Orange Almond Granola' (Golden Temple)	1 oz	133	4.0	19.0	25	2.0	4.0	0
'Oregon Blueberry Crunch' honeysweet gourmet (Breadshop)	1 oz	125	3.5	18.0	2	2.5	5.0	na
'Organic Amaranth Flakes' (Health Valley)	1 oz	90	3.0	20.0	10	3.0	0.0	0
'Original' toasted oatmeal (Quaker)	1 oz	100	3.0	22.0	160	2.1	1.0	0
'Peach Pecan Müesli' (Ralston)	1.45 oz	150	4.0	30.0	150	3.0	3.0	0
'Peaches 'N Cream' nectarsweet gourmet (Breadshop)	1 oz	115	3.5	18.5	2	2.5	3.0	na
'Post Toasties Corn Flakes' (Post)	1 oz	110	2.0	24.0	310	(tr)	0.0	0
'Product 19' corn and other grains (Kellogg's)	1 oz	108	2.8	23.6	325	1.2	0.2	0
'Puffed Corn' (Arrowhead Mills)	.5 oz	50	3.0	11.0	1	3.0	0.0	na
'Puffed Kamut' (Arrowhead Mills)	.5 oz	40	2.0	10.0	0	2.0	0.0	na
'Puffed Rice' (Arrowhead Mills)	.5 oz	50	1.0	12.0	1	3.0	0.0	na
'Puffed Rice' (Malt•O•Meal)	.5 oz	50	1.0	12.0	0	0	0.0	0
'Puffed Wheat' (Arrowhead Mills)	.5 oz	50	2.0	11.0	1	6.0	0.0	na
'Puffed Wheat' (Malt•O•Meal)	.5 oz	50	2.0	10.0	0	1.0	0.0	0
'Quisp' corn and oat	1 oz	118	1.4	23.7	228	.5	2.0	0
'Raisin Apricot-Date Granola' (Golden Temple)	1 oz	127	3.0	20.0	25	2.0	3.5	0
'Raisin Bran' (Barbara's Bakery)	1 oz	170	3.0	36.0	80	na	1.0	0
'Raisin Bran' (Erewhon)	1 oz	100	3.0	22.0	80	3.0	0.0	0
'Raisin Bran' (Krusteaz)	3/4 cup	120	3.0	30.0	210	4.0	1.0	0
'Raisin Bran' wheat (Kellogg's)	1.3 oz	115	4.0	27.9	204	4.0	0.7	0
'Raisin Bran' wheat (Post)	1 oz	87	2.6	21.5	185	4.0	0.5	0
'Raisin Bran' wheat (Ralston)	1 1/3 oz	120	3.0	31.4	328	>1.1 c	0.2	0
'Raisin Bran Flakes' (Malt•O•Meal)	1.4 oz	130	3.0	30.0	200	5.0	2.0	0
'Raisin Grape-Nuts' (Post)	1 oz	100	3.0	23.0	140	2.0	0.0	0
'Raisin Squares' (Kellogg's)	1 oz	90	2.0	23.0	0	2.0	0.0	0
'Raspberry Almond Müesli' (Ralston)	1.45 oz	150	4.0	30.0	140	3.0	3.0	0
'Raspberry 'N Cream' nectar sweet gourmet (Breadshop)	1 oz	115	3.8	18.5	2	2.5	3.0	na
'Rice Chex' (Ralston)	1 oz	112	1.5	25.3	237	>.1 c	0.1	0
'Rice Krispies' (Kellogg's)	1 oz	112	1.9	24.8	341	.4	0.2	0
'Rice Krispies Treats' (Kellogg's)	1 oz	110	1.0	24.0	160	0	1.0	na
'Rice Mini Puffs' (Glenny's)	1 oz	109	4.0	20.0	30	na	<.5	na
'Right Start' (Erewhon)	1 oz	90	3.0	24.0	80	5.0	0.0	0
'Right Start With Raisins' (Erewhon)	1 oz	90	3.0	22.0	80	5.0	0.0	0
'Ripple Crisp' (General Mills)	1 oz	110	1.0	24.0	280	1.0	<1.0	0
'Ripple Crisp' honey bran (General Mills)	1 oz	100	2.0	24.0	210	3.0	<1.0	0
'Shredded Wheat' (Barbara's Bakery)	1.4 oz	140	4.0	31.0	0	na	1.0	0
'Shredded Wheat' (Nabisco)	1 biscuit	80	2.0	19.0	0	3.0	1.0	0
'Shredded Wheat 'n Bran' (Nabisco)	1 oz	90	3.0	23.0	0	4.0	0.0	0

Food Name	Serv. Size	Total Cal.	Prot. GMS	Carbs GMS	Sod. MGS	Fiber GMS	Fat GMS	Chol. MGS
'Shredded Wheat With Oat Bran' (Nabisco)	1 oz	100	3.0	22.0	0	4.0	1.0	0
'6-Grain Crisp' fruit and flaxseed (Golden Temple)	1 oz	118	3.0	20.0	73	2.0	3.5	0
'Smacks' (Kellogg's)	1 oz	110	2.0	25.0	70	1.0	1.0	0
'Smacks' wheat (Kellogg's)	1 oz	106	2.0	24.8	75	.4	0.5	0
'S'Mores Grahams' (General Mills)	1 oz	120	1.0	24.0	230	na	2.0	0
'Smurf-Magic Berries' (Post)	1 oz	120	2.0	26.0	60	(tr)	1.0	0
'Special K' rice and wheat (Kellogg's)	1 oz	111	5.6	21.3	266	.7	0.1	0
'Spelt Flakes' (Arrowhead Mills)	1 oz	100	4.0	21.0	60	na	1.0	0
'Spoon Size Shredded Wheat' (Nabisco)	1 oz	90	3.0	23.0	0	3.0	1.0	0
'Sprinkle Spangles' corn puffs, sprinkles (General Mills)	1 oz	110	1.0	25.0	130	na	1.0	0
'Sprouts 7' bananas and Hawaiian fruit (Health Valley)	1 oz	90	3.0	16.0	0	4.3	0.0	0
'Sprouts 7' raisins, fat-free (Health Valley)	1 oz	90	4.0	16.0	0	4.7	0.0	0
'Startoons' cocoa (Barbara's Bakery)	1 cup	110	2.0	26.0	140	na	0.5	0
'Startoons' honey (Barbara's Bakery)	1 cup	110	2.0	26.0	50	na	0.0	0
'Strawberry 'N Cream' nectarsweet gourmet (Breadshop)	1 oz	110	3.0	16.0	5	3.0	4.0	na
'Strawberry Squares' (Kellogg's)	1 oz	90	2.0	23.0	5	3.0	0.0	0
'Sugar Corn Pops' (Kellogg's)	1 oz	108	1.4	25.7	104	.2	0.1	0
'Sugar Frosted Flakes' (Krusteaz)	1 oz	110	1.0	26.0	230	1.0	0.0	0
'Sugar Frosted Flakes' (Malt•O•Meal)	1 oz	110	1.0	26.0	170	1.0	0.0	0
'Sugar Puffs' (Malt•O•Meal)	1 oz	110	2.0	25.0	25	na	0.0	0
'Sunflakes Multi-Grain' (Ralston)	1 oz	100	2.0	24.0	240	0	1.0	0
'Super Nutty Granola' (Golden Temple)	1 oz	135	4.0	19.0	25	3.0	5.0	0
'Super O's' (Erewhon)	1 oz	110	3.0	24.0	5	4.0	0.0	0
'Super Sugar Crisp' wheat (Post)	1 oz	106	1.9	25.6	25	.4	0.3	0
'Supernatural' honeysweet gourmet (Breadshop)	1 oz	100	3.5	17.5	2	3.5	5.0	na
'Supernatural New England' honeysweet gourmet (Breadshop)	1 oz	130	3.0	18.0	2	2.0	5.0	na
'Sweet Home Farm Almond' (Golden Temple)	1 oz	123	3.0	18.0	14	2.0	4.0	0
'Sweet Home Farm Crunchy Müesli' low fat (Golden Temple)	1 oz	105	3.0	21.0	98	2.0	2.0	0
'Sweet Home Farm Granola' low fat (Golden Temple)	1 oz	110	3.0	22.0	65	2.0	2.0	0
'Sweet Home Farm Raisin' (Golden Temple)	1 oz	120	3.0	19.0	13	2.0	4.0	0
'Sweetened Puffed Wheat' (Malt•O•Meal)	1 oz	110	2.0	25.0	25	1.0	0.0	0
'Swiss Style Müesli' (Golden Temple)	1 oz	105	3.0	19.0	15	3.0	1.5	0
'Tasteeos' oat and other grains	1 oz	112	3.6	22.5	216	3.0	0.8	0
'Team' rice and other grains (Nabisco)	1 oz	111	1.8	24.4	176	.4	0.5	0

Food Name	Serv. Size	Total Cal.	Prot. GMS	Carbs GMS	Sod. MGS	Fiber GMS	Fat GMS	Chol. MGS
'Team Flakes' *(Nabisco)*	1 oz	110	2.0	24.0	180	na	1.0	0
'Teenage Mutant Ninja Turtles' *(Ralston)*	1 oz	110	1.0	26.0	190	na	0.0	0
'35% Fruit Müesli' *(Golden Temple)*	1 oz	97	3.0	19.0	16	3.0	1.0	0
'Toasted Oat' 100%natural *(Nature Valley)*	1 oz	130	2.0	20.0	50	1.0	5.0	0
'Toasted Oats' *(Krusteaz)*	1 oz	110	4.0	22.0	290	2.0	1.0	0
'Toasted Oats' *(Malt•O•Meal)*	1 oz	110	4.0	20.0	240	2.0	2.0	0
'Toasties' corn *(Post)*	1 oz	110	2.3	24.4	298	1.0	0.1	0
'Tootie Fruities' *(Malt•O•Meal)*	1 oz	110	2.0	25.0	120	na	1.0	0
'Total Corn Flakes' *(General Mills)*	1 oz	110	2.0	24.0	200	na	1.0	0
'Total Raisin Bran' *(General Mills)*	1.5 oz	140	3.0	33.0	190	4.0	1.0	0
'Total' wheat *(General Mills)*	1 oz	100	2.8	22.4	281	3.7	0.6	0
'Triples' *(General Mills)*	1 oz	110	2.0	24.0	200	na	1.0	0
'Triples' breakfast pack *(General Mills)*	1 oz	110	2.0	23.0	190	na	1.0	0
'Trix' corn and other grains *(General Mills)*	1 oz	109	1.5	25.2	181	.3	0.4	0
'Uncle Sam' *(US Mills)*	1 oz	110	4.0	20.0	65	7.0	1.0	0
'Urkel-O's' *(Ralston)*	1 oz	110	1.0	25.0	160	na	1.0	0
'Waffelos' wheat and other grains	1 oz	115	1.6	24.5	118	>.1 c	1.2	0
'Wheat Chex' *(Ralston)*	1 oz	104	2.8	23.3	190	>.6 c	0.7	0
'Wheat Flakes' *(Erewhon)*	1 oz	110	3.0	22.0	75	3.5	0.0	0
'Wheat 'n Raisin Chex' *(Ralston)*	1 1/3 oz	130	3.5	30.1	214	>.6 c	0.3	0
'Wheaties' *(General Mills)*	1 oz	99	2.7	22.6	270	>.5 c	0.5	0
'Wheaties Honey Gold' *(General Mills)*	1 oz	100	2.0	25.0	200	1.0	1.0	0
'Whole-Grain Shredded Wheat' *(Kellogg's)*	1 oz	90	3.0	23.0	0	4.0	0.0	0
'Whole-Grain Wheat Chex' *(Ralston)*	1 oz	100	3.0	23.0	230	3.0	1.0	30
CEREAL SNACK. See also GRANOLA AND CEREAL BAR; GRANOLA SNACK.								
'Cheerios-to-Go' *(General Mills)*	1 pouch	80	3.0	15.0	220	2.0	2.0	0
'Cheerios-to-Go' apple cinnamon *(General Mills)*	1 pouch	110	2.0	22.0	180	1.5	2.0	0
'Cheerios-to-Go' honey nut *(General Mills)*	1 pouch	110	3.0	23.0	250	1.5	1.0	0
'Fingos' cinnamon *(General Mills)*	1 oz	110	1.0	22.0	170	2.0	3.0	0
'Fingos' honey toasted oat *(General Mills)*	1 oz	110	2.0	21.0	210	1.5	3.0	0
CHARD. See SWISS CHARD.								
CHAYOTE								
boiled, drained	4 oz	27	0.7	5.8	1	>.7 c	0.5	0
boiled, drained, 1-inch pieces	1/2 cup	19	0.5	4.1	1	>.5 c	.0.4	0
raw, approx 7.2 oz	1 med	49	1.8	11.0	8	>1.4 c	0.6	0
raw, 1-inch pieces	1/2 cup	16	0.6	3.6	3	>.5 c	0.2	0
raw, trimmed	1 oz	7	0.3	1.5	1	>.2 c	0.1	0
raw, untrimmed	1 lb	108	4.0	24.3	18	>3.1 c	1.4	0
CHEDDARWURST								
'Bun Size' *(Hillshire Farm)*	2 oz	200	8.0	1.0	480	(tr)	18.0	(mq)
'Links' *(Hillshire Farm)*	2 oz	190	8.0	1.0	480	(tr)	17.0	(mq)

Food Name	Serv. Size	Total Cal.	Prot. GMS	Carbs GMS	Sod. MGS	Fiber GMS	Fat GMS	Chol. MGS
CHEESE. See also CHEESE, ALTERNATIVE; CHEESE BALL; CHEESE FOOD; CHEESE LOG; CHEESE NUGGET; CHEESE NUT; CHEESE PRODUCT; CHEESE SPREAD; CHEESE STICK.								
AMERICAN								
(Borden) fat-free, low-cholesterol	1 oz	40	6.0	4.0	380	na	0.0	5
(Borden) 'Light'	1 oz	70	6.0	1.0	420	na	4.0	15
(Borden) 'Loaf'	1 oz	110	6.0	1.0	40	0	9.0	(mq)
(Borden) 'Slices'	1 oz	110	6.0	1.0	40	0	9.0	(mq)
(Borden) slices 'Premium'	1 oz	110	6.0	1.0	460	na	9.0	na
(Dorman's)	1 oz	110	6.0	1.0	440	0	9.0	(mq)
(Dorman's) 'Loaf Low Sodium'	1 oz	110	6.0	1.0	140	0	9.0	(mq)
(Healthy Favorites)	2/3 oz	45	4.0	2.0	260	na	2.0	10
(Hoffman's)	1 oz	110	6.0	1.0	400	0	9.0	(mq)
(Kraft) 'Deluxe Loaf'	1 oz	110	6.0	1.0	430	0	9.0	25
(Kraft) 'Deluxe Slices'	1 oz	110	6.0	1.0	450	0	9.0	25
(Land O'Lakes)	1 oz	110	6.0	<1.0	405	0	9.0	25
(Land O'Lakes) sharp	1 oz	100	6.0	1.0	360	na	9.0	30
(Old English) sharp 'Loaf'	1 oz	110	6.0	1.0	400	0	9.0	30
(Old English) sharp 'Slices'	1 oz	110	6.0	1.0	440	0	9.0	30
(Sargento) hot pepper	1 oz	110	6.0	0.5	410	(tr)	9.0	27
ASIAGO *(Frigo)* wheel	1 oz	110	7.0	1.0	400	0	9.0	(mq)
BABYBEL								
(Laughing Cow)	1 oz	91	7.0	tr	227	0	7.0	22
(Laughing Cow) mini	3/4 oz	74	4.7	tr	170	0	6.0	18
BLUE								
crumbled, not packed	1 cup	477	28.9	3.2	1884	0	38.8	102
(Dorman's) 'Castello 70%'	1 oz	134	3.7	0.1	286	0	12.3	29
(Dorman's) 'Danablu 60%'	1 oz	108	4.8	0.3	200	0	9.7	31
(Dorman's) 'Danablu 50%'	1 oz	100	6.4	0.3	200	0	8.2	23
(Dorman's) 'Saga 70%'	1 oz	134	3.7	0.1	286	0	12.3	29
(Frigo)	1 oz	100	6.0	1.0	400	0	8.0	(mq)
(Hickory Farms) 'Domestic'	1 oz	101	6.1	0.7	396	0	8.3	21
(Kraft)	1 oz	100	6.0	1.0	330	0	9.0	30
(Sargento)	1 oz	100	6.0	1.0	400	0	8.0	21
BONBEL								
(Laughing Cow)	1 oz	100	6.0	tr	227	0	8.0	24
(Laughing Cow) mini, 3/4 oz	1 oz	74	4.7	tr	170	0	6.0	18
BONBINO *(Laughing Cow)*	1 oz	103	7.0	tr	227	0	9.0	27
BRICK								
(Dorman's)	1 oz	110	7.0	1.0	180	0	8.0	(mq)
(Kraft)	1 oz	110	7.0	0.0	180	0	9.0	30
(Land O'Lakes)	1 oz	110	7.0	1.0	160	0	8.0	25
BRIE								
(Dorman's)	1 oz	81	5.1	0.3	229	0	6.6	20

Food Name	Serv. Size	Total Cal.	Prot. GMS	Carbs GMS	Sod. MGS	Fiber GMS	Fat GMS	Chol. MGS
(Sargento)	1 oz	100	6.0	0.1	180	0	8.0	28
BURGER *(Sargento)*	1 oz	110	6.0	0.5	410	0	9.0	27
BUTTERNIP *(Hickory Farms)*	1 oz	110	5.2	1.1	82	0	9.4	25
CAJUN *(Sargento)*	1 oz	110	7.0	0.3	165	0	9.0	28
CALJACK *(Churny)*	1 oz	100	6.0	1.0	(mq)	0	8.0	(mq)
CAMEMBERT								
domestic	1 oz	84	5.5	0.1	236	0	6.8	20
(Dorman's) '50%'	1 oz	89	5.6	0.3	285	0	7.3	23
(Dorman's) '45%'	1 oz	82	6.0	0.3	226	0	6.3	17
(Hickory Farms)	1 oz	90	6.0	0.1	239	0	7.0	26
(Sargento)	1 oz	90	6.0	0.1	240	0	7.0	20
CARAWAY	1 oz	105	7.1	0.9	193	0	8.2	26
CHEDDAR								
American domestic	1 oz	113	7.0	0.4	174	0	9.3	29
American domestic, shredded, not packed	1 cup	455	28.1	1.5	701	0	37.5	119
(Alpine Lace) 'Cheddar Flavored'	1 oz	100	7.0	1.0	95	0	8.0	25
(Alpine Lace) shredded 'Ched-R-Lo' milk cheese	1 oz	80	7.0	1.0	95	na	5.0	20
(Alta•Dena) mild	1 oz	110	7.0	1.0	200	na	9.0	na
(Alta•Dena) sharp	1 oz	110	7.0	1.0	200	na	9.0	na
(Axelrod) extra sharp	1 oz	110	7.0	1.0	200	0	9.0	30
(Boar's Head) sliced	1 oz	110	7.0	1.0	100	0	9.0	18
(Darigold)	1 oz	110	7.0	<1.0	170	0	9.0	29
(Dorman's)	1 oz	110	7.0	1.0	200	0	9.0	(mq)
(Dorman's) 'Chedda-Delite'	1 oz	90	7.0	1.0	100	0	7.0	(mq)
(Dorman's) reduced fat 'Low Sodium'	1 oz	80	8.0	1.0	100	0	5.0	20
(Dorman's) w/Monterey Jack 'Chedda-Jack'	1 oz	90	7.0	1.0	100	0	7.0	(mq)
(Featherweight) 'Low Sodium'	1 oz	110	7.0	1.0	5	0	9.0	(mq)
(Frigo)	1 oz	110	7.0	1.0	200	0	9.0	(mq)
(Golden Balance) mild, shredded 'Natural Shreds'	1 oz	90	8.0	1.0	150	na	6.0	20
(Golden Balance) sharp, shredded 'Natural Shreds'	1 oz	90	8.0	1.0	130	na	6.0	20
(Healthy Choice) shredded, fat-free	1 oz	40	9.0	1.0	200	na	0.0	5
(Healthy Favorites) mild, fancy shredded	1 oz	70	8.0	0.0	220	na	4.0	15
(Hickory Farms)	1 oz	110	7.0	1.0	176	0	9.0	30
(Hickory Farms) raw milk 'Light Choice Low Sodium'	1 oz	114	6.0	0.0	100	0	8.0	30
(Hoffman's) super sharp processed	1 oz	110	6.0	2.0	390	0	8.0	(mq)
(Kraft)	1 oz	110	7.0	1.0	180	0	9.0	30
(Kraft) mild, finely shredded 'Light Naturals'	1 oz	80	8.0	1.0	220	na	5.0	20
(Kraft) mild, reduced fat 'Light Naturals'	1 oz	80	9.0	0.0	220	0	5.0	20
(Kraft) mild, shredded 'Light Naturals'	1 oz	80	9.0	0.0	220	na	5.0	20

Food Name	Serv. Size	Total Cal.	Prot. GMS	Carbs GMS	Sod. MGS	Fiber GMS	Fat GMS	Chol. MGS
(Kraft) sharp, shredded 'Light Naturals'	1 oz	80	9.0	1.0	220	na	5.0	20
(Land O'Lakes)	1 oz	110	7.0	<1.0	175	0	9.0	30
(Land O'Lakes) 'Chedarella'	1 oz	100	7.0	<1.0	180	na	8.0	25
(Laughing Cow)	1 oz	110	7.0	tr	227	0	9.0	28
(Sargento)	1 oz	110	7.0	0.4	176	0	9.0	30
(Sargento) mild, fancy shredded 'Preferred Light'	1 oz	90	8.0	1.0	210	na	5.0	15
(Sargento) 'New York'	1 oz	110	7.0	0.4	180	0	9.0	30
(Weight Watchers) mild, 'Natural'	1 oz	80	8.0	1.0	150	0	5.0	15
(Weight Watchers) mild, 'Natural Low Sodium'	1 oz	80	8.0	1.0	70	0	5.0	15
(Weight Watchers) mild, shredded 'Natural'	1 oz	80	8.0	1.0	150	0	5.0	15
CHESHIRE	1 oz	108	6.5	1.3	196	0	8.6	29
CHUTTER *(Hickory Farms)* 'Cold Pack'	1 oz	87	6.0	2.6	213	0	5.8	46
COLBY								
(Alpine Lace) 'Colby-Lo'	1 oz	80	7.0	1.0	85	0	5.0	20
(Dorman's)	1 oz	110	7.0	1.0	190	0	9.0	(mq)
(Hickory Farms) 'Light Choice Low Sodium'	1 oz	100	8.0	1.0	4	0	6.0	20
(Hickory Farms) 'Longhorn'	1 oz	112	6.7	0.7	171	0	8.6	27
(Hickory Farms) lowfat, calcium-enriched 'Light Choice'	1 oz	100	7.0	1.0	180	0	8.0	(mq)
(Kraft)	1 oz	110	7.0	1.0	180	0	9.0	30
(Kraft) reduced fat 'Light Naturals'	1 oz	80	9.0	0.0	220	0	5.0	20
(Kraft) w/Monterey Jack, reduced fat 'Light Naturals'	1 oz	80	8.0	1.0	220	0	5.0	20
(Land O'Lakes)	1 oz	110	7.0	1.0	170	0	9.0	25
(Sargento)	1 oz	110	7.0	1.0	170	0	9.0	27
(Sargento) Jack	1 oz	110	7.0	0.5	160	0	9.0	27
(Weight Watchers) 'Natural'	1 oz	80	8.0	1.0	130	0	5.0	15
COTTAGE CHEESE								
Creamed								
large curd	4 oz	117	14.1	3.0	457	0	5.1	17
large curd, not packed	1 cup	217	26.2	5.6	850	0	9.5	31
lowfat 1%	1 oz	20	3.5	0.8	115	0	0.3	1
lowfat 2%	1 oz	25	3.9	1.0	115	0	0.5	2
small curd	4 oz	117	14.1	3.0	457	0	5.1	17
small curd, not packed	1 cup	217	26.2	5.6	850	0	9.5	31
(Bison) chive	1/2 cup	120	14.0	4.0	420	(tr)	5.0	20
(Bison) 4% fat	1/2 cup	120	14.0	4.0	420	0	5.0	20
(Bison) garden salad	1/2 cup	110	12.0	4.0	420	(mq)	4.0	15
(Bison) lowfat 1%	1/2 cup	90	14.0	4.0	350	0	2.0	5
(Bison) w/pineapple	1/2 cup	140	10.0	18.0	340	(mq)	4.0	15
(Borden) 4% fat	1/2 cup	120	14.0	4.0	400	0	5.0	(mq)

Food Name	Serv. Size	Total Cal.	Prot. GMS	Carbs GMS	Sod. MGS	Fiber GMS	Fat GMS	Chol. MGS
(Borden) 4% fat, unsalted	1/2 cup	120	14.0	4.0	40	0	5.0	(mq)
(Breakstone's)	4 oz	110	13.0	3.0	370	0	5.0	25
(Breakstone's) lowfat 2%	4 oz	100	14.0	4.0	510	0	2.0	15
(Carnation) 4% fat, large curd	1/2 cup	115	14.0	4.0	440	na	5.0	na
(Carnation) 4% fat, small curd	1/2 cup	115	14.0	4.0	440	na	5.0	na
(Carnation) 4% fat, w/pineapple	1/2 cup	130	10.0	12.0	430	na	5.0	na
(Crowley) 4% fat	1/2 cup	120	14.0	4.0	390	0	5.0	15
(Crowley) 4% fat, w/peaches	1/2 cup	140	10.0	17.0	340	(mq)	3.0	10
(Crowley) 4% fat, w/pineapple	1/2 cup	140	11.0	15.0	330	(mq)	4.0	15
(Crowley) lowfat 1%	1/2 cup	90	14.0	4.0	390	0	1.0	5
(Crowley) lowfat 1%, calcium-fortified	1/2 cup	90	14.0	4.0	390	0	1.0	5
(Crowley) lowfat 1% 'No Salt Added'	1/2 cup	90	14.0	4.0	50	0	1.0	5
(Crowley) lowfat 1%, w/pineapple	1/2 cup	110	11.0	15.0	330	(mq)	1.0	5
(Darigold) 4% fat	4 oz	120	14.0	4.0	510	0	4.2	17
(Darigold) lowfat 2% 'Trim'	4 oz	100	14.0	4.0	510	0	3.2	17
(Friendship) 'California Style 4%'	1/2 cup	120	14.0	4.0	380	0	5.0	17
(Friendship) 4% fat, w/pineapple	1/2 cup	140	11.0	15.0	300	(mq)	4.0	17
(Friendship) lowfat 1%	1/2 cup	90	14.0	4.0	350	0	1.0	5
(Friendship) lowfat 1%, lactose-reduced	1/2 cup	90	14.0	4.0	350	0	1.0	5
(Friendship) lowfat 1% 'No Salt Added'	1/2 cup	90	14.0	4.0	31	0	1.0	5
(Friendship) lowfat 1%, w/pineapple	1/2 cup	110	11.0	15.0	300	(mq)	1.0	5
(Friendship) lowfat 2%, pot style, large curd	1/2 cup	100	14.0	4.0	405	0	2.0	9
(Knudsen) 4% fat, large curd	4 oz	120	14.0	4.0	340	0	5.0	20
(Knudsen) 4% fat, small curd	4 oz	120	14.0	4.0	370	0	5.0	20
(Knudsen) 4% fat, w/pineapple	4 oz	140	10.0	14.0	260	(mq)	5.0	25
(Lite-Line) lowfat 1.5%	1/2 cup	90	14.0	4.0	400	0	2.0	(mq)
(Weight Watchers) lowfat 1%	1/2 cup	90	14.0	4.0	460	0	1.0	(mq)
(Weight Watchers) lowfat 2%	1/2 cup	100	14.0	4.0	460	0	2.0	(mq)
Lowfat								
1%, not packed	1 cup	164	28.0	6.2	918	0	2.3	10
2%, not packed	1 cup	203	31.0	8.2	918	0	4.4	19
(Carnation) 1.5% 'Slender'	1/2 cup	90	14.0	4.0	440	na	2.0	na
(Knudsen) 2%	4 oz	100	14.0	4.0	370	0	2.0	15
(Knudsen) 2%, w/fruit cocktail	4 oz	130	11.0	16.0	330	(mq)	2.0	10
(Knudsen) 2%, w/Mandarin orange	4 oz	110	11.0	11.0	320	(mq)	2.0	10
(Knudsen) 2%, w/peach	6 oz	170	16.0	19.0	270	(mq)	2.0	15
(Knudsen) 2%, w/pear	4 oz	110	11.0	12.0	320	(mq)	2.0	10
(Knudsen) 2%, w/pineapple	6 oz	170	16.0	18.0	300	(mq)	2.0	15
(Knudsen) 2%, w/spiced apple	6 oz	180	16.0	20.0	280	(mq)	2.0	15
(Knudsen) 2%, w/strawberry	6 oz	170	16.0	19.0	320	(mq)	2.0	15
(Light n' Lively) 1%	4 oz	80	14.0	4.0	370	0	2.0	10
(Light n' Lively) 1%, garden salad	4 oz	80	18.0	5.0	350	(mq)	2.0	10

Food Name	Serv. Size	Total Cal.	Prot. GMS	Carbs GMS	Sod. MGS	Fiber GMS	Fat GMS	Chol. MGS
(Sealtest) 2%	4 oz	100	14.0	4.0	340	0	2.0	15
Nonfat								
(Knudsen)	4 oz	70	15.0	3.0	420	0	0.0	5
(Light n' Lively)	4 oz	90	14.0	7.0	400	na	0.0	10
Uncreamed								
dry, large curd	4 oz	96	19.5	2.1	14	0	0.5	8
dry, large curd, not packed	1 cup	123	25.0	2.7	19	0	0.6	10
dry, small curd	4 oz	96	19.5	2.1	14	0	0.5	8
dry, small curd, not packed	1 cup	123	25.0	2.7	19	0	0.6	10
dry curd, unsalted (Borden)	1/2 cup	80	18.0	3.0	20	0	1.0	(mq)
dry curd, unsalted (Darigold)	4 oz	80	18.0	3.0	15	0	1.0	10
dry curd, unsalted, nonfat (Breakstone's)	4 oz	90	16.0	6.0	65	0	0.0	10
CREAM CHEESE								
natural	1 oz	98	2.1	0.7	83	0	9.8	31
(Alta•Dena) pasteurized	1 oz	100	2.0	2.0	110	na	10.0	na
(Crowley)	1 oz	110	2.0	1.0	100	0	9.0	30
(Darigold)	1 oz	99	2.2	0.8	84	0	9.9	31
(Dorman's) '70%'	1 oz	102	2.7	0.6	200	0	9.9	30
(Dorman's) '65%'	1 oz	90	3.0	0.6	200	0	8.4	26
(Healthy Choice) fat-free	1 oz	30	6.0	2.0	200	na	0.0	5
(Healthy Choice) herb and garlic, fat-free	1 oz	30	6.0	2.0	200	na	0.0	5
(Healthy Favorites)	1 oz	60	3.0	2.0	110	na	5.0	15
(Philadelphia Brand)	1 oz	100	2.0	1.0	90	0	10.0	30
(Philadelphia Brand) 'Free'	1 oz	25	4.0	1.0	170	na	0.0	5
(Philadelphia Brand) pasteurized process 'Light'	1 oz	60	3.0	2.0	160	na	5.0	10
(Philadelphia Brand) w/chives	1 oz	90	2.0	1.0	125	(tr)	9.0	30
(Philadelphia Brand) w/olive and pimento, fat-free	1 oz	90	2.0	2.0	160	na	8.0	na
(Philadelphia Brand) w/pimento	1 oz	90	2.0	1.0	150	(tr)	9.0	30
Soft								
(Friendship)	1 oz	103	1.5	0.8	70	0	10.0	31
(Philadelphia Brand)	1 oz	100	1.0	2.0	100	0	10.0	30
(Philadelphia Brand) w/chives and onion	1 oz	100	2.0	2.0	100	(tr)	9.0	30
(Philadelphia Brand) w/herb and garlic	1 oz	100	1.0	2.0	160	(tr)	9.0	25
(Philadelphia Brand) w/olives and pimento	1 oz	90	2.0	2.0	160	(tr)	8.0	25
(Philadelphia Brand) w/pineapple	1 oz	90	1.0	4.0	90	(tr)	8.0	25
(Philadelphia Brand) w/smoked salmon	1 oz	90	2.0	1.0	180	0	9.0	25
(Philadelphia Brand) w/strawberries	1 oz	90	1.0	4.0	75	(tr)	8.0	20
Whipped								
(Philadelphia Brand)	1 oz	100	2.0	1.0	85	0	10.0	30
(Philadelphia Brand) w/chives	1 oz	90	2.0	1.0	150	(tr)	8.0	30
(Philadelphia Brand) w/onions	1 oz	90	2.0	2.0	170	(tr)	8.0	25

Food Name	Serv. Size	Total Cal.	Prot. GMS	Carbs GMS	Sod. MGS	Fiber GMS	Fat GMS	Chol. MGS
(Philadelphia Brand) w/smoked salmon ...	1 oz	90	2.0	2.0	170	0	8.0	30
(Temp-Tee)	1 oz	100	2.0	1.0	85	na	10.0	30
DANBO								
(Dorman's) 20%	1 oz	62	8.9	0.3	200	0	2.8	9
(Dorman's) 45%	1 oz	98	7.3	0.3	200	0	7.5	23
EDAM								
(Dorman's)	1 oz	100	7.0	1.0	200	0	8.0	(mq)
(Dorman's) 45%	1 oz	91	6.7	0.3	200	0	7.0	21
(Hickory Farms) 'Domestic'	1 oz	100	6.0	0.9	182	0	8.4	24
(Kaukauna)	1 oz	100	7.0	<1.0	275	0	8.0	25
(Kraft)	1 oz	90	8.0	0.0	310	0	7.0	20
(Land O'Lakes)	1 oz	100	7.0	<1.0	275	0	8.0	25
(Laughing Cow)	1 oz	100	6.0	tr	227	0	8.0	26
(May-Bud)	1 oz	100	7.0	0.0	275	0	8.0	(mq)
(Sargento)	1 oz	100	7.0	0.4	270	0	8.0	25
EFORT, sheep's milk	1 oz	314	18.3	1.7	1538	0	26.0	76
FARMER								
(Friendship)	1/2 cup	160	16.0	4.0	356	0	12.0	40
(Friendship) 'No Salt Added'	1/2 cup	160	16.0	4.0	8	0	12.0	40
(Hickory Farms)	1 oz	90	6.0	1.0	210	0	7.0	20
(Hickory Farms) 'Light Choice'	1 oz	90	6.0	1.0	150	0	7.0	20
(Kaukauna)	1 oz	100	7.0	<1.0	(mq)	0	8.0	25
(May-Bud)	1 oz	90	6.0	1.0	210	0	7.0	20
(Sargento)	1 oz	100	7.0	1.0	130	0	8.0	26
FETA								
sheep's milk	1 oz	75	4.0	1.2	316	0	6.0	25
(Churny) 'Natural'	1 oz	75	4.7	1.2	316	0	6.5	25
(Dorman's) 45%	1 oz	91	5.9	0.4	(mq)	0	7.3	(mq)
(Sargento)	1 oz	80	4.0	1.0	320	0	6.0	25
FONTINA *(Sargento)*	1 oz	110	7.0	0.4	(mq)	0	9.0	33
FRENCH ONION *(Alouette)*	1 oz	95	2.0	2.0	205	na	9.0	31
GJETOST								
goat's milk, fresh	1 oz	82	4.5	0.9	180	0	6.8	20
(Sargento)	1 oz	130	3.0	12.0	170	0	8.0	(mq)
GOAT								
hard type	1 oz	128	8.6	0.6	98	0	10.1	30
semisoft type	1 oz	103	6.1	0.7	146	0	8.5	22
soft type	1 oz	76	5.3	0.3	104	0	6.0	13
GOUDA								
(Dorman's)	1 oz	100	7.0	1.0	210	0	8.0	(mq)
(Kaukauna)	1 oz	100	7.0	1.0	230	0	8.0	30
(Kaukauna) w/caraway seed	1 oz	100	7.0	<1.0	230	(tr)	8.0	30
(Kaukauna) w/hickory smoke flavor	1 oz	100	7.0	<1.0	230	0	8.0	25

Food Name	Serv. Size	Total Cal.	Prot. GMS	Carbs GMS	Sod. MGS	Fiber GMS	Fat GMS	Chol. MGS
(Kraft)	1 oz	110	7.0	0.0	200	0	9.0	30
(Land O'Lakes)	1 oz	100	7.0	1.0	230	0	8.0	30
(Laughing Cow)	1 oz	110	7.0	tr	227	0	9.0	28
(Laughing Cow) mini	3/4 oz	80	5.3	tr	170	0	6.4	21
(May-Bud)	1 oz	100	7.0	1.0	230	0	8.0	(mq)
(Sargento)	1 oz	100	7.0	1.0	230	0	8.0	32
GRATED. See also PARMESAN; ROMANO.								
(Polly-O)	1 oz	130	11.0	1.0	530	0	10.0	25
(Sargento) Italian style	1 oz	110	8.0	1.0	105	0	8.0	26
GRUYERE	1 oz	116	8.4	0.1	94	0	9.1	31
HAVARTI								
(Casino)	1 oz	120	6.0	0.0	140	0	11.0	35
(Dorman's) 45%	1 oz	91	6.7	0.3	200	0	7.0	21
(Dorman's) 60%	1 oz	118	5.4	0.3	200	0	10.6	31
(Hickory Farms) 'Danish Special'	1 oz	117	5.1	0.3	198	0	10.5	31
(Sargento)	1 oz	120	5.0	0.3	200	0	11.0	31
HORSERADISH (Kaukauna) hearty, cold pack 'Cup'	1 oz	100	6.0	3.0	250	(tr)	7.0	25
HOT PEPPER (Hickory Farms)	1 oz	106	6.3	0.5	406	(tr)	8.9	27
JARLSBERG								
(Hickory Farms)	1 oz	100	7.0	1.0	130	0	7.0	16
(Norseland)	1 oz	97	7.0	1.0	135	0	7.0	18
LIMBURGER								
(Mohawk Valley) 'Little Gem'	1 oz	90	6.0	0.0	250	0	8.0	25
(Sargento)	1 oz	90	6.0	0.1	230	0	8.0	26
MASCARPONE 'Imported' (Galbani)	1 oz	128	1.5	1.2	17	0	13.1	39
MONTEREY	1 oz	105	6.8	0.2	150	0	8.5	25
MONTEREY JACK								
(Alpine Lace) 'Monti-Jack-Lo'	1 oz	80	7.0	1.0	75	0	5.0	15
(Alpine Lace) 'Monti-Jack-Lo' sliced	1 oz	80	7.0	1.0	75	na	5.0	15
(Alta•Dena)	1 oz	100	7.0	1.0	180	na	8.0	na
(Alta•Dena) w/jalapeño pepper	1 oz	100	7.0	1.0	180	na	8.0	na
(Axelrod)	1 oz	100	6.0	1.0	150	0	8.0	30
(Axelrod) w/jalapeño pepper	1 oz	100	6.0	1.0	220	(tr)	8.0	30
(Darigold)	1 oz	110	7.0	<1.0	150	0	8.0	25
(Dorman's)	1 oz	100	6.0	1.0	180	0	8.0	(mq)
(Dorman's) reduced fat 'Low Sodium'	1 oz	80	8.0	1.0	90	0	5.0	18
(Hickory Farms) 'Light Choice Low Sodium'	1 oz	110	6.0	0.0	100	0	8.0	30
(Kaukauna)	1 oz	110	7.0	<1.0	150	0	9.0	25
(Kraft)	1 oz	110	6.0	0.0	190	0	9.0	30
(Kraft) reduced fat 'Light Naturals'	1 oz	80	9.0	1.0	220	0	5.0	20
(Kraft) reduced fat 'Light Naturals' w/peppers	1 oz	80	8.0	1.0	220	(tr)	5.0	20
(Kraft) 'Singles'	1 oz	90	5.0	2.0	390	0	7.0	25

Food Name	Serv. Size	Total Cal.	Prot. GMS	Carbs GMS	Sod. MGS	Fiber GMS	Fat GMS	Chol. MGS
(Kraft) w/caraway	1 oz	100	7.0	1.0	180	(tr)	8.0	30
(Kraft) w/jalapeño pepper	1 oz	110	7.0	1.0	190	(tr)	9.0	30
(Land O'Lakes)	1 oz	110	7.0	<1.0	150	0	9.0	20
(Land O'Lakes) hot pepper	1 oz	110	7.0	<1.0	150	na	9.0	20
(Land O'Lakes) processed 'Jalapeño Jack'	1 oz	90	5.0	1.0	430	na	8.0	20
(May-Bud)	1 oz	110	7.0	0.0	150	0	9.0	(mq)
(Sargento)	1 oz	110	7.0	0.2	150	0	9.0	25
(Weight Watchers) 'Natural'	1 oz	80	8.0	1.0	120	0	5.0	15
MOZZARELLA. See also CHEESE NUGGET.								
(Dorman's)	1 oz	90	7.0	1.0	190	0	6.0	(mq)
(Healthy Choice) fat-free, chunk	1 oz	40	9.0	1.0	200	na	0.0	5
(Hickory Farms)	1 oz	72	6.9	0.8	132	0	4.5	16
(Hickory Farms) 'Light Choice Low Sodium'	1 oz	80	8.0	1.0	90	0	5.0	15
(Kraft)	1 oz	90	6.0	1.0	190	0	7.0	20
(Polly-O) 'Fior di Latte'	1 oz	80	5.0	1.0	20	0	6.0	20
(Polly-O) 'Lite'	1 oz	70	7.0	1.0	200	0	4.0	15
(Weight Watchers) 'Natural'	1 oz	70	8.0	1.0	150	0	4.0	15
Part skim milk								
(Alpine Lace) low moisture	1 oz	70	7.0	1.0	75	0	5.0	15
(Crowley)	1 oz	70	8.0	1.0	240	0	4.0	15
(Dorman's) low moisture 'Low Sodium'	1 oz	80	8.0	1.0	90	0	5.0	15
(Frigo) low moisture	1 oz	80	7.0	1.0	190	0	5.0	10
(Frigo) low moisture, reduced fat	1 oz	60	8.0	1.0	150	0	3.0	10
(Kraft) low moisture	1 oz	80	8.0	1.0	200	0	5.0	15
(Kraft) w/jalapeño pepper	1 oz	80	8.0	1.0	230	(tr)	5.0	20
(Land O'Lakes) low moisture	1 oz	80	8.0	1.0	150	0	5.0	15
(Polly-O)	1 oz	80	6.0	1.0	280	0	5.0	15
(Sargento) low moisture	1 oz	80	8.0	1.0	150	0	5.0	15
Reduced fat								
(Dorman's) 'Low Sodium'	1 oz	80	9.0	1.0	90	0	4.0	17
(Kraft) 'Light Naturals'	1 oz	80	8.0	1.0	200	0	4.0	15
Shredded								
(Alpine Lace)	1 oz	70	7.0	1.0	75	na	5.0	15
(Alpine Lace) sliced	1 oz	70	7.0	1.0	75	na	5.0	15
(Healthy Choice) fat-free	1 oz	40	9.0	1.0	200	na	0.0	5
(Kraft) 'Light Naturals'	1 oz	80	8.0	1.0	150	na	4.0	15
(Sargento) fancy 'Preferred Light'	1 oz	60	8.0	<1.0	150	na	3.0	10
(Weight Watchers) 'Natural'	1 oz	80	8.0	1.0	150	0	4.0	15
Whole milk								
(Crowley)	1 oz	90	5.0	1.0	240	0	7.0	25
(Frigo) low moisture	1 oz	90	6.0	1.0	190	0	7.0	15
(Sargento)	1 oz	90	6.0	1.0	120	0	7.0	25
(Polly-O)	1 oz	90	5.0	1.0	280	0	6.0	20

Food Name	Serv. Size	Total Cal.	Prot. GMS	Carbs GMS	Sod. MGS	Fiber GMS	Fat GMS	Chol. MGS
MOZZARELLA CHEDDAR								
(Precious) shredded 'Pizza Cheese'	1 oz	95	7.0	1.0	180	na	7.0	na
MUENSTER								
(Alpine Lace)	1 oz	100	7.0	1.0	85	0	8.0	30
(Alpine Lace) sliced 'Low Sodium'	1 oz	100	7.0	1.0	85	na	9.0	25
(Dorman's)	1 oz	110	7.0	0.0	190	0	9.0	(mq)
(Dorman's) 50%	1 oz	100	6.4	0.3	200	0	8.2	24
(Dorman's) 'Low Sodium'	1 oz	110	7.0	0.0	95	0	9.0	(mq)
(Dorman's) reduced fat 'Low Sodium'	1 oz	80	8.0	0.0	140	0	5.0	18
(Hickory Farms)	1 oz	100	6.6	0.3	180	0	8.5	25
(Hickory Farms) 'Light Choice Low Sodium'	1 oz	110	7.0	0.0	95	0	9.0	27
(Kaukauna)	1 oz	110	7.0	<1.0	180	0	9.0	25
(Land O'Lakes)	1 oz	100	7.0	<1.0	180	0	9.0	25
(Sargento) red rind	1 oz	100	7.0	0.3	180	0	9.0	27
NEUFCHATEL								
(Hickory Farms) chocolate	1 oz	110	2.0	8.0	90	(tr)	8.0	33
(Hickory Farms) orange	1 oz	100	2.0	4.0	75	(tr)	8.0	45
(Hickory Farms) peach	1 oz	90	2.0	3.0	85	(tr)	8.0	39
(Hickory Farms) pineapple	1 oz	90	2.0	2.0	60	(tr)	8.0	33
(Hickory Farms) rum date nut	1 oz	100	2.0	4.0	80	(tr)	8.0	31
(Hickory Farms) strawberry	1 oz	90	2.0	3.0	70	(tr)	8.0	32
(Kaukauna) garden vegetable	1 oz	80	3.0	1.0	200	(tr)	7.0	25
(Kaukauna) garlic and herbs	1 oz	80	3.0	1.0	150	(tr)	7.0	25
(Philadelphia Brand) 'Light'	1 oz	80	3.0	1.0	115	0	7.0	25
NEW HOLLAND (Hickory Farms) w/herbs								
'Light Choice'	1 oz	90	7.0	1.0	100	(tr)	8.0	27
PARMESAN								
natural, piece	1 oz	110	10.0	0.9	448	0	7.2	19
natural, shredded	1 oz	116	10.6	1.0	475	0	7.7	20
natural, shredded	1 tbsp	21	1.9	0.2	85	0	1.4	4
(Churny) 'Natural'	1 oz	110	10.0	1.0	455	na	7.0	20
(Hickory Farms)	1 oz	110	10.0	1.0	350	0	7.0	(mq)
(Kraft)	1 oz	100	9.0	1.0	290	0	7.0	20
(Sargento) fresh	1 oz	110	10.0	1.0	450	0	7.0	19
Grated								
natural	1 oz	128	11.6	1.0	521	0	8.4	22
natural	1 tbsp	23	2.1	0.2	93	0	1.5	4
(Frigo)	1 oz	130	12.0	1.0	510	0	9.0	(mq)
(Frigo) fresh	1 oz	110	10.0	1.0	350	0	7.0	(mq)
(Kraft)	1 oz	130	12.0	1.0	430	0	9.0	30
(Polly-O)	1 oz	130	11.0	1.0	530	0	9.0	20
(Progresso)	1 tbsp	23	2.0	<1.0	95	0	2.0	4
(Sargento)	1 oz	130	12.0	2.0	530	0	9.0	22

Food Name	Serv. Size	Total Cal.	Prot. GMS	Carbs GMS	Sod. MGS	Fiber GMS	Fat GMS	Chol. MGS
Hard	1 oz	111	10.1	0.9	454	0	7.3	19
Wheel *(Frigo)*	1 oz	110	10.0	1.0	350	0	7.0	(mq)
W/Romano cheese, grated								
(Frigo)	1 oz	130	12.0	1.0	510	0	9.0	(mq)
(Sargento)	1 oz	110	10.0	1.0	400	0	7.0	24
PARMESAN REGGIANO *(Galbani)* 'Imported'	1 oz	105	10.1	1.0	188	0	7.1	21
PIZZA								
(Frigo) shredded	1 oz	90	6.0	1.0	190	0	7.0	20
(Frigo) shredded, lowfat	1 oz	65	9.0	1.0	150	0	3.0	10
(Healthy Choice) fancy, shredded, fat-free	1 oz	40	9.0	1.0	200	na	0.0	5
PORT DU SALUT	1 oz	98	6.7	0.2	150	0	7.9	34
PORT WINE *(Hickory Farms)*	1 oz	97	5.6	2.4	262	0	6.9	18
POT *(Sargento)*	1 oz	25	5.0	1.0	1	0	0.2	(mq)
PRIMAVERA *(Bel Paese)* 'Lite'	1 oz	68	6.0	2.0	165	(tr)	4.0	14
PROVOLONE								
(Alpine Lace) 'Provo-Lo'	1 oz	70	7.0	1.0	85	0	5.0	15
(Dorman's)	1 oz	90	7.0	1.0	290	0	7.0	(mq)
(Frigo)	1 oz	100	7.0	1.0	230	0	7.0	(mq)
(Frigo) smoked	1 oz	100	7.0	1.0	230	0	7.0	(mq)
(Hickory Farms) 'Light Choice Low Sodium'	1 oz	90	7.0	1.0	140	0	7.0	20
(Kraft)	1 oz	100	7.0	1.0	260	0	7.0	25
(Land O'Lakes)	1 oz	100	7.0	1.0	250	0	8.0	20
(Sargento)	1 oz	100	7.0	1.0	250	0	8.0	20
PUB *(Hickory Farms)*	1 oz	94	5.6	2.4	237	0	6.9	18
QUESO BLANCO *(Sargento)*	1 oz	100	7.0	0.3	180	0	9.0	27
QUESO DE PAPA *(Sargento)*	1 oz	110	7.0	0.4	180	0	9.0	30
QUESO DE TACO *(Hickory Farms)*	1 oz	106	6.3	0.5	450	0	8.9	27
RICOTTA								
Light/lowfat								
(Gardenia) '95% Fat-free'	1 oz	30	3.0	2.0	130	na	1.0	na
(Polly-O) 'Lite'	2 oz	80	7.0	3.0	65	0	4.0	15
(Precious) 'Lowfat'	1 oz	40	3.0	2.0	20	na	2.0	10
(Sargento) 'Lite'	1 oz	23	3.0	1.0	20	0	1.0	4
Part skim milk								
(Crowley)	2 oz	80	7.0	3.0	50	0	4.0	15
(Frigo)	1 oz	45	3.0	1.0	100	0	3.0	10
(Frigo) 'Truly Lite' fat-free	1 oz	20	4.0	2.0	15	na	0.0	3
(Polly-O)	2 oz	90	7.0	2.0	45	0	6.0	20
(Sargento)	1 oz	30	3.0	1.0	30	0	2.0	10
Whole milk								
(Breakstone's)	4 oz	200	12.0	6.0	95	na	15.0	55
(Crowley)	2 oz	100	6.0	3.0	50	0	7.0	25
(Frigo)	1 oz	50	3.0	1.0	100	0	4.0	15

Food Name	Serv. Size	Total Cal.	Prot. GMS	Carbs GMS	Sod. MGS	Fiber GMS	Fat GMS	Chol. MGS
(Polly-O)	2 oz	100	7.0	2.0	45	0	7.0	20
ROMANO								
Grated								
(Frigo)	1 oz	130	12.0	1.0	510	0	9.0	(mq)
(Kraft)	1 oz	130	11.0	1.0	350	0	9.0	30
(Kraft) 'Natural'	1 oz	100	8.0	1.0	250	0	7.0	20
(Polly-O)	1 oz	130	11.0	1.0	530	0	10.0	30
(Progresso)	1 tbsp	23	2.0	<1.0	70	0	2.0	6
(Sargento)	1 oz	110	9.0	1.0	340	0	8.0	29
Loaf *(Hickory Farms)*	1 oz	110	9.0	1.0	350	0	8.0	(mq)
Wedge *(Frigo)*	1 oz	110	9.0	1.0	350	0	8.0	(mq)
ROQUEFORT								
	1 oz	103	6.0	0.6	507	0	8.6	25
sheep's milk	1 oz	105	6.1	0.6	513	0	8.7	26
SLIM JACK *(Dorman's)*	1 oz	90	6.0	1.0	90	0	7.0	(mq)
SMOKED								
(Hickory Farms) 'Light Choice Smoky Lyte'	1 oz	80	7.0	1.0	449	0	6.0	5
(Hoffman's) sharp, processed	1 oz	110	6.0	1.0	440	0	9.0	(mq)
(Sargento) 'Smokestick'	1 oz	100	7.0	1.0	390	0	7.0	24
STRING								
(Frigo)	1 oz	80	7.0	1.0	190	0	5.0	(mq)
(Kraft) low moisture	1 oz	80	8.0	1.0	230	0	5.0	20
(Polly-O)	1 oz	90	7.0	2.0	200	0	6.0	15
(Sargento)	1 oz	80	8.0	1.0	150	0	5.0	15
(Sargento) smoked	1 oz	80	8.0	1.0	150	0	5.0	15
SWISS								
domestic	1 oz	105	8.0	1.0	73	0	7.7	26
domestic	1-inch cube	56	4.3	0.5	39	0	4.1	14
(Boar's Head) 'Domestic'	1 oz	110	7.0	1.0	75	0	8.0	25
(Boar's Head) 'No Salt Added'	1 oz	100	8.0	<1.0	12	0	8.0	26
(Casino)	1 oz	110	8.0	1.0	35	0	8.0	30
(Cracker Barrel) baby 'Natural'	1 oz	110	7.0	0.0	65	0	9.0	25
(Dorman's)	1 oz	100	8.0	0.0	80	0	8.0	(mq)
(Dorman's) 'No Salt Added'	1 oz	100	8.0	0.0	8	0	8.0	(mq)
(Hickory Farms) creamy 'Cold Pack'	1 oz	92	5.6	2.5	237	0	7.2	24
(Hickory Farms) 'Domestic'	1 oz	110	8.1	1.0	75	0	7.8	25
(Hickory Farms) 'Light Choice Lorraine'	1 oz	100	8.0	0.0	35	0	7.8	25
(Hickory Farms) 'Light Choice Low Sodium'	1 oz	100	8.0	0.0	8	0	8.0	26
(Kraft)	1 oz	110	8.0	1.0	40	0	8.0	25
(Kraft) aged	1 oz	110	8.0	1.0	45	0	8.0	25
(Kraft) 'Light Naturals'	1 oz	90	10.0	1.0	45	0	5.0	20
(Land O'Lakes)	1 oz	110	8.0	1.0	75	0	8.0	25
(Sargento) 'Finland'	1 oz	110	8.0	1.0	75	0	8.0	26

Food Name	Serv. Size	Total Cal.	Prot. GMS	Carbs GMS	Sod. MGS	Fiber GMS	Fat GMS	Chol. MGS
(Weight Watchers) 'Natural'	1 oz	90	9.0	1.0	50	0	5.0	15
Processed								
(Alpine Lace) sliced, milk cheese 'Swiss-Lo'	1 oz	90	8.0	1.0	35	na	6.0	20
(Alpine Lace) 'Swiss-Lo'	1 oz	100	8.0	1.0	35	0	7.0	20
(Borden)	1 oz	100	7.0	1.0	380	0	8.0	(mq)
(Borden) fat-free, low-cholesterol	1 oz	40	6.0	4.0	na	na	0.0	5
(Dorman's) 'Reduced Fat'	1 oz	90	10.0	0.0	80	0	5.0	17
(Dorman's) smoked	1 oz	100	7.0	1.0	390	0	7.0	(mq)
(Healthy Favorites) sliced, reduced fat	1 oz	80	9.0	1.0	70	na	4.0	15
(Hoffman's) smoky, w/cheddar	1 oz	110	7.0	1.0	410	0	8.0	(mq)
(Kraft) 'Deluxe'	1 oz	90	7.0	1.0	420	0	7.0	25
(Kraft) 'Light'	1 oz	70	6.0	2.0	350	na	3.0	15
(Kraft) reduced fat 'Light Naturals'	1 oz	90	10.0	1.0	70	0	5.0	20
(Kraft) %75% Very Low Sodium'	1 oz	110	8.0	1.0	10	0	8.0	25
(Sargento)	1 oz	110	8.0	1.0	75	0	8.0	26
TACO								
(Frigo) shredded	1 oz	110	7.0	1.0	200	0	9.0	(mq)
(Kraft) shredded	1 oz	110	7.0	1.0	190	0	9.0	30
(Sargento)	1 oz	110	7.0	0.5	160	0	9.0	27
TALEGGIO *(Tal-Fino)* 'Brand Imported'	1 oz	89	5.4	0.2	176	0	7.4	(mq)
TILSIT								
whole milk	1 oz	95	6.8	0.5	211	0	7.3	29
(Sargento)	1 oz	100	7.0	1.0	210	0	7.0	29
TYBO								
(Dorman's) 45%	1 oz	98	7.3	0.3	200	0	7.5	23
(Sargento) red wax	1 oz	100	7.0	0.3	200	0	7.0	23
VERMONT *(Churny)*	1 oz	110	7.0	1.0	180	0	9.0	30
CHEESE, ALTERNATIVE								
(Cheeztwin)	1 oz	90	5.0	3.0	400	0	6.0	na
American cheddar style *(Soya Kaas)*	1 oz	79	6.2	1.6	250	na	5.4	na
American style *(Delicia)*	1 oz	80	6.0	1.0	300	0	6.0	3
American style *(Golden Image)*	1 oz	90	7.0	2.0	360	0	6.0	5
American style, hickory smoked *(Delicia)*	1 oz	80	6.0	0.0	470	0	6.0	1
American style, lactose-free, singles								
(Formägg)	3/4 oz	70	5.0	<1.0	280	na	5.0	0
American style, 'Low Sodium Slices'								
(Weight Watchers)	1 oz	50	7.0	2.0	120	0	2.0	5
American style, 'Slices' *(Weight Watchers)*	1 oz	50	6.0	2.0	400	0	2.0	5
American style, w/caraway *(Delicia)*	1 oz	80	6.0	1.0	275	(tr)	6.0	3
American style, w/hot pepper *(Delicia)*	1 oz	80	6.0	1.0	300	(tr)	6.0	3
American style, w/salami *(Delicia)*	1 oz	80	6.0	1.0	370	(tr)	6.0	3
California cheddar style 'AlmondRella'								
(Sharon's Finest)	1 oz	50	7.0	1.0	170	.4	1.4	0

Food Name	Serv. Size	Total Cal.	Prot. GMS	Carbs GMS	Sod. MGS	Fiber GMS	Fat GMS	Chol. MGS
California cheddar style 'Zero-Fat Rella'								
(Sharon's Finest)	1 oz	45	8.0	3.0	170	0	0.0	0
cheddar style (Frigo)	1 oz	90	5.0	1.0	280	0	7.0	0
cheddar style (Sargento)	1 oz	90	7.0	<1.0	350	0	6.0	2
cheddar style, fancy shredded (Formägg)	1 oz	70	7.0	1.0	70	na	5.0	0
cheddar style, shredded 'Ched-O-Mate'								
(Fisher)	1 oz	90	6.0	1.0	330	0	7.0	na
colby style (Golden Image)	1 oz	110	7.0	1.0	190	0	9.0	5
colby style 'LoChol' (Dorman's)	1 oz	90	7.0	1.0	140	0	6.0	1
colby style, Longhorn style (Delicia)	1 oz	80	6.0	1.0	550	0	6.0	3
cream cheese style (Soya Kaas)	1 oz	90	2.3	0.1	60	na	9.4	na
cream cheese style (Weight Watchers)	1 oz	35	3.0	1.0	40	0	2.0	na
cream cheese style, all flavors 'Better								
than Cream Cheese' (Tofutti)	1 oz	80	1.0	1.0	200	(mq)	8.0	0
garlic-herb style 'AlmondRella'								
(Sharon's Finest)	1 oz	50	7.0	1.0	170	.4	1.4	0
'Heart Beat' (Nucoa)	1 oz	50	7.0	2.0	280	0	2.0	0
jalapeño jack style 'Zero-Fat Rella'								
(Sharon's Finest)	1 oz	45	8.0	3.0	170	0	0.0	0
'Jalapeño Mexi Kaas' (Soya Kaas)	1 oz	77	6.8	0.3	160	na	5.3	na
'Low Cholesterol' (Lite-Line)	1 oz	90	5.0	2.0	430	0	7.0	na
mild cheddar style (Golden Image)	1 oz	110	7.0	0.0	190	0	9.0	5
mild cheddar style 'TofuRella'								
(Sharon's Finest)	1 oz	80	8.0	1.0	170	na	5.0	0
mild cheddar style 'TofuRella' slices								
(Sharon's Finest)	3/4 oz	60	5.0	1.0	280	na	4.0	0
mozzarella style (Frigo)	1 oz	90	6.0	1.0	240	0	7.0	0
mozzarella style (Sargento)	1 oz	80	7.0	<1.0	310	0	6.0	2
mozzarella style (Soya Kaas)	1 oz	78	6.7	1.8	155	na	5.6	na
mozzarella style 'AlmondRella'								
(Sharon's Finest)	1 oz	50	7.0	1.0	170	.4	1.4	0
mozzarella style, shredded 'Pizza-Mate'								
(Fisher)	1 oz	90	6.0	1.0	310	0	7.0	na
mozzarella style 'TofuRella'								
(Sharon's Finest)	1 oz	80	8.0	1.0	170	na	5.0	0
mozzarella style 'TofuRella' slices								
(Sharon's Finest)	3/4 oz	60	5.0	1.0	280	na	4.0	0
mozzarella style 'Zero-Fat Rella'								
(Sharon's Finest)	1 oz	45	8.0	3.0	170	0	0.0	0
Muenster style 'LoChol' (Dorman's)	1 oz	100	7.0	1.0	140	0	7.0	1
'Sandwich-Mate' (Fisher)	1 oz	90	5.0	3.0	400	0	6.0	na
sharp cheddar style 'Slices'								
(Weight Watchers)	1 oz	50	6.0	2.0	400	0	2.0	5

Food Name	Serv. Size	Total Cal.	Prot. GMS	Carbs GMS	Sod. MGS	Fiber GMS	Fat GMS	Chol. MGS
Swiss style, lactose-free, singles								
(Formägg)	3/4 oz	70	5.0	<1.0	280	na	5.0	0
Swiss style 'LoChol' (Dorman's)	1 oz	100	7.0	1.0	140	0	7.0	1
Swiss style 'Slices' (Weight Watchers)	1 oz	50	6.0	2.0	400	0	2.0	15
CHEESE BALL								
cheddar, w/almonds and bacon (Kaukauna)	1 oz	100	6.0	3.0	250	(mq)	7.0	25
green onion flavor, w/almonds (Kaukauna)	1 oz	100	6.0	3.0	250	(mq)	7.0	25
Port wine, w/almonds (Kaukauna)	1 oz	100	6.0	3.0	250	(mq)	7.0	25
sharp cheddar, w/almonds (Kaukauna)	1 oz	100	6.0	3.0	250	(mq)	7.0	25
CHEESE BLINTZ. See BLINTZ.								
CHEESE FLAVORED SNACKS								
(Barbara's Bakery)								
'Pinta Puffs' tangy triple cheese	1 oz	70	2.0	10.0	100	na	2.0	5
puff lights	1 oz	40	1.0	3.0	55	na	3.0	na
(Bearitos) puffs, cheddar, baked, original	.5 oz	80	1.0	7.0	2	na	5.0	130
(Chee•tos)								
cheddar valley	1 oz	160	2.0	16.0	240	1.0	9.0	0
crunchy	1 oz	150	1.0	17.0	310	1.0	9.0	0
crunchy, light	1 oz	140	2.0	19.0	360	(mq)	6.0	0
curls	1 oz	150	1.0	17.0	270	1.0	9.0	0
flamin' hot	1 oz	150	2.0	16.0	240	1.0	9.0	0
light	1 oz	140	2.0	19.0	280	1.0	6.0	0
paws	1 oz	160	1.0	15.0	310	1.0	10.0	0
puffed balls	1 oz	160	2.0	16.0	360	1.0	10.0	0
puffs	1 oz	160	1.0	16.0	330	1.0	9.0	0
(Flavor Tree) sticks, cheddar	1/4 cup	129	2.7	11.9	335	>.1 c	8.1	na
(Health Valley)								
'Cheddar Lite' puffs, w/organic corn, baked	.25 oz	40	1.0	4.0	35	na	2.0	0
puffs, fat-free	1 oz	100	3.0	21.0	75	.1	0.0	0
puffs, w/chili, fat-free	1 oz	100	3.0	21.0	75	.1	0.0	0
puffs, w/green onion, fat-free	1 oz	100	3.0	21.0	75	.1	0.0	0
(Keebler) 'RC Ricers' zesty cheddar	1 oz	140	2.0	17.0	200	na	8.0	0
(Planter)								
'Cheez Balls'	1 oz	160	2.0	14.0	270	(mq)	11.0	5
'Cheez Balls' Nacho	1 oz	160	2.0	15.0	290	na	10.0	5
'Cheez Curls'	1 oz	160	2.0	14.0	290	(mq)	11.0	5
'Cheez Curls' Nacho	1 oz	160	2.0	15.0	290	na	10.0	5
(Weight Watchers) curls, crunchy	.5-oz pkg	70	1.0	10.0	45	na	2.0	0
(Wise)								
'Cheez Doodles' baked, puffed	1 oz	150	2.0	16.0	360	na	9.0	na
'Cheez Doodles' fried, crunchy	1 oz	160	2.0	16.0	230	na	10.0	na
'Cheez Waffies'	1 oz	140	3.0	14.0	420	(mq)	8.0	na
corn spirals, nacho	1 oz	160	2.0	16.0	190	(mq)	10.0	na

Food Name	Serv. Size	Total Cal.	Prot. GMS	Carbs GMS	Sod. MGS	Fiber GMS	Fat GMS	Chol. MGS
corn twists, nacho, crispy	1 oz	160	2.0	16.0	190	na	10.0	na

CHEESE FOOD
AMERICAN
(Darigold)	1 oz	80	5.0	2.0	381	0	6.0	16
cold pack	1 oz	94	5.6	2.4	274	0	6.9	18
colored (Hoffman's)	1 oz	100	5.0	3.0	490	0	7.0	(mq)
grated (Kraft)	1 oz	130	8.0	8.0	740	0	7.0	25
'Light' (Kraft)	1 oz	70	6.0	2.0	420	na	4.0	15
sharp, 'Singles' (Borden)	1 oz	90	5.0	2.0	470	0	7.0	(mq)
'Singles' (Borden)	1 oz	90	5.0	3.0	350	0	7.0	(mq)
'Singles' (Kraft)	1 oz	90	5.0	2.0	390	0	7.0	25
'Slices' (Borden)	1 oz	100	6.0	2.0	420	0	7.0	(mq)
white, 'Singles' (Kraft)	1 oz	90	5.0	2.0	400	0	7.0	20
w/Swiss cheese (Land O'Lakes)	1 oz	100	7.0	1.0	400	na	8.0	25

BACON
(Cracker Barrel)	1 oz	90	5.0	3.0	280	0	7.0	20
'Chees'N Bacon' (Hoffman's)	1 oz	90	6.0	3.0	540	0	6.0	(mq)
'Cheez'N Bacon' (Kraft)	1 oz	90	6.0	2.0	400	0	7.0	25
CARAWAY, 'Swisson Rye' (Hoffman's)	1 oz	90	6.0	2.0	400	(tr)	7.0	(mq)

CHEDDAR
extra sharp (Cracker Barrel)	1 oz	90	5.0	3.0	240	0	7.0	20
extra sharp (Land O'Lakes)	1 oz	100	6.0	1.0	370	na	9.0	30
extra sharp, cold pack 'Cup' (Kaukauna) ..	1 oz	100	6.0	3.0	250	0	7.0	25
'La Chedda' (Land O'Lakes)	1 oz	90	6.0	2.0	335	0	7.0	20
nacho, cold pack, 'Cup' (Kaukauna)	1 oz	100	6.0	3.0	250	0	7.0	25
Port wine (Cracker Barrel)	1 oz	100	4.0	3.0	230	0	7.0	20
sharp (Cracker Barrel)	1 oz	100	4.0	4.0	230	0	7.0	20
sharp, cold pack (Wispride)	1 oz	100	5.0	2.0	210	0	7.0	25
sharp, cold pack 'Cup' (Kaukauna)	1 oz	100	6.0	3.0	250	0	7.0	25
sharp, cup 'Lite 50' (Kaukauna)	1 oz	70	5.0	5.0	190	na	3.0	15
sharp 'Lite' (Kaukauna)	1 oz	70	5.0	5.0	230	0	4.0	15
smoky 'Lite' (Kaukauna)	1 oz	70	5.0	5.0	230	0	4.0	15
w/bacon (Land O'Lakes)	1 oz	110	6.0	1.0	350	na	9.0	25
w/bacon and horseradish, cold pack, 'Cup'								
(Kaukauna)	1 oz	100	6.0	3.0	250	(tr)	7.0	25
GARLIC (Kraft)	1 oz	90	5.0	2.0	370	(tr)	7.0	20
ITALIAN HERB (Land O'Lakes)	1 oz	90	6.0	2.0	430	na	7.0	20

JALAPEÑO
(Hoffman's)	1 oz	90	5.0	2.0	580	(tr)	7.0	(mq)
(Kraft)	1 oz	90	5.0	2.0	390	(tr)	7.0	20
(Land O'Lakes)	1 oz	90	6.0	2.0	400	na	7.0	20
hot, 'Mexican' (Velveeta)	1 oz	100	6.0	3.0	430	(tr)	7.0	25
mild, 'Mexican' (Velveeta)	1 oz	100	6.0	3.0	420	(tr)	7.0	25

Food Name	Serv. Size	Total Cal.	Prot. GMS	Carbs GMS	Sod. MGS	Fiber GMS	Fat GMS	Chol. MGS
'Singles' (Kraft)	1 oz	90	5.0	2.0	450	(tr)	7.0	25
MEXICAN								
hot, shredded (Velveeta)	1 oz	100	6.0	3.0	430	(tr)	7.0	25
mild, shredded (Velveeta)	1 oz	100	6.0	3.0	420	(tr)	7.0	25
ONION								
(Land O'Lakes)	1 oz	90	6.0	2.0	330	(tr)	7.0	15
'Chees'N Onion' (Hoffman's)	1 oz	100	5.0	3.0	490	(tr)	7.0	(mq)
PEPPPERONI (Land O'Lakes)	1 oz	90	6.0	1.0	395	0	7.0	20
PIMIENTO								
'Deluxe' (Kraft)	1 oz	100	6.0	1.0	440	(tr)	8.0	25
'Singles' (Kraft)	1 oz	90	5.0	2.0	390	(tr)	7.0	25
PORT WINE								
cold pack (Wispride)	1 oz	100	5.0	3.0	210	0	7.0	25
cold pack, 'Cup' (Kaukauna)	1 oz	100	6.0	3.0	250	0	7.0	25
cup, 'Lite 50' (Kaukauna)	1 oz	70	5.0	5.0	190	na	3.0	15
PROCESSED								
(Land O'Lakes)	1 oz	90	5.0	2.0	350	na	6.0	20
singles, fat-free (Healthy Choice)	1 oz	40	6.0	3.0	390	na	0.0	5
singles, 'Free' (Kraft)	1 oz	45	6.0	4.0	430	na	0.0	5
slices (Land O'Lakes)	3/4 oz	70	4.0	2.0	260	na	5.0	15
slices (Land O'Lakes)	2/3 oz	60	4.0	2.0	230	na	4.0	15
SALAMI								
(Land O'Lakes)	1 oz	90	6.0	2.0	410	0	7.0	20
'Chees'N Salami' (Hoffman's)	1 oz	90	5.0	3.0	560	0	6.0	(mq)
SHARP, 'Singles' (Kraft)	1 oz	100	6.0	1.0	400	0	8.0	25
SHREDDED (Velveeta)	1 oz	100	6.0	3.0	410	0	7.0	20
SMOKY, cold pack, 'Cup' (Kaukauna)	1 oz	100	6.0	3.0	250	0	7.0	25
SWISS								
(Velveeta)	1 oz	100	6.0	3.0	410	0	7.0	20
almond, cup, 'Lite 50' (Kaukauna)	1 oz	70	5.0	5.0	180	na	3.0	15
country, cold pack,'Cup' (Kaukauna)	1 oz	100	6.0	3.0	250	0	7.0	25
country, 'Lite' (Kaukauna)	1 oz	70	6.0	5.0	200	0	4.0	15
singles (Kraft)	1 oz	90	6.0	2.0	440	0	7.0	25
singles, 'Free' (Kraft)	1 oz	45	6.0	4.0	390	na	0.0	5
slices, 'Singles' (Borden)	1 oz	100	6.0	2.0	420	na	7.0	na
CHEESE LOG								
hickory smoke/white sharp cheddar, double (Kaukauna)	1 oz	100	6.0	3.0	250	(mq)	7.0	25
Port wine (Sargento)	1 oz	100	6.0	3.0	250	(mq)	7.0	18
Port wine, w/almonds (Kaukauna)	1 oz	100	6.0	3.0	250	(mq)	7.0	25
sharp cheddar (Sargento)	1 oz	100	6.0	3.0	250	(mq)	7.0	18
sharp cheddar, w/almonds (Cracker Barrel)	1 oz	90	5.0	4.0	410	(mq)	6.0	15
sharp cheddar, w/almonds (Kaukauna)	1 oz	100	6.0	3.0	250	(mq)	7.0	25

Food Name	Serv. Size	Total Cal.	Prot. GMS	Carbs GMS	Sod. MGS	Fiber GMS	Fat GMS	Chol. MGS
smoky, w/almonds *(Cracker Barrel)*	1 oz	90	5.0	4.0	410	(mq)	6.0	15
Swiss almond *(Sargento)*	1 oz	90	6.0	2.0	350	(mq)	7.0	21
Swiss almond, w/almonds *(Kaukauna)*	1 oz	100	6.0	3.0	250	(mq)	7.0	25
white sharp cheddar/green onion, double *(Kaukauna)*	1 oz	100	6.0	3.0	250	(mq)	7.0	25
CHEESE NUGGET								
mozzarella, breaded, frozen 'Hot Bites' *(Banquet)*	2.63 oz	240	14.0	16.0	530	(mq)	13.0	(mq)
CHEESE NUT								
Port wine *(Cracker Barrel)*	1 oz	90	5.0	4.0	260	(mq)	6.0	15
sharp, w/bell and jalapeño peppers *(Kaukauna)*	1 oz	100	6.0	3.0	250	(mq)	7.0	25
sharp cheddar *(Cracker Barrel)*	1 oz	100	5.0	4.0	250	(mq)	7.0	20
CHEESE PASTRY, pocket *(Tastykake)*	3 oz	325	4.4	40.8	231	1.3	16.7	11
CHEESE PRODUCT								
(Alpine Lace)	1 oz	90	6.0	2.0	200	0	7.0	20
'Free N' Lean' singles *(Alpine Lace)*	1 oz	40	8.0	1.0	260	na	0.0	5
'Free Singles' *(Kraft)*	1 oz	45	7.0	4.0	420	0	0.0	5
'Light' *(Velveeta)*	1 oz	70	6.0	3.0	470	0	4.0	15
sandwich slices *(Lunch Wagon)*	1 oz	90	5.0	2.0	370	0	7.0	5
'Singles' fat-free *(Borden)*	1 oz	40	6.0	4.0	380	na	0.0	5
'Slices' *(Velveeta)*	1 oz	90	5.0	3.0	400	0	6.0	20
slices, fat-free *(Lite-Line)*	1 slice	25	4.0	3.0	250	na	0.0	5
AMERICAN FLAVOR								
(Harvest Moon)	1 oz	70	6.0	2.0	420	0	4.0	15
(Lite-Line)	1 oz	50	7.0	1.0	410	0	2.0	(mq)
'Light' *(Borden)*	1 oz	70	6.0	1.0	420	0	5.0	(mq)
'Light Singles' *(Kraft)*	1 oz	70	6.0	2.0	420	0	4.0	15
'Reduced Sodium' *(Lite-Line)*	1 oz	70	6.0	2.0	90	0	4.0	(mq)
'Singles' *(Light n' Lively)*	1 oz	70	6.0	2.0	420	0	4.0	15
'Sodium Lite' *(Lite-Line)*	1 oz	70	6.0	2.0	200	0	4.0	(mq)
white 'Light Singles' *(Kraft)*	1 oz	70	6.0	2.0	410	0	4.0	15
white 'Singles' *(Light n' Lively)*	1 oz	70	6.0	2.0	410	0	4.0	15
CHEDDAR FLAVOR								
medium-sharp *(Spreadery)*	1 oz	70	5.0	3.0	250	0	4.0	15
mild *(Lite-Line)*	1 oz	50	7.0	1.0	380	0	2.0	(mq)
sharp *(Lite-Line)*	1 oz	50	7.0	1.0	440	0	2.0	(mq)
sharp *(Spreadery)*	1 oz	70	5.0	3.0	240	0	4.0	15
sharp, 'Free' *(Kraft)*	1 oz	45	6.0	4.0	390	0	0.0	5
sharp, 'Light' *(Kraft)*	1 oz	70	6.0	2.0	380	0	4.0	15
sharp, 'Singles' *(Kraft)*	1 oz	100	6.0	1.0	400	0	8.0	25
sharp, 'Singles' *(Light n' Lively)*	1 oz	70	6.0	2.0	380	0	4.0	15
sharp, slices *(Lite-Line)*	1 slice	35	4.0	1.0	300	na	2.0	5
Vermont white *(Spreadery)*	1 oz	70	5.0	3.0	230	0	4.0	15

Food Name	Serv. Size	Total Cal.	Prot. GMS	Carbs GMS	Sod. MGS	Fiber GMS	Fat GMS	Chol. MGS
CREAM CHEESE FLAVOR 'Light'								
(Philadelphia Brand)	1 oz	60	3.0	2.0	160	0	5.0	10
MEXICAN FLAVOR mild, w/jalapeños								
(Spreadery)	1 oz	70	5.0	3.0	260	(tr)	4.0	15
MOZZARELLA FLAVOR (Lite-Line)	1 oz	50	7.0	1.0	340	0	2.0	(mq)
MUENSTER FLAVOR (Lite-Line)	1 oz	50	7.0	1.0	450	0	2.0	(mq)
NACHO FLAVOR (Spreadery)	1 oz	70	5.0	3.0	240	0	4.0	15
NEUFCHATEL								
classic ranch (Spreadery)	1 oz	70	2.0	1.0	190	(tr)	7.0	20
French onion (Spreadery)	1 oz	70	2.0	2.0	135	(tr)	6.0	20
garden vegetable (Spreadery)	1 oz	70	2.0	2.0	220	(tr)	6.0	20
garlic and herb (Spreadery)	1 oz	70	2.0	1.0	140	(tr)	6.0	20
w/strawberries (Spreadery)	1 oz	70	2.0	1.0	270	(tr)	5.0	15
PORT WINE FLAVOR (Spreadery)	1 oz	70	5.0	3.0	250	0	4.0	15
SWISS FLAVOR								
(Lite-Line)	1 oz	50	7.0	1.0	380	0	2.0	(mq)
'Free Singles' (Kraft)	1 oz	45	6.0	4.0	390	na	0.0	5
'Light' (Kraft)	1 oz	70	6.0	2.0	350	0	3.0	15
'Singles' (Light n' Lively)	1 oz	70	6.0	2.0	350	0	3.0	15
CHEESE SPREAD								
AMERICAN								
(Kraft)	1 oz	80	4.0	2.0	470	0	6.0	15
'Easy Cheese American' (Nabisco)	1 oz	80	4.0	2.0	350	na	6.0	na
sharp 'Cracker Snacks' (Sargento)	1 oz	110	6.0	0.5	410	0	9.0	27
w/pimiento 'Cracker Snacks' (Sargento)	1 oz	110	6.0	0.5	410	(tr)	9.0	27
BACON								
(Kraft)	1 oz	80	5.0	1.0	560	0	7.0	20
(Squeez-A-Snak)	1 oz	80	5.0	1.0	509	0	7.0	20
BLUE (Roka)	1 oz	70	3.0	2.0	270	0	6.0	20
BRICK 'Cracker Snacks' (Sargento)	1 oz	100	6.0	1.0	430	0	9.0	25
CHEDDAR								
'Easy Cheese Cheddar' (Nabisco)	1 oz	80	4.0	2.0	370	na	6.0	na
'Easy Cheese Cheddar 'n Bacon' (Nabisco)	1 oz	80	4.0	2.0	350	na	6.0	na
'Easy Cheese Sharp Cheddar' (Nabisco)	1 oz	80	4.0	2.0	320	na	6.0	na
sharp, 'Cup' (Weight Watchers)	1 oz	70	4.0	7.0	190	0	3.0	10
FRENCH ONION (Alouette)	1 oz	95	2.0	2.0	205	na	9.0	31
GARLIC								
(Squeez-A-Snak)	1 oz	80	5.0	1.0	430	(tr)	7.0	20
and herbs, soft 'Lite' (Rondel)	1 oz	70	3.0	2.0	170	na	6.0	15
and spices (Alouette)	1 oz	95	2.0	2.0	165	na	9.0	31
HERB								
and garlic, soft 'Light' (Alouette)	1 oz	60	3.0	2.0	130	na	4.5	15
soft, 'Fines Herbes' (Rondel)	1 oz	90	3.0	2.0	170	na	8.0	na

Food Name	Serv. Size	Total Cal.	Prot. GMS	Carbs GMS	Sod. MGS	Fiber GMS	Fat GMS	Chol. MGS
HICKORY (Squeez-A-Snak)	1 oz	80	5.0	1.0	440	0	7.0	20
HORSERADISH, and chive (Alouette)	1 oz	85	2.0	1.0	130	na	8.0	28
JALAPEÑO								
(Cheez Whiz)	1 oz	80	4.0	2.0	430	(tr)	6.0	20
(Kraft)	1 oz	70	2.0	3.0	95	(tr)	5.0	15
(Squeez-A-Snak)	1 oz	80	5.0	1.0	510	(tr)	6.0	20
loaf (Kraft)	1 oz	80	5.0	2.0	470	(tr)	6.0	20
LIMBURGER (Mohawk Valley)	1 oz	70	4.0	0.0	420	0	6.0	20
MEXICAN								
'Easy Cheese Nacho' (Nabisco)	1 oz	80	4.0	2.0	340	na	6.0	na
hot (Velveeta)	1 oz	80	5.0	3.0	520	(tr)	6.0	20
mild (Cheez Whiz)	1 oz	80	4.0	2.0	430	(tr)	6.0	20
mild (Velveeta)	1 oz	80	5.0	3.0	440	(tr)	6.0	20
OLIVE, and pimiento (Kraft)	1 oz	60	2.0	2.0	160	(tr)	5.0	15
PIMIENTO								
(Kraft)	1 oz	70	2.0	3.0	120	(tr)	5.0	15
(Velveeta)	1 oz	80	5.0	3.0	400	(tr)	6.0	20
PINEAPPLE (Kraft)	1 oz	70	2.0	4.0	15	(tr)	5.0	75
PORT WINE, 'Cup' (Weight Watchers)	1 oz	70	4.0	7.0	190	0	3.0	10
SALMON (Alouette)	1 oz	70	2.0	2.0	140	na	6.0	20
SHARP								
(Old English)	1 oz	80	5.0	1.0	480	0	7.0	20
(Squeez-A-Snak)	1 oz	80	5.0	1.0	440	0	7.0	20
SPINACH, creamy (Alouette)	1 oz	90	2.0	2.0	125	na	8.0	na
SWISS, 'Cracker Snacks' (Sargento)	1 oz	100	7.0	1.0	390	0	7.0	24
VEGETABLE								
garden, soft (Rondele)	1 oz	90	3.0	3.0	160	na	8.0	na
spring, soft 'Light' (Alouette)	1 oz	60	3.0	1.0	120	na	4.5	15
CHEESE STICK								
cheddar, breaded, frozen (Farm Rich)	3 oz	300	10.9	19.0	740	(mq)	21.0	(mq)
cheddar, snack (Flavor Tree)	1/4 cup	129	2.7	11.9	335	>.1 c	8.1	na
hot pepper, breaded, frozen (Farm Rich)	3 oz	260	8.0	20.0	700	(mq)	17.0	(mq)
mozzarella, breaded, frozen (Farm Rich)	3 oz	240	10.0	19.0	570	(mq)	13.0	(mq)
provolone, breaded, frozen (Farm Rich)	3 oz	270	10.0	22.0	820	(mq)	16.0	(mq)
CHEESE STRAW								
made w/lard, 5 x 3/8 x 3/8 inches	10 straws	272	6.7	20.7	433	>.1 c	17.9	32
made w/vegetable shortening, 5 x 3/8 x 3/8 inches	10 straws	272	6.7	20.7	433	>.1 c	17.9	19
CHEESE TOPPING, cheddar, w/bacon								
(Tone's)	1 tsp	10	0.5	0.7	81	0	1.0	1
CHEESECAKE. See CAKE.								
CHEESECAKE FILLING								
'No-Bake' lite (Royal)	1/8 pie	130	4.0	22.0	230	na	3.0	5

Food Name	Serv. Size	Total Cal.	Prot. GMS	Carbs GMS	Sod. MGS	Fiber GMS	Fat GMS	Chol. MGS
'No-Bake' real *(Royal)*	1/8 pie	160	4.0	29.0	250	na	3.0	na

CHERIMOYA. See CUSTARD APPLE.

CHERRY

SOUR, RED

trimmed, w/pits	1 cup	52	1.0	12.6	3	1.2	0.3	0
trimmed, w/pits	1 oz	14	0.3	3.5	1	(mq)	0.1	0
trimmed, w/o pits	1 cup	78	1.5	18.9	5	1.9	0.5	0
untrimmed	1 lb	203	4.1	49.7	13	(mq)	1.2	0

SWEET

trimmed, w/pits	1 cup	104	1.7	24.0	0	3.3	1.4	0
trimmed, w/pits	1 oz	20	0.3	4.7	tr	.4	0.3	0
trimmed, w/pits, approx 2.6 oz	10 med	49	0.8	11.3	0	1.6	0.7	0
untrimmed	1 lb	293	4.9	67.6	2	6.3	3.9	0
untrimmed *(Dole)*	1 cup	90	1.0	19.0	0	3.0	1.0	na

CHERRY, CANNED

SOUR, RED

(A&P)	1/2 cup	50	<1.0	12.0	5	(mq)	<1.0	0
in extra heavy syrup	1/2 cup	148	0.9	38.0	9	>.1 c	0.1	0
in heavy syrup	1/2 cup	116	0.9	29.8	9	1.0	0.1	0
in light syrup	1/2 cup	94	0.9	24.3	9	>.1 c	0.1	0
in water	1/2 cup	44	0.9	10.9	9	1.0	0.1	0

Pitted

in extra heavy syrup	1/2 cup	129	0.8	33.1	8	>.1 c	0.1	0
in heavy syrup	1/2 cup	103	0.8	26.4	8	>.1 c	0.1	0
in light syrup	1/2 cup	85	0.8	21.9	8	>.1 c	0.1	0
in water	1/2 cup	41	0.8	10.0	8	>.1 c	0.1	0
in water *(Stokely)*	1/2 cup	45	1.0	10.0	15	(mq)	0.0	0
tart *(Lucky Leaf)*	4 oz	50	1.0	11.0	0	(mq)	0.0	0
tart *(Musselman's)*	4 oz	50	1.0	11.0	0	(mq)	0.0	0
(White House)	3.5 oz	43	0.0	11.0	5	(mq)	0.0	0

SWEET

dark *(Del Monte)*	1/2 cup	90	0.0	23.0	10	(mq)	0.0	0
in extra heavy syrup	1/2 cup	116	0.7	29.7	3	>.4 c	0.2	0
in heavy syrup	1/2 cup	94	0.7	24.1	3	>.4 c	0.2	0
in juice	1/2 cup	61	1.0	15.7	3	>.3 c	<.1	0
in light syrup	1/2 cup	76	0.7	19.6	3	>.4 c	0.2	0
in light syrup *(Del Monte)*	1/2 cup	100	0.0	26.0	10	(mq)	0.0	0
in water	1/2 cup	52	0.9	13.3	1	>.2 c	0.1	0

Pitted

dark *(Del Monte)*	1/2 cup	90	0.0	24.0	10	(mq)	0.0	0
in extra heavy syrup	1/2 cup	133	0.8	34.1	4	>.4 c	0.2	0
in heavy syrup	1/2 cup	107	0.8	27.4	4	.9	0.2	0
in juice	1/2 cup	68	1.1	17.3	4	.9	0.0	0

Food Name	Serv. Size	Total Cal.	Prot. GMS	Carbs GMS	Sod. MGS	Fiber GMS	Fat GMS	Chol. MGS
in light syrup	1/2 cup	84	0.8	21.8	4	.9	0.2	0
in water	1/2 cup	57	1.0	14.6	1	.9	0.2	0
CHERRY, FROZEN								
SOUR, RED								
unsweetened	4 oz	52	1.0	12.5	1	1.3	0.5	0
unsweetened	1/2 cup	36	0.7	8.5	1	1.0	0.3	0
SWEET								
sweetened	10-oz pkg	253	3.3	63.5	3	2.8	0.4	0
sweetened	1 cup	231	3.0	57.9	3	2.6	0.3	0
sweetened	4 oz	101	1.3	25.4	1	1.1	0.1	0
sweetened (Lucky Leaf)	4 oz	130	1.0	31.0	150	(mq)	0.0	0
CHERRY, MARASCHINO, in jar, w/liquid	1 oz	33	0.1	8.3	na	>.1 c	0.1	0
CHERRY, PUERTO RICAN								
approx .2 oz	1 med	2	<.1	0.4	tr	>.1 c	<.1	0
trimmed	1/2 cup	16	0.2	3.8	4	>.2 c	0.1	0
trimmed	1 oz	9	0.1	2.2	2	>.1 c	0.1	0
untrimmed	1 lb	114	1.5	27.9	26	>1.5 c	1.1	0
CHERRY CIDER (Knudsen & Sons)	8 oz	100	<1.0	24.0	na	na	0.0	na
CHERRY DRINK								
(Hi-C) aseptic box	6 oz	100	0.0	24.0	25	na	0.0	na
(Hi-C) chilled	6 oz	100	0.0	24.0	25	na	0.0	na
(Kool-Aid) 'Koolers'	8.45 oz	140	0.0	38.0	10	na	0.0	0
(Squeezit) 'Chucklin Cherry'	6.75 oz	110	0.0	27.0	5	na	0.0	na
CHERRY DRINK MIX								
(Finast) prepared	8 oz	80	0.0	21.0	15	(tr)	0.0	0
(Kool-Aid) sugar-sweetened, prepared	8 oz	80	0.0	20.0	0	na	0.0	0
(Kool-Aid) unsweetened, prepared w/sugar	8 oz	100	0.0	25.0	0	na	0.0	0
(Kool-Aid) unsweetened, prepared w/o sugar	8 oz	2	0.0	0.0	0	na	0.0	0
(Kool-Aid) w/NutraSweet, prepared	8 oz	4	0.0	0.0	0	na	0.0	0
(Pathmark) 'No Frills' prepared	8 oz	90	0.0	22.0	65	(tr)	0.0	0
(Wyler's) 'Fruit Slush' prepared	4 oz	157	0.0	39.3	10	(tr)	0.0	0
CHERRY JUICE								
(Dole) 'Pure and Light Mountain Cherry'	6 oz	87	0.2	22.0	8	(mq)	0.1	0
(Juicy Juice) bottled	6 oz	90	1.0	23.0	10	na	0.0	na
(Juicy Juice) boxed	8.45 oz	130	1.0	32.0	10	na	0.0	na
(Knudsen & Sons) tart	8 oz	125	<1.0	30.0	na	na	0.0	na
(Santa Cruz Natural) 'Cruz' organic	8 oz	125	1.0	29.0	na	na	<1.0	na
(Welch's) 'Orchard'	6 oz	180	0.0	45.0	10	(tr)	0.0	0
CHERRY JUICE DRINK								
(Hi-C)	8.45 oz	141	0.2	34.8	24	(tr)	0.1	0
(Hi-C)	6 oz	100	0.1	24.7	17	(tr)	0.1	0
(Tang) 'Fruit Box'	8.45 oz	130	0.0	34.0	10	na	0.0	0

Food Name	Serv. Size	Total Cal.	Prot. GMS	Carbs GMS	Sod. MGS	Fiber GMS	Fat GMS	Chol. MGS
CHERRY LEMONADE								
(Knudsen & Sons)	8 oz	105	<1.0	31.0	na	na	0.0	na
(Santa Cruz natural) dark, sweet, organic	8 oz	60	<1.0	20.0	na	na	<1.0	na
CHERRY PASTRY								
(Hormel) frozen 'Cherry Dulcita'	4 oz	300	5.0	48.0	345	(mq)	9.0	na
(Tastykake) pocket	3 oz	325	4.4	40.8	231	1.3	16.7	11
CHERRY PIE FILLING. See PIE FILLING.								
CHERRY STRUDEL, individual								
(Aunt Fanny's)	3 oz	320	4.0	39.0	190	na	16.0	5
CHERVIL								
dried	1 oz	67	6.6	13.9	24	3.2	1.1	0
dried	1 tbsp	4	0.4	0.9	2	.2	0.1	0
dried	1 tsp	1	0.1	0.3	1	.1	0.0	0
CHESTNUT, CHINESE								
boiled or steamed	1 oz	43	0.8	9.6	1	>.3 c	0.2	0
dried	1 oz	103	1.9	22.6	1	>.8 c	0.5	0
raw	1 oz	64	1.2	13.9	1	>.5 c	0.3	0
raw, in shell	1 lb	852	16.0	187.0	13	>6.2 c	4.2	0
roasted	1 oz	68	1.3	14.9	1	>.5 c	0.3	0
CHESTNUT, EUROPEAN/Italian chestnut/sweet chestnut								
boiled or steamed, shelled	1 oz	37	0.8	7.9	8	>.2 c	0.4	0
dried, in shell	1 lb	1357	23.2	280.5	135	>19.8 c	16.1	0
dried, shelled, peeled	1 oz	105	1.4	22.3	11	>1.4 c	1.1	0
dried, shelled, unpeeled	1 oz	106	1.8	22.0	11	3.3	1.3	0
raw, in shell	1 lb	714	8.1	152.8	9	33.3	7.6	0
raw, shelled, peeled	1 oz	56	0.5	12.5	1	>.3 c	0.4	0
raw, shelled, unpeeled	1 cup	309	3.5	66.0	4	11.7	3.3	0
raw, shelled, unpeeled	1 oz	60	0.7	12.9	1	2.3	0.6	0
roasted, in shell	1 lb	700	9.1	151.3	6	33.4	6.3	0
roasted, in shell	1 cup	350	4.5	75.7	3	18.4	3.2	0
roasted, in shell	1 oz	70	0.9	15.0	1	3.7	0.6	0
roasted, shelled	1 oz	70	0.9	15.0	1	3.3	0.6	0
roasted, shelled, approx 17 nuts	1 cup	350	4.3	75.7	3	16.7	3.2	0
CHESTNUT, ITALIAN. See CHESTNUT, EUROPEAN.								
CHESTNUT, JAPANESE								
boiled or steamed	1 oz	16	0.2	3.6	1	>.1 c	0.1	0
dried, in shell	1 lb	1078	15.7	243.7	101	>6.8 c	3.7	0
dried, shelled	1 oz	102	1.5	23.1	10	>.6 c	0.4	0
dried, shelled	1 cup	558	8.1	126.2	53	>3.5 c	1.9	0
raw, in shell	1 lb	462	6.7	104.5	43	>2.9 c	1.6	0
raw, shelled	1 oz	44	0.6	9.9	4	>.3 c	0.2	0
roasted	1 oz	57	0.8	12.8	5	>.3 c	0.2	0
CHESTNUT, SWEET. See CHESTNUT, EUROPEAN.								

Food Name	Serv. Size	Total Cal.	Prot. GMS	Carbs GMS	Sod. MGS	Fiber GMS	Fat GMS	Chol. MGS
CHESTNUT FLOUR	100 gm	362	6.1	76.2	11	>2.0 c	3.7	0
CHEWING GUM. See CANDY.								
CHIA SEEDS, dried	1 oz	134	4.7	13.6	11	>7.2 c	7.4	0
CHICK PEA. See GARBANZO BEAN.								
CHICK PEA FLOUR. See GARBANZO FLOUR.								
CHICKEN. For fresh chicken see CHICKEN, BROILER-FRYER; CHICKEN, CAPON; CHICKEN, ROASTER; CHICKEN, STEWING.								
CHICKEN, ALTERNATIVE								
(Heartline) 'Chicken Fillet Style'	2 oz	176	19.0	9.0	260	na	7.0	0
(Heartline) 'Chicken Fillet Style' lite	.5 oz	22	5.0	1.0	135	3.0	0.0	0
Canned								
(Worthington) diced, drained	1/4 cup	90	4.0	2.0	330	(mq)	8.0	0
(Worthington) 'FriChik' 1.6-oz pieces ..	2 pieces	180	11.0	4.0	610	(mq)	13.0	0
(Worthington) sliced, drained, 1.05-oz slices	2 slices	90	4.0	2.0	330	(mq)	8.0	0
Frozen								
(Morningstar Farms) nuggets, homestyle 'Country Crisps'	3 oz	250	8.0	18.0	480	(mq)	16.0	0
(Morningstar Farms) nuggets, zesty 'Country Crisps'	3 oz	280	9.0	17.0	740	(mq)	19.0	0
(Morningstar Farms) patty 'Country Crisps'	2.5 oz	220	8.0	13.0	620	(mq)	15.0	0
(Worthington) 'Crispy Chik'	3 oz	280	10.0	17.0	500	(mq)	19.0	0
(Worthington) diced 'Meatless Chicken'	1/2 cup	190	13.0	5.0	680	(mq)	13.0	0
(Worthington) patty 'Crispy Chik'	2.5 oz	220	8.0	13.0	620	(mq)	15.0	0
(Worthington) roll 'Chic-ketts'	1/2 cup	160	19.0	6.0	640	(mq)	7.0	0
(Worthington) roll 'Meatless Chicken'	2.5 oz	150	11.0	4.0	570	(mq)	10.0	0
(Worthington) sliced 'Meatless Chicken' 1-oz slices.......................	2 slices	130	9.0	3.0	460	(mq)	9.0	0
(Worthington) sticks 'Chik Stiks' approx 1.7-oz pieces	1 stick	110	9.0	4.0	390	(mq)	7.0	0
CHICKEN, BONELESS BREAST, PREPARED								
(Hillshire Farm) smoked 'Deli Select'	1 oz	31	6.0	<1.0	290	0	0.2	(mq)
(Louis Rich) hickory-smoked	1 oz	30	5.1	0.6	356	0	0.8	14
(Louis Rich) hickory-smoked, 97% fat-free	1 oz	30	5.0	<1.0	370	na	<1.0	15
(Louis Rich) oven-roasted 'Deluxe'	1 oz	30	4.9	0.6	332	0	0.8	14
(Louis Rich) oven-roasted, 'Deluxe' 96% fat-free	1 oz	30	5.0	<1.0	330	na	1.0	15
(Oscar Mayer) oven-roasted	1 oz	29	5.2	0.6	414	0	0.7	15
(Oscar Mayer) smoked	1 oz	25	5.3	0.2	397	0	0.4	15
CHICKEN, BROILER-FRYER								
BACK MEAT AND SKIN								
fried, flour-coated	4 oz	375	31.5	7.4	102	>.1 c	23.5	101

Food Name	Serv. Size	Total Cal.	Prot. GMS	Carbs GMS	Sod. MGS	Fiber GMS	Fat GMS	Chol. MGS
raw	1 oz	90	4.0	0.0	18	0	8.1	22
roasted	4 oz	340	29.4	0.0	99	0	23.8	100
stewed	4 oz	293	25.2	0.0	73	0	20.6	88
BACK MEAT ONLY								
raw	1 lb	624	88.0	0.0	400	0	28.8	400
raw	1 oz	39	5.5	0.0	23	0	1.7	23
roasted	4 oz	271	32.0	0.0	109	0	14.9	102
stewed	4 oz	237	28.7	0.0	76	0	12.7	96
BREAST MEAT AND SKIN								
fried, batter-dipped	4 oz	295	28.2	10.2	312	.4	15.0	96
fried, flour-coated	4 oz	252	36.1	1.9	86	>.1 c	10.1	101
raw	1 lb	784	94.4	0.0	288	0	41.6	288
raw	1 oz	49	5.9	0.0	18	0	2.6	18
roasted	4 oz	223	33.8	0.0	81	0	8.8	95
stewed	4 oz	209	31.1	0.0	70	0	8.4	85
BREAST MEAT ONLY								
raw	1 lb	496	104.0	0.0	288	0	6.4	256
raw	1 oz	31	6.5	0.0	18	0	0.4	16
roasted	4 oz	187	35.2	0.0	84	0	4.0	96
stewed	4 oz	171	32.9	0.0	71	0	3.4	87
DARK MEAT AND SKIN								
fried, batter-dipped	4 oz	338	24.8	10.6	335	>.1 c	21.1	101
fried, flour-coated	4 oz	323	30.9	4.6	101	>.1 c	19.2	104
raw	1 lb	1072	75.2	0.0	336	0	83.2	368
raw	1 oz	67	4.7	0.0	21	0	5.2	23
roasted	4 oz	287	29.4	0.0	99	0	17.9	103
stewed	4 oz	264	26.6	0.0	79	0	16.6	93
DARK MEAT ONLY								
fried, chopped or diced	1 cup	335	40.6	3.6	136	0	16.3	134
raw	1 lb	560	96.0	0.0	384	0	19.2	368
raw	1 oz	35	6.0	0.0	24	0	1.2	23
roasted	1 cup	287	38.3	0.0	130	0	13.6	130
roasted	4 oz	232	31.0	0.0	105	0	11.0	105
roasted, chopped or diced	1 cup	286	38.3	0.0	130	0	13.6	130
stewed	1 cup	269	36.4	0.0	104	0	12.6	123
stewed	4 oz	218	29.4	0.0	84	0	10.2	100
stewed, chopped or diced	1 cup	269	36.4	0.0	104	0	12.6	123
DRUMSTICK MEAT AND SKIN								
fried, batter-dipped	4 oz	304	24.9	9.4	305	>.1 c	17.9	98
fried, flour-coated	4 oz	278	30.6	1.8	101	>.1 c	15.6	102
raw	1 lb	736	88.0	0.0	384	0	40.0	368
raw	1 oz	46	5.5	0.0	24	0	2.5	23
roasted	4 oz	245	30.7	0.0	102	0	12.6	103

Food Name	Serv. Size	Total Cal.	Prot. GMS	Carbs GMS	Sod. MGS	Fiber GMS	Fat GMS	Chol. MGS
stewed	4 oz	231	28.7	0.0	86	0	12.1	94
DRUMSTICK MEAT ONLY								
raw	1 lb	544	92.8	0.0	400	0	16.0	352
raw	1 oz	34	5.8	0.0	25	0	1.0	22
roasted	4 oz	195	32.1	0.0	108	0	6.4	105
stewed	4 oz	192	31.2	0.0	91	0	6.5	100
LEG MEAT AND SKIN								
fried, batter-dipped	4 oz	310	24.7	9.9	316	>.1 c	18.3	102
fried, flour-coated	4 oz	285	30.1	2.8	99	>.1 c	16.2	105
raw	1 lb	848	81.6	0.0	352	0	54.4	384
raw	1 oz	53	5.1	0.0	22	0	3.4	24
stewed	4 oz	249	27.4	0.0	83	0	14.7	95
LEG MEAT ONLY								
raw	1 lb	544	91.2	0.0	384	0	17.6	368
raw	1 oz	34	5.7	0.0	24	0	1.1	23
roasted	4 oz	217	30.7	0.0	103	0	9.6	107
stewed	4 oz	210	29.8	0.0	88	0	9.1	101
LIGHT MEAT AND SKIN								
fried, batter-dipped	4 oz	312	26.6	10.7	324	>.1 c	17.4	94
fried, flour-coated	4 oz	279	34.5	2.1	87	>.1 c	13.7	99
raw	1 lb	848	91.2	0.0	288	0	49.6	304
raw	1 oz	53	5.7	0.0	18	0	3.1	19
roasted	4 oz	252	32.9	0.0	85	0	12.3	95
stewed	4 oz	228	29.6	0.0	71	0	11.3	84
LIGHT MEAT ONLY								
fried	8 oz	269	46.0	0.6	113	0	7.8	126
raw	1 lb	512	105.6	0.0	304	0	8.0	256
raw	1 oz	32	6.6	0.0	19	0	0.5	16
roasted	1 cup	242	43.3	0.0	108	0	6.3	119
roasted	4 oz	196	35.1	0.0	87	0	5.1	96
roasted, chopped or diced	1 cup	242	43.3	0.0	108	0	6.3	118
stewed, chopped or diced	1 cup	223	40.4	0.0	91	0	5.6	107
stewed	4 oz	180	32.7	0.0	74	0	4.5	87
NECK MEAT AND SKIN								
fried, batter-dipped	4 oz	374	22.5	9.9	313	>.1 c	26.7	103
fried, flour-coated	4 oz	376	27.2	4.8	93	>.1 c	26.8	107
raw	1 lb	1344	64.0	0.0	288	0	118.4	448
raw	1 oz	84	4.0	0.0	18	0	7.4	28
simmered	4 oz	280	22.2	0.0	59	0	20.5	79
NECK MEAT ONLY								
raw	1 lb	704	80.0	0.0	368	0	40.0	384
raw	1 oz	44	5.0	0.0	23	0	2.5	24
simmered	4 oz	203	27.9	0.0	73	0	9.3	90

Food Name	Serv. Size	Total Cal.	Prot. GMS	Carbs GMS	Sod. MGS	Fiber GMS	Fat GMS	Chol. MGS
SKIN ONLY								
fried, batter-dipped	1 oz	112	2.9	6.6	165	>.1 c	8.2	21
roasted	1 oz	129	5.8	0.0	18	0	11.5	24
stewed	1 oz	103	4.3	0.0	16	0	9.4	18
THIGH MEAT AND SKIN								
fried, batter-dipped	4 oz	314	24.5	10.3	327	>.1 c	18.7	105
fried, flour-coated	4 oz	297	30.3	3.6	100	>.1 c	17.0	110
raw	1 lb	960	78.4	0.0	352	0	68.8	384
raw	1 oz	60	4.9	0.0	22	0	4.3	24
roasted	4 oz	280	28.4	0.0	95	0	17.6	105
stewed	4 oz	263	26.4	0.0	81	0	16.7	95
THIGH MEAT ONLY								
raw	1 lb	544	89.6	0.0	384	0	17.6	384
raw	1 oz	34	5.6	0.0	24	0	1.1	24
roasted	4 oz	237	29.4	0.0	100	0	12.3	108
stewed	4 oz	221	28.4	0.0	85	0	11.1	102
WING MEAT AND SKIN								
fried, batter-dipped	4 oz	367	22.5	12.4	363	>.1 c	24.7	90
fried, flour-coated	4 oz	364	29.6	2.7	87	>.1 c	25.1	92
raw	1 lb	1008	83.2	0.0	336	0	72.0	352
raw	1 oz	63	5.2	0.0	21	0	4.5	22
roasted	4 oz	329	30.5	0.0	93	0	22.1	95
stewed	4 oz	282	25.8	0.0	76	0	19.1	79
WING MEAT ONLY								
raw	1 lb	576	99.2	0.0	368	0	16.0	256
raw	1 oz	36	6.2	0.0	23	0	1.0	16
roasted	4 oz	230	34.5	0.0	104	0	9.2	96
stewed	4 oz	205	30.8	0.0	83	0	8.1	84
CHICKEN, CANNED								
Chunk								
(Featherweight)	3 oz	90	16.0	0.0	60	0	3.0	65
(Hormel) breast	6.75 oz	350	41.0	0.0	855	0	20.0	(mq)
(Hormel) breast	2.5 oz	90	15.0	0.0	310	na	3.0	30
(Hormel) breast, no salt	2.5 oz	90	16.0	0.0	25	na	3.0	35
(Hormel) dark	6.75 oz	327	42.0	0.0	933	0	18.0	(mq)
(Hormel) white and dark	6.75 oz	340	39.0	0.0	857	0	20.0	(mq)
(Hormel) white and dark, unsalted	6.75 oz	330	42.0	0.0	75	0	18.0	(mq)
(Swanson) 'Mixin' Chicken'	2.5 oz	130	13.0	1.0	230	0	8.0	(mq)
(Swanson) white and dark	2.5 oz	100	16.0	0.0	240	0	4.0	40
Loaf (Hormel)	2 oz	130	7.0	0.0	608	0	10.0	(mq)
White (Swanson)	2.5 oz	100	15.0	0.0	235	0	4.0	35

Food Name	Serv. Size	Total Cal.	Prot. GMS	Carbs GMS	Sod. MGS	Fiber GMS	Fat GMS	Chol. MGS
CHICKEN, CAPON								
GIBLETS								
raw	1 lb	592	83.2	6.4	352	0	24.0	1328
raw	1 oz	37	5.2	0.4	.22	0	1.5	83
simmered	1 cup	238	38.3	1.1	80	0	7.8	629
simmered	4 oz	186	29.9	0.9	62	0	6.1	492
MEAT AND SKIN								
raw	1 lb	1056	84.8	0.0	208	0	76.8	336
raw	1 oz	66	5.3	0.0	13	0	4.8	21
roasted	4 oz	260	32.8	0.0	56	0	13.2	98
CHICKEN, FROZEN. See also CHICKEN DINNER/ENTRÉE, FROZEN.								
BREAST								
Boneless								
(Pilgrim's Pride)	3 oz	195	15.1	10.8	450	(mq)	10.2	26
(Tyson)	3 oz	190	13.0	15.0	400	(mq)	9.0	25
(Tyson) barbecue	3 oz	110	14.0	6.0	310	na	3.0	35
(Tyson) chunks	3 oz	240	13.0	10.0	430	(mq)	17.0	30
(Tyson) grilled	2.75 oz	100	15.0	4.0	410	na	3.0	45
(Tyson) hot and spicy	2.75 oz	110	14.0	7.0	490	na	3.0	35
(Tyson) skinless, wholesale club item	3.5 oz	110	23.0	1.0	380	na	2.0	55
Halves, wholesale club item (Tyson)	3.5 oz	230	27.0	0.0	50	na	13.0	90
Pieces								
(Banquet) fried	5.75 oz	220	16.0	13.0	710	(mq)	11.0	(mq)
(Tyson) mesquite, wholesale club item	3.5 oz	170	27.0	1.0	540	na	7.0	70
Portions (Swanson) fried, 'Plump & Juicy'	4.5 oz	360	23.0	21.0	800	(mq)	20.0	(mq)
Strips (Weaver)	3.3 oz	200	13.0	14.0	500	na	10.0	na
Tenders								
(Banquet) Southern fried	2.25 oz	160	10.0	13.0	340	(mq)	7.0	(mq)
(Pilgrim's Pride)	3 oz	181	12.7	11.1	430	(mq)	9.5	26
(Tyson) blanched, wholesale club item	3.5 oz	200	18.0	12.0	340	na	8.0	30
(Tyson) breaded, wholesale club item	3.5 oz	200	18.0	12.0	340	na	8.0	30
(Tyson) Southern fried	3 oz	220	14.0	15.0	630	(mq)	11.0	25
(Tyson) unbreaded, wholesale club item	3.5 oz	120	28.0	0.0	55	na	1.0	50
Whole								
(Tyson) wholesale club item	3.5 oz	210	26.0	0.0	50	na	12.0	80
(Weaver)	4.5 oz	270	20.0	18.0	520	na	13.0	na
(Weaver) batter-dipped	4.4 oz	310	20.0	13.0	220	na	20.0	na
CHUNKS								
(Country Pride)	3 oz	240	10.0	15.0	560	(mq)	15.0	(mq)
(Country Pride) Southern fried	3 oz	280	10.0	14.0	690	(mq)	20.0	(mq)
(Tyson) diced	3 oz	150	26.0	1.0	50	0	5.0	70
(Tyson) mesquite flavor 'Hors D'Oeuvres'	3.5 oz	100	22.0	1.0	600	na	1.0	45
(Tyson) microwave, boneless	3.5 oz	220	10.0	11.0	na	na	15.0	na

Food Name	Serv. Size	Total Cal.	Prot. GMS	Carbs GMS	Sod. MGS	Fiber GMS	Fat GMS	Chol. MGS
LEG MEAT								
(Banquet) thighs and drumsticks, fried	6.25 oz	250	14.0	14.0	790	(mq)	14.0	(mq)
(Pilgrim's Pride) drumsters	3 oz	200	11.5	10.5	320	(mq)	12.5	38
(Tyson) drums and thighs, wholesale club item	3.5 oz	270	28.0	0.0	110	na	17.0	130
(Tyson) 'Julienne Leg Meat' wholesale club item	3.5 oz	160	25.0	0.0	60	na	6.0	105
(Tyson) thighs, skinless, wholesale club item	3.5 oz	200	26.0	0.0	70	na	10.0	105
(Weaver) batter-dipped	3 oz	210	11.0	11.0	220	na	14.0	na
(Weaver) drums and thighs, 'Crispy Dutch Frye'	3.5 oz	290	16.0	14.0	640	na	19.0	na
NUGGETS								
(Country Pride)	3 oz	250	11.0	14.0	460	(mq)	16.0	(mq)
(Pilgrim's Pride)	3 oz	202	12.4	10.4	370	(mq)	12.3	31
(Weaver)	2.6 oz	190	10.0	10.0	450	na	12.0	na
(Weight Watchers)	5.9 oz	220	16.0	23.0	500	na	7.0	40
PORTIONS								
(Pilgrim's Pride) fried	3 oz	255	12.0	11.9	480	(mq)	17.7	38
(Swanson) 'Homestyle Recipe'	7 oz	390	18.0	33.0	1100	(mq)	21.0	(mq)
(Swanson) 'Take-Out Pre-Fried'	3.25 oz	270	15.0	16.0	650	(mq)	16.0	(mq)
ROASTER *(Tyson)* wholesale club item	3.5 oz	230	27.0	0.0	80	na	13.0	105
WINGS								
(Pilgrim's Pride) Southern fried	3 oz	228	13.3	5.1	480	(mq)	17.2	51
(Pilgrim's Pride) 'Wing Zappers'	3 oz	187	16.1	1.8	340	na	12.8	90
(Tyson) all varieties, 'Flyers'	3.5 oz	220	23.0	0.0	400	0	14.0	(mq)
(Tyson) drummettes, wholesale club item	3.5 oz	260	25.0	2.0	80	na	17.0	135
(Tyson) barbecue 'Hors D'Oeuvres' wholesale club item	3.5 oz	210	24.0	3.0	430	na	12.0	130
(Tyson) raw, hot, wholesale club item	3.5 oz	280	26.0	1.0	80	na	19.0	135
(Tyson) roaster 'Hors D'Oeuvres' wholesale club item	3.5 oz	210	25.0	0.0	280	na	12.0	135
(Weaver) batter-dipped	4 oz	400	16.0	20.0	520	na	28.0	na
(Weaver) 'Crispy Dutch Frye'	4 oz	400	16.0	20.0	520	na	28.0	na
(Weaver) hot	2.7 oz	170	17.0	1.0	670	na	11.0	na
CHICKEN, ROASTER								
DARK MEAT ONLY								
raw	1 lb	512	84.8	0.0	432	0	16.0	320
raw	1 oz	32	5.3	0.0	27	0	1.0	20
roasted	4 oz	202	26.4	0.0	108	0	9.9	85
GIBLETS, simmered	1 cup	239	38.8	1.3	87	0	7.6	518
LIGHT MEAT ONLY								
raw	1 lb	496	100.8	0.0	224	0	8.0	256

Food Name	Serv. Size	Total Cal.	Prot. GMS	Carbs GMS	Sod. MGS	Fiber GMS	Fat GMS	Chol. MGS
raw	1 oz	31	6.3	0.0	14	0	0.5	16
roasted	1 cup	214	38.0	0.0	71	0	5.7	105
roasted	4 oz	174	30.8	0.0	58	0	4.6	85
MEAT AND SKIN								
raw	1 lb	976	78.4	0.0	304	0	72.0	336
raw	1 oz	61	4.9	0.0	19	0	4.5	21
roasted	4 oz	253	27.2	0.0	83	0	15.2	86
CHICKEN, STEWING								
DARK MEAT ONLY								
raw	1 lb	720	89.6	0.0	464	0	36.8	352
raw	1 oz	45	5.6	0.0	29	0	2.3	22
stewed	1 cup	361	39.4	0.0	133	0	21.4	133
stewed	4 oz	293	31.9	0.0	108	0	17.3	108
GIBLETS								
raw	1 lb	560	81.6	8.0	352	0	20.8	1184
raw	1 oz	35	5.1	0.5	22	0	1.3	74
simmered	1 cup	281	37.3	0.2	81	0	13.5	515
LIGHT MEAT ONLY								
raw	1 lb	624	104.0	0.0	240	0	19.2	208
raw	1 oz	39	6.5	0.0	15	0	1.2	13
stewed	1 cup	298	46.3	0.0	81	0	11.2	98
stewed	4 oz	242	37.5	0.0	66	0	9.0	79
MEAT AND SKIN								
raw	1 lb	1168	80.0	0.0	320	0	92.8	320
raw	1 oz	73	5.0	0.0	20	0	5.8	20
stewed	4 oz	323	30.5	0.0	83	0	21.4	90
CHICKEN DINNER/ENTRÉE, CANNED								
(Featherweight) and dumplings	7.5 oz	160	12.0	18.0	115	(mq)	5.0	(mq)
(LaChoy)								
chow mein	3/4 cup	240	8.0	47.0	1420	1.0	2.0	19
chow mein 'Bi-Pack'	8.642 oz	97	7.7	9.5	1199	3.2	3.8	17
chow mein 'Bi-Pack'	3/4 cup	80	7.0	8.0	980	1.0	3.0	18
Oriental 'Bi-Pack'	3/4 cup	240	9.0	47.0	1400	1.0	2.0	(mq)
Oriental w/noodles 'Bi-Pack'	9 oz	160	10.6	23.0	1163	3.9	3.8	13
sweet and sour	3/4 cup	240	8.0	47.0	1420	1.0	2.0	19
sweet and sour 'Bi-Pack'	8.959 oz	161	7.6	28.6	745	3.3	2.5	18
sweet and sour 'Bi-Pack'	3/4 cup	120	7.0	18.0	440	2.0	2.0	13
teriyaki 'Bi-Pack'	8.642 oz	110	7.4	14.9	1226	2.9	3.0	15
teriyaki 'Bi-Pack'	3/4 cup	85	8.0	8.0	850	1.0	2.0	20
(Luck's) and dumplings	7.25 oz	240	16.0	18.0	605	(mq)	11.0	(mq)
(Swanson)								
à la king	5 1/4 oz	190	10.0	9.0	690	(mq)	12.0	(mq)
and dumplings	7.5 oz	220	11.0	19.0	980	(mq)	11.0	(mq)

Food Name	Serv. Size	Total Cal.	Prot. GMS	Carbs GMS	Sod. MGS	Fiber GMS	Fat GMS	Chol. MGS
CHICKEN DINNER/ENTRÉE, FROZEN								
(Armour)								
à la king 'Classics Lite'	11.25 oz	290	19.0	38.0	630	(mq)	7.0	55
and noodles 'Classics'	11 oz	230	19.0	23.0	660	(mq)	7.0	50
breast, Marsala 'Classics Lite'	10.5 oz	250	20.0	27.0	930	(mq)	7.0	80
Burgundy 'Classics Lite'	10 oz	210	23.0	25.0	780	(mq)	2.0	45
fettuccini 'Classics'	11 oz	260	17.0	28.0	660	(mq)	9.0	50
glazed 'Classics'	10.75 oz	300	15.0	24.0	960	(mq)	16.0	60
mesquite 'Classics'	9.5 oz	370	15.0	42.0	660	(mq)	16.0	55
Oriental 'Classics Lite'	10 oz	180	18.0	24.0	660	(mq)	1.0	35
parmigiana 'Classics'	11.5 oz	370	22.0	27.0	1060	(mq)	19.0	75
sweet and sour 'Classics Lite'	11 oz	240	18.0	39.0	820	(mq)	2.0	35
w/wine and mushroom sauce 'Classics'	10.75 oz	280	22.0	24.0	900	(mq)	11.0	50
(Banquet)								
à la king 'Cookin' Bags'	4 oz	110	8.0	9.0	na	na	5.0	(mq)
and dumplings	10 oz	430	17.0	34.0	940	(mq)	24.0	45
and dumplings 'Family Entrées'	7 oz	280	12.0	28.0	(mq)	(mq)	14.0	(mq)
drumsnackers 'Platters'	7 oz	430	20.0	49.0	690	(mq)	19.0	(mq)
fettuccini 'Healthy Balance'	11.25 oz	320	17.0	47.0	650	na	7.0	35
fried	10 oz	400	15.0	45.0	1100	(mq)	22.0	(mq)
fried 'Extra Helping'	16 oz	570	20.0	70.0	1470	(mq)	28.0	(mq)
fried, white meat 'Extra Helping'	16 oz	570	20.0	70.0	1470	(mq)	28.0	(mq)
fried, white meat 'Platter'	9 oz	430	38.0	21.0	(mq)	(mq)	22.0	105
fried, white meat, hot'n spicy 'Platter'	9 oz	430	38.0	21.0	(mq)	(mq)	22.0	105
hot'n spicy 'Snack'n'	3.75 oz	140	6.0	8.0	480	(mq)	9.0	(mq)
nuggets, breast, Southern fried w/barbecue sauce	4.5 oz	370	19.0	20.0	930	(mq)	23.0	(mq)
nuggets, hot'n spicy, w/barbecue sauce	4.5 oz	360	20.0	23.0	820	(mq)	21.0	(mq)
nuggets, 'Platters'	6.4 oz	430	17.0	46.0	630	(mq)	21.0	(mq)
nuggets, Southern fried, w/barbecue sauce	4.5 oz	370	19.0	20.0	930	(mq)	23.0	(mq)
nuggets, w/barbecue sauce 'Extra Helping'	10 oz	640	29.0	56.0	1390	(mq)	36.0	(mq)
nuggets, w/sweet and sour sauce 'Extra Helping'	10 oz	650	28.1	64.0	(mq)	(mq)	34.0	(mq)
nuggets, w/sweet and sour sauce 'Microwave'	4.5 oz	360	20.0	22.0	770	(mq)	21.0	(mq)
parmesan, w/vermicelli 'Healthy Balance'	10.8 oz	290	19.0	30.0	710	na	10.0	55
patties, breast, Southern fried, w/biscuit	4 oz	320	12.0	37.0	980	(mq)	14.0	(mq)
patties 'Platters'	7.5 oz	380	15.0	34.0	760	(mq)	21.0	(mq)
pie	7 oz	550	15.0	39.0	860	(mq)	36.0	35
pie 'Supreme Microwave'	7 oz	430	15.0	30.0	740	(mq)	28.0	40

Food Name	Serv. Size	Total Cal.	Prot. GMS	Carbs GMS	Sod. MGS	Fiber GMS	Fat GMS	Chol. MGS
primavera and vegetable 'Cookin' Bags'	4 oz	100	6.0	14.0	(mq)	(mq)	2.0	(mq)
primavera and vegetable 'Family Entrées'	7 oz	140	9.0	18.0	(mq)	(mq)	3.0	(mq)
sweet and sour 'Cookin' Bags'	4 oz	130	5.0	22.0	na	na	2.0	(mq)
(Budget Gourmet)								
and egg noodles, w/broccoli	10 oz	450	23.0	31.0	1110	(mq)	26.0	130
cacciatore	11 oz	300	20.0	27.0	810	(mq)	13.0	60
Marsala	10 oz	250	15.0	37.0	660	(mq)	5.0	65
Mexicana	12.8 oz	510	23.0	70.0	1210	(mq)	15.0	40
Oriental, and vegetables 'Light and Healthy'	9 oz	280	19.0	44.0	690	na	6.0	20
roast	11.2 oz	280	19.0	34.0	1110	(mq)	7.0	40
sweet and sour, w/rice	10 oz	350	18.0	53.0	640	(mq)	7.0	40
teriyaki	12 oz	360	20.0	44.0	610	(mq)	12.0	55
w/fettuccini	10 oz	400	23.0	29.0	740	(mq)	21.0	100
(Celentano)								
parmigiana	9 oz	330	32.0	15.0	560	(mq)	20.0	(mq)
primavera	11.5 oz	270	25.0	18.0	580	(mq)	10.0	(mq)
(Chun King)								
chow mein	13 oz	370	25.0	53.0	1560	(mq)	6.0	(mq)
imperial	13 oz	300	17.0	54.0	1540	(mq)	1.0	(mq)
walnut, crunchy	13 oz	310	16.0	49.0	1700	(mq)	5.0	(mq)
(Country Pride) primavera sticks	3 oz	240	10.0	16.0	400	(mq)	15.0	(mq)
(Dining Lite)								
à la king	9 oz	240	14.0	30.0	780	(mq)	7.0	40
and noodles	9 oz	240	17.0	28.0	570	(mq)	7.0	50
chow mein	9 oz	180	10.0	31.0	650	(mq)	2.0	30
glazed	9 oz	220	17.0	30.0	680	(mq)	4.0	45
(Freezer Queen)								
à la king 'Cook-In-Pouch'	4 oz	70	9.0	6.0	460	na	1.0	(mq)
à la king, w/rice 'Single Serve'	9 oz	270	20.0	37.0	520	(mq)	5.0	(mq)
cacciatore 'Single Serve'	9 oz	270	20.0	33.0	710	(mq)	6.0	(mq)
croquettes, breaded, w/gravy 'Family Suppers'	7 oz	240	12.0	20.0	1000	(mq)	12.0	(mq)
nuggets 'Deluxe Family Suppers'	3 oz	270	14.0	15.0	770	(mq)	17.0	(mq)
nuggets platter	6 oz	410	14.0	36.0	950	(mq)	23.0	(mq)
pattie 'Platter'	7.5 oz	360	17.0	33.0	1160	(mq)	17.0	(mq)
primavera, sliced, w/gravy 'Cook-In-Pouch'	5 oz	80	7.0	6.0	820	na	3.0	(mq)
sweet and sour, w/rice 'Single Serve'	9 oz	300	20.0	48.0	700	(mq)	4.0	(mq)
(Green Giant) and broccoli 'Entrées'	9.5 oz	340	23.0	28.0	890	(mq)	15.0	(mq)
(Healthy Choice)								
à l'orange	9 oz	260	23.0	38.0	340	na	2.0	40
and pasta divan	11.5 oz	300	25.0	41.0	520	na	4.0	50
and vegetables	11.5 oz	210	20.0	31.0	490	na	1.0	35

Food Name	Serv. Size	Total Cal.	Prot. GMS	Carbs GMS	Sod. MGS	Fiber GMS	Fat GMS	Chol. MGS
breast, glazed	8.5 oz	220	21.0	27.0	510	na	3.0	45
cacciatore 'Classics'	12.5 oz	310	26.0	47.0	430	na	3.0	35
chow mein	9 oz	240	20.0	29.0	530	na	5.0	45
chow mein, low fat, low cholesterol	9 oz	240	20.0	29.0	530	na	5.0	45
Dijon	11 oz	260	22.0	38.0	420	na	3.0	45
herb roasted	11 oz	380	26.0	56.0	470	na	7.0	60
honey mustard, low fat, low cholesterol	9.5 oz	250	24.0	37.0	480	na	3.0	40
Mandarin	10 oz	240	21.0	35.0	370	na	2.0	45
mesquite	10.5 oz	300	21.0	54.0	390	na	3.0	40
Oriental	11.25 oz	200	19.0	32.0	440	na	1.0	35
parmigiana	11.5 oz	290	23.0	41.0	340	na	6.0	55
roasted	12.3 oz	290	25.0	39.0	430	na	4.0	50
'Salsa Chicken Dinner'	11.25 oz	240	20.0	36.0	450	na	2.0	50
southwestern style, low fat, low cholesterol	12.5 oz	340	25.0	51.0	550	na	5.0	60
stir fry, w/vermicelli 'Extra Portion'	12 oz	300	23.0	42.0	550	na	5.0	30
sweet and sour	11.5 oz	280	20.0	52.0	320	na	2.0	35
teriyaki, low fat, low cholesterol	12.25 oz	290	24.0	39.0	560	na	4.0	55
w/barbecue sauce, low fat, low cholesterol	12.75 oz	410	24.0	65.0	550	na	6.0	55
(Hot Bites)								
drumsnackers	2.63 oz	220	10.0	13.0	530	(mq)	15.0	(mq)
nuggets	2.63 oz	210	11.0	11.0	550	(mq)	14.0	(mq)
nuggets, hot'n spicy	2.63 oz	250	10.0	10.0	380	(mq)	19.0	(mq)
nuggets, Southern fried	2.63 oz	220	10.0	13.0	530	(mq)	14.0	(mq)
nuggets, w/cheddar	2.63 oz	250	11.0	11.0	560	(mq)	18.0	(mq)
primavera sticks	2.63 oz	220	10.0	11.0	350	(mq)	15.0	(mq)
tenders, breast	2.25 oz	150	11.0	12.0	280	(mq)	6.0	(mq)
tenders, breast 'Microwave'	4 oz	260	19.0	24.0	560	(mq)	10.0	(mq)
(Kid Cuisine)								
fried	7.25 oz	420	15.0	41.0	1050	(mq)	22.0	(mq)
fried 'Mega Meal'	10.8 oz	720	34.0	53.0	1400	na	41.0	na
nuggets	6.25 oz	400	11.0	46.0	610	(mq)	19.0	60
nuggets 'Mega Meal'	8.4 oz	470	21.0	51.0	1010	na	20.0	na
(LaChoy)								
almond, w/rice and vegetables 'Fresh & Lite'	9.75 oz	270	14.0	40.1	1092	3.0	8.0	42
imperial, w/rice 'Fresh & Lite'	11 oz	260	13.0	45.0	1269	3.1	6.0	46
Oriental, spicy 'Fresh & Lite'	9.75 oz	270	11.0	52.0	560	4.0	4.0	42
sweet and sour, w/rice and vegetables 'Fresh & Lite'	10 oz	260	13.0	50.1	601	3.7	3.0	53
(LeMenu)								
à la king	10.25 oz	330	23.0	29.0	830	(mq)	13.0	(mq)

Food Name	Serv. Size	Total Cal.	Prot. GMS	Carbs GMS	Sod. MGS	Fiber GMS	Fat GMS	Chol. MGS
à la king, w/seasoned rice 'LightStyle'	8.25 oz	240	19.0	29.0	670	(mq)	5.0	30
breast, glazed 'LightStyle'	10 oz	230	25.0	25.0	430	(mq)	3.0	55
breast, herb roasted, w/rice and vegetables	7.75 oz	260	22.0	29.0	500	(mq)	6.0	45
cordon bleu	11 oz	460	23.0	47.0	850	(mq)	20.0	(mq)
Dijon, w/pasta and vegetables 'LightStyle'	8.5 oz	240	22.0	21.0	500	(mq)	7.0	40
empress, w/seasoned rice 'LightStyle'	8.25 oz	210	16.0	26.0	690	(mq)	5.0	30
herb-roasted 'LightStyle'	10 oz	240	27.0	18.0	400	(mq)	7.0	70
in wine sauce	10 oz	280	26.0	27.0	680	(mq)	7.0	(mq)
Kiev	8 oz	530	20.0	24.0	780	(mq)	39.0	(mq)
parmigiana	11.75 oz	410	26.0	31.0	1030	(mq)	20.0	(mq)
sweet and sour	11.25 oz	400	19.0	41.0	1020	(mq)	18.0	(mq)
sweet and sour 'LightStyle'	10 oz	250	18.0	29.0	530	(mq)	7.0	2
(Mrs. Paterson's) 'Aussie Pie'	5.5 oz	440	13.0	43.0	760	na	24.0	80
(Myers)								
à la gratin	3.5 oz	129	9.0	9.0	276	(mq)	7.0	(mq)
à la king	3.5 oz	137	9.0	6.0	357	na	9.0	(mq)
and noodles	3.5 oz	136	8.0	9.0	399	(mq)	8.0	(mq)
creamed	3.5 oz	151	12.0	5.0	372	na	10.0	(mq)
croquettes	3.5 oz	168	16.0	10.0	364	na	7.0	(mq)
pie	3.5 oz	129	7.0	10.0	253	(mq)	7.0	(mq)
(Pilgrim's Pride) Cajun style	3 oz	241	13.3	8.6	480	(mq)	17.0	51
(Pillsbury)								
and cheese casserole 'Microwave Classic'	1 pkg	480	21.0	33.0	940	(mq)	29.0	(mq)
casserole 'Microwave Classic'	1 pkg	400	21.0	30.0	890	(mq)	22.0	(mq)
(Right Course)								
Italiano, w/fettuccini and vegetables	9 5/8 oz	280	24.0	29.0	560	(mq)	8.0	45
sesame primavera	10 oz	320	25.0	34.0	590	(mq)	9.0	50
tenderloins in barbecue sauce	8.75 oz	270	20.0	35.0	590	(mq)	6.0	40
tenderloins in peanut sauce	9.25 oz	330	27.0	32.0	570	(mq)	10.0	50
(Shanghai) stir fry	10.3 oz	190	22.0	19.0	1220	na	3.0	30
(Smart Ones)								
a l'orange	8 oz	190	12.0	34.0	530	na	<1.0	15
chow mein	9 oz	170	14.0	27.0	470	na	1.0	20
fiesta, w/Spanish rice	8 oz	210	14.0	37.0	390	na	1.0	20
Francais, w/garlic vegetables	8.5 oz	150	15.0	18.0	400	na	1.0	5
grilled, glazed, and sauce	8 oz	130	12.0	17.0	540	na	1.0	20
honey mustard, and sauce	7.5 oz	140	11.0	20.0	220	na	1.0	10
Mirabella	9.2 oz	160	13.0	26.0	420	na	1.0	10
piccata, lemon herb	7.5 oz	160	13.0	25.0	500	na	1.0	5
(Stouffer's)								
à la king, w/rice	9.5 oz	270	18.0	38.0	800	na	5.0	na

Food Name	Serv. Size	Total Cal.	Prot. GMS	Carbs GMS	Sod. MGS	Fiber GMS	Fat GMS	Chol. MGS
a l'orange, w/almond rice, 'Lean Cuisine' ..	8 oz	280	27.0	33.0	290	na	4.0	55
and noodles, homestyle	10 oz	290	22.0	21.0	1040	na	13.0	na
and vegetables, w/vermicelli 'Lean Cuisine'	11.75 oz	240	18.0	30.0	500	na	5.0	30
breaded, baked, w/parsleyed potatoes and vegetables, 'Lean Cuisine'	8 oz	200	17.0	21.0	480	na	5.0	35
breast, baked, in gravy, w/potato, homestyle	8 7/8 oz	250	22.0	18.0	550	na	10.0	na
breast, fried, and whipped potatoes, homestyle	7 1/8 oz	350	17.0	30.0	900	na	18.0	na
breast, grilled, in barbecue sauce, homestyle	7 5/8 oz	210	23.0	14.0	550	na	7.0	na
breast, Marsala, w/vegetables, 'Lean Cuisine'	8 1/8 oz	180	22.0	13.0	430	na	4.0	55
breast, Parmesan, w/rib meat, 'Lean Cuisine'	10 7/8 oz	260	24.0	25.0	580	na	7.0	60
cacciatore, w/vermicelli, 'Lean Cuisine'	10 7/8 oz	280	22.0	31.0	570	na	7.0	45
chow mein, w/rice	10.75 oz	250	13.0	39.0	720	na	5.0	na
chow mein, w/rice, 'Lean Cuisine'	9 oz	240	14.0	34.0	530	na	5.0	30
creamed	6.5 oz	300	19.0	8.0	690	na	21.0	(mq)
divan	8 oz	220	24.0	11.0	610	na	10.0	na
escalloped, and noodles	10 oz	420	21.0	30.0	840	na	24.0	na
fettuccini, 'Lean Cuisine'	9 oz	280	23.0	33.0	500	na	6.0	35
fettuccini, w/vegetable medley, homestyle	9.5 oz	350	23.0	27.0	780	na	17.0	na
fiesta, 'Lean Cuisine'	8.5 oz	240	19.0	30.0	560	na	5.0	40
glazed, w/vegetable rice, 'Lean Cuisine' .	8.5 oz	250	21.0	24.0	590	na	7.0	50
honey mustard, 'Lean Cuisine'	7.5 oz	230	18.0	30.0	540	na	4.0	40
in barbecue sauce, w/rice pilaf, 'Lean Cuisine'	8.75 oz	260	20.0	32.0	500	na	6.0	50
Italiano, w/fettuccini 'Lean Cuisine'	9 oz	270	22.0	33.0	590	na	6.0	40
Oriental, w/vermicelli, 'Lean Cuisine'	9 oz	280	22.0	31.0	480	na	7.0	35
parmigiana and pasta Alfredo, homestyle	9 7/8 oz	360	31.0	24.0	990	na	15.0	na
pie	10 oz	440	16.0	32.0	750	na	27.0	na
sweet-n-sour, w/rice, 'Lean Cuisine'	9 oz	280	17.0	39.0	490	na	6.0	50
tenderloins in herb sauce, 'Lean Cuisine'	9.5 oz	240	29.0	19.0	490	na	5.0	60
tenderloins in peanut sauce, 'Lean Cuisine'	9 oz	290	23.0	33.0	530	na	7.0	45
tenders, breaded, w/potatoes, homestyle	8 3/8 oz	430	20.0	46.0	950	na	18.0	na
(Swanson) boneless 'Hungry Man'	17.75 oz	700	48.0	65.0	1530	(mq)	28.0	(mq)

Food Name	Serv. Size	Total Cal.	Prot. GMS	Carbs GMS	Sod. MGS	Fiber GMS	Fat GMS	Chol. MGS
cacciatore 'Homestyle Recipe'	10.95 oz	260	15.0	33.0	1030	(mq)	8.0	(mq)
fried, barbecue flavored	10 oz	540	25.0	61.0	1160	(mq)	22.0	(mq)
fried, dark meat	9.75 oz	560	22.0	55.0	1130	(mq)	28.0	(mq)
fried, dark meat 'Hungry Man'	1 pkg	860	36.0	77.0	1660	(mq)	45.0	(mq)
fried, white meat	10.25 oz	550	22.0	60.0	1460	(mq)	25.0	(mq)
fried, white meat 'Hungry Man'	1 pkg	870	35.0	80.0	2150	(mq)	46.0	(mq)
grilled, white meat in garlic sauce, almonds	10 oz	310	17.0	39.0	630	na	9.0	30
nibbles 'Homestyle Recipe'	4.25 oz	340	10.0	29.0	730	(mq)	20.0	(mq)
nibbles 'Plump & Juicy'	3.25 oz	300	12.0	19.0	690	(mq)	19.0	(mq)
nuggets	8.75 oz	470	19.0	47.0	650	(mq)	23.0	(mq)
nuggets 'Plump & Juicy'	3 oz	230	13.0	14.0	360	(mq)	14.0	(mq)
parmigiana 'Budget'	10 oz	300	7.0	35.0	780	na	15.0	na
pie 'Homestyle Recipe'	8 oz	410	15.0	41.0	1030	(mq)	21.0	(mq)
pie 'Hungry Man'	16 oz	630	22.0	57.0	1600	(mq)	35.0	(mq)
thighs/drumsticks 'Plump & Juicy'	3.25 oz	290	15.0	17.0	610	(mq)	18.0	(mq)
(Swift)								
cordon bleu 'International'	6 oz	360	30.0	23.0	1010	(mq)	17.0	(mq)
Kiev 'International'	6 oz	420	27.0	22.0	1030	(mq)	24.0	(mq)
(Tyson)								
a l'orange 'Gourmet Selection'	9.5 oz	300	21.0	36.0	670	(mq)	8.0	(mq)
and beef luau 'Gourmet Selection'	10.5 oz	330	18.0	42.0	1030	(mq)	10.0	(mq)
'Barbecue Chicken Meal'	12.5 oz	400	27.0	56.0	600	na	8.0	50
breast, boneless, barbecue marinated	3.75 oz	120	22.0	5.0	400	na	3.0	(mq)
breast, boneless, butter garlic marinated	3.75 oz	160	21.0	3.0	320	na	7.0	(mq)
breast, boneless, Italian marinated	3.75 oz	130	22.0	6.0	320	na	2.0	(mq)
breast, boneless, lemon pepper marinated	3.75 oz	120	22.0	4.0	210	na	2.0	(mq)
breast, boneless, teriyaki marinated	3.75 oz	130	22.0	6.0	290	na	2.0	(mq)
breast strips, Oriental, boneless	2.75 oz	110	14.0	6.0	250	na	3.0	40
'Chick'n Cheddar'	2.6 oz	220	11.0	11.0	310	(mq)	15.0	40
'Chick'n Chunks'	2.6 oz	220	10.0	11.0	500	(mq)	15.0	35
'Chick'n Chunks' Southern fried	2.6 oz	220	10.0	11.0	540	(mq)	15.0	35
'Chicken Marinara Meal'	13.75 oz	340	31.0	37.0	590	na	7.0	45
'Classic Colonial' wholesale club item	3.5 oz	180	13.0	11.0	190	na	9.0	40
'Cordon Bleu' wholesale club item	7 oz	480	40.0	28.0	1030	na	22.0	na
'Cordon Bleu' wholesale club item	5 oz	340	28.0	20.0	740	na	16.0	na
Dijon 'Gourmet Selection'	8.5 oz	310	17.0	22.0	840	(mq)	17.0	(mq)
Français 'Gourmet Selection'	9.5 oz	280	19.0	20.0	1130	(mq)	14.0	(mq)
glazed, w/sauce 'Gourmet Selections'	9.25 oz	240	22.0	29.0	930	na	4.0	44
grilled, 'Gourmet Selections'	7.75 oz	220	26.0	22.0	520	na	3.0	55
grilled, Italian 'Gourmet Selections'	9 oz	210	28.0	19.0	420	na	3.0	40
'Herb Chicken Meal'	13.75 oz	340	32.0	43.0	550	na	4.0	50

Food Name	Serv. Size	Total Cal.	Prot. GMS	Carbs GMS	Sod. MGS	Fiber GMS	Fat GMS	Chol. MGS
'Honey Mustard Chicken Meal'	13.75 oz	390	31.0	52.0	520	na	6.0	50
honey roasted 'Gourmet Selections'	9 oz	220	26.0	23.0	500	na	4.0	48
'Italian Style Chicken Meal'	13.75 oz	310	30.0	38.0	600	na	4.0	50
Kiev 'Gourmet Selection'	9.25 oz	520	16.0	40.0	1200	(mq)	33.0	(mq)
'Looney Tunes Bugs Bunny' chunks	7.7 oz	290	17.0	31.0	480	na	11.0	28
'Looney Tunes Road Runner'	6.7 oz	300	8.0	42.0	490	na	11.0	24
'Looney Tunes Tazmanian Devil' drummettes	8 oz	310	14.0	31.0	480	na	14.0	40
'Looney Tunes Yosemite Sam' barbecue glazed	7.38 oz	230	12.0	28.0	510	na	8.0	45
Marsala 'Gourmet Selection'	10.5 oz	300	19.0	26.0	900	(mq)	13.0	(mq)
mesquite breast tenders, boneless	2.75 oz	110	17.0	4.0	420	na	3.0	45
'Mesquite Chicken Meal'	13.25 oz	330	34.0	38.0	600	na	5.0	45
mesquite 'Gourmet Selections'	9 oz	320	23.0	39.0	660	na	8.0	55
'Mini Cordon Bleu' wholesale club item	1 piece	90	8.0	5.0	210	na	4.0	17
nuggets 'Microwave'	3.5 oz	220	10.0	11.0	(mq)	(mq)	15.0	(mq)
Oriental 'Gourmet Selection'	10.25 oz	270	20.0	32.0	1140	(mq)	7.0	(mq)
parmigiana 'Gourmet Selection'	11.25 oz	380	19.0	37.0	1100	(mq)	17.0	(mq)
piccata 'Gourmet Selection'	9 oz	240	19.0	19.0	680	(mq)	10.0	(mq)
pie, premium	9 oz	390	16.0	36.0	1065	na	20.0	43
pie, white meat, premium	9 oz	400	22.0	33.0	783	na	20.0	56
roasted 'Gourmet Selections'	9 oz	200	21.0	21.0	430	na	2.0	42
'Salsa Chicken Meal'	13.75 oz	370	34.0	52.0	470	na	6.0	45
'Sesame Chicken Meal'	13.5 oz	400	27.0	59.0	450	na	6.0	45
sesame 'Healthy Portions'	13.5 oz	390	27.0	58.0	410	na	5.0	45
stir fry w/vegetables, wholesale club item	3.5 oz	130	11.0	13.0	710	na	5.0	45
supreme 'Gourmet Selections'	9 oz	230	21.0	23.0	480	na	6.0	51
sweet and sour 'Gourmet Selection'	11 oz	420	22.0	50.0	850	na	15.0	(mq)
tenders 'Microwave'	3.5 oz	230	16.0	19.0	(mq)	(mq)	11.0	(mq)
'Wings of Fire' wholesale club item	3.5 oz	220	26.0	2.0	390	na	12.0	105
(Ultimate 200)								
barbecue, glazed, w/vegetables	7 oz	200	19.0	22.0	450	na	6.0	30
cordon bleu, w/vegetables	7.7 oz	170	19.0	15.0	560	na	5.0	40
grilled, glazed	7.5 oz	150	15.0	17.0	520	na	2.0	20
imperial	8.5 oz	200	18.0	25.0	430	na	3.0	25
Kiev, w/vegetables and rice	7 oz	190	14.0	22.0	470	na	5.0	15
patty, Southern baked, w/vegetables	6.3 oz	170	17.0	10.0	520	na	7.0	45
teriyaki	7.6 oz	150	21.0	7.0	590	na	4.0	50
(Weaver)								
batter-dipped, assorted pieces	3.6 oz	290	16.0	16.0	550	na	18.0	na
crispy, light, skinless	2.9 oz	170	14.0	9.0	320	na	9.0	na
'Crispy Dutch Frye' assorted pieces	3.6 oz	290	16.0	16.0	550	na	18.0	na
'Crispy Dutch Frye' breast	4.5 oz	350	22.0	17.0	520	na	22.0	na

Food Name	Serv. Size	Total Cal.	Prot. GMS	Carbs GMS	Sod. MGS	Fiber GMS	Fat GMS	Chol. MGS
crispy mini drums	3 oz	210	13.0	13.0	480	na	12.0	na
croquettes	2 pieces	280	14.0	22.0	780	na	16.0	na
mini drums, herb and spice	3 oz	200	13.0	13.0	320	na	11.0	na
'Rondolet, Cheese'	2.6 oz	190	11.0	12.0	520	na	11.0	na
'Rondolet, Italian'	2.6 oz	190	11.0	11.0	560	na	11.0	na
'Rondolet, Original'	3 oz	190	13.0	13.0	610	na	10.0	na
'Tenders, Honey Batter'	3 oz	220	13.0	14.0	500	na	12.0	na
'Tenders, Premium'	3 oz	170	12.0	11.0	500	na	9.0	na
(Weight Watchers)								
fettuccini, w/Parmesan sauce	8.25 oz	280	22.0	25.0	590	na	9.0	40
ginger, w/vegetable, Hunan 'Stir Fry'	9 oz	160	15.0	21.0	430	na	2.0	15
grilled, Suiza, w/Spanish rice 'Mexican Style'	8.6 oz	220	21.0	18.0	590	na	7.0	60
orange glazed, w/rice 'Stir Fry'	9 oz	170	14.0	25.0	360	na	2.0	10
Polynesian 'Stir Fry'	9 oz	190	12.0	34.0	240	na	1.0	20
sesame, w/lo mein noodles 'Stir Fry'	9 oz	200	19.0	23.0	420	na	4.0	10
teriyaki, w/spring vegetables 'Stir Fry'	9 oz	140	13.0	16.0	470	na	3.0	20
'Tex Mex' w/Spanish rice 'Mexican Style'	8.3 oz	250	18.0	33.0	590	na	5.0	35

CHICKEN DINNER/ENTRÉE, PACKAGED

Food Name	Serv. Size	Total Cal.	Prot. GMS	Carbs GMS	Sod. MGS	Fiber GMS	Fat GMS	Chol. MGS
(Chicken By George)								
Cajun	5 oz	180	25.0	4.0	890	na	8.0	80
Caribbean grill	5 oz	200	25.0	10.0	610	na	6.0	80
Italian blue cheese	5 oz	180	26.0	2.0	890	na	8.0	85
lemon herb	5 oz	170	24.0	6.0	870	na	6.0	70
lemon oregano	5 oz	160	26.0	4.0	580	na	4.0	75
mesquite barbecue	5 oz	170	25.0	6.0	790	na	6.0	70
mustard dill	5 oz	180	26.0	3.0	640	na	7.0	80
roasted	5 oz	150	26.0	2.0	710	na	4.0	70
teriyaki	5 oz	180	25.0	9.0	740	na	5.0	70
tomato herb, w/basil	5 oz	190	25.0	7.0	800	na	7.0	80
(Chicken Helper) 'Skillet Dinner'								
cheesy broccoli, dry	1/5 pkg	160	4.0	32.0	700	na	2.0	5
cheesy broccoli, prepared	7 oz	310	24.0	34.0	790	na	9.0	65
creamy chicken, dry	1/5 pkg	170	6.0	26.0	720	na	5.0	40
creamy chicken, prepared	8.25 oz	330	26.0	29.0	820	na	13.0	100
creamy mushroom, dry	1/5 pkg	170	5.0	28.0	720	na	4.0	30
creamy mushroom, prepared	8 oz	320	25.0	31.0	810	na	11.0	90
fettuccini Alfredo, dry	1/5 pkg	160	6.0	25.0	690	na	4.0	10
fettuccini Alfredo, prepared	7.5 oz	320	26.0	27.0	780	na	12.0	70
stir fry, dry	1/5 pkg	170	4.0	36.0	800	na	<1.0	0
stir fry, prepared	7 oz	370	25.0	36.0	950	na	14.0	145
(Dinty Moore) and dumplings, microwave cup	7.5 oz	190	15.0	20.0	680	na	6.0	30

Food Name	Serv. Size	Total Cal.	Prot. GMS	Carbs GMS	Sod. MGS	Fiber GMS	Fat GMS	Chol. MGS
(LaChoy)								
sweet and sour, 'Dinner Classics'								
prepared	3/4 cup	310	32.0	30.0	860	<1.0	6.0	50
sweet and sour, w/noodles	9.383 oz	256	9.4	49.4	697	1.8	3.1	10
(Libby's)								
chow mein 'Diner' microwave cup	7.75 oz	130	5.0	19.0	830	2.4	4.0	10
w/pasta spirals 'Diner' microwave cup	7.75 oz	120	8.0	16.0	910	2.2	3.0	15
(Lipton) 'Microeasy'								
barbecue style, dry	1/4 pkg	110	2.0	24.0	980	(mq)	<1.0	na
barbecue style, prepared	1/4 pkg	220	16.0	24.0	1020	(mq)	6.0	(mq)
country style, dry	1/4 pkg	80	3.0	15.0	840	(mq)	<1.0	na
country style, prepared	1/4 pkg	190	18.0	15.0	880	(mq)	6.0	(mq)
(Lunch Bucket)								
and dumplings, microwave cup	7.5 oz	140	4.0	25.0	880	na	2.0	na
w/beans and rice 'Light'n Healthy'								
micro cup	7.5 oz	170	7.0	28.0	600	na	3.0	10
(Top Shelf)								
à la king	10 oz	360	18.0	49.0	890	na	10.0	37
Acapulco	1 serving	390	28.0	41.0	1320	(mq)	13.0	55
breast, glazed	10 oz	170	19.0	19.0	780	na	2.0	35
breast, w/Spanish rice	10 oz	400	27.0	38.0	810	na	15.0	75
'Cacciatore'	10 oz	210	21.0	25.0	810	na	3.0	50
sweet and sour	1 serving	270	24.0	41.0	280	(mq)	1.0	60
(Ultra Slim Fast)								
and vegetables	12 oz	290	24.0	45.0	850	na	3.0	30
chow mein	12 oz	320	25.0	43.0	580	na	6.0	60
fettuccini	12 oz	390	31.0	38.0	980	na	12.0	65
mesquite	12 oz	350	29.0	61.0	300	na	1.0	65
roasted, in mushroom sauce	12 oz	280	25.0	30.0	830	na	6.0	55
sweet and sour	12 oz	330	20.0	57.0	340	na	2.0	45
CHICKEN ENTRÉE, ALTERNATIVE								
(Worthington) pie, frozen	8 oz	380	7.0	43.0	1200	(mq)	20.0	0
CHICKEN FAT								
	1 cup	1846	0.0	0.0	0	0	204.6	174
	1 oz	178	1.1	0.0	9	0	19.3	16
	1 tbsp	115	0.0	0.0	0	0	12.8	11
CHICKEN FRYING MIX, dry mix *(Golden Dipt)*	1 oz	90	2.0	20.0	1430	(mq)	0.0	0
CHICKEN GIBLETS								
fried	1 cup	402	47.2	6.3	164	0	19.5	647
simmered	1 cup	228	37.5	1.4	84	0	6.9	570
CHICKEN GIZZARD								
all classes, simmered	1 cup	222	39.4	1.6	97	0	5.3	281
broiler-fryer, raw, approx 1.3 oz	1 med	44	6.7	0.2	28	0	1.6	48

Food Name	Serv. Size	Total Cal.	Prot. GMS	Carbs GMS	Sod. MGS	Fiber GMS	Fat GMS	Chol. MGS
broiler-fryer, simmered, approx .8 oz ... 1 med	34	6.0	0.3	15	0	0.8	43

CHICKEN HEART

Food Name	Serv. Size	Total Cal.	Prot. GMS	Carbs GMS	Sod. MGS	Fiber GMS	Fat GMS	Chol. MGS
all classes, simmered	1 cup	268	38.3	0.2	70	0	11.5	351
broiler-fryer, raw, 1 heart	2 oz	9	1.0	<.1	5	0	0.6	8
broiler-fryer, simmered	4 oz	210	29.9	0.1	54	0	9.0	275

CHICKEN LIVER

Food Name	Serv. Size	Total Cal.	Prot. GMS	Carbs GMS	Sod. MGS	Fiber GMS	Fat GMS	Chol. MGS
all classes, simmered	1 cup	220	34.1	1.2	71	0	7.6	883
broiler-fryer, chopped, simmered	1 cup	219	34.1	1.2	71	0	7.6	883
broiler-fryer, raw, approx 1.1 oz	1 liver	40	5.8	1.1	25	0	1.2	140
broiler-fryer, simmered	4 oz	178	27.6	1.0	58	0	6.2	716
CHICKEN POT PIE (Swanson), frozen	7 oz	380	11.0	35.0	760	(mq)	22.0	(mq)

CHICKEN SALAD

Food Name	Serv. Size	Total Cal.	Prot. GMS	Carbs GMS	Sod. MGS	Fiber GMS	Fat GMS	Chol. MGS
(Longacre)	1 oz	64	3.0	3.0	110	na	5.0	15
(Longacre) 'Saladfest'	1 oz	47	4.0	1.0	150	na	3.0	15

CHICKEN SALAD SPREAD, 'Spreadables'

Food Name	Serv. Size	Total Cal.	Prot. GMS	Carbs GMS	Sod. MGS	Fiber GMS	Fat GMS	Chol. MGS
(Libby's)	1.9 oz	90	5.0	5.0	230	1.9	6.0	15

CHICKEN SEASONING MIX

Food Name	Serv. Size	Total Cal.	Prot. GMS	Carbs GMS	Sod. MGS	Fiber GMS	Fat GMS	Chol. MGS
(Featherweight) dry mix	1/4 pkg	18	1.0	8.0	30	(mq)	0.0	0
(Schilling) 'Bag 'n Season'	1 pkg	134	3.0	19.0	4771	na	5.0	1
(Schilling) dry mix, for fried chicken	1/4 tsp	1	0.1	0.2	132	na	<.1	na

CHICKEN SPREAD, CANNED

Food Name	Serv. Size	Total Cal.	Prot. GMS	Carbs GMS	Sod. MGS	Fiber GMS	Fat GMS	Chol. MGS
(Hormel)	.5 oz	30	2.0	0.0	(mq)	0	2.0	(mq)
(Underwood) chunky	2 1/8 oz	150	10.0	2.0	440	na	9.0	40
(Underwood) 'Light'	2 1/8 oz	80	11.0	2.0	330	na	3.0	30
(Underwood) smoky	2 1/8 oz	150	10.0	10.0	290	na	8.0	40

CHICKEN STEW

Food Name	Serv. Size	Total Cal.	Prot. GMS	Carbs GMS	Sod. MGS	Fiber GMS	Fat GMS	Chol. MGS
(Dinty Moore) canned	7.5 oz	260	11.0	15.0	850	na	18.0	80
(Dinty Moore) microwave cup	7.5 oz	260	11.0	15.0	850	na	18.0	80
(Featherweight) w/wild rice, canned	7.5 oz	140	10.0	23.0	400	(mq)	1.0	20
(Heinz) w/dumplings, canned	7.5 oz	210	9.0	22.0	850	(mq)	9.0	(mq)
(Mountain House) freeze-dried, prepared	1 cup	230	9.0	30.0	209	(mq)	8.0	(mq)
(Swanson) canned	7 5/8 oz	160	9.0	15.0	990	(mq)	7.0	(mq)

CHICORY, WITLOOF

Food Name	Serv. Size	Total Cal.	Prot. GMS	Carbs GMS	Sod. MGS	Fiber GMS	Fat GMS	Chol. MGS
raw	1/2 cup	8	0.4	1.8	1	1.4	0.0	0
raw, approx 2.1 oz	1 head	9	0.5	2.1	1	1.6	0.1	0
trimmed	1 oz	4	0.3	0.9	2	(mq)	<.1	0
untrimmed	1 lb	61	4.0	12.9	28	(mq)	0.4	0

CHICORY GREENS

Food Name	Serv. Size	Total Cal.	Prot. GMS	Carbs GMS	Sod. MGS	Fiber GMS	Fat GMS	Chol. MGS
trimmed	1 oz	7	0.5	1.3	13	(mq)	0.1	0
trimmed, chopped	1/2 cup	21	1.5	4.2	41	3.6	0.3	0
untrimmed	1 lb	87	6.3	17.5	167	(mq)	1.1	0

CHICORY ROOT

Food Name	Serv. Size	Total Cal.	Prot. GMS	Carbs GMS	Sod. MGS	Fiber GMS	Fat GMS	Chol. MGS
raw, approx 2.6 oz	1 root	44	0.8	10.5	30	>1.2 c	0.1	0

Food Name	Serv. Size	Total Cal.	Prot. GMS	Carbs GMS	Sod. MGS	Fiber GMS	Fat GMS	Chol. MGS
raw, 1-inch pieces	1/2 cup	33	0.6	7.9	23	>.9 c	0.1	0
trimmed	1 oz	21	0.4	5.0	14	>.6 c	0.1	0
untrimmed	1 lb	272	5.2	65.1	186	>7.3 c	0.7	0
CHILI, CANNED								
beef, w/beans *(Cimmaron)*	7.5 oz	230	17.0	21.0	na	na	9.0	35
chicken, w/beans *(Cimmaron)*	7.5 oz	180	12.0	22.0	970	na	5.0	60
chicken, w/beans *(Stagg)*	7.5 oz	200	14.0	21.0	na	na	6.0	na
'Chili Con Carne' *(Heinz)*	7.75 oz	350	15.0	27.0	1000	(mq)	21.0	(mq)
'Chili Mac' *(Chef Boyardee)*	7.5 oz	230	8.0	26.0	1410	(mq)	11.0	(mq)
'Chili Mac' *(Heinz)*	7.5 oz	250	10.0	26.0	860	(mq)	12.0	(mq)
country, w/beans *(Stagg)*	7.5 oz	270	14.0	25.0	na	na	12.0	na
plain *(Gebhardt)*	1 cup	530	21.0	20.0	990	1.0	41.0	150
vegetarian *(Gebhardt)*	4 oz	219	9.6	6.9	555	(mq)	17.1	0
vegetarian *(Worthington)*	2/3 cup	190	10.0	15.0	550	(mq)	10.0	0
vegetarian, plain *(Gebhardt)*	4.339 oz	232	7.3	11.1	736	3.1	18.5	42
vegetarian, plain *(Open Range)*	4.409 oz	176	8.8	9.4	608	2.8	12.8	24
vegetarian, spicy *(Hain)*	7.5 oz	160	7.0	29.0	1060	(mq)	1.0	0
vegetarian, spicy *(Hain)* 'Reduced Sodium'	7.5 oz	170	7.0	31.0	200	(mq)	1.0	0
vegetarian, spicy *(Natural Touch)*	2/3 cup	230	12.0	19.0	890	(mq)	12.0	0
vegetarian, 3-bean, mild, fat-free *(Health Valley)*	5 oz	90	10.0	12.0	180	9.0	0.0	0
vegetarian, w/beans *(Gebhardt)*	4.444 oz	195	7.4	18.3	694	4.8	12.0	23
vegetarian, w/beans *(Just Rite)*	4.55 oz	190	8.8	15.3	616	6.0	13.3	18
vegetarian, w/beans *(Open Range)*	4.5 oz	136	8.6	12.6	645	5.2	8.0	13
vegetarian, w/beans, 'Longhorn' *(Gebhardt)*	4.55 oz	225	9.1	16.0	545	4.1	15.7	16
vegetarian, w/beans, mild *(Health Valley)*	4 oz	130	8.0	16.0	730	8.2	3.0	0
vegetarian, w/beans, mild *(Health Valley)* 'No Salt Added'	4 oz	130	8.0	16.0	25	8.2	3.0	0
vegetarian, w/beans, spicy *(Health Valley)*	4 oz	130	8.0	16.0	430	8.2	3.0	0
vegetarian, w/beans, spicy *(Health Valley)* 'No Salt Added'	4 oz	130	8.0	16.0	25	8.2	3.0	0
vegetarian, w/black beans, mild, fat-free *(Health Valley)*	5 oz	140	11.0	23.0	290	12.2	0.0	0
vegetarian, w/black beans, spicy, fat-free *(Health Valley)*	5 oz	70	7.0	9.0	180	8.0	0.0	0
vegetarian, w/lentils, mild *(Health Valley)*	4 oz	130	8.0	16.0	200	8.2	3.0	0
vegetarian, w/lentils, mild *(Health Valley)* 'No Salt Added'	4 oz	130	8.0	16.0	50	8.2	3.0	0
vegetarian, w/tempeh, spicy *(Hain)*	7.5 oz	160	7.0	24.0	1350	(mq)	4.0	0
w/beans	1/2 cup	143	7.3	15.2	668	5.6	7.0	22
w/beans *(Armour)*	6 oz	320	10.0	21.0	870	na	22.0	na

Food Name	Serv. Size	Total Cal.	Prot. GMS	Carbs GMS	Sod. MGS	Fiber GMS	Fat GMS	Chol. MGS
w/beans (Armour)	7.5 oz	390	13.0	27.0	1080	na	26.0	na
w/beans (Estee)	7.5 oz	370	16.0	27.0	125	(mq)	20.0	60
w/beans (Featherweight)	7.5 oz	280	19.0	29.0	440	(mq)	10.0	30
w/beans (Gebhardt)	1 cup	495	20.0	47.0	1010	6.0	28.0	92
w/beans (Just Rite)	4 oz	200	10.0	16.0	500	1.0	11.0	33
w/beans (Nalley's)	7.5 oz	260	17.0	27.0	880	(mq)	9.0	(mq)
w/beans (Van Camp's)	1 cup	352	14.9	20.9	1215	>2.3 c	23.2	(mq)
w/beans (Wolf Brand)	8 oz	345	15.0	21.8	1013	>2.3 c	22.0	(mq)
w/beans '15-oz' (Dennison's)	7.5 oz	310	16.0	27.0	875	8.0	15.0	(mq)
w/beans '15-oz' (Hormel)	7.5 oz	310	17.0	23.0	1127	(mq)	17.0	(mq)
w/beans '15-oz' (Libby's)	7.5 oz	270	13.0	25.0	810	(mq)	13.0	(mq)
w/beans '9.2 oz' (Quincy's)	1 serving	346	20.0	32.0	1380	(mq)	16.0	(mq)
w/beans '24-oz' (Libby's)	8 oz	290	14.0	27.0	860	(mq)	14.0	(mq)
w/beans '25-oz' (Hormel)	8 1/3 oz	350	18.0	30.0	1202	(mq)	20.0	(mq)
w/beans '30-oz' (Dennison's)	7.5 oz	310	16.0	30.0	840	8.0	15.0	(mq)
w/beans '40-oz' (Dennison's)	8 oz	340	17.0	30.0	1050	8.0	17.0	(mq)
w/beans '40-oz' (Hormel)	8 oz	320	17.0	25.0	1135	(mq)	17.0	(mq)
w/beans, beef (Chef Boyardee)	7.5 oz	330	15.0	30.0	1005	(mq)	17.0	(mq)
w/beans, chunky (Dennison's)	7.5 oz	310	16.0	28.0	780	10.0	14.0	(mq)
w/beans, chunky (Hormel)	7.5 oz	290	15.0	25.0	780	na	14.0	50
w/beans 'Cook-Off' (Dennison's)	7.5 oz	340	17.0	25.0	915	8.0	19.0	(mq)
w/beans, extra spicy (Wolf Brand)	7.75 oz	324	14.1	20.6	926	>2.2 c	20.6	(mq)
w/beans, hot (Armour)	7.5 oz	390	13.0	27.0	1080	na	26.0	na
w/beans, hot (Gebhardt)	1 cup	470	16.0	47.0	1000	6.0	27.0	65
w/beans, hot (Gebhardt)	4 oz	189	7.1	9.2	497	2.1	14.2	17
w/beans, hot (Heinz)	7.75 oz	330	15.0	30.0	1140	(mq)	16.0	(mq)
w/beans, hot (Just Rite)	4 oz	195	11.0	16.0	495	1.0	10.0	33
w/beans, hot (Nalley's)	7.5 oz	280	17.0	30.0	810	(mq)	10.0	(mq)
w/beans, hot '15 oz' (Hormel)	7.5 oz	310	16.0	24.0	1121	(mq)	16.0	(mq)
w/beans, hot '15 oz' (Dennison's)	7.5 oz	310	16.0	26.0	910	7.0	16.0	(mq)
w/beans, hot '40 oz' (Dennison's)	8 oz	350	17.0	29.0	950	7.0	19.0	(mq)
w/beans, hot, jalapeño (Nalley's)	7.5 oz	260	14.0	29.0	920	(mq)	10.0	(mq)
w/beans 'Laredo' (Stagg)	7.5 oz	260	15.0	22.0	na	na	12.0	na
w/beans 'Micro-Cup' (Hormel)	7.5 oz	250	15.0	20.0	980	(mq)	11.0	65
w/beans 'Premium Lite' (Armour)	7.5 oz	260	16.0	27.0	1110	na	10.0	na
w/beans 'Thick' (Nalley's)	7.5 oz	260	16.0	29.0	840	(mq)	9.0	(mq)
w/chicken, spicy (Hain)	7.5 oz	130	11.0	19.0	1030	(mq)	2.0	40
w/o beans (Armour)	7.5 oz	390	13.0	14.0	1150	na	31.0	na
w/o beans (Hormel)	10.5 oz	540	24.0	19.0	1384	(mq)	41.0	(mq)
w/o beans (Just Rite)	4 oz	180	13.0	9.0	515	<1.0	11.0	41
w/o beans (Libby's)	7.5 oz	390	18.0	11.0	800	(mq)	30.0	(mq)
w/o beans (Van Camp's)	1 cup	412	15.4	12.1	1499	>1.6 c	33.5	(mq)
w/o beans (Wolf Brand)	8 oz	387	20.7	16.2	1042	>2.0 c	26.6	(mq)

Food Name	Serv. Size	Total Cal.	Prot. GMS	Carbs GMS	Sod. MGS	Fiber GMS	Fat GMS	Chol. MGS
w/o beans 'Big Chunk' *(Nalley's)*	7.5 oz	270	17.0	14.0	810	(mq)	16.0	(mq)
w/o beans 'Chili-Mac' *(Wolf Brand)*	7.75 oz	317	11.5	22.9	854	>1.1 c	19.9	(mq)
w/o beans '15 oz' *(Dennison's)*	7.5 oz	300	17.0	15.0	1380	(mq)	19.0	(mq)
w/o beans '15 oz' *(Hormel)*	7.5 oz	370	17.0	12.0	1012	(mq)	28.0	(mq)
w/o beans '15 oz' *(Libby's)*	7.5 oz	390	18.0	11.0	800	na	30.0	na
w/o beans '19 oz' *(Dennison's)*	9.5 oz	380	22.0	18.0	1335	(mq)	24.0	(mq)
w/o beans 'Steak House' *(Stagg)*	7.5 oz	300	16.0	17.0	na	na	19.0	na
w/o beans '25 oz' *(Hormel)*	8 1/3 oz	430	20.0	13.0	1070	(mq)	33.0	(mq)
w/o beans, extra spicy *(Wolf Brand)*	7.5 oz	363	19.4	15.3	962	>1.9 c	24.9	(mq)
w/o beans, hot '15 oz' *(Hormel)*	7.5 oz	370	17.0	12.0	985	(mq)	28.0	(mq)
w/o beans, w/franks 'Chilee Weenee' *(Van Camp's)*	1 cup	309	14.4	27.6	1057	>2.2 c	15.7	(mq)

CHILI, FREEZE-DRIED

Food Name	Serv. Size	Total Cal.	Prot. GMS	Carbs GMS	Sod. MGS	Fiber GMS	Fat GMS	Chol. MGS
w/beans, prepared *(Mountain House)*	1 cup	390	20.0	38.0	153	(mq)	16.0	(mq)
w/beef 'Chili Mac' prepared *(Mountain House)*	1 cup	250	12.0	31.0	115	(mq)	8.0	(mq)

CHILI, FROZEN

Food Name	Serv. Size	Total Cal.	Prot. GMS	Carbs GMS	Sod. MGS	Fiber GMS	Fat GMS	Chol. MGS
con carne 'Homestyle Recipe' *(Swanson)*	8.25 oz	270	20.0	26.0	740	(mq)	10.0	(mq)
con carne, w/beans *(Stouffer's)*	8.75 oz	260	19.0	24.0	1270	(mq)	10.0	(mq)
vegetarian *(Right Course)*	9.75 oz	280	9.0	45.0	590	(mq)	7.0	0

CHILI, MICROWAVE

Food Name	Serv. Size	Total Cal.	Prot. GMS	Carbs GMS	Sod. MGS	Fiber GMS	Fat GMS	Chol. MGS
'Chili Mac' micro cup *(Hormel)*	7.5 oz	192	10.0	18.0	977	na	9.0	22
w/beans *(Armour)*	7.5 oz	300	16.0	26.0	1120	na	14.0	na
w/beans, 'Diner' microwave cup *(Libby's)*	7.75 oz	280	15.0	29.0	820	4.3	12.0	40
w/beans, hot, micro cup *(Hormel)*	7.38 oz	250	15.0	24.0	977	na	11.0	49
w/beans, microwave *(Lunch Bucket)*	7.5 oz	300	16.0	26.0	1120	na	14.0	45
w/o beans, micro cup *(Hormel)*	7.38 oz	290	18.0	15.0	830	na	17.0	60

CHILI BEAN, CANNED. See also KIDNEY BEAN, CANNED; PINTO BEAN.

Food Name	Serv. Size	Total Cal.	Prot. GMS	Carbs GMS	Sod. MGS	Fiber GMS	Fat GMS	Chol. MGS
(Gebhardt)	4.586 oz	134	7.1	30.7	630	7.2	1.0	0
(Hunt's)	4 oz	102	5.7	18.1	488	(mq)	0.0	0
(Hunt's)	4.48 oz	87	6.0	17.1	597	5.7	1.0	0
(S&W)	1/2 cup	130	7.0	23.0	520	(mq)	1.0	na
baked style, hot *(Campbell's)*	7.75 oz	180	10.0	38.0	870	(mq)	4.0	na
caliente style *(Green Giant)*	1/2 cup	100	6.0	20.0	700	7.0	1.0	0
caliente style *(Joan of Arc)*	1/2 cup	100	6.0	20.0	700	7.0	1.0	0
extra spicy *(Green Giant)*	1/2 cup	100	7.0	21.0	580	6.0	1.0	0
extra spicy *(Joan of Arc)*	1/2 cup	100	7.0	21.0	580	6.0	1.0	0
50% less salt *(Green Giant)*	1/2 cup	100	7.0	21.0	310	7.0	1.0	0
50% less salt *(Joan of Arc)*	1/2 cup	100	7.0	21.0	310	7.0	1.0	0
hot *(A&P)*	1/2 cup	140	8.0	24.0	440	(mq)	1.0	na
hot *(Allens)*	1/2 cup	90	5.0	17.0	420	(mq)	<1.0	na
hot *(Bush's Best)*	1/2 cup	70	5.0	20.0	420	6.0	0.0	na

Food Name	Serv. Size	Total Cal.	Prot. GMS	Carbs GMS	Sod. MGS	Fiber GMS	Fat GMS	Chol. MGS
in chili gravy (Dennison's)	7.5 oz	180	12.0	30.0	770	12.0	1.0	na
in sauce (Hormel)	5 oz	130	6.0	19.0	453	(mq)	3.0	na
Mexican style (Allens)	1/2 cup	135	8.0	24.0	430	(mq)	<1.0	na
Mexican style (Van Camp's)	1 cup	210	11.4	39.0	730	(mq)	2.4	na
spiced (Gebhardt)	4 oz	113	7.5	19.7	590	6.7	1.1	0
spicy 'Dry Beans in Sauce' (Green Giant)	1/2 cup	100	7.0	21.0	620	7.0	1.0	0
spicy 'Dry Beans in Sauce' (Joan of Arc)	1/2 cup	100	7.0	21.0	620	7.0	1.0	0
CHILI MIX								
'Chili Quick' dry (Gebhardt)	1.5-oz pkt	82	2.5	16.8	2784	3.0	1.1	0
'Chili con Carne' prepared (Old El Paso)	1 cup	162	19.0	8.0	510	1.5	7.0	47
'Homestyle Chili Fixins' (Hunt's)	4.656 oz	84	5.6	18.5	858	6.0	1.2	0
vegetarian, w/beans, prepared (Fantastic Foods)	1/2 cup	104	8.0	19.0	180	(mq)	0.8	0
w/beans, prepared (Old El Paso)	1 cup	217	15.0	17.0	480	6.0	10.0	32
CHILI POWDER								
(Durkee)	1 tsp	11	0.0	0.0	0	0	0.01	na
(Laurel Leaf)	1 tsp	11	0.0	0.0	0	0	0.01	na
CHILI SAUCE. See SAUCE.								
CHILI SEASONING								
(Gebhardt)	1 tsp	6	0.0	1.0	30	(mq)	0.0	0
(Gebhardt)	.0106 oz	1	0.0	0.1	0	.1	0.0	0
(Gebhardt) mix 'Chili Quick'	1 tsp	10	<1.0	2.0	165	<1.0	<1.0	0
(Hain) hot	1/4 pkg	30	1.0	5.0	370	(mq)	1.0	0
(Hain) medium	1/4 pkg	30	1.0	5.0	300	(mq)	1.0	0
(Hain) mild	1/2 pkg	30	1.0	5.0	330	(mq)	1.0	0
(Lawry's) 'Seasoning Blends'	1 pkg	143	4.9	26.6	2291	>2.1 c	1.8	0
(Old El Paso)	1/5 pkg	21	1.0	4.0	717	1.0	1.0	0
(Schilling)	1/4 pkg	27	1.0	4.5	290	(mq)	0.5	na
(Tio Sancho)	1.23 oz	109	4.1	6.0	832	>4.2 c	2.2	na
CHIMICHANGA								
beef 'Primera' (Marquez)	1 chimichanga	380	13.0	42.0	890	2.0	17.0	30
CHIMICHANGA DINNER, FROZEN								
bean and cheese (Old El Paso)	1 pkg	380	12.0	40.0	610	(mq)	19.0	20
beef (Old El Paso)	1 piece	370	12.0	34.0	470	(mq)	21.0	(mq)
beef and cheese 'Festive Dinners' (Old El Paso)	11 oz	510	22.0	53.0	1400	(mq)	23.0	(mq)
beef and pork (Old El Paso)	1 pkg	340	13.0	35.0	700	(mq)	16.0	(mq)
beef 'Festive Dinners' (Old El Paso)	11 oz	540	23.0	65.0	1200	(mq)	21.0	(mq)
chicken (Old El Paso)	1 piece	360	13.0	33.0	470	(mq)	20.0	(mq)

CHINESE APPLE. See POMEGRANATE.

CHINESE CABBAGE. See CABBAGE, NAPA.

Food Name	Serv. Size	Total Cal.	Prot. GMS	Carbs GMS	Sod. MGS	Fiber GMS	Fat GMS	Chol. MGS
CHINESE DATE								
dried	1 oz	81	1.0	20.1	3	>.9 c	0.3	0
raw, seeded	1 oz	22	0.3	5.7	1	>.4 c	0.1	0
raw, w/seeds	1 lb	331	5.1	85.3	11	>5.9 c	0.8	0
CHINESE FUNGUS/Jew's ear								
approx .2 oz	1 piece	2	0.0	0.4	0	0	(tr)	0
sliced	1/2 cup	13	0.2	3.3	5	0	(tr)	0
trimmed	1 oz	7	0.1	1.9	3	0	na	0
untrimmed	1 lb	111	2.1	30.0	41	0	0.2	0
CHINESE GOOSEBERRY. See KIWI FRUIT.								
CHINESE NOODLE. See NOODLE, CHINESE.								
CHINESE PARSLEY. See CORIANDER.								
CHINESE PARSLEY LEAF. See CORIANDER LEAF.								
CHINESE PARSLEY SEED. See CORIANDER SEED.								
CHINESE RADISH								
boiled, drained	4 oz	19	0.8	3.9	15	>.6 c	0.3	0
boiled, drained, sliced	1/2 cup	13	0.5	2.5	10	1.2	0.2	0
dried	1/2 cup	157	4.6	36.8	161	>4.9 c	0.4	0
dried	1 oz	77	2.2	18.0	79	>2.4 c	0.2	0
raw, 7 inches long, 2 1/4 inches diam,								
approx 15.1 oz	1 med	62	2.0	13.9	71	5.4	0.3	0
raw, trimmed	1 oz	5	0.2	1.2	6	>.2 c	<.1	0
raw, trimmed (Frieda's)	1 lb	86	4.1	19.1	(mq)	(mq)	0.5	0
raw, trimmed (Frieda's)	1 oz	5	0.3	1.2	(mq)	(mq)	<.1	0
raw, trimmed, sliced	1/2 cup	8	0.3	1.8	9	.7	<.1	0
raw, untrimmed	1 lb	65	2.2	14.7	75	>2.3 c	0.4	0
CHINESE WATERMELON								
boiled, drained	4 oz	15	0.5	3.4	121	>.6 c	0.2	0
boiled, drained, cubes	1/2 cup	11	0.4	2.6	93	>.4 c	0.2	0
raw, cubes	1 cup	17	0.5	4.0	147	>.7 c	0.3	0
raw, trimmed	1 oz	4	0.1	0.9	31	.2	0.1	0
raw, untrimmed	1 lb	42	1.3	9.7	358	1.9	0.6	0
CHINESE YAM. See JICAMA.								
CHIVES								
	1 oz	7	0.8	1.1	2	.9	0.2	0
freeze-dried	1 tbsp	1	0.0	0.1	0	tr	0.0	0
freeze-dried	1/4 cup	2	0.2	0.5	1	>.1 c	0.0	0
raw, chopped	1 tbsp	1	0.1	0.1	0	.1	0.0	0
raw, chopped	1 tsp	0	0.0	0.0	0	na	0.0	0
CHOCOLATE, BAKING								
Bar								
semi-sweet (Baker's)	1 oz	140	1.0	17.0	0	na	9.0	0
semi-sweet (Nestlé)	1 oz	160	2.0	16.0	0	(mq)	9.0	na

Food Name	Serv. Size	Total Cal.	Prot. GMS	Carbs GMS	Sod. MGS	Fiber GMS	Fat GMS	Chol. MGS
semi-sweet 'Premium' (Hershey's)	1 oz	140	1.0	16.0	0	(mq)	8.0	na
sweet 'German' (Baker's)	1 oz	140	1.0	17.0	0	(mq)	10.0	na
unsweetened (Baker's)	1 oz	140	3.0	9.0	0	na	15.0	0
unsweetened (Hershey's)	1 oz	190	4.0	7.0	5	(mq)	16.0	0
unsweetened (Nestlé)	1 oz	180	4.0	9.0	0	(mq)	14.0	na
unsweetened 'Premium' (Hershey's)	1 oz	190	4.0	7.0	5	na	16.0	0
white 'Premier' (Nestlé)	1 oz	150	2.0	18.0	15	(mq)	9.0	na
Chips								
milk chocolate (Baker's)	1 oz	140	2.0	18.0	25	(mq)	8.0	5
milk chocolate (Hershey's)	1/4 cup	220	2.0	27.0	55	na	12.0	10
milk chocolate (Hershey's)	1 oz	150	2.0	27.0	55	(mq)	12.0	10
milk chocolate 'Big Chips' (Baker's)	1/4 cup	240	3.0	30.0	40	na	13.0	10
mint chocolate (Hershey's)	1.5 oz	230	2.0	28.0	<1	(mq)	12.0	na
semi-sweet (Baker's)	1/4 cup	200	2.0	30.0	30	(mq)	9.0	0
semi-sweet 'Big Chips' (Baker's)	1/4 cup	220	2.0	31.0	0	na	13.0	0
semi-sweet, mini, approx 1/4 cup (Hershey's)	1.5 oz	220	2.0	26.0	5	(mq)	12.0	0
semi-sweet, real chocolate (Baker's)	1/4 cup	200	2.0	28.0	0	na	11.0	0
semi-sweet, regular (Hershey's)	1.5 oz	220	2.0	27.0	0	na	12.0	0
vanilla 'White' milk (Hershey's)	1.5 oz	240	3.0	25.0	65	(mq)	14.0	na
Chunks								
milk chocolate, 12 pieces (Hershey's)	1 oz	160	2.0	16.0	25	na	9.0	10
semi-sweet (Hershey's)	1 oz	140	1.0	15.0	na	(mq)	8.0	na
white 'Premier Treasures' (Nestlé)	1 oz	160	2.0	15.0	25	(mq)	10.0	na
Grated, bitter	1 cup	667	14.1	38.2	5	20.3	70.0	0
Powder								
cocoa, 100% (Nestlé)	1 oz	80	7.0	5.0	5	1.0	5.0	na
cocoa 'Premium' (Saco Foods)	1 tbsp	15	1.6	3.6	51	na	0.9	0
Premelted, unsweetened 'Choco Bake' (Nestlé)	1 oz	190	4.0	7.0	na	(mq)	16.0	0
Squares								
unsweetened, grated	1 cup	689	13.6	37.4	18	20.3	73.0	0
unsweetened, 1 oz	1 square	148	2.9	8.0	4	4.4	15.7	0
CHOCOLATE FLAVOR DRINK. See also DIET DRINK.								
Canned								
(Frostee)	8 oz	200	2.0	30.0	160	(tr)	8.0	na
Dutch 'Lite' (Sego)	10 oz	150	11.0	20.0	480	(tr)	3.0	5
liquid food, nutritionally complete (Sustacal)	8 oz	240	14.5	33.0	220	na	5.5	na
liquid nutrition (Ensure)	8 oz	250	9.3	33.8	200	na	8.8	5
liquid nutrition 'Plus' (Ensure)	8 oz	355	13.5	46.8	250	na	12.6	5
liquid nutrition, w/fiber (Ensure)	8 oz	260	9.9	37.8	200	na	8.8	5
'Lite' (Sego)	10 oz	150	11.0	20.0	480	(tr)	3.0	5
malt 'Very Chocolate' (Sego)	10 oz	225	11.0	43.0	450	(tr)	1.0	5

Food Name	Serv. Size	Total Cal.	Prot. GMS	Carbs GMS	Sod. MGS	Fiber GMS	Fat GMS	Chol. MGS
'Very Chocolate' (Sego)	10 oz	225	11.0	43.0	450	(tr)	1.0	5
Mix/powder								
approx 2-3 heaping tsp	.8 oz	75	0.7	19.5	45	1.3	0.7	0
approx 2-3 heaping tsp, prepared w/1 cup 1% milk	1 cup	177	8.7	31.2	168	>.2 c	3.3	10
approx 2-3 heaping tsp, prepared w/1 cup 2% milk	1 cup	196	8.8	31.2	167	3.8	5.4	18
approx 2-3 heaping tsp, prepared w/1 cup skim milk	1 cup	161	9.1	31.4	171	>.2 c	1.1	4
'Chocolate Milk Maker' (Swiss Miss)	.6702 oz	73	0.5	17.1	55	.4	0.3	0
classic chocolate chip (Nestlé)	1.13 oz	90	7.0	12.0	170	6.0	2.0	na
classic chocolate chip, prepared (Nestlé)	8 oz	180	15.0	24.0	300	6.0	2.0	na
creamy milk chocolate (Nestlé)	1.13 oz	90	7.0	12.0	150	6.0	2.0	na
creamy milk chocolate, prepared (Nestlé)	8 oz	180	15.0	24.0	280	6.0	2.0	na
dairy, reduced calorie, w/aspartame	.75-oz pkt	63	5.3	10.7	166	.3	0.6	2
'Hershey's Chocolate Milk Mix' (Hershey's)	3 heaping tsp	90	<1.0	22.0	40	na	<1.0	0
protein powder, prepared w/lowfat milk (Turbo Nutrition)	8 oz	330	36.0	34.0	450	na	6.0	na
'Quik' (Nestlé)	1 heaping tsp	90	1.0	20.0	25	(mq)	1.0	0
'Quik' prepared w/skim milk (Nestlé)	1 cup	170	9.0	31.0	150	(mq)	1.0	(mq)
'Quik' prepared w/2% milk (Nestlé)	1 cup	210	9.0	31.0	150	(mq)	5.0	(mq)
'Quik' prepared w/whole milk (Nestlé)	1 cup	230	9.0	31.0	150	(mq)	9.0	(mq)
'Quik' sugar-free, approx 1 heaping tsp (Nestlé)	.2 oz	18	1.0	3.0	35	(mq)	<1.0	na
'Quik' sugar-free, prepared w/2% milk (Nestlé)	1 cup	140	9.0	15.0	150	(mq)	5.0	(mq)
weight gain protein powder, (Turbo Nutrition)	2 oz	210	28.0	22.0	320	na	1.0	na
Refrigerated								
'Hershey's Genuine' (Hershey's)	8 oz	150	5.0	28.0	85	na	2.0	na
(Yoo-Hoo)	9 oz	140	3.0	27.0	130	0	1.0	(tr)
CHOCOLATE MILK								
whole	1 cup	208	7.9	25.8	149	>.2 c	8.5	30
whole	1 oz	26	1.0	3.2	19	(mq)	1.1	4
whole (Hershey's)	1 cup	210	7.0	28.0	120	(mq)	9.0	(mq)
whole (Nestlé Quik)	1 cup	230	7.0	31.0	120	0.0	9.0	30
3.5% fat (Hershey's)	1 cup	210	7.0	28.0	120	na	8.0	na
2% fat	1 cup	179	8.0	26.0	150	(mq)	5.0	17
2% fat (Darigold)	1 cup	190	8.0	28.0	210	(mq)	5.0	17
2% fat (Lucerne)	1 cup	200	8.0	29.0	200	0.0	5.0	25
2% fat (Hershey's)	1 cup	190	8.0	29.0	130	(mq)	5.0	20
2% fat 'Dutch Brand' (Borden)	1 cup	180	8.0	25.0	180	(mq)	5.0	(mq)

Food Name	Serv. Size	Total Cal.	Prot. GMS	Carbs GMS	Sod. MGS	Fiber GMS	Fat GMS	Chol. MGS
1% fat	1 cup	158	8.1	26.1	152	(mq)	2.5	7
CHOCOLATE SAUCE. See SAUCE.								
CHOCOLATE SYRUP								
chocolate-flavored *(Hershey's)*	2 tbsp	103	0.9	23.9	19	<1.0	.4	0
'Choco-Syp' *(Estee)*	1 tbsp	20	0.0	5.0	5	na	0.0	0
fudge-type	1 cup	1176	15.0	200.3	442	>8.2 c	45.6	41
fudge type	1 oz	124	1.9	20.3	33	>.2 c	5.1	0
fudge-type	1 tbsp	73	0.9	12.4	27	>.5 c	2.8	3
'Quik' *(Nestlé)*	1.22 oz	100	1.0	22.0	45	(mq)	1.0	0
unsweetened, 1 oz	1 pkt	134	3.4	9.6	3	>.9 c	13.5	0
w/added nutrients	1 cup	735	5.4	197.4	459	5.4	3.9	0
w/added nutrients	1 oz	92	0.7	24.7	57	>.2 c	0.5	0
w/added nutrients	1 tbsp	46	0.3	12.4	29	.3	0.2	0
w/o added nutrients	1 cup	654	5.7	176.7	288	5.4	2.7	0
w/o added nutrients	1 oz	82	0.7	22.1	36	.7	0.3	0
CHOCOLATE TOPPING								
(Kraft)	1 tbsp	50	1.0	11.0	15	(mq)	0.0	0
(Mrs. Richardson's) dark chocolate fudge	2 tbsp	130	1.0	19.0	55	na	6.0	0
(Mrs. Richardson's) dark, fudge, microwavable	2 tbsp	130	1.0	19.0	55	na	6.0	0
(Nestlé) milk chocolate, w/almonds 'Candytops'	1.25 oz	230	2.0	14.0	15	(mq)	18.0	(mq)
(Nestlé) milk chocolate, w/crisps 'Crunch Candytops'	2 tbsp	220	2.0	16.0	40	(mq)	17.0	(mq)
(Nestlé) white chocolate, w/almonds 'Candytops'	1.25 oz	230	3.0	12.0	20	(mq)	19.0	na
(Smucker's) chocolate fudge 'Magic Shell'	2 tbsp	190	1.0	16.0	50	na	15.0	na
(Smucker's) dark chocolate 'Special Recipe'	2 tbsp	130	1.0	31.0	45	(mq)	1.0	na
(Smucker's) flavored syrup	2 tbsp	130	1.0	27.0	35	(mq)	2.0	na
(Smucker's) 'Magic Shell'	2 tbsp	190	1.0	16.0	25	na	15.0	na
(Smucker's) milk chocolate fudge, Swiss	2 tbsp	140	3.0	31.0	70	(mq)	1.0	na
(Smucker's) nut 'Magic Shell'	2 tbsp	200	2.0	25.0	40	(mq)	16.0	na
CHORIZO								
	1 oz	129	6.8	0.5	350	0	10.9	25
4 inches	1 link	273	14.5	1.1	741	0	23.0	53
(Carmelita) beef	2.5 oz	250	8.0	5.0	510	0	23.0	80
(Carmelita) pork	2.5 oz	250	8.0	3.0	500	0	23.0	110
CHOW MEIN								
chicken, w/o noodles, can	1 cup	95	6.5	17.7	725	>.8 c	0.3	8
vegetarian, Mandarin, prepared w/tofu *(Tofu Classics)*	1/2 cup	110	8.0	14.0	390	(mq)	6.0	0

Food Name	Serv. Size	Total Cal.	Prot. GMS	Carbs GMS	Sod. MGS	Fiber GMS	Fat GMS	Chol. MGS
CHOW MEIN NOODLE								
with almonds (Chun King)	1/3 cup	140	4.0	15.0	380	1	7.0	0
with sesame bits (Chun King)	1/3 cup	140	3.0	16.0	460	1	7.0	0
CHRYSANTHEMUM GARLAND								
boiled, drained	4 oz	23	1.9	4.9	60	>1.3 c	0.1	0
boiled, drained, 1-inch pieces	1/2 cup	10	0.8	2.2	27	1.2	0.1	0
raw, 1 stem, 8.75 inches long	.5 oz	2	0.2	0.6	7	.4	<.1	0
raw, 1-inch pieces	1 cup	4	0.4	1.1	13	.7	0.0	0
raw, 8.75 inches long	1 stem	2	0.2	0.6	7	>.1 c	0.0	0
raw, trimmed	1 oz	5	0.4	1.2	15	>.3 c	<.1	0
raw, untrimmed	1 lb	76	6.8	19.0	225	>3.9 c	0.8	0
CHUB/cisco								
raw	1 lb	446	86.1	0.0	249	0	8.7	(mq)
raw	1 oz	28	5.4	0.0	16	0	0.5	(mq)
smoked	1 oz	50	4.6	0.0	135	0	3.3	9
smoked	1 oz	50	4.6	0.0	135	0	3.3	9
CILANTRO								
approx .8 oz	9 plants	4	0.5	0.5	6	>.2 c	0.1	0
trimmed	1 oz	6	0.7	0.7	8	>.2 c	0.2	0
trimmed	1/4 cup	1	0.1	0.1	1	>.1 c	<.1	0
untrimmed	1 lb	77	9.1	10.0	108	>3.1 c	2.3	0
CILANTRO LEAF								
dried	1 oz	79	6.2	14.8	60	>2.9 c	1.3	0
dried	1 tbsp	5	0.4	0.9	4	>.2 c	0.1	0
dried	1 tsp	2	0.1	0.3	1	>.1 c	<.1	0
CILANTRO SEED								
whole	1 oz	84	3.5	15.6	10	>8.3 c	5.0	0
whole	1 tbsp	15	0.6	2.8	2	>1.5 c	0.9	0
whole	1 tsp	5	0.2	1.0	1	>.5 c	0.3	0
whole (Spice Islands)	1 tsp	6	0.2	0.8	<1	>.4 c	0.3	0
CINNAMON								
ground	1 oz	74	1.1	22.6	7	>6.9 c	0.9	0
ground	1 tbsp	18	0.3	5.4	2	3.7	0.2	0
ground	1 tsp	6	0.1	1.8	1	1.3	0.1	0
ground (Durkee)	1 tsp	8	0.0	0.0	0	0	tr	na
ground (Laurel Leaf)	1 tsp	8	0.0	0.0	0	0	tr	na
ground (Spice Islands)	1 tsp	6	0.1	1.4	<1	>.3 c	<.1	0
CISCO. See CHUB.								
CITRON, candied	1 oz	88	0.1	22.5	81	>.4 c	0.1	0
CITRUS COOLER DRINK (Gatorade)								
'Thirst Quencher'	8 oz	50	0.0	14.0	110	na	0.0	na
CITRUS DRINK								
(Five Alive) chilled	6 oz	90	0.0	22.0	20	na	0.0	na

Food Name	Serv. Size	Total Cal.	Prot. GMS	Carbs GMS	Sod. MGS	Fiber GMS	Fat GMS	Chol. MGS
(Fruitopia) 'Citrus Consciousness' real fruit	8 oz	120	0.0	30.0	25	na	0.0	na
CITRUS DRINK MIX								
(Crystal Light) blend, sugar-free,								
w/NutraSweet	8 oz	4	0.0	0.0	0	na	0.0	0
(Five Alive) frozen, diluted	6 oz	90	0.0	22.0	na	na	0.0	na
CITRUS FRUIT JUICE DRINK								
frozen concentrate	12-oz can	685	5.1	170.5	13	>.4 c	0.4	0
frozen concentrate, diluted	1 cup	114	0.7	28.5	7	0	0.0	0
(Five Alive) aseptic box	8.45 oz	123	0.8	30.7	32	(tr)	0.0	0
(Five Alive) chilled or frozen, berry, diluted	6 oz	88	0.2	22.1	21	(tr)	0.1	0
(Five Alive) chilled or frozen, diluted	6 oz	87	0.6	21.8	23	(tr)	0.0	0
(Five Alive) chilled or frozen, tropical, diluted	6 oz	85	0.4	21.3	19	(tr)	0.1	0
(Hi-C) 'Citrus Cooler'	6 oz	95	0.1	23.3	17	(tr)	<.1	0
CITRUS GRILL MARINADE *(Lawry's)*	2 tbsp	34	3.8	3.4	3350	.1	0.4	0
CITRUS JUICE *(Santa Cruz Natural)*								
organic 'Cruz'	8 oz	125	1.0	29.0	na	na	<1.0	0
CITRUS PUNCH								
(Minute Maid) can or bottle 'Juices To Go'	6 oz	90	0.0	23.0	20	na	0.0	na
(Minute Maid) chilled	6 oz	90	0.0	23.0	20	na	0.0	na
(Tampico) 2% orange, tangerine, and								
lemon juice	8 oz	120	<1.0	30.0	10	0	0.0	0
CITRUS PUNCH DRINK								
(Sunny Delight) 'California Style'	8 oz	100	0.0	23.0	95	na	0.0	na
(Sunny Delight) 'Florida Citrus Punch'	8 oz	120	0.0	27.0	125	na	<1.0	na
(Sunny Delight) 'Florida Citrus Punch'								
plus calcium	8 oz	130	0.0	32.0	125	na	<1.0	na
CITRUS PUNCH MIX *(Minute Maid)* frozen,								
concentrate	6 oz	90	0.0	22.0	0	na	0.0	na
CITRUS SALAD *(Florigold)*	8 oz	120	2.7	27.2	3	(mq)	0.0	0
CLAM, CANNED								
chopped *(Gorton's)*	3.25 oz	40	7.0	2.0	5.90	na	<1.0	20
chopped *(Progresso)*	1/2 cup	70	12.0	2.0	140	0	<1.0	31
chopped, w/liquid *(Doxsee)*	6.5 oz	100	14.0	8.0	1160	0	<1.0	(mq)
chopped, w/liquid *(Orleans)*	6.5 oz	100	14.0	8.0	1160	0	<1.0	(mq)
minced *(Gorton's)*	3.25 oz	40	7.0	2.0	5.90	na	<1.0	20
minced *(Progresso)*	1/2 cup	70	12.0	2.0	140	0	<1.0	31
minced, w/liquid *(Doxsee)*	6.5 oz	100	14.0	8.0	1160	0	<1.0	(mq)
minced, w/liquid *(Orleans)*	6.5 oz	100	14.0	8.0	1160	0	<1.0	(mq)
mixed species, drained	1 cup	237	40.9	8.2	179	0	3.1	107
mixed species, drained	4 oz	168	29.0	5.8	127	0	2.2	76
mixed species, drained	3 oz	126	21.7	4.4	95	0	1.7	57
mixed species, liquid only	1 cup	5	1.0	0.2	516	0	0.1	7
mixed species, liquid only	3 oz	2	0.3	0.1	183	0	0.0	3

Food Name	Serv. Size	Total Cal.	Prot. GMS	Carbs GMS	Sod. MGS	Fiber GMS	Fat GMS	Chol. MGS
CLAM, MIXED SPECIES								
boiled	4 oz	168	29.0	5.8	127	0	2.2	76
breaded and fried	20 small	380	26.8	19.4	684	>.3 c	21.0	115
breaded and fried	4 oz	229	16.1	11.7	413	>.2 c	12.6	69
breaded and fried	3 oz	172	12.1	8.8	309	>.1 c	9.5	52
moist-heat cooked	20 small	133	23.0	4.6	101	0	1.8	60
moist-heat cooked	3 oz	126	21.7	4.4	95	0	1.7	57
poached	4 oz	168	29.0	5.8	127	0	2.2	76
raw	1 lb	335	57.9	11.6	253	0	4.4	152
raw	1 oz	21	3.6	0.7	16	0	0.3	10
raw	20 small	133	23.0	4.6	101	0	1.8	61
raw	9 large	133	23.0	4.6	101	0	1.8	61
raw	3 oz	63	10.9	2.2	48	0	0.8	29
steamed	4 oz	168	29.0	5.8	127	0	2.2	76
CLAM, STUFFED, New England style								
(Matlaw's)	2 clams	180	8.0	21.0	730	3.0	8.0	0
CLAM JUICE								
(Doxsee)	3 oz	4	<1.0	0.0	110	0	0.0	na
(Snow's)	3 oz	4	<1.0	0.0	110	0	0.0	na
CLAM SAUCE. See SAUCE.								
CLAM TOMATO JUICE, canned	5.5 oz	76	1.0	18.1	664	>.2 c	0.2	0
CLARIFIED BUTTER. See GHEE.								
CLEARMALT. See ALCOHOLIC BEVERAGES.								
CLOVES								
ground	1 tbsp	21	0.4	4.0	16	2.3	1.3	0
ground	1 tsp	7	0.1	1.3	5	.7	0.4	0
ground (Durkee)	1 tsp	9	0.0	0.0	0	0	<0.1	na
ground (Laurel Leaf)	1 tsp	9	0.0	0.0	0	0	<0.1	na
ground (Spice Islands)	1 tsp	7	0.1	1.2	4	.7	0.2	0
CLUB SODA. See SOFT DRINKS AND MIXERS.								
COATING MIX. See SEASONING AND COATING MIX.								
COBBLER								
Fresh								
apple (Stilwell)	4 oz	200	2.0	4.0	225	(mq)	4.0	na
apple, deep dish (Awrey's)	1/8 pie	320	2.0	48.0	300	1.0	14.0	0
blueberry, deep dish (Awrey's)	1/8 pie	310	2.0	45.0	360	2.0	14.0	0
Frozen								
apple, 4.33 oz (Pet-Ritz)	1/6 pkg	290	1.0	50.0	(mq)	(mq)	9.0	na
blackberry (Stilwell)	4 oz	280	3.0	50.0	220	(mq)	8.0	na
blackberry, 4.33 oz (Pet-Ritz)	1/6 pkg	250	2.0	39.0	(mq)	(mq)	10.0	na
blueberry, 4.33 oz (Pet-Ritz)	1/6 pkg	370	3.0	50.0	(mq)	(mq)	12.0	na
cherry (Stilwell)	4 oz	250	3.0	46.0	205	(mq)	6.0	na
cherry, 4.33 oz (Pet-Ritz)	1/6 pkg	280	2.0	46.0	(mq)	(mq)	10.0	na

Food Name	Serv. Size	Total Cal.	Prot. GMS	Carbs GMS	Sod. MGS	Fiber GMS	Fat GMS	Chol. MGS
peach *(Stilwell)*	4 oz	270	2.0	55.0	200	(mq)	5.0	na
peach, 4.33 oz *(Pet-Ritz)*	1/6 pkg	260	2.0	46.0	(mq)	(mq)	10.0	na
strawberry, 4.33 oz *(Pet-Ritz)*	1/6 pkg	290	1.0	50.0	(mq)	(mq)	9.0	na

COBNUT, SHELLED. See HAZELNUT, SHELLED.

COCKTAIL ONION. See ONION, COCKTAIL.

COCKTAIL SAUCE. See SAUCE.

COCOA BUTTER OIL

Food Name	Serv. Size	Total Cal.	Prot. GMS	Carbs GMS	Sod. MGS	Fiber GMS	Fat GMS	Chol. MGS
....	1 cup	1927	0.0	0.0	0	0	218.0	0
....	1 oz	251	0.0	0.0	0	0	28.4	0
....	1 tbsp	120	0.0	0.0	0	0	13.6	0

COCOA MIX

Food Name	Serv. Size	Total Cal.	Prot. GMS	Carbs GMS	Sod. MGS	Fiber GMS	Fat GMS	Chol. MGS
Amaretto creme flavor *(Swiss Miss)*	1.25 oz	150	2.0	29.0	220	(mq)	3.0	na
Bavarian chocolate, hot cocoa *(Swiss Miss)*	1 oz	110	1.0	20.0	170	0	3.0	2
chocolate, w/marshmallows *(Carnation)*	1 oz	110	1.0	24.0	120	.2	1.2	2
chocolate almond mocha *(Swiss Miss)*	1.235 oz	144	1.9	28.0	207	1.5	2.7	1
chocolate and mint 'Cocoa Classics' *(Land O'Lakes)*	1 envelope	160	4.0	24.0	160	na	5.0	na
chocolate and raspberry 'Cocoa Classics' *(Land O'Lakes)*	1 envelope	160	4.0	25.0	160	na	5.0	na
chocolate Bavarian mint *(Swiss Miss)*	1.235 oz	142	1.9	28.3	231	1.5	2.3	1
chocolate English toffee *(Swiss Miss)*	1.235 oz	142	1.8	28.5	223	na	2.3	1
chocolate flavor *(Pathmark)*	1 oz	110	2.0	24.0	110	(mq)	1.0	na
chocolate flavor *(Swiss Miss)*	1 oz	110	1.0	24.0	125	(mq)	1.0	na
chocolate flavor 'Sugar-free' *(Swiss Miss)*	.5 oz	50	2.0	9.0	130	(mq)	1.0	<1
chocolate fudge flavor *(Carnation)*	1-oz pkt	110	1.0	24.0	135	.3	1.3	11
chocolate praline and creme *(Swiss Miss)*	1.235 oz	142	2.8	28.5	223	1.5	2.3	1
chocolate raspberry truffle *(Swiss Miss)*	1.235 oz	144	1.8	27.8	220	1.5	2.8	1
chocolate supreme 'Cocoa Classics' *(Land O'Lakes)*	1 envelope	160	4.0	25.0	160	na	5.0	na
dark chocolate truffle *(Swiss Miss)*	1.235 oz	142	2.0	27.9	225	1.5	2.5	1
diet *(Swiss Miss)*	.26 oz	20	2.0	3.0	180	0	<1.0	1
diet 'Hot Cocoa Mix' *(Swiss Miss)*	.26 oz	22	1.9	3.8	205	.7	0.2	0
double rich chocolate flavor *(Swiss Miss)*	1 oz	110	2.0	24.0	125	(mq)	1.0	0
fat-free 'Hot Cocoa Mix' *(Swiss Miss)*	.5 oz	50	3.3	9.0	197	.7	0.3	2
lite *(Swiss Miss)*	.75 oz	70	1.0	17.0	160	0	<1.0	1
lite 'Hot Cocoa Mix' *(Swiss Miss)*	.7407 oz	74	1.5	17.1	197	1.6	0.5	0
marshmallow lovers 'Hot Cocoa Mix' *(Swiss Miss)*	1.199 oz	132	1.6	23.6	167	.9	1.5	2
milk chocolate flavor *(Alba '66)*	.68 oz	60	6.0	10.0	160	na	0.0	na
milk chocolate flavor *(Saco Foods)*	1 oz	110	2.0	24.0	150	na	1.0	na
milk chocolate flavor *(Swiss Miss)*	1-oz pkt	110	1.0	20.0	170	(mq)	3.0	<1

Food Name	Serv. Size	Total Cal.	Prot. GMS	Carbs GMS	Sod. MGS	Fiber GMS	Fat GMS	Chol. MGS
milk chocolate flavor 'Sugar-free'								
(Swiss Miss) .... .5 oz		60	3.0	10.0	125	(mq)	0.0	na
milk chocolate flavor, w/marshmallows								
(Alba '66) .... .68 oz		60	6.0	10.0	160	na	0.0	na
milk chocolate 'Hot Cocoa Mix'								
(Swiss Miss) .... 1.199 oz		133	1.7	28.9	169	.9	1.5	2
milk chocolate 'Hot Cocoa Mix'								
(Swiss Miss) .... 1 oz		110	1.4	23.9	139	.8	1.3	1
milk chocolate w/mini marshmallows								
'Hot Cocoa Mix' (Swiss Miss) .... 1.199 oz		132	1.8	28.5	181	.9	1.5	1
milk chocolate w/mini marshmallows								
'Hot Cocoa Mix' (Swiss Miss) .... 1 oz		109	1.5	23.5	149	.8	1.3	1
milk flavor (Carnation) .... 1-oz pkt		110	2.0	24.0	130	.2	1.1	1
mini (Pathmark) .... 1 oz		110	2.0	24.0	140	(mq)	1.0	na
mint flavor (Featherweight) .... .44 oz		50	2.0	8.0	110	(mq)	1.0	0
mocha flavor 'Sugar-free' (Carnation) .... 1 pkt		50	3.0	9.0	140	.1	0.3	2
reduced calorie, aspartame sweetened ... 1 oz		8	0.6	1.4	(mq)	(mq)	0.1	na
regular (Finast) .... 6 oz		110	2.0	24.0	150	(mq)	1.0	na
rich, sugar-free 'Hot Cocoa Mix'								
(Swiss Miss) .... .5 oz		50	2.6	10.0	165	.8	0.3	0
rich chocolate 'Hot Cocoa Mix'								
(Swiss Miss) .... 1 oz		110	1.8	23.5	166	.8	1.2	1
rich milk flavor (Carnation) .... 1-oz pkt		110	1.0	24.0	120	.2	1.1	1
rich milk flavor 'Sugar-free' (Carnation) ... 1 pkt		50	4.0	8.0	160	.1	0.4	3
rich milk flavor, w/marshmallows								
(Weight Watchers) .... 1 pkt		60	6.0	10.0	160	(mq)	0.0	0
'70-Calorie' (Carnation) .... 1 pkt		70	3.0	16.0	135	>.2 c	0.3	1
'Sugar-free' (Hills Bros) .... 3 tbsp		60	2.0	9.0	145	(mq)	2.0	na
sugar-free 'Hot Cocoa Mix'								
(Swiss Miss) .... .7055 oz		67	3.2	13.6	242	.9	0.3	1
sugar-free 'Hot Cocoa Mix' (Swiss Miss) .. .5 oz		49	2.4	10.0	179	.7	0.2	0
sugar-free, sweetened w/NutraSweet								
(Saco Foods) .... 1 pkt		50	3.0	9.0	150	na	1.0	na
sugar-free, w/mini marshmallows								
'Hot Cocoa Mix' (Swiss Miss) .... .7055 oz		68	1.9	13.9	210	.9	0.8	2
sugar-free, w/mini marshmallows								
'Hot Cocoa Mix' (Swiss Miss) .... .5 oz		51	1.4	10.5	159	.7	0.6	1
vending 'Hot Cocoa Mix' (Swiss Miss) .. 1.34 oz		146	1.8	31.7	185	1.0	1.7	2
white chocolate 'Hot Cocoa Mix'								
(Swiss Miss) .... 1 oz		111	3.0	21.4	130	.1	1.4	1
w/added nutrients .... 1-oz pkt		120	1.9	24.0	201	>.2 c	3.0	1
w/added nutrients, prepared .... 1 pkt		119	1.9	24.0	207	>.2 c	2.9	0
w/aspartame .... .53-oz pkt		48	3.8	8.4	104	.4	0.4	2

Food Name	Serv. Size	Total Cal.	Prot. GMS	Carbs GMS	Sod. MGS	Fiber GMS	Fat GMS	Chol. MGS
w/aspartame, w/added calcium and								
potassium .... .53-oz pkt		48	3.8	8.5	98	.4	0.5	1
w/aspartame, w/added sodium and								
vitamin A .... .53-oz pkt		48	3.8	8.5	168	.4	0.5	1
w/marshmallows *(Carnation)* .... 1-oz pkt		110	1.0	24.0	120	.2	1.0	1
w/mini marshmallows *(Finast)* .... 6 oz		110	2.0	24.0	150	(mq)	1.0	na
w/mini marshmallows *(Swiss Miss)* ...... 1 oz		110	1.0	23.0	140	(mq)	1.0	na
w/mini marshmallows 'Sugar-free'								
(Swiss Miss) .... .5-oz pkt		50	3.0	9.0	120	(mq)	<1.0	na
w/o added nutrients .... 1-oz pkt		103	3.1	22.5	143	.3	1.1	1
w/o added nutrients, prepared .. 3-4 heaping tsp		103	3.1	22.5	148	2.5	1.2	2
COCOA POWDER. See also CHOCOLATE, BAKING.								
(Bensdorp) .... 1 oz		130	6.0	8.0	5	(mq)	7.0	<1
(Hershey's) approx 1/3 cup .... 1 oz		120	7.0	13.0	10	(mq)	4.0	0
(Hershey's) 'European' .... 1 oz		90	7.0	8.0	15	(mq)	3.0	0
(Hershey's) unsweetened, European style 1 cup		170	16.6	48.8	52	>4.5 c	8.3	0
(Hershey's) unsweetened, European style 1 tbsp		10	1.0	2.8	3	>.3 c	0.5	0
(Nestlé) .... 1.5 oz		180	11.0	21.0	6	(mq)	6.0	na
COCONUT								
mature kernel, in shell .... 1 lb		834	7.9	35.9	47	21.2	79.0	0
mature kernel, shelled .... 1 oz		100	0.9	4.3	6	2.6	9.5	0
mature kernel, shelled, grated, packed .. 1 cup		460	4.3	19.8	26	11.7	43.5	0
meat, raw, 2 x 2 x 1/2 inch .... 1 piece		159	1.5	6.8	9	4.1	15.1	0
meat, raw, shredded .... 1 cup		283	2.7	12.2	16	7.2	26.8	0
COCONUT, DRIED								
creamed .... 1 oz		194	1.5	6.1	11	>1.1 c	19.6	0
sweetened, flaked, canned .... 4 oz		505	3.8	46.6	23	5.1	36.1	0
sweetened, flaked, canned .... 1 cup		341	2.6	31.5	15	3.5	24.4	0
sweetened, flaked, canned .... 1 oz		126	0.9	11.6	6	>.6 c	9.0	0
sweetened, flaked, canned 'Angel Flake'								
(Baker's) .... 1/3 cup		110	1.0	10.0	5	(mq)	9.0	0
sweetened, flaked, packaged .... 7-oz pkg		943	6.5	94.7	509	8.6	64.0	0
sweetened, flaked, packaged .... 1 cup		351	2.4	35.2	189	3.2	23.8	0
sweetened, flaked, packaged .... 1 oz		134	0.9	13.5	73	>.6 c	9.1	0
sweetened, flaked, packaged 'Angel Flake'								
(Baker's) .... 1/3 cup		120	1.0	10.0	75	(mq)	8.0	0
sweetened, flaked, packaged 'Snowflake'								
(Finast) .... 1 oz		137	1.0	12.0	<1	(mq)	9.0	0
sweetened, flaked, packaged, toasted								
(Baker's) .... 1/3 cup		200	2.0	17.0	85	(mq)	17.0	0
sweetened, shredded .... 7-oz pkg		997	5.7	94.9	521	9.0	70.6	0
sweetened, shredded .... 1 cup		466	2.7	44.3	244	4.2	33.0	0
sweetened, shredded .... 1 oz		142	0.8	13.5	74	>.6 c	10.1	0

Food Name	Serv. Size	Total Cal.	Prot. GMS	Carbs GMS	Sod. MGS	Fiber GMS	Fat GMS	Chol. MGS
sweetened, shredded 'Premium Shred'								
(Baker's) .... 1/3 cup		140	1.0	12.0	85	(mq)	9.0	0
sweetened, shredded, toasted .... 1 oz		168	1.5	12.6	11	>.7 c	13.4	0
sweetened, shredded, toasted 'Angel Flake'								
(Baker's) .... 1/3 cup		200	2.0	17.0	85	na	17.0	0
unsweetened .... 1 oz		187	2.0	6.7	11	3.2	18.3	0
COCONUT CREAM								
Canned								
liquid expressed from grated meat ...... 1 cup		568	8.0	24.7	148	>6.9 c	52.5	0
liquid expressed from grated meat ..... 1 tbsp		36	0.5	1.6	10	>.4 c	3.4	0
sweetened .... 1 oz		54	0.8	2.4	14	(mq)	5.0	0
sweetened (Coco Lopez) .... 2 tbsp		120	0.0	20.0	10	(mq)	5.0	0
sweetened (Holland House) .... 1 oz		81	0.0	18.0	21	(mq)	(mq)	0
Raw								
liquid expressed from grated meat ...... 1 cup		792	8.7	16.0	10	>8.9 c	83.2	0
liquid expressed from grated meat ..... 1 tbsp		49	0.5	1.0	1	>.6 c	5.2	0
liquid expressed from grated meat ...... 1 oz		94	1.0	1.9	1	(mq)	9.8	0
COCONUT MILK								
canned .... 1 cup		445	4.6	6.3	29	>4.9 c	48.2	0
canned .... 1 oz		56	0.6	0.8	4	(mq)	6.0	0
canned .... 1 tbsp		30	0.3	0.4	2	>.3 c	3.2	0
frozen .... 1 cup		485	3.9	13.4	29	>5.5 c	49.9	0
frozen .... 1 oz		57	0.5	1.6	3	(mq)	5.9	0
frozen .... 1 tbsp		30	0.2	0.8	2	>.3 c	3.1	0
raw .... 1 cup		552	5.5	13.3	36	>6.3 c	57.2	0
raw .... 1 oz		65	0.6	1.6	4	(mq)	6.8	0
raw .... 1 tbsp		35	0.3	0.8	2	>.4 c	3.6	0
COCONUT NECTAR (Knudsen & Sons) ... 8 oz		150	<1.0	29.0	na	na	0.0	na
COCONUT OIL								
.... 1/2 cup		964	0.0	0.0	0	0	109.0	0
.... 1 oz		251	0.0	0.0	0	0	28.4	0
.... 1 tbsp		120	0.0	0.0	0	0	13.6	0
(Hain) .... 1 tbsp		120	0.0	0.0	0	0	14.0	0
COCONUT PINEAPPLE NECTAR, can or								
bottle (Kern's) .... 6 oz		140	1.0	26.0	25	na	4.0	na
COCONUT VEGETABLE OIL								
.... 1 cup		1879	0.0	0.0	0	0	218.0	0
.... 1 tbsp		117	0.0	0.0	0	0	13.6	0
COCONUT WATER								
.... 1 cup		46	1.7	8.9	252	2.6	0.5	0
.... 1 oz		5	0.2	1.1	30	>.1 c	0.1	0
.... 1 tbsp		3	0.1	0.6	16	.2	0.0	0

Food Name	Serv. Size	Total Cal.	Prot. GMS	Carbs GMS	Sod. MGS	Fiber GMS	Fat GMS	Chol. MGS
COD, ALASKAN								
raw	1 oz	55	3.8	0.0	16	0	4.3	14
raw, 6.8 oz	1/2 fillet	377	25.9	0.0	108	0	29.5	95
smoked	4 oz	291	20.0	0.0	836	0	22.8	73
COD, ATLANTIC								
baked	4 oz	119	25.9	0.0	88	0	1.0	62
broiled	4 oz	119	25.9	0.0	88	0	1.0	62
dried and salted	3 oz	247	53.4	0.0	5973	0	2.0	129
dried and salted	1 oz	81	17.6	0.0	1968	0	0.7	42
dry-heat cooked	3 oz	89	19.4	0.0	66	0	0.7	47
microwaved	4 oz	119	25.9	0.0	88	0	1.0	62
raw	1 lb	372	80.8	0.0	246	0	3.1	195
raw	3 oz	70	15.1	0.0	46	0	0.6	37
raw	1 oz	23	5.0	0.0	15	0	0.2	12
COD, BLACK								
raw	1 lb	886	60.8	0.0	254	0	69.4	222
raw	1 oz	55	3.8	0.0	16	0	4.3	14
smoked	1 oz	73	5.0	0.0	209	0	5.7	18
COD, FROZEN								
breaded 'Light' *(Mrs. Paul's)*	1 piece	240	15.0	22.0	430	(mq)	11.0	(mq)
breaded 'Light' *(Van de Kamp's)*	1 piece	250	17.0	20.0	510	(mq)	11.0	35
breaded, lemon thyme crumb 'Select' *(Gorton's)*	1 fillet	90	12.0	5.0	240	na	2.0	45
fillet *(Booth)*	4 oz	89	20.0	0.0	350	0	1.0	(mq)
fillet *(Finast)*	4 oz	80	18.0	0.0	200	0	1.0	(mq)
fillet *(SeaPak)*	4 oz	90	20.0	0.0	135	0	1.0	(mq)
fillet 'Fishmarket Fresh' *(Gorton's)*	5 oz	110	26.0	0.0	90	0	1.0	(mq)
fillet 'Individually Wrapped' *(Booth)*	4 oz	90	20.0	0.0	80	0	1.0	(mq)
fillet, light *(Van de Kamp's)*	1 piece	250	17.0	20.0	510	na	11.0	35
fillet, natural *(Van de Kamp's)*	4 oz	90	20.0	0.0	90	0	1.0	25
natural *(Van de Kamp's)*	4 oz	90	20.0	0.0	90	na	1.0	25
COD, PACIFIC								
dry-heat cooked	3 oz	89	19.5	0.0	77	0	0.7	40
fillets, raw *(Peter Pan Seafoods)*	3.5 oz	80	17.0	na	71	na	0.6	37
raw	1 lb	372	81.2	0.0	322	0	2.9	168
raw	3 oz	70	15.2	0.0	60	0	0.5	31
raw	1 oz	23	5.1	0.0	20	0	0.2	10
COD CAKE, CANNED, 2 cakes *(Gorton's)*	4 oz	100	8.0	16.0	640	na	<1.0	15
COD ENTRÉE, FROZEN								
fillet, au gratin *(Booth)*	9.5 oz	280	27.0	18.0	1160	(mq)	11.0	(mq)
fillet, Florentine *(Booth)*	9.5 oz	244	20.0	29.0	880	(mq)	6.0	(mq)
fillet, w/lemon butter sauce and rice *(Booth)*	9.5 oz	567	22.0	27.0	1330	(mq)	38.0	(mq)
fillet, w/mushroom sauce and rice *(Booth)*	9.5 oz	280	27.0	19.0	1010	(mq)	11.0	(mq)

Food Name	Serv. Size	Total Cal.	Prot. GMS	Carbs GMS	Sod. MGS	Fiber GMS	Fat GMS	Chol. MGS
COD LIVER OIL								
cherry *(Hain)*	1 tbsp	120	0.0	0.0	0	0	14.0	75
mint *(Hain)*	1 tbsp	120	0.0	0.0	0	0	14.0	85
regular	1 cup	1966	0.0	0.0	0	0	218.0	1243
regular	1 tbsp	123	0.0	0.0	0	0	13.6	78
regular *(Hain)*	1 tbsp	120	0.0	0.0	0	0	14.0	85
COD NUGGETS, FROZEN								
minced, crunchy 'Bunch O'Crunch' 4 oz								
(Frionor)	8 pieces	320	14.0	19.0	411	<1.0	21.0	(mq)
COFFEE								
brewed	6 oz	4	0.2	0.7	2	0	0.0	0
brewed 'Regular' *(Chock Full o'Nuts)*	6 oz	2	(mq)	(mq)	0	0	0.0	0
freeze-dried, prepared, dark roast 'Maragor' *(Taster's Choice)*	8 oz	4	<1.0	1.0	0	0	<1.0	0
freeze-dried, prepared 'Colombian Select' *(Taster's Choice)*	8 oz	4	<1.0	1.0	0	0	<1.0	0
freeze-dried, prepared 'Original' *(Taster's Choice)*	8 oz	4	<1.0	1.0	0	0	<1.0	0
COFFEE, ALTERNATIVE								
cereal grain beverage, powder *(Pero)*	1 serving	4	<1.0	<1.0	2	(tr)	0.0	0
cereal grain beverage, powder *(Pionier)*	1 serving	6	0.0	1.4	0	(tr)	0.0	0
cereal grain beverage, powder, dry	1 tsp	9	0.1	1.9	2	0	0.1	0
cereal grain beverage, powder,'Instant,' prepared *(Postum)*	6 oz	12	0.0	3.0	0	na	0.0	0
cereal grain beverage, prepared w/water	1 tsp	9	0.2	1.8	7	0	0.0	0
cereal grain beverage, prepared w/skim milk	6 oz	74	6.4	10.8	97	(tr)	0.4	3
cereal grain beverage, prepared w/1% milk	6 oz	86	6.1	10.6	94	(tr)	2.0	8
cereal grain beverage, prepared w/2% milk	6 oz	100	6.2	10.7	94	(tr)	3.6	14
cereal grain beverage, prepared w/whole milk	6 oz	120	6.1	10.4	91	0	6.1	24
cereal grain beverage, w/o added ingredients *(Kaffree Roma)*	8 oz	6	0.0	1.0	(mq)	na	0.0	0
COFFEE, DECAFFEINATED								
(Chock Full o'Nuts)	6 oz	2	(mq)	(mq)	0	0	0.0	0
freeze-dried, prepared, dark roast 'Maragor' *(Taster's Choice)*	8 oz	4	<1.0	1.0	0	0	<1.0	0
freeze-dried, prepared 'Original' *(Taster's Choice)*	8 oz	4	<1.0	1.0	0	0	<1.0	0
instant, powder	1 round tsp	4	0.2	0.8	0	0	0.0	0
instant, powder, prepared	6 oz	4	0.2	0.7	5	0	0.0	0
instant, prepared 'Decaf' *(Nescafé)*	8 oz	4	<1.0	1.0	0	0	<1.0	0

Food Name	Serv. Size	Total Cal.	Prot. GMS	Carbs GMS	Sod. MGS	Fiber GMS	Fat GMS	Chol. MGS
instant, w/chicory, prepared								
(Mountain Blend)	8 oz	6	<1.0	1.0	0	0	<1.0	0
'Suisse Mocha International'								
(General Foods)	6 oz	50	0.0	7.0	30	na	3.0	0
'Suisse Mocha International' sugar-free								
(General Foods)	6 oz	30	0.0	3.0	30	na	2.0	0
COFFEE, FLAVORED								
'Cafe Amaretto International' prepared								
(General Foods)	6 oz	50	0.0	7.0	20	(tr)	2.0	0
'Cafe Français International' prepared								
(General Foods)	6 oz	60	0.0	6.0	25	(tr)	3.0	0
'Cafe Français International' sugar-free								
prepared (General Foods)	6 oz	35	0.0	3.0	30	(tr)	2.0	0
'Cafe Irish Creme International' prepared								
(General Foods)	6 oz	50	0.0	8.0	15	(tr)	2.0	0
'Cafe Vienna Cafe Coffees' prepared								
(Hills Bros)	6 oz	60	1.0	9.0	35	(tr)	2.0	na
'Cafe Vienna International' prepared								
(General Foods)	6 oz	60	0.0	10.0	110	(tr)	2.0	0
'Cafe Vienna International' sugar-free,								
prepared (General Foods)	6 oz	30	0.0	3.0	80	(tr)	2.0	0
'Cappio Cinnamon Iced Cappuccino'								
(Maxwell House)	8 oz	130	2.0	25.0	70	na	3.0	15
'Cappio Coffee Iced Cappuccino'								
(Maxwell House)	8 oz	120	2.0	23.0	75	na	3.0	15
'Cappio Mocha Iced Cappuccino'								
(Maxwell House)	8 oz	130	2.0	25.0	65	na	2.0	15
'Cinnamon Hot Cappuccino'								
(Maxwell House)	6 oz	60	2.0	11.0	100	na	1.0	0
'Coffee Hot Cappuccino' (Maxwell House)	6 oz	60	1.0	12.0	110	na	1.0	0
'Double Dutch Chocolate International'								
prepared (General Foods)	6 oz	50	0.0	8.0	15	(tr)	2.0	0
'Dutch Chocolate Mint International'								
prepared (General Foods)	6 oz	50	0.0	8.0	80	(tr)	2.0	0
'French Vanilla Cafe International' prepared								
(General Foods)	6 oz	60	0.0	9.0	50	na	3.0	0
'Hazelnut Belgian Cafe International'								
prepared (General Foods)	6 oz	60	0.0	10.0	55	na	2.0	0
mocha, banana nut 'Sugar-free' prepared								
(MJB)	6 oz	39	0.8	4.9	60	(tr)	1.8	na
mocha, cherry, prepared (MJB)	6 oz	53	0.5	9.7	17	(tr)	1.4	na
mocha, fudge 'Sugar-free' prepared (MJB)	6 oz	39	1.2	4.5	88	(tr)	1.8	na
mocha, mint, prepared (MJB)	6 oz	53	0.4	9.9	16	(tr)	1.3	na

Food Name	Serv. Size	Total Cal.	Prot. GMS	Carbs GMS	Sod. MGS	Fiber GMS	Fat GMS	Chol. MGS
mocha, mint 'Sugar-free' prepared (MJB) ..	6 oz	37	0.7	5.6	43	(tr)	1.3	na
mocha, prepared (MJB)	6 oz	52	0.6	9.5	54	(tr)	1.3	na
mocha, Swiss 'Cafe Coffees' prepared (Hills Bros)	6 oz	60	1.0	8.0	10	(tr)	2.0	na
mocha, Swiss 'Cafe Coffees Sugar-free' prepared (Hills Bros)	6 oz	40	1.0	5.0	25	(tr)	2.0	na
mocha, vanilla 'Sugar-free' prepared (MJB)	6 oz	39	0.7	5.2	50	(tr)	1.7	na
'Mocha Hot Cappuccino' (Maxwell House)	6 oz	70	2.0	12.0	80	na	2.0	0
orange, Capri 'Cafe Coffees' prepared (Hills Bros)	6 oz	60	1.0	9.0	30	(tr)	2.0	na
'Orange Cappuccino International' prepared (General Foods)	6 oz	60	0.0	10.0	100	(tr)	2.0	0
'Orange Cappuccino International, sugar-free, prepared (General Foods)	6 oz	30	0.0	3.0	60	(tr)	2.0	0
'Suisse Mocha International' prepared (General Foods)	6 oz	50	0.0	7.0	15	na	3.0	0
'Suisse Mocha International' sugar-free, prepared (General Foods)	6 oz	30	0.0	3.0	15	na	2.0	0
'Viennese Chocolate Cafe International' prepared (General Foods)	6 oz	50	0.0	8.0	20	na	2.0	0
COFFEE, INSTANT								
'Brava' prepared (Nescafé)	8 oz	4	<1.0	1.0	0	0	<1.0	0
'Classic' prepared (Nescafé)	8 oz	4	<1.0	1.0	0	0	<1.0	0
powder (Kava)	1 tsp	2	0.0	1.0	5	0	0.0	0
prepared (Nescafé)	8 oz	4	<1.0	1.0	0	0	<1.0	0
regular powder	1 oz	68	3.5	11.7	10	0	0.1	0
regular, powder	1 round tsp	4	0.2	0.7	1	0	0.0	0
regular, prepared	6 oz	4	0.2	0.7	5	0	0.0	0
'Silka' prepared (Nescafé)	8 oz	4	<1.0	1.0	0	0	<1.0	0
w/chicory, powder	1 round tsp	6	0.2	1.3	5	0	0.0	0
w/chicory, prepared	6 oz	7	0.2	1.3	11	0	0.0	0
w/chicory, prepared (Sunrise)	8 oz	6	<1.0	1.0	0	0	<1.0	0
w/chicory 'Mountain Blend' prepared (Nescafé)	8 oz	6	<1.0	1.0	0	0	<1.0	0
w/sugar, cappuccino flavor, powder	2 round tsp	62	0.4	10.7	98	0	2.1	0
w/sugar, cappuccino flavor, prepared	6 oz	61	0.4	10.8	104	0	2.1	0
w/sugar, French flavor, powder	2 round tsp	57	0.5	6.6	24	0	3.4	0
w/sugar, French flavor, prepared	6 oz	57	0.6	6.6	30	0	3.4	0
w/sugar, mocha flavor, powder	2 round tsp	51	0.5	8.4	31	.1	1.9	0
w/sugar, mocha flavor, prepared	6 oz	51	0.6	8.5	36	0	1.9	0
COFFEE FLAVOR DRINK, canned, liquid nutrition (Ensure)	8 oz	250	8.8	34.3	na	na	8.8	na

COFFEE LIQUEUR. See ALCOHOLIC BEVERAGES.

Food Name	Serv. Size	Total Cal.	Prot. GMS	Carbs GMS	Sod. MGS	Fiber GMS	Fat GMS	Chol. MGS
COLA BEVERAGE. See SOFT DRINKS AND MIXERS.								
COLD CUTS. See LUNCHEON MEATS.								
COLE. See KALE.								
COLESLAW								
fresh	4 oz	78	1.5	14.1	26	>.7 c	3.0	9
fresh	1/2 cup	41	0.8	7.4	14	>.4 c	1.6	5
fresh	1 tbsp	6	0.1	1.0	2	>.1 c	0.2	1
COLESLAW DRESSING								
(Kraft)	1 tbsp	70	0.0	4.0	200	na	6.0	10
(Kraft) 'Miracle Whip'	1 tbsp	70	0.0	3.0	105	na	6.0	5
(Litehouse) refrigerated	1 tbsp	80	0.0	2.0	41	na	8.0	na
(T. Marzetti) light	1 tbsp	50	0.0	6.0	240	na	3.0	na
(T. Marzetti) original	1 tbsp	79	<1.0	3.0	180	na	7.0	14
(T. Marzetti) 'South Recipe'	1 tbsp	66	0.0	6.0	93	na	5.0	9
COLEWORT. See KALE.								
COLLARDS								
boiled, drained	4 oz	31	1.5	7.0	18	>.6 c	0.2	0
boiled, drained, chopped	1/2 cup	17	0.9	3.9	161	1.3	0.1	0
raw, chopped	1/2 cup	6	0.3	1.3	4	.7	0.0	0
raw, trimmed	1 oz	9	0.4	2.0	6	>.2 c	0.1	0
raw, untrimmed	1 lb	80	4.1	18.4	51	>1.5 c	0.6	0
Canned								
chopped (Allens)	1/2 cup	20	2.0	2.0	15	(mq)	<1.0	0
chopped, greens (Bush's Best)	1/2 cup	30	2.0	5.0	320	na	0.0	na
chopped, w/pork (Luck's)	7.5 oz	90	2.0	7.0	420	(mq)	7.0	(mq)
Frozen								
boiled, drained	4 oz	41	3.4	8.1	57	>1.2 c	0.5	0
chopped (Seabrook)	3.3 oz	25	3.0	4.0	45	>1.0 c	0.0	0
chopped (Southern)	3.5 oz	30	2.7	4.6	60	(mq)	0.4	0
chopped, boiled, drained	1/2 cup	31	2.5	6.0	43	>.9 c	0.4	0
chopped, unprepared	10-oz pkg	94	7.6	18.3	136	5.7	1.0	0
COLORADO PINYON PINE NUT. See PINE NUT.								
CONCORD PUNCH, 'Juices To Go' (Minute Maid)	6 oz	90	0.0	23.0	20	na	0.0	na
CONDIMENTS. See individual listings.								
COOKIE								
ALMOND								
(Health Valley) date 'Fruit Jumbos'	1 cookie	70	2.0	10.0	30	1.1	3.0	0
(Mother's) shortbread	2 cookies	120	1.0	13.0	50	na	7.0	na
(Natures Warehouse) butter, approx 1 oz	2 cookies	122	2.0	19.2	41	na	4.1	na
(Stella D'oro) 'Breakfast Treats'	1 cookie	101	1.6	15.4	(mq)	(mq)	3.6	na
(Stella D'oro) 'Chinese Dessert'	1 cookie	169	2.4	19.5	(mq)	(mq)	8.9	na
(Stella D'oro) toast 'Mandel'	1 cookie	58	1.3	10.2	(mq)	(mq)	1.4	na

Food Name	Serv. Size	Total Cal.	Prot. GMS	Carbs GMS	Sod. MGS	Fiber GMS	Fat GMS	Chol. MGS
AMARANTH *(Health Valley)* .... 1 cookie		90	2.0	12.0	30	2.3	3.0	0
ANGEL WINGS *(Stella D'oro)* .... 1 cookie		74	1.1	7.0	(mq)	(mq)	4.7	na
ANIMAL CRACKERS								
(FFV) .... 1.25-oz pkg		160	2.0	26.0	150	(mq)	6.0	0
(Finast) 15 pieces .... 1 oz		120	2.0	22.0	110	(mq)	3.0	na
(Grandma's) candied, 5 cookies ...... 1 oz		140	1.0	20.0	80	na	6.0	0
(Keebler) approx .5 oz .... 5 cookies		70	1.0	11.0	75	(mq)	2.0	0
(Mother's) circus animal .... 4 cookies		110	1.0	14.0	40	na	6.0	na
(Nabisco) 'Barnum's Animals' 5								
1/2 pieces .... .5 oz		60	1.0	11.0	70	0	2.0	0
(Sunshine) .... 13 cookies		130	2.0	21.0	160	(mq)	4.0	0
ANISE								
(Stella D'oro) 'Anisette Sponge' .... 1 cookie		51	1.1	9.9	(mq)	(mq)	0.8	na
(Stella D'oro) 'Anisette Toast' .... 1 cookie		46	0.8	9.3	(mq)	(mq)	0.6	na
(Stella D'oro) 'Anisette Toast Jumbo' .. 1 cookie		109	2.0	23.0	(mq)	(mq)	1.0	na
APPLE								
(Archway) n' raisin .... 1 cookie		120	2.0	20.0	169	1.0	3.0	10
(Bakery Wagon) cinnamon .... 1 cookie		100	1.0	17.0	100	na	3.0	2
(Bakery Wagon) filled oatmeal .... 1 cookie		90	1.0	14.0	115	na	4.0	2
(Bakery Wagon) walnut raisin .... 1 cookie		100	2.0	17.0	110	na	3.0	2
(Break Cake) sandwich .... 1 cookie		90	1.0	15.0	70	na	3.0	5
(Estee) cinnamon 'Snack Crisps'								
new blue pkg .... .66 oz		80	1.0	15.0	75	na	2.0	0
(Frookie) cinnamon oat bran .... 1 cookie		45	1.0	6.5	35	na	2.0	0
(Frookie) 'Fruitins' .... 1 cookie		60	1.0	12.0	25	na	1.0	0
(Frookie) spice, fat-free .... 1 cookie		50	1.0	11.0	80	1.0	0.0	0
(Great Cakes) .... 4.5 oz		260	10.0	40.0	20	21.0	6.0	0
(Health Valley) cinnamon 'Mini Fruit								
Centers' fat-free .... 3 cookies		75	2.0	17.0	60	3.0	0.0	0
(Health Valley) 'Fruit Centers' fat-free .. 1 cookie		80	2.0	17.0	80	2.0	0.0	0
(Health Valley) raisin 'Fruit Chunks' ...3 cookies		85	2.0	19.0	80	3.0	0.0	0
(Health Valley) raisin 'Jumbos' fat-free 1 cookie		80	2.0	17.0	80	3.5	0.0	0
(Health Valley) spice, fat-free ...... 3 cookies		80	2.0	18.0	80	3.0	0.0	0
(Healthy Times) 'Hugga Bears' organic .... 1 oz		120	2.0	17.0	38	na	3.0	0
(Nabisco) 'Newtons' 1.25 oz .... 1 cookie		120	1.0	24.0	110	(mq)	3.0	0
(Nabisco) 'Newtons' .75 oz .... 1 cookie		70	1.0	15.0	70	na	2.0	0
(Nabisco) 'Newtons' fat-free, .75 oz ... 1 cookie		70	1.0	16.0	45	0	0.0	0
(Stella D'oro) bar, Dutch .... 1 cookie		112	1.4	18.9	(mq)	(mq)	3.3	na
(Stella D'oro) pastry, dietetic .... 1 cookie		86	1.0	13.0	10	(mq)	3.3	na
(Weight Watchers) fruit filled .... 1 cookie		80	<1.0	21.0	35	na	<1.0	0
(Weight Watchers) raisin bar .... 1 cookie		100	1.0	18.0	115	(mq)	3.0	0

Food Name	Serv. Size	Total Cal.	Prot. GMS	Carbs GMS	Sod. MGS	Fiber GMS	Fat GMS	Chol. MGS
APRICOT								
(Health Valley) almond								
'Fancy Fruit Chunks'	2 cookies	90	2.0	14.0	45	1.8	4.0	0
(Health Valley) apple 'Fruit Chunks'	3 cookies	85	2.0	19.0	80	3.0	0.0	0
(Health Valley) delight, fat-free	3 cookies	80	2.0	18.0	80	3.0	0.0	0
(Health Valley) 'Fruit Centers' fat-free	1 cookie	80	2.0	17.0	80	2.0	0.0	0
(Pepperidge Farm) raspberry								
'Fruit Cookies'	2 cookies	100	1.0	15.0	50	(mq)	4.0	10
(Pepperidge Farm) raspberry 'Zurich'	1 cookie	60	1.0	10.0	30	(mq)	2.0	0
ARROWROOT *(Nabisco)* 'National Arrowroot								
Biscuit' 6 pieces	1 oz	130	2.0	21.0	85	0	4.0	10
ASSORTED								
(Archway) 'Select Assortment'	1 cookie	50	1.0	7.0	40	(mq)	2.0	5
(Fifty 50) wafers, creme filled, w/o sugar	1 wafer	35	<1.0	4.0	10	na	2.0	0
(Stella D'oro) 'Hostess'	1 cookie	42	0.5	5.5	(mq)	(mq)	2.0	na
(Stella D'oro) 'Lady Stella'	1 cookie	42	0.6	5.5	(mq)	(mq)	2.0	na
BANANA								
(Break Cake) creme	1 cookie	240	2.0	37.0	200	na	9.0	5
(Frookie) fat-free	1 cookie	45	1.0	10.0	90	1.0	0.0	0
(Health Valley) spice 'Fruit Chunks'	3 cookies	85	2.0	19.0	80	3.0	0.0	0
(Natures Warehouse) wheat-free, fat-free	1 oz	90	1.6	20.5	84	na	0.7	0
BLUEBERRY *(Great Cakes)*	4.5 oz	260	10.0	40.0	20	21.0	6.0	0
BROWNIE								
(Break Cake) creme	1 cookie	240	2.0	38.0	150	na	8.0	5
(Pepperidge Farm) chocolate nut								
'Old Fashioned'	2 pieces	110	1.0	11.0	45	(mq)	7.0	5
(Pepperidge Farm) cream sandwich								
'Capri'	1 cookie	80	0.0	10.0	45	(mq)	5.0	0
BUTTER								
(Barbara's Bakery) pecan bites								
'Small Indulgences'	1 oz	140	2.0	16.0	95	na	8.0	20
(Delicious) frosted, made w/Land O'Lakes								
butter	1 cookie	88	1.0	11.0	44	0	5.0	10
(Fifty 50) fructose sweetened,								
low sodium	1 cookie	40	<1.0	5.0	20	na	2.0	5
(Keebler) flavor, chocolate coated								
'Baby Bear' .5 oz	3 cookies	70	1.0	10.0	55	(mq)	2.0	0
(Keebler) flavor, chocolate coated								
'E.L. Fudge' .5 oz	2 cookies	80	<1.0	10.0	40	(mq)	4.0	5
(Lu) 'Little Schoolboy'	1 cookie	70	1.0	8.0	35	na	4.0	na
(Lu) 'Petite Beurre'	1 cookie	40	1.0	7.0	45	na	1.0	na
(Mother's) flavored	5 cookies	140	2.0	20.0	130	na	6.0	na
(Pepperidge Farm) flavor 'Chessmen'	2 cookies	90	1.0	12.0	60	(mq)	4.0	10

Food Name	Serv. Size	Total Cal.	Prot. GMS	Carbs GMS	Sod. MGS	Fiber GMS	Fat GMS	Chol. MGS
(Stella D'oro) 'Como Delight'	1 cookie	145	2.1	17.9	(mq)	(mq)	7.2	na
CANDY *(Oven Lovin')*	1 cookie	70	0.0	10.0	40	na	3.0	0
CARAMEL								
(FFV) patties, approx 1 oz	2 cookies	150	1.0	20.0	125	(mq)	7.0	na
(Keebler) apple oatmeal 'Elfin Delights'	1 cookie	65	<1.0	12.0	55	na	2.0	0
(Natures Warehouse) crisp, wheat-free, fat-free	1 oz	90	1.6	20.5	84	na	0.7	0
CAROB								
(Health Valley) 'Healthy Chips' fat-free	3 cookies	80	2.0	18.0	80	2.0	0.0	0
(Natures Warehouse) fudge, approx 1 oz	2 cookies	116	1.4	20.5	78	na	3.1	na
(Westbrae) 'Rice Malt Snap'	1 oz	140	2.0	18.0	70	na	7.0	0
CARROT WALNUT 'Wholesome Choice'								
(Pepperidge Farm)	1 piece	60	1.0	11.0	45	(mq)	1.0	0
CHERRY								
(Great Cakes) carob	4.5 oz	280	10.0	40.0	20	21.0	8.0	0
(Natures Warehouse) wheat-free, fat-free	1 oz	90	1.6	20.5	84	na	0.7	0
CHIPS AND CREME								
(Break Cake)	1 cookie	140	1.0	21.0	130	na	6.0	2
(Frookie) and vanilla sandwich 'Frookwich'	1 cookie	50	<1.0	7.0	30	na	2.0	0
CHOCOLATE								
(Barbara's Bakery) raspberry 'Cookies & Creme'	2 cookies	120	2.0	18.0	80	na	5.0	15
(Barbara's Bakery) vanilla 'Cookies & Creme'	2 cookies	120	2.0	18.0	80	na	5.0	15
(Betty Crocker) w/peanut butter creme 'Dunkaroos'	1 tray	140	3.0	15.0	140	na	8.0	0
(Drake's) approx 1 oz	2 cookies	130	2.0	19.0	85	(mq)	5.0	0
(Estee) 'Snack Crisps'	.66 oz	80	1.0	15.0	65	na	2.0	0
(Featherweight) creme wafer	1 cookie	20	0.0	3.0	0	(mq)	1.0	0
(Frookie) 'Animal Frackers'	6 cookies	60	1.0	9.0	70	na	2.0	0
(Frookie) 'Funky Monkeys'	8 cookies	60	1.0	10.0	60	na	2.0	0
(Grandma's) 'Chocolate Cookie Bits' 8 cookies	1 oz	140	2.0	19.0	180	na	6.0	0
(Lu) 'Chocolatiers'	2 cookies	85	1.0	10.0	10	na	4.0	na
(Lu) 'Chocolatiers' dipped	2 cookies	105	1.0	12.0	15	na	6.0	na
(Nabisco) 'Chocolate Snap' 4 pieces	.5 oz	70	1.0	10.0	80	na	2.0	0
(Nabisco) 'Pure Chocolate Middles'	.5 oz cookie	80	1.0	9.0	35	0	5.0	5
(Pepperidge Farm) walnut 'Beacon Hill'	1 cookie	120	2.0	14.0	65	1.0	7.0	5
(Stella D'oro) 'Castelets'	1 cookie	64	0.8	9.0	(mq)	(mq)	2.8	na
(Stella D'oro) 'Margherite'	1 cookie	72	0.9	10.2	(mq)	(mq)	3.1	na
(Tastykake) 'Soft 'n Chewy'	1.4 oz	171	2.1	26.2	111	1.1	7.0	3

Food Name	Serv. Size	Total Cal.	Prot. GMS	Carbs GMS	Sod. MGS	Fiber GMS	Fat GMS	Chol. MGS
(Weight Watchers)	3 cookies	80	1.0	13.0	70	(mq)	3.0	na
CHOCOLATE CHIP								
(Almost Home)	.5 oz	60	1.0	8.0	45	na	3.0	2
(Archway)	1 cookie	50	1.0	7.0	40	(mq)	3.0	5
(Barbara's Bakery)	1 oz	130	2.0	16.0	60	na	6.0	0
(Barbara's Bakery) crisp								
'Small Indulgences'	1 oz	140	2.0	18.0	105	na	7.0	15
(Break Cake) approx 1 oz	5 cookies	140	2.0	20.0	115	na	6.0	5
(Chips Ahoy!)	.5 oz	50	1.0	7.0	35	0	2.0	0
(Chips Ahoy!) 'Chewy'	.5 oz	60	1.0	7.0	40	0	3.0	0
(Chips Ahoy!) 'Mini'	.5 oz	70	1.0	9.0	50	0	3.0	0
(Chips Ahoy!) pecan 'Selections'	.5 oz	100	1.0	10.0	65	0	6.0	10
(Chips Ahoy!) 'Rockers'	1 cookie	60	1.0	8.0	40	na	3.0	0
(Chips Ahoy!) 'Sprinkled'	.5 oz	60	1.0	8.0	40	0	3.0	0
(Chips Ahoy!) 'Striped'	.5 oz	90	1.0	10.0	45	0	5.0	0
(Chips Ahoy!) walnut 'Selections'	.5 oz	100	1.0	9.0	70	0	6.0	5
(Chips Ahoy!) white fudge chunk	1 cookie	90	1.0	11.0	75	na	5.0	5
(Drake's) approx 1 oz	2 cookies	140	1.0	18.0	110	(mq)	6.0	0
(Duncan Hines)	2 cookies	110	1.0	15.0	85	na	5.0	na
(Entenmann's)	3 cookies	140	1.0	19.0	85	na	7.0	na
(Estee)	3 cookies	110	1.0	13.0	20	na	5.0	0
(Featherweight)	1 cookie	45	1.0	6.0	0	(mq)	2.0	0
(Fifty 50) fructose sweetened	1 cookie	35	<1.0	4.0	10	na	2.0	0
(Finast)	1 oz	90	1.0	18.0	60	(mq)	7.0	0
(Frookie)	1 cookie	45	1.0	6.5	35	na	2.0	0
(Frookie) Mandarin	1 cookie	45	1.0	6.5	35	na	2.0	0
(Frookie) mint	1 cookie	45	1.0	6.5	35	na	2.0	0
(Grandma's) 'Big Cookies' 2.75 oz	2 cookies	370	4.0	50.0	270	(mq)	17.0	5
(Grandma's) 'Rich'N Chewy' 3 cookies	1 oz	140	1.0	20.0	80	na	6.0	5
(Keebler) bakery crisp 'Chips Deluxe' ..	1 cookie	60	1.0	7.0	45	na	3.0	0
(Keebler) chewy 'Elfin Delights'	1 cookie	65	<1.0	11.0	55	na	2.0	0
(Keebler) 'Chips Deluxe' approx .5 oz .	1 cookie	80	<1.0	10.0	75	(mq)	4.0	5
(Keebler) 'Coconut Chocolate Drop' ..	1 cookie	80	1.0	10.0	60	na	5.0	0
(Keebler) deluxe 'Bakery Crisp'	1 cookie	60	1.0	7.0	45	na	3.0	0
(Keebler) 'Rainbow Chips Deluxe' .5 oz	1 cookie	80	1.0	11.0	45	(mq)	3.0	5
(Keebler) 'Soft Batch' approx .5 oz	1 cookie	80	<1.0	10.0	70	(mq)	4.0	0
(Mother's)	1 cookie	70	1.0	10.0	55	na	3.0	na
(Mother's) angel	2 cookies	120	1.0	14.0	45	na	8.0	na
(Nabisco) bite size 'Snack Wells'	.5 oz	60	<1.0	11.0	85	na	1.0	0
(Nabisco) 'Chocolate Chip Snaps' 3 pieces .5 oz		70	1.0	11.0	50	0	2.0	0
(Oven Lovin')	1 cookie	70	0.0	9.0	50	na	3.0	5
(Pepperidge Farm) 'Family Request' ..	2 cookies	90	1.0	15.0	55	na	5.0	5
(Pepperidge Farm) 'Old Fashioned' ..	2 cookies	100	1.0	12.0	45	(mq)	5.0	5

Food Name	Serv. Size	Total Cal.	Prot. GMS	Carbs GMS	Sod. MGS	Fiber GMS	Fat GMS	Chol. MGS
(Pepperidge Farm) w/macadamia nuts								
'Big, Soft and Chewy'	1 cookie	130	1.0	16.0	45	na	7.0	10
(Pepperidge Farm) w/macadamia nuts								
'Sausalito'	1 cookie	120	1.0	14.0	65	(mq)	7.0	5
(Tastykake) bar, 1.5 oz	1 cookie	193	3.0	28.3	97	1.0	8.4	4
(Tastykake) 'Soft 'n Chewy'	1.4 oz	174	2.3	25.5	168	.9	7.3	10
(Weight Watchers)	2 cookies	90	1.0	18.0	65	na	2.0	0
CHOCOLATE CHOCOLATE CHIP								
(Barbara's Bakery)	1 oz	125	2.0	17.0	50	na	5.0	0
(Natures Warehouse) approx 1 oz	2 cookies	130	2.8	16.4	69	na	6.1	na
(Pepperidge Farm) walnut, big,								
soft & chewy	1 cookie	130	1.0	17.0	45	na	6.0	5
(Pillsbury's Best)	1 cookie	70	1.0	9.0	35	na	3.0	0
CHOCOLATE CHUNK								
(Chips Ahoy!) 'Chunky'	1 cookie	80	1.0	11.0	60	1.0	4.0	10
(Chips Ahoy!) 'Selections'	.5 oz	90	1.0	10.0	65	0	5.0	10
(Dunkin' Donuts) 1.5 oz	1 cookie	200	3.0	25.0	110	1.0	10.0	30
(Dunkin' Donuts) w/nuts, 1.5 oz	1 cookie	210	3.0	23.0	100	2.0	11.0	30
(Pepperidge Farm) 'Big, Soft								
and Chewy'	1 cookie	130	2.0	17.0	45	na	6.0	10
CHOCOLATE-FILLED SANDWICH								
(Keebler) 'E.L. Fudge'	1 cookie	60	<1.0	8.0	35	(mq)	3.0	5
(Pepperidge Farm) 'Brussels'	2 cookies	110	1.0	13.0	65	(mq)	5.0	0
(Pepperidge Farm) 'Brussels Mint'	2 cookies	130	1.0	17.0	40	(mq)	7.0	0
(Pepperidge Farm) 'Double Chocolate								
Milano'	2 cookies	150	2.0	18.0	45	na	8.0	10
(Pepperidge Farm) 'Hazelnut Milano'	2 cookies	130	2.0	15.0	30	na	8.0	5
(Pepperidge Farm) 'Lido'	1 cookie	90	1.0	10.0	30	(mq)	5.0	5
(Pepperidge Farm) 'Milano'	2 cookies	120	1.0	15.0	45	(mq)	6.0	5
(Pepperidge Farm) 'Mint Milano'	2 cookies	150	1.0	17.0	60	(mq)	7.0	5
(Pepperidge Farm) 'Orange Milano'	2 cookies	150	1.0	17.0	60	(mq)	7.0	5
(Pepperidge Farm) 'Orleans'	2 cookies	120	1.0	14.0	40	(mq)	8.0	0
CHOCOLATE GRAHAM								
(Keebler) 'Thin Bits' approx .5 oz	12 cookies	70	1.0	9.0	75	(mq)	3.0	0
(Nabisco) approx .5 oz	11 cookies	60	1.0	10.0	90	(mq)	2.0	0
(Nabisco) 'Bugs Bunny'	.5 oz	60	1.0	10.0	80	na	2.0	0
(Nabisco) 'Chocolate Grahams'	.5 oz	150	3.0	17.0	80	0	7.0	0
(Teddy Grahams) 'Bearwichs'	.5 oz	70	1.0	10.0	60	na	3.0	0
(Teddy Grahams) w/vanilla creme								
'Bearwichs'	4 cookies	70	1.0	10.0	60	(mq)	3.0	0
CHOCOLATE SANDWICH								
(Estee)	1 cookie	50	<1.0	7.0	15	(mq)	2.0	0
(Frookie) 'Frookwich'	1 cookie	50	<1.0	7.0	30	na	2.0	0

Food Name	Serv. Size	Total Cal.	Prot. GMS	Carbs GMS	Sod. MGS	Fiber GMS	Fat GMS	Chol. MGS
(Keebler) 'Chocolate Creme Sandwich' .... .5 oz		80	1.0	12.0	70	(mq)	4.0	0
(Keebler) 'E.L. Fudge' .... 1 cookie		70	<1.0	9.0	50	(mq)	3.0	0
(Keebler) fudge creme 'Elfin Delights' .. 1 cookie		55	<1.0	10.0	50	na	2.0	0
(Keebler) peanut butter 'E.L. Fudge' ... 1 cookie		50	1.0	7.0	50	(mq)	3.0	0
(Little Debbie) .... 1.8 oz		250	3.0	35.0	260	(mq)	12.0	<1
(Oreo) 'Big Stuf' .... .25 oz		200	2.0	27.0	220	1.0	9.0	5
(Oreo) 'Double Stuf' 2 cookies .... 1 oz		70	1.0	9.0	75	na	4.0	na
(Oreo) fudge covered .... .75 oz		110	1.0	13.0	80	(mq)	6.0	2
(Oreo) 'Halloween Treats' 1 oz ...... 2 cookies		140	1.0	20.0	150	1.0	7.0	0
(Oreo) 2 1/2 cookies .... 1 oz		140	1.0	20.0	170	0	6.0	0
(Oreo) white fudge covered .... .75 oz		110	1.0	14.0	75	(mq)	6.0	2
(Weight Watchers) .... 2 cookies		90	1.0	15.0	90	na	3.0	0
CHUNK								
(Pepperidge Farm) 'Nantucket' ...... 1 cookie		120	1.0	15.0	60	1.0	6.0	5
(Pepperidge Farm) pecan 'Chesapeake' .... 1 cookie		120	1.0	14.0	60	1.0	7.0	5
(Pepperidge Farm) pecan 'Special Collection' .... 1 cookie		70	0.0	8.0	25	(mq)	4.0	10
CINNAMON								
(Frookie) 'Animal Frackers' .... 6 cookies		60	1.0	9.0	45	na	2.0	0
(Mother's) dinosaur, mini .... 7 cookies		70	1.0	9.0	40	na	2.0	na
(Mother's) dinosaur grahams .... 1 cookie		80	1.0	12.0	50	na	3.0	na
CINNAMON GRAHAM								
(Honey Maid) approx .5 oz .... 2 cookies		60	1.0	12.0	85	(mq)	1.0	0
(Keebler) 'Alpha Grahams' .... 6 cookies		70	1.0	10.0	55	(mq)	2.0	0
(Keebler) 'Cinnamon Crisp' .5 oz .... 4 cookies		70	1.0	11.0	85	(mq)	2.0	0
(Keebler) fudge covered 'Deluxe' .5 oz .... 2 cookies		90	<1.0	11.0	60	(mq)	4.0	0
(Keebler) 'Thin Bits' approx .5 oz ... 12 cookies		70	1.0	10.0	50	(mq)	3.0	0
(Nabisco) 'Bugs Bunny' .... .5 oz		60	1.0	11.0	80	na	3.0	0
(Nabisco) fat-free 'Snack Wells' .... .5 oz		50	1.0	12.0	45	na	0.0	0
(Nabisco) w/fudge 'Cookies'N Fudge' .. 1 cookie		45	<1.0	6.0	35	(mq)	2.0	0
(Natures Warehouse) approx 1 oz ... 2 cookies		113	1.2	18.8	71	na	3.6	na
(Pepperidge Farm) sugar 'Family Request' .... 2 cookies		80	1.0	12.0	40	na	4.0	15
(Sunshine) .... 1 cookie		70	1.0	11.0	95	(mq)	3.0	0
(Teddy Grahams) 'Bearwichs' .... .5 oz		70	1.0	10.0	60	na	3.0	0
COCOA								
(Westbrae) chip 'Rice Malt Snap' .... 1 oz		130	2.0	18.0	60	na	7.0	0
(Westbrae) 'Rice Malt Snap' .... 1 oz		140	2.0	17.0	70	na	7.0	0
COCONUT								
(Break Cake) macaroons .... 2 cookies		270	2.0	34.0	160	na	14.0	0
(Drake's) approx 1 oz .... 2 cookies		130	2.0	20.0	95	(mq)	5.0	0

Food Name	Serv. Size	Total Cal.	Prot. GMS	Carbs GMS	Sod. MGS	Fiber GMS	Fat GMS	Chol. MGS
(Estee) .... 3 cookies		110	1.0	14.0	15	na	5.0	0
(Glenny's) almonds, raisins 'Nookie Bar' 1.15 oz		138	2.0	18.0	na	na	3.0	na
(Mother's) cocadas	4 cookies	120	2.0	17.0	150	na	6.0	na
(Mother's) macaroons	1 cookie	80	1.0	8.0	40	na	5.0	na
(Natures Warehouse) approx 1 oz ...	2 cookies	130	1.4	13.9	20	na	7.6	na
(Pepperidge Farm) chocolate-filled 'Tahiti'	1 cookie	90	0.0	9.0	25	(mq)	6.0	5
(Stella D'oro) dietetic	1 cookie	52	0.8	6.8	10	(mq)	2.4	na
(Stella D'oro) macaroon	1 cookie	60	0.7	6.6	(mq)	(mq)	3.4	na
COFFEE								
(Barbara's Bakery) coffee cake crunch								
'Small Indulgences' .... 1 oz		130	2.0	18.0	140	na	6.0	20
(Pepperidge Farm)	1 cookie	50	0.0	6.0	20	(mq)	3.0	5
CRANBERRY								
(Frookie) orange, fat-free	1 cookie	45	1.0	10.0	75	1.0	0.0	0
(Nabisco) 'Newtons' fat-free	1 cookie	70	1.0	16.0	70	na	0.0	0
(Pepperidge Farm) honey, soft								
'Wholesome Choice'	1 cookie	60	1.0	11.0	50	na	2.0	0
CROKINE (Lu)	2 cookies	35	1.0	7.0	70	na	0.0	na
DATE								
(Bakery Wagon) filled oatmeal	1 cookie	90	1.0	15.0	100	na	3.0	2
(Break Cake) creme	1 cookie	140	1.0	21.0	140	na	5.0	2
(Health Valley) delight, fat-free	3 cookies	80	2.0	18.0	80	3.0	0.0	0
(Health Valley) 'Fruit Centers' fat-free ..	1 cookie	70	1.0	16.0	35	3.5	0.0	0
(Health Valley) pecan 'Fancy Fruit Chunks'	2 cookies	90	2.0	15.0	45	1.7	4.0	0
(Pepperidge Farm) pecan 'Kitchen Hearth'	2 cookies	110	1.0	15.0	40	(mq)	5.0	10
DEVIL'S FOOD								
(Break Cake) creme	1 cookie	130	1.0	20.0	120	na	5.0	0
(FFV) 'Trolley Cakes' 2 oz	2 cookies	120	2.0	25.0	80	(mq)	2.0	na
(Nabisco) cakes	1 cookie	70	1.0	15.0	40	(mq)	1.0	0
DUPLEX SANDWICH (Mother's)	2 cookies	105	1.0	15.0	70	na	5.0	na
EGG BISCUIT								
(Estee) 'Original Sandwich'	1 cookie	45	<1.0	6.0	5	(mq)	2.0	0
(FFV) 'Kreem Pilot Bread'	1 cookie	60	1.0	9.0	60	(mq)	2.0	na
(FFV) 'Royal Dainty' .7 oz	2 cookies	120	1.0	14.0	90	(mq)	6.0	na
(FFV) 'T.C. Rounds' approx 1 oz	2 cookies	160	1.0	20.0	65	(mq)	8.0	na
(FFV) 'Tango' 1.2 oz	2 cookies	160	1.0	26.0	50	(mq)	5.0	na
(Stella D'oro)	1 cookie	43	1.6	6.7	(mq)	(mq)	1.1	na
(Stella D'oro) 'Anginetti'	1 cookie	31	0.5	4.9	(mq)	(mq)	1.0	na
(Stella D'oro) dietetic	1 cookie	43	1.7	6.5	10	(mq)	1.1	na
(Stella D'oro) dietetic 'Kitchen'	1 cookie	8	0.2	0.7	10	(mq)	0.5	na
(Stella D'oro) 'Jumbo'	1 cookie	47	1.0	9.1	(mq)	(mq)	0.7	na
(Stella D'oro) 'Roman'	1 cookie	137	2.7	20.4	(mq)	(mq)	5.0	na
(Stella D'oro) sugared	1 cookie	75	1.6	14.3	(mq)	(mq)	1.4	na

Food Name	Serv. Size	Total Cal.	Prot. GMS	Carbs GMS	Sod. MGS	Fiber GMS	Fat GMS	Chol. MGS
ENGLISH TEA (Mother's) sandwich ...	1 cookie	100	1.0	14.0	60	na	4.0	na
FIG								
(Estee) bar	2 cookies	90	<1.0	21.0	60	na	1.0	0
(FFV) bar, vanilla	1 cookie	70	1.0	12.0	55	(mq)	1.0	0
(FFV) bar, whole wheat	1 cookie	70	1.0	11.0	50	(mq)	2.0	0
(Frookie) 'Fruitins'	1 cookie	60	1.0	12.0	25	na	1.0	0
(Frookie) 'Fruitins' fat-free	2 cookies	90	1.0	21.0	75	1.0	0.0	0
(Keebler) bar	1 cookie	60	1.0	11.0	70	(mq)	2.0	0
(Mother's) bar	2 cookies	110	1.0	23.0	85	na	2.0	na
(Mother's) whole wheat	2 cookies	120	2.0	25.0	105	na	2.0	na
(Nabisco) 'Newtons'	.5 oz	60	1.0	11.0	6	(mq)	1.0	0
(Nabisco) 'Newtons'	1.25 oz	120	1.0	24.0	110	(mq)	3.0	0
(Nabisco) 'Newtons Cookie Variety' ...	1 oz	120	1.0	24.0	110	na	3.0	0
(Nabisco) 'Newtons' fat-free, 1 piece ...	.75 oz	70	1.0	15.0	80	<1.0 c	0.0	0
(Natures Warehouse) bar, apple cinnamon, wheat-free	1 oz	98	1.0	19.0	18	na	2.0	na
(Natures Warehouse) bar, raspberry, wheat-free	1 oz	98	1.0	19.0	18	na	2.0	na
(Natures Warehouse) bar, wheat-free	1 oz	98	1.0	19.0	18	na	2.0	na
(Natures Warehouse) bar, whole wheat ...	1 oz	98	1.0	19.0	18	na	2.0	na
(Stella D'oro) pastry, dietetic	1 cookie	89	1.0	13.0	10	(mq)	3.7	na
FORTUNE								
(LaChoy)	1 oz	112	1.5	26.3	11	.7	0.2	0
(LaChoy)	1 cookie	15	<1.0	4.0	1	<1.0	<1.0	0
FRUIT								
(Barbara's Bakery) and nut	1 oz	140	2.0	18.0	55	na	6.0	0
(Health Valley) 'Fruit & Fitness'	5 cookies	200	4.0	40.0	249	4.0	6.0	0
(Health Valley) Hawaiian, fat-free ...	3 cookies	80	2.0	18.0	80	3.0	0.0	0
(Health Valley) tropical 'Fancy Fruit Chunks'	2 cookies	80	2.0	13.0	45	1.7	3.0	0
(Health Valley) tropical 'Fruit Centers' fat-free	1 cookie	80	2.0	17.0	80	2.0	0.0	0
(Health Valley) tropical 'Fruit Jumbos' ..	1 cookie	70	1.0	10.0	26	1.5	2.0	0
(Stella D'oro) slices	1 cookie	60	1.1	8.7	(mq)	(mq)	2.2	na
FUDGE								
(Almost Home)	.5 oz	70	1.0	9.0	50	(mq)	3.0	2
(Almost Home) chocolate chip	.5 oz	70	1.0	9.0	50	0	3.0	2
(Chips Ahoy!) mini bites 'Little Fudgies' ...	1 oz	230	3.0	27.0	105	0	12.0	0
(Estee)	1 cookie	30	<1.0	4.0	0	(mq)	1.0	0
(Fifty 50) brownie, fructose sweetened	1 cookie	35	<1.0	5.0	0	na	2.0	0
(Grandma's) 'Big Cookies' 2.75 oz ...	2 cookies	350	4.0	54.0	380	(mq)	13.0	5
(Keebler) mint 'Grasshopper' approx .5 oz	2 cookies	70	<1.0	10.0	35	(mq)	3.0	0

Food Name	Serv. Size	Total Cal.	Prot. GMS	Carbs GMS	Sod. MGS	Fiber GMS	Fat GMS	Chol. MGS
(M&M/Mars) 'Twix'	1 bar	100	1.0	11.0	35	na	6.0	na
(Mother's) double fudge sandwich	2 cookies	100	2.0	15.0	75	na	4.0	na
(Mother's) wafer 'Flaky Flix'	2 cookies	130	1.0	14.0	30	na	9.0	30
(Nabisco) caramel, peanut								
'Heyday Bars' 1 piece	.75 oz	110	2.0	13.0	40	1.0	6.0	0
(Nabisco) middles	.5 oz	80	1.0	9.0	35	(mq)	5.0	5
(Nabisco) wafer 'Famous Wafers'								
2 1/2 pieces	.5 oz	70	1.0	11.0	110	(mq)	2.0	2
(Nabisco) snaps, approx .5 oz	4 cookies	70	1.0	11.0	75	(mq)	2.0	2
(Stella D'oro) 'Swiss Fudge Cookie'	1 cookie	68	0.8	8.5	(mq)	(mq)	3.4	na
(Tastykake) bar	1.8 oz	205	2.3	35.0	155	1.4	6.8	6
GINGER								
(FFV) boys	1.25-oz pkg	150	2.0	26.0	210	(mq)	5.0	0
(Frookie) spice	1 cookie	45	1.0	6.5	35	na	2.0	0
(Pepperidge Farm) 'Gingerman'	2 cookies	70	1.0	10.0	50	(mq)	3.0	5
(Westbrae) 'Rice Malt Snap'	1 oz	130	2.0	20.0	140	na	5.0	0
GINGERSNAPS								
(Archway) '80/pkg'	1 cookie	25	1.0	4.0	20	(mq)	<1.0	0
(Archway) '54/pkg'	1 cookie	35	0.0	6.0	30	(mq)	1.0	0
(Break Cake) approx 1 oz	5 cookies	130	2.0	20.0	110	na	5.0	0
(Delicious)	.5 oz	64	0.8	11.3	78	na	1.7	<1
(FFV) approx 1 oz	5 cookies	130	2.0	22.0	140	(mq)	4.0	0
(Nabisco) 'Old Fashioned'	.25 oz	30	<1.0	6.0	45	(mq)	1.0	0
(Sunshine)	5 cookies	100	1.0	16.0	120	(mq)	3.0	0
GRAHAM. See also HONEY GRAHAM.								
(Betty Crocker) w/chocolate frosting								
'Dunkaroos'	1 tray	130	1.0	19.0	70	na	5.0	0
(Betty Crocker) w/vanilla frosting								
'Dunkaroos'	1 tray	130	<1.0	21.0	60	na	5.0	0
(Keebler) chocolate 'Selects'	4 cookies	60	1.0	9.0	55	na	3.0	0
(Keebler) honey nut 'Selects'	4 cookies	60	1.0	9.0	70	na	3.0	0
(Mother's) dinosaur, original	1 cookie	70	1.0	12.0	50	na	2.0	na
(Mother's) dinosaur, mini	7 cookies	60	1.0	9.0	40	na	1.0	na
(Nabisco) 'Bugs Bunny' 5 pieces	.5 oz	60	1.0	11.0	70	na	2.0	0
(Pepperidge Farm) cinnamon 'Goldfish'	1 oz	130	2.0	19.0	130	na	7.0	10
(Pepperidge Farm) 'Goldfish'	1 oz	140	2.0	18.0	140	na	7.0	10
(Teddy Grahams) snacks, chocolate	.5 oz	60	1.0	10.0	80	0	2.0	0
(Teddy Grahams) snacks, cinnamon	.75-oz bag	100	1.0	16.0	120	0	3.0	0
(Teddy Grahams) snacks, honey, 11 pieces	.5 oz	60	1.0	11.0	90	na	2.0	0
(Teddy Grahams) vanilla honey								
'Bearwichs'	4 cookies	70	1.0	10.0	65	(mq)	3.0	0

Food Name	Serv. Size	Total Cal.	Prot. GMS	Carbs GMS	Sod. MGS	Fiber GMS	Fat GMS	Chol. MGS
GRANOLA								
(Betty Crocker) chocolate filling								
'Incredibites'	1 pouch	170	2.0	24.0	150	na	7.0	0
(Betty Crocker) peanut butter								
'Incredibites'	1 pouch	170	2.0	23.0	160	na	8.0	0
(Betty Crocker) vanilla creme								
'Incredibites'	1 pouch	170	2.0	24.0	180	na	7.0	0
(Health Valley) 'Healthy'	3 cookies	75	2.0	17.0	60	3.0	0.0	0
'HERMIT' (Break Cake)	1 cookie	230	3.0	38.0	280	na	7.0	10
'HOB-NOBS' (Carr's)	1 cookie	72	1.1	9.6	78	(mq)	3.2	na
HONEY								
(Bakery Wagon) fruit bar	1 cookie	100	1.0	16.0	70	na	3.0	2
(Health Valley) cinnamon, crisp								
'Honey Jumbos'	1 cookie	70	1.0	10.0	35	2.6	2.0	0
(Health Valley) oat bran, fancy								
'Honey Jumbos'	1 cookie	70	1.0	10.0	22	1.6	2.0	0
(Health Valley) peanut butter, crisp								
'Honey Jumbos'	1 cookie	70	2.0	10.0	24	1.5	2.0	0
(Stella D'oro) 'Royal Nuggets'	1 cookie	2	0.1	0.1	na	na	0.1	na
HONEY GRAHAM								
(Carafection) 'Original' carob coated	1 oz	139	2.0	17.0	26	na	7.0	na
(Carr's) wheat 'Home Wheat Graham'	1 cookie	74	1.0	10.9	<1	(mq)	3.3	na
(Health Valley) 'Fancy'	7 cookies	130	3.0	21.0	89	3.5	5.0	0
(Health Valley) oat bran	7 cookies	130	3.0	25.0	47	3.4	2.0	0
(Honey Maid) .5 oz	2 pieces	60	1.0	11.0	90	(mq)	1.0	0
(Honey Maid) honey'n oat bran								
'Graham Bites'	.5 oz	60	1.0	11.0	55	(mq)	2.0	0
(Keebler) approx .5 oz	4 cookies	70	1.0	12.0	85	(mq)	2.0	0
(Nabisco) vanilla, approx .5 oz	11 cookies	60	1.0	10.0	75	(mq)	2.0	0
(Pepperidge Farm) hazelnut								
'Old Fashioned'	2 cookies	110	1.0	15.0	75	(mq)	6.0	0
(Sunshine)	1 piece	60	1.0	10.0	90	(mq)	2.0	0
JELLY								
(Delicious) top	.8 oz	112	1.7	14.3	34	na	5.3	<1
(FFV) tarts	1 cookie	60	<1.0	11.0	55	(mq)	2.0	0
LEMON								
(Barbara's Bakery) almond delights								
'Small Indulgences'	1 oz	140	2.0	18.0	135	na	6.0	20
(Delicious) sugar wafer	1 wafer	35	<1.0	4.0	3	na	2.0	0
(Estee)	3 cookies	100	1.0	14.0	15	na	5.0	0
(Estee) 'Snack Crisps'	.66 oz	80	1.0	15.0	75	na	2.0	0
(Featherweight)	1 cookie	45	1.0	6.0	0	(mq)	2.0	0
(Frookie) sandwich 'Frookwich'	1 cookie	50	<1.0	7.0	30	na	2.0	0

Food Name	Serv. Size	Total Cal.	Prot. GMS	Carbs GMS	Sod. MGS	Fiber GMS	Fat GMS	Chol. MGS
(Pepperidge Farm) nut crunch								
'Old Fashioned'	2 cookies	110	1.0	13.0	50	(mq)	7.0	5
(Westbrae) 'Rice Malt Snap'	1 oz	130	2.0	20.0	70	na	6.0	0
MARSHMALLOW								
(Nabisco) cake 'Mallomars'	1 cookie	60	1.0	8.0	20	na	3.0	0
(Nabisco) fudge cake 'Puffs'	.75 oz	90	1.0	14.0	45	(mq)	4.0	0
(Nabisco) fudge cake 'Twirls'	1 oz	140	1.0	20.0	70	(mq)	6.0	0
(Nabisco) fudge graham								
'Suddenly S'Mores'	.75 oz	100	1.0	15.0	90	na	4.0	0
(Nabisco) 'Pinwheels'	1 cookie	130	1.0	20.0	35	0	5.0	0
(Pinwheels) chocolate cake	1 oz	130	1.0	20.0	40	(mq)	5.0	0
MINI-CREME *(Delicious)*	1 wafer	24	<1.0	3.0	2	na	1.0	0
MINT								
(Carafection) honey graham, carob coated	1 oz	139	2.0	17.0	26	na	7.0	na
(FFV) sandwich, approx 1.1 oz	2 cookies	160	2.0	22.0	50	(mq)	7.0	na
(Girl Scout Cookies) thin mints	4 cookies	160	1.0	20.0	140	2.0	9.0	0
(Keebler) 'Soft Batch'	1 cookie	80	1.0	10.0	70	(mq)	4.0	0
(Nabisco) sandwich 'Mystic Mint'	.5 oz	90	1.0	11.0	65	0	4.0	0
MOLASSES								
(Archway)	1 cookie	100	1.0	18.0	155	2.0	2.0	10
(Bakery Wagon) iced	1 cookie	100	1.0	17.0	120	na	4.0	5
(Grandma's) 'Old Time Big Cookies'	2 cookies	320	4.0	58.0	520	(mq)	9.0	5
(Nabisco) 'Pantry'	.5 oz	80	1.0	13.0	75	(mq)	3.0	0
(Pepperidge Farm) crisps 'Old Fashioned'	2 cookies	70	1.0	8.0	50	(mq)	3.0	0
MÜESLI *(Carr's)*	1 cookie	84	1.1	10.8	30	(mq)	4.1	na
OAT BRAN								
(Awrey's) raisin	1 cookie	100	1.0	14.0	115	1.0	4.0	0
(Frookie) muffin	1 cookie	45	1.0	6.5	35	na	2.0	0
(Health Valley) animal cookies	7 cookies	110	3.0	20.0	50	3.0	4.0	0
(Health Valley) fruit and nut	2 cookies	110	3.0	17.0	70	2.8	4.0	0
(Health Valley) fruit 'Oat Bran Fruit Jumbos'	1 cookie	70	1.0	10.0	22	1.5	2.0	0
(Health Valley) raisin 'Fancy Fruit Chunks'	2 cookies	90	2.0	15.0	95	1.6	3.0	0
(Natures Warehouse) chocolate chip, approx 1 oz	2 cookies	139	3.5	16.6	55	na	6.0	na
(Natures Warehouse) wheat-free, approx 1 oz	2 cookies	129	2.3	16.0	54	na	6.2	na
OATMEAL								
(Almost Home) raisin	.5 oz	70	1.0	10.0	40	1.0	3.0	2
(Archway)	1 cookie	110	2.0	19.0	90	1.0	3.0	5
(Archway) apple filled	1 cookie	90	1.0	18.0	115	1.0	1.0	5
(Archway) date filled	1 cookie	100	1.0	18.0	105	1.0	2.0	5
(Archway) iced	1 cookie	140	2.0	22.0	107	1.7	5.0	5
(Archway) 'Ruth's Golden'	1 cookie	120	2.0	20.0	122	1.2	4.0	5

Food Name	Serv. Size	Total Cal.	Prot. GMS	Carbs GMS	Sod. MGS	Fiber GMS	Fat GMS	Chol. MGS
(Bakers Bonus)	.5 oz	80	1.0	12.0	65	na	3.0	0
(Bakery Wagon) chocolate chunk	1 cookie	100	2.0	17.0	80	na	3.0	2
(Bakery Wagon) soft	1 cookie	100	2.0	15.0	105	na	5.0	2
(Bakery Wagon) walnut raisin	1 cookie	100	2.0	16.0	80	na	4.0	2
(Barbara's Bakery) raisin	1 oz	100	2.0	19.0	50	na	2.0	0
(Break Cake) approx 1 oz	5 cookies	140	1.0	20.0	60	na	6.0	0
(Chips Ahoy!) chocolate chip 'Selections'	.5 oz	90	1.0	10.0	60	na	5.0	5
(Drake's) approx 1 oz	2 cookies	120	2.0	19.0	50	(mq)	4.0	0
(Dunkin' Donuts) pecan, raisin	1 cookie	200	3.0	28.0	100	na	9.0	25
(Duncan Hines) raisin	2 cookies	110	1.0	15.0	85	na	5.0	na
(Entemann's) chocolatey chip 'Fat-Free Cholesterol-Free'	2 cookies	80	1.0	19.0	110	1.0	0.0	0
(Entenmann's) raisin	2 cookies	30	1.0	17.0	120	na	0.0	0
(Estee) raisin	3 cookies	100	2.0	14.0	15	na	4.0	0
(FFV) approx 1 oz	5 cookies	130	2.0	20.0	150	(mq)	4.0	0
(Fifty 50) hearty oatmeal, fructose sweetened	1 cookie	35	<1.0	5.0	15	na	1.0	0
(Frookie) raisin	1 cookie	45	1.0	6.5	35	na	2.0	0
(Frookie) raisin, fat-free	1 cookie	50	1.0	11.0	75	1.0	0.0	0
(Frookie) 7-grain oatmeal	1 cookie	45	1.0	6.5	35	na	2.0	0
(Glenny's) wheat-free 'Noah 'N Friends Animal'	.5 oz	65	1.0	10.0	20	na	2.0	na
(Grandma's) apple spice 'Big Cookies' 2.75 oz	2 cookies	330	5.0	51.0	570	(mq)	12.0	10
(Health Valley) raisin cinnamon 'Fruit Chunks'	3 cookies	85	2.0	19.0	80	3.0	0.0	0
(Keebler) 'Old Fashion' approx .5 oz	1 cookie	80	1.0	12.0	110	(mq)	3.0	0
(Keebler) w/chocolate 'Magic Middles' .5 oz	1 cookie	80	1.0	8.0	30	(mq)	5.0	0
(Keebler) w/raisins, chewy 'Raisin Ruckus'	1 cookie	70	1.0	10.0	45	na	3.0	0
(Little Debbie)	2.75 oz	340	5.0	52.0	440	(mq)	12.0	2
(Mother's)	1 cookie	60	1.0	8.0	80	na	3.0	na
(Mother's) chocolate chip	1 cookie	70	1.0	10.0	85	na	3.0	na
(Mother's) iced	1 cookie	70	1.0	10.0	70	na	3.0	na
(Mother's) walnut chocolate chip	1 cookie	70	1.0	9.0	60	na	3.0	na
(Nabisco) raisin, 'Snack Wells'	1 cookie	60	1.0	10.0	65	na	1.0	0
(Natures Warehouse) raisin, approx 1 oz	2 cookies	135	2.0	17.3	44	na	6.4	na
(Pepperidge Farm) chocolate chunk 'Dakota'	1 cookie	110	1.0	15.0	70	1.0	6.0	5
(Pepperidge Farm) 'Family Request'	2 cookies	90	1.0	13.0	70	na	4.0	10

Food Name	Serv. Size	Total Cal.	Prot. GMS	Carbs GMS	Sod. MGS	Fiber GMS	Fat GMS	Chol. MGS
(Pepperidge Farm) Irish 'Old Fashioned'	2 cookies	90	1.0	13.0	80	(mq)	5.0	5
(Pepperidge Farm) raisin, soft, low-fat 'Wholesome Choice'	1 cookie	60	1.0	11.0	50	na	1.0	0
(Weight Watchers) raisin	2 cookies	90	1.0	20.0	75	na	<1.0	0
(Weight Watchers) spice	3 cookies	80	1.0	13.0	75	na	2.0	na
(Westbrae) 'Rice Malt Snap'	1 oz	130	2.0	19.0	130	na	5.0	0
ORANGE-PINEAPPLE								
(Health Valley) 'Mini Fruit Centers' fat-free	3 cookies	75	2.0	17.0	60	3.0	0.0	0
PEACH *(Great Cakes)*	4.5 oz	260	10.0	40.0	20	21.0	6.0	0
PEACH-APRICOT								
(FFV) bar, vanilla	1 cookie	70	<1.0	14.0	50	(mq)	1.0	0
(FFV) bar, whole wheat	1 cookie	70	<1.0	11.0	50	(mq)	2.0	0
(Health Valley) 'Mini Fruit Centers' fat-free	3 cookies	75	2.0	17.0	60	3.0	0.0	0
(Stella D'oro) pastry	1 cookie	93	1.2	13.6	(mq)	(mq)	3.8	na
(Stella D'oro) pastry, dietetic	1 cookie	87	1.2	12.3	10	(mq)	3.7	na
PEANUT *(Health Valley)* 'Fancy Peanut Chunks'	2 cookies	100	2.0	14.0	585	2.3	3.0	0
PEANUT BUTTER								
(Bakery Wagon) oatmeal	1 cookie	110	3.0	12.0	150	na	7.0	2
(Break Cake)	1 cookie	140	2.0	18.0	110	na	7.0	0
(Break Cake) wafer	1 wafer	180	2.0	24.0	75	na	9.0	0
(Delicious) and jelly sandwich 'Skippy & Welchs'	1 cookie	120	2.0	15.0	90	<1.0	6.0	0
(Delicious) made w/Skippy peanut butter	1 cookie	80	2.0	7.0	65	.5	5.0	0
(Estee) sandwich	1 cookie	50	1.0	5.0	35	(mq)	3.0	0
(Featherweight)	1 cookie	40	1.0	5.0	10	(mq)	2.0	0
(Featherweight) creme wafer	1 cookie	25	1.0	3.0	0	(mq)	1.0	0
(FFV) sandwich, approx 1.1 oz	2 cookies	170	2.0	21.0	110	(mq)	8.0	na
(Fifty 50) fructose sweetened	1 cookie	40	<1.0	5.0	10	na	2.0	0
(Frookie) sandwich 'Frookwich'	1 cookie	50	<1.0	7.0	30	na	2.0	0
(Glenny's) 'Noah 'N Friends Animal Cookies'	.5 oz	65	1.0	9.0	35	na	3.0	na
(Grandma's) 'Big Cookies' 2.75 oz	2 cookies	410	7.0	43.0	410	(mq)	30.0	10
(Grandma's) cookie bits, 8 cookies	1 oz	140	3.0	19.0	125	na	6.0	0
(Great Cakes) and jelly	4.5 oz	280	10.0	40.0	20	21.0	8.0	0
(Keebler) chocolate chip 'Soft Batch' .5 oz	1 cookie	80	1.0	9.0	55	(mq)	5.0	0
(Keebler) nut 'Soft Batch' approx .5 oz	1 cookie	80	11.0	9.0	60	(mq)	4.0	0
(Mother's) sandwich 'Gaucho'	1 cookie	90	1.0	12.0	75	na	5.0	na
(Nabisco) 'Ideal Bars'	.5 oz cookie	90	1.0	10.0	80	na	5.0	0

Food Name	Serv. Size	Total Cal.	Prot. GMS	Carbs GMS	Sod. MGS	Fiber GMS	Fat GMS	Chol. MGS
(Nabisco) 'Nutter Butter Peanut Sandwich'	.5 oz	70	1.0	9.0	50	0	3.0	0
(Natures Warehouse) approx 1 oz	2 cookies	128	3.6	18.2	29	na	6.1	na
(Natures Warehouse) chocolate chip, approx 1 oz	2 cookies	139	4.1	13.9	50	na	8.5	na
(Pepperidge Farm) chocolate chunk 'Cheyenne'	1 cookie	110	2.0	13.0	80	1.0	6.0	5
(Pepperidge Farm) chocolate filled 'Nassau'	1 cookie	80	1.0	9.0	45	(mq)	5.0	5
(Pepperidge Farm) 'Family Request'	2 cookies	80	2.0	10.0	65	(mq)	5.0	5
(Pitter Patter) cream filled, approx .5 oz	1 cookie	90	2.0	12.0	115	(mq)	4.0	0
(Planters) crispy cookie 'P.B. Crisps'	1 oz	140	3.0	17.0	125	na	7.0	0
PEANUT CREME *(Nabisco)* 'Nutter Butter Patties'	.5 oz	80	2.0	8.0	45	na	4.0	0
PECAN								
(Archway) crunch	1 cookie	60	1.0	8.0	45	(mq)	3.0	5
(Dunkin' Donuts) raisin cookie, 1.6 oz	1 cookie	200	3.0	28.0	100	1.0	9.0	25
PRALINE PECAN *(FFV)*	1 cookie	40	<1.0	10.0	40	(mq)	2.0	5
PRUNE, PASTRY, DIETETIC *(Stella D'oro)*	1 cookie	95	1.2	15.0	10	(mq)	3.4	na
RAISIN								
(Almost Home)	.5 oz	70	1.0	10.0	40	(mq)	3.0	2
(Archway)	1 cookie	100	2.0	18.0	107	.9	3.0	5
(Archway) bran	1 cookie	100	2.0	18.0	95	1.0	3.0	5
(Archway) oatmeal	1 cookie	50	1.0	7.0	20	(mq)	2.0	0
(Break Cake) creme	1 cookie	140	1.0	22.0	120	na	5.0	2
(Entenmann's)	2 cookies	80	1.0	17.0	120	(mq)	0.0	0
(Featherweight)	1 cookie	45	1.0	6.0	0	(mq)	2.0	0
(Grandma's) soft 'Big Cookies' approx 2.75 oz	2 cookies	320	3.0	54.0	280	(mq)	10.0	10
(Health Valley) apple 'Fruit Centers' fat-free	1 cookie	70	2.0	16.0	35	3.5	0.0	0
(Health Valley) 'Jumbos' fat-free	1 cookie	80	2.0	17.0	80	3.5	0.0	0
(Health Valley) nut 'Fruit Jumbos'	1 cookie	70	2.0	16.0	35	.9	3.0	0
(Health Valley) oatmeal, fat-free	3 cookies	80	2.0	18.0	80	3.0	0.0	0
(Keebler) bar, iced	1 cookie	80	1.0	10.0	85	(mq)	4.0	0
(Keebler) 'Soft Batch' approx .5 oz	1 cookie	70	1.0	10.0	65	(mq)	3.0	0
(Mother's) iced	1 cookie	80	1.0	11.0	45	na	4.0	na
(Nabisco) nut 'Newtons'	.5 oz	60	1.0	11.0	50	(mq)	2.0	0
(Pepperidge Farm) bran 'Kitchen Hearth'	2 cookies	110	1.0	13.0	55	(mq)	5.0	5
(Pepperidge Farm) 'Old Fashioned'	2 cookies	110	1.0	15.0	115	(mq)	5.0	10
(Pepperidge Farm) 'Santa Fe'	1 cookie	100	1.0	16.0	70	1.0	4.0	5
(Stella D'oro) 'Golden Bars'	1 cookie	109	1.6	16.0	(mq)	(mq)	4.3	na

Food Name	Serv. Size	Total Cal.	Prot. GMS	Carbs GMS	Sod. MGS	Fiber GMS	Fat GMS	Chol. MGS
(Sunshine) .... 2 cookies	110	1.0	16.0	125	(mq)	5.0	0
(Tastykake) bar .... 1.8 oz	212	3.2	31.8	255	1.2	8.3	17
(Tastykake) 'Soft'n Chewy' .... 1.4 oz	161	3.4	26.8	158	1.0	5.4	3
(Weight Watchers) spice .... 3 cookies	80	1.0	13.0	75	(mq)	2.0	na
RASPBERRY							
(Bakery Wagon) filled .... 1 cookie	90	1.0	16.0	125	na	3.0	2
(Frookie) 'Fruitins' fat-free .... 2 cookies	90	1.0	21.0	75	1.0	0.0	0
(Great Cakes) .... 4.5 oz	260	10.0	40.0	20	21.0	6.0	0
(Health Valley) apple 'Fruit Chunks' .. 3 cookies	85	2.0	19.0	80	3.0	0.0	0
(Health Valley) apple 'Mini Fruit Centers' fat-free .... 3 cookies	75	2.0	17.0	60	3.0	0.0	0
(Health Valley) 'Fruit Centers' fat-free .. 1 cookie	80	2.0	17.0	80	2.0	0.0	0
(Health Valley) 'Jumbos' fat-free ...... 1 cookie	80	2.0	17.0	80	3.5	0.0	0
(Lu) 'Pims' .... 2 cookies	95	1.0	18.0	25	na	2.0	na
(Nabisco) 'Newtons' .75 oz .... 1 cookie	80	1.0	15.0	70	(mq)	2.0	0
(Nabisco) 'Newtons' fat-free .... 1 cookie	60	1.0	16.0	75	na	0.0	0
(Natural Nectar) swirl 'Incredible Edible Novelties' .... 1 cookie	220	4.0	33.0	115	na	8.0	20
(Natures Warehouse) wheat-free, fat-free .. 1 oz	90	1.6	20.5	84	na	0.7	0
(Pepperidge Farm) filled 'Chantilly' .... 1 cookie	80	1.0	14.0	35	(mq)	2.0	5
(Pepperidge Farm) filled, chocolate 'Chantilly' .... 1 cookie	90	1.0	14.0	35	(mq)	3.0	5
(Pepperidge Farm) filled 'Linzer' ...... 1 cookie	120	2.0	20.0	55	(mq)	4.0	5
(Pepperidge Farm) tart, low fat 'Wholesome Choice' .... 1 cookie	60	1.0	11.0	35	na	1.0	0
(Weight Watchers) fruit filled .... 1 cookie	80	<1.0	22.0	45	na	<1.0	0
REESE'S PIECES (Oven Lovin') ...... 1 cookie	70	1.0	9.0	50	na	3.0	5
SESAME							
(Glenny's) 'Nookie' bite size .... .5 oz	60	1.0	6.0	8	na	4.0	na
(Stella D'oro) dietetic 'Regina' .... 1 cookie	41	0.8	5.1	10	(mq)	2.0	na
(Stella D'oro) 'Regina' .... 1 cookie	48	0.9	6.1	(mq)	(mq)	2.2	na
SHORTBREAD							
(Break Cake) approx 1 oz .... 5 cookies	140	1.0	19.0	70	na	6.0	5
(Estee) .... 3 cookies	100	2.0	16.0	100	na	3.0	0
(FFV) country .... 1 cookie	70	1.0	9.0	45	(mq)	4.0	5
(Keebler) covered 'Fudge'n Caramel' . 1 cookie	60	1.0	8.0	30	na	3.0	0
(Keebler) fudge covered 'Toffee Toppers' .... 2 cookies	60	<1.0	10.0	50	na	4.0	0
(Keebler) fudge striped 'Fudge Stripes' .5 oz .... 1 cookie	50	<1.0	7.0	55	(mq)	3.0	0
(Keebler) 'Pecan Sandies' approx .5 oz 1 cookie	80	<1.0	9.0	75	(mq)	5.0	5
(Keebler) 'Pecan Sandies' bite size .. 4 cookies	90	1.0	9.0	50	na	5.0	5

Food Name	Serv. Size	Total Cal.	Prot. GMS	Carbs GMS	Sod. MGS	Fiber GMS	Fat GMS	Chol. MGS
(Keebler) w/chocolate center								
'Magic Middles' .5 oz .... 1 cookie		80	1.0	9.0	25	(mq)	5.0	5
(Keebler) w/toffee pieces								
'Toffee Sandies' .... 1 cookie		70	1.0	8.0	45	na	4.0	0
(Lorna Doone) .5 oz .... 3 cookies		70	1.0	9.0	65	(mq)	4.0	5
(Mother's) striped .... 2 cookies		100	1.0	14.0	55	na	5.0	na
(Nabisco) fudge striped								
'Cookies 'n Fudge' .... .5 oz		60	1.0	7.0	50	(mq)	3.0	0
(Nabisco) pecan supreme,								
low cholesterol .... 1 cookie		80	1.0	9.0	45	na	5.0	2
(Pepperidge Farm) 'Old Fashioned' .. 2 cookies		150	1.0	17.0	85	(mq)	8.0	5
(Pepperidge Farm) pecan								
'Old Fashioned' .... 1 cookie		70	1.0	7.0	15	(mq)	5.0	0
(Weight Watchers) .... 3 cookies		80	1.0	13.0	95	(mq)	2.0	na
SNACK, for weight control *(Spicer's)* .... 1 oz		100	3.0	12.0	70	9.0	4.0	0
SPICE *(Stella D'oro)* 'Pfeffernusse' ...... 1 piece		35	0.5	6.7	(mq)	(mq)	0.8	na
STRAWBERRY								
(Healthy Times) 'Hugga Bears' organic ... 1 oz		120	2.0	17.0	38	na	3.0	0
(Health Valley) 'Mini Fruit Centers'								
fat-free .... 3 cookies		75	2.0	17.0	60	3.0	0.0	0
(Nabisco) 'Newtons' .... 1.25 oz		120	1.0	24.0	110	(mq)	3.0	0
(Nabisco) 'Newtons' .75 oz .... 1 cookie		70	1.0	15.0	70	na	2.0	0
(Nabisco) 'Newtons' fat-free .... 1 cookie		60	1.0	16.0	80	na	0.0	0
(Nabisco) 'Suddenly S'Mores' .... .75 oz		100	1.0	15.0	90	(mq)	4.0	0
(Natural Nectar) swirl 'Incredible Edible								
Novelties' .... 1 cookie		220	4.0	33.0	115	na	8.0	20
(Pepperidge Farm) 'Fruit Cookies' ... 2 cookies		100	1.0	15.0	50	(mq)	5.0	10
SUGAR								
(Almost Home) .... .5 oz		70	1.0	10.0	80	na	3.0	0
(Almost Home) 'Old Fashioned' .... .5 oz		70	1.0	10.0	80	(mq)	3.0	2
(Mother's) .... 1 cookie		70	1.0	8.0	35	na	4.0	na
(Pepperidge Farm) 'Old Fashioned' .. 2 cookies		100	1.0	13.0	55	(mq)	5.0	10
(Stella D'oro) 'Holiday Trinkets' ...... 1 cookie		38	0.6	4.6	(mq)	(mq)	1.9	na
TAFFY *(Mother's)* sandwich .... 1 cookie		100	1.0	12.0	60	na	6.0	na
TEA BISCUIT *(Nabisco)* 'Social Tea Biscuit'								
3 pieces .... .5 oz		60	1.0	11.0	60	0	2.0	5
TOFFEE								
(Chips Ahoy!) chunk, Heath 'Selections' 1 cookie		90	1.0	5.0	85	0	5.0	5
(Delicious) w/Heath English toffee .... 1 cookie		90	1.0	10.0	45	1.0	5.0	8
(Pepperidge Farm) 'Old Fashioned' .. 2 cookies		100	1.0	12.0	75	(mq)	5.0	5
TOFU *(Health Valley)* 'The Great Tofu								
Cookie' .... 2 cookies		90	2.0	16.0	29	1.4	3.0	0

Food Name	Serv. Size	Total Cal.	Prot. GMS	Carbs GMS	Sod. MGS	Fiber GMS	Fat GMS	Chol. MGS
VANILLA								
(Barbara's Bakery) animal cookies ...... 1 oz		145	2.0	18.0	85	na	7.0	0
(Barbara's Bakery) 'Cookies & Creme' 2 cookies		120	1.0	18.0	75	na	5.0	15
(Barbara's Bakery) raspberry 'Cookies & Creme' .... 2 cookies		120	1.0	18.0	75	na	5.0	15
(Estee) .... 3 cookies		100	1.0	14.0	15	na	5.0	0
(Estee) sandwich .... 2 cookies		110	1.0	17.0	20	na	4.0	0
(Featherweight) .... 1 cookie		45	1.0	6.0	0	(mq)	2.0	0
(Frookie) 'Funky Monkeys' .... 8 cookies		60	1.0	10.0	60	na	2.0	0
(Frookie) sandwich 'Frookwich' ...... 1 cookie		50	<1.0	7.0	30	na	2.0	0
(Frookie) 'Trolls' .... 11 cookies		60	1.0	10.0	65	na	2.0	0
(Glenny's) 'Noah 'N Friends Animal Cookies' .... .5 oz		65	1.0	10.0	35	na	2.0	na
(Grandma's) cookie bits, artificially flavored .... 1 oz		140	2.0	20.0	75	na	6.0	5
(Keebler) creme sandwich 'French' .5 oz .... 1 cookie		80	<1.0	12.0	80	(mq)	4.0	0
(Lu) 'Marie Lu' .... 1 cookie		50	1.0	8.0	45	na	2.0	na
(Lu) 'Marie Lu' mini .... 5 cookies		50	1.0	8.0	45	na	2.0	na
(Nabisco) creme sandwich 'Cameo' ...... .5 oz		70	1.0	10.0	50	(mq)	3.0	0
(Nabisco) creme sandwich 'Cookie Break' .... 1 cookie		50	1.0	7.0	35	0	2.0	0
(Nabisco) creme sandwich 'Giggles' 2 pieces .... 1 oz		60	1.0	8.0	20	(mq)	3.0	2
(Nabisco) reduced fat 'Snack Wells' .... .5 oz		50	1.0	10.0	50	na	1.0	0
(Pepperidge Farm) 'Bordeaux' .... 2 cookies		70	1.0	11.0	40	(mq)	3.0	0
(Pepperidge Farm) chocolate coated 'Orleans' .... 3 cookies		90	0.0	11.0	30	(mq)	6.0	0
(Pepperidge Farm) chocolate laced 'Pirouettes' .... 2 cookies		70	1.0	8.0	20	(mq)	4.0	5
(Pepperidge Farm) chocolate nut coated 'Geneva' .... 2 cookies		130	1.0	14.0	50	(mq)	6.0	0
(Pepperidge Farm) 'Goldfish' .... 1 oz		140	2.0	19.0	50	na	7.0	15
(Pepperidge Farm) 'Pirouettes' .... 2 cookies		70	0.0	9.0	35	(mq)	4.0	5
(Stella D'oro) 'Angelica Goodies' .... 1 cookie		106	1.7	15.7	(mq)	(mq)	4.0	na
(Stella D'oro) 'Castelets' .... 1 cookie		72	1.0	10.0	(mq)	(mq)	3.1	na
(Stella D'oro) 'Margherite' .... 1 cookie		72	1.0	10.8	(mq)	(mq)	2.8	na
(Tastykake) creme sandwich, shortbread .. .4 oz		55	0.7	6.4	31	.1	3.0	na
(Weight Watchers) sandwich .... 2 cookies		90	1.0	15.0	50	na	3.0	0
WAFER								
(Archway) vanilla .... 1 wafer		30	0.0	6.0	30	(mq)	<1.0	0
(Biscos) sugar, 4 pieces .... .5 oz		70	0.0	10.0	20	na	3.0	0
(Biscos) waffle creme .... 1 wafers		45	0.0	6.0	10	0	2.0	6

Food Name	Serv. Size	Total Cal.	Prot. GMS	Carbs GMS	Sod. MGS	Fiber GMS	Fat GMS	Chol. MGS
(Break Cake) chocolate, sugar	4 wafers	200	2.0	30.0	95	na	9.0	0
(Break Cake) strawberry, sugar	4 wafers	220	1.0	28.0	100	na	11.0	0
(Break Cake) 'Striper Wafer'	1 wafer	190	2.0	23.0	80	na	10.0	0
(Break Cake) vanilla, sugar	4 wafers	220	1.0	28.0	105	na	11.0	0
(Delicious) chocolate strawberry, sugar	1 wafer	35	<1.0	3.0	4	na	2.0	0
(Delicious) chocolate, sugar	1 wafer	34	<1.0	2.0	5	na	2.0	0
(Delicious) strawberry, sugar	1 wafer	35	<1.0	4.0	3	na	2.0	0
(Delicious) sugar, assorted	.25 oz	38	<1.0	4.0	<1	na	2.0	2
(Delicious) vanilla	.5 oz	70	0.8	10.5	41	na	2.2	<1
(Delicious) vanilla, sugar	.25 oz	37	<1.0	4.0	<1	na	2.0	2
(Delicious) vanilla, sugar	1 wafer	35	<1.0	4.0	3	na	2.0	0
(Estee) chocolate creme	4 wafers	90	<1.0	11.0	0	na	5.0	0
(Estee) strawberry	3 wafers	100	<1.0	14.0	0	na	5.0	0
(Estee) vanilla	3 wafers	100	<1.0	14.0	0	na	5.0	0
(Estee) vanilla creme	4 wafers	90	<1.0	12.0	0	na	4.0	0
(Featherweight) strawberry creme	1 wafer	20	0.0	3.0	0	(mq)	1.0	0
(Featherweight) vanilla creme	1 wafers	20	0.0	3.0	0	(mq)	1.0	0
(FFV) vanilla, approx 1 oz	8 wafers	130	1.0	19.0	100	(mq)	5.0	5
(Fifty 50) chocolate creme filled, w/o sugar	1 wafer	35	<1.0	4.0	10	na	2.0	0
(Fifty 50) vanilla, creme filled, w/o sugar	1 wafer	35	<1.0	4.0	5	na	2.0	0
(Keebler) vanilla, golden	4 wafers	80	<1.0	10.0	60	(mq)	3.0	0
(Lu) cream	3 cookies	110	1.0	11.0	50	na	7.0	na
(Mother's) checkerboard	5 wafers	85	1.0	13.0	15	na	4.0	na
(Mother's) vanilla, 'Flaky Flix'	2 wafers	115	1.0	18.0	na	na	5.0	25
(Nabisco) 'Brown Edge Wafers' 2 1/2 wafers	.5 oz	70	1.0	10.0	45	0	3.0	2
(Nabisco) 'Famous Chocolate Wafers' 2 1/2 wafers	.5 oz	60	1.0	11.0	100	na	2.0	5
(Nabisco) striped wafer 'Cookies 'N Fudge'	1 wafer	70	1.0	8.0	25	0	4.0	0
(Nabisco) vanilla, cinnamon 'Nilla Wafers' .5 oz	3 1/2 wafers	60	1.0	11.0	45	(mq)	2.0	5
(Nabisco) vanilla, 'Nilla Wafers' approx .5 oz	3 1/2 wafers	60	1.0	11.0	45	(mq)	2.0	5
(Tastykake) vanilla, sugar	10 wafers	34	0.3	4.1	11	<.1	1.9	0
(Weider) 'Victory Explosive Workout'	6 wafers	30	<1.0	6.0	60	na	0.0	na
(Westbrae) 5-spice	4 1/2 wafers	40	1.0	8.0	30	na	0.0	0
WALNUT								
(Keebler) 'Soft Batch' approx .5 oz	1 cookie	80	1.0	10.0	70	(mq)	4.0	0
(Lu) whole wheat and cinnamon 'Marie Lu'	1 cookie	45	1.0	8.0	55	na	1.0	na
(Mother's) fudge	1 cookie	70	1.0	8.0	50	na	4.0	na

Food Name	Serv. Size	Total Cal.	Prot. GMS	Carbs GMS	Sod. MGS	Fiber GMS	Fat GMS	Chol. MGS
COOKIE DOUGH, PREPARED								
chocolate chip	1 oz	126	1.3	17.4	59	na	5.8	7
chocolate chip	1 cookie	71	0.7	9.8	33	na	3.3	4
chocolate chip (Pillsbury)	1 cookie	70	1.0	9.0	55	(mq)	3.0	5
chocolate chip, baked	1 oz	139	1.4	19.3	66	na	6.4	8
chocolate chip, baked	1 cookie	59	0.6	8.2	28	na	2.7	3
chocolate chip 'Ready To Bake' (Toll House)	1.2 oz	150	1.0	20.0	115	(mq)	7.0	na
chocolate chip 'Ready To Bake' w/nuts (Toll House)	1.2 oz	160	2.0	19.0	90	(mq)	8.0	na
double chocolate chip 'Ready To Bake' 1.2 oz (Toll House)	2 cookies	150	2.0	19.0	60	(mq)	7.0	na
oatmeal	1 oz	120	1.5	16.7	83	na	5.4	7
oatmeal	1 cookie	68	0.9	9.5	47	na	3.0	4
oatmeal, baked	1 oz	134	1.7	18.6	93	na	5.9	7
oatmeal, baked	1 cookie	57	0.7	7.9	39	na	2.5	3
oatmeal raisin (Pillsbury)	1 cookie	60	1.0	9.0	55	(mq)	3.0	0
oatmeal raisin 'Ready To Bake' 2 cookies (Toll House)	1.2 oz	130	2.0	21.0	55	(mq)	5.0	na
peanut butter (Pillsbury)	1 cookie	70	1.0	9.0	75	(mq)	3.0	5
sugar	1 oz	124	1.2	16.7	120	na	5.9	8
sugar	1 cookie	70	0.7	9.4	68	na	3.3	5
sugar (Pillsbury)	1 cookie	70	1.0	9.0	70	(mq)	3.0	5
sugar, baked	1 oz	137	1.3	18.6	133	na	6.6	9
COOKIE MIX								
chocolate chip (Duncan Hines)	2 cookies	130	1.0	20.0	85	(mq)	5.0	na
chocolate chip (Finast)	2 cookies	110	1.0	16.0	290	(mq)	5.0	na
chocolate chip, 2-inch diam each (Estee)	2 cookies	90	1.0	13.0	80	na	4.0	0
chocolate chip 'Big Batch' (Betty Crocker)	2 cookies	120	1.0	16.0	100	(mq)	6.0	(mq)
'Deluxe' 2-inch diam (Krusteaz)	1 cookie	120	1.0	16.0	126	na	5.0	11
golden sugar (Duncan Hines)	2 cookies	130	1.0	17.0	70	(mq)	6.0	na
oatmeal raisin (Duncan Hines)	2 cookies	130	2.0	18.0	70	(mq)	6.0	na
peanut butter (Duncan Hines)	2 cookies	140	3.0	15.0	120	(mq)	7.0	na
COOKING SPRAY								
(Mazola) corn oil 'No Stick'	2.5-sec spray	6	0.0	0.0	0	0	1.0	0
(Pam) for 1/3 of 10-inch skillet	1 spray	2	0.0	0.0	0	0	1.0	0
(Weight Watchers) 'Buttery Spray' butter flavor	1-sec spray	2	0.0	0.0	0	0	<1.0	0
(Weight Watchers) canola oil spray	.33 grams	2	0.0	0.0	0	na	<1.0	0
(Weight Watchers) 'Cooking Spray'	1-sec spray	2	0.0	0.0	0	0	1.0	0
(Wesson) lite	.27 grams	<1	0.0	0.0	0	0	<1.0	0

Food Name	Serv. Size	Total Cal.	Prot. GMS	Carbs GMS	Sod. MGS	Fiber GMS	Fat GMS	Chol. MGS
(Wesson) no-stick	.25 gram	2	0.0	0.0	0	0	0.3	0
COOL WHIP. See CREAM TOPPING, NONDAIRY.								
CORIANDER/Chinese parsley								
raw	1 tbsp	5	0.4	0.9	4	>.2 c	0.1	0
raw	1 tsp	2	0.1	0.3	1	>.1 c	0.0	0
raw, approx .8 oz	9 plants	4	0.5	0.5	6	.5	0.1	0
trimmed	1 oz	6	0.7	0.7	8	>.2 c	0.2	0
untrimmed	1 lb	77	9.1	10.0	108	>3.1 c	2.3	0
CORIANDER LEAF/Chinese parsley leaf								
dried	1 oz	79	6.2	14.8	60	>2.9 c	1.3	0
dried	1 tbsp	5	0.4	.9	4	.2	0.1	0
dried	1 tsp	2	0.1	0.3	1	.1	<.1	0
CORIANDER SEED/Chinese parsley seed								
whole	1 oz	84	3.5	15.6	10	>8.3 c	5.0	0
whole	1 tbsp	15	0.6	2.8	2	>1.5 c	0.9	0
whole	1 tsp	5	0.2	1.0	1	>.5 c	0.3	0
whole *(Durkee)*	1 tsp	8	0.0	0.0	0	0	<0.1	na
whole *(Laurel Leaf)*	1 tsp	8	0.0	0.0	0	0	<0.1	na
whole *(Spice Islands)*	1 tsp	6	0.2	0.8	<1	>.4 c	0.3	0
CORN								
cooked	1/2 cup	88	1.8	19.5	0	3.4	0.5	0
dry	1 cup	375	7.8	83.2	3	11.6	2.2	0
dry	2 oz	203	4.3	45.2	2	6.3	1.2	0
sweet, boiled, drained	4 oz	122	3.8	28.5	19	4.2	1.5	0
sweet, raw, trimmed	1 oz	24	0.9	5.4	4	.9	0.3	0
sweet, raw, untrimmed	1 lb	140	5.3	31.1	25	5.2	1.9	0
sweet, white, boiled, drained, cut	1/2 cup	89	2.7	20.6	14	4.7	1.0	0
sweet, white, kernels, boiled, drained	1 ear	83	2.6	19.3	13	4.4	1.0	0
sweet, white, kernels from cob, raw	1 ear	77	2.9	17.1	14	2.9	1.1	0
sweet, white, raw, cut	1/2 cup	66	2.5	14.7	12	2.5	0.9	0
sweet, yellow, boiled, drained, cut	1/2 cup	89	2.7	20.6	14	3.0	1.0	0
sweet, yellow, kernels, boiled, drained	1 ear	83	2.6	19.3	13	2.8	1.0	0
sweet, yellow, kernels from cob, raw	1 ear	77	2.9	17.1	14	2.9	1.1	0
sweet, yellow, raw, cut	1/2 cup	66	2.5	14.7	12	2.5	0.9	0
white	1/2 cup	303	7.8	61.6	29	>2.4 c	3.9	0
yellow	1/2 cup	303	7.8	61.6	29	>2.4 c	3.9	0
CORN, CANNED								
cream style	1/2 cup	93	2.2	23.2	365	1.3	0.5	0
cream style	4 oz	82	2.0	20.6	323	1.1	0.5	0
cream style *(A&P)*	1/2 cup	100	2.0	25.0	330	(mq)	1.0	0
cream style *(Finast)*	1/2 cup	105	2.0	25.0	350	(mq)	1.0	0
cream style *(Green Giant)*	1/2 cup	100	2.0	24.0	390	2.0	<1.0	0
cream style *(S&W Nutradiet)*	1/2 cup	100	3.0	21.0	0	(mq)	1.0	0

Food Name	Serv. Size	Total Cal.	Prot. GMS	Carbs GMS	Sod. MGS	Fiber GMS	Fat GMS	Chol. MGS
cream style, golden *(Del Monte)*	1/2 cup	80	2.0	18.0	355	(mq)	1.0	0
cream style, golden *(Pathmark)*	1/2 cup	100	2.0	25.0	350	(mq)	1.0	0
cream style, golden *(Stokely)*	1/2 cup	100	2.0	23.0	380	(mq)	0.0	0
cream style, golden, low-sodium	4 oz	82	2.0	20.6	3	>.6 c	0.5	0
cream style, golden 'No Salt Added' *(Del Monte)*	1/2 cup	80	2.0	20.0	10	(mq)	1.0	0
cream style, golden, white *(Stokely)*	1/2 cup	100	2.0	23.0	380	(mq)	0.0	0
cream style 'No Frills' *(Pathmark)*	1 cup	210	5.0	51.0	700	(mq)	1.0	0
cream style 'Premium Homestyle No Starch Added' *(S&W)*	1/2 cup	120	3.0	24.0	285	(mq)	1.0	0
cream style 'Premium Homestyle Starch Added' *(S&W)*	1/2 cup	105	2.0	25.0	435	(mq)	1.0	0
cream style, white *(Del Monte)*	1/2 cup	90	2.0	21.0	355	(mq)	0.0	0
'Crisp 'N Sweet' vacuum packed *(Freshlike)*	1/2 cup	80	2.0	18.0	5	na	1.0	na
'Delicorn' *(Green Giant)*	1/2 cup	80	2.0	19.0	350	2.0	<1.0	0
golden *(Pathmark)*	1/2 cup	90	2.0	19.0	330	(mq)	1.0	0
golden *(Stokely)*	1/2 cup	90	2.0	20.0	300	(mq)	0.0	0
golden, cream style *(Freshlike)*	1/2 cup	110	2.0	25.0	290	na	1.0	na
golden, cream style *(Veg•All)*	1/2 cup	110	2.0	25.0	290	na	1.0	na
golden, cream style, no salt added *(Freshlike)*	1/2 cup	110	2.0	25.0	15	na	1.0	na
golden, 50% less salt *(Green Giant)*	1/2 cup	70	2.0	16.0	175	2.0	<1.0	0
golden 'No Salt Added' *(Del Monte)*	1/2 cup	80	2.0	18.0	10	(mq)	1.0	0
golden 'No Salt or Sugar Added' *(Green Giant)*	1/2 cup	80	3.0	18.0	0	2.0	<1.0	0
golden 'No Salt or Sugar Added' *(Stokely)*	1/2 cup	80	2.0	16.0	5	(mq)	0.0	0
golden 'Pantry Express' *(Green Giant)*	1/2 cup	80	2.0	18.0	210	1.0	<1.0	0
golden, sweet *(IGA)*	1/2 cup	70	2.0	16.0	10	(mq)	1.0	0
golden, vacuum pack *(Green Giant)*	1/2 cup	80	2.0	20.0	330	2.0	0.0	0
golden, vacuum pack *(Stokely)*	1/2 cup	90	3.0	22.0	300	(mq)	0.0	0
golden, whole kernel *(Veg•All)*	1/2 cup	80	2.0	19.0	320	na	1.0	na
golden, whole kernel, vacuum packed *(Freshlike)*	1/2 cup	100	3.0	22.0	260	na	1.0	na
golden, whole kernel, vacuum packed *(Veg•All)*	1/2 cup	100	3.0	22.0	260	na	1.0	na
golden, whole kernel, water packed, w/o salt *(Freshlike)*	1/2 cup	80	2.0	19.0	5	na	1.0	na
golden, whole kernel, water packed, w/o sugar and salt *(Freshlike)*	1/2 cup	80	2.0	19.0	5	na	1.0	na
golden, w/liquid *(Del Monte)*	1/2 cup	70	2.0	17.0	355	(mq)	1.0	0
in brine, w/liquid *(Green Giant)*	1/2 cup	70	2.0	18.0	350	2.0	0.0	0

Food Name	Serv. Size	Total Cal.	Prot. GMS	Carbs GMS	Sod. MGS	Fiber GMS	Fat GMS	Chol. MGS
kernel, w/liquid	4 oz	69	2.2	16.8	287	.9	0.5	0
kernel, w/liquid (A&P)	1/2 cup	80	2.0	20.0	350	(mq)	1.0	0
kernel, w/liquid (Featherweight)	1/2 cup	80	2.0	16.0	10	(mq)	1.0	0
kernel, w/liquid (Finast)	1/2 cup	90	2.0	20.0	390	(mq)	1.0	0
kernel, w/liquid (Green Giant)	1/2 cup	80	2.0	18.0	280	2.7	0.0	0
kernel, w/liquid (S&W Nutradiet)	1/2 cup	80	2.0	15.0	0	(mq)	1.0	0
kernel, w/liquid, drained	4 oz	92	3.0	21.1	(mq)	1.5	1.1	0
kernel, w/liquid, 50% less salt, no sugar (Green Giant)	1/2 cup	50	2.0	11.0	140	2.0	1.0	0
kernel, w/liquid, low-sodium	4 oz	69	2.2	16.8	3	.9	0.5	0
kernel, w/liquid 'No Frills' (Pathmark)	1 cup	160	5.0	38.0	550	(mq)	1.0	0
kernel, w/liquid 'No Salt Added' (A&P)	1/2 cup	80	2.0	18.0	10	(mq)	<1.0	0
kernel, w/liquid 'No Salt Added' (Finast)	1/2 cup	80	3.0	19.0	10	(mq)	1.0	0
kernel, w/liquid 'No Salt Added' (Pathmark)	1/2 cup	70	2.0	16.0	10	(mq)	1.0	0
niblets (Green Giant)	1/2 cup	80	2.0	20.0	310	2.0	0.0	0
niblets, no salt, no sugar added (Green Giant)	1/2 cup	80	2.0	18.0	0	2.0	<1.0	0
sweet, select (Green Giant)	1/2 cup	60	2.0	15.0	280	3.0	<1.0	0
sweet, white, brine pack, drained solids	1/2 cup	66	2.2	15.2	265	1.2	0.8	0
sweet, white, brine pack, regular, w/liquid	1/2 cup	78	2.5	19.0	324	>.6 c	0.6	0
sweet, white, brine pack, dietary, w/liquid	1/2 cup	78	2.5	19.0	4	>.6 c	0.6	0
sweet, white, cream style, regular pack	1/2 cup	92	2.2	23.2	365	1.5	0.5	0
sweet, white, cream style, special dietary pack	1/2 cup	92	2.2	23.2	4	>.6 c	0.5	0
sweet, white, vacuum pack, regular pack	1/2 cup	83	2.5	20.4	286	>.8 c	0.5	0
sweet, white, vacuum pack, special dietary pack	1/2 cup	83	2.5	20.4	3	>.8 c	0.5	0
sweet, yellow, brine pack, drained solids	1/2 cup	66	2.2	15.2	265	1.1	0.8	0
sweet, yellow, brine pack, regular, w/liquid	1/2 cup	78	2.5	19.0	324	1.0	0.6	0
sweet, yellow, brine pack, dietary, w/liquid	1/2 cup	78	2.5	19.0	4	1.0	0.6	0
sweet, yellow, cream style, regular pack	1/2 cup	92	2.2	23.2	365	1.5	0.5	0
sweet, yellow, cream style, special dietary pack	1/2 cup	92	2.2	23.2	4	7.0	0.5	0
sweet, yellow, vacuum pack, regular pack	1/2 cup	83	2.5	20.4	286	6.0	0.5	0
sweet, yellow, vacuum pack, special dietary pack	1/2 cup	83	2.5	20.4	3	6.0	0.5	0

Food Name	Serv. Size	Total Cal.	Prot. GMS	Carbs GMS	Sod. MGS	Fiber GMS	Fat GMS	Chol. MGS
vacuum pack, w/liquid *(Del Monte)*	1/2 cup	90	3.0	22.0	355	(mq)	1.0	0
vacuum pack, w/liquid 'No Salt Added' *(Del Monte)*	1/2 cup	90	3.0	22.0	10	(mq)	1.0	0
white *(Green Giant)*	1/2 cup	80	2.0	20.0	310	2.0	0.0	0
white *(Stokely)*	1/2 cup	90	3.0	21.0	290	(mq)	0.0	0
white, vacuum pack *(A&P)*	1/2 cup	100	2.0	25.0	300	(mq)	1.0	0
white, vacuum pack *(Finast)*	4 oz	90	5.0	20.0	150	(mq)	1.0	0
white, vacuum pack *(Green Giant)*	1/2 cup	80	2.0	20.0	290	2.0	0.0	0
white, vacuum pack *(Pathmark)*	1/2 cup	120	3.0	25.0	350	(mq)	1.0	0
white, vacuum pack 'Niblets' *(Green Giant)*	1/2 cup	80	3.0	16.0	280	1.7	1.0	0
white, w/liquid *(Del Monte)*	1/2 cup	70	2.0	16.0	355	(mq)	0.0	0
white, young, tender 'Premium' *(S&W)*	1/2 cup	90	2.0	20.0	295	(mq)	1.0	0
whole kernel, golden, sweet *(Green Giant)*	1/2 cup	70	2.0	18.0	360	2.0	0.0	0
whole kernel, golden, sweet,50% less salt *(Green Giant)*	1/2 cup	70	2.0	16.0	180	2.0	<1.0	0
w/peppers 'Mexicorn' *(Green Giant)*	1/2 cup	80	2.0	19.0	450	2.0	<1.0	0
CORN, FROZEN								
(Health Valley)	1/2 cup	76	2.0	17.0	4	1.7	0.0	0
cream style *(Green Giant)*	1/2 cup	110	3.0	25.0	370	2.5	1.0	0
freeze-dried, prepared *(Mountain House)*	1/2 cup	90	2.0	18.0	<1	(mq)	1.0	0
golden, in butter sauce *(Green Giant)*	1/2 cup	100	3.0	19.0	310	2.0	2.0	5
in butter sauce *(Finast)*	1/2 cup	170	4.0	30.0	390	(mq)	4.0	na
in butter sauce 'Niblets' *(Green Giant)*	1/2 cup	100	2.0	18.0	280	2.0	2.0	na
in butter sauce 'Niblets One Serving' *(Green Giant)*	4.5 oz	120	3.0	24.0	350	3.0	2.0	5
in butter sauce 'Side Dish' *(Budget Gourmet)*	5.5 oz	190	4.0	31.0	310	(mq)	6.0	15
in butter sauce 'Singles' *(Stokely)*	4 oz	110	3.0	23.0	230	(mq)	1.0	5
in sauce, country style 'Side Dish' *(Budget Gourmet)*	5.75 oz	140	4.0	19.0	290	na	5.0	15
kernel *(A&P)*	3.3 oz	80	3.0	18.0	0	(mq)	<1.0	0
kernel *(Finast)*	3.3 oz	80	3.0	20.0	5	(mq)	1.0	0
kernel, cut *(Frosty Acres)*	3.3 oz	80	3.0	20.0	3	>1.0 c	1.0	0
kernel, cut *(Seabrook)*	3.3 oz	80	3.0	20.0	3	>1.0 c	1.0	0
kernel, cut *(Southern)*	3.5 oz	98	3.1	21.3	20	(mq)	0.7	0
kernel, cut, petite 'Deluxe' *(Birds Eye)*	2.6 oz	70	2.0	16.0	0	2.0	1.0	0
kernel, cut 'Portion Pack' *(Birds Eye)*	3 oz	70	3.0	18.0	0	2.0	1.0	0
kernel, cut 'Singles' *(Stokely)*	3 oz	75	3.0	18.0	5	(mq)	1.0	0
kernel 'Harvest Fresh Niblets' *(Green Giant)*	1/2 cup	80	2.0	17.0	40	2.0	1.0	0
kernel 'Niblets' *(Green Giant)*	1/2 cup	90	2.0	19.0	5	2.0	<1.0	0

Food Name	Serv. Size	Total Cal.	Prot. GMS	Carbs GMS	Sod. MGS	Fiber GMS	Fat GMS	Chol. MGS
kernel 'Niblets Supersweet'								
(Green Giant)	1/2 cup	60	2.0	13.0	5	2.0	1.0	0
kernel 'Sweet' (Birds Eye)	3.3 oz	80	3.0	20.0	0	2.0	1.0	0
kernel 'Tender Sweet Deluxe'								
(Birds Eye)	3.3 oz	80	3.0	20.0	0	2.0	1.0	0
niblets 'Butter Sauce' (Green Giant)	1/2 cup	100	3.0	19.0	310	2.0	2.0	5
niblets 'Plain Polybag' (Green Giant)	1/2 cup	90	2.0	19.0	5	2.0	<1.0	0
on the cob (A&P)	1 ear	120	4.0	28.0	0	(mq)	1.0	0
on the cob (Birds Eye)	1 ear	120	4.0	29.0	0	na	1.0	0
on the cob (Frosty Acres)	1 ear	120	4.0	29.0	0	(mq)	1.0	0
on the cob (Seabrook)	5-inch ear	120	4.0	29.0	4	>1.0 c	1.0	0
on the cob (Southern)	5-inch ear	140	5.0	30.0	na	(mq)	1.0	0
on the cob, baby 'Deluxe' (Birds Eye)	2.6 oz	25	2.0	4.0	10	2.0	0.0	0
on the cob 'Big Ears' (Birds Eye)	1 ear	160	4.0	37.0	0	na	1.0	0
on the cob, boiled, drained, kernels								
from ear	4 oz	59	2.0	14.1	3	>.4 c	0.5	0
on the cob 'Cob Treats' (A&P)	2 ears	130	5.0	28.0	5	(mq)	1.0	0
on the cob, 5.3 oz edible portion (Ore-Ida)	1 ear	180	5.0	39.0	40	(mq)	2.0	0
on the cob, in butter sauce 'Singles'								
(Stokely)	1 ear	70	2.0	16.0	200	(mq)	1.0	5
on the cob, kernels from ear	8 oz	123	4.1	29.4	6	>.9 c	1.0	0
on the cob 'Little Ears' (Birds Eye)	2 ears	130	4.0	30.0	0	na	1.0	0
on the cob, miniature 'Mini-Gold'								
(Ore-Ida)	2 ears	180	5.0	39.0	40	(mq)	2.0	0
on the cob 'Nibblers, 6-ear pkg'								
(Green Giant)	2 ears	120	4.0	27.0	10	2.0	1.0	0
on the cob 'Nibblers Supersweet'								
(Green Giant)	2 ears	90	3.0	19.0	10	2.0	2.0	0
on the cob 'Niblet Ears' (Green Giant)	1 ear	120	4.0	27.0	10	2.0	1.0	0
on the cob 'Niblet Ears Supersweet'								
(Green Giant)	1 ear	90	3.0	19.0	10	2.0	2.0	0
on the cob 'One Serving'								
(Green Giant)	2 half ears	120	4.0	26.0	10	2.0	1.0	0
on the cob 'Sweet Select' (Green Giant)	1 ear	90	3.0	19.0	10	2.0	2.0	0
on the cob 'Sweet Select' half ears								
(Green Giant)	2 half ears	90	3.0	19.0	10	2.0	2.0	0
sweet (Birds Eye)	3.3 oz	80	3.0	20.0	0	2.0	1.0	0
sweet, select 'Plain Polybag'								
(Green Giant)	1/2 cup	60	2.0	13.0	5	2.0	1.0	0
sweet, tender 'Butter Sauce Combination'								
(Birds Eye)	3.3 oz	90	2.0	17.0	250	2.0	2.0	5
sweet, tender 'Deluxe' (Birds Eye)	3.3 oz	80	3.0	20.0	0	2.0	1.0	0
sweet, white, kernels, boiled, drained	1 ear	59	2.0	14.1	3	3.6	0.5	0

Food Name	Serv. Size	Total Cal.	Prot. GMS	Carbs GMS	Sod. MGS	Fiber GMS	Fat GMS	Chol. MGS
sweet, white, kernels, boiled, drained	1/2 cup	76	2.5	18.3	3	4.7	0.6	0
sweet, white, kernels, unprepared	1/2 cup	72	2.5	17.1	2	4.7	0.6	0
sweet, yellow, kernels, boiled, drained	1 ear	59	2.0	14.1	3	3.6	0.5	0
sweet, yellow, kernels, boiled, drained	1/2 cup	76	2.5	18.3	3	>.5 c	0.6	0
sweet, yellow, kernels, unprepared	1/2 cup	72	2.5	17.1	2	2.0	0.6	0
white (Green Giant)	1/2 cup	90	2.0	19.0	5	2.0	1.0	0
white (Seabrook)	3.3 oz	80	3.0	19.0	3	>1.0 c	1.0	0
white, in butter sauce (Green Giant)	1/2 cup	100	2.0	20.0	280	2.3	2.0	5
white, shoepeg 'Butter Sauce' (Green Giant)	1/2 cup	100	2.0	20.0	280	2.0	2.0	5
white, shoepeg 'Harvest Fresh' (Green Giant)	1/2 cup	90	3.0	19.0	60	2.0	1.0	0
white, shoepeg 'Select' (Green Giant)	1/2 cup	90	2.0	19.0	5	2.0	<1.0	0
whole kernel, 'Portion Pack' (Birds Eye)	3 oz	70	3.0	18.0	0	2.0	1.0	0
CORN AND PEPPERS, CANNED								
red and green peppers, solid and liquid	1/2 cup	86	2.7	20.7	396	>.7 c	0.6	0
vacuum packed (Freshlike)	1/2 cup	90	3.0	23.0	300	na	1.0	na
vacuum packed (Veg•All)	1/2 cup	90	3.0	23.0	300	na	1.0	na
CORN BRAN								
crude	1 cup	170	6.3	65.1	5	65.4	0.7	0
crude	1 oz	64	2.4	24.3	2	24.0	0.3	0
CORN CAKE								
apple cinnamon flavor (Roman Meal)	1 cake	49	<1.0	10.5	<5	na	<1.0	0
caramel, fat-free (Quaker)	1 cake	50	1.0	12.0	30	na	0.0	0
caramel flavor, fat-free (Roman Meal)	1 cake	50	<1.0	11.0	5	0	0.0	0
cheddar flavor (Roman Meal)	1 cake	43	<1.0	9.0	14	na	<1.0	0
natural butter flavor, fat-free (Roman Meal)	1 cake	40	<1.0	8.0	35	0	0.0	0
plain	1 cake	35	0.7	7.5	44	.2	0.2	0
popcorn	1 cake	38	1.0	8.0	29	.3	0.3	0
popcorn, butter flavor (Chico-San)	1 cake	40	1.0	8.0	45	na	0.0	0
popcorn, caramel (Chico-San)	1 cake	50	1.0	10.0	55	na	0.0	0
popcorn, lightly salted (Chico-San)	1 cake	40	1.0	8.0	45	na	0.0	0
popcorn, white cheddar cheese (Chico-San)	1 cake	50	1.0	9.0	65	na	1.0	0
popped, butter flavor (Quaker)	1 cake	35	1.0	7.0	55	na	0.0	0
popped, white cheddar flavor (Quaker)	1 cake	40	1.0	8.0	110	na	0.0	0
very low sodium	1 cake	24	0.0	6.3	5	0	0.0	0
white cheddar flavor, fat-free (Roman Meal)	1 cake	45	<1.0	9.0	15	0	0.0	0
CORN CHIPS AND SNACKS. See also TORTILLA CHIPS.								
barbecue (Bachman)	1 oz	150	<1.0	17.0	230	(mq)	9.0	0
barbecue 'Rowdy Rustlers' 34 chips (Fritos)	1 oz	150	2.0	17.0	300	1.1	9.0	0

Food Name	Serv. Size	Total Cal.	Prot. GMS	Carbs GMS	Sod. MGS	Fiber GMS	Fat GMS	Chol. MGS
'Bar-B-Q Fritos' 34 pieces (Fritos)	1 oz	150	2.0	16.0	320	(mq)	9.0	0
bare bean 'Garden Vegetable Chips' (Harry's)	1 oz	144	2.7	17.0	<1	2.4	7.0	0
bare bean 'Offbeat Originals' (Peddlers) ...	1 oz	144	2.7	17.0	<1	2.4	7.0	0
beet garlic 'Garden Vegetable Chips' (Harry's)	1 oz	134	2.2	20.0	43	2.2	5.0	0
beet garlic 'Offbeat Originals' (Peddlers) ..	1 oz	134	2.2	20.0	43	2.2	5.0	0
bell pepper 'Garden Vegetable Chips' (Harry's)	1 oz	140	2.0	19.0	40	2.0	6.0	0
bell pepper 'Offbeat Originals' (Peddlers) ..	1 oz	140	2.0	19.0	40	2.0	6.0	0
blue corn 'Corn Curls' (Arrowhead Mills) ..	1 oz	120	3.0	22.0	54	4.0	2.0	0
blue corn 'Corn Curls Unsalted' (Arrowhead Mills)	1 oz	120	3.0	22.0	1	4.0	2.0	0
blue corn, no salt added (Barbara's Bakery)	1 oz	140	2.0	18.0	15	na	7.0	0
blue corn, regular (Barbara's Bakery)	1 oz	140	2.0	18.0	120	na	7.0	0
blue garlic 'Garden Vegetable Chips' (Harry's)	1 oz	129	2.6	21.0	28	3.0	4.0	0
blue garlic 'Offbeat Originals' (Peddlers) ...	1 oz	129	2.6	21.0	28	3.0	4.0	0
caramel corn puffs, apple cinnamon, fat-free (Health Valley)	1 oz	100	3.0	21.0	50	.1	0.0	0
caramel corn puffs, original style, fat-free (Health Valley)	1 oz	100	3.0	21.0	45	.1	0.0	0
caramel corn puffs, peanut flavor, fat-free (Health Valley)	1 oz	100	3.0	21.0	65	.1	0.0	0
carrot caraway 'Garden Vegetable Chips' (Harry's)	1 oz	131	2.4	20.0	31	1.5	4.0	0
carrot caraway 'Offbeat Originals' (Peddlers)	1 oz	131	2.4	20.0	31	1.5	4.0	0
cheddar cheese (Health Valley)	1 oz	160	3.0	15.0	120	1.0	10.0	2
cheese 'Baked' (Jax)	1 oz	140	2.0	17.0	290	(mq)	7.0	na
cheese 'Baked, Corn Puffs' (Cheez Doodles)	1 oz	150	2.0	17.0	360	(mq)	8.0	na
cheese 'Cheese Curls Low Salt' (Featherweight)	1 oz	150	2.0	16.0	81	(mq)	9.0	0
cheese 'Crunchy' (Jax)	1 oz	160	2.0	14.0	250	(mq)	11.0	na
cheese curls 'Great Tasting' (Ultra Slim Fast)	1 oz	110	2.0	20.0	360	3.0	3.0	0
cheese 'Fried Corn Puffs' (Cheez Doodles)	1 oz	160	2.0	15.0	220	(mq)	10.0	na
chili cheese, 34 chips (Fritos)	1 oz	160	2.0	15.0	300	1.1	10.0	0
cones, nacho-flavor	1 oz	152	1.8	16.2	270	>.1 c	9.0	1
cones, plain	1 oz	145	1.6	17.8	290	>.2 c	7.6	0
cool ranch (Doritos)	1 oz	140	2.0	18.0	115	0	7.0	0
corn chips (Wise)	1 oz	160	2.0	15.0	180	(mq)	10.0	0

Food Name	Serv. Size	Total Cal.	Prot. GMS	Carbs GMS	Sod. MGS	Fiber GMS	Fat GMS	Chol. MGS
corn crunchies (Wise)	1 oz	160	2.0	15.0	180	(mq)	10.0	0
corn nuggets, toasted (Fritos)	1.38 oz	170	3.0	29.0	265	na	5.0	0
corn ridgies (Wise)	1 oz	160	2.0	15.0	180	(mq)	10.0	0
corn spirals, toasted (Wise)	1 oz	160	2.0	15.0	125	(mq)	10.0	0
corn twists, crispy (Wise)	1 oz	160	2.0	15.0	125	na	10.0	na
'Crisp 'N Thin' 18 chips (Fritos)	1 oz	160	2.0	16.0	210	1.1	10.0	0
curls, barbecue flavored (Weight Watchers)	.5 oz	60	1.0	10.0	110	na	2.0	0
curls, pizza flavored (Weight Watchers)	.5 oz	60	1.0	10.0	130	na	2.0	0
curls, ranch flavored (Weight Watchers)	.5 oz	60	1.0	9.0	170	na	2.0	0
'Dip Size Fritos' 13 pieces (Fritos)	1 oz	150	2.0	17.0	210	(mq)	9.0	0
'Fritos' 34 pieces (Fritos)	1 oz	150	1.0	16.0	230	(mq)	9.0	0
'Low Salt' (Featherweight)	1 oz	170	2.0	15.0	3	(mq)	11.0	0
mild bean 'Garden Vegetable Chips' (Harry's)	1 oz	144	2.7	17.0	74	2.4	7.0	0
mild bean 'Offbeat Originals' (Peddlers)	1 oz	144	2.7	17.0	74	2.4	7.0	0
nacho cheese (Bugles)	1 oz	160	2.0	17.0	250	(mq)	9.0	na
nacho cheese (Corn Snackers)	.5-oz pkg	60	1.0	10.0	240	(mq)	2.0	na
nacho cheese flavor (Doritos)	1 oz	140	2.0	18.0	150	0	7.0	0
nacho cheese 'Non-Stop' 34 chips (Fritos)	1 oz	150	2.0	16.0	220	1.1	9.0	1
'No Salt Added' (Health Valley)	1 oz	160	1.0	13.0	1	1.0	11.0	0
onion-flavor	1 oz	142	2.2	18.5	278	1.1	6.4	0
'Pinta Blues' picante (Barbara's Bakery)	1 oz	130	2.0	18.0	250	na	6.0	0
'Pinta Blues' regular (Barbara's Bakery)	1 oz	140	2.0	20.0	110	na	6.0	0
'Pinta Puffs' salsa (Barbara's Bakery)	1 oz	70	2.0	10.0	130	na	2.0	0
'Pinta' regular (Barbara's Bakery)	1 oz	138	2.0	18.0	100	na	6.0	0
plain	1 oz	153	1.9	16.1	179	1.4	9.5	0
plain (Bachman)	1 oz	160	2.0	15.0	160	(mq)	10.0	0
plain (Bugles)	1 oz	150	2.0	18.0	290	(mq)	8.0	0
plain (Corn Snackers)	.5-oz pkg	60	1.0	10.0	190	(mq)	2.0	0
plain (Health Valley)	1 oz	160	1.0	13.0	90	1.0	11.0	0
plain (Planters)	1 oz	160	2.0	15.0	160	(mq)	10.0	0
plain (Snyder's)	1 oz	160	2.0	14.0	150	(mq)	11.0	0
'Potilla' chipotle chili (Barbara's Bakery)	1 oz	140	2.0	18.0	180	na	8.0	0
'Potilla' regular (Barbara's Bakery)	1 oz	140	2.0	18.0	120	na	8.0	0
puffs, cheese-flavor	1 oz	157	2.2	15.2	298	.3	9.8	1
puffs, cheese-flavor, enriched	1 oz	110	2.3	23.6	8	>.2 c	0.7	0
ranch (Bugles)	1 oz	150	2.0	16.0	290	na	9.0	na
'Rippled Corn Chips' (Dipsy Doodles)	1 oz	160	2.0	15.0	180	(mq)	10.0	0
toasted corn, crunchy, barbecue (Cornuts)	2 oz	247	5.1	40.7	553	4.8	8.1	0
toasted corn, crunchy, barbecue (Cornuts)	1 oz	124	2.5	20.3	277	2.4	4.1	0
toasted corn, crunchy, chili picante (Cornuts)	1 oz	120	2.0	22.0	260	2.2	4.0	0
toasted corn, crunchy, nacho (Cornuts)	2 oz	248	5.3	40.6	359	4.5	8.1	1

Food Name	Serv. Size	Total Cal.	Prot. GMS	Carbs GMS	Sod. MGS	Fiber GMS	Fat GMS	Chol. MGS
toasted corn, crunchy, nacho (Cornuts)	1 oz	124	2.7	20.3	180	2.3	4.0	1
toasted corn, crunchy, original (Cornuts) ...	2 oz	249	4.8	41.6	311	3.9	8.0	0
toasted corn, crunchy, original (Cornuts) ...	1 oz	124	2.4	20.8	156	2.0	4.0	0
toasted corn, crunchy, ranch (Cornuts)	1 oz	120	2.0	20.0	190	1.7	4.0	0
toasted corn, crunchy, unsalted (Cornuts) ..	1 oz	120	2.0	19.0	30	2.7	4.0	0
'Unsalted' (Azteca)	1 oz	140	2.0	18.0	110	(mq)	7.0	0
veggie 'Garden Vegetable Chips' (Harry's)	1 oz	141	2.2	18.0	40	2.5	7.0	0
veggie 'Offbeat Originals' (Peddlers)	1 oz	141	2.2	18.0	40	2.5	7.0	0
wild bean 'Garden Vegetable Chips'								
(Harry's)	1 oz	141	2.9	17.8	51	2.6	6.0	0
wild bean 'Offbeat Originals' (Peddlers) ...	1 oz	141	2.9	17.8	51	2.6	6.0	0
'Wild 'N Mild' 32 chips (Fritos)	1 oz	160	2.0	16.0	240	1.1	9.0	0
yellow 'Corn Chips' (Arrowhead Mills)	.75 oz	90	2.0	18.0	31	3.0	1.0	0
yellow, w/cheese 'Corn Chips'								
(Arrowhead Mills)	.75 oz	90	2.0	15.0	30	3.0	2.0	na
CORN FLAKE CRUMBS (Kellogg's)	1 oz	100	2.0	24.0	290	1.0	0.0	0
CORN FLOUR								
masa	1 oz	103	2.6	21.6	1	>.5 c	1.1	0
masa, enriched, white	1 cup	416	10.6	86.9	6	10.9	4.3	0
masa, enriched, yellow	1 cup	416	10.6	86.9	6	>1.9 c	4.3	0
'Masa Harina De Maiz' approx 1/3 cup								
(Quaker)	1.3 oz	137	3.5	27.4	5	2.7	1.5	0
'Masa Trigo' approx 1/3 cup (Quaker) ...	1.3 oz	149	3.5	24.7	794	1.0	4.0	0
whole-grain	1 oz	102	2.0	21.8	1	3.8	1.1	0
whole-grain, white	1/2 cup	209	4.0	44.6	3	5.6	2.2	0
whole-grain, yellow	1/2 cup	209	4.0	44.6	3	7.8	2.2	0
CORN FRITTER, frozen (Mrs. Paul's) ..	2 pieces	240	5.0	35.0	560	(mq)	9.0	10
CORN GRITS. See GRITS.								
CORN NUGGETS, FROZEN								
breaded, fried 'Quickkrisp' (Stilwell)	3 oz	210	3.0	30.0	420	(mq)	8.0	1
CORN OIL								
....	1/2 cup	964	0.0	0.0	0	0	109.0	0
....	1 oz	251	0.0	0.0	0	0	28.4	0
....	1 tbsp	120	0.0	0.0	0	0	13.6	0
(Crisco)	1 tbsp	120	0.0	0.0	0	0	14.0	0
(Crisco) 'Puritan'	1 tbsp	120	0.0	0.0	0	0	14.0	0
(Hain)	1 tbsp	120	0.0	0.0	0	0	14.0	0
(Kroger)	1 tbsp	122	0.0	0.0	0	0	13.6	0
(Mazola)	1 tbsp	120	0.0	0.0	0	0	14.0	0
(Pathmark)	1 tbsp	130	0.0	0.0	0	0	14.0	0
(Pathmark) 'No Frills'	1 tbsp	130	0.0	0.0	0	0	14.0	0
(Spectrum Naturals)	1 tbsp	120	0.0	0.0	0	(tr)	14.0	(tr)
(Wesson)	1 tbsp	120	0.0	0.0	0	0	14.0	0

Food Name	Serv. Size	Total Cal.	Prot. GMS	Carbs GMS	Sod. MGS	Fiber GMS	Fat GMS	Chol. MGS
CORN OIL SPRAY. See COOKING SPRAY.								
CORN OIL SPREAD								
(Fleischmann's) 60% oil 'Light'	1 tbsp	80	0.0	0.0	70	na	8.0	0
(Fleischmann's) 40% oil 'Extra Light'	1 tbsp	50	0.0	0.0	55	na	6.0	0
CORN SALAD, raw	1/2 cup	6	0.6	1.0	1	>.2 c	0.1	
CORN SOUFFLÉ, FROZEN, 1 pkg								
(Stouffer's)	6 oz	240	7.0	27.0	760	na	11.0	na
CORN SYRUP								
dark	1 cup	925	0.0	251.3	508	0	0.0	0
dark	1 tbsp	56	0.0	15.3	31	0	0.0	0
dark (Karo)	1 tbsp	60	0.0	15.0	40	0	0.0	0
high-fructose	1 cup	871	0.0	235.6	6	0	0.0	0
high-fructose	1 tbsp	53	0.0	14.4	0	0	0.0	0
light	1 cup	925	0.0	251.3	397	0	0.0	0
light	1 tbsp	56	0.0	15.3	24	0	0.0	0
light (Karo)	1 tbsp	60	0.0	15.0	30	0	0.0	0
table blends, refiner, and sugar	1 cup	1008	0.0	265.1	224	0	0.0	0
table blends, refiner, and sugar	1 tbsp	64	0.0	16.8	14	0	0.0	0
CORNBREAD. See BREAD.								
CORNMEAL								
	1 cup	605	15.6	123.3	58	>4.8 c	7.9	0
	1 oz	103	2.7	21.1	10	>.8 c	1.3	0
blue, whole-grain (Arrowhead Mills)	2 oz	210	6.0	41.0	1	5.6	3.0	0
degermed	1 oz	104	8.5	22.0	1	1.5	0.5	0
degermed, enriched, white	1 cup	505	11.7	107.2	4	10.2	2.3	0
degermed, enriched, yellow	1 cup	505	11.7	107.2	4	10.2	2.3	0
degermed, unenriched, white	1 cup	505	11.7	107.2	4	10.2	2.3	0
degermed, unenriched, yellow	1 cup	505	11.7	107.2	4	10.2	2.3	0
white, bolted (Aunt Jemima)	1 oz	99	2.4	20.8	337	(mq)	0.7	0
white, bolted, enriched (Aunt Jemima)	1 oz	99	2.3	20.4	382	(mq)	0.9	0
white, dry (Albers)	1 oz	100	2.0	22.0	0	1.5	1.0	0
white, enriched, approx 3 tbsp (Aunt Jemima)	1 oz	102	2.4	22.2	1	1.2	0.5	0
white, whole-grain	1 cup	442	9.9	93.8	43	8.9	4.4	0
whole-grain	1 oz	103	2.3	21.8	10	3.1	1.0	0
whole-grain, hi-lysine (Arrowhead Mills)	2 oz	210	4.0	43.0	1	6.8	2.0	0
yellow, dry (Albers)	1 oz	100	2.0	22.0	0	1.5	1.0	0
yellow, enriched (Aunt Jemima)	1 oz	102	2.4	22.2	1	1.2	0.5	0
yellow, whole-grain	1 cup	442	9.9	93.8	43	8.9	4.4	0
yellow, whole-grain (Arrowhead Mills)	2 oz	210	4.0	43.0	1	6.8	2.0	0
CORNMEAL, SELF-RISING								
bolted	1 oz	95	2.3	19.9	353	>.3 c	1.0	0
bolted, w/wheat flour	1 oz	99	2.4	20.8	374	>.2 c	0.8	0

Food Name	Serv. Size	Total Cal.	Prot. GMS	Carbs GMS	Sod. MGS	Fiber GMS	Fat GMS	Chol. MGS
degermed	1 oz	101	2.4	21.2	382	>.2 c	0.5	0
white (Aunt Jemima)	1 oz	98	2.3	21.1	381	>.2 c	0.5	0
white, bolted (Aunt Jemima)	1 oz	98	2.3	21.1	381	>.2 c	0.5	0
white, bolted, enriched (Aunt Jemima)	1 oz	99	2.3	20.4	382	(mq)	0.9	0
white, bolted, plain, enriched	1 cup	407	10.1	85.7	1521	>1.3 c	4.2	0
white, bolted, wheat flour added, enriched	1 cup	592	14.3	124.8	2242	>1.3 c	4.8	0
white, buttermilk (Aunt Jemima)	3 tbsp	101	2.5	20.2	439	(mq)	1.1	0
white, degermed, enriched	1 cup	490	11.6	103.2	1860	>.7 c	2.4	0
yellow (Aunt Jemima)	3 tbsp	100	2.0	21.0	490	(mq)	1.0	0
yellow, bolted, plain, enriched	1 cup	407	10.1	85.7	1521	>1.3 c	4.2	0
yellow, bolted, wheat flour added, enriched	1 cup	592	14.3	124.8	2242	>1.3 c	4.8	0
yellow, degermed, enriched	1 cup	490	11.6	103.2	1860	>.7 c	2.4	0
CORNED BEEF. See BEEF, CORNED.								
CORNISH GAME HEN								
frozen (Tyson)	3.5 oz	240	28.0	0.0	70	0	14.0	75
frozen, w/skin (Tyson)	3.5 oz	250	27.0	1.0	80	na	15.0	155
w/wild rice, wholesale club item (Tyson)	3.5 oz	190	19.0	6.0	125	na	11.0	85
CORNSTARCH								
	1 cup	488	0.3	116.8	12	1.1	0.1	0
	1 oz	108	0.1	25.9	3	.3	<.1	0
	1 tbsp	30	<.1	7.3	1	.1	tr	0
(Argo)	1 tbsp	30	0.0	7.0	0	tr	0.0	0
(Cream)	1 tbsp	29	tr	7.0	tr	na	tr	0
(Kingsford)	1 tbsp	30	0.0	7.0	0	tr	0.0	0
COTTAGE CHEESE. See CHEESE.								
COTTONSEED FLOUR								
lowfat	1 oz	94	14.1	10.2	10	>.7 c	0.4	0
partially defatted	1 cup	337	38.5	38.1	33	2.8	5.8	0
partially defatted	1 oz	102	11.6	11.5	10	.8	1.8	0
partially defatted	1 tbsp	18	2.0	2.0	2	>.1 c	0.3	0
COTTONSEED KERNELS								
roasted	1 cup	754	48.6	32.6	37	8.2	54.1	0
roasted	1 oz	143	9.2	6.2	7	1.6	10.3	0
roasted	1 tbsp	51	3.3	2.2	3	.6	3.6	0
COTTONSEED MEAL, partially defatted	1 oz	104	13.9	10.9	11	>.7 c	1.4	0
COTTONSEED OIL								
	1 cup	1927	0.0	0.0	0	0	218.0	0
	1/2 cup	964	0.0	0.0	0	0	109.0	0
	1 tbsp	120	0.0	0.0	0	0	13.6	0
(Wesson)	1 tbsp	122	0.0	0.0	0	0	13.6	0
COUSCOUS								
cooked	1/2 cup	101	3.4	20.8	4.5	1.3	0.1	0

Food Name	Serv. Size	Total Cal.	Prot. GMS	Carbs GMS	Sod. MGS	Fiber GMS	Fat GMS	Chol. MGS
cooked	4 oz	127	4.3	26.3	6	1.6	0.2	0
dry	1/2 cup	346	11.7	71.2	9	4.6	0.6	0
dry	1 oz	107	3.6	22.0	3	1.4	0.2	0
mix, dry *(Near East)*	1.25 oz	120	4.0	26.0	5	(mq)	0.0	0
mix, prepared w/2 tbsp salted butter *(Fantastic Foods)*	1/2 cup	122	3.0	22.0	35	(mq)	3.0	(mq)
mix, prepared w/o added ingredients *(Fantastic Foods)*	1/2 cup	105	3.0	22.0	1	(mq)	0.0	0
mix, whole-wheat *(Fantastic Foods)*	1/2 cup	94	3.5	20.0	0	(mq)	0.0	0
mix, whole-wheat, prepared w/2 tbsp salted butter *(Fantastic Foods)*	1/2 cup	111	3.5	20.0	23	(mq)	2.0	(mq)
COUSCOUS PILAF MIX								
(Casbah) dry	1 oz	100	4.0	20.0	na	(mq)	0.0	0
(Casbah) prepared w/o added ingredients	1/2 cup	100	4.0	20.0	na	(mq)	0.0	0
(Quick Pilaf) savory, prepared w/2 tbsp salted butter	1/2 cup	124	4.0	19.0	254	(mq)	3.0	(mq)
(Quick Pilaf) savory, prepared w/o added ingredients	1/2 cup	94	4.0	19.0	215	(mq)	0.0	0
COWPEA. See BLACK-EYED PEAS.								
CRAB								
ALASKAN KING								
boiled	4 oz	110	21.9	0.0	1216	0	1.7	60
boiled, approx 4.7 oz	1 leg	129	25.9	0.0	1436	0	1.7	72
moist-heat cooked	3 oz	82	16.5	0.0	911	0	1.3	45
poached	4 oz	110	21.9	0.0	1216	0	1.7	60
poached, approx 4.7 oz	1 leg	129	25.9	0.0	1436	0	1.7	72
raw	1 lb	379	83.0	0.0	3792	0	2.7	189
raw	3 oz	71	15.6	0.0	711	0	0.5	36
raw	1 oz	24	5.2	0.0	237	0	0.2	12
steamed	4 oz	110	21.9	0.0	1216	0	1.7	60
steamed, approx 4.7 oz	1 leg	129	25.9	0.0	1436	0	1.7	72
BLUE								
boiled	4 oz	116	22.9	0.0	316	0	2.0	113
boiled, approx 4.75 oz	1 cup	138	27.3	0.0	376	0	2.4	135
cake, fried	4 oz	176	22.9	0.5	374	>.6 c	8.5	170
cake, fried, approx 2.1 oz	1 med	93	12.1	0.3	198	>.1 c	4.5	90
canned	1 cup	134	27.7	0.0	450	0	1.7	120
canned	4 oz	112	23.3	0.0	378	0	1.4	101
canned	3 oz	84	17.4	0.0	283	0	1.0	76
moist-heat cooked	1 cup	138	27.3	0.0	377	0	2.4	135
moist-heat cooked	3 oz	87	17.2	0.0	237	0	1.5	85
poached	4 oz	116	22.9	0.0	316	0	2.0	113
poached, approx 4.75 oz	1 cup	138	27.3	0.0	376	0	2.4	135

Food Name	Serv. Size	Total Cal.	Prot. GMS	Carbs GMS	Sod. MGS	Fiber GMS	Fat GMS	Chol. MGS
raw	1 lb	395	81.9	0.2	1329	0	4.9	355
raw	3 oz	74	15.3	0.0	249	0	0.9	66
raw	1 oz	25	5.1	<.1	83	0	0.3	22
steamed	4 oz	116	22.9	0.0	316	0	2.0	113
steamed, approx 4.75 oz	1 cup	138	27.3	0.0	376	0	2.4	135
DUNGENESS								
canned *(S&W)*	3.25 oz	81	18.0	1.0	920	0	2.0	(mq)
moist-heat cooked	3 oz	94	19.0	0.8	321	0	1.0	65
raw	1 lb	391	79.0	3.3	1340	0	4.4	269
raw	3 oz	73	14.8	0.6	251	0	0.8	50
raw	1 oz	24	4.9	0.2	84	0	0.3	17
IMPERIAL	1 cup	323	32.1	8.6	1602	0	16.7	308
QUEEN								
moist-heat cooked	100 gm	115	23.7	0.0	691	0	1.5	71
moist-heat cooked	3 oz	98	20.2	0.0	587	0	1.3	60
raw	1 lb	407	83.9	0.0	2445	0	5.4	248
raw	3 oz	77	15.7	0.0	458	0	1.0	47
raw	1 oz	26	5.2	0.0	153	0	0.3	16
SNOW								
frozen *(Wakefield)*	3 oz	60	13.0	0.0	270	0	1.0	(mq)
raw, Opilio, clusters *(Peter Pan Seafoods)*	3.5 oz	91	20.6	na	539	na	1.2	55
raw, Opilio, 'Snap 'n' Eat' scored *(Peter Pan Seafoods)*	3.5 oz	91	20.6	na	539	na	1.2	55
SOFTSHELL								
boiled	4 oz	116	22.9	0.0	316	0	2.0	113
boiled, approx 4.75 oz	1 cup	138	27.3	0.0	376	0	2.4	135
cake, fried	4 oz	176	22.9	0.5	374	>.6 c	8.5	170
cake, fried, approx 2.1 oz	1 med	93	12.1	0.3	198	>.1 c	4.5	90
poached	4 oz	116	22.9	0.0	316	0	2.0	113
poached, approx 4.75 oz	1 cup	138	27.3	0.0	376	0	2.4	135
raw	1 lb	395	81.9	0.2	1329	0	4.9	355
raw	1 oz	25	5.1	<.1	83	0	0.3	22
raw, approx .7 oz	1 crab	18	3.8	<.1	62	0	0.2	16
steamed	4 oz	116	22.9	0.0	316	0	2.0	113
steamed, approx 4.75 oz	1 cup	138	27.3	0.0	376	0	2.4	135
CRAB, ALTERNATIVE								
	1 lb	463	54.5	46.4	3815	0	5.9	89
	1 oz	29	3.4	3.0	238	0	0.4	6
Alaskan King, made from surimi	3 oz	87	10.2	8.7	715	0	1.1	17
(Icicle Brand)	3.5 oz	99	12.0	11.0	900	0	0.1	10
CRAB, DEVILED								
	1 cup	451	27.4	31.9	2081	0	22.6	245
breaded, frozen, cake *(Mrs. Paul's)*	3 oz	180	8.0	18.0	480	(mq)	9.0	20

Food Name	Serv. Size	Total Cal.	Prot. GMS	Carbs GMS	Sod. MGS	Fiber GMS	Fat GMS	Chol. MGS
breaded, frozen, miniature *(Mrs. Paul's)*	3.5 oz	240	9.0	25.0	540	(mq)	12.0	20
CRAB AND SHRIMP, frozen *(Wakefield)*	3 oz	60	13.0	0.0	210	0	1.0	(mq)
CRAB CAKE								
....	100 gm	147	26.2	3.9	504	0	2.1	169
....	1 cake	88	15.7	2.3	302	0	1.3	101
blue crab	1 cake	93	12.1	0.3	198	0	4.5	90
CRABAPPLE								
raw	100 gm	76	0.4	20.0	1	>.6 c	0.3	0
raw, slices, w/skin	1 cup	84	0.4	21.9	1	>.7 c	0.3	0
trimmed, w/skin	1 oz	22	0.1	5.7	<1	>.2 c	0.1	0
trimmed, w/skin, sliced	1/2 cup	42	0.2	11.0	1	>.3 c	0.2	0
untrimmed	1 lb	316	1.7	83.2	4	>2.5 c	1.3	0
CRABAPPLE, CANNED								
spiced *(Lucky Leaf)*	4 oz	110	0.0	28.0	(mq)	(mq)	0.0	0
spiced *(Musselman's)*	4 oz	110	0.0	28.0	(mq)	(mq)	0.0	0
CRACKER								
apple cinnamon 'Orchard Crisps' *(Nabisco)*	.5 oz	60	1.0	11.0	40	na	2.0	0
bacon flavor *(Delicious)*	.5 oz	70	1.0	10.0	190	na	3.0	0
bacon flavor 'Bacon Flavored Thins' .5 oz *(Nabisco)*	7 crackers	70	1.0	9.0	210	(mq)	4.0	0
bacon flavor 'Toasteds' approx .5 oz *(Keebler)*	4 crackers	60	1.0	8.0	125	(mq)	3.0	0
banana walnut 'Orchard Crisps' *(Nabisco)*	.5 oz	60	1.0	11.0	40	na	2.0	0
barbecue wheat, for weight control *(Spicer's)*	1 oz	100	5.0	12.0	75	9.0	5.0	0
bar-b-que, tater crisps *(Mr. Phipps)*	.5 oz	60	1.0	10.0	160	na	2.0	0
bite size *(Delicious)*	.5 oz	70	1.0	9.0	90	na	3.0	0
bite size, low sodium *(Delicious)*	.5 oz	70	1.0	9.0	55	na	3.0	0
'Bits' approx .5 oz *(Triscuit)*	15 crackers	60	1.0	10.0	85	na	3.0	0
bran *(FiberRich)*	1 cracker	18	1.0	6.0	10	2.8	<1.0	0
bran, toasted 'Bran Thins' *(Nabisco)*	7 crackers	60	1.0	9.0	70	(mq)	3.0	0
butter, country flavor *(McCrakens)*	1 oz	140	2.0	18.0	170	na	8.0	0
butter flavor *(Ritz)*	4 crackers	70	1.0	9.0	140	0	4.0	0
butter flavor, approx .5 oz *(Escort)*	3 crackers	70	1.0	9.0	115	(mq)	4.0	0
butter flavor 'Club Low Salt' approx .5 oz *(Keebler)*	4 crackers	60	1.0	9.0	75	(mq)	3.0	0
butter flavor, dairy, .5 oz *(American Classic)*	4 crackers	70	1.0	9.0	140	(mq)	3.0	2
butter flavor 'Flutters' *(Pepperidge Farm)*	.75 oz	100	2.0	15.0	150	(mq)	4.0	5
butter flavor 'Ritz Bits' 22 pieces *(Ritz)*	.5 oz	70	1.0	9.0	120	(mq)	4.0	0
butter flavor 'Ritz Bits Low Salt' 22 pieces *(Ritz)*	.5 oz	70	1.0	9.0	60	(mq)	4.0	0

Food Name	Serv. Size	Total Cal.	Prot. GMS	Carbs GMS	Sod. MGS	Fiber GMS	Fat GMS	Chol. MGS
butter flavor 'Ritz Low Salt' approx .5 oz *(Ritz)*	4 crackers	70	1.0	9.0	60	(mq)	4.0	0
butter flavor 'Ritz' approx .5 oz *(Ritz)*	4 crackers	70	1.0	9.0	120	(mq)	4.0	0
butter flavor 'Toasteds Buttercrisp' .5 oz *(Keebler)*	4 crackers	60	1.0	8.0	125	(mq)	3.0	0
butter flavor 'Town House Low Salt' .5 oz *(Keebler)*	4 crackers	70	1.0	8.0	60	(mq)	4.0	0
butter flavor 'Town House' approx .5 oz *(Keebler)*	4 crackers	70	1.0	8.0	120	(mq)	4.0	0
butter flavor, thins 'Distinctive' *(Pepperidge Farm)*	4 crackers	70	1.0	10.0	115	(mq)	3.0	5
cheese *(Combos)*	1.8 oz	240	5.0	34.0	580	(mq)	10.0	na
cheese *(Delicious)*	.5 oz	70	1.0	9.0	135	na	3.0	<1
cheese 'Better Cheddars' *(Nabisco)*	.5 oz	70	2.0	8.0	130	0	4.0	0
cheese 'Better Cheddars' low salt *(Nabisco)*	.5 oz	70	2.0	8.0	65	0	4.0	2
cheese, bite size *(Delicious)*	.5 oz	70	1.0	9.0	135	na	3.0	<1
cheese, cheddar, approx 13-16 crackers *(Frito-Lay's)*	.5 oz	70	1.0	8.0	150	0	4.0	0
cheese, cheddar, baked, cracker chips 'Zings' *(Nabisco)*	.5 oz	70	1.0	9.0	140	na	3.0	2
cheese, cheddar 'Crackups' *(Nabisco)*	.5 oz	70	1.0	10.0	100	na	3.0	0
cheese, cheddar 'Goldfish' *(Pepperidge Farm)*	1 oz	120	4.0	19.0	230	1.0	4.0	5
cheese, cheddar 'Goldfish Thins' *(Pepperidge Farm)*	4 crackers	50	1.0	8.0	160	(mq)	2.0	0
cheese, cheddar 'Guppies' 12 pieces *(Pepperidge Farm)*	.5 oz	40	1.0	5.0	95	(mq)	2.0	na
cheese, cheddar 'Original Goldfish' *(Pepperidge Farm)*	1 oz	130	3.0	18.0	190	1.0	5.0	0
cheese, cheddar 'Snorkels' *(Nabisco)*	.5 oz	70	2.0	9.0	150	na	2.0	0
cheese, cheddar, tangy *(McCrakens)*	1 oz	140	2.0	18.0	170	na	8.0	0
cheese, cheddar 'Town House Jrs.' 8 pieces *(Keebler)*	.5 oz	80	1.0	8.0	95	(mq)	4.0	5
cheese 'Cheddar Wedges' 31 pieces *(Nabisco)*	.5 oz	70	1.0	9.0	150	0	3.0	0
cheese 'Cheese Nips' 13 pieces *(Nabisco)*	.5 oz	70	1.0	9.0	130	0	3.0	0
cheese 'Cheese Peanut Butter Sandwich' 4 pieces *(Nabisco)*	1 oz	130	3.0	15.0	320	na	7.0	0
cheese 'Cheese Ritz Bite Mini Ritz' 22 pieces *(Ritz)*	.5 oz	70	1.0	8.0	130	0	4.0	0
cheese 'Cheez-Its' *(Sunshine)*	12 crackers	70	2.0	7.0	135	(mq)	4.0	2

Food Name	Serv. Size	Total Cal.	Prot. GMS	Carbs GMS	Sod. MGS	Fiber GMS	Fat GMS	Chol. MGS
cheese 'Cheez-Its Low Salt' (Sunshine) .... 12 crackers		70	2.0	7.0	65	(mq)	4.0	2
cheese, Parmesan 'Goldfish' (Pepperidge Farm) .... 1 oz		120	4.0	19.0	330	1.0	4.0	5
cheese, reduced fat 'Snack Wells' 18 pieces (Nabisco) .... .5 oz		60	2.0	11.0	160	na	1.0	0
cheese 'Ritz Bits Sandwiches' approx .5 oz (Ritz) .... 6 crackers		80	1.0	7.0	135	0	5.0	0
cheese, sandwich-type w/peanut butter filling .... .5 oz		68	1.8	8.1	141	.2	3.3	1
cheese, Swiss 'Naturally Flavored' .5 oz (Nabisco) .... 7 crackers		70	1.0	9.0	170	na	3.0	0
cheese 'Tid-Bits' 15 pieces (Nabisco) .... .5 oz		70	1.0	8.0	200	<1.0	4.0	5
cheese, white cheddar 'Cheez-Its' (Sunshine) .... .5 oz		76	1.0	9.0	160	na	4.0	2
cheese flavor (Hain) .... 1 oz		130	3.0	17.0	180	(mq)	6.0	na
cheese flavor, organic, fat-free (Health Valley) .... .5 oz		40	1.0	9.0	80	1.9	0.0	0
cheese flavor, 25 pieces (Rokeach) ...... 1 oz		140	3.0	16.0	(mq)	(mq)	8.0	na
cheese sandwich, and cheese 'Handi-Snacks' (Kraft) .... 1 pkg		120	4.0	9.0	360	(mq)	8.0	20
cheese sandwich, and peanut butter, .5 oz (Keebler) .... 2 crackers		70	2.0	9.0	150	(mq)	3.0	0
cheese sandwich, cheddar 'Town House' .5 oz (Keebler) ..... 1 cracker		70	1.0	6.0	105	(mq)	4.0	5
cheese sandwich, wheat and American cheese, .5 oz Keebler) .... 1 cracker		70	1.0	7.0	85	(mq)	4.0	5
cheese-filled, 6 crackers (Frito-Lay's) .... 1.5 oz		210	4.0	24.0	470	0	10.0	5
chicken flavor 'Chicken in a Biskit' 7 pieces (Nabisco) .... .5 oz		80	1.0	8.0	130	(mq)	5.0	0
cinnamon graham (Delicious) .... .5 oz		60	1.0	11.0	50	na	2.0	0
cinnamon graham, fat-free 'Snack Wells' (Nabisco) .... .5 oz		50	1.0	12.0	45	na	0.0	0
cracked pepper, fat-free 'Snack Wells' (Nabisco) .... .5 oz		60	1.0	12.0	160	na	0.0	0
cracked pepper 'Gourmet' fat-free (Frookie) .... 4 crackers		35	1.0	7.0	40	na	0.0	0
cracked wheat, approx .5 oz (American Classic) .... 4 crackers		70	1.0	8.0	140	(mq)	4.0	0
cracked wheat 'Distinctive' (Pepperidge Farm) .... 3 crackers		100	2.0	14.0	180	1.0	4.0	0
cracked wheat 'Wafers' (Hickory Farms) .... 8 crackers		100	2.0	17.0	290	(mq)	3.0	na

Food Name	Serv. Size	Total Cal.	Prot. GMS	Carbs GMS	Sod. MGS	Fiber GMS	Fat GMS	Chol. MGS
'Crackerbread' (Crisp & Light)	1 slice	17	1.0	3.0	25	(mq)	<1.0	0
'Crackerbread Salt Free' (Crisp & Light)	1 slice	17	1.0	3.0	<1	(mq)	<1.0	0
'Crackerdiles' (Delicious)	.5 oz	70	1.0	9.0	135	na	3.0	<1
crispbread (Dar-Vida)	1 cracker	20	1.0	4.0	40	(mq)	<1.0	0
crispbread 'Breakfast' (Wasa)	1 cracker	50	2.0	8.0	65	.7	1.0	0
crispbread, dark (Finn Crisp)	2 crackers	38	1.0	9.0	130	1.6	<1.0	0
crispbread 'Extra Crisp' (Wasa)	1 cracker	25	1.0	5.0	40	(mq)	0.0	0
crispbread 'Fiber Plus' (Wasa)	1 cracker	35	1.0	5.0	65	2.8	1.0	0
crispbread, garlic flavor (Weight Watchers)	2 crackers	30	<1.0	7.0	55	(mq)	0.0	0
crispbread, high fiber 'Crisp Bread' (Ryvita)	1 cracker	23	0.9	4.0	10	2.0	<1.0	0
crispbread, high fiber 'Snackbread' (Ryvita)	1 cracker	14	0.6	3.0	25	1.0	<1.0	0
crispbread, regular (Finn Crisp)	2 crackers	38	1.0	9.0	130	1.6	<1.0	0
crispbread, thick (Kavli Norwegian)	1 slice	35	1.0	7.5	31	1.9	0.3	0
crispbread, thin (Kavli Norwegian)	2 slices	40	1.0	8.0	32	6.0	0.3	0
crispbread, w/caraway (Finn Crisp)	2 slices	38	1.0	9.0	130	1.6	<1.0	0
5-spice wafer (Westbrae)	4.5 wafers	40	1.0	8.0	30	na	0.0	0
garlic 'Discos' (Delicious)	.5 oz	78	1.0	6.0	184	na	5.0	0
garlic 'Garlic Tams' (Manischewitz)	10 crackers	153	2.0	19.0	165	(mq)	8.0	0
garlic and herb 'Gourmet' fat-free (Frookie)	8 crackers	70	2.0	16.0	170	1.0	0.0	0
graham, chocolate 'Selects' (Keebler)	4 crackers	60	1.0	9.0	55	na	3.0	0
graham, honey nut 'Selects' (Keebler)	4 crackers	60	1.0	9.0	70	na	3.0	0
graham cracker 'Amaranth Graham Crackers' (Health Valley)	7 crackers	110	3.0	25.0	110	3.1	3.0	0
graham cracker, apple cinnamon 'Graham Bites' (Honey Maid)	11 crackers	60	1.0	11.0	80	(mq)	2.0	0
graham cracker, approx .5 oz (Keebler)	4 crackers	70	1.0	12.0	85	(mq)	2.0	0
graham cracker, approx 1 oz (Regal)	2 crackers	140	1.0	19.0	120	(mq)	7.0	na
graham cracker, approx 1 oz (Rokeach)	8 crackers	120	2.0	21.0	(mq)	(mq)	3.0	na
graham cracker, brown sugar 'Graham Bites' .5 oz (Honey Maid)	11 crackers	60	1.0	11.0	80	(mq)	2.0	0
graham cracker 'Grahamy Bears' (Sunshine)	9 crackers	130	2.0	21.0	160	(mq)	5.0	0
graham cracker, 2 pieces (Nabisco)	.5 oz	60	1.0	11.0	90	1.0	1.0	0
grain, 6 pieces (Harvest Crisps)	.5 oz	60	1.0	10.0	135	1.0	2.0	0
hearty wheat 'Distinctive' (Pepperidge Farm)	4 crackers	100	2.0	13.0	140	1.0	5.0	0

Food Name	Serv. Size	Total Cal.	Prot. GMS	Carbs GMS	Sod. MGS	Fiber GMS	Fat GMS	Chol. MGS
herb, garden 'Flutters' (Pepperidge Farm)	.75 oz	100	2.0	14.0	190	(mq)	4.0	0
herb, organic, fat-free (Health Valley)	.5 oz	40	1.0	9.0	80	1.9	0.0	0
herb 'Stoned Wheat' (Health Valley)	13 crackers	120	3.0	17.0	160	3.5	6.0	0
herb 'Stoned Wheat No Salt Added' (Health Valley)	13 crackers	120	3.0	17.0	30	3.5	6.0	0
honey graham (Delicious)	.5 oz	60	1.0	11.0	50	na	2.0	0
hot and spicy 'Cheez-Its' approx 12 crackers (Sunshine)	.5 oz	70	1.0	8.0	160	na	4.0	2
'Low Salt' (Featherweight)	2 crackers	30	0.0	5.0	1	(mq)	1.0	0
matzo, American board (Manischewitz)	1 oz	115	2.9	22.0	na	(mq)	1.9	0
matzo 'Daily Unsalted' board (Manischewitz)	1 oz	110	3.0	24.0	1	.1	0.3	0
matzo, dietetic, thin board (Manischewitz)	.8 oz	91	2.6	19.0	<1	.1	0.4	0
matzo, egg	.5 oz	55	1.7	11.1	3	na	0.3	12
matzo, egg, 1 oz	1 matzo	111	3.5	22.3	6	na	0.6	25
matzo, egg, miniature 'Passover' approx 1 oz (Manischewitz)	10 crackers	108	3.0	20.0	10	(mq)	2.0	20
matzo, egg 'Passover' board (Manischewitz)	1.2 oz	132	4.0	27.0	5	(mq)	2.0	25
matzo, egg and onion	.5 oz	55	1.4	10.9	40	.7	0.6	8
matzo, egg and onion, 1 oz	1 matzo	111	2.8	21.9	81	1.4	1.1	15
matzo, egg n' onion, board (Manischewitz)	1 oz	112	3.1	23.0	180	(mq)	1.0	15
matzo, miniature (Manischewitz)	10 crackers	90	2.0	20.0	10	(mq)	<1.0	0
matzo 'Passover' board (Manischewitz)	1.1 oz	129	3.3	27.0	5	(mq)	0.4	0
matzo, plain	.5 oz	56	1.4	11.9	0	.4 ns	0.2	0
matzo, plain, 1 oz	1 matzo	112	2.8	23.7	1	.9	0.4	0
matzo, tea 'Daily' thin board (Manischewitz)	.9 oz	103	3.0	22.0	1	.1	0.3	0
matzo, thin board (Manischewitz)	.9 oz	100	3.0	21.0	0	.1	0.3	na
matzo, whole-wheat	.5 oz	50	1.9	11.2	0	1.6	0.2	0
matzo, whole-wheat, 1 oz	1 matzo	100	3.7	22.4	1	3.3	0.4	0
matzo, whole wheat, w/bran, board (Manischewitz)	1 oz	110	4.0	21.0	1	.6	0.6	0
melba toast, bacon 'Rounds' (Old London)	.5 oz	53	2.1	10.1	126	.9	1.0	0
melba toast, garlic 'Rounds' (Old London)	.5 oz	56	2.1	9.9	132	.6	1.2	0
melba toast, honey bran (Devonsheer)	1 cracker	16	1.0	3.0	25	.2	0.4	0
melba toast, honey bran 'Rounds' (Devonsheer)	.5 oz	52	2.1	10.2	98	.9	0.9	0
melba toast, oat, .5 oz (Harvest Crisps)	6 crackers	60	1.0	10.0	135	(mq)	2.0	0
melba toast, onion 'Rounds' (Devonsheer)	.5 oz	51	1.9	10.7	120	.8	0.6	0
melba toast, onion 'Rounds' (Old London)	.5 oz	52	2.0	10.2	121	.7	0.8	0
melba toast, plain	.5 oz	55	1.7	10.9	118	.9	0.5	0

Food Name	Serv. Size	Total Cal.	Prot. GMS	Carbs GMS	Sod. MGS	Fiber GMS	Fat GMS	Chol. MGS
melba toast, plain *(Devonsheer)*	1 cracker	16	1.0	3.0	30	.2	0.4	0
melba toast, plain 'Rounds' *(Devonsheer)*	.5 oz	53	2.0	11.0	111	.8	0.6	0
melba toast, plain 'Unsalted' *(Devonsheer)* ...	1 cracker	16	1.0	3.0	5	.2	0.4	0
melba toast, plain 'Unsalted Rounds' *(Devonsheer)*	.5 oz	52	1.8	10.9	5	.8	0.6	0
melba toast, plain, w/o salt	.5 oz	55	1.7	10.9	3	.9	0.5	0
melba toast, pumpernickel *(Old London)* ..	.5 oz	54	1.6	11.0	156	.8	0.6	0
melba toast, rye	.5 oz	55	1.6	11.0	127	1.1	0.5	0
melba toast, rye *(Devonsheer)*	1 cracker	16	1.0	3.0	30	.2	0.4	0
melba toast, rye *(Old London)*	.5 oz	52	1.8	10.9	132	.8	0.7	0
melba toast, rye, .5 oz *(Devonsheer)* .	1 cracker	16	1.0	3.0	30	.2	0.4	0
melba toast, rye 'Rounds' *(Devonsheer)* ...	.5 oz	53	1.8	10.7	130	.9	0.6	0
melba toast, rye 'Rounds' *(Old London)*	.5 oz	52	1.7	10.8	132	.9	0.7	0
melba toast, rye 'Unsalted' *(Devonsheer)*	1 cracker	16	1.0	3.0	5	.2	0.4	0
melba toast, sesame *(Devonsheer)* ...	1 cracker	16	1.0	3.0	25	.2	0.5	ე
melba toast, sesame *(Old London)*	.5 oz	55	2.3	8.9	148	.9	1.8	0
melba toast, sesame 'Rounds' *(Devonsheer)*	.5 oz	57	2.3	9.0	131	.9	1.8	0
melba toast, sesame 'Rounds' *(Old London)*	.5 oz	56	2.3	8.9	149	.9	1.8	0
melba toast, sesame 'Unsalted' *(Old London)*	.5 oz	55	2.3	8.9	5	1.0	1.8	0
melba toast, vegetable *(Devonsheer)*	1 cracker	16	1.0	3.0	25	.2	0.4	0
melba toast, wheat	.5 oz	53	1.8	10.8	119	1.0	0.3	0
melba toast, wheat *(Old London)*	.5 oz	51	2.1	10.5	121	.9	0.7	0
melba toast, wheat '6-calorie' *(Estee)*	1 cracker	6	<1.0	1.0	5	(mq)	<1.0	0
melba toast, wheat 'Snax' *(Estee)*	1 oz	100	4.0	22.0	15	(mq)	<1.0	0
melba toast, white *(Old London)*	.5 oz	51	2.0	10.4	111	.8	0.6	0
melba toast, white 'Rounds' *(Old London)*	.5 oz	48	2.0	9.8	111	.8	0.6	0
melba toast, white 'Unsalted' *(Old London)*	.5 oz	51	1.8	10.7	4	.8	0.6	0
melba toast, whole grain *(Old London)*	.5 oz	52	2.1	10.1	116	.8	0.9	0
melba toast, whole grain 'Rounds' *(Old London)*	.5 oz	54	2.1	9.9	102	.9	1.2	0
melba toast, whole grain 'Unsalted' *(Old London)*	.5 oz	53	2.1	10.0	4	.9	1.0	0
melba toast, whole wheat *(Devonsheer)*	1 cracker	16	1.0	3.0	30	.2	0.4	0
melba toast, whole wheat 'Unsalted' *(Devonsheer)*	1 cracker	16	1.0	3.0	5	.2	0.4	0
milk	.5 oz	65	1.1	9.9	84	na	2.2	2
multi-grain *(Premium)*	.5 oz	60	1.0	10.0	140	na	2.0	0

Food Name	Serv. Size	Total Cal.	Prot. GMS	Carbs GMS	Sod. MGS	Fiber GMS	Fat GMS	Chol. MGS
multi-grain 'Wheat Thins' (Nabisco) ...... .5 oz		60	1.0	10.0	135	na	2.0	0
nacho cheese flavor (Delicious) .... .5 oz		89	1.0	8.0	150	na	5.0	0
natural, for weight control (Spicer's) ..... 1 oz		100	4.0	11.0	65	9.0	4.0	0
nutty wheat 'Wheat Thins' approx .5 oz								
(Nabisco) .... 7 crackers		70	1.0	9.0	170	(mq)	4.0	0
oat 'Oat Krisp' (Ralston) .... .5 oz		50	1.0	7.0	140	3.0	2.0	0
oat 'Oat Thins' approx .5 oz								
(Nabisco) .... 8 crackers		70	1.0	10.0	90	(mq)	3.0	0
oat, .5 oz (Harvest Crisps) .... 6 crackers		60	1.0	10.0	135	1.0	2.0	0
oat bran 'Oat Bran Krisps' (Ralston) ..... .5 oz		60	1.0	9.0	140	3.2	3.0	0
'Old Fashioned' (Hickory Farms) .. 10 crackers		90	2.0	16.0	170	(mq)	3.0	na
onion (Delicious) .... .5 oz		70	1.0	10.0	180	na	3.0	0
onion 'Discos' (Delicious) .... .5 oz		76	1.0	7.0	156	na	5.0	0
onion, minced, approx .5 oz								
(American Classic) .... 4 crackers		70	1.0	10.0	120	(mq)	3.0	0
onion, organic, fat-free (Health Valley) ... .5 oz		40	1.0	9.0	80	1.9	0.0	0
onion flavor (Hain) .... 1 oz		130	3.0	17.0	160	(mq)	6.0	na
onion flavor 'No Salt Added' (Hain) ...... 1 oz		130	3.0	17.0	5	(mq)	6.0	na
onion flavor 'Onion Tams'								
(Manischewitz) .... 10 crackers		150	2.0	18.0	157	(mq)	8.0	0
onion flavor 'Toasteds' approx								
.5 oz (Keebler) .... 4 crackers		60	1.0	9.0	140	(mq)	3.0	0
onion garlic wafer (Westbrae) ...... 4.5 crackers		40	1.0	8.0	50	na	0.0	0
oyster .... .5 oz		62	1.3	10.1	185	.4	1.7	0
oyster (OTC) .... 1 cracker		25	1.0	4.0	65	(mq)	1.0	0
oyster (Premium) .... 20 crackers		60	1.0	10.0	210	0	1.0	0
oyster (Sunshine) .... 16 crackers		60	1.0	11.0	190	(mq)	1.0	0
oyster, approx .5 oz (Dandy) ...... 20 crackers		60	1.0	10.0	220	(mq)	2.0	0
oyster, low salt .... .5 oz		62	1.3	10.1	90	.4	1.7	0
oyster 'Oysterettes' approx .5 oz								
(Nabisco) .... 18 crackers		60	1.0	10.0	140	(mq)	1.0	0
oyster, unsalted tops .... .5 oz		62	1.3	10.1	109	.4	1.7	0
peanut butter (Combos) .... 1.8 oz		240	6.0	30.0	360	(mq)	10.0	na
peanut butter, cheese (Little Debbie) ... 1.4 oz		190	6.0	23.0	390	(mq)	9.0	<1
peanut butter, cheese (Little Debbie) ... .93 oz		130	4.0	14.0	260	(mq)	6.0	<1
peanut butter, cheese sandwich								
(Handi-Snacks) .... 1 pkg		190	6.0	11.0	180	(mq)	14.0	0
peanut butter 'Ritz Bits Sandwiches'								
1 oz (Ritz) .... 12 crackers		80	2.0	8.0	80	na	4.0	0
peanut butter, toast, approx .5 oz								
(Keebler) .... 2 crackers		70	2.0	9.0	120	(mq)	3.0	<1
peanut butter 'Toast Sandwich'								
4 pieces (Nabisco) .... 1 oz		130	3.0	15.0	300	na	7.0	0

Food Name	Serv. Size	Total Cal.	Prot. GMS	Carbs GMS	Sod. MGS	Fiber GMS	Fat GMS	Chol. MGS
peanut butter, toasty *(Little Debbie)*	1.4 oz	200	6.0	21.0	380	(mq)	12.0	<1
peanut butter, toasty *(Little Debbie)*	.93 oz	140	4.0	14.0	250	(mq)	7.0	<1
peanut butter bar *(Frito-Lay's)*	1.75 oz	270	2.0	30.0	65	na	16.0	0
peanut butter-filled, 6 crackers								
(Frito-Lay's)	1.5 oz	210	6.0	24.0	450	0	10.0	0
pizza 'Goldfish' *(Pepperidge Farm)*	1 oz	130	4.0	19.0	220	1.0	5.0	5
poppy, toasted, approx .5 oz								
(American Classic)	4 crackers	70	1.0	9.0	140	(mq)	3.0	0
pumpernickel *(Delicious)*	.5 oz	70	1.0	9.0	160	na	3.0	0
pumpernickel 'Snack Sticks'								
(Pepperidge Farm)	8 crackers	140	3.0	20.0	330	1.0	6.0	0
ranch, baked, cracker chips 'Zings'								
(Nabisco)	.5 oz	70	1.0	9.0	140	na	3.0	2
ranch 'Snack Crisps' *(Estee)*	.66 oz	80	2.0	13.0	135	na	2.0	0
'Regency' *(Delicious)*	.5 oz	70	1.0	9.0	100	na	<3.0	0
rice, approx .5 oz *(Harvest Crisps)* ..	6 crackers	60	1.0	11.0	135	1.0	2.0	0
rice, harvest 'Crispbread'								
(Weight Watchers)	2 crackers	30	<1.0	7.0	55	(mq)	0.0	0
rice bran *(Health Valley)*	7 crackers	130	4.0	19.0	64	1.5	4.0	0
'Rich' *(Hain)*	1 oz	130	3.0	18.0	160	(mq)	5.0	na
'Rich, No Salt Added' *(Hain)*	1 oz	130	3.0	18.0	15	(mq)	5.0	na
'Royal Lunch Milk Crackers' .5 oz								
(Nabisco)	1 cracker	60	1.0	10.0	80	1.0	2.0	0
rusk toast	.5 oz	58	1.9	10.2	36	na	1.0	4
rye	.5 oz	52	1.1	11.6	37	2.3	0.2	0
rye *(Hain)*	1 oz	120	3.0	19.0	200	(mq)	4.0	0
rye, BBQ 'Rounds O' Rye' *(Hickory Farms)*	1 oz	153	2.7	13.0	60	(mq)	10.6	na
rye, dark 'Crisp Bread' *(Ryvita)*	1 cracker	26	0.7	6.0	35	1.3	<1.0	0
rye, garlic 'Rounds O' Rye' *(Hickory Farms)*	1 oz	147	2.7	14.5	126	(mq)	8.9	na
rye, golden 'Crispbread' *(Wasa)*	1 cracker	35	1.0	7.0	55	1.4	0.0	0
rye, hearty 'Crispbread' *(Wasa)*	1 cracker	45	2.0	9.0	70	2.6	0.0	0
rye, light 'Crisp Bread' *(Ryvita)*	1 cracker	26	0.7	6.0	20	1.3	<1.0	0
rye, light 'Crispbread Lite' *(Wasa)* ...	1 cracker	25	1.0	5.0	40	1.2	0.0	0
rye, light 'Hi-Fiber' *(Finn Crisp)*	1 cracker	35	1.0	8.0	60	(mq)	1.0	0
rye, natural 'Rounds O' Rye'								
(Hickory Farms)	1 oz	156	3.1	12.2	93	(mq)	10.9	na
rye 'No Salt Added' *(Hain)*	1 oz	120	3.0	19.0	10	(mq)	4.0	0
rye, original 'Hi-Fiber' *(Finn Crisp)* ...	1 cracker	40	1.0	10.0	95	(mq)	0.0	0
rye 'RyKrisp' *(Ralston)*	.5 oz	40	1.0	11.0	75	na	0.0	0
rye 'Rykrisp Twindividuals' 2 triple								
pieces *(Ralston)*	.5 oz	45	1.0	11.0	105	3.0	1.0	0
rye 'Salt Free' *(Hickory Farms)*	8 crackers	90	2.0	18.0	na	(mq)	1.0	0
rye, sandwich-type w/cheese filling	.5 oz	68	1.3	8.6	148	na	3.2	1

Food Name	Serv. Size	Total Cal.	Prot. GMS	Carbs GMS	Sod. MGS	Fiber GMS	Fat GMS	Chol. MGS
rye, seasoned 'Rykrisp' (Ralston)	.5 oz	45	1.0	11.0	105	3.0	1.0	0
rye, sesame 'Rykrisp' 2 triple pieces (Ralston)	.5 oz	50	1.0	10.0	105	3.0	2.0	0
rye, sesame, toasted 'Crisp Bread' (Ryvita)	1 cracker	31	1.1	5.0	10	1.4	<1.0	0
rye, sour cream 'Rounds O'Rye' (Hickory Farms)	1 oz	155	2.7	12.6	130	(mq)	10.7	na
rye 'Toasteds' approx .5 oz (Keebler)	4 crackers	60	1.0	8.0	140	(mq)	3.0	0
rye 'Wafers' (Hickory Farms)	8 crackers	90	2.0	17.0	250	(mq)	2.0	na
rye wafers, plain	.5 oz	47	1.4	11.4	113	na	0.1	0
rye wafers, seasoned	.5 oz	54	1.3	10.5	126	na	1.3	0
salsa 'Crackups' (Nabisco)	.5 oz	70	1.0	9.0	100	na	3.0	0
salt sticks, Vienna bread type, 6.5 inches long	1 stick	106	3.3	20.3	548	>.1 c	1.1	1
saltine, approx .5 oz (Zesta)	5 crackers	60	1.0	10.0	190	(mq)	2.0	0
saltine 'Bits Mini Saltine Crackers' .5 oz (Premium)	16 crackers	70	1.0	9.0	160	0	3.0	0
saltine, crumbs, not packed	1 cup	303	6.3	50.0	770	>.3 c	8.4	0
saltine 'Fat-Free' .5 oz (Premium) ..	4 crackers	50	1.0	12.0	115	0	0.0	0
saltine 'Krispy' (Sunshine)	5 crackers	60	1.0	11.0	210	(mq)	1.0	0
saltine 'Krispy Unsalted Tops' (Sunshine)	5 crackers	60	1.0	11.0	120	(mq)	1.0	0
saltine, low salt	.5 oz	62	1.3	10.1	90	.4	1.7	0
saltine 'Low Salt' approx .5 oz (Premium)	5 crackers	60	1.0	10.0	115	0	2.0	0
saltine 'Low Salt' approx .5 oz (Zesta)	5 crackers	60	1.0	10.0	95	(mq)	2.0	0
saltine, mild cheddar 'Krispy' (Sunshine)	5 crackers	60	2.0	10.0	180	na	2.0	2
saltine, 1 7/8-inch square	10 crackers	123	2.6	20.3	312	>.1 c	3.4	0
saltine, original, .5 oz (Premium) ...	5 crackers	60	1.0	10.0	180	0	2.0	0
saltine, 10 pieces (Rokeach)	1 oz	120	2.0	20.0	na	(mq)	3.0	0
saltine, unsalted tops	.5 oz	62	1.3	10.1	109	.4	1.7	0
saltine 'Unsalted' (Estee)	4 crackers	60	1.0	9.0	0	(mq)	2.0	0
saltine 'Unsalted Tops' approx .5 oz (Premium)	5 crackers	60	1.0	10.0	135	(mq)	2.0	0
saltine 'Unsalted Tops' approx .5 oz (Zesta)	5 crackers	60	1.0	10.0	85	(mq)	2.0	0
saltine, wheat, approx .5 oz (Zesta) ..	5 crackers	60	1.0	10.0	190	(mq)	2.0	0
saltine, wheat 'Whole Wheat Premium Plus' .5 oz (Premium)	4 crackers	60	1.0	10.0	130	1.0	2.0	0
sandwich, peanut-cheese, 6 sandwiches ..	1 pkt	206	6.4	23.6	417	>.2 c	10.0	7
sandwich, peanut-cheese, 4 sandwiches ..	1 pkt	137	4.3	15.7	278	>.1 c	6.7	4

Food Name	Serv. Size	Total Cal.	Prot. GMS	Carbs GMS	Sod. MGS	Fiber GMS	Fat GMS	Chol. MGS
sandwich, w/cheese filling .... .5 oz	.5 oz	68	1.3	8.8	199	na	3.0	0
sandwich, w/peanut butter filling .... .5 oz	.5 oz	69	1.6	8.3	134	na	3.4	0
'Schooners' 33 pieces (FFV) .... .5 oz	.5 oz	60	1.0	10.0	130	(mq)	2.0	0
sesame (Hain) .... 1 oz	1 oz	140	3.0	16.0	210	(mq)	7.0	na
sesame, bread wafer, approx .5 oz (Meal Mates) .... 3 crackers	3 crackers	70	1.0	9.0	160	(mq)	3.0	0
sesame 'Crisp' (FFV) .... 1 cracker	1 cracker	60	1.0	10.0	120	(mq)	2.0	0
sesame 'Crispbread' (Dar-Vida) ..... 1 cracker	1 cracker	22	1.0	4.0	40	(mq)	1.0	0
sesame 'Distinctive' (Pepperidge Farm) .... 4 crackers	4 crackers	80	2.0	12.0	140	2.0	4.0	0
sesame, golden (American Classic) 4 crackers	4 crackers	70	1.0	9.0	120	(mq)	3.0	0
sesame, golden, .5 oz (American Classic) .... 4 crackers	4 crackers	70	1.0	9.0	120	(mq)	3.0	0
sesame, golden 'Flutters' (Pepperidge Farm) .... .75 oz	.75 oz	110	2.0	13.0	150	(mq)	5.0	0
sesame 'No Salt Added' (Hain) .... 1 oz	1 oz	140	3.0	16.0	5	(mq)	7.0	na
sesame 'RyKrisp' (Ralston) .... .5 oz	.5 oz	50	1.0	9.0	105	3.0	2.0	0
sesame, savory 'Crispbread' (Wasa) .. 1 cracker	1 cracker	30	2.0	4.0	40	2.4	1.0	0
sesame 'Snack Sticks' (Pepperidge Farm) .... 8 crackers	8 crackers	140	4.0	19.0	280	1.0	5.0	0
sesame 'Toasteds' approx .5 oz (Keebler) .... 4 crackers	4 crackers	60	1.0	8.0	130	(mq)	3.0	0
sesame, wafer 'Crisp' approx .5 oz (FFV) .... 4 crackers	4 crackers	60	2.0	9.0	140	(mq)	2.0	0
sesame and cheese 'Twigs Snack Sticks' .5 oz (Nabisco) .... 5 crackers	5 crackers	70	1.0	8.0	140	(mq)	4.0	2
sesame chips (Flavor Tree) .... 1/4 cup	1/4 cup	163	3.2	10.6	380	>.1 c	9.2	0
sesame wafer (Westbrae) .... 4.5 crackers	4.5 crackers	40	1.0	8.0	60	na	0.0	0
sesame wheat (Delicious) .... .5 oz	.5 oz	80	1.0	9.0	170	na	4.0	0
sesame wheat 'Crispbread' (Wasa) .. 1 cracker	1 cracker	50	2.0	8.0	65	.6	2.0	0
sesame wheat 'Stoned Wheat' (Health Valley) .... 13 crackers	13 crackers	130	3.0	16.0	150	2.6	6.0	0
sesame wheat 'Stoned Wheat No Salt Added' (Health Valley) .... 13 crackers	13 crackers	130	3.0	17.0	20	2.6	6.0	0
seven grain 'Stoned Wheat' (Health Valley) .... 13 crackers	13 crackers	120	3.0	17.0	125	2.8	5.0	0
seven grain 'Stoned Wheat No Salt Added' (Health Valley) .... 13 crackers	13 crackers	120	3.0	17.0	20	2.8	5.0	0
seven-grain vegetable, organic, fat-free (Health Valley) .... .5 oz	.5 oz	40	1.0	9.0	80	1.9	0.0	0
seven-grain vegetable, organic, no salt added (Health Valley) .... .5 oz	.5 oz	40	1.0	9.0	80	1.9	0.0	0

Food Name	Serv. Size	Total Cal.	Prot. GMS	Carbs GMS	Sod. MGS	Fiber GMS	Fat GMS	Chol. MGS
snack, approx .5 oz *(Finast)* . . . . . . .12 crackers		70	1.0	9.0	135	(mq)	3.0	na
snack, approx .5 oz *(Rokeach)* . . . . . 9 crackers		130	2.0	19.0	(mq)	(mq)	5.0	na
'Snack N' Cracker' *(Delicious)* . . . . .5 oz		70	1.0	10.0	180	na	3.0	0
'Snackers' *(Delicious)* . . . . .5 oz		70	1.0	9.0	90	na	3.0	0
'Sociables' approx .5 oz *(Nabisco)* . . 6 crackers		70	1.0	9.0	135	0	4.0	0
soda *(Sailor Boy Pilot)* . . . . 1 cracker		100	2.0	17.0	125	(mq)	3.0	0
soda 'Distinctive English Water Biscuit'								
(Pepperidge Farm) . . . . 4 crackers		70	2.0	13.0	100	(mq)	1.0	0
soda 'English' *(North Castles)* . . . . . . 1 cracker		10	0.0	3.0	14	(mq)	0.0	0
soda, .5 oz *(Crown Pilot)* . . . . 1 cracker		70	1.0	11.0	70	(mq)	2.0	0
soda, low salt . . . . .5 oz		62	1.3	10.1	90	.4	1.7	0
soda, 'Lunch' 1 cracker *(Royal)* . . . . .5 oz		60	1.0	17.0	125	(mq)	3.0	0
soda 'Ocean Crisps' *(FFV)* . . . . 1 cracker		60	1.0	10.0	120	(mq)	2.0	0
soda, unsalted tops . . . . .5 oz		62	1.3	10.1	109	.4	1.7	0
soup, low salt . . . . .5 oz		62	1.3	10.1	90	.4	1.7	0
soup, unsalted tops . . . . .5 oz		62	1.3	10.1	109	.4	1.7	0
sour cream and chive *(Hain)* . . . . 1 oz		130	3.0	15.0	150	(mq)	6.0	na
sour cream and chive 'No Salt Added'								
(Hain) . . . . 1 oz		130	3.0	15.0	25	(mq)	6.0	na
sour cream and chive flavor *(McCrakens)* . . 1 oz		140	2.0	18.0	170	na	8.0	0
sour cream and onion 'Discos' *(Delicious)* .5 oz		79	1.0	6.0	162	na	5.0	0
sour cream and onion, for weight control								
(Spicer's) . . . . 1 oz		100	4.0	12.0	150	6.0	4.0	0
sour cream and onion 'Mr. Phipp's Tater								
Crisps' *(Nabisco)* . . . . .5 oz		60	1.0	10.0	150	na	2.0	0
sourdough *(Delicious)* . . . . .5 oz		70	1.0	9.0	160	na	3.0	0
sourdough *(Hain)* . . . . .5 oz		65	2.0	9.0	100	(mq)	3.0	0
sourdough 'Low Salt' *(Hain)* . . . . 1 oz		130	3.0	18.0	10	(mq)	5.0	0
sticks 'Snack Sticks'								
(Pepperidge Farm) . . . . 8 crackers		130	4.0	19.0	400	1.0	5.0	0
'Tam Tams' *(Manischewitz)* . . . . .10 crackers		147	2.0	17.0	171	(mq)	8.0	0
'Tam Tams No Salt' *(Manischewitz)* 10 crackers		138	2.0	18.0	10	(mq)	7.0	0
tamari wafer *(Westbrae)* . . . . 4.5 crackers		40	1.0	8.0	60	na	0.0	0
'Uneeda Biscuits Unsalted Tops'								
approx .5 oz *(Nabisco)* . . . . .2 crackers		60	1.0	10.0	100	na	2.0	0
vegetable *(Hain)* . . . . 1 oz		130	3.0	10.0	180	(mq)	5.0	0
vegetable, garden *(Delicious)* . . . . .5 oz		70	1.0	10.0	220	na	3.0	0
vegetable 'Garden Crisps' *(Nabisco)* . . . . .5 oz		60	1.0	11.0	135	na	2.0	0
vegetable 'No Salt Added' *(Hain)* . . . . 1 oz		130	3.0	10.0	50	(mq)	5.0	0
'Vegetable Thins' *(Nabisco)* . . . . 7 crackers		70	1.0	8.0	140	(mq)	4.0	0
wafer, no salt *(Westbrae)* . . . . 4.5 wafers		40	1.0	8.0	0	na	0.0	0
water *(Sailor Boy Pilot)* . . . . 1 cracker		100	2.0	17.0	125	(mq)	3.0	0

Food Name	Serv. Size	Total Cal.	Prot. GMS	Carbs GMS	Sod. MGS	Fiber GMS	Fat GMS	Chol. MGS
water 'Distinctive English Water Biscuit'								
(Pepperidge Farm) .... 4 crackers		70	2.0	13.0	100	(mq)	1.0	0
water 'English' (North Castles) ...... 1 cracker		10	0.0	3.0	14	(mq)	0.0	0
water, .5 oz (Crown Pilot) .... 1 cracker		70	1.0	11.0	70	(mq)	2.0	0
water 'Gourmet' fat-free (Frookie) ... 4 crackers		35	1.0	7.0	60	na	0.0	0
water, 'Lunch' 1 cracker (Royal) .... .5 oz		60	1.0	17.0	125	(mq)	3.0	0
water 'Ocean Crisps' (FFV) .... 1 cracker		60	1.0	10.0	120	(mq)	2.0	0
water 'Table Water, Bite Size' (Carr's) 2 crackers		25	1.0	5.0	15	(mq)	1.0	na
'Waverly Crackers' approx .5 oz								
(Nabisco) .... 4 crackers		70	1.0	10.0	160	na	3.0	0
'Waverly Crackers Low Salt' approx								
.5 oz (Nabisco) .... 4 crackers		70	1.0	10.0	80	(mq)	3.0	0
'Waverly Wafer' approx .5 oz								
(Nabisco) .... 4 crackers		70	1.0	10.0	160	(mq)	3.0	0
wheat (Delicious) .... .5 oz		70	1.0	9.0	85	na	3.0	0
wheat, approx .5 oz (Sociables) .... 6 crackers		70	1.0	9.0	135	(mq)	3.0	0
wheat 'Bits' approx .5 oz (Triscuit) .. 8 crackers		60	1.0	10.0	75	(mq)	2.0	0
wheat 'Crispy Wafer' approx .5 oz								
(FFV) .... 6 crackers		70	1.0	9.0	80	(mq)	3.0	na
wheat, low salt .... .5 oz		67	1.2	9.2	40	.8	2.9	0
wheat 'Low Salt' approx .5 oz								
(Triscuit) .... 3 crackers		60	1.0	10.0	35	(mq)	2.0	0
'Wheat On' (Delicious) .... .5 oz		68	1.0	8.0	86	na	3.0	0
wheat 'Original Snackbread' (Ryvita) .. 1 cracker		20	0.5	4.0	20	.2	<1.0	0
wheat 'Original Wheat Thins' approx								
.5 oz (Nabisco) .... 8 crackers		70	1.0	9.0	120	<1.0	3.0	0
wheat, regular .... .5 oz		67	1.2	9.2	113	.8	2.9	0
wheat, sandwich, w/cheese filling .... .5 oz		70	1.4	8.3	129	na	3.5	1
wheat, sandwich, w/peanut butter filling .. .5 oz		70	1.9	7.6	114	na	3.8	0
wheat 'Snack Wells' (Nabisco) .... .5 oz		50	1.0	11.0	160	na	0.0	0
wheat 'Snacks' approx .5 oz (Finast) 7 crackers		70	1.0	9.0	85	(mq)	3.0	na
wheat 'Stone Ground' approx .5 oz								
(Wheatsworth) .... 4 crackers		70	1.0	9.0	135	(mq)	3.0	0
wheat 'Stoned Wheat' (Health Valley) 13 crackers		120	3.0	17.0	85	3.9	6.0	0
wheat 'Stoned Wheat No Salt Added'								
(Health Valley) .... 13 crackers		120	3.0	17.0	10	3.9	6.0	0
wheat 'Stoned Wheat Wafer' approx								
.5 oz (FFV) .... 4 crackers		60	1.0	10.0	170	(mq)	2.0	0
wheat 'Stoned Wheat Wafers Salt Free'								
(Hickory Farms) .... 8 crackers		100	2.0	18.0	0	(mq)	2.0	na
wheat toasted (McCrakens) .... 1 oz		140	2.0	18.0	170	na	8.0	0
wheat, toasted 'Distinctive'								
(Pepperidge Farm) .... 4 crackers		80	2.0	12.0	140	(mq)	3.0	0

Food Name	Serv. Size	Total Cal.	Prot. GMS	Carbs GMS	Sod. MGS	Fiber GMS	Fat GMS	Chol. MGS
wheat, toasted 'Flutters' (Pepperidge Farm) .75 oz		110	2.0	13.0	170	(mq)	5.0	0
wheat 'Wheat Krisp' (Ralston) .5 oz		50	2.0	11.0	220	na	1.0	0
wheat 'Wheat Mill Wafers Salt Free' (Hickory Farms)	4 crackers	50	1.0	9.0	na	(mq)	1.0	0
wheat 'Wheat Tams' (Manischewitz)	10 crackers	150	2.0	18.0	180	(mq)	8.0	0
wheat 'Wheat Thins' (Nabisco)	8 crackers	70	1.0	9.0	120	(mq)	3.0	0
wheat 'Wheat Thins Low Salt' approx .5 oz (Nabisco)	8 crackers	70	1.0	9.0	60	(mq)	3.0	0
wheat 'Wheats' (Sunshine)	8 crackers	70	1.0	9.0	170	(mq)	4.0	0
wheat 'Whole Wheat'N Bran Wafers' (Triscuit)	3 crackers	60	1.0	10.0	75	na	2.0	0
'Wheatine' bits (Barbara's Bakery) .5 oz		60	2.0	9.0	132	na	2.0	0
'Wheatines' cracked pepper (Barbara's Bakery) .5 oz		60	2.0	9.0	132	na	2.0	0
'Wheatines' lightly salted tops (Barbara's Bakery) .5 oz		60	2.0	9.0	132	na	2.0	0
'Wheatines' sesame (Barbara's Bakery) .5 oz		60	2.0	9.0	132	na	2.0	0
'Wheatines' unsalted tops (Barbara's Bakery) .5 oz		60	2.0	9.0	45	na	2.0	0
wheatstone (Delicious) .5 oz		70	2.0	9.0	180	na	3.0	0
whole grain 'Crispbread' approx .35 oz (Wasa)	1 slice	30	2.0	4.0	40	2.4	1.0	0
whole grain 'Harvest Wheats' approx .5 oz (Keebler)	4 crackers	60	1.0	8.0	95	(mq)	3.0	0
whole wheat .5 oz		63	1.3	9.7	93	1.5	2.4	0
whole wheat (Carr's)	2 crackers	70	1.0	12.0	15	(mq)	1.0	(mq)
whole wheat (Manischewitz)	10 crackers	90	3.0	18.0	10	(mq)	1.0	0
whole wheat, approx .5 oz (Ritz)	5 crackers	70	1.0	9.0	135	0	3.0	0
whole wheat 'Gourmet' fat-free (Frookie)	4 crackers	35	1.0	7.0	60	na	0.0	0
whole wheat, low salt .5 oz		63	1.3	9.7	35	1.5	2.4	0
whole wheat, organic, fat-free (Health Valley) .5 oz		40	1.0	9.0	80	1.9	0.0	0
whole wheat 'Wheatables' approx .5 oz (Keebler)	12 crackers	70	1.0	9.0	140	(mq)	3.0	0
w/bacon and cheese (Handi-Snacks)	1 pkg	130	4.0	8.0	410	(mq)	9.0	20
zesty Italian, approx 13-16 crackers (Frito-Lay's) .5 oz		70	1.0	9.0	115	0	3.0	0
zwieback	1 oz	121	2.9	21.0	66	.7	2.8	6
'Zwieback Teething Toast' approx .5 oz (Nabisco)	2 crackers	60	2.0	10.0	20	na	1.0	na

Food Name	Serv. Size	Total Cal.	Prot. GMS	Carbs GMS	Sod. MGS	Fiber GMS	Fat GMS	Chol. MGS
CRACKER CRUMBS AND MEAL								
meal	1 cup	440	10.7	93.0	32	na	2.0	0
meal	1 oz	109	2.6	22.9	8	na	0.5	0
(Golden Dipt) meal	1 oz	100	3.0	22.0	0	(mq)	0.0	0
(Manischewitz) matzo 'Farfel'	1 cup	280	6.8	60.0	2	.2	0.8	0
(Manischewitz) matzo meal 'Daily'	1 cup	514	13.0	109.0	3	.5	1.4	0
(Nabisco) meal	1/4 cup	110	3.0	24.0	10	1.0	0.0	0
(Premium) fat-free	2 tbsp	50	1.0	11.0	0	na	0.0	0
CRANBERRY								
raw (Ocean Spray) approx 2 oz	1/2 cup	25	0.0	6.0	0	(mq)	0.0	0
raw, chopped	1 cup	54	0.4	14.0	1	4.6	0.2	0
raw, whole	1 cup	47	0.4	12.0	1	4.0	0.2	0
trimmed	1 oz	14	0.1	3.6	<1	1.2	0.1	0
trimmed, chopped	1/2 cup	27	0.2	7.0	1	2.3	0.1	0
trimmed, whole	1/2 cup	23	0.2	6.0	1	2.0	0.1	0
w/stems	1 lb	210	1.7	54.6	5	18.0	0.9	0
CRANBERRY APPLE COCKTAIL								
(Minute Maid) 'Juices To Go'	6 oz	120	0.0	30.0	20	na	0.0	na
(Welch's) frozen, diluted	6 oz	120	0.0	30.0	0	0	0.0	0
CRANBERRY APPLE DRINK								
	6 oz	123	0.2	31.5	4	0	0.0	0
(A&P)	6 oz	130	<1.0	32.0	<1	(tr)	(tr)	0
(Ocean Spray) 'Cran•Apple'	6 oz	120	0.0	31.0	15	(tr)	0.0	0
(Ocean Spray) 'Cran•Apple Low Calorie'	6 oz	35	0.0	9.0	15	(tr)	0.0	0
(P&Q)	6 oz	130	<1.0	32.0	<1	(tr)	(tr)	0
(Pathmark)	6 oz	130	0.0	32.0	10	(tr)	0.0	0
CRANBERRY APPLESAUCE, 'Cran•Fruit'								
(Ocean Spray)	2 oz	100	0.0	23.0	10	(mq)	0.0	0
CRANBERRY APRICOT DRINK								
	6 oz	118	0.4	29.8	4	.2	0.0	0
'Cranicot' (Ocean Spray)	6 oz	120	0.0	29.0	15	(tr)	0.0	0
CRANBERRY BEAN/borlotti/Roman bean/rose coco								
boiled	1 cup	241	16.5	43.3	2	>1.8 c	0.8	0
boiled	1/2 cup	120	8.2	21.5	1	3.0	0.4	0
boiled	4 oz	154	10.6	27.7	1	3.9	0.5	0
raw	1 cup	653	44.9	117.1	12	>4.9 c	2.4	0
raw	1/2 cup	328	22.6	58.9	6	9.1	1.2	0
raw	1 oz	95	6.5	17.0	2	2.6	0.3	0
CRANBERRY BEAN, CANNED								
	1 cup	216	14.4	39.3	863	>2.4 c	0.7	0
(Progresso)	1/2 cup	110	7.0	18.0	420	12.0	<1.0	0
w/liquid	1/2 cup	108	7.2	19.7	431	>1.2 c	0.4	0
w/liquid	4 oz	94	6.3	17.1	376	>1.0 c	0.3	0

Food Name	Serv. Size	Total Cal.	Prot. GMS	Carbs GMS	Sod. MGS	Fiber GMS	Fat GMS	Chol. MGS
CRANBERRY BLUEBERRY JUICE								
(Knudsen & Sons)	8 oz	115	<1.0	36.0	na	na	0.0	na
CRANBERRY COCKTAIL JUICE								
(J. Hungerford)	9.03 oz	141	0.8	35.5	0	0	0.0	0
(J. Hungerford) 50% juice	9.03 oz	134	0.1	34.8	7	0	0.1	0
(J. Hungerford) 100% juice	9.03 oz	133	0.0	33.0	19	0	0.0	0
CRANBERRY DRINK								
(Ocean Spray) citrus 'Refreshers'	6 oz	100	0.0	26.0	15	na	0.0	0
(Ocean Spray) 'Cran•Blueberry'	6 oz	120	0.0	31.0	10	(tr)	0.0	0
(Ocean Spray) 'Cran•Raspberry'	6 oz	110	0.0	27.0	15	(tr)	0.0	0
(Ocean Spray) 'Cran•Raspberry Low Calorie'	6 oz	40	0.0	9.0	15	(tr)	0.0	0
(Ocean Spray) 'Cran•Strawberry'	6 oz	110	0.0	27.0	15	na	0.0	na
(Tropicana) 'Cranberry Orchard Juice Sparkler'	8 oz	120	(tr)	30.0	20	(tr)	0.0	0
CRANBERRY GRAPE COCKTAIL								
frozen, prepared (Welch's)	6 oz	110	0.0	27.0	0	0	0.0	0
CRANBERRY GRAPE DRINK								
(Finast)	6 oz	103	0.0	26.0	5	(tr)	0.0	0
(Ocean Spray) 'Cran•Grape'	6 oz	120	0.0	31.0	15	(tr)	0.0	0
(Pathmark)	6 oz	103	0.0	26.0	5	(tr)	0.0	0
CRANBERRY JUICE								
(Knudsen & Sons) 'Just Cranberry'	8 oz	40	<1.0	10.0	na	na	0.0	na
(Knudsen & Sons) 'Yankee'	8 oz	125	<1.0	31.0	na	na	0.0	na
(Lucky Leaf)	6 oz	110	0.0	26.0	10	(tr)	0.0	0
(Ocean Spray) 'Cran•tastic'	6 oz	100	0.0	26.0	15	(tr)	0.0	0
(Santa Cruz Natural) organic 'Sparkling'	8 oz	90	<1.0	22.0	na	na	<1.0	0
(Snapple) 'Cranberry Royale'	8 oz	150	0.0	37.0	25	na	0.0	0
CRANBERRY JUICE COCKTAIL								
	1 cup	144	0.0	36.4	5	0	0.3	0
	6 oz	108	0.0	27.4	4	0	0.2	0
(A&P)	6 oz	100	<1.0	26.0	0	(tr)	<1.0	0
(Ocean Spray)	6 oz	110	0.0	26.0	10	(tr)	0.0	0
(Ocean Spray) 'Low Calorie'	6 oz	40	0.0	9.0	15	(tr)	0.0	0
(P&Q)	6 oz	100	<1.0	24.0	0	(tr)	<1.0	0
(Pathmark)	6 oz	100	0.0	26.0	10	(tr)	0.0	0
(Pathmark) 'No Frills'	6 oz	100	0.0	26.0	10	(tr)	0.0	0
(Sunkist)	6 oz	110	0.1	28.2	8	(tr)	0.1	0
(Sunkist) frozen, prepared	6 oz	110	0.1	28.2	0	(tr)	0.1	0
(Veryfine)	8 oz	160	<1.0	40.0	10	(tr)	0.0	0
(Welch's) frozen 'No Sugar Added' prepared	6 oz	40	0.0	10.0	5	0	0.0	0
(Welch's) frozen, prepared	6 oz	100	0.0	26.0	0	0	0.0	0

Food Name	Serv. Size	Total Cal.	Prot. GMS	Carbs GMS	Sod. MGS	Fiber GMS	Fat GMS	Chol. MGS
(Welch's) frozen, w/blueberry, prepared ...	6 oz	110	0.0	27.0	0	0	0.0	0
(Welch's) frozen, w/raspberry, prepared ...	6 oz	110	0.0	28.0	0	0	0.0	0
CRANBERRY JUICE DRINK								
citrus 'Refreshers' *(Ocean Spray)*	6 oz	100	0.0	26.0	15	na	0.0	na
CRANBERRY LEMONADE								∢
(Knudsen & Sons)	8 oz	115	<1.0	29.0	na	na	0.0	na
(Santa Cruz Natural) organic	8 oz	100	<1.0	24.0	na	na	<1.0	na
CRANBERRY NECTAR								
(Knudsen & Sons)	8 oz	110	<1.0	28.0	na	na	0.0	na
(Santa Cruz Natural) organic	8 oz	110	<1.0	28.0	na	na	<1.0	na
CRANBERRY RASPBERRY DRINK								
(Tropicana) w/strawberry 'Twister'	6 oz	110	<1.0	27.0	4	na	<1.0	na
(Tropicana) w/strawberry 'Twister Light' w/NutraSweet	6 oz	30	<1.0	7.0	15	na	<1.0	na
CRANBERRY RASPBERRY JUICE								
(Knudsen & Sons)	8 oz	100	<1.0	25.0	na	na	0.0	na
CRANBERRY RASPBERRY SAUCE								
'Cran•Fruit' *(Ocean Spray)*	2 oz	100	0.0	23.0	10	(mq)	0.0	0
CRANBERRY SAUCE								
canned *(A&P)*	2 oz	100	<1.0	25.0	15	(mq)	<1.0	0
canned *(Knudsen & Sons)*	1 oz	30	<1.0	8.0	na	na	<1.0	na
canned, sweetened	1 cup	418	0.6	107.7	80	>.8 c	0.4	0
canned, sweetened	4 oz	171	0.2	44.1	33	>.3 c	0.2	0
jellied *(Finast)*	2 oz	90	0.0	22.0	10	(mq)	0.0	0
jellied *(Ocean Spray)*	2 oz	80	0.0	22.0	10	(mq)	0.0	0
jellied *(Pathmark)*	2 oz	90	0.0	22.0	10	(mq)	0.0	0
jellied 'Old Fashioned' *(S&W)*	1/2 cup	90	0.0	22.0	20	(mq)	0.0	0
whole berry *(Finast)*	2 oz	90	0.0	22.0	10	(mq)	0.0	0
whole berry *(Ocean Spray)*	2 oz	80	0.0	21.0	10	(mq)	0.0	0
whole berry 'Old Fashioned' *(S&W)*	1/2 cup	90	0.0	22.0	20	(mq)	0.0	0
CRANBERRY STRAWBERRY SAUCE								
crushed, for chicken 'Cran•Fruit' *(Ocean Spray)*	2 oz	90	0.0	22.0	10	na	0.0	na
CRAPPIE. See SUNFISH.								
CRAWFISH ENTRÉE, frozen, étouffée *(Cajun Cookin')*	12 oz	390	23.0	51.0	1110	na	10.0	(mq)
CRAYFISH, MIXED SPECIES								
farmed, moist-heat cooked	100 gm	87	17.5	0.0	97	0	1.3	137
farmed, moist-heat cooked	3 oz	74	14.9	0.0	82	0	1.1	116
farmed, raw	3 oz	61	12.6	0.0	53	0	0.8	91
farmed, raw	8 crayfish	19	4.0	0.0	17	0	0.3	29
wild, moist-heat cooked	100 gm	88	16.8	0.0	94	0	1.2	133
wild, moist-heat cooked	3 oz	75	14.2	0.0	80	0	1.0	113

Food Name	Serv. Size	Total Cal.	Prot. GMS	Carbs GMS	Sod. MGS	Fiber GMS	Fat GMS	Chol. MGS
wild, raw	3 oz	65	13.6	0.0	49	0	0.8	97
wild, raw	8 crayfish	21	4.3	0.0	16	0	0.3	31
CREAM								
half and half	1 cup	315	7.2	10.4	98	0	27.8	89
half and half	1 oz	37	0.8	1.2	12	0	3.3	10
half and half	1 tbsp	20	0.4	0.7	6	0	1.7	6
half and half *(Crowley)*	1 oz	35	1.0	1.0	10	0	3.0	15
half and half *(Darigold)*	8 oz	310	8.0	11.0	120	0	27.0	89
half and half *(Knudsen)*	4 oz	150	4.0	5.0	60	0	13.0	(mq)
half and half *(Rockview)*	2 tbsp	35	1.0	0.0	15	0	3.0	15
heavy, whipping	1 cup	821	4.9	6.6	89	0	88.1	326
heavy, whipping	1 tbsp	52	0.3	0.4	6	0	5.6	21
light, whipping	1 cup	699	5.2	7.1	82	0	73.9	265
light, whipping	1 tbsp	44	0.3	0.4	5	0	4.6	17
light, coffee or table	1 cup	469	6.5	8.8	95	0	46.3	159
light, coffee or table	1 oz	55	0.8	1.0	11	0	5.5	19
light, coffee or table	1 tbsp	29	0.4	0.6	6	0	2.9	10
medium, 25% fat	1 cup	583	5.9	8.3	88	0	59.7	209
medium, 25% fat	1 oz	69	0.7	1.0	10	0	7.1	25
medium, 25% fat	1 tbsp	37	0.4	0.5	6	0	3.8	13
CREAM CHEESE. See CHEESE.								
CREAM NUT. See BRAZIL NUT.								
CREAM OF TARTAR	1 tsp	8	0.0	1.8	2	na	0.0	0
CREAM SODA. See SOFT DRINKS AND MIXERS.								
CREAM TOPPING								
creamy white 'Dolci Frutta Crema Bianca' *(Saco Foods)*	1 box	900	6.7	98.4	110	na	50.1	0
dark chocolate 'Dolci Frutta Con Cioccolatta' *(Saco Foods)*	1 box	886	8.6	110.5	107	na	52.8	0
frozen, whipped *(La Creme)*	1 tbsp	16	0.0	1.0	5	0	1.0	<1
frozen, whipped 'Real Cream' *(Kraft)*	1/4 cup	30	0.0	2.0	5	0	2.0	10
pressurized can, whipped	1 cup	154	1.9	7.5	78	0	13.3	46
pressurized can, whipped	1 oz	73	0.9	3.5	37	0	6.3	22
pressurized can, whipped	1 tbsp	8	0.1	0.4	4	0	0.7	2
pressurized can, whipped *(Crowley)*	1 tbsp	20	<1.0	<1.0	10	0	1.0	5
whipping, heavy	1 oz	98	0.6	0.8	11	0	10.5	39
whipping, heavy *(Crowley)*	1 oz	110	1.0	1.0	10	0	11.0	40
whipping, heavy *(Darigold)*	1 cup	790	6.0	8.0	90	0	81.0	290
whipping, heavy 'Classic' *(Darigold)*	1 cup	858	5.1	6.9	77	0	90.0	334
whipping, heavy 'UHT' *(Darigold)*	1 cup	790	6.0	8.0	90	0	81.0	290
whipping, heavy, whipped	2 cups	821	4.9	6.6	89	0	90.0	326
whipping, heavy, whipped	2 tbsp	52	0.3	0.4	6	0	5.6	21
whipping, light	1 oz	83	0.6	0.8	10	0	8.8	31

Food Name	Serv. Size	Total Cal.	Prot. GMS	Carbs GMS	Sod. MGS	Fiber GMS	Fat GMS	Chol. MGS
whipping, light, whipped	2 cups	699	5.2	7.1	82	0	5.6	265
whipping, light, whipped	2 tbsp	44	0.3	0.4	5	0	8.8	17
CREAM TOPPING, NONDAIRY								
frozen	1 cup	239	0.9	17.3	19	0	19.0	0
frozen	1 oz	90	0.4	6.5	7	0	7.2	0
frozen	1 tbsp	13	0.1	0.9	1	0	1.0	0
frozen, chocolate 'Cool Whip' (Birds Eye)	1 tbsp	12	0.0	1.0	0	na	1.0	na
frozen 'Cool Whip' (Birds Eye)	1 tbsp	12	0.0	1.0	0	0	1.0	0
frozen 'Cool Whip Lite' (Birds Eye)	1 tbsp	8	0.0	1.0	0	0	<1.0	0
frozen, extra creamy 'Cool Whip Dairy Recipe' (Birds Eye)	1 tbsp	14	0.0	1.0	0	0	1.0	0
frozen, semisolid	1 cup	239	0.9	17.3	19	0	19.0	0
frozen, semisolid	1 tbsp	13	0.1	0.9	1	0	1.0	0
frozen 'Whip' (Pet)	1 tbsp	14	0.0	1.0	0	0	1.0	0
frozen 'Whipped Topping' (Kraft)	1/4 cup	35	0.0	2.0	10	0	3.0	0
mix, dry	1.5 oz	245	2.1	22.3	52	0	17.0	0
mix, prepared (D-Zerta)	1 tbsp	8	0.0	0.0	5	0	1.0	0
mix, prepared (Featherweight)	1 tbsp	4	0.0	0.0	5	na	0.0	0
mix, prepared (Dream Whip)	1 tbsp	10	0.0	1.0	0	na	0.0	0
pressurized can	1 cup	184	0.7	11.3	43	0	15.6	0
pressurized can	1 oz	75	0.3	4.6	18	0	6.3	0
pressurized can	1 tbsp	11	<.1	0.6	2	0	0.9	0
pressurized can 'Richwhip' (Rich's)	.25 oz	20	1.0	1.0	5	0	2.0	0
prewhipped (Estee)	1 tbsp	4	<1.0	<1.0	0	0	<1.0	0
prewhipped 'Richwhip' (Rich's)	1 tbsp	12	0.0	1.0	0	0	1.0	0
reduced calorie (D-Zerta)	1 tbsp	8	0.0	0.0	5	na	1.0	0
unwhipped 'Richwhip' (Rich's)	.25 oz	20	0.0	1.0	10	0	2.0	0
CREAMER, NONDAIRY								
Liquid								
frozen	1/2 cup	164	1.2	13.7	95	0	12.0	0
frozen	1 oz	39	0.3	3.2	22	0	2.8	0
frozen	1 tbsp	20	0.2	1.7	12	0	1.5	0
w/hydrogenated vegetable oil and soy protein	1/2 cup	163	1.2	13.7	95	0	12.0	0
w/hydrogenated vegetable oil and soy protein	1/2 oz	20	0.2	1.7	12	0	1.5	0
w/lauric acid oil and sodium caseinate	1/2 cup	164	1.2	13.7	95	0	12.0	0
w/lauric acid oil and sodium caseinate	1/2 oz	20	0.2	1.7	12	0	1.5	0
(Coffee-Mate)	1 tbsp	16	0.0	2.0	5	0	1.0	0
(Coffee-Mate) 'Amaretto'	1 tbsp	40	0.0	5.0	5	na	2.0	na
(Coffee-Mate) 'Cinnamon Creme'	1 tbsp	40	0.0	5.0	5	na	2.0	na
(Coffee-Mate) fat-free	1 tbsp	10	0.0	2.0	0	0	0.0	0
(Coffee-Mate) 'Hazelnut'	1 tbsp	40	0.0	5.0	5	na	2.0	na

Food Name	Serv. Size	Total Cal.	Prot. GMS	Carbs GMS	Sod. MGS	Fiber GMS	Fat GMS	Chol. MGS
(Coffee-Mate) 'Irish Creme'	1 tbsp	40	0.0	5.0	5	na	2.0	na
(Crowley)	.5 oz	16	<1.0	1.0	5	0	1.0	5
(Diehl)	1 tsp	10	0.0	1.0	0	0	<1.0	0
(Finast) frozen	.5 oz	20	0.0	2.0	10	0	2.0	0
(IGA)	1 tsp	10	0.0	2.0	5	0	<1.0	0
(N-Rich)	1 tsp	10	0.1	2.0	2	0	0.6	0
(Pathmark) 'No Frills'	1 tsp	10	0.0	1.0	5	0	0.0	0
(Rich's) frozen 'Coffee Rich'	.5 oz	20	0.0	2.0	10	0	2.0	0
(Rich's) frozen 'Farm Rich'	.5 oz	20	0.0	1.0	5	0	2.0	0
(Rich's) frozen 'Poly Rich'	.5 oz	20	0.0	2.0	5	0	1.0	0
(Saco Foods) 'kwik kream'	1 tbsp	10	0.0	2.0	0	na	<1.0	0
(Westbrae)	1 tbsp	10	<1.0	2.0	10	na	<1.0	0
Powder								
	1/2 cup	257	2.3	16.7	85	0	25.8	0
	1 oz	155	1.4	15.6	51	0	10.1	0
	1 tsp	11	0.1	1.1	4	0	0.7	0
(Coffee-Mate)	1 tsp	10	<1.0	1.0	5	0	<1.0	0
(Coffee-Mate) 'Amaretto'	2 tsp	60	0.0	9.0	15	na	3.0	0
(Coffee-Mate) 'Hazelnut'	2 tsp	60	0.0	0.0	15	na	3.0	0
(Coffee-Mate) 'Irish Creme'	2 tsp	60	0.0	9.0	15	na	3.0	0
(Coffee-Mate) 'Lite'	1 tsp	8	<1.0	2.0	0	0	<1.0	0
(Cremora)	1 tsp	10	0.0	1.0	5	0	<1.0	0
CREME DE MENTHE. See ALCOHOLIC BEVERAGES.								
CR/PE MIX, 7-inch crêpes (Krusteaz)	2 crêpes	80	2.0	14.0	110	na	1.0	0
CRESS, GARDEN								
boiled, drained	4 oz	26	2.2	4.3	9	>1.0 c	0.7	0
boiled, drained	1/2 cup	16	1.3	2.6	5	.5	0.4	0
raw	1/2 cup	8	0.7	1.4	4	.3	0.2	0
raw, trimmed	1 oz	9	0.7	1.6	4	>.3 c	0.2	0
raw, untrimmed	1 lb	103	8.4	17.7	45	>3.5 c	2.3	0
CROAKER, ATLANTIC								
raw	1 lb	474	80.7	0.0	252	0	14.4	277
raw	3 oz	88	15.1	0.0	48	0	2.7	52
raw	1 oz	29	5.0	0.0	16	0	0.9	17
raw, approx 2.8 oz	1 fillet	82	14.1	0.0	44	0	2.5	48
CROISSANT								
almond, 3.7 oz (Dunkin' Donuts)	1 croissant	420	8.0	38.0	280	3.0	27.0	0
butter (Awrey's)	3 oz	300	5.0	32.0	280	1.0	17.0	45
butter (Awrey's)	2 oz	200	3.0	21.0	190	1.0	11.0	30
butter (Awrey's)	1 oz	100	2.0	10.0	90	0	6.0	15
frozen, butter, 1.5 oz (Sara Lee)	1 croissant	170	4.0	19.0	250	(mq)	9.0	(mq)
frozen, butter, petite (Pepperidge Farm)	1 croissant	140	3.0	13.0	160	(mq)	7.0	(mq)

Food Name	Serv. Size	Total Cal.	Prot. GMS	Carbs GMS	Sod. MGS	Fiber GMS	Fat GMS	Chol. MGS
frozen, butter, petite 1 oz *(Sara Lee)*	1 croissant	120	3.0	13.0	160	(mq)	6.0	(mq)
margarine *(Awrey's)*	2.5 oz	250	4.0	26.0	360	1.0	14.0	5
margarine *(Awrey's)*	1.25 oz	120	2.0	13.0	180	0	7.0	5
plain, 2.5 oz *(Dunkin' Donuts)*	1 croissant	310	7.0	27.0	240	2.0	19.0	0
'Sandwich Quartet' *(Pepperidge Farm)*	1 croissant	170	4.0	22.0	250	tr	7.0	0
wheat *(Awrey's)*	2.5 oz	240	4.0	24.0	390	1.0	14.0	5

CROOKNECK SQUASH. See SQUASH, CROOKNECK.

CROUTONS

Food Name	Serv. Size	Total Cal.	Prot. GMS	Carbs GMS	Sod. MGS	Fiber GMS	Fat GMS	Chol. MGS
Caesar salad *(Brownberry)*	.5 oz	62	1.8	8.0	165	.5	2.6	<1
Caesar salad *(Reese)*	.5 oz	60	2.0	9.0	130	na	2.0	na
cheddar and Romano cheese *(Pepperidge Farm)*	.5 oz	60	2.0	10.0	200	(mq)	2.0	0
cheddar cheese *(Brownberry)*	.5 oz	63	1.8	8.3	155	.3	2.8	3
cheese and garlic *(Pepperidge Farm)*	.5 oz	70	2.0	9.0	180	(mq)	3.0	0
onion and garlic *(Brownberry)*	.5 oz	60	1.6	8.0	190	.4	2.2	1
onion and garlic *(Pepperidge Farm)*	.5 oz	70	2.0	9.0	160	(mq)	3.0	0
plain	1 cup	122	3.6	22.0	209	1.5	2.0	0
plain	.5 oz	58	1.7	10.4	99	.7	0.9	0
seasoned	1 cup	186	4.3	25.4	495	2.0	7.3	1
seasoned	.5 oz	66	1.5	9.0	175	.7	2.6	0
seasoned *(Brownberry)*	.5 oz	59	1.6	8.5	155	.5	2.2	<1
seasoned *(Pepperidge Farm)*	.5 oz	70	2.0	9.0	180	(mq)	3.0	0
seasoned *(Weight Watchers)*	1 pouch	30	1.0	5.0	120	(mq)	0.0	na
sour cream and chive *(Pepperidge Farm)*	.5 oz	70	2.0	9.0	170	(mq)	3.0	0
toasted *(Brownberry)*	.5 oz	56	1.7	9.7	145	.4	1.4	0

CRUMPET

Food Name	Serv. Size	Total Cal.	Prot. GMS	Carbs GMS	Sod. MGS	Fiber GMS	Fat GMS	Chol. MGS
blueberry, low-fat, cholestrol-free *(Wolferman's)*	1 crumpet	90	3.0	21.0	250	1.0	<1.0	0
brown sugar cinnamon, low-fat *(Wolferman's)*	1 crumpet	110	3.0	21.0	220	2.0	2.0	0
raspberry, low-fat, cholestrol-free *(Wolferman's)*	1 crumpet	90	3.0	20.0	260	1.0	1.0	0

CUCUMBER

Food Name	Serv. Size	Total Cal.	Prot. GMS	Carbs GMS	Sod. MGS	Fiber GMS	Fat GMS	Chol. MGS
raw, approx 10.9 oz	1 med	39	2.1	8.3	6	2.4	0.4	0
raw, slices	1/2 cup	7	0.4	1.4	1	.4	0.1	0
raw, w/peel, trimmed	1 oz	4	0.2	0.8	1	.3	<.1	0
raw, w/peel, untrimmed	1 lb	56	2.4	12.8	9	4.4	0.6	0

CUMIN SEED

Food Name	Serv. Size	Total Cal.	Prot. GMS	Carbs GMS	Sod. MGS	Fiber GMS	Fat GMS	Chol. MGS
whole	1 oz	106	5.0	12.5	48	>3.0 c	6.3	0
whole	1 tbsp	22	1.1	2.7	10	.6	1.3	0
whole	1 tsp	8	0.4	0.9	4	.2	0.5	0
whole *(Durkee)*	1 tsp	10	0.0	0.0	0	0	<0.1	na
whole *(Laurel Leaf)*	1 tsp	10	0.0	0.0	0	0	<0.1	na

Food Name	Serv. Size	Total Cal.	Prot. GMS	Carbs GMS	Sod. MGS	Fiber GMS	Fat GMS	Chol. MGS
whole (Spice Islands)	1 tsp	7	0.3	0.7	3	>.1 c	0.4	0
CUPU ASSU OIL								
....	1/2 cup	964	0.0	0.0	0	0	109.0	0
....	1 oz	251	0.0	0.0	0	0	28.4	0
....	1 tbsp	120	0.0	0.0	0	0	13.6	0
CUPU ASSU PUNCH, 'Rain Forest'								
(Knudsen & Sons)	8 oz	110	<1.0	25.0	na	na	0.0	na
CURRANT, BLACK/European currant								
raw	1 cup	71	1.6	17.2	2	>2.7 c	0.5	0
trimmed	1 oz	18	0.4	4.4	1	1.5	0.1	0
untrimmed	1 lb	282	6.2	68.4	8	24.1	1.8	0
CURRANT, RED								
raw	1 cup	63	1.6	15.5	1	4.8	0.2	0
trimmed	1 oz	16	0.4	3.9	<1	>1.0 c	0.1	0
untrimmed	1 lb	249	6.2	61.3	5	>15.1 c	0.9	0
CURRANT, WHITE								
raw	1 cup	63	1.6	15.5	1	4.8	0.2	0
trimmed	1/2 cup	31	0.8	7.7	1	>1.9 c	0.1	0
trimmed	1 oz	16	0.4	3.9	<1	>1.0 c	0.1	0
untrimmed	1 lb	249	6.2	61.3	5	>15.1 c	0.9	0
CURRANT, ZANTE								
dried	1 lb	1282	18.5	336.0	35	30.8	1.2	0
dried	1 cup	408	5.9	106.7	12	9.8	0.4	0
dried	1 oz	80	1.2	21.0	2	1.9	0.1	0
dried (Del Monte)	1/2 cup	200	2.0	53.0	10	(mq)	0.0	0
CURRY POWDER								
ground	1 oz	92	3.6	16.5	15	9.7	3.9	0
ground	1 tbsp	20	0.8	3.7	3	2.1	0.9	0
ground	1 tsp	7	0.3	1.2	1	.7	0.3	0
CUSK/torsk/tusk								
dry-heat cooked	3 oz	95	20.7	0.0	34	0	0.8	45
raw	1 lb	396	86.2	0.0	143	0	3.1	186
raw	3 oz	74	16.1	0.0	26	0	0.6	35
raw	1 oz	25	5.4	0.0	9	0	0.2	12
raw, approx 4.3 oz	1 fillet	106	23.2	0.0	38	0	0.8	50
CUSTARD. See PUDDING MIX; PUDDING/PIE FILLING, MIX.								
CUSTARD APPLE/bullock's heart/cherimoya								
raw	100 gm	101	1.7	25.2	4	>3.4 c	0.6	0
trimmed	1 oz	29	0.5	7.1	1	>1.0 c	0.2	0
untrimmed	1 lb	267	4.5	66.3	11	>9.0 c	1.6	0
CUTTLEFISH, MIXED SPECIES								
moist-heat cooked	100 gm	158	32.5	1.6	744	0	1.4	224
moist-heat cooked	3 oz	134	27.6	1.4	632	0	1.2	190

	Serv.	Total	Prot.	Carbs	Sod.	Fiber	Fat	Chol.
raw	1 lb	359	73.7	3.7	1686	0	3.2	507
raw	3 oz	67	13.8	0.7	316	0	0.6	95
raw	1 oz	22	4.6	0.2	105	0	0.2	32

CYMLING. See SQUASH, SCALLOP.

D

Food Name	Serv. Size	Total Cal.	Prot. GMS	Carbs GMS	Sod. MGS	Fiber GMS	Fat GMS	Chol. MGS
DAIKON/mullangi/Oriental radish								
boiled, drained	4 oz	19	0.8	3.9	15	>.6 c	0.3	0
boiled, drained, sliced	1/2 cup	13	0.5	2.5	10	>.4 c	0.2	0
dried	1/2 cup	157	4.6	36.8	161	>4.9 c	0.4	0
dried	1 oz	77	2.2	18.0	79	>2.4 c	0.2	0
raw, trimmed	1 oz	5	0.2	1.2	6	>.2 c	<.1	0
raw, trimmed (Frieda's)	1 lb	86	4.1	19.1	(mq)	(mq)	0.5	0
raw, trimmed (Frieda's)	1 oz	5	0.3	1.2	(mq)	(mq)	<.1	0
raw, trimmed, sliced	1/2 cup	8	0.3	1.8	9	>.3 c	<.1	0
raw, untrimmed	1 lb	65	2.2	14.7	75	>2.3 c	0.4	0
DAIQUIRI. See ALCOHOLIC BEVERAGES.								
DANDELION GREENS								
boiled, drained	4 oz	37	2.3	7.3	50	>1.5 c	0.7	0
boiled, drained, chopped	1 cup	35	2.1	6.7	46	3.1	0.6	0
raw, chopped	1 oz	13	0.8	2.6	22	>.5 c	0.2	0
raw, trimmed	1 lb	204	12.3	41.7	345	>7.3 c	3.2	0
DANISH CABBAGE. See CABBAGE, DANISH.								
DANISH PASTRY								
APPLE								
(Awrey's)								
filled, 'Miniature' 1.7 oz	1 piece	160	2.0	21.0	170	0	8.0	5
filled 'Round' 4.5 oz	1 piece	390	4.0	50.0	390	1.0	20.0	10
filled 'Round' 2.75 oz	1 piece	270	3.0	34.0	310	1.0	14.0	5
filled 'Square' 3 oz	1 piece	220	3.0	34.0	230	1.0	8.0	10
(Pepperidge Farm) frozen, 2.25 oz	1 piece	220	2.0	35.0	130	(mq)	8.0	na
(Sara Lee)								
frozen 'Free & Light'	1/8 pkg	130	2.0	30.0	120	(mq)	0.0	0
frozen 'Individual' 1.3 oz	1 piece	120	2.0	15.0	120	(mq)	6.0	na
frozen twist	1/8 pkg	190	3.0	22.0	200	(mq)	10.0	10
CARAMEL (Pillsbury) w/nuts, refrigerated	1 piece	160	2.0	19.0	240	(mq)	8.0	0

Food Name	Serv. Size	Total Cal.	Prot. GMS	Carbs GMS	Sod. MGS	Fiber GMS	Fat GMS	Chol. MGS
CHEESE								
(Awrey's)								
filled, 'Miniature' 1.7 oz	1 piece	170	2.0	21.0	200	4.0	9.0	5
filled 'Round' 4.5 oz	1 piece	420	5.0	52.0	530	1.0	22.0	15
filled 'Round' 2.75 oz	1 piece	280	3.0	34.0	350	1.0	15.0	10
filled 'Square' 2.5 oz	1 piece	210	4.0	25.0	300	1.0	11.0	15
(Pepperidge Farm) frozen, 2.25 oz	1 piece	240	3.0	25.0	230	(mq)	14.0	(mq)
(Sara Lee) frozen, 'Individual' 1.3 oz	1 piece	130	2.0	13.0	130	(mq)	8.0	na
CINNAMON *(Sara Lee)* twist, frozen	1/8 pkg	200	3.0	21.0	270	(mq)	12.0	15
CINNAMON-RAISIN								
(Awrey's)								
filled 'Square' 3 oz	1 piece	290	3.0	41.0	280	1.0	12.0	15
filled 'Miniature' 1.5 oz	1 piece	160	2.0	21.0	150	1.0	8.0	5
(Pepperidge Farm) frozen, 2.25 oz	1 piece	250	3.0	35.0	170	(mq)	11.0	na
(Pillsbury) w/icing, refrigerated	1 piece	150	2.0	20.0	230	(mq)	7.0	0
(Sara Lee) frozen, 'Individual' 1.3 oz	1 piece	150	2.0	17.0	140	(mq)	8.0	na
CINNAMON-WALNUT *(Awrey's)* 'Round'								
2.75 oz	1 piece	300	4.0	31.0	290	1.0	18.0	5
LEMON *(Entenmann's)* twist	1.2 oz	140	2.0	17.0	140	na	7.0	na
ORANGE *(Pillsbury)* w/icing, refrigerated	1 piece	150	2.0	19.0	250	(mq)	7.0	0
PECAN RING *(Entenmann's)*	1.5 oz	190	3.0	19.0	130	na	12.0	na
PINEAPPLE *(Awrey's)* filled, 'Miniature'								
1.7 oz	1 piece	157	2.0	21.0	180	1.0	8.0	5
RASPBERRY								
(Awrey's) filled 'Square' 3 oz	1 piece	260	3.0	45.0	210	1.0	8.0	10
(Entenmann's) twist	1.2 oz	140	2.0	18.0	120	na	7.0	na
(Pepperidge Farm) frozen, 2.25 oz	1 piece	220	3.0	31.0	140	(mq)	9.0	na
(Sara Lee) twist, frozen	1/8 pkg	200	3.0	25.0	220	(mq)	9.0	15
RING *(Entenmann's)*	1.5 oz	180	3.0	18.0	160	na	10.0	na
STRAWBERRY								
(Awrey's)								
filled 'Miniature' 1.7 oz	1 piece	160	2.0	21.0	180	0	8.0	5
filled 'Round' 4.5 oz	1 piece	400	4.0	53.0	410	1.0	20.0	10
filled 'Round' 2.75 oz	1 piece	270	3.0	34.0	320	1.0	14.0	5
WALNUT RING *(Entenmann's)*	1.5 oz	190	3.0	19.0	130	na	12.0	na
DASHEEN								
cooked	4 oz	161	0.6	39.2	11	>1.0 c	0.1	0
cooked, sliced	1/2 cup	94	0.3	22.8	10	>.6 c	0.1	0
raw, sliced	1/2 cup	56	0.8	13.8	6	>.4 c	0.1	0
raw, trimmed	1 oz	30	0.4	7.5	3	>.2 c	0.1	0
raw, untrimmed	1 lb	419	5.9	103.2	43	>3.1 c	0.8	0
DASHEEN LEAF								
raw	1/2 cup	6	0.7	0.9	1	>.3 c	0.1	0

Food Name	Serv. Size	Total Cal.	Prot. GMS	Carbs GMS	Sod. MGS	Fiber GMS	Fat GMS	Chol. MGS
raw, trimmed	1 oz	12	1.4	1.9	1	>.6 c	0.2	0
raw, untrimmed	1 lb	115	13.5	18.3	8	>5.5 c	2.0	0
steamed	1/2 cup	18	2.0	3.0	2	>.4 c	0.3	0
steamed	4 oz	27	3.1	4.6	2	>.6 c	0.5	0
DASHEEN SHOOTS								
cooked	4 oz	16	0.8	3.6	2	>.6 c	0.1	0
cooked, sliced	1/2 cup	10	0.5	2.2	1	>.4 c	0.1	0
raw, sliced	1/2 cup	5	0.4	1.0	<1	>.3 c	<.1	0
raw, trimmed	1 oz	3	0.3	0.7	<1	>.2 c	<.1	0
raw, untrimmed	1 lb	45	3.7	9.3	4	>2.3 c	0.4	0
DATE								
Domestic, natural and dry								
chopped	1/2 cup	245	1.8	65.4	3	4.5	0.4	0
w/pits	1 lb	1123	8.0	300.1	10	20.8	1.8	0
w/o pits	1 oz	78	0.6	20.8	1	1.4	0.1	0
w/o pits, 2.9 oz	10 dates	228	1.6	61.0	2	4.2	0.4	0
w/o pits *(Dole)*	1/2 cup	280	5.0	62.0	0	(mq)	0.0	0
Imported, pitted								
(Amport Foods) chopped	1.5 oz	135	0.0	36.0	0	5	0.0	0
(Amport Foods) whole	1.5 oz	135	0.0	36.0	0	5	0.0	0
(Bordo)	2 oz	204	1.2	47.2	5	>1.5 c	1.2	0
(Bordo) diced	2 oz	203	1.0	47.5	5	>1.2 c	1.1	0
(Dromedary) approx 1 oz	5 dates	100	1.0	23.0	0	(mq)	0.0	0
(Dromedary) chopped	1/4 cup	130	1.0	31.0	0	(mq)	0.0	0
DEER								
raw	1 lb	544	104.1	0.0	231	na	11.0	386
raw	1 oz	34	6.4	0.0	14	na	0.7	24
roasted	3 oz	134	25.7	0.0	46	na	2.7	95
DIET BAR. See also SNACK BAR.								
(Figurines)								
chocolate	1 bar	100	2.0	11.0	50	1.0	5.0	0
chocolate caramel	1 bar	100	2.0	11.0	65	1.0	6.0	0
chocolate caramel '100'	1 bar	100	2.0	10.0	55	(mq)	6.0	na
chocolate peanut butter	1 bar	100	3.0	10.0	55	1.0	6.0	0
'S'mores'	1 bar	100	2.0	11.0	55	1.0	5.0	0
vanilla	1 bar	100	2.0	11.0	55	1.0	6.0	0
(Nestlé)								
chewy chocolate brownie 'Sweet Success'	1 bar	120	2.0	18.0	35	3.0	4.0	na
chewy chocolate chip 'Sweet Success'	1 bar	120	2.0	18.0	35	3.0	4.0	na
chewy chocolate peanut butter 'Sweet Success'	1 bar	120	2.0	18.0	35	3.0	4.0	na
(Ultra Slim Fast) chocolate chip crunch	1 bar	120	2.0	19.0	30	3.0	4.0	0

Food Name	Serv. Size	Total Cal.	Prot. GMS	Carbs GMS	Sod. MGS	Fiber GMS	Fat GMS	Chol. MGS
DIET DRINK								
(Nestlé)								
chocolate mocha, ready to drink,								
'Sweet Success'	10 oz	200	11.0	32.0	230	6.0	3.0	na
chocolate raspberry truffle, powder,								
'Sweet Success'	1.13 oz	90	7.0	11.0	150	6.0	2.0	na
chocolate raspberry truffle, prepared,								
'Sweet Success'	8 oz	180	15.0	23.0	na	6.0	2.0	280
creamy milk chocolate, canned,								
'Sweet Success'	10 oz	200	11.0	32.0	230	6.0	3.0	na
dark chocolate fudge, canned,								
'Sweet Success'	10 oz	200	11.0	32.0	210	6.0	3.0	na
dark chocolate fudge, powder,								
'Sweet Success'	1.13 oz	90	7.0	11.0	na	6.0	2.0	150
dark chocolate fudge, prepared,								
'Sweet Success'	8 oz	180	15.0	23.0	280	6.0	2.0	na
rich chocolate almond, powder,								
'Sweet Success'	1.13 oz	90	7.0	12.0	150	6.0	2.0	na
rich chocolate almond, prepared,								
'Sweet Success'	8 oz	180	15.0	24.0	280	6.0	2.0	na
(Ultra Slim Fast)								
cafe mocha powder	1 scoop	100	5.0	24.0	130	6.0	<1.0	na
cafe mocha powder, prepared								
w/skim milk	8 oz	200	15.0	38.0	280	6.0	1.0	na
chocolate fantasy 'Plus' powder	1 scoop	120	3.0	33.0	140	8.0	1.0	na
chocolate fantasy 'Plus' powder,								
prepared w/skim milk	12 oz	250	15.0	50.0	330	8.0	2.0	na
French vanilla powder	1 scoop	100	5.0	24.0	120	4.0	<1.0	na
French vanilla powder, prepared								
w/skim milk	8 oz	190	14.0	36.0	250	4.0	1.0	na
'French Vanilla' canned	12 oz	220	13.0	38.0	240	5.0	1.0	na
piña colada 'Plus' powder	1 scoop	90	5.0	24.0	120	6.0	<1.0	na
piña colada 'Plus' powder, prepared								
w/skim milk	8 oz	190	15.0	38.0	260	6.0	<1.0	na
strawberry jubilee 'Plus' powder	1 scoop	110	3.0	32.0	140	8.0	1.0	na
strawbery jubilee 'Plus' powder, prepared								
w/skim milk	12 oz	240	15.0	50.0	330	8.0	2.0	na
DILL SEASONING, 'Parsley Patch It's								
a Dilly' *(Schilling)*	1 tsp	11	0.4	2.0	5	(tr)	0.4	0
DILL SEED								
whole	1 oz	86	4.5	15.6	6	>6.0 c	4.1	0
whole	1 tbsp	20	1.0	3.6	1	1.4	1.0	0
whole	1 tsp	6	0.3	1.2	0	.4	0.3	0

Food Name	Serv. Size	Total Cal.	Prot. GMS	Carbs GMS	Sod. MGS	Fiber GMS	Fat GMS	Chol. MGS
whole (Durkee)	1 tsp	9	0.0	0.0	0	0	<0.1	na
whole (Laurel Leaf)	1 tsp	9	0.0	0.0	0	0	<0.1	na
whole (Spice Islands)	1 tsp	9	0.3	1.2	<1	.4	0.4	0
DILL WEED								
dried	1 oz	72	5.7	15.8	79	>3.4 c	1.2	0
dried	1 tbsp	8	0.6	1.7	6	>.4 c	0.1	0
dried	1 tsp	3	0.2	0.6	2	>.1 c	0.0	0
fresh, sprigs	1 cup	4	0.3	0.6	5	na	0.1	0
DIP								
ACAPULCO (Ortega)	1 oz	8	0.0	2.0	0	na	0.0	0
AVOCADO (Kraft)	2 tbsp	50	1.0	3.0	210	na	4.0	0
BACON AND HORSERADISH								
(Breakstone's)	2 tbsp	70	1.0	2.0	270	na	6.0	15
(Kraft)	2 tbsp	60	1.0	3.0	200	na	5.0	0
(Kraft) 'Premium'	2 tbsp	50	1.0	2.0	270	na	5.0	15
(Sealtest)	2 tbsp	70	1.0	2.0	270	na	6.0	15
BACON AND ONION								
(Breakstone's) 'Gourmet'	2 tbsp	70	1.0	2.0	210	na	6.0	15
(Kraft) 'Premium'	2 tbsp	60	1.0	2.0	170	na	5.0	15
BEAN								
(Chi-Chi's) 'Fiesta'	1 oz	30	1.0	4.0	126	na	1.0	3
(Hain) hot	4 tbsp	70	4.0	10.0	250	(mq)	1.0	5
BLACK BEAN								
(Guiltless Gourmet) barbeque, mild	1 oz	23	1.0	4.0	100	2.0	0.0	0
(Guiltless Gourmet) barbeque, spicy	1 oz	23	1.0	4.0	100	2.0	0.0	0
(Guiltless Gourmet) mild	1 oz	23	1.0	4.0	100	2.0	0.0	0
(Guiltless Gourmet) spicy	1 oz	23	1.0	4.0	100	2.0	0.0	0
(Tostitos) fat free, medium	2 tbsp	30	2.0	6.0	210	2.0	0.0	0
BLUE CHEESE								
(Kraft) 'Premium'	2 tbsp	50	1.0	2.0	210	0	4.0	10
(Litehouse) 'Lite' and dressing, refrigerated	1 tbsp	33	1.0	1.0	86	na	3.0	na
(Litehouse) 'Original' and dressing, refrigerated	1 tbsp	77	1.0	0.0	82	na	8.0	na
CAESAR (Litehouse) and dressing, refrigerated	1 tbsp	57	0.0	0.0	84	na	6.0	na
CHEDDAR CHEESE								
(Frito-Lay's)	1 oz	45	1.0	3.0	180	na	3.0	1
(Guiltless Gourmet) queso, mild	1 oz	20	1.0	5.0	150	0	0.0	0
(Guiltless Gourmet) queso, spicy	1 oz	20	1.0	5.0	150	0	0.0	0
CHEESE (Chi-Chi's) 'Fiesta'	1 oz	41	1.0	3.0	296	na	3.0	9
CHILI (La Victoria)	1 tbsp	6	<1.0	1.0	90	na	<1.0	na

Food Name	Serv. Size	Total Cal.	Prot. GMS	Carbs GMS	Sod. MGS	Fiber GMS	Fat GMS	Chol. MGS
CLAM								
(Breakstone's)	2 tbsp	50	1.0	2.0	220	na	4.0	15
(Breakstone's) 'Gourmet Chesapeake'	2 tbsp	50	1.0	2.0	200	na	4.0	20
(Kraft)	2 tbsp	60	1.0	3.0	240	na	4.0	10
(Kraft) 'Premium'	2 tbsp	45	1.0	2.0	210	na	4.0	20
(Sealtest)	2 tbsp	50	1.0	2.0	220	na	4.0	15
COUNTRY BLUE CHEESE								
(Litehouse) and dressing, refrigerated	1 tbsp	76	1.0	0.0	84	na	8.0	na
COUNTRY RANCH (Litehouse) and								
dressing, refrigerated	1 tbsp	61	0.0	1.0	75	na	7.0	na
CUCUMBER (Kraft) creamy 'Premium'	2 tbsp	50	1.0	2.0	130	(tr)	4.0	10
CUCUMBER AND ONION								
(Breakstone's)	2 tbsp	50	1.0	2.0	160	na	4.0	15
(Sealtest)	2 tbsp	50	1.0	2.0	160	na	4.0	15
DILL (Nasoya) creamy 'Vegi-Dip'	1 oz	60	2.0	4.0	100	na	4.0	0
FRENCH ONION								
(Bison)	1 oz	60	1.0	2.0	180	na	5.0	20
(Breakstone's)	2 tbsp	50	1.0	2.0	140	na	5.0	15
(Frito-Lay's)	1 oz	50	1.0	3.0	180	na	3.0	3
(Heluva Good) real sour cream	2 tbsp	50	1.0	2.0	160	0	5.0	20
(Kraft)	2 tbsp	60	1.0	3.0	140	na	4.0	0
(Kraft) 'Premium'	2 tbsp	45	1.0	2.0	150	na	4.0	10
(Lucerne)	2 tbsp	70	1.0	2.0	160	0	6.0	5
(Nasoya) 'Vegi-Dip'	1 oz	50	2.0	4.0	100	na	3.0	0
(Sealtest)	2 tbsp	50	1.0	2.0	140	na	5.0	15
GARLIC (Life) and dressing, w/tofu								
'All Natural'	1 tbsp	70	<1.0	1.4	75	(mq)	7.1	0
GARLIC AND HERB (Nasoya) 'Vegi-Dip'	1 oz	50	2.0	6.0	100	(mq)	2.0	0
GUACAMOLE								
(Kraft)	2 tbsp	50	1.0	3.0	210	na	4.0	0
(Lucerne)	2 tbsp	80	1.0	1.0	170	0	8.0	5
HONEY MUSTARD (Litehouse) and								
dressing, refrigerated	1 tbsp	67	0.0	2.0	55	na	7.0	na
HUMMUS (Fantastic Foods)	2 oz	111	4.0	9.5	263	(mq)	6.5	0
ITALIAN (Litehouse) and dressing, creamy,								
refrigerated	1 tbsp	60	0.0	0.0	76	na	6.0	na
JALAPEÑO								
(Breakstone's) cheddar 'Gourmet'	2 tbsp	70	2.0	2.0	90	na	6.0	15
(Frito-Lay's)	1 oz	30	1.0	4.0	115	na	1.0	0
(Hain) medium	4 tbsp	70	4.0	10.0	150	na	1.0	5
(Kraft)	2 tbsp	50	1.0	3.0	160	na	4.0	0
(Kraft) cheese 'Premium'	2 tbsp	50	1.0	3.0	160	na	4.0	15

Food Name	Serv. Size	Total Cal.	Prot. GMS	Carbs GMS	Sod. MGS	Fiber GMS	Fat GMS	Chol. MGS
(Litehouse) ranch, and dressing, refrigerated	1 tbsp	60	0.0	1.0	80	na	6.0	na
(Old El Paso)	1 tbsp	14	1.0	2.0	53	1.0	0.0	0
(Price's) nacho	1 oz	80	2.6	2.0	(mq)	na	7.1	na
(Wise)	2 tbsp	25	1.0	5.0	100	na	0.0	0
MEXICAN BEAN *(Hain)*	4 tbsp	60	4.0	9.0	260	na	1.0	5
MUSHROOM AND HERB *(Breakstone's)* 'Gourmet'	2 tbsp	50	1.0	2.0	150	na	4.0	10
NACHO CHEESE								
(Kraft) 'Premium'	2 tbsp	55	2.0	2.0	200	0	4.0	10
(Tio Sancho) 'Microwave Snacks' cheese sauce mix	3.5 oz	247	14.5	2.3	995	>.4 c	20.0	(mq)
ONION								
(Breakstone's) toasted 'Gourmet'	2 tbsp	50	1.0	2.0	170	na	5.0	10
(Hain) bean	4 tbsp	70	4.0	10.0	270	(mq)	1.0	5
(Kraft) creamy 'Premium'	2 tbsp	45	1.0	2.0	160	na	4.0	10
(Kraft) green	2 tbsp	60	1.0	3.0	170	na	4.0	0
PEPPERCORN *(Litehouse)* and dressing, refrigerated	1 tbsp	67	0.0	0.0	66	na	7.0	na
PICANTE SAUCE								
(Frito-Lay's)	1 oz	10	0.0	3.0	160	na	0.0	0
(Wise)	2 tbsp	12	0.0	3.0	130	na	0.0	na
PINTO BEAN								
(Guiltless Gourmet) barbeque, mild	1 oz	27	2.0	5.0	100	2.0	0.0	0
(Guiltless Gourmet) barbeque, spicy	1 oz	27	2.0	5.0	100	2.0	0.0	0
(Guiltless Gourmet) mild	1 oz	27	2.0	5.0	100	2.0	0.0	0
(Guiltless Gourmet) spicy	1 oz	27	2.0	5.0	100	2.0	0.0	0
POPPYSEED *(Litehouse)* and dressing, refrigerated	1 tbsp	65	0.0	3.0	83	na	6.0	na
RANCH								
(Heluva Good) real sour cream	2 tbsp	60	1.0	2.0	180	0	5.0	20
(Litehouse) and dressing, refrigerated	1 tbsp	59	0.0	1.0	67	na	6.0	na
(Litehouse) 'Lite' and dressing, refrigerated	1 tbsp	35	1.0	1.0	80	na	3.0	na
(Litehouse) 'Vegi-Dip' refrigerated	1 tbsp	60	0.0	1.0	68	na	7.0	na
(Lucerne)	2 tbsp	110	1.0	2.0	160	0	11.0	10
SALSA								
(Pace) 'Chunky' medium	2 tbsp	4	<1.0	<1.0	102	na	<1.0	na
(Pace) 'Chunky' mild	2 tbsp	4	<1.0	<1.0	101	na	<1.0	na
SOUR CREAM AND CHIVES								
(Litehouse) vinaigrette, and dressing, refrigerated	1 tbsp	63	0.0	1.0	72	na	7.0	na

Food Name	Serv. Size	Total Cal.	Prot. GMS	Carbs GMS	Sod. MGS	Fiber GMS	Fat GMS	Chol. MGS
TACO								
(Hain) and sauce	4 tbsp	25	1.0	5.0	350	na	1.0	5
(Wise)	2 tbsp	12	0.0	3.0	115	na	0.0	0
THOUSAND ISLAND (Litehouse) and								
dressing, refrigerated	1 tbsp	65	0.0	1.0	99	na	7.0	na
VEGETABLE (T. Marzetti) and dressing	1 tbsp	88	0.0	1.0	120	na	10.0	2
DISHCLOTH GOURD. See GOURD, DISHCLOTH.								
DOCK								
boiled, drained	4 oz	23	2.1	3.3	3	>.8 c	0.7	0
boiled, drained	100 gm	20	1.8	2.9	3	>.7 c	0.6	0
raw, chopped	1/2 cup	15	1.3	2.1	3	1.94	0.5	0
raw, trimmed	1 oz	6	0.6	0.9	1	>.2 c	0.2	0
raw, untrimmed	1 lb	70	6.4	10.2	13	>2.5 c	2.2	0
DOLLARFISH								
raw	1 lb	663	78.4	0.0	401	0	36.4	295
raw	1 oz	41	4.9	0.0	25	0	2.3	18
DOLPHIN FISH. See MAHI MAHI.								
DONUT								
(Awrey's)								
crunch	1 donut	600	7.0	65.0	730	2.0	34.0	40
plain	1 donut	490	6.0	48.0	650	1.0	30.0	35
sugared	1 donut	610	7.0	68.0	735	2.0	35.0	40
(Break Cake)								
chocolate, 1 oz	1 donut	130	1.0	14.0	115	na	8.0	5
chocolate, gem, .5 oz	1 donut	70	1.0	7.0	60	na	4.0	5
chocolate, gem, .5 oz	6 donuts	400	4.0	42.0	340	na	24.0	15
cinnamon, 1 oz	1 donut	120	1.0	15.0	130	na	6.0	5
cinnamon, gem, .5 oz	1 donut	60	1.0	8.0	70	na	3.0	5
dunkin stix, .5 oz	2 stix	420	3.0	43.0	320	na	27.0	0
powdered, 1 oz	1 donut	120	1.0	16.0	135	na	5.0	5
powdered, gem, .5 oz	1 donut	60	1.0	8.0	70	na	3.0	5
powdered, gem, .5 oz	6 donuts	350	4.0	47.0	400	na	16.0	15
(Dunkin' Donuts)								
apple filled, w/cinnamon sugar, 2.8 oz	1 donut	250	5.0	33.0	280	1.0	11.0	0
Bavarian filled, w/chocolate frosting,								
2.8 oz	1 donut	240	5.0	32.0	260	2.0	11.0	0
blueberry filled, 2.4 oz	1 donut	210	4.0	29.0	240	2.0	8.0	0
'Boston Kreme'	1 donut	240	4.0	30.0	250	na	11.0	0
cinnamon, apple filled	1 donut	190	4.0	25.0	220	na	9.0	0
coffee roll, glazed, 2.9 oz	1 donut	280	5.0	37.0	310	2.0	12.0	0
cruller, French, glazed, 1.3 oz	1 donut	140	2.0	16.0	130	0	8.0	30
cruller, honey dipped	1 donut	260	4.0	36.0	330	na	11.0	0
jelly filled, 2.4 oz	1 donut	220	4.0	31.0	230	1.0	9.0	0

Food Name	Serv. Size	Total Cal.	Prot. GMS	Carbs GMS	Sod. MGS	Fiber GMS	Fat GMS	Chol. MGS
lemon filled, 2.8 oz	1 donut	260	4.0	33.0	280	1.0	12.0	0
plain, cake w/handle	1 donut	240	4.0	26.0	370	na	14.0	0
ring, buttermilk, glazed, 2.6 oz	1 donut	290	4.0	37.0	370	1.0	14.0	10
ring, chocolate, glazed, 2.5 oz	1 donut	324	3.5	34.0	383	1.9	21.0	2
ring, plain, cake	1 donut	262	3.0	23.0	330	na	18.0	0
ring, plain, cake, 2.2 oz	1 donut	270	4.0	25.0	330	1.0	17.0	10
ring, powdered, cake	1 donut	270	3.0	28.0	340	na	16.0	0
ring, whole wheat, glazed, 2.9 oz	1 donut	330	4.0	39.0	380	na	18.0	5
ring, yeast, chocolate frosted, 1.9 oz	1 donut	200	4.0	25.0	190	na	10.0	0
ring, yeast, glazed, 1.9 oz	1 donut	200	4.0	26.0	230	na	9.0	0
(Entenmann's)								
crumb topped	1 donut	260	3.0	34.0	220	na	12.0	na
devil's food crumb	1 donut	250	3.0	34.0	200	na	12.0	na
rich, frosted	1 donut	280	3.0	27.0	210	na	18.0	na
(Hostess)								
cinnamon, 'Donette Gems'	1 donut	60	1.0	7.0	70	.3	3.0	5
cinnamon, 'Family Pack'	1 donut	120	2.0	14.0	140	.5	6.0	5
crumb	1 donut	160	1.0	16.0	140	.9	10.0	10
crumb, 'Donette Gems'	1 donut	80	1.0	8.0	70	.4	5.0	5
frosted, 1.5 oz	1 donut	190	2.0	20.0	180	1.1	12.0	5
frosted, 'Donette Gems'	1 donut	80	1.0	8.0	70	.4	5.0	5
glazed, 'Old Fashioned'	1 donut	250	3.0	33.0	230	1.4	12.0	15
glazed whirl	1 donut	190	3.0	27.0	230	.9	7.0	5
honey wheat	1 donut	250	3.0	32.0	280	1.2	12.0	25
plain, 'Old Fashioned'	1 donut	170	3.0	21.0	230	.9	9.0	10
(Little Debbie) stick 1.67 oz	1 stick	230	2.0	26.0	180	(mq)	13.0	<1
(Rich's)								
frozen, glazed 'Ever Fresh' 1.2 oz	1 donut	141	2.4	17.2	(mq)	(mq)	7.0	na
frozen, jelly 'Ever Fresh' 2.17 oz	1 donut	213	3.6	26.0	(mq)	(mq)	9.5	na
(Tastykake)								
cinnamon, 'Assorted' 1.6 oz	1 donut	179	2.6	24.5	211	.8	8.2	11
cinnamon, mini	1 donut	48	0.7	6.4	54	.3	2.4	4
frosted, rich, 2 oz	1 donut	258	3.6	28.2	196	3.3	16.0	9
frosted, rich, mini	1 donut	61	0.9	7.7	59	.5	3.2	4
honey wheat, 2 oz	1 donut	209	2.3	33.3	190	.9	7.5	15
honey wheat, mini	1 donut	40	0.6	7.2	48	.2	1.2	3
orange glazed, 2 oz	1 donut	219	2.7	32.1	178	.8	9.1	10
plain, 'Assorted' 1.6 oz	1 donut	185	3.0	21.6	171	.9	10.1	12
powdered sugar, 'Assorted' 1.6 oz	1 donut	188	2.6	24.4	221	.8	8.6	10
powdered sugar, mini	1 donut	42	0.6	6.9	71	.2	1.3	4

DRAGON'S EYE. See LONGAN.

DREAM WHIP. See CREAM TOPPING, NONDAIRY.

DRESSING. See SALAD DRESSING.

Food Name	Serv. Size	Total Cal.	Prot. GMS	Carbs GMS	Sod. MGS	Fiber GMS	Fat GMS	Chol. MGS

DRINKS. See ALCOHOL-FREE BEVERAGES; ALCOHOLIC BEVERAGES; COFFEE; DIET DRINK;
MILK; SOFT DRINKS AND MIXERS; SPORTS DRINK; TEA; WATER; and individual listings.
DRINK MIX. See individual drink mix flavors.

DRUM, FRESHWATER

Food Name	Serv. Size	Total Cal.	Prot. GMS	Carbs GMS	Sod. MGS	Fiber GMS	Fat GMS	Chol. MGS
dry-heat cooked	3 oz	130	19.1	0.0	82	0	5.4	70
raw	1 lb	541	79.5	0.0	340	0	22.4	290
raw	3 oz	101	14.9	0.0	64	0	4.2	54
raw	1 oz	34	5.0	0.0	21	0	1.4	18

DUCK, DOMESTICATED

Meat and skin

raw	1 oz	115	3.3	0.0	18	0	11.2	22
roasted	4 oz	382	21.5	0.0	67	0	32.1	95

Meat only

raw	1 oz	37	5.2	0.0	21	0	1.7	22
roasted	4 oz	228	26.6	0.0	74	0	12.7	101

DUCK, WILD

Breast meat, raw	1 oz	35	5.6	0.0	16	0	1.2	(mq)
Meat and skin, raw	1 oz	60	4.9	0.0	16	0	4.3	123

DUCK FAT

	1 cup	1846	0.0	0.0	0	0	204.6	205
	1 oz	255	0.0	0.0	0	0	28.3	28
	1 tbsp	115	0.0	0.0	0	0	12.8	13

DUCK LIVER, domesticated, raw	1 oz	39	5.3	1.0	(mq)	0	1.3	146
DULSE, raw	100 gm	0	0.0	0.0	2085	>1.2 c	3.2	0

E

Food Name	Serv. Size	Total Cal.	Prot. GMS	Carbs GMS	Sod. MGS	Fiber GMS	Fat GMS	Chol. MGS

EEL, MIXED SPECIES

broiled	4 oz	268	26.8	0.0	74	0	17.0	183
dry-heat cooked	3 oz	201	20.1	0.0	55	0	12.7	137
raw	1 lb	834	83.7	0.0	231	0	52.9	571
raw	1 oz	52	5.2	0.0	14	0	3.3	36

EGG, ALTERNATIVE

Frozen

(Fleischmann's) 'Egg Beaters' cheese omelet	1/2 cup	110	14.0	2.0	480	na	5.0	5
(Fleischmann's) 'Egg Beaters' vegetable omelet	1/2 cup	50	7.0	5.0	170	na	0.0	0
(Morningstar Farms) 'Scramblers'	1/4 cup	60	6.0	3.0	(mq)	0	3.0	0
(Tofutti) 'Egg Watchers'	2 oz	50	7.0	2.0	100	na	2.0	0

Food Name	Serv. Size	Total Cal.	Prot. GMS	Carbs GMS	Sod. MGS	Fiber GMS	Fat GMS	Chol. MGS
Refrigerated								
(Featherweight)	2 eggs	120	9.0	2.0	250	0	8.0	15
(Fleischmann's) 'Egg Beaters'	1/4 cup	25	5.0	1.0	80	0	0.0	0
Mix								
(Healthy Choice) 'Cholesterol Free								
Egg Product'	1.9-oz serving	30	5.0	1.0	90	na	0.0	0
(Tofu Scrambler) prepared w/tofu	1/2 cup	98	11.0	7.0	252	(mq)	5.0	0
EGG, CHICKEN. See also EGG WHITE, CHICKEN; EGG YOLK, CHICKEN.								
Cooked								
fried	1 large	91	6.2	0.6	162	0	6.9	211
hard-boiled	1 oz	44	3.6	0.3	35	0	3.0	120
hard-boiled, chopped	1 cup	211	17.1	1.5	169	0	14.4	577
poached	1 large	74	6.2	0.6	140	0	5.0	212
poached	1 oz	42	3.5	0.3	79	0	2.8	120
scrambled	1 cup	365	24.4	4.8	616	0	26.9	774
scrambled	1 large	100	6.7	1.3	168	0	7.3	211
Dried								
	1 oz	168	13.0	1.4	148	0	11.9	544
	1 tbsp	30	2.3	0.2	26	0	2.1	96
sifted	1 cup	505	39.0	4.1	443	0	35.5	1631
stabilized, glucose reduced	1 oz	174	13.7	0.7	155	0	12.5	572
stabilized, glucose reduced	1 tbsp	31	2.4	0.1	27	0	2.2	101
stabilized, glucose reduced, sifted	1 cup	523	40.9	2.0	466	0	37.4	1714
Pickled (Penrose)	1 large	80	8.0	1.0	230		5.0	(mq)
Raw								
fresh or frozen	1 cup	363	30.4	3.0	307	0	24.3	1033
fresh or frozen	1 large	75	6.3	0.6	63	0	5.0	213
fresh or frozen	1 oz	42	3.5	0.3	36	0	2.8	120
EGG, DUCK								
raw	1 large	130	9.0	1.0	102	0	9.6	619
raw	1 oz	52	3.6	0.4	41	0	3.9	251
EGG, GOOSE								
raw	1 large	267	20.0	1.9	199	0	19.1	1227
raw	1 oz	52	3.9	0.4	na	0	3.8	(mq)
EGG, QUAIL								
raw	1 oz	45	3.7	0.1	na	0	3.1	239
raw	1 large	14	1.2	0.0	13	0	1.0	76
EGG, TURKEY								
raw	1 large	135	10.8	0.9	120	0	9.4	737
raw	1 oz	48	3.9	0.3	na	0	3.4	265
EGG BREAKFAST, ALTERNATIVE, FROZEN								
vegetarian, w/hash browns and links								
'Scramblers' (Morningstar Farms)	7 oz	360	16.0	22.0	660	(mq)	23.0	0

Food Name	Serv. Size	Total Cal.	Prot. GMS	Carbs GMS	Sod. MGS	Fiber GMS	Fat GMS	Chol. MGS
vegetarian, w/pancakes and links								
'Scramblers' *(Morningstar Farms)*	6.8 oz	380	18.0	33.0	900	(mq)	19.0	0

EGG BREAKFAST, FREEZE-DRIED

(Mountain House)

Food Name	Serv. Size	Total Cal.	Prot. GMS	Carbs GMS	Sod. MGS	Fiber GMS	Fat GMS	Chol. MGS
cheese omelet, prepared	1/2 pkg	180	13.0	8.0	207	na	9.0	(mq)
w/bacon, prepared	1/2 pkg	170	12.0	7.0	165	na	10.0	(mq)
w/butter, prepared	1/2 pkg	160	11.0	8.0	174	na	8.0	(mq)

EGG BREAKFAST, SCRAMBLED, FROZEN

Food Name	Serv. Size	Total Cal.	Prot. GMS	Carbs GMS	Sod. MGS	Fiber GMS	Fat GMS	Chol. MGS
w/bacon and home fried potatoes								
(Swanson)	5.6 oz	340	11.0	16.0	690	(mq)	26.0	(mq)
w/cheddar cheese and fried potatoes								
(Aunt Jemima)	5.9 oz	250	11.0	22.0	910	(mq)	13.0	(mq)
w/ham and hash browns *(Downyflake)*	6.25 oz	360	13.0	17.0	730	(mq)	26.0	(mq)
w/ham and pecan twirl *(Downyflake)*	6.25 oz	470	15.0	40.0	670	(mq)	28.0	(mq)
w/hash browns and sausage link								
(Downyflake)	6.25 oz	420	12.0	17.0	790	(mq)	34.0	(mq)
w/home fried potatoes 'Great Starts'								
Budget Breakfast *(Swanson)*	4.6 oz	260	7.0	14.0	380	(mq)	19.0	(mq)
w/sausages and hash browns								
(Aunt Jemima)	5.7 oz	290	12.0	14.0	810	(mq)	20.0	(mq)
w/sausages and hash browns *(Swanson)*	6.5 oz	430	13.0	19.0	760	(mq)	34.0	(mq)
w/sausages and pancakes *(Aunt Jemima)*	5.2 oz	270	13.0	21.0	880	(mq)	14.0	(mq)
w/sausages and pecan twirl *(Downyflake)*	6.25 oz	510	16.0	39.0	710	(mq)	33.0	(mq)

EGG FOO YUNG

Food Name	Serv. Size	Total Cal.	Prot. GMS	Carbs GMS	Sod. MGS	Fiber GMS	Fat GMS	Chol. MGS
(LaChoy) mix, prepared	8.8 oz	164	8.2	19.2	1250	(mq)	7.0	na
(LaChoy) packaged 'Dinner Classics'								
prepared	2 patties	170	8.0	20.0	1390	1.0	7.0	275

EGG NOODLE. See NOODLE, EGG.

EGG ROLL

Frozen

(Chun King)

Food Name	Serv. Size	Total Cal.	Prot. GMS	Carbs GMS	Sod. MGS	Fiber GMS	Fat GMS	Chol. MGS
chicken	3.6 oz	220	5.0	32.0	600	(mq)	8.0	(mq)
meat and shrimp	3.6 oz	220	6.0	31.0	680	(mq)	8.0	(mq)
pork 'Restaurant Style'	3 oz	180	6.0	23.0	450	(mq)	6.0	(mq)
shrimp	3.6 oz	200	4.0	31.0	480	(mq)	6.0	(mq)

(Jeno's)

Food Name	Serv. Size	Total Cal.	Prot. GMS	Carbs GMS	Sod. MGS	Fiber GMS	Fat GMS	Chol. MGS
chicken 'Snacks' approx 6 rolls	3 oz	190	5.0	21.0	350	(mq)	9.0	(mq)
meat and shrimp 'Snacks' approx 6 rolls	3 oz	200	5.0	21.0	420	(mq)	11.0	(mq)
shrimp and cheese 'Snacks' approx 6 rolls	3 oz	190	7.0	22.0	290	(mq)	8.0	(mq)

(LaChoy)

Food Name	Serv. Size	Total Cal.	Prot. GMS	Carbs GMS	Sod. MGS	Fiber GMS	Fat GMS	Chol. MGS
almond chicken	3 oz	120	5.0	19.0	290	na	3.0	5
chicken 'Snack'	1.45 oz	90	3.0	12.0	140	na	3.0	<1
lobster 'Snack'	1.45 oz	75	2.0	12.0	150	na	2.0	<1

Food Name	Serv. Size	Total Cal.	Prot. GMS	Carbs GMS	Sod. MGS	Fiber GMS	Fat GMS	Chol. MGS
meat and shrimp 'Snack'	1.45 oz	80	3.0	11.0	115	na	3.0	4
pork 'Restaurant Style'	3 oz	150	7.0	20.0	480	na	5.0	7
shrimp 'Restaurant Style'	3 oz	130	5.0	19.0	260	na	4.0	5
shrimp 'Snack'	1.45 oz	75	2.0	12.0	120	na	2.0	4
sweet and sour chicken	3 oz	150	4.0	24.0	280	na	4.0	5
(Worthington) vegetarian roll, frozen	3 oz	160	6.0	20.0	530	(mq)	6.0	0
Refrigerated								
(Chung's)								
chicken, white meat	3 oz	150	8.0	21.0	560	4.0	6.0	9
pork	3 oz	190	7.0	20.0	590	3.0	10.0	10
shrimp	3 oz	170	5.0	22.0	496	10.0	7.0	11
vegetable	3 oz	180	4.0	23.0	510	15.0	8.0	0
EGG ROLL WRAPPER								
(Azumaya Pasta)	2 pieces	130	4.0	26.0	200	1.0	0.0	<5
(Nasoya)	1 piece	23	1.0	4.5	19	(mq)	0.0	0
EGG WHITE, CHICKEN								
Dried								
stabilized, glucose reduced, flakes	1 oz	100	21.8	1.2	328	0	<.1	0
stabilized, glucose reduced, powder	1 cup	402	88.2	4.8	1325	0	<.1	0
stabilized, glucose reduced, powder	1 oz	107	23.4	1.3	351	0	<.1	0
Raw								
fresh or frozen	1 cup	122	25.6	2.5	399	0	0.0	na
fresh or frozen	1 large	17	3.5	0.3	55	0	0.0	na
fresh or frozen	1 oz	14	3.0	0.3	46	0	0.0	0
EGG WHITE STABILIZER *(Tone's)*	1 tsp	12	<.1	3.0	1	.1	(tr)	0
EGG YOLK, CHICKEN								
Dried								
sifted	1 cup	460	20.5	0.3	61	0	41.1	1962
sifted	1 oz	195	8.7	0.1	26	0	17.4	830
sifted	1 tbsp	27	1.2	0.0	4	0	2.5	117
Raw								
fresh	1 cup	870	40.7	4.3	104	0	75.0	3113
fresh	1 oz	101	4.8	0.5	12	0	8.8	363
fresh	1 large	59	2.8	0.3	7	0	5.1	213
frozen, salted	100 gm	278	14.2	1.5	3932	0	23.4	973
frozen, sugared	100 gm	317	14.2	11.5	56	0	23.4	973
frozen, sugared	1 oz	92	3.7	2.7	16	0	7.2	328
EGGNOG, NON-ALCOHOLIC								
Canned *(Borden)*	1/2 cup	160	3.0	16.0	80	0	9.0	(mq)
Chilled								
(Crowley)	6 oz	270	6.0	34.0	200	0	13.0	100
(Darigold)	8 oz	350	6.0	43.0	120	0	17.0	(mq)
(Darigold) 'Classic'	8 oz	390	10.0	48.0	170	0	17.0	(mq)

Food Name	Serv. Size	Total Cal.	Prot. GMS	Carbs GMS	Sod. MGS	Fiber GMS	Fat GMS	Chol. MGS
(Ensure) liquid nutrition	8 oz	250	8.8	34.3	na	na	8.8	na
EGGNOG MIX								
dry, 2 heaping tsp	1 oz	111	0.1	27.7	44	0	0.3	7
1 oz powder, prepared w/whole milk	1 cup	261	8.2	38.9	163	0	8.4	33
1 oz powder, prepared w/2% milk	1 cup	232	8.2	39.4	166	0	5.0	18
1 oz powder, prepared w/1% milk	1 cup	213	8.1	39.4	167	0	2.9	10
1 oz powder, prepared w/skim milk	1 cup	197	8.5	39.6	170	0	0.7	4
EGGPLANT/aubergine								
boiled, drained	4 oz	32	0.9	7.5	3	>1.1 c	0.3	0
boiled, drained, 1-inch cubes	1 cup	27	0.8	6.4	3	2.4	0.2	0
raw, 1-inch pieces	1/2 cup	11	0.4	2.5	1	1.0	0.1	0
raw, peeled, approx 1 lb	1 eggplant	119	4.7	27.8	14	11.5	0.8	0
raw, trimmed	1 oz	7	0.3	1.8	1	.4	<.1	0
raw, untrimmed	1 lb	95	4.0	23.0	13	5.5	0.4	0
EGGPLANT APPETIZER, 'Caponata'								
(Progresso)	1/2 can	70	2.0	4.0	260	(mq)	4.0	0
EGGPLANT ENTRÉE, FROZEN								
(Celentano)								
parmigiana	10 oz	350	18.0	29.0	500	(mq)	19.0	(mq)
parmigiana	8 oz	280	14.0	23.0	400	(mq)	15.0	(mq)
parmigiana	6.25 oz	260	9.0	36.0	220	(mq)	10.0	(mq)
rollettes	11 oz	320	14.0	36.0	210	(mq)	14.0	na
(Mrs. Paul's) parmigiana	5 oz	240	6.0	18.0	600	(mq)	16.0	15
ELBOW MACARONI. See PASTA.								
ELDERBERRY								
fresh	1 lb	329	3.0	83.5	na	>31.8 c	2.3	0
fresh	1 oz	21	0.2	5.2	na	>2.0 c	0.1	0
fresh	1 cup	106	1.0	26.7	na	>10.1 c	0.7	0
ENCHILADA *(Gebhardt)*	2 enchiladas	310	5.0	20.0	460	2.0	24.0	58
ENCHILADA DINNER, FROZEN. See also ENCHILADA ENTRÉE, FROZEN.								
BEEF								
(Banquet)	12 oz	500	19.0	72.0	1810	(mq)	15.0	(mq)
(Banquet) chili and gravy 'Family Entrées'	7 oz	270	10.0	28.0	(mq)	(mq)	13.0	(mq)
(Healthy Choice)	13.4 oz	370	15.0	66.0	450	na	5.0	30
(Old El Paso) 'Festive Dinners'	11 oz	390	24.0	56.0	1200	(mq)	8.0	(mq)
(Patio)	13.25 oz	520	16.0	59.0	1810	(mq)	24.0	40
(Swanson)	13.75 oz	480	17.0	55.0	1350	(mq)	21.0	(mq)
(Van de Kamp's) 'Mexican Dinner'	1/2 pkg	200	8.0	27.0	740	(mq)	7.0	(mq)
CHEESE								
(Banquet)	12 oz	550	22.0	71.0	2170	(mq)	19.0	(mq)
(Patio)	12.25 oz	380	14.0	59.0	2010	(mq)	10.0	20
(Old El Paso) 'Festive Dinners'	11 oz	590	24.0	51.0	1200	(mq)	31.0	(mq)
(Van de Kamp's) 'Mexican Dinner'	1/2 pkg	220	8.0	26.0	620	(mq)	9.0	(mq)

Food Name	Serv. Size	Total Cal.	Prot. GMS	Carbs GMS	Sod. MGS	Fiber GMS	Fat GMS	Chol. MGS
CHICKEN								
(Healthy Choice)	13.4 oz	340	14.0	61.0	470	na	5.0	30
(Healthy Choice)	9.5 oz	310	14.0	44.0	480	na	9.0	35
(Old El Paso) 'Festive Dinners'	11 oz	460	21.0	54.0	770	(mq)	18.0	(mq)
(Weight Watchers) nacho grande								
'Mexican Style'	9 oz	280	14.0	38.0	590	na	8.0	20
ENCHILADA DINNER, MIX								
(Old El Paso) prepared	1 enchilada	145	7.0	11.0	325	2.0	3.0	21
(Tio Sancho) 'Dinner Kit'	1 shell	80	1.3	10.8	2	>.6 c	3.5	na
(Tio Sancho) 'Dinner Kit' and sauce mix	3 oz	278	4.5	62.0	4058	>1.8 c	1.5	na
ENCHILADA ENTRÉE, FROZEN. See also ENCHILADA DINNER, FROZEN.								
BEEF								
(Hormel)	1 enchilada	140	6.0	17.0	573	(mq)	(mq)	(mq)
(Old El Paso)	1 pkg	210	8.0	16.0	720	(mq)	13.0	10
(Ultimate 200) Ranchero	9.12 oz	190	18.0	18.0	500	na	5.0	20
(Van de Kamp's) 'Mexican Entrées'	1 pkg	270	11.0	30.0	1040	(mq)	12.0	(mq)
(Van de Kamp's) 'Mexican Entrées Family Pack'	1/4 pkg	150	7.0	19.0	530	(mq)	5.0	(mq)
(Van de Kamp's) shredded, 'Mexican Entrées'	1 pkg	360	20.0	40.0	1010	(mq)	14.0	(mq)
BLACK BEAN-VEGETABLE								
(Amy's Kitchen)	4.75 oz	135	4.0	20.0	290	2.0	4.0	0
CHEESE								
(Amy's Kitchen) organic	4.75 oz	210	11.0	16.0	290	2.0	9.0	19
(Hormel)	1 enchilada	151	6.0	18.0	676	(mq)	(mq)	(mq)
(Old El Paso)	1 pkg	250	10.0	24.0	830	(mq)	12.0	(mq)
(Stouffer's)	9.75 oz	490	23.0	33.0	550	na	29.0	na
(Van de Kamp's) 'Mexican Entrées'	1 pkg	300	11.0	31.0	980	(mq)	15.0	(mq)
(Van de Kamp's) 'Mexican Entrées Family Pack'	1/4 pkg	200	7.0	19.0	460	(mq)	10.0	(mq)
CHICKEN								
(Le Menu) 'Light Style'	8 oz	280	21.0	32.0	530	(mq)	8.0	35
(Old El Paso)	1 pkg	220	8.0	20.0	740	(mq)	12.0	(mq)
(Old El Paso) w/sour cream sauce	1 pkg	280	10.0	18.0	520	(mq)	19.0	(mq)
(Stouffer's)	10 oz	490	21.0	31.0	860	na	31.0	na
(Van de Kamp's) 'Mexican Entrées'	1 pkg	260	13.0	27.0	1010	(mq)	11.0	(mq)
RANCHERO *(Van de Kamp's)* 'Mexican Entrées'	1/2 pkg	260	11.0	26.0	630	(mq)	12.0	(mq)
SUIZA								
(Van de Kamp's) 'Mexican Entrées'	1 pkg	230	12.0	23.0	390	(mq)	10.0	(mq)
(Weight Watchers)	9 oz	230	16.0	25.0	530	na	7.0	40
VEGETABLE *(Legume)* w/tofu and sauce	11 oz	270	14.0	36.0	390	10.3	8.0	0

Food Name	Serv. Size	Total Cal.	Prot. GMS	Carbs GMS	Sod. MGS	Fiber GMS	Fat GMS	Chol. MGS
ENCHILADA SEASONING MIX								
(Old El Paso)	1/8 pkg	6	0.0	1.0	80	0	0.0	0
(Lawry's) 'Seasoning Blends'	1 pkg	152	5.3	29.9	1723	1.2	1.2	na
ENDIVE								
approx 1.3 lb	1 head	87	6.4	17.2	113	15.9	1.0	0
chopped	1/2 cup	4	0.3	0.8	6	.8	0.1	0
trimmed	1 oz	5	0.4	0.9	6	>.3 c	0.1	0
untrimmed	1 lb	65	4.9	13.1	87	>3.5 c	0.8	0
ENGLISH MUFFIN								
(Earth Grains)								
oat bran, 12-oz pkg	1 muffin	120	5.0	24.0	410	2.0	1.0	0
plain, 12.5-oz pkg	1 muffin	130	5.0	26.0	410	1.0	1.0	0
plain, 12-oz pkg	1 muffin	120	5.0	25.0	390	1.0	1.0	0
raisin, 14-oz pkg	1 muffin	160	5.0	33.0	300	1.0	2.0	0
raisin, 'Sun Maid' 15-oz pkg	1 muffin	160	5.0	34.0	180	2.0	1.0	0
sourdough, 12.5-oz pkg	1 muffin	130	5.0	26.0	410	1.0	1.0	0
sourdough, 12-oz pkg	1 muffin	120	5.0	25.0	390	1.0	1.0	0
whole wheat, 15-oz pkg	1 muffin	140	6.0	28.0	450	4.0	2.0	0
whole wheat, 14-oz pkg	1 muffin	130	6.0	26.0	420	4.0	1.0	0
(Hi Fiber)								
cinnamon raisin	1 muffin	110	4.0	21.0	275	5.0	1.0	0
multigrain	1 muffin	120	4.0	23.0	240	4.0	1.0	0
plain	1 muffin	110	5.0	21.0	280	5.0	1.0	0
(Oatmeal Goodness)								
cinnamon and raisin oatmeal	1 muffin	140	5.0	26.0	160	1.5	2.0	0
honey and oatmeal	1 muffin	140	5.0	26.0	160	1.5	2.0	0
(Oroweat)								
extra crisp	1 muffin	130	4.0	26.0	260	na	1.0	na
health nut	1 muffin	170	6.0	29.0	220	1.0	4.0	0
sourdough	1 muffin	140	4.0	27.0	370	na	1.0	na
(Pepperidge Farm)								
cinnamon apple	1 muffin	140	4.0	27.0	210	(mq)	1.0	0
cinnamon chip	1 muffin	160	4.0	28.0	180	(mq)	3.0	0
cinnamon raisin	1 muffin	150	4.0	29.0	200	(mq)	2.0	0
plain	1 muffin	140	5.0	27.0	220	(mq)	1.0	0
sourdough	1 muffin	135	4.0	27.0	260	(mq)	1.0	0
(Roman Meal)								
honey nut and oat bran, refrigerated	1/2 muffin	81	2.5	14.7	114	1.1	1.3	0
plain, 'Original'	1 muffin	146	6.4	28.5	350	2.7	1.8	0
wheatberry, 14-oz pkg	1 muffin	140	6.0	28.0	470	2.0	1.0	0
(Thomas')								
honey wheat	1 muffin	129	5.0	24.0	200	>.4 c	1.1	0
oat bran	1 muffin	116	4.2	26.0	192	2.9	1.2	0

Food Name	Serv. Size	Total Cal.	Prot. GMS	Carbs GMS	Sod. MGS	Fiber GMS	Fat GMS	Chol. MGS
plain	1 muffin	130	4.3	25.4	206	(mq)	1.3	0
raisin	1 muffin	153	4.5	30.4	200	>.2 c	1.5	0
rye	1 muffin	120	5.0	27.0	210	3.0	1.0	0
(Wonder) plain	1 muffin	130	4.0	26.0	280	1.2	1.0	0
ENSURE NUTRITION DRINK. See individual flavors.								
ENTRÉES. See individual entrées.								
EPPAW, raw	1/2 cup	75	2.3	15.8	6	>2.0 c	0.9	0
EQUAL. See SUGAR SUBSTITUTE.								
EUCHALON. See CANDLEFISH.								

F

Food Name	Serv. Size	Total Cal.	Prot. GMS	Carbs GMS	Sod. MGS	Fiber GMS	Fat GMS	Chol. MGS
FAJITA ENTRÉE, refrigerated								
(Chicken By George)	5 oz	170	28.0	2.0	370	na	6.0	85
FAJITA ENTRÉE, FROZEN								
beef (Healthy Choice)	7 oz	210	19.0	26.0	250	na	4.0	35
chicken (Healthy Choice)	7 oz	200	17.0	25.0	310	na	3.0	35
FAJITA ENTRÉE KIT								
(Tyson)	4 oz	80	7.0	2.0	240	na	2.0	na
(Tyson) wholesale club item	3.5 oz	160	10.0	18.0	420	na	5.0	30
FAJITA MARINADE (Old El Paso)	1/8 jar	14	0.0	3.0	450	0	0.0	0
FAJITA SAUCE. See SAUCE.								
FAJITA SEASONING MIX, 'Seasoning								
Blends' (Lawry's)	1 pkg	63	2.0	14.0	2118	>.5 c	0.4	na
FALAFEL								
(Casbah) mix, dry	1 oz	103	7.0	15.0	na	(mq)	2.0	0
(Fantastic Foods) mix 'Falafil' prepared	3 oz	129	8.0	20.0	188	(mq)	2.0	0
(Near East) mix, prepared	3 patties	270	13.0	22.0	680	(mq)	15.0	na
FARINA. See CEREAL, HOT.								
FAT, ALTERNATIVE, 'Neutral Nyafat'								
(Rokeach)	1 tbsp	99	0.0	0.0	0	0	11.0	0
FATHEAD. See SHEEPSHEAD.								
FAVA BEAN/horse bean/jack bean								
boiled, drained	4 oz	64	5.4	11.5	47	>2.2 c	0.6	0
mature seeds, boiled	1/2 cup	94	6.5	16.7	4	>.8 c	0.3	0
mature seeds, raw	1/2 cup	256	19.6	43.7	10	18.75	1.1	0
raw, trimmed	1/2 cup	40	3.1	6.4	28	>1.2 c	0.4	0
raw, trimmed	1 oz	20	1.6	3.3	14	>.6 c	0.2	0
raw, untrimmed	1 lb	317	24.6	51.5	220	>9.7 c	2.6	0
Canned								
mature seeds	1/2 cup	91	7.0	15.9	580	>.5 c	0.3	0

Food Name	Serv. Size	Total Cal.	Prot. GMS	Carbs GMS	Sod. MGS	Fiber GMS	Fat GMS	Chol. MGS
mature seeds, w/liquid	4 oz	81	6.2	14.1	514	>.5 c	0.2	0
Dried								
mature seeds, boiled	4 oz	125	8.6	22.3	6	5.8	0.5	0
mature seeds, boiled	1/2 cup	93	6.5	16.7	4	4.3	0.3	0
mature seeds, raw	1/2 cup	256	19.6	43.7	9	10.9	1.2	0
mature seeds, raw	1 oz	97	7.4	16.5	4	4.1	0.4	0
FEIJAO								
raw	1 fruit	25	0.6	5.3	2	na	0.4	0
raw, purée	1 cup	119	3.0	25.8	7	na	1.9	0
FENNEL/finocchio								
(Frieda's)	1 lb	68	5.0	11.8	408	(mq)	0.5	0
(Frieda's)	1 oz	4	0.3	0.7	26	(mq)	<.1	0
raw, bulb	1 bulb	73	2.9	17.1	122	na	0.5	0
raw, leaves	100 gm	28	2.8	5.1	9	>.5 c	0.4	0
raw, sliced	1 cup	27	1.1	6.3	45	na	0.2	0
FENNEL SEED								
whole	1 oz	98	4.8	14.8	25	>4.4 c	4.2	0
whole	1 tbsp	20	0.9	3.0	5	>.9 c	0.9	0
whole	1 tsp	7	0.3	1.0	2	>.3 c	0.3	0
whole (Durkee)	1 tsp	7	0.0	0.0	0	0	tr	na
whole (Laurel Leaf)	1 tsp	7	0.0	0.0	0	0	tr	na
whole (Spice Islands)	1 tsp	8	0.2	1.3	2	>.4 c	0.2	0
FENUGREEK SEED								
whole	1 oz	92	6.5	16.5	19	>2.9 c	1.8	0
whole	1 tbsp	36	2.5	6.5	7	>1.1 c	0.7	0
whole	1 tsp	12	0.9	2.2	2	>.4 c	0.2	0
FETTUCCINE ENTRÉE, FROZEN								
Alfredo (Healthy Choice)	8 oz	240	10.0	36.0	370	na	7.0	45
Alfredo (Lean Cuisine)	9 oz	280	14.0	41.0	570	na	7.0	15
Alfredo (Weight Watchers)	8 oz	230	15.0	28.0	550	na	7.0	25
Alfredo, 10-oz pkg (Stouffer's)	5 oz	245	8.0	22.0	400	na	14.0	na
Alfredo, w/broccoli 'Lowfat' (Weight Watchers)	8 oz	230	15.0	28.0	550	na	7.0	25
chicken (Healthy Choice)	8.5 oz	240	22.0	29.0	370	na	4.0	45
primavera (Green Giant)	1 pkg	230	13.0	26.0	610	6.0	8.0	25
primavera (Lean Cuisine)	10 oz	260	14.0	32.0	510	na	8.0	45
primavera 'Microwave Garden Gourmet' (Green Giant)	1 pkg	260	17.0	25.0	640	6.0	13.0	na
w/broccoli (Dining Lite)	9 oz	290	12.0	33.0	1020	(mq)	12.0	35
w/meat sauce (Budget Gourmet)	10 oz	290	16.0	34.0	980	(mq)	10.0	25
FETTUCCINE ENTRÉE, MIX								
Alfredo 'Pasta & Cheese' prepared (Kraft)	1/2 cup	180	7.0	19.0	590	(mq)	9.0	30

FIG 305

Food Name	Serv. Size	Total Cal.	Prot. GMS	Carbs GMS	Sod. MGS	Fiber GMS	Fat GMS	Chol. MGS
Alfredo 'Pasta & Sauce' (Hain)	1/4 pkg	180	5.0	27.0	420	(mq)	4.0	na
FETTUCCINE LUNCH, FROZEN								
Alfredo sauce 'Lunch Express' w/chicken								
(Lean Cuisine)	10.25 oz	240	16.0	31.0	540	6.0		22%
FIELD PEAS, CANNED								
'Fresh' (Allens)	1/2 cup	100	7.0	18.0	370	(mq)	<1.0	0
'Fresh' w/snaps (Allens)	1/2 cup	100	5.0	20.0	370	(mq)	<1.0	0
tiny, 'Fresh' w/snaps (Allens)	1/2 cup	70	6.0	13.0	340	(mq)	<1.0	0
w/snaps (Bush's Best)	1/2 cup	80	6.0	16.0	550	3.0	0.0	na
FIG								
candied	100 gm	299	3.5	73.7	34	>5.6 c	0.2	0
raw, w/o stem	1 large	47	0.5	12.3	1	2.1	0.2	0
raw, w/o stem	1 med	37	0.4	9.6	1	1.6	0.2	0
trimmed	1 oz	21	0.2	5.4	<1	>.3 c	0.1	0
w/stems	1 lb	333	3.4	86.1	5	>5.4 c	1.4	0
Canned								
in extra heavy syrup	4 oz	121	0.4	31.6	1	>.6 c	0.1	0
in extra heavy syrup, solid and liquid	1 cup	279	1.0	72.7	3	>1.4 c	0.3	0
in extra heavy syrup, w/1.75 tbsp liquid	3 fruits	91	0.3	23.7	1	>.5 c	0.1	0
in heavy syrup	4 oz	100	0.4	26.0	1	>.6 c	0.1	0
in heavy syrup, solid and liquid	1 cup	228	1.0	59.3	3	5.7	0.3	0
in heavy syrup, whole (Del Monte)	1/2 cup	100	0.0	28.0	10	(mq)	0.0	0
in heavy syrup, whole, Kadota 'Fancy'								
(S&W)	1/2 cup	100	0.0	28.0	10	(mq)	0.0	0
in heavy syrup, w/1.75 tbsp liquid	3 fruits	75	0.3	19.5	1	1.9	0.1	0
in light syrup	1/2 cup	87	0.5	22.6	2	2.2	0.1	0
in light syrup	4 oz	78	0.4	20.4	1	>.6 c	0.1	0
in light syrup, solid and liquid	1 cup	174	1.0	45.2	3	>1.4 c	0.3	0
in light syrup, w/1.75 tbsp liquid	3 fruits	59	0.3	15.3	1	1.5	0.1	0
in water	1/2 cup	65	0.5	17.3	2	>.7 c	0.1	0
in water	4 oz	60	0.5	15.9	1	>.6 c	0.1	0
in water, solid and liquid	1 cup	131	1.0	34.7	2	5.5	0.3	0
in water, w/1.75 tbsp liquid	3 fruits	42	0.3	11.2	1	1.8	0.1	0
Dried								
cooked	4 oz	122	1.5	31.3	6	>2.3 c	0.6	0
stewed	1/2 cup	140	1.7	35.8	7	6.2	0.6	0
uncooked	1 cup	507	6.1	130.1	22	18.5	2.3	0
uncooked	4 oz	289	3.5	74.1	15	10.5	1.3	0
uncooked, Calimyrna (Blue Ribbon)	1/2 cup	250	3.0	58.0	10	(mq)	2.0	0
uncooked, Calimyrna (Sun•Maid)	1/2 cup	250	3.0	58.0	10	(mq)	2.0	0
uncooked, Mission (Blue Ribbon)	1/2 cup	210	3.0	1.0	20	(mq)	(mq)	0
uncooked, Mission (Sun•Maid)	1/2 cup	210	3.0	1.0	20	(mq)	(mq)	0
uncooked, trimmed	10 fruits	477	5.7	122.2	21	17.4	2.2	0

Food Name	Serv. Size	Total Cal.	Prot. GMS	Carbs GMS	Sod. MGS	Fiber GMS	Fat GMS	Chol. MGS
FILBERT, SHELLED. See HAZELNUT, SHELLED.								
FILBERT BUTTER, roasted								
(Maranatha Natural)	2 tbsp	180	5.0	6.0	5	na	16.0	na
FILO DOUGH. See PHYLLO DOUGH.								
FINNAN HADDIE, smoked	4 oz	132	28.6	0.0	865	0	1.1	87
FINOCCHIO. See FENNEL.								
FISH. See individual listings.								
FISH CAKE								
fried	1 cake	103	8.8	5.6	106	0	4.8	25
fried, bite size	5 cakes	103	8.8	5.6	106	0	4.8	25
frozen (Mrs. Paul's)	2 pieces	190	9.0	24.0	690	(mq)	7.0	20
FISH DINNER, FROZEN								
(Healthy Choice) lemon pepper, 10.7 oz	1 serving	300	13.0	52.0	370	na	5.0	40
(Kid Cuisine) nuggets	7 oz	320	13.0	33.0	750	(mq)	15.0	45
(Morton)	9.75 oz	370	18.0	46.0	910	(mq)	13.0	65
(Swanson) n' chips	10 oz	500	20.0	60.0	960	(mq)	21.0	(mq)
FISH ENTRÉE								
Canned, Dijon 'Light' (Mrs. Paul's)	8.75 oz	200	21.0	17.0	650	(mq)	5.0	60
Frozen								
fillet of, divan (Lean Cuisine)	10 3/8 oz	210	27.0	13.0	490	na	5.0	65
fillet of, Florentine (Lean Cuisine)	9 5/8 oz	220	26.0	13.0	590	na	7.0	65
fillet of, Florentine 'Light' (Mrs. Paul's)	8 oz	220	25.0	10.0	820	(mq)	8.0	95
fish 'n fries 'Home Style Recipe'								
(Swanson)	6.5 oz	340	11.0	37.0	670	(mq)	16.0	(mq)
gems, fancy style (Wakefield)	4 oz	80	11.0	11.0	(mq)	(mq)	1.0	(mq)
gems, salad style (Wakefield)	3 oz	70	10.0	8.0	(mq)	na	1.0	(mq)
in herb sauce (Gorton's)	1 pkg	190	26.0	3.0	450	(mq)	8.0	90
Mornay 'Light' (Mrs. Paul's)	9 oz	230	24.0	12.0	670	(mq)	10.0	80
oven baked, w/vegetable medley								
(Ultimate 200)	6.64 oz	120	16.0	10.0	390	na	2.0	0
'Platters' (Banquet)	8.75 oz	450	31.0	33.0	(mq)	(mq)	22.0	95
salmon, Keta (Libby's)	3.7 oz	130	20.0	0.0	450	na	6.0	40
sticks 'Looney Tunes Sylvester' (Tyson)	7.5 oz	290	13.0	36.0	510	na	11.0	17
FISH FILLET, ALTERNATIVE								
vegetarian, frozen (Worthington)								
1.5-oz pieces	2 pieces	180	15.0	9.0	910	(mq)	9.0	0
FISH FILLET, FROZEN								
battered (Mrs. Paul's)	2 pieces	330	16.0	28.0	650	(mq)	17.0	60
battered (Van de Kamp's)	1 piece	170	7.0	13.0	350	(mq)	10.0	20
battered 'Crispy Batter' (Gorton's)	2 pieces	290	11.0	18.0	550	(mq)	19.0	35
battered 'Crispy Batter' large (Gorton's)	1 piece	320	12.0	20.0	680	(mq)	21.0	(mq)
battered 'Crunchy' (Gorton's)	2 pieces	230	13.0	16.0	420	(mq)	13.0	40
battered 'Crunchy' (Mrs. Paul's)	2 pieces	280	12.0	26.0	730	(mq)	14.0	22

Food Name	Serv. Size	Total Cal.	Prot. GMS	Carbs GMS	Sod. MGS	Fiber GMS	Fat GMS	Chol. MGS
battered 'Crunchy Microwave' (Gorton's)	2 pieces	340	10.0	17.0	400	(mq)	26.0	30
battered 'Crunchy Microwave' large (Gorton's)	1 piece	320	11.0	20.0	500	(mq)	22.0	35
battered, minced 'Portions' (Mrs. Paul's)	2 pieces	300	11.0	21.0	540	(mq)	19.0	33
battered 'Potato Crisp' (Gorton's)	2 pieces	300	12.0	18.0	360	(mq)	20.0	30
battered, tempura 'Light Recipe' (Gorton's)	1 piece	200	10.0	8.0	400	(mq)	14.0	30
battered 'Value Pack Portions' (Gorton's)	1 piece	180	7.0	13.0	490	(mq)	11.0	(mq)
breaded (Van de Kamp's)	2 pieces	280	11.0	18.0	280	(mq)	18.0	35
breaded 'Crisp and Healthy' baked (Van de Kamp's)	2 pieces	150	12.0	18.0	350	na	3.0	25
breaded 'Crispy Crunchy' (Mrs. Paul's)	2 pieces	220	13.0	23.0	380	(mq)	9.0	22
breaded, crispy 'Microwave' (Van de Kamp's)	1 piece	140	6.0	9.0	210	(mq)	9.0	15
breaded, crispy 'Microwave' large (Van de Kamp's)	1 piece	290	12.0	21.0	640	(mq)	17.0	25
breaded, 8 fillets (Healthy Choice)	2.5 oz	120	9.0	11.0	250	na	4.0	20
breaded, 4 fillets (Healthy Choice)	3 oz	140	10.0	14.0	300	na	4.0	25
breaded 'Light Recipe' (Gorton's)	1 piece	180	11.0	16.0	380	(mq)	8.0	30
breaded, minced 'Crispy Crunchy Portions' (Mrs. Paul's)	2 pieces	230	10.0	14.0	300	(mq)	15.0	25
breaded, reheated, 2 oz	1 piece	155	8.9	13.5	332	>.2 c	7.0	64
breaded 'Snack Pack' (Van de Kamp's)	2 pieces	220	8.0	13.0	280	na	10.0	20
breaded, 2 fillets (Healthy Choice)	3.5 oz	160	12.0	16.0	350	na	5.0	30
coated, ranch 'Specialty Microwave' (Gorton's)	1 piece	330	12.0	24.0	520	(mq)	21.0	(mq)
crispy, microwave (Van de Kamp's)	1 piece	140	6.0	9.0	210	na	9.0	15
crispy, microwave large (Van de Kamp's)	1 piece	290	12.0	21.0	640	na	17.0	25
in butter sauce 'Light' (Mrs. Paul's)	1 piece	140	20.0	1.0	520	na	6.0	40
marinated, Cajun style, catfish 'Select' (Gorton's)	1 fillet	220	22.0	3.0	560	na	13.0	90
FISH LOAF, cooked	1 loaf	1507	171.3	88.7	2151	0	45.0	486
FISH NUGGET, FROZEN, battered (Van de Kamp's)	4 pieces	130	5.0	8.0	310	na	9.0	10
FISH OIL								
herring	1 cup	1966	0.0	0.0	0	0	218.0	1670
herring	1 tbsp	123	0.0	0.0	0	0	13.6	104
menhaden	1 cup	1966	0.0	0.0	0	0	218.0	1136
menhaden	1 tbsp	123	0.0	0.0	0	0	13.6	71
menhaden, fully hydrogenated	1 cup	1849	0.0	0.0	0	0	205.0	1025

Food Name	Serv. Size	Total Cal.	Prot. GMS	Carbs GMS	Sod. MGS	Fiber GMS	Fat GMS	Chol. MGS
menhaden, fully hydrogenated	1 tbsp	113	0.0	0.0	0	0	12.5	63
salmon	1 cup	1966	0.0	0.0	0	0	218.0	1057
salmon	1 tbsp	123	0.0	0.0	0	0	13.6	66
sardine	1 cup	1966	0.0	0.0	0	0	218.0	1548
sardine	1 tbsp	123	0.0	0.0	0	0	13.6	97
FISH PASTE CAKE								
Japanese, block, steamed 'Kamoboko' ...	4 oz	111	13.6	11.0	1134	na	1.0	(mq)
Japanese, stick, grilled 'Chikuwa'	4 oz	143	13.8	15.3	1134	na	2.4	(mq)
FISH SEASONING MIX. See SEAFOOD SEASONING MIX.								
FISH STICKS, FROZEN								
battered *(Mrs. Paul's)*	4 pieces	210	7.0	15.0	590	(mq)	12.0	25
battered *(Van de Kamp's)*	4 pieces	160	8.0	12.0	350	(mq)	9.0	20
battered 'Crispy Batter' *(Gorton's)*	4 pieces	260	9.0	16.0	480	(mq)	18.0	25
battered 'Crunchy' *(Gorton's)*	4 pieces	210	7.0	15.0	240	(mq)	13.0	25
battered, minced *(Mrs. Paul's)*	4 pieces	220	8.0	20.0	630	(mq)	13.0	20
battered 'Potato Crisp' *(Gorton's)*	4 pieces	260	8.0	21.0	390	(mq)	16.0	20
battered 'Value Pack' *(Gorton's)*	4 pieces	190	9.0	17.0	420	(mq)	9.0	(mq)
breaded *(Healthy Choice)*	2.4 oz	120	8.0	14.0	350	na	4.0	20
breaded *(Van de Kamp's)*	4 pieces	200	9.0	15.0	290	(mq)	12.0	20
breaded 'Bunch o' Crunch' approx 2.7 oz *(Frionor)*	4 pieces	210	9.0	13.0	267	<.1	14.0	(mq)
breaded 'Crisp and Healthy' baked *(Van de Kamp's)*	4 pieces	120	9.0	17.0	330	na	2.0	15
breaded 'Crispy Crunchy' *(Mrs. Paul's)*	4 pieces	140	7.0	14.0	340	(mq)	6.0	20
breaded, crispy 'Microwave' *(Van de Kamp's)*	3 pieces	130	7.0	11.0	280	(mq)	7.0	15
breaded, minced 'Crispy Crunchy' *(Mrs. Paul's)*	4 pieces	190	9.0	18.0	560	(mq)	8.0	25
breaded 'Snack Pack' *(Van de Kamp's)*	4 pieces	170	8.0	13.0	270	na	10.0	20
breaded 'Value Pack' *(Van de Kamp's)*	4 pieces	170	8.0	13.0	270	(mq)	10.0	20
breaded w/whole wheat 'Microwave' *(Booth)*	2 oz	150	6.0	14.0	210	(mq)	8.0	(mq)
FIVE-SPICE, Oriental spice *(Tone's)*	1 tsp	9	0.3	1.9	2	.5	0.3	0
FLAN. See PUDDING MIX.								
FLATFISH. See FLOUNDER; HALIBUT SOLE.								
FLAX OIL								
(Spectrum Naturals) organic 'Veg-Omega 3'	1 tbsp	120	0.0	0.0	0	(tr)	14.0	(tr)
(Spectrum Naturals) organic 'Veg-Omega 3' cinnamon flavored ...	1 tbsp	120	0.0	0.0	0	(tr)	14.0	(tr)
FLAXSEED *(Arrowhead Mills)*	1 oz	140	5.0	11.0	<1	6.0	10.0	0

Food Name	Serv. Size	Total Cal.	Prot. GMS	Carbs GMS	Sod. MGS	Fiber GMS	Fat GMS	Chol. MGS
FLOUNDER								
dry-heat cooked	3 oz	99	20.5	0.0	89	0	1.3	58
raw	3 oz	77	16.0	0.0	69	0	1.0	41
FLOUNDER, FROZEN								
(Booth) Atlantic	4 oz	90	19.0	0.0	180	0	1.0	(mq)
(Finast)	4 oz	90	19.0	0.0	150	0	1.0	(mq)
(Gorton's) crunch breaded, fillet 'Select'								
approx. 2.9 oz	1 fillet	190	10.0	17.0	420	na	9.0	30
(Gorton's) 'Fishmarket Fresh'	5 oz	110	23.0	1.0	170	0	1.0	(mq)
(Mrs. Paul's) battered, fillets 'Crunchy'	2 pieces	220	12.0	23.0	560	(mq)	9.0	40
(Mrs. Paul's) breaded, fillets 'Light'	1 piece	240	16.0	20.0	450	(mq)	10.0	50
(SeaPak)	4 oz	90	20.0	0.0	120	0	1.0	(mq)
(Van de Kamp's) breaded fillets 'Light'	1 piece	260	18.0	21.0	480	(mq)	12.0	45
(Van de Kamp's) fillet 'Light'	1 piece	260	18.0	21.0	480	na	12.0	45
(Van de Kamp's) 'Natural'	4 oz	100	22.0	0.0	100	0	2.0	35
FLOUNDER ENTRÉE, FROZEN								
stuffed 'Microwave Entrees' *(Gorton's)* ...	1 pkg	350	25.0	21.0	850	(mq)	18.0	120
FLOUR. See also individual listings.								
all-purpose, 4 oz *(Gold Medal)*	1 cup	400	11.0	87.0	0	na	1.0	na
all-purpose, 4 oz *(Red Band)*	1 cup	290	10.0	85.0	0	na	1.0	na
all-purpose, 4 oz *(Robin Hood)*	1 cup	400	13.0	85.0	0	na	1.0	na
'Better for Bread' 4 oz *(Gold Medal)*	1 cup	400	14.0	83.0	0	na	1.0	na
'Drifted Snow' 4 oz *(Red Band)*	1 cup	400	11.0	87.0	0	na	1.0	na
'La Piña' 4 oz *(Red Band)*	1 cup	400	10.0	87.0	0	na	1.0	na
self-rising, 4 oz *(Gold Medal)*	1 cup	380	10.0	83.0	1520	na	1.0	na
self-rising, 4 oz *(Red Band)*	1 cup	380	9.0	83.0	1520	na	1.0	na
self-rising, 4 oz *(Robin Hood)*	1 cup	380	10.0	83.0	1520	na	1.0	na
'Softasilk' 1 oz *(Red Band)*	1/4 cup	100	2.0	23.0	0	na	0.0	na
unbleached, 4 oz *(Gold Medal)*	1 cup	400	11.0	87.0	0	na	1.0	na
unbleached, 4 oz *(Robin Hood)*	1 cup	400	13.0	85.0	0	na	1.0	na
'Wondra' 4 oz *(Red Band)*	1 cup	400	11.0	87.0	0	na	1.0	na
FLYING FISH								
raw	1 lb	413	95.3	0.0	(mq)	0	0.9	(mq)
raw	1 oz	26	6.0	0.0	(mq)	0	<.1	(mq)
FON GOOT YAM. See JICAMA.								
FONDANT. See CANDY.								
FORMULA, INFANT. See BABY FOOD.								
FRANKFURTER								
beef and pork, 1 oz	1 frank	91	3.2	0.7	318	0	8.3	14
cheesefurter/cheese smokie, 1 oz	1 frank	93	4.0	0.4	307	0	8.2	19
cheesefurter/cheese smokie, approx								
1.5 oz	1 frank	141	6.0	0.6	465	0	12.5	29
chicken, 1 oz	1 frank	73	3.7	1.9	388	0	5.5	29

Food Name	Serv. Size	Total Cal.	Prot. GMS	Carbs GMS	Sod. MGS	Fiber GMS	Fat GMS	Chol. MGS
raw, beef and pork, 2 oz	1 frank	182	6.4	1.5	638	0	16.6	28
raw, w/nonfat dry milk and cereal, 2 oz	1 frank	156	8.1	0.0	627	0	12.4	37
turkey, 1 oz	1 frank	64	4.1	0.4	404	0	5.0	30
(Ball Park)								
beef 'Lite'	1 frank	140	7.0	1.0	na	na	12.0	na
beef, pork and chicken 'Lite'	1 frank	140	7.0	1.0	na	na	12.0	na
(Boar's Head)								
beef, 1 oz	1 frank	80	4.0	<1.0	(mq)	0	7.0	15
pork and beef, 1 oz	1 frank	80	4.0	<1.0	250	0	7.0	15
(Butterball) turkey	1 frank	140	7.0	2.0	610	0	11.0	(mq)
(Eckrich)								
beef 'Jumbo'	1 frank	190	6.0	2.0	520	0	17.0	(mq)
beef '1-lb pkg'	1 frank	150	5.0	2.0	400	0	14.0	(mq)
'Bunsize'	1 frank	190	6.0	2.0	500	0	17.0	(mq)
cheesefurter/cheese smokie	1 frank	180	7.0	2.0	530	0	16.0	(mq)
'Jumbo Lean Supreme'	1 frank	140	7.0	2.0	490	0	12.0	(mq)
'1-lb pkg'	1 frank	160	5.0	2.0	420	0	14.0	(mq)
(Health Valley)								
chicken 'Weiners'	1 frank	96	5.0	1.0	90	0	8.0	49
turkey 'Weiners'	1 frank	96	5.0	1.0	112	0	8.0	35
(Healthy Choice) turkey, pork, and beef								
'Jumbo' lowfat	1 frank	70	8.0	5.0	570	na	2.0	20
(Healthy Favorites) w/turkey, 2 oz	1 frank	57	8.5	2.1	572	0	1.6	24
(Hebrew National) beef, 1.7 oz	1 frank	149	5.8	<1.0	497	0	14.0	15
(Hillshire Farm)								
beef 'Bun Size Wieners' 2 oz	1 frank	180	7.0	2.0	560	0	16.0	(mq)
beef 'Hot Links' 2 oz	1 frank	190	8.0	1.0	560	0	17.0	(mq)
cheesefurter/cheese smokie 'Bun Size Wieners' 2 oz	1 frank	180	7.0	2.0	530	0	16.0	(mq)
'Hot Links' 2 oz	1 frank	190	8.0	2.0	530	0	16.0	(mq)
natural casing 'Wieners' 2 oz	1 frank	180	6.0	2.0	470	0	17.0	(mq)
(Hormel)								
batter-wrapped, frozen 'Corn Dogs'	1 frank	220	7.0	21.0	656	(mq)	12.0	(mq)
batter-wrapped, frozen 'Tater Dogs'	1 frank	210	6.0	15.0	170	(mq)	14.0	(mq)
beef '1-lb pkg'	1 frank	140	5.0	1.0	463	0	13.0	(mq)
beef '12-oz pkg'	1 frank	100	4.0	1.0	362	0	10.0	(mq)
chili 'Frank 'n Stuff'	1 frank	165	7.0	2.0	517	na	15.0	(mq)
'Light & Lean 97' 1.6 oz	1 frank	45	6.0	2.0	390	na	1.0	15
Mexicali Dogs' 5 oz	1 frank	400	14.0	41.0	952	na	21.0	(mq)
'1-lb pkg'	1 frank	140	5.0	1.0	486	0	13.0	(mq)
smoked, beef 'Wranglers'	1 frank	170	7.0	2.0	619	0	15.0	(mq)
smoked 'Range Brand Wranglers'	1 frank	170	7.0	1.0	600	0	16.0	(mq)
smoked, w/cheese 'Wranglers'	1 frank	180	8.0	1.0	546	0	16.0	(mq)

Food Name	Serv. Size	Total Cal.	Prot. GMS	Carbs GMS	Sod. MGS	Fiber GMS	Fat GMS	Chol. MGS
'12-oz pkg'	1 frank	110	4.0	1.0	378	0	10.0	(mq)
(Hygrade) chicken 'Grillmaster'	1 frank	130	7.0	3.0	na	na	11.0	na
(JM)								
beef, 1.2 oz	1 frank	100	4.0	1.0	350	0	9.0	20
beef 'Jumbo' 2 oz	1 frank	180	6.0	2.0	600	0	16.0	33
beef '10 per lb pkg' 1.6 oz	1 frank	140	5.0	1.0	480	0	13.0	26
cheesefurter/cheese smokie 'Cheese								
Franks' 1.6 oz	1 frank	140	5.0	2.0	540	0	13.0	(mq)
'German Brand' 2 oz	1 frank	160	7.0	1.0	620	0	14.0	(mq)
1.2 oz	1 frank	110	4.0	1.0	370	0	10.0	16
'10 per lb' 1.6 oz	1 frank	140	5.0	1.0	490	0	13.0	22
w/cheese 'German Brand' 2 oz	1 frank	160	8.0	2.0	620	0	14.0	37
(Kahn's)								
beef	1 frank	140	5.0	2.0	500	0	13.0	(mq)
beef 'Bun Size Franks'	1 frank	190	6.0	3.0	560	0	17.0	(mq)
beef 'Jumbo'	1 frank	190	6.0	3.0	560	0	18.0	(mq)
beef w/cheddar 'Beef n' Cheddar'	1 frank	180	7.0	2.0	640	0	16.0	(mq)
cheesefurter/cheese smokie								
'Cheese Wiener'	1 frank	150	6.0	1.0	490	0	13.0	(mq)
smoked, beef 'Bun Size Beef Smokey'	1 frank	190	7.0	2.0	530	0	17.0	(mq)
smoked 'Big Red Smokey'	1 frank	170	8.0	2.0	550	0	14.0	(mq)
smoked 'Bun Size Smokey'	1 frank	180	8.0	2.0	550	0	15.0	(mq)
'Wieners'	1 frank	140	5.0	2.0	500	0	13.0	(mq)
(King Kold) beef, 2 oz	1 frank	173	9.0	1.0	815	0	16.3	(mq)
(Longacre)								
chicken	1 frank	63	4.0	1.0	230	0	5.0	30
turkey	1 frank	66	4.0	0.0	260	0	6.0	30
(Louis Rich)								
turkey 'Bun Length' 2 oz	1 frank	128	7.2	1.5	640	0	10.4	53
turkey, cheese, 1.6 oz	1 frank	109	6.1	1.3	523	0	8.9	44
turkey, 1.6 oz	1 frank	101	5.7	1.2	505	0	8.2	42
(Mr. Turkey)								
turkey, 1.6 oz	1 frank	106	5.5	0.9	440	0	8.9	31
turkey, cheese, 1.6 oz	1 frank	109	5.9	0.9	526	0	9.1	29
(OHSE)								
beef, 1 oz	1 frank	85	3.0	1.0	280	0	8.0	(mq)
chicken, beef, and pork, 1 oz	1 frank	85	3.0	1.0	260	0	8.0	(mq)
'Wieners' 1 oz	1 frank	90	3.0	1.0	300	0	8.0	(mq)
(Oscar Mayer)								
bacon and cheddar cheese 'Hot Dogs'								
1.6 oz	1 frank	137	6.3	1.0	501	0	12.0	29
beef 'Bun-Length Franks' 2 oz	1 frank	182	6.3	1.4	568	0	16.8	34
beef, deli 'Big & Juicy' 2.7 oz	1 frank	249	8.9	0.5	677	0	23.5	49

Food Name	Serv. Size	Total Cal.	Prot. GMS	Carbs GMS	Sod. MGS	Fiber GMS	Fat GMS	Chol. MGS
beef 'Franks' 2 oz	1 frank	181	6.3	1.4	583	0	16.7	35
beef, garlic 'Big & Juicy' 2.7 oz	1 frank	239	9.0	0.2	652	0	22.5	51
beef 'Light Franks' 2 oz	1 frank	131	6.8	0.9	594	0	11.1	23
beef, quarter lb, bun length 'Big & Juicy' 4 oz	1 frank	359	12.8	1.6	1146	0	33.5	64
beef w/cheddar 'Franks' 2 oz	1 frank	163	7.5	1.1	655	0	14.3	36
'Bun-Length Wieners' 2 oz	1 frank	184	6.3	1.4	571	0	16.9	34
cheesefurter/cheese smokie 'Hot Dogs' 1.6 oz	1 frank	143	5.4	1.1	480	0	12.9	30
cocktail 'Little Wieners' .3 oz	1 frank	28	1.1	0.2	92	0	2.6	5
hot and spicy 'Big & Juicy' 2.7 oz	1 frank	224	9.5	0.6	773	0	20.4	46
'Hot Dogs' 1.6 oz	1 frank	137	6.3	1.0	501	0	12.0	29
'Light Wieners' 2 oz	1 frank	127	7.3	0.3	623	0	10.8	30
97% fat free, turkey, beef 'Healthy Favorites'	1 frank	60	9.0	2.0	570	na	1.5	25
original 'Big & Juicy' 2.7 oz	1 frank	244	8.9	0.0	690	0	23.2	43
'Wieners' 2 oz	1 frank	181	6.3	1.4	576	0	16.9	36
(Pilgrim's Pride)								
'1-lb pkg' 2-oz frank	1 frank	118	7.8	1.1	456	0	8.8	31
'12-oz pkg' 1.5-oz frank	1 frank	88	5.8	0.8	342	0	6.6	24
(Quick Meal) w/chili, and cheese, 4.5 oz	1 frank	340	14.0	25.0	540	na	20.0	80
(State Fair) beef, batter-wrapped, on stick 'Corn Dogs' 2.67 oz	1 frank	210	6.0	24.0	na	na	10.0	na
(Tyson)								
chicken	1 frank	115	6.0	1.0	700	na	10.0	na
chicken, batter-wrapped 'Corn Dogs' 3.5 oz	1 frank	280	9.0	28.0	70	(mq)	14.0	75
w/cheese	1 frank	145	7.0	1.0	680	na	11.0	na
FRANKFURTER, ALTERNATIVE								
(Smart Dog) 'Lightlife' fat-free, 1.5 oz	1 frank	40	8.2	1.1	290	na	0.0	0
(White Wave Soyfood) 'Healthy' 1.5 oz	1 frank	120	7.0	5.0	340	na	8.0	0
(Worthington)								
canned 'Super-Links' 1.7 oz	1 frank	100	7.0	3.0	440	(mq)	7.0	0
canned 'Veja-Links'	2 franks	140	8.0	4.0	330	(mq)	10.0	0
frozen 'Leanies' 1.4 oz	1 frank	100	8.0	2.0	440	(mq)	6.0	0
frozen, on a stick 'Dixie Dogs' 2.5 oz	1 frank	200	8.0	21.0	640	(mq)	10.0	0
FRENCH ARTICHOKE. See ARTICHOKES, FRENCH.								
FRENCH BEAN								
boiled	4 oz	146	8.0	27.2	7	>1.6 c	0.9	0
dried, boiled	1/2 cup	111	6.1	20.7	5	>1.2 c	0.7	0
raw	1/2 cup	316	17.3	59.0	17	>3.4 c	1.9	0
raw, dried	1 oz	97	5.3	18.2	5	>1.1 c	0.6	0

Food Name	Serv. Size	Total Cal.	Prot. GMS	Carbs GMS	Sod. MGS	Fiber GMS	Fat GMS	Chol. MGS
FRENCH TOAST, FROZEN								
(Aunt Jemima) cinnamon swirl	3 oz	171	6.7	27.5	516	1.3	4.3	41
(Aunt Jemima) 'Original'	3 oz	166	6.7	26.5	554	1.3	4.4	46
(Aunt Jemima) sticks, and syrup 'Homestyle'	5.2 oz	400	7.0	48.0	640	(mq)	20.0	(mq)
(Aunt Jemima) wedges, and sausages 'Homestyle'	5.3 oz	360	13.0	40.0	780	(mq)	17.0	(mq)
(Downyflake)	2 slices	270	6.0	34.0	380	(mq)	12.0	73
(Downyflake) 'Extra Thick'	1 slice	150	5.0	11.0	340	(mq)	9.0	(mq)
(Downyflake) Texas style, and sausage	4.25 oz	400	10.0	37.0	550	(mq)	24.0	(mq)
(Krusteaz) cinnamon swir	2 slices	270	10.0	46.0	370	na	5.0	120
(Krusteaz) regular	2 slices	250	11.0	38.0	380	na	6.0	120
(Morningstar Farms) vegetarian, cinnamon swirl, w/patties	6.5 oz	380	24.0	37.0	1220	4.0	15.0	0
(Swanson) cinnamon swirl, w/sausages 'Great Starts'	5.5 oz	390	12.0	37.0	530	(mq)	21.0	(mq)
(Swanson) mini, w/sausage 'Great Starts'	2.5 oz	190	6.0	22.0	320	(mq)	9.0	(mq)
(Swanson) oatmeal, w/lite links 'Great Starts'	4.65 oz	310	13.0	35.0	500	(mq)	13.0	(mq)
(Swanson) w/sausages 'Great Starts'	5.5 oz	380	12.0	35.0	550	(mq)	21.0	(mq)
FRENCH TOAST, STICKS								
apple cinnamon (Farm Rich)	3 oz	310	6.0	39.0	300	(mq)	15.0	na
blueberry (Farm Rich)	3 oz	310	6.0	37.0	280	(mq)	14.0	na
original (Farm Rich)	3 oz	300	5.0	37.0	280	(mq)	15.0	na
FRENCH FRY SEASONING (Tone's)	1 tsp	5	0.2	1.0	1551	.2	0.1	0
FROG'S LEGS								
raw	100 gm	73	16.4	0.0	58	0	.0.3	50
raw	1 oz	21	4.6	0.0	(mq)	0	<1.0	(mq)
FROGFISH. See MONKFISH.								
FROSTING MIX								
(Betty Crocker)								
cherry 'Creamy' prepared w/margarine	1/12 pkg	180	0.0	31.0	100	(tr)	6.0	0
chocolate fudge 'Creamy' dry	1/12 pkg	140	<1.0	30.0	25	na	2.0	0
chocolate fudge 'Creamy' prepared w/butter	1/12 pkg	180	<1.0	30.0	70	na	6.0	10
chocolate fudge 'Creamy' prepared w/margarine	1/12 pkg	180	<1.0	30.0	70	na	6.0	0
coconut pecan 'Creamy' dry	1/12 pkg	110	1.0	19.0	5	na	4.0	0
coconut pecan 'Creamy' prepared w/butter, 2% milk	1/12 pkg	150	<1.0	19.0	50	na	8.0	10
coconut pecan 'Creamy' prepared w/margarine, skim milk	1/12 pkg	150	<1.0	19.0	50	na	8.0	0

Food Name	Serv. Size	Total Cal.	Prot. GMS	Carbs GMS	Sod. MGS	Fiber GMS	Fat GMS	Chol. MGS
milk chocolate 'Creamy' prepared								
w/margarine	1/12 pkg	170	1.0	29.0	40	(tr)	5.0	0
rainbow chip 'Creamy' prepared								
w/margarine	1/12 pkg	190	<1.0	32.0	50	(tr)	7.0	0
sour cream, chocolate fudge 'Creamy'								
prepared w/margarine	1/12 pkg	180	1.0	30.0	75	(tr)	6.0	0
sour cream, white 'Creamy' prepared								
w/margarine	1/12 pkg	170	0.0	31.0	100	(tr)	5.0	0
vanilla 'Creamy' dry	1/12 pkg	150	0.0	32.0	5	na	2.0	0
vanilla 'Creamy' prepared w/butter	1/12 pkg	170	0.0	32.0	50	na	5.0	10
vanilla 'Creamy' prepared w/margarine	1/12 pkg	170	0.0	32.0	50	na	5.0	0
white 'Fluffy'	1/12 pkg	70	<1.0	16.0	40	(tr)	0.0	0
(Estee)	1 tbsp	65	0.0	13.0	28	na	1.5	0
FROSTING, READY-TO-SPREAD								
(Betty Crocker)								
amaretto almond 'Creamy Deluxe'	1/12 tub	160	0.0	27.0	50	(tr)	6.0	0
butter pecan 'Creamy Deluxe'	1/12 tub	170	0.0	26.0	50	na	7.0	0
cherry 'Creamy Deluxe'	1/12 tub	160	0.0	27.0	50	na	6.0	0
chocolate 'Creamy Deluxe'	1/12 tub	160	<1.0	24.0	60	na	7.0	0
chocolate 'Creamy Deluxe Light'	1/12 tub	130	<1.0	28.0	60	na	2.0	0
chocolate chip 'Creamy Deluxe'	1/12 tub	170	<1.0	27.0	30	na	7.0	0
chocolate chip, coated								
'Creamy Deluxe Party'	1/12 tub	160	<1.0	24.0	60	(tr)	7.0	0
chocolate chip, double 'Creamy Deluxe'	1/12 tub	170	<1.0	24.0	60	(tr)	8.0	0
chocolate coconut almond								
'Creamy Deluxe'	1/12 tub	160	1.0	21.0	55	(tr)	8.0	0
chocolate w/dinosaurs								
'Creamy Deluxe Party'	1/12 tub	160	<1.0	24.0	60	na	7.0	0
chocolate w/red gel								
'Creamy Deluxe Party'	1/12 tub	160	<1.0	24.0	50	na	7.0	0
chocolate w/turbo racers								
'Creamy Deluxe Party'	1/12 tub	160	<1.0	24.0	50	na	7.0	0
coconut pecan 'Creamy Deluxe'	1/12 tub	160	<1.0	20.0	60	na	9.0	0
cream cheese 'Creamy Deluxe'	1/12 tub	170	0.0	26.0	70	na	7.0	0
dark Dutch fudge 'Creamy Deluxe'	1/12 tub	160	1.0	22.0	70	na	7.0	0
lemon 'Creamy Deluxe'	1/12 tub	170	0.0	28.0	70	na	6.0	0
milk chocolate 'Creamy Deluxe'	1/12 tub	160	<1.0	25.0	55	na	6.0	0
milk chocolate 'Creamy Deluxe Light'	1/12 tub	140	<1.0	29.0	60	na	2.0	0
rainbow chip 'Creamy Deluxe'	1/12 tub	170	<1.0	27.0	30	na	7.0	0
rocky road 'Creamy Deluxe'	1/12 tub	150	<1.0	20.0	50	(tr)	8.0	0
sour cream chocolate 'Creamy Deluxe'	1/12 tub	160	<1.0	23.0	100	na	7.0	0
sour cream white 'Creamy Deluxe'	1/12 tub	160	0.0	27.0	50	na	6.0	0
vanilla 'Creamy Deluxe'	1/12 tub	160	0.0	27.0	25	na	6.0	0

Food Name	Serv. Size	Total Cal.	Prot. GMS	Carbs GMS	Sod. MGS	Fiber GMS	Fat GMS	Chol. MGS
vanilla 'Creamy Deluxe Light'	1/12 tub	140	0.0	30.0	30	na	2.0	0
vanilla w/blue gel 'Creamy Deluxe Party'	1/12 tub	160	0.0	27.0	30	na	6.0	0
vanilla w/teddy bears 'Creamy Deluxe Party'	1/12 tub	160	0.0	27.0	25	na	6.0	0
(Duncan Hines)								
chocolate	1/12 tub	160	0.0	24.0	90	(tr)	7.0	na
cream cheese	1/12 tub	160	0.0	24.0	120	na	8.0	na
cream cheese 'Homestyle'	1/12 tub	160	0.0	26.0	75	na	6.0	0
dark chocolate 'Homestyle'	1/12 tub	160	0.0	25.0	75	na	6.0	0
Dutch fudge	1/12 tub	160	0.0	24.0	95	(tr)	7.0	na
lemon	1/12 tub	120	0.0	18.0	60	na	6.0	na
milk chocolate	1/12 tub	160	0.0	24.0	85	(tr)	7.0	na
milk chocolate 'Homestyle'	1/12 tub	160	0.0	25.0	75	na	6.0	0
vanilla	1/12 tub	160	0.0	24.0	80	(tr)	7.0	na
vanilla 'Homestyle'	1/12 tub	160	0.0	26.0	75	na	6.0	0
(Finast) milk chocolate	1/12 tub	160	0.0	25.0	105	(tr)	6.0	na
(Lovin' Lites)								
chocolate fudge	1/12 tub	130	1.0	28.0	95	1.0	2.0	0
milk chocolate	1/12 tub	130	1.0	28.0	95	1.0	2.0	0
vanilla	1/12 tub	130	0.0	29.0	70	0	2.0	0
(Pathmark)								
chocolate, creamy	1/12 tub	160	0.0	25.0	95	(tr)	6.0	na
fudge, creamy	1/12 tub	160	0.0	25.0	100	(tr)	7.0	na
white, creamy	1/12 tub	160	0.0	25.0	95	(tr)	6.0	na
(Pillsbury)								
butter fudge 'Frosting Supreme'	1/12 tub	140	1.0	22.0	50	na	6.0	0
caramel pecan 'Frosting Supreme'	1/12 tub	150	0.0	20.0	70	0	8.0	0
chocolate chip 'Frosting Supreme'	1/12 tub	150	0.0	27.0	70	(tr)	5.0	na
chocolate fudge 'Frosting Supreme'	1/12 tub	150	0.0	22.0	85	na	6.0	na
chocolate fudge 'Funfetti'	1/12 tub	140	0.0	23.0	80	na	6.0	0
chocolate, double Dutch 'Frosting Supreme'	1/12 tub	140	1.0	22.0	45	(tr)	6.0	na
coconut almond 'Frosting Supreme'	1/12 tub	150	1.0	17.0	60	(tr)	9.0	na
coconut pecan 'Frosting Supreme'	1/12 tub	160	0.0	17.0	60	(tr)	10.0	na
cream cheese 'Frosting Supreme'	1/12 tub	160	0.0	26.0	115	(tr)	6.0	na
decorator, all flavors except chocolate	1 tbsp	70	0.0	12.0	na	(tr)	2.0	0
decorator, chocolate	1 tbsp	60	0.0	11.0	na	(tr)	2.0	0
double Dutch 'Frosting Supreme'	1/12 tub	140	1.0	22.0	50	na	6.0	0
fudge 'Frosting Supreme'	1/12 tub	150	<1.0	24.0	80	(tr)	6.0	na
lemon 'Frosting Supreme'	1/12 tub	160	0.0	26.0	80	(tr)	6.0	na
milk chocolate 'Frosting Supreme'	1/12 tub	150	0.0	23.0	65	na	6.0	0

Food Name	Serv. Size	Total Cal.	Prot. GMS	Carbs GMS	Sod. MGS	Fiber GMS	Fat GMS	Chol. MGS
milk chocolate w/fudge swirl								
'Frosting Supreme'	1/12 tub	150	0.0	23.0	65	na	6.0	0
mint 'Frosting Supreme'	1/12 tub	150	<1.0	24.0	80	(tr)	7.0	na
mocha 'Frosting Supreme'	1/12 tub	150	<1.0	24.0	60	(tr)	6.0	na
sour cream vanilla 'Frosting Supreme'	1/12 tub	160	0.0	27.0	80	(tr)	6.0	na
strawberry 'Frosting Supreme'	1/12 tub	160	.0.0	26.0	75	(tr)	6.0	na
vanilla 'Frosting Supreme'	1/12 tub	160	0.0	26.0	75	(tr)	6.0	na
vanilla 'Funfetti'	1/12 tub	150	0.0	25.0	75	0	6.0	0
vanilla 'Funfetti Sunshine'	1/12 tub	150	0.0	25.0	75	0	6.0	0
vanilla, pink and white 'Funfetti'	1/12 tub	150	0.0	24.0	70	(tr)	6.0	na
vanilla w/fudge swirl 'Frosting Supreme'	1/12 tub	150	0.0	25.0	75	0	6.0	0
white, fluffy	1/12 tub	60	0.0	15.0	65	(tr)	0.0	0
FRUCTOSE								
(Estee)	1 tsp	16	0.0	4.0	0	na	0.0	0
(Estee) packet	1 pkt	12	0.0	3.0	0	na	0.0	0
(Featherweight)	1 tsp	12	0.0	3.0	0	0	0.0	0
FRUIT. See individual listings.								
FRUIT, MIXED								
Canned								
(A&P) in light syrup	1/2 cup	75	<1.0	20.0	10	(mq)	<1.0	0
(Del Monte) chunky	1/2 cup	80	0.0	23.0	10	(mq)	0.0	0
(Del Monte) chunky 'Lite'	1/2 cup	50	0.0	14.0	10	(mq)	0.0	0
(Del Monte) 'Fruit Cup'	5 oz	100	0.0	27.0	10	(mq)	0.0	0
(Del Monte) tropical	1/2 cup	90	0.0	26.0	10	(mq)	0.0	0
(Dole) pineapple and Mandarin orange								
segments	1/2 cup	80	0.0	19.0	5	na	<1.0	na
(Dole) tropical fruit salad	1/2 cup	70	0.0	17.0	10	na	0.0	na
(Finast) in heavy syrup, chunky	1/2 cup	70	0.0	18.0	10	(mq)	0.0	0
(Kraft) salad 'Pure'	1/2 cup	80	1.0	18.0	10	(mq)	0.0	0
(Libby's) in juice, chunky 'Lite'	1/2 cup	50	1.0	14.0	5	(mq)	0.0	0
(Pathmark) in juice, chunky	1/2 cup	50	1.0	14.0	15	(mq)	0.0	0
(Pathmark) in light syrup 'No Frills'	1 cup	150	1.0	39.0	20	(mq)	0.0	0
(S&W) in juice, chunky, sweetened,								
clarified	1/2 cup	90	1.0	21.0	5	(mq)	0.0	0
(S&W Nutradiet) chunky	1/2 cup	40	0.0	10.0	5	(mq)	0.0	0
(Sun Fresh) jar, chilled, in light syrup								
'Tropical Salad'	3.5 oz	88	1.2	18.7	39	2.3	0.9	1
Dried								
(Del Monte)	2 oz	130	1.0	34.0	10	(mq)	0.0	0
(SunSweet)	2 oz	150	1.0	39.0	20	(mq)	0.0	0
(SunSweet) bits	2 oz	150	2.0	40.0	50	(mq)	<1.0	0
(Sun•Maid)	2 oz	150	1.0	39.0	20	(mq)	0.0	0
(Sun•Maid) bits	2 oz	150	2.0	40.0	50	(mq)	<1.0	0

Food Name	Serv. Size	Total Cal.	Prot. GMS	Carbs GMS	Sod. MGS	Fiber GMS	Fat GMS	Chol. MGS
Frozen *(Birds Eye)* in syrup								
'Quick Thaw pouch'	5 oz	120	1.0	31.0	5	1.0	0.0	0
FRUIT AND NUT MIX								
(Estee)	14 pieces	70	2.0	6.0	15	na	5.0	0
(Estee)	4 pieces	35	1.0	3.0	0	(mq)	2.0	<1
(Planters) 'Caribbean Crunch'	1 oz	150	3.0	14.0	130	na	10.0	30
(Planters) 'Fruit 'n Nut'	1 oz	150	5.0	13.0	90	(mq)	9.0	0
FRUIT BAR, FROZEN. See also ICE BARS AND DESSERTS; SHERBET; SORBET.								
all flavors 'Fruit Juicee' *(Minute Maid)*	1 bar	60	0.0	14.0	0	na	0.0	0
blueberry and cream 'Fruit & Cream' *(Dole)*	1 bar	90	1.0	19.4	20	na	1.4	5
cherry 'Fresh Lites' *(Dole)*	1 bar	25	<1.0	6.0	6	na	<1.0	0
cherry and yogurt 'Fruit & Yogurt' *(Dole)*	1 bar	80	2.0	17.0	22	na	<1.0	(mq)
chocolate/banana and cream 'Fruit & Cream'								
(Dole)	1 bar	175	2.0	22.0	20	na	9.0	na
chocolate/strawberry and cream								
'Fruit & Cream' *(Dole)*	1 bar	140	2.0	23.0	20	na	8.0	0
coconut *(Sunkist)*	1 bar	170	3.0	15.0	70	(mq)	10.0	0
grape 'SunTops' *(Dole)*	1 bar	40	<1.0	9.0	5	na	<1.0	0
lemon 'Fresh Lites' *(Dole)*	1 bar	25	<1.0	6.0	16	na	<1.0	0
lemonade *(Sunkist)*	1 bar	90	0.0	24.0	5	na	0.0	0
lemonade 'SunTops' *(Dole)*	1 bar	40	<1.0	9.0	5	na	<1.0	0
orange 'Juice Bar' *(Sunkist)*	1 bar	100	0.0	25.0	0	na	0.0	0
orange, tropical 'SunTops' *(Dole)*	1 bar	40	<1.0	9.0	5	na	<1.0	0
peach and cream 'Fruit & Cream' *(Dole)*	1 bar	90	1.0	19.4	19	na	1.4	5
pineapple 'Fruit 'n Juice' *(Dole)*	1 bar	70	0.3	17.0	4	na	<.1	0
pineapple-orange 'Fresh Lites' *(Dole)*	1 bar	25	<1.0	6.0	7	na	<1.0	0
piña colada 'Fruit 'n Juice' *(Dole)*	1 bar	90	1.0	16.0	2	na	3.0	0
punch 'SunTops' *(Dole)*	1 bar	40	<1.0	9.0	5	na	<1.0	0
raspberry 'Fresh Lites' *(Dole)*	1 bar	25	<1.0	6.0	6	na	<1.0	0
raspberry 'Fruit 'n Juice' *(Dole)*	1 bar	70	0.2	16.0	14	na	<.1	0
raspberry and cream 'Fruit & Cream' *(Dole)*	1 bar	90	1.0	20.0	23	na	1.4	5
strawberry and cream *(Sunkist)*	1 bar	90	0.0	19.0	30	na	1.0	na
strawberry and cream 'Fruit & Cream'								
(Dole)	1 bar	90	1.0	19.3	22	na	1.4	5
raspberry and yogurt 'Fruit & Yogurt' *(Dole)*	1 bar	70	1.0	17.0	18	na	<1.0	(mq)
strawberry and yogurt 'Fruit & Yogurt'								
(Dole)	1 bar	70	1.0	17.0	16	na	<1.0	(mq)
strawberry 'Fruit 'n Juice' *(Dole)*	1 bar	70	0.2	16.0	6	na	<.1	0
wildberry *(Sunkist)*	1 bar	140	0.0	33.0	15	na	0.0	0
FRUIT COCKTAIL, CANNED								
(Del Monte)	1/2 cup	80	0.0	23.0	10	(mq)	0.0	0
(Hunt's)	4 oz	90	<1.0	23.0	7	<1.0	<1.0	0
fruit for salad *(Del Monte)*	1/2 cup	90	0.0	22.0	10	(mq)	0.0	0

Food Name	Serv. Size	Total Cal.	Prot. GMS	Carbs GMS	Sod. MGS	Fiber GMS	Fat GMS	Chol. MGS
in extra heavy syrup	4 oz	98	0.4	26.0	7	>.5 c	0.1	0
in extra heavy syrup, solid and liquid	1/2 cup	114	0.5	29.8	8	>.6 c	0.1	0
in extra light syrup	4 oz	51	0.5	13.2	5	>.5 c	0.1	0
in extra light syrup, solid and liquid	1/2 cup	55	0.5	14.3	5	>.6 c	0.1	0
in heavy syrup	4 oz	83	0.4	21.4	7	>.5 c	0.1	0
in heavy syrup (A&P)	1/2 cup	90	<1.0	24.0	15	(mq)	<1.0	0
in heavy syrup (Finast)	1/2 cup	90	0.0	24.0	9	(mq)	0.0	0
in heavy syrup (Pathmark)	1 cup	180	1.0	48.0	35	(mq)	0.0	0
in heavy syrup (S&W)	1/2 cup	90	1.0	24.0	15	(mq)	0.0	0
in heavy syrup, solid and liquid	1/2 cup	93	0.5	24.2	8	1.4	0.1	0
in juice	4 oz	52	0.5	13.4	5	.7	<.1	0
in juice (Featherweight)	1/2 cup	50	1.0	14.0	10	(mq)	0.0	0
in juice (IGA)	1/2 cup	60	1.0	15.0	10	(mq)	0.0	0
in juice (S&W)	1/2 cup	90	1.0	21.0	5	(mq)	0.0	0
in juice 'Lite' (Libby's)	1/2 cup	50	1.0	13.0	10	(mq)	0.0	0
in juice, solid and liquid	1/2 cup	57	0.6	14.7	5	1.4	0.1	0
in light syrup	4 oz	65	0.5	16.9	7	>.5 c	0.1	0
in light syrup, solid and liquid	1/2 cup	72	0.5	18.8	8	1.4	0.1	0
in pear juice (A&P)	1/2 cup	50	1.0	14.0	15	(mq)	<1.0	0
in water	4 oz	36	0.5	9.7	5	>.5 c	0.1	0
in water, solid and liquid	1/2 cup	39	0.5	10.4	5	1.3	0.1	0
'Lite' (Del Monte)	1/2 cup	50	0.0	15.0	10	(mq)	0.0	0
'No Sugar Added' (Finast)	1/2 cup	50	1.0	14.0	10	(mq)	0.0	0
'Regulars Unsweetened' (S&W Nutradiet)	1/2 cup	40	0.0	10.0	5	(mq)	0.0	0
FRUIT DRINK								
(Finast)	8 oz	80	0.0	21.0	15	(tr)	0.0	0
(Fruitopia) 'Fruit Integration' real fruit	8 oz	120	0.0	31.0	25	na	0.0	na
(Hi-C) 'Bubble Gum' aseptic box or chilled	6 oz	90	0.0	22.0	20	na	0.0	na
(Hi-C) 'Double Fruit Cooler'	6 oz	93	<.1	22.9	18	(tr)	<.1	0
(Hi-C) 'Double Fruit Cooler' aseptic box	6 oz	90	0.0	22.0	25	na	0.0	na
(Hi-C) 'Ecto Cooler'	6 oz	95	0.1	23.3	17	(tr)	<.1	0
(Hi-C) 'Ecto Cooler' aseptic box	6 oz	90	0.0	23.0	20	na	0.0	na
(Hi-C) 'Hula Cooler'	6 oz	97	0.1	23.9	17	(tr)	<.1	0
FRUIT JUICE								
(Juicy Juice) bottled	6 oz	100	1.0	23.0	10	na	0.0	na
(Juicy Juice) boxed	8.45 oz	140	1.0	33.0	10	na	0.0	na
(McCain) mixed fruit, 100% juice 'Junior'	4.2 oz	60	0.0	15.0	5	na	0.0	na
FRUIT JUICE COCKTAIL								
'Orchard Harvest Blend' (Welch's)	6 oz	110	0.0	27.0	20	0	0.0	0
'Orchard Harvest Blend' 'Cocktails-In-A-Box' (Welch's)	8.45 oz	150	0.0	38.0	20	0	0.0	0
'Orchard Harvest Blend' frozen, prepared (Welch's)	6 oz	110	0.0	27.0	10	0	0.0	0

Food Name	Serv. Size	Total Cal.	Prot. GMS	Carbs GMS	Sod. MGS	Fiber GMS	Fat GMS	Chol. MGS
FRUIT JUICE DRINK, mixed 'Fruit Box'								
(Tang)	8.45 oz	140	0.0	36.0	10	na	0.0	0
FRUIT JUICE DRINK MIX								
'Mixes w/Fruit Juice' powder								
(Ultra Slim Fast)	1 scoop	90	10.0	17.0	75	6.0	0.0	na
'Mixes w/Fruit Juice' prepared								
w/orange juice								
(Ultra Slim Fast)	8 oz	200	11.0	43.0	80	6.0	<1.0	na
FRUIT JUICE PUNCH DRINK								
concentrate, prepared w/water	1 cup	124	0.3	30.3	12	>.3 c	0.5	0
concentrate, prepared w/water	1 oz	15	0.0	3.8	2	(tr)	0.1	0
concentrate, undiluted	12 oz	739	1.2	182.1	41	(tr)	3.0	0
(Veryfine) can, bottle, or box								
'100% Juice Punch'	8 oz	122	<1.0	30.0	10	(tr)	0.0	0
FRUIT PUNCH								
(Bright & Early) frozen 'Bright & Early Fruit Punch'								
prepared	6 oz	90	0.0	22.0	5	na	0.0	na
(Juicy Juice) can, bottle, or box	6 oz	100	1.0	23.0	10	(tr)	0.0	0
(Minute Maid) aseptic box, canned,								
or chilled	6 oz	90	0.0	22.0	20	na	0.0	na
(Minute Maid) frozen, concentrate,								
prepared	6 oz	90	0.0	23.0	0	na	0.0	na
(Pathmark) can, bottle, or box	6 oz	90	0.0	22.0	0	(tr)	0.0	0
(Snapple)	8 oz	120	0.0	29.0	5	na	0.0	0
FRUIT PUNCH DRINK								
(All Sport) thirst quencher, caffeine-free	8 oz	80	0.0	21.0	55	na	0.0	na
(Bama)	8.45 oz	130	0.0	32.0	15	(tr)	0.0	0
(Crowley)	8 oz	130	0.0	32.0	15	(tr)	0.0	0
(Gatorade) low sodium, no caffeine	8 oz	50	0.0	14.0	110	na	0.0	0
(Hawaiian Punch) island fruit	6 oz	90	0.0	22.0	30	(tr)	0.0	0
(Hawaiian Punch) red 'Fruit Juicy'	6 oz	90	0.0	22.0	20	(tr)	0.0	0
(Hawaiian Punch) red 'Fruit Juicy Lite'	6 oz	60	0.0	15.0	30	(tr)	0.0	0
(Hawaiian Punch) tropical	6 oz	90	0.0	22.0	30	(tr)	0.0	0
(Hawaiian Punch) tropical, wild fruit	6 oz	90	0.0	23.0	35	(tr)	0.0	0
(Hi-C)	6 oz	96	0.1	23.7	17	(tr)	<.1	0
(Hi-C) aseptic box or chilled	6 oz	90	0.0	23.0	20	na	0.0	na
(Hi-C) 'Hula Punch'	6 oz	87	0.1	21.4	17	(tr)	<.1	0
(Hi-C) 'Hula Punch Drink' aseptic box	6 oz	90	0.0	23.0	20	na	0.0	na
(J. Hungerford) 20% juice	9.03 oz	43	0.0	11.2	32	0	0.0	0
(J. Hungerford) 50% juice	9.03 oz	107	0.3	26.6	7	0	0.0	0
(J. Hungerford) 100% juice	9.03 oz	116	0.5	29.5	11	0	0.0	0
(Mott's)	10 oz	170	0.0	42.0	4	(tr)	0.0	0
(Mott's)	9.5 oz	161	0.0	40.0	4	(tr)	0.0	0

Food Name	Serv. Size	Total Cal.	Prot. GMS	Carbs GMS	Sod. MGS	Fiber GMS	Fat GMS	Chol. MGS
(PowerAde) thirst quencher, high energy	8 oz	70	0.0	19.0	70	na	0.0	na
(10-K)	8 oz	60	0.0	15.0	55	na	0.0	na
(Tropicana)	6 oz	90	<1.0	21.0	15	na	<1.0	na
(Tropicana) 'Single Serve'	10 oz	148	(tr)	37.0	3	(tr)	0.0	0
(Welch's) 'Orchard Fruit Harvest Punch'	10 oz	180	0.0	45.0	0	0	0.0	0
(Wyler's)	6 oz	84	0.0	21.3	8	(tr)	0.1	0
(Wyler's) tropical	6 oz	157	0.0	39.3	10	0	0.0	0
(Wyler's) tropical 'Fruit Slush'	4 oz	157	0.0	39.3	10	(tr)	0.0	0
FRUIT PUNCH DRINK MIX								
frozen concentrate, prepared	12 oz	677	0.8	173.0	33	0	0.0	0
frozen, prepared w/water	1 cup	114	0.0	28.9	10	0	0.0	0
frozen, prepared w/water	1 oz	14	0.0	3.6	1	0	0.0	0
instant 'Thirst Quencher' prepared								
(Gatorade)	8 oz	60	0.0	15.0	110	na	0.0	na
'No Frills' prepared *(Pathmark)*	8 oz	90	0.0	22.0	85	(tr)	0.0	0
powder, w/added sodium, dry	2 rounded tbsp	97	0.0	24.8	30	0	0.0	0
powder, w/added sodium, prepared	8 oz	97	0.0	24.9	37	0	0.0	0
powder, w/o added sodium, dry	2 rounded tbsp	97	0.0	24.8	11	0	0.0	0
powder, w/o added sodium, prepared	8 oz	97	0.0	24.9	10	0	0.0	0
sugar-free, prepared *(Crystal Light)*	8 oz	4	0.0	0.0	0	0	0.0	0
sugar-free, w/NutraSweet, prepared								
(Crystal Light)	8 oz	4	0.0	0.0	0	na	0.0	0
tropical 'Crystals' prepared *(Wyler's)*	8 oz	85	0.0	21.1	18	(tr)	0.1	0

FRUIT ROLL. See FRUIT SNACK.

FRUIT SALAD, CANNED. See FRUIT COCKTAIL, CANNED.

FRUIT SNACK

Food Name	Serv. Size	Total Cal.	Prot. GMS	Carbs GMS	Sod. MGS	Fiber GMS	Fat GMS	Chol. MGS
all flavors 'Berry Bears' *(Betty Crocker)*	1 pouch	100	<1.0	22.0	20	na	<1.0	0
all flavors 'Fruit Roll-Ups Peel-Outs'								
(Betty Crocker)	1 roll	50	<1.0	12.0	40	(mq)	<1.0	0
all flavors 'Shark Bites' *(Betty Crocker)*	1 pouch	100	<1.0	22.0	20	na	<1.0	0
apple *(Weight Watchers)*	1 pouch	50	<1.0	13.0	75	na	<1.0	0
apple chips *(Weight Watchers)*	.75 oz	70	0.0	19.0	110	na	0.0	na
apple roll *(Flavor Tree)*	1 piece	75	0.2	18.5	17	(mq)	0.0	0
apricot roll *(Flavor Tree)*	1 piece	76	0.3	17.7	17	(mq)	0.5	0
assorted flavors, all shapes 'Fun Fruits'								
(Sunkist)	1 pouch	100	0.1	21.8	10	na	1.4	0
assorted flavors 'Bugs Bunny and								
Friends' *(Betty Crocker)*	1 pouch	90	<1.0	21.0	30	na	1.0	na
assorted flavors 'Chip 'N Dale Rescue								
Rangers' *(Fruit Parade)*	1 pouch	100	0.0	22.0	10	na	1.0	na
assorted flavors 'Darkwing Duck'								
(Fruit Parade)	1 pouch	100	0.0	22.0	10	na	1.0	na
assorted flavors 'Dinosaurs' *(Farley's)*	1 oz	90	1.0	22.0	0	na	<1.0	na

Food Name	Serv. Size	Total Cal.	Prot. GMS	Carbs GMS	Sod. MGS	Fiber GMS	Fat GMS	Chol. MGS
assorted flavors 'Fruit Circus Fruit Bears'								
(Flavor Tree)	1.05 oz	117	0.1	25.4	12	na	1.6	0
assorted flavors 'Tale Spin' (Fruit Parade)	1 pouch	100	0.0	22.0	10	na	1.0	na
assorted flavors 'Tasmanian Devil'								
(Betty Crocker)	1 pouch	90	<1.0	21.0	30	na	1.0	na
assorted flavors 'Teenage Mutant Ninja								
Turtles' (Farley's)	1 oz	90	1.0	22.0	0	na	<1.0	na
assorted flavors 'Trolls' (Farley's)	1 oz	90	1.0	22.0	0	na	<1.0	na
berry 'Fun Fruits Berry Bunch' (Sunkist)	1 pouch	100	0.1	21.8	10	na	1.4	0
cherry 'Fruit by the Foot' (Betty Crocker) ..	1 roll	80	<1.0	17.0	45	na	2.0	na
cherry 'Fruit Roll-Ups' (Betty Crocker)	.5-oz roll	50	<1.0	12.0	40	na	<1.0	na
cherry 'Fun Fruits' (Sunkist)	1 pouch	100	0.1	21.8	10	na	1.4	0
cherry 'Wild Cherry Gushers' w/juicy								
centers (Betty Crocker)	1 pouch	90	<1.0	21.0	40	na	1.0	na
cherry roll (Flavor Tree)	1 piece	75	0.3	18.3	18	(mq)	0.1	0
cinnamon flavor (Weight Watchers) ...	1 pouch	50	<1.0	13.0	75	na	<1.0	0
compote (Rokeach)	4 oz	120	1.0	31.0	4	(mq)	1.0	0
crazy colors 'Fruit Roll-Ups'								
(Betty Crocker)	.5-oz roll	50	<1.0	12.0	40	na	<1.0	0
'Fun Fruits Fantastic Fruit' (Sunkist) ...	1 pouch	100	0.1	21.8	10	na	1.4	0
'Garfield and Friends' 'Wild Blue'								
(Betty Crocker)	1 roll	50	<1.0	12.0	20	(mq)	<1.0	0
grape 'Fruit by the Foot' (Betty Crocker) ..	1 roll	80	<1.0	17.0	45	na	2.0	na
grape 'Fruit Roll-Ups' (Betty Crocker) ..	.5-oz roll	50	<1.0	12.0	40	na	<1.0	na
grape 'Fun Fruits' (Sunkist)	1 pouch	100	0.1	21.8	10	na	1.4	0
grape 'Gushin Grape Gushers'								
(Betty Crocker)	1 pouch	90	<1.0	21.0	45	na	<1.0	na
grape roll (Flavor Tree)	1 piece	76	0.2	18.5	13	(mq)	0.1	0
orange 'Fun Fruits' (Sunkist)	1 pouch	100	0.1	21.8	10	na	1.4	0
peach (Weight Watchers)	.5 oz	50	<1.0	13.0	75	na	<1.0	na
raspberry 'Fruit Roll-Ups'								
(Betty Crocker)	.5-oz roll	50	<1.0	12.0	40	na	<1.0	na
raspberry roll (Flavor Tree)	1 piece	75	0.2	18.3	20	(mq)	0.1	0
strawberry (Weight Watchers)	1 pouch	50	<1.0	13.0	75	na	<1.0	0
strawberry 'Fruit by the Foot'								
(Betty Crocker)	1 roll	80	<1.0	17.0	45	na	2.0	na
strawberry 'Fruit Roll-Ups'								
(Betty Crocker)	.5-oz roll	50	<1.0	12.0	40	na	<1.0	na
strawberry 'Fun Fruits' (Sunkist)	1 pouch	100	0.1	21.8	10	na	1.4	0
strawberry roll (Flavor Tree)	1 piece	74	0.2	18.0	11	(mq)	0.1	0
strawberry 'Strawberry Splash Gushers'								
(Betty Crocker)	1 pouch	90	<1.0	21.0	45	na	1.0	na

Food Name	Serv. Size	Total Cal.	Prot. GMS	Carbs GMS	Sod. MGS	Fiber GMS	Fat GMS	Chol. MGS
strawberry, yogurt coated								
'Creme Supremes' (Sunkist)	1 pouch	114	0.2	20.1	19	na	3.6	na
FRUIT SPREAD								
all flavors 'Homestyle' (Smucker's)	1 tsp	15	0.0	3.0	0	na	0.0	na
all flavors 'Slenderella' (Smucker's)	1 tsp	7	0.0	2.0	0	0	0.0	0
apple, no sugar added (Fifty 50)	1 tsp	2	0.0	<1.0	5	0	0.0	0
apricot 'All Fruit Spreadable Fruit' (Polaner)	1 tsp	14	0.0	4.0	0	na	0.0	na
apricot 'Light' w/NutraSweet (Smucker's)	1 tsp	7	0.0	2.0	0	na	0.0	na
apricot, low sugar (Smucker's)	1 tsp	8	0.0	2.0	10	na	0.0	na
apricot 'Simply Fruit' (Smucker's)	1 tsp	16	0.0	4.0	0	na	0.0	na
apricot-pineapple (Knott's Berry Farm)	1 tsp	16	0.0	4.0	0	na	0.0	na
apricot-pineapple 'Light' w/NutraSweet								
(Knott's Berry Farm)	1 tsp	8	0.0	2.0	0	na	0.0	na
apricot-pineapple, portion pack								
(Knott's Berry Farm)	.5 oz	35	0.0	9.0	0	0.0		0%
black cherry 'All Fruit Spreadable Fruit'								
(Polaner)	1 tsp	14	0.0	4.0	0	na	0.0	na
black raspberry 'Simply Fruit' (Smucker's)	1 tsp	16	0.0	4.0	0	na	0.0	na
blackberry (Knott's Berry Farm)	1 tsp	16	0.0	4.0	0	na	0.0	na
blackberry 'Light' w/NutraSweet								
(Knott's Berry Farm)	1 tsp	8	0.0	2.0	0	na	0.0	na
blackberry, low sugar (Smucker's)	1 tsp	8	0.0	2.0	10	na	0.0	na
blackberry, portion pack								
(Knott's Berry Farm)	.5 oz	35	0.0	9.0	0	na	0.0	na
blackberry 'Simply Fruit' (Smucker's)	1 tsp	16	0.0	4.0	0	na	0.0	na
blueberry 'All Fruit Spreadable Fruit'								
(Polaner)	1 tsp	14	0.0	4.0	0	na	0.0	na
blueberry 'Simply Fruit' (Smucker's)	1 tsp	16	0.0	4.0	0	na	0.0	na
boysenberry (Knott's Berry Farm)	1 tsp	16	0.0	4.0	0	na	0.0	na
boysenberry 'Light' w/NutraSweet								
(Knott's Berry Farm)	1 tsp	8	0.0	2.0	0	na	0.0	na
boysenberry 'Light' w/NutraSweet								
(Smucker's)	1 tsp	7	0.0	2.0	0	na	0.0	na
boysenberry, low sugar (Smucker's)	1 tsp	8	0.0	2.0	10	na	0.0	na
boysenberry, portion pack								
(Knott's Berry Farm)	.5 oz	35	0.0	9.0	0	na	0.0	na
calamansi 'Tropical Rainforest'								
(Knudsen & Sons)	2 tsp	35	0.0	8.0	0	na	0.0	na
grape (Weight Watchers)	1 tsp	8	0.0	2.0	0	na	0.0	na
grape 'All Fruit Spreadable Fruit' (Polaner)	1 tsp	14	0.0	4.0	0	na	0.0	na
grape, Concord, low sugar (Smucker's)	1 tsp	8	0.0	2.0	0	na	0.0	na
grape 'Imitation' (Smucker's)	1 tsp	2	0.0	1.0	2	0	0.0	0
grape, no sugar added (Fifty 50)	1 tsp	2	0.0	<1.0	5	0	0.0	0

Food Name	Serv. Size	Total Cal.	Prot. GMS	Carbs GMS	Sod. MGS	Fiber GMS	Fat GMS	Chol. MGS
grape 'Simply Fruit' (Smucker's)	1 tsp	16	0.0	4.0	0	na	0.0	na
guanabana 'Tropical Rainforest' (Knudsen & Sons)	2 tsp	35	0.0	8.0	0	na	0.0	na
orange 'All Fruit Spreadable Fruit' (Polaner)	1 tsp	14	0.0	4.0	0	na	0.0	na
orange marmalade (Knott's Berry Farm)	1 tsp	16	0.0	4.0	0	na	0.0	na
orange marmalade 'Light' w/NutraSweet (Knott's Berry Farm)	1 tsp	8	0.0	2.0	0	na	0.0	na
orange marmalade 'Light' w/NutraSweet (Smucker's)	1 tsp	7	0.0	2.0	0	na	0.0	na
orange marmalade, low sugar (Smucker's)	1 tsp	8	0.0	2.0	10	na	0.0	na
orange marmalade, no sugar added (Fifty 50)	1 tsp	2	0.0	<1.0	5	0	0.0	0
orange marmalade, portion pack (Knott's Berry Farm)	.5 oz	35	0.0	9.0	0	na	0.0	na
orange marmalade 'Simply Fruit' (Smucker's)	1 tsp	16	0.0	4.0	0	na	0.0	na
peach 'Simply Fruit' (Smucker's)	1 tsp	16	0.0	4.0	0	na	0.0	na
raspberry (Weight Watchers)	1 tsp	8	0.0	2.0	0	na	0.0	na
raspberry 'All Fruit Spreadable Fruit' (Polaner)	1 tsp	14	0.0	4.0	0	na	0.0	na
raspberry 'All Fruit Spreadable Fruit' seedless (Polaner)	1 tsp	14	0.0	4.0	0	na	0.0	na
raspberry, no sugar added (Fifty 50)	1 tsp	2	0.0	<1.0	5	0	0.0	0
red raspberry (Knott's Berry Farm)	1 tsp	16	0.0	4.0	0	na	0.0	na
red raspberry 'Light' w/NutraSweet (Knott's Berry Farm)	1 tsp	8	0.0	2.0	0	na	0.0	na
red raspberry 'Light' w/NutraSweet (Smucker's)	1 tsp	7	0.0	2.0	0	na	0.0	na
red raspberry, low sugar (Smucker's)	1 tsp	8	0.0	2.0	0	na	0.0	na
red raspberry, portion pack (Knott's Berry Farm)	.5 oz	35	0.0	9.0	0	na	0.0	na
red raspberry 'Simply Fruit' (Smucker's)	1 tsp	16	0.0	4.0	0	na	0.0	na
strawberry (Weight Watchers)	1 tsp	8	0.0	2.0	0	na	0.0	na
strawberry 'All Fruit Spreadable Fruit' (Polaner)	1 tsp	14	0.0	4.0	0	na	0.0	na
strawberry 'Imitation' (Smucker's)	1 tsp	2	0.0	1.0	2	na	0.0	0
strawberry 'Light' w/NutraSweet (Knott's Berry Farm)	1 tsp	8	0.0	2.0	0	na	0.0	na
strawberry 'Light' w/NutraSweet (Smucker's)	1 tsp	7	0.0	2.0	0	na	0.0	na
strawberry, low sugar (Smucker's)	1 tsp	8	0.0	2.0	0	na	0.0	na
strawberry, no sugar added (Fifty 50)	1 tsp	2	0.0	<1.0	5	0	0.0	0

Food Name	Serv. Size	Total Cal.	Prot. GMS	Carbs GMS	Sod. MGS	Fiber GMS	Fat GMS	Chol. MGS
strawberry 'Simply Fruit' (Smucker's)	1 tsp	16	0.0	4.0	0	na	0.0	na
FRUIT SYRUP								
all flavors (Smucker's)	2 tbsp	100	0.0	26.0	0	na	0.0	0
'Fruit 'n Maple' (Knudsen & Sons)	1 oz	105	<1.0	26.0	na	na	<1.0	na
'Fruit 'n Maple' pourable (Knudsen & Sons)	1 oz	105	0.0	26.0	0	na	0.0	na
raspberry, pourable (Knudsen & Sons) ...	1 oz	75	0.0	18.0	0	na	1.0	na
strawberry, pourable (Knudsen & Sons) ...	1 oz	75	0.0	18.0	0	na	1.0	na
FUDGE TOPPING								
(Hershey's)	2 tbsp	100	1.0	14.0	30	(mq)	4.0	5
(Kraft) hot	1 tbsp	70	1.0	11.0	50	(mq)	2.0	0
(Mrs. Richardson's) hot	2 tbsp	140	1.0	20.0	75	na	7.0	0
(Mrs. Richardson's) hot, microwavable ..	2 tbsp	140	1.0	20.0	75	na	7.0	0
(Smucker's)	2 tbsp	130	1.0	31.0	50	(mq)	1.0	0
(Smucker's) hot	2 tbsp	110	1.0	18.0	55	(mq)	4.0	0
(Smucker's) hot 'Light'	2 tbsp	70	2.0	19.0	35	na	0.0	0
(Smucker's) hot 'Special Recipe'	2 tbsp	150	2.0	23.0	60	(mq)	5.0	0
(Smucker's) 'Magic Shell'	2 tbsp	190	1.0	16.0	50	(mq)	15.0	0

FUKI. See BUTTERBUR.

G

Food Name	Serv. Size	Total Cal.	Prot. GMS	Carbs GMS	Sod. MGS	Fiber GMS	Fat GMS	Chol. MGS
GARBANZO BEAN/ceci/chick pea								
boiled	4 oz	186	10.0	31.1	8	4.0	2.9	0
boiled	1/2 cup	134	7.3	22.5	6	>2.0 c	2.1	0
raw	1/2 cup	364	19.3	60.7	24	17.4	6.0	0
raw	1 oz	103	5.5	17.2	7	1.8	1.7	0
raw (Arrowhead Mills)	2 oz	200	12.0	35.0	9	7.0	3.0	0
Canned								
(A&P)	1/2 cup	100	6.0	17.0	270	(mq)	1.0	0
(Allens)	1/2 cup	110	5.0	18.0	320	(mq)	<1.0	0
(Bush's Best)	1/2 cup	80	5.0	21.0	350	6.0	0.0	na
(Eden Foods) organic, very low sodium, no salt added	1/2 cup	90	6.0	17.0	10	4.0	1.0	0
(Eden Foods) organic, w/liquid	1/2 cup	110	6.0	17.0	15	4.0	2.0	0
(Finast)	8 oz	210	10.0	35.0	250	(mq)	3.0	0
(Green Giant)	1/2 cup	90	6.0	18.0	320	5.0	2.0	0
(Green Giant) 50% less salt	1/2 cup	90	6.0	18.0	160	5.0	2.0	0
(Joan of Arc) 50% less salt	1/2 cup	90	6.0	18.0	160	5.0	2.0	0
(Old El Paso)	1/2 cup	190	5.0	16.0	250	(mq)	<1.0	0
(Progresso)	1/2 cup	110	9.0	22.0	200	6.0	1.0	0
(S&W) large, 50% less salt 'Lite'	1/2 cup	110	6.0	21.0	295	(mq)	1.0	0

Food Name	Serv. Size	Total Cal.	Prot. GMS	Carbs GMS	Sod. MGS	Fiber GMS	Fat GMS	Chol. MGS
(S&W Nutradiet)	1/2 cup	100	5.0	19.0	5	(mq)	1.0	0
GARBANZO FLOUR/chick pea flour								
(Arrowhead Mills)	2 oz	200	12.0	35.0	9	7.4	3.0	0
GARDEN SALAD								
(Joan of Arc) canned	1/2 cup	70	2.0	17.0	500	2.4	0.0	0
(Read) canned	1/2 cup	70	2.0	17.0	500	2.4	0.0	0
(S&W) refrigerated marinated	1/2 cup	60	2.0	11.0	670	(mq)	0.0	0
(Trader Joe's) refrigerated fresh vegetables, no-oil vinaigrette	1 container	90	3.0	17.0	770	2.0	1.0	5
(Trader Joe's) refrigerated w/eggless egg salad, no-oil vinaigrette	1 container	140	11.0	8.0	340	2.0	7.0	0
GARLIC								
trimmed	1 oz	42	1.8	9.4	5	>.4 c	0.1	0
untrimmed	1 lb	587	25.1	130.5	67	>5.9 c	2.0	0
GARLIC BREAD. See BREAD.								
GARLIC BREAD SEASONING								
'Garlic Bread Sprinkle' *(Schilling)*	1/4 tsp	5	<.1	0.1	25	na	0.4	na
GARLIC BREAD SPREAD *(Lawry's)*	1/2 tbsp	47	0.2	1.0	15	>.1 c	4.6	na
GARLIC PEPPER, 'Spice Blends' *(Lawry's)*	1 tsp	11	0.2	2.0	292	.1	<.1	0
GARLIC POWDER								
dry	1 oz	94	4.8	20.6	7	.5	0.2	0
dry	1 tbsp	28	1.4	6.1	2	.2	0.1	0
dry	1 tsp	9	0.5	2.0	1	.1	0.0	0
dry *(Durkee)*	1 tsp	10	0.0	0.1	0	0	tr	na
dry *(Laurel Leaf)*	1 tsp	10	0.0	0.1	0	0	tr	na
dry *(Lawry's)* w/parsley	1 tsp	12	0.5	2.3	5	.1	0.9	0
dry *(Spice Islands)*	1 tsp	5	0.3	1.1	<1	<.1	tr	0
GARLIC SALT								
(Lawry's)	1 tsp	4	0.1	0.8	968	<.1	<.1	0
(Morton)	1 tsp	3	<1.0	<1.0	1300	(mq)	<.1	0
GARLIC SEASONING								
(Gilroy) crushed	1 tsp	8	0.3	2.0	4	na	0.0	na
(Gilroy) minced	1 tsp	23	0.3	2.0	4	na	1.0	na
(Golden Dipt)	2 grams	8	0.0	1.0	87	na	0.0	0
(Schilling) 'Parsley Patch'	1 tsp	13	0.5	2.0	1	(mq)	0.5	0
(Schilling) 'Season All'	1/4 tsp	2	<.1	0.1	163	na	(tr)	0
GARLIC SPREAD, concentrate *(Lawry's)*	1 tbsp	15	0.0	0.2	21	0	1.6	0
GATORADE. See individual flavors.								
GEFILTE FISH								
Hors d'oeuvres *(Rokeach)*	8 balls	60	8.0	4.0	(mq)	(mq)	1.0	(mq)
In jelled broth								
(Mother's) 'Old Fashioned' 24-oz jar	1 ball	70	9.0	5.0	(mq)	(mq)	1.0	(mq)
(Mother's) 'Old Fashioned' 12-oz jar	1 ball	54	7.0	4.0	(mq)	(mq)	0.8	(mq)

Food Name	Serv. Size	Total Cal.	Prot. GMS	Carbs GMS	Sod. MGS	Fiber GMS	Fat GMS	Chol. MGS
(Mother's) 'Old World'	1 ball	70	8.0	7.0	(mq)	(mq)	1.0	(mq)
(Mother's) 'Unsalted'	1 ball	45	5.0	2.0	(mq)	(mq)	1.0	(mq)
(Rokeach) 'Old Vienna' 31-oz jar	3 oz	81	9.0	9.0	(mq)	(mq)	1.0	(mq)
(Rokeach) 'Old Vienna' 24-oz jar	2.6 oz	70	8.0	8.0	(mq)	(mq)	1.0	(mq)
(Rokeach) 'Old Vienna' 12-oz jar	2 oz	54	6.0	6.0	(mq)	(mq)	1.0	(mq)
(Rokeach) 'Redi-Jelled'	4 oz	92	12.0	6.0	444	(mq)	2.0	(mq)
(Rokeach) 'Redi-Jelled'	3 oz	65	9.0	5.0	333	(mq)	1.0	(mq)
(Rokeach) 'Redi-Jelled'	2 oz	46	6.0	3.0	222	(mq)	1.0	(mq)
In liquid								
(Mother's) 'Old Fashioned' 24- or 31-oz jar	1 ball	70	9.0	7.0	(mq)	(mq)	1.0	(mq)
(Mother's) 'Old Fashioned' 12-oz jar	1 ball	54	7.0	5.0	(mq)	(mq)	0.8	(mq)
In natural broth								
(Rokeach) 24-oz jar	4 oz	60	8.0	4.0	835	(mq)	1.0	(mq)
(Rokeach) 24-oz jar	2.6 oz	50	7.0	4.0	(mq)	(mq)	1.0	(mq)
Sweet (Mother's) 'Old World'	1 ball	54	6.0	5.0	(mq)	(mq)	0.8	(mq)
WHITEFISH								
In jelled broth								
(Mother's) 24- or 31-oz jar	1 ball	60	9.0	4.0	(mq)	(mq)	1.0	(mq)
(Mother's) 12-oz jar	1 ball	46	7.0	3.0	(mq)	(mq)	0.8	(mq)
In liquid								
(Mother's) 24- or 31-oz jar	1 ball	70	9.0	7.0	(mq)	(mq)	1.0	(mq)
(Mother's) 12-oz jar	1 ball	54	7.0	5.0	(mq)	(mq)	0.8	(mq)
WHITEFISH AND PIKE								
In jelled broth								
(Mother's) 24- or 31-oz jar	1 ball	60	9.0	4.0	(mq)	(mq)	1.0	(mq)
(Mother's) 12-oz jar	1 ball	46	7.0	3.0	(mq)	(mq)	0.8	(mq)
(Mother's) 'Old World'	1 ball	54	6.0	5.0	(mq)	(mq)	0.8	(mq)
(Rokeach)	2.6 oz	60	9.0	4.0	(mq)	(mq)	1.0	(mq)
(Rokeach)	2 oz	46	7.0	3.0	(mq)	(mq)	1.0	(mq)
In liquid (Mother's)	1 ball	70	9.0	7.0	(mq)	(mq)	1.0	(mq)
GELATIN, JAPANESE								
raw	1 lb	116	2.5	30.6	40	>2.0 c	0.1	0
raw	1 oz	7	0.2	1.9	3	>.1 c	tr	0
GELATIN, UNFLAVORED (Knox)	1 pkt	25	6.0	0.0	10	0	0.0	0
GELATIN DESSERT								
PREPARED FROM MIX								
(D-Zerta)								
all flavors	1/2 cup	8	2.0	0.0	0	0	0.0	0
all flavors, low calorie, w/aspartame	1/2 cup	8	2.0	0.0	0	na	0.0	0
(Featherweight)								
all flavors except lemon	1/2 cup	10	2.0	1.0	5	0	0.0	0
lemon	1/2 cup	10	2.0	1.0	4	0	0.0	0

Food Name	Serv. Size	Total Cal.	Prot. GMS	Carbs GMS	Sod. MGS	Fiber GMS	Fat GMS	Chol. MGS
(Jell-O)								
berry blue	1/2 cup	80	2.0	19.0	50	na	0.0	0
black raspberry	1/2 cup	80	2.0	19.0	35	(tr)	0.0	0
cherry	1/2 cup	80	2.0	19.0	70	(tr)	0.0	0
cherry, sugar-free	1/2 cup	8	1.0	0.0	80	na	0.0	0
Concord grape	1/2 cup	80	2.0	19.0	35	(tr)	0.0	0
lemon	1/2 cup	80	2.0	19.0	75	(tr)	0.0	0
lemon, sugar-free	1/2 cup	8	1.0	0.0	60	na	0.0	0
lime	1/2 cup	80	2.0	19.0	55	(tr)	0.0	0
lime, sugar-free	1/2 cup	8	1.0	0.0	65	na	0.0	0
orange, sugar-free	1/2 cup	8	1.0	0.0	55	na	0.0	0
orange-pineapple	1/2 cup	80	2.0	19.0	65	(tr)	0.0	0
raspberry, sugar-free	1/2 cup	8	1.0	0.0	55	na	0.0	0
strawberry, sugar-free	1/2 cup	8	1.0	0.0	65	na	0.0	0
strawberry banana, sugar-free	1/2 cup	8	1.0	0.0	55	na	0.0	0
watermelon	1/2 cup	80	2.0	20.0	50	na	0.0	0
wild strawberry	1/2 cup	80	2.0	19.0	75	(tr)	0.0	0
(Royal)								
apple	1/2 cup	80	2.0	19.0	95	na	0.0	na
blackberry	1/2 cup	80	2.0	19.0	95	na	0.0	na
cherry	1/2 cup	80	2.0	19.0	95	na	0.0	na
cherry, sugar-free	1/2 cup	8	1.0	1.0	90	na	0.0	na
Concord grape	1/2 cup	80	2.0	19.0	130	na	0.0	na
fruit punch	1/2 cup	80	2.0	19.0	90	na	0.0	na
lemon	1/2 cup	80	2.0	19.0	125	na	0.0	0
lemon-lime	1/2 cup	80	2.0	19.0	95	na	0.0	na
lime	1/2 cup	80	2.0	19.0	125	na	0.0	0
lime, sugar-free	1/2 cup	8	1.0	1.0	100	na	0.0	na
mixed berry	1/2 cup	80	2.0	19.0	90	na	0.0	0
orange	1/2 cup	80	2.0	19.0	95	na	0.0	na
orange, sugar-free	1/2 cup	10	1.0	1.0	90	na	0.0	na
peach	1/2 cup	80	2.0	19.0	95	na	0.0	na
pineapple	1/2 cup	80	2.0	19.0	95	na	0.0	na
raspberry	1/2 cup	80	2.0	19.0	125	na	0.0	0
raspberry, sugar-free	1/2 cup	8	1.0	1.0	90	na	0.0	na
strawberry	1/2 cup	80	2.0	19.0	105	na	0.0	0
strawberry, sugar-free	1/2 cup	8	1.0	1.0	90	na	0.0	na
strawberry banana	1/2 cup	80	2.0	19.0	105	na	0.0	na
strawberry banana, sugar-free	1/2 cup	8	1.0	1.0	85	na	0.0	na
strawberry orange	1/2 cup	80	2.0	19.0	110	na	0.0	na
tropical fruit	1/2 cup	80	2.0	19.0	110	na	0.0	na
READY TO SERVE								
(Estee)	1/2 cup	8	1.0	<1.0	0	(tr)	0.0	0

Food Name	Serv. Size	Total Cal.	Prot. GMS	Carbs GMS	Sod. MGS	Fiber GMS	Fat GMS	Chol. MGS
(Jell-O) berry blue, six pack	3.5 oz	80	1.0	18.0	40	na	0.0	0
(Jell-O) cherry, six pack	3.5 oz	80	1.0	18.0	40	na	0.0	0
(Jell-O) strawberry, six pack	3.5 oz	80	1.0	18.0	40	na	0.0	0
GELATIN DRINK MIX								
orange flavor	1 oz	108	10.0	17.1	47	(tr)	0.3	na
orange flavor *(Knox)*	1 envelope	39	5.7	4.0	17	(tr)	0.1	0
GERMAN SAUSAGE. See also individual listings.								
(Hickory Farms)	1 oz	100	5.0	1.0	385	0	8.0	20
GHEE/clarified butter	1 oz	249	0.0	0.0	na	0	28.4	(mq)
GIN. See ALCOHOLIC BEVERAGES.								
GINGER								
ground	1 oz	98	2.6	20.1	9	>1.7 c	1.7	0
ground	1 tbsp	19	0.5	3.8	2	.7	0.3	0
ground	1 tsp	6	0.2	1.3	1	.2	0.1	0
ground *(Durkee)*	1 tsp	7	0.0	0.0	0	0	tr	na
ground *(Laurel Leaf)*	1 tsp	7	0.0	0.0	0	0	tr	na
ground *(Spice Islands)*	1 tsp	6	0.1	1.2	1	.2	0.1	0
GINGER, PICKLED, Japanese	1 oz	10	0.1	2.1	105	(mq)	<.1	0
GINGER ALE. See SOFT DRINKS AND MIXERS.								
GINGER ROOT								
candied, crystallized	1 lb	1544	1.4	395.4	272	>3.2 c	0.9	0
candied, crystallized	1 oz	95	0.1	24.4	17	>.2 c	0.1	0
raw, slices, 1-inch diam	1/4 cup	17	0.4	3.6	3	.5	0.2	0
raw, slices, 1-inch diam	5 slices	8	0.2	1.7	1	.2	0.1	0
trimmed	1 oz	20	0.5	4.3	4	>.3 c	0.2	0
untrimmed	1 lb	291	7.4	63.6	53	>4.3 c	3.1	0
GINGER TERIYAKI MARINADE *(Golden Dipt)*	1 oz	120	1.0	12.0	920	na	7.0	0
GINGERBREAD. See BREAD.								
GINKGO NUT								
canned	1 cup	172	3.5	34.3	476	14.4	2.5	0
canned, approx 9 large, 14 medium, or 22 small	1 oz	32	0.7	6.3	87	>.5 c	0.5	0
dried	1 oz	99	2.9	20.6	4	>.3 c	0.6	0
dried, in shell	1 lb	1198	35.7	249.8	46	>3.4 c	6.9	0
raw	1 oz	52	1.2	10.7	2	>.1 c	0.5	0
raw, in shell	1 lb	628	14.9	129.6	24	>1.7 c	5.8	0
GLOBE ARTICHOKE. See ARTHICHOKES, GLOBE.								
GLUTEN. See WHEAT GLUTEN.								
GOA BEAN. See WINGED BEAN.								
GOAT								
raw	1 lb	494	93.4	0.0	372	na	10.5	259
raw	1 oz	31	5.8	0.0	23	na	0.7	16
roasted	4 oz	162	30.7	0.0	98	0	3.4	85

Food Name	Serv. Size	Total Cal.	Prot. GMS	Carbs GMS	Sod. MGS	Fiber GMS	Fat GMS	Chol. MGS
roasted, diced	1 cup	200	37.9	0.0	120	0	4.2	105
GOATFISH								
raw	1 lb	435	92.5	0.0	(mq)	0	4.5	(mq)
raw	1 oz	27	5.8	0.0	(mq)	0	0.3	(mq)
GOBO. See BURDOCK ROOT.								
GOOSE, DOMESTICATED								
meat and skin, raw	1 oz	105	4.5	0.0	21	0	9.5	23
meat and skin, roasted	4 oz	346	28.5	0.0	79	0	24.9	103
meat only, raw	1 oz	46	6.4	0.0	25	0	2.0	24
meat only, roasted	4 oz	270	32.9	0.0	86	0	14.4	109
GOOSE FAT								
	1/2 cup	923	0.0	0.0	0	0	102.3	103
	1 oz	255	0.0	0.0	0	0	28.3	28
	1 tbsp	115	0.0	0.0	0	0	12.8	13
GOOSE GIBLETS, raw	100 gm	156	21.1	0.6	70	0	7.0	350
GOOSE GIZZARD, raw	100 gm	139	21.4	0.0	65	0	5.3	145
GOOSE LIVER, raw	1 lb	15	1.8	0.7	15	0	0.5	57
GOOSEBERRY								
whole	1 lb	202	4.0	46.2	4	>8.6 c	2.6	0
whole	1 oz	12	0.2	2.9	<1	>.5 c	0.2	0
whole	1 cup	66	1.3	15.3	2	6.4	0.9	0
GOOSEBERRY, CANNED, in light syrup	4 oz	83	0.7	21.3	2	>1.4 c	0.2	0
GOOSEFISH. See MONKFISH.								
GOURD, BOTTLE/calabash gourd/white-flowered gourd								
boiled, drained	4 oz	17	0.7	4.2	2	>.7 c	<.1	0
boiled, drained, 1-inch cubes	1/2 cup	11	0.4	2.7	1	>.5 c	<.1	0
raw, approx 2.4 lb	1 med	106	5.0	26.1	19	8.5	0.2	0
raw, 1-inch cubes	1/2 cup	8	0.4	2.0	1	.6	<.1	0
raw, trimmed	1 oz	4	0.2	1.0	1	.3	tr	0
raw, untrimmed	1 lb	44	2.0	10.8	8	3.5	0.1	0
GOURD, CALABASH. See GOURD, BOTTLE.								
GOURD, DISHCLOTH/loofah gourd/rag gourd/sponge gourd/towel gourd/vegetable sponge								
boiled, drained	4 oz	64	0.7	16.3	24	.5	0.4	0
boiled, drained, 1-inch slices	1/2 cup	50	0.6	12.8	19	>.3 c	0.3	0
raw, approx 8.6 oz	1 med	36	2.1	7.8	5	>.9 c	0.4	0
raw, 1-inch slices	1 cup	19	1.1	4.1	3	>.5 c	0.2	0
raw, trimmed	1 oz	6	0.3	1.2	1	>.1 c	0.1	0
raw, untrimmed	1 lb	67	4.0	14.4	11	>1.7 c	0.7	0
GOURD, RAG. See GOURD, DISHCLOTH.								
GOURD, SPONGE. See GOURD, DISHCLOTH.								
GOURD, WAX								
boiled, drained	4 oz	15	0.5	3.4	121	>.6 c	0.2	0
boiled, drained, cubes	1/2 cup	11	0.4	2.6	93	.9	0.2	0

Food Name	Serv. Size	Total Cal.	Prot. GMS	Carbs GMS	Sod. MGS	Fiber GMS	Fat GMS	Chol. MGS
raw, cubes	1 cup	17	0.5	4.0	147	3.8	0.3	0
raw, trimmed	1 oz	4	0.1	0.9	31	.2	0.1	0
raw, untrimmed	1 lb	42	1.3	9.7	358	1.9	0.6	0
GOURD, WHITE/tunka								
boiled, drained	4 oz	15	0.5	3.4	121	>.6 c	0.2	0
boiled, drained, cubes	1/2 cup	11	0.4	2.6	93	.9	0.2	0
raw, cubes	1 cup	17	0.5	4.0	147	3.8	0.3	0
raw, trimmed	1 oz	4	0.1	0.9	31	.2	0.1	0
raw, untrimmed	1 lb	42	1.3	9.7	358	1.9	0.6	0
GOURD, WHITE-FLOWERED. See GOURD, BOTTLE.								
GOVERNOR PLUM, trimmed	1 oz	31	0.1	8.4	na	>.1 c	0.0	0
GRANADILLA. See PASSION FRUIT.								
GRANOLA. See CEREAL, READY-TO-SERVE.								
GRANOLA AND CEREAL BAR. See also GRANOLA SNACKS.								
(Barbara's Bakery)								
cinnamon and oats, 2 oz	1 bar	281	6.0	31.0	na	na	15.0	0
coconut almond, 2 oz	1 bar	306	8.0	23.0	na	na	20.0	0
peanut butter, 2 oz	1 bar	275	7.0	28.0	na	na	15.0	0
(Bear Valley)								
carob-cocoa, food bar 'Pemmican' 3.75 oz	1 bar	440	16.0	68.0	80	7.0	12.0	0
coconut almond, food bar 'Meal Pack' 3.75 oz	1 bar	400	16.0	56.0	80	6.0	12.0	0
sesame lemon, food bar 'Meal Pack' 3.75 oz	1 bar	410	17.0	57.0	85	4.0	13.0	0
fruit 'n nut, food bar 'Pemmican' 3.75 oz	1 bar	420	17.0	59.0	90	9.0	13.0	0
(Glenny's)								
apple, 'Original Fruit Bar'	1 bar	100	2.0	15.0	15	4.0	3.0	0
'Bee Pollen Sunrise' 1.5 oz	1 bar	190	5.0	22.0	na	na	8.0	na
carob mint w/oat bran 'Brown Rice Treats'	1 bar	180	3.0	37.0	20	1.7	2.0	na
cinnamon and raisin 'Brown Rice Treats' 1.75 oz	1 bar	170	2.0	38.0	30	na	1.0	na
coconut amandine 'Moist and Chewy' 1.5 oz	1 bar	190	3.0	22.0	20	na	10.0	na
'Ginseng Sunrise' 1.5 oz	1 bar	160	1.0	24.0	na	na	7.0	na
oatmeal raisin 'Moist and Chewy' 1.5 oz	1 bar	160	3.0	30.0	25	na	3.0	na
peanut and raisin 'Brown Rice Treats' 2 oz	1 bar	210	4.0	39.0	29	na	5.0	na
peanut snack 'Moist and Chewy' 1.5 oz	1 bar	180	5.0	24.0	20	na	7.0	na
plain and fancy 'Brown Rice Treats' 1.25 oz	1 bar	120	1.0	28.0	29	na	1.0	na
raisin bran 'Brown Rice Treats' 1.75 oz	1 bar	170	2.0	38.0	17	na	1.0	na
'Spirulina Sunrise' 1.5 oz	1 bar	140	3.0	21.0	na	na	5.0	na
sunflower 'Moist and Chewy' 1.5 oz	1 bar	180	5.0	24.0	15	na	7.0	na

Food Name	Serv. Size	Total Cal.	Prot. GMS	Carbs GMS	Sod. MGS	Fiber GMS	Fat GMS	Chol. MGS
toasted almond w/oat bran								
'Brown Rice Treats'	1 bar	200	4.0	34.0	20	1.6	5.0	na
(Golden Temple)								
cashew almond 'Wha Guru Chew Bar'	1 bar	164	3.0	15.0	63	1.0	11.0	0
peanut cashew 'Wha Guru Chew Bar'	1 bar	167	4.0	14.0	62	1.0	11.0	0
sesame almond 'Wha Guru Chew Bar'	1 bar	160	3.0	15.0	61	1.0	10.0	0
(Health Valley)								
blueberry apple, fat-free	1 bar	140	3.0	33.0	10	3.7	0.0	0
date almond flavor, fat-free	1 bar	140	3.0	33.0	10	3.7	0.0	0
raspberry, fat-free	1 bar	140	3.0	33.0	10	3.7	0.0	0
(Hershey's)								
chocolate chip, chocolate coated, 1.2 oz	1 bar	170	2.0	22.0	50	(mq)	8.0	na
cocoa creme, chocolate coated, 1.2 oz	1 bar	180	2.0	22.0	50	(mq)	9.0	5
cookies and creme, chocolate coated,								
1.2 oz	1 bar	170	2.0	22.0	50	(mq)	8.0	na
peanut butter, chocolate coated, 1.2 oz	1 bar	180	4.0	19.0	65	(mq)	10.0	5
raspberry filled 'Common Sense								
Smart Start'	1 bar	170	2.0	28.0	160	1.0	6.0	0
(Kudo's)								
chocolate chip	1 bar	180	3.0	21.0	60	(mq)	9.0	na
chocolate chunk 'Simply Kudos'	1 bar	100	1.0	13.0	50	na	4.0	na
fudge, nutty	1 bar	190	4.0	19.0	60	(mq)	11.0	na
honey nut 'Simply Kudos'	1 bar	100	2.0	13.0	55	na	4.0	na
oatmeal raisin 'Simply Kudos'	1 bar	90	1.0	13.0	55	na	4.0	na
peanut butter, chocolate coated, 1.3 oz	1 bar	190	4.0	18.0	70	(mq)	12.0	na
(Natural Nectar)								
almond, 'Treat Yourself Right'	1 bar	150	3.0	22.0	40	5.0	5.0	0
apple-oatmeal spice, 'Fi-Bar A.M.'	1 bar	150	3.0	27.0	25	5.0	3.0	0
banana nut, 'Fi-Bar A.M.'	1 bar	150	2.0	26.0	20	5.0	4.0	0
cocoa almond, 'Fi-Bar Chewy & Nutty'	1 bar	130	3.0	21.0	20	4.0	4.0	0
cocoa almond crunch, 'Canadian Chewy								
& Nutty'	1 bar	130	3.0	21.0	20	2.0	4.0	0
cocoa peanut, 'Fi-Bar Chewy & Nutty'	1 bar	130	3.0	20.0	20	4.0	1.0	0
cocoa peanut butter crunch, 'Chewy								
& Nutty'	1 bar	130	3.0	20.0	20	2.0	4.0	0
coconut	1 bar	120	2.0	20.0	30	6.0	4.0	0
cranberry, w/wild berries 'Original Fruit Bar'	1 bar	120	2.0	23.0	15	4.0	2.0	0
lemon 'Original Fruit Bar'	1 bar	100	2.0	15.0	15	4.0	3.0	0
Mandarin orange 'Original Fruit Bar'	1 bar	100	2.0	15.0	15	4.0	3.0	0
peanut butter	1 bar	130	3.0	20.0	30	6.0	4.0	0
peanut butter 'Treat Yourself Right'	1 bar	150	4.0	18.0	55	5.0	5.0	0
raisin nut bran, 'Fi-Bar A.M.'	1 bar	150	3.0	26.0	30	5.0	4.0	0
raspberry 'Canadian'	1 bar	120	2.0	21.0	15	3.0	3.0	0

Food Name	Serv. Size	Total Cal.	Prot. GMS	Carbs GMS	Sod. MGS	Fiber GMS	Fat GMS	Chol. MGS
raspberry 'Original Fruit Bar'	1 bar	120	2.0	23.0	15	4.0	2.0	0
strawberry 'Canadian'	1 bar	120	2.0	21.0	15	3.0	3.0	0
strawberry 'Original Fruit Bar'	1 bar	120	2.0	23.0	15	4.0	2.0	0
strawberry-oatmeal w/almonds, 'Fi-Bar A.M.'	1 bar	150	3.0	24.0	30	5.0	4.0	0
vanilla almond, 'Fi-Bar Chewy & Nutty'	1 bar	130	3.0	21.0	20	4.0	4.0	0
vanilla almond crunch, 'Canadian Chewy & Nutty'	1 bar	130	3.0	21.0	20	2.0	4.0	0
vanilla peanut, 'Fi-Bar Chewy & Nutty'	1 bar	130	3.0	20.0	20	4.0	4.0	0
wild cranberry 'Canadian'	1 bar	120	2.0	21.0	15	3.0	3.0	0
(Nature Valley)								
cinnamon, .8 oz	1 bar	120	2.0	17.0	70	1.0	5.0	0
oat bran-honey graham, .8 oz	1 bar	110	2.0	16.0	90	1.0	4.0	0
oats and honey, .8 oz	1 bar	120	2.0	17.0	65	1.0	5.0	0
peanut butter, .8 oz	1 bar	120	2.0	15.0	70	1.0	6.0	0
(Nature's Choice)								
carob chip, .75 oz	1 bar	90	2.0	15.0	15	na	3.0	0
cinnamon-raisin, .75 oz	1 bar	90	2.0	15.0	10	na	3.0	0
oats 'n honey, .75 oz	1 bar	90	2.0	15.0	15	na	3.0	0
peanut butter, .75 oz	1 bar	90	2.0	14.0	25	na	3.0	0
(Nutri Grain)								
blueberry 'Smart Start' 1.5 oz	1 bar	180	2.0	26.0	170	1.0	8.0	0
corn flakes, mixed berry-filled 'Smart Start'	1 bar	170	2.0	27.0	160	1.0	7.0	0
raisin bran 'Smart Start' 1.5 oz	1 bar	160	2.0	28.0	170	2.0	5.0	0
rice krispies w/almonds 'Smart Start' 1 oz	1 bar	130	2.0	18.0	65	1.0	6.0	0
strawberry 'Smart Start' 1.5 oz	1 bar	180	2.0	26.0	170	1.0	8.0	0
(Quaker)								
apple berry 'Chewy'	1 bar	120	2.0	20.0	95	na	4.0	0
caramel nut 'Granola Dipps' 1 oz	1 bar	148	1.9	20.9	81	.7	6.4	2
chocolate chip 'Chewy'	1 bar	128	2.0	19.3	90	1.4	4.7	0
chocolate chip 'Granola Dipps' 1 oz	1 bar	139	1.8	18.7	78	1.0	6.3	1
chocolate fudge 'Granola Dipps' 1 oz	1 bar	160	2.1	20.0	74	(mq)	7.9	na
chunky nut and raisin 'Chewy' 1 oz	1 bar	131	2.5	17.2	86	1.6	5.8	0
honey and oats 'Chewy' 1 oz	1 bar	125	2.3	19.1	95	1.3	4.4	<1
peanut butter 'Chewy' 1 oz	1 bar	128	3.1	17.8	116	1.2	4.9	1<1
peanut butter, chocolate chip 'Chewy' 1 oz	1 bar	131	3.1	17.0	112	1.2	5.7	0
peanut butter, chocolate chip 'Granola Dipps'	1 bar	174	3.6	17.4	102	(mq)	10.0	na
peanut butter 'Granola Dipps' 1 oz	1 bar	170	3.6	18.5	74	1.0	9.1	2
raisin and cinnamon 'Chewy' 1 oz	1 bar	128	2.2	18.6	92	1.2	5.0	<1
S'mores 'Chewy' 1 oz	1 bar	126	1.9	19.7	108	1.1	4.4	10
trail mix 'Chewy' 1 oz	1 bar	130	2.0	18.0	105	na	5.0	0

Food Name	Serv. Size	Total Cal.	Prot. GMS	Carbs GMS	Sod. MGS	Fiber GMS	Fat GMS	Chol. MGS
(Sunbelt)								
apple bar, baked, 1.31 oz	1 bar	130	1.0	28.0	130	1.0	2.0	na
chocolate chip, chewy, 1.25 oz	1 bar	150	3.0	23.0	75	(mq)	7.0	<1
chocolate chip, fudge dipped, chewy,								
1.63 oz	1 bar	220	2.0	29.0	60	(mq)	11.0	<1
chocolate chip, fudge dipped, chewy,								
1.5 oz	1 bar	210	2.0	26.0	55	4.0	10.0	2
oats and honey, chewy, 1 oz	1 bar	130	2.0	18.0	35	(mq)	5.0	<1
oats and honey, fudge dipped, chewy,								
1.38 oz	1 bar	190	2.0	24.0	55	(mq)	10.0	<1
w/almonds, chewy, 1 oz	1 bar	120	3.0	18.0	65	(mq)	6.0	<1
w/chocolate chips, chewy, 1.75 oz	1 bar	220	4.0	32.0	105	(mq)	9.0	<1
w/peanuts, fudge dipped, chewy, 2.25 oz	1 bar	300	6.0	36.0	90	(mq)	18.0	<1
w/peanuts, fudge dipped, chewy, 1.38 oz	1 bar	190	2.0	24.0	55	(mq)	10.0	<1
w/raisins, chewy, 1.25 oz	1 bar	150	2.0	24.0	65	(mq)	6.0	<1
w/raisins, fudge dipped, chewy, 1.5 oz	1 bar	200	4.0	24.0	60	(mq)	12.0	<1
GRANOLA SNACKS. See also GRANOLA AND CEREAL BAR.								
(Natural Nectar)								
almond butter crunch 'Nectar Nuggets'	1 cup	120	3.0	11.0	30	5.0	7.0	0
almond cappuccino crunch								
'Nectar Nuggets'	1 cup	110	2.0	14.0	30	5.0	5.0	0
coconut almond crunch 'Nectar Nuggets'	1 cup	110	2.0	15.0	20	4.0	5.0	0
peanut butter crunch 'Nectar Nuggets'	1 cup	120	4.0	11.0	30	5.0	7.0	0
(Nature Valley)								
apple-cinnamon 'Granola Bites'	1 pkg	170	3.0	25.0	100	2.0	7.0	0
honey nut 'Granola Bites'	1 pkg	170	3.0	24.0	120	2.0	8.0	0
variety pack 'Granola Bites'	1 pkg	170	3.0	24.0	120	2.0	8.0	0
(Nature's Choice)								
chocolate chip 'Grrr-Nola Treats'	.75 oz	80	1.0	15.0	5	na	2.0	0
cinnamon toast 'Grrr-Nola Treats'	.75 oz	80	1.0	15.0	5	na	2.0	0
peanut butter and jelly 'Grrr-Nola Treats'	.75 oz	80	1.0	14.0	5	na	3.0	0
tutti-frutti 'Grrr-Nola Treats'	.75 oz	75	1.0	15.0	5	na	2.0	0
GRAPE								
AMERICAN (Concord, Delaware, Niagara)								
(Dole)	1.5 cup	85	1.0	24.0	3	2.0	0.0	na
Slipskin								
peeled and seeded	1 oz	18	0.2	4.9	<1	>.2 c	0.1	0
trimmed	10 fruits	15	0.2	4.1	0	>.2 c	0.1	0
untrimmed	1 lb	165	1.7	45.1	4	>2.0 c	0.9	0
untrimmed	1 cup	58	0.6	15.8	2	>.9 c	0.3	0
EUROPEAN (Muskat, Tokay, Thompson)								
Adherent skin								
trimmed	10 fruits	35	0.3	8.9	1	.5	0.3	0

Food Name	Serv. Size	Total Cal.	Prot. GMS	Carbs GMS	Sod. MGS	Fiber GMS	Fat GMS	Chol. MGS
untrimmed	1 lb	287	2.7	72.0	7	2.8	2.3	0
untrimmed	1 cup	114	1.1	28.4	3	1.6	0.9	0
untrimmed w/o seeds	1 lb	309	2.9	77.4	7	3.0	2.5	0
w/seeds	1/2 cup	57	0.5	14.2	2	.6	0.5	0
w/seeds	1 oz	20	0.2	5.0	1	.2	0.2	0
w/o seeds	1/2 cup	57	0.5	14.2	2	.6	0.5	0
w/o seeds	1 oz	20	0.2	5.0	1	.2	0.2	0
w/o seeds, approx 1.75 oz	10 grapes	36	0.3	8.9	1	.4	0.3	0
GRAPE, CANNED								
THOMPSON, seedless								
in heavy syrup	1 cup	187	1.2	50.3	13	1.0	0.3	0
in heavy syrup	4 oz	83	0.5	22.3	6	>.2 c	0.1	0
in heavy syrup (S&W)	1/2 cup	100	0.0	25.0	5	(mq)	0.0	0
in water	1 cup	98	1.2	25.2	15	2.5	0.3	0
in water	4 oz	45	0.6	11.7	7	>.2 c	0.1	0
GRAPE APPLE DRINK, bottle (Mott's)	10 oz	167	0.0	42.0	<1	0	0.0	0
GRAPE DRINK								
Can, bottle, or box								
(A&P)	6 oz	100	<1.0	25.0	0	0	<1.0	0
(All Sport) thirst quencher, caffeine-free	8 oz	70	0.0	20.0	55	na	0.0	na
(Bama)	8.45 oz	120	0.0	29.0	25	0	0.0	0
(Bright & Early) frozen, diluted	6 oz	100	0.0	24.0	0	na	0.0	0
(Crowley)	8 oz	130	0.0	32.0	15	0	0.0	0
(Fruitopia) 'The Grape Beyond' real fruit	8 oz	130	0.0	32.0	25	na	0.0	na
(Gatorade) low sodium, no caffeine	8 oz	50	0.0	14.0	110	na	0.0	na
(Hi-C) aseptic box	6 oz	90	0.0	23.0	25	na	0.0	0
(J. Hungerford)	9.03 oz	41	0.0	10.9	31	0	0.0	0
(Kool-Aid) 'Koolers'	8.45 oz	140	0.0	35.0	10	0	0.0	0
(Pathmark)	6 oz	90	0.0	22.0	0	0	0.0	0
(Squeezit) 'Grumpy Grape'	6.75 oz	120	0.0	30.0	5	na	0.0	na
(10-K) 'Clear'	8 oz	60	0.0	15.0	55	na	0.0	na
(Tropicana)	6 oz	90	<1.0	22.0	10	na	<1.0	0
(Veryfine)	8 oz	130	0.1	34.0	10	0	0.0	0
(Wyler's) 'Fruit Slush'	4 oz	157	0.0	39.3	10	0	0.0	0
Prepared from mix								
(Finast)	8 oz	80	0.0	21.0	15	0	0.0	0
(Gatorade) instant 'Thirst Quencher'	8 oz	60	0.0	15.0	110	na	0.0	na
(Kool-Aid) sugar-sweetened	8 oz	80	0.0	20.0	25	na	0.0	0
(Kool-Aid) unsweetened, prepared w/sugar	8 oz	100	0.0	25.0	0	na	0.0	0
(Kool-Aid) unsweetened, prepared w/o sugar	8 oz	2	0.0	0.0	0	na	0.0	0
(Kool-Aid) w/NutraSweet	8 oz	4	0.0	0.0	0	na	0.0	0
(Pathmark) 'No Frills'	8 oz	90	0.0	22.0	20	0	0.0	0

Food Name	Serv. Size	Total Cal.	Prot. GMS	Carbs GMS	Sod. MGS	Fiber GMS	Fat GMS	Chol. MGS
(Pathmark) 'No Frills Sodium Free'	6 oz	80	0.0	22.0	0	0	0.0	0
GRAPE JUICE								
Can, bottle, or box								
(IGA) 'Unsweetened'	6 oz	120	0.0	30.0	5	0	0.0	0
(J. Hungerford)	9.03 oz	160	0.2	40.2	0	.1	0.0	0
(J. Hungerford) 100% juice	9.03 oz	155	0.5	39.2	11	.4	0.0	0
(J. Hungerford) 50% juice	9.03 oz	135	0.2	33.7	0	0	0.0	0
(J. Hungerford) 20% juice	9.03 oz	41	0.0	10.9	31	0	0.0	0
(Juicy Juice) blend	6 oz	100	0.0	25.0	5	0	0.0	0
(Juicy Juice) bottled	6 oz	90	1.0	22.0	5	na	0.0	na
(Juicy Juice) boxed	8.45 oz	130	1.0	31.0	10	na	0.0	na
(Knudsen & Sons)	8 oz	130	1.0	32.0	na	na	0.0	na
(Knudsen & Sons) Concord	8 oz	130	1.0	32.0	na	na	0.0	na
(Kraft) 'Pure 100% Unsweetened'	6 oz	104	1.0	25.0	0	0	0.0	0
(Pathmark) 'No Frills'	6 oz	113	0.0	27.0	10	0	0.0	0
(Lucky Leaf)	6 oz	130	0.0	32.0	0	0	0.0	0
(Minute Maid) aseptic box	6 oz	100	1.0	24.0	20	na	1.0	na
(Pathmark) 'Unsweetened'	6 oz	120	0.0	30.0	10	0	0.0	0
(S&W) Concord 'Unsweetened'	6 oz	100	1.0	25.0	9	0	0.0	0
(Sippin' Pak)	8.45 oz	130	1.0	32.0	25	0	0.0	0
(Squeezit 100) 'Caped Grape' 100% natural fruit juice	6.75 oz	100	0.0	24.0	20	na	0.0	na
(Veryfine) '100%'	8 oz	153	1.0	37.0	20	0	0.0	0
(Welch's) purple	6 oz	120	0.0	30.0	10	0	0.0	0
(Welch's) red	8.45 oz	170	0.0	43.0	20	0	0.0	0
(Welch's) red	6 oz	120	0.0	30.0	15	0	0.0	0
(Welch's) sparkling red	6 oz	128	0.0	30.0	30	0	0.0	0
(Welch's) sparkling white	6 oz	120	0.0	30.0	30	0	0.0	0
(Welch's) 'USDA'	6 oz	120	0.0	30.0	10	0	0.0	0
(Welch's) white	8.45 oz	160	0.0	39.0	20	0	0.0	0
(Welch's) white	6 oz	120	0.0	30.0	15	0	0.0	0
Frozen, diluted as directed								
(Minute Maid)	6 oz	90	0.0	24.0	0	na	0.0	na
(Sunkist)	6 oz	69	0.3	17.1	3	0	0.1	0
(Welch's) 'No Sugar Added'	6 oz	40	0.0	10.0	5	0	0.0	0
(Welch's) 'Orchard'	10 oz	170	0.0	43.0	10	0	0.0	0
(Welch's) 'Orchard'	6 oz	110	0.0	27.0	20	0	0.0	0
(Welch's) 'Orchard Cocktails-In-A-Box'	8.45 oz	150	0.0	38.0	20	0	0.0	0
(Welch's) purple	6 oz	100	0.0	25.0	0	0	0.0	0
(Welch's) white	6 oz	100	0.0	25.0	0	0	0.0	0
GRAPE JUICE DRINK								
(Hi-C)	8.45 oz	136	0.1	33.4	24	0	0.1	0
(Hi-C)	6 oz	96	0.1	23.7	17	0	0.1	0

Food Name	Serv. Size	Total Cal.	Prot. GMS	Carbs GMS	Sod. MGS	Fiber GMS	Fat GMS	Chol. MGS
(Sunkist) frozen, diluted	6 oz	69	0.3	17.0	3	0	0.1	0
(Tang) 'Fruit Box'	8.45 oz	130	0.0	34.0	10	na	0.0	0
GRAPE PUNCH								
(Minute Maid) chilled	6 oz	90	0.0	23.0	20	na	0.0	na
(Minute Maid) frozen concentrate	6 oz	90	0.0	23.0	0	na	0.0	na
GRAPEFRUIT								
PINK AND RED								
Arizona/California								
fresh, 3.75-inch diam	1/2 fruit	46	0.6	11.9	1	>.3 c	0.1	0
sections w/juice	1 cup	85	1.1	22.3	2	>.5 c	0.2	0
trimmed	1 oz	11	0.1	2.7	<1	>.1 c	<.1	0
untrimmed	1 lb	86	1.2	22.4	1	>.5 c	0.2	0
Florida								
fresh *(Ocean Spray)*	1/2 med	50	1.0	13.0	0	(mq)	0.0	0
fresh, 3.75-inch diam	1/2 fruit	37	0.7	9.2	0	1.4	0.1	0
sections w/juice	1 cup	69	1.3	17.3	0	2.5	0.2	0
trimmed	1 oz	9	0.2	2.1	tr	>.1 c	<.1	0
untrimmed	1 lb	69	1.3	17.4	1	>.5 c	0.2	0
WHITE								
California								
fresh, 3.75-inch diam	1/2 fruit	44	1.0	10.7	0	>.2 c	0.1	0
sections w/juice	1 cup	85	2.0	20.9	0	>.5 c	0.2	0
trimmed	1 oz	10	0.2	2.6	tr	>.1 c	<.1	0
untrimmed	1 lb	81	2.0	20.2	1	>.4 c	0.2	0
Florida								
fresh *(Ocean Spray)*	1/2 med	45	1.0	12.0	0	(mq)	0.0	0
fresh, 3.75-inch diam	1/2 fruit	38	0.7	9.7	0	1.3	0.1	0
sections w/juice	1 cup	74	1.5	18.8	0	2.5	0.2	0
trimmed	1 oz	9	0.2	2.3	tr	<.1	<.1	0
GRAPEFRUIT, CANNED								
(Featherweight) in juice	1/2 cup	40	0.0	9.0	10	(mq)	0.0	0
(Finast) in light syrup	1/2 cup	80	0.0	20.0	10	(mq)	<.1	0
(Kraft) chilled 'Pure'	1/2 cup	50	1.0	12.0	0	(mq)	0.0	0
(S&W) in light syrup	1/2 cup	80	<1.0	24.0	0	(mq)	0.0	0
(S&W) 'Unsweetened'	1/2 cup	40	0.0	9.0	10	(mq)	0.0	0
(S&W Nutradiet)	1/2 cup	40	0.0	9.0	0	(mq)	0.0	0
(Stokely) in light syrup	1/2 cup	90	1.0	23.0	5	(mq)	1.0	0
GRAPEFRUIT JUICE								
Can, bottle, or box								
(Del Monte)	6 oz	70	1.0	17.0	10	tr	0.0	0
(J. Hungerford) regular	9.03 oz	120	0.3	29.8	0	.1	0.0	0
(J. Hungerford) 100% juice	9.03 oz	98	0.8	24.2	6	.3	0.0	0
(J. Hungerford) 50% juice	9.03 oz	109	0.7	26.9	0	0	0.0	0

Food Name	Serv. Size	Total Cal.	Prot. GMS	Carbs GMS	Sod. MGS	Fiber GMS	Fat GMS	Chol. MGS
(Knudsen & Sons)	8 oz	70	1.0	17.0	na	na	0.0	na
(Knudsen & Sons) pink	8 oz	80	1.0	18.0	na	na	0.0	na
(Kraft) '100% pure'	6 oz	70	1.0	16.0	0	tr	0.0	0
(Libby's)	6 oz	70	1.0	17.0	na	na	0.0	0
(Minute Maid)	6 oz	70	1.0	17.0	20	na	0.0	na
(Minute Maid) 'Juices to Go'	6 oz	70	1.0	17.0	20	na	0.0	na
(Mott's)	9.5 oz	118	1.0	29.0	5	tr	0.0	0
(Mott's)	10 oz	124	1.0	30.0	5	tr	0.0	0
(Ocean Spray)	6 oz	70	1.0	16.0	10	tr	0.0	0
(Ocean Spray) 100%	6 oz	60	0.0	18.0	15	na	0.0	na
(Ocean Spray) pink 'Pink Premium'	6 oz	60	1.0	15.0	10	tr	0.0	0
(Ocean Spray) 'Ruby Red'	6 oz	100	0.0	24.0	15	na	0.0	na
(S&W)	6 oz	80	1.0	18.0	10	tr	0.0	0
(Snapple)	8 oz	110	1.0	25.0	45	na	0.0	0
(Stokely)	6 oz	76	1.0	18.0	5	tr	1.0	0
(Sunkist) 'Fresh Squeezed'	8 oz	96	1.2	22.7	3	tr	0.2	0
(Tree Top)	6 oz	80	1.0	19.0	0	tr	0.0	0
(TreeSweet) pink	6 oz	72	0.0	17.0	15	tr	0.0	0
(TreeSweet) regular	6 oz	72	0.0	17.0	15	tr	0.0	0
(Tropicana) 100% pure	6 oz	70	1.0	14.0	20	na	<1.0	na
(Tropicana) 'Ruby Red 100% pure'	6 oz	70	1.0	14.0	20	na	<1.0	na
(Veryfine) '100%'	8 oz	101	1.4	23.0	10	tr	0.0	0
Fresh								
juice from one 3.75-inch diam fruit	6 oz	76	1.0	18.0	2	(mq)	0.2	0
pink	1 cup	96	1.2	22.7	2	na	0.3	0
white	1 cup	96	1.2	22.7	2	0	0.3	0
Frozen, diluted as directed								
(A&P)	6 oz	80	<1.0	18.0	0	tr	<1.0	0
(Minute Maid)	6 oz	80	1.0	18.0	0	na	0.0	na
(Minute Maid) pink	6 oz	80	0.0	20.0	0	na	0.0	na
(Sunkist)	6 oz	56	0.8	13.3	1	tr	0.2	0
(TreeSweet)	6 oz	78	1.0	18.0	15	tr	0.0	0
GRAPEFRUIT JUICE COCKTAIL								
(IGA)	6 oz	80	0.0	20.0	15	(tr)	0.0	0
(Minute Maid) 'Juices To Go'	6 oz	80	0.0	20.0	20	na	0.0	na
(Ocean Spray)	6 oz	80	0.0	20.0	15	(tr)	0.0	0
(Pathmark)	6 oz	80	0.0	20.0	15	(tr)	0.0	0
(TreeSweet) 'Lite'	6 oz	40	1.0	10.0	15	(tr)	0.0	0
(Tropicana) 'Twister'	8 oz	110	(tr)	28.0	1	(tr)	0.0	0
(Tropicana) 'Twister Light' w/NutraSweet	6 oz	30	<1.0	6.0	20	na	<1.0	na
(Veryfine)	8 oz	120	<1.0	29.0	15	(tr)	0.0	0
GRAPEFRUIT JUICE DRINK								
(Citrus Hill) 'Plus Calcium'	6 oz	70	<1.0	19.0	10	(tr)	<1.0	0

Food Name	Serv. Size	Total Cal.	Prot. GMS	Carbs GMS	Sod. MGS	Fiber GMS	Fat GMS	Chol. MGS
(Tropicana) 'Juice Sparkler'	8 oz	110	(tr)	26.0	50	(tr)	0.0	0
(Wyler's) 'Fruit Slush'	4 oz	157	0.0	39.3	10	(tr)	0.0	0
GRAPESEED OIL								
	1 cup	1927	0.0	0.0	0	0	218.0	0
	1 oz	251	0.0	0.0	0	0	28.4	0
	1 tbsp	120	0.0	0.0	0	0	13.6	0
GRAVY. See also SAUCE.								
AU JUS								
Canned or in jars								
(Franco-American)	2 oz	10	0.0	2.0	330	na	0.0	0
(Heinz) 'HomeStyle'	1/4 cup	18	0.0	2.0	350	na	1.0	na
Prepared from mix								
(French's)	1/4 cup	10	0.0	2.0	260	na	0.0	0
(Lawry's)	1 cup	84	6.3	11.1	3454	>.2 c	1.6	na
(McCormick/Schilling)	1/4 cup	20	1.0	3.5	786	na	0.3	na
BEEF								
Canned								
(Franco-American)	2 oz	25	0.0	4.0	340	na	1.0	(mq)
(Hormel) w/chunky beef 'Great Beginnings'	5 oz	136	12.0	7.0	904	na	7.0	(mq)
BROWN								
Canned or in jars								
(Heinz) 'HomeStyle'	1/4 cup	25	1.0	3.0	320	na	1.0	na
(Heinz) 'HomeStyle' w/onions	1/4 cup	25	1.0	3.0	330	(mq)	1.0	na
(LaChoy)	1/2 tsp	15	<1.0	4.0	15	<1.0	<1.0	0
Prepared from mix								
(French's)	1/4 cup	20	1.0	4.0	250	na	1.0	na
(Lawry's)	1 cup	94	3.8	16.5	1500	>.1 c	1.4	na
(McCormick/Schilling)	1/3 cup	30	0.7	4.7	417	na	1.0	na
(McCormick/Schilling)	1/4 cup	23	0.5	3.5	313	na	0.8	na
(McCormick/Schilling) 'Lite'	1/4 cup	10	<1.0	2.0	450	na	1.0	na
(Pillsbury)	1/4 cup	15	<1.0	3.0	300	na	0.0	0
(Weight Watchers)	1/4 cup	10	1.0	2.0	360	na	0.0	na
(Weight Watchers) w/mushrooms	1/4 cup	10	1.0	2.0	270	na	0.0	na
(Weight Watchers) w/onions	1/4 cup	10	1.0	2.0	310	na	0.0	na
CHICKEN								
Canned or in jars								
(Franco-American)	2 oz	45	0.0	3.0	240	na	4.0	na
(Franco-American) giblet	2 oz	30	1.0	3.0	310	na	2.0	na
(Heinz) 'HomeStyle'	1/4 cup	35	1.0	3.0	350	na	2.0	(mq)
(Heinz) 'Homestyle' w/mushrooms and onions	1/4 cup	35	1.0	3.0	330	na	2.0	1
(Hormel) 'Great Beginnings' w/chunky chicken	5 oz	147	14.0	5.0	567	na	8.0	(mq)

Food Name	Serv. Size	Total Cal.	Prot. GMS	Carbs GMS	Sod. MGS	Fiber GMS	Fat GMS	Chol. MGS
(Weight Watchers)	1/4 cup	10	1.0	2.0	410	na	0.0	na
Prepared from mix								
(French's)	1/4 cup	25	1.0	4.0	270	na	1.0	na
(Lawry's)	1 cup	99	2.5	15.5	980	>.1 c	2.8	na
(McCormick/Schilling)	1/4 cup	22	0.8	3.7	300	na	0.4	na
(Pillsbury)	1/4 cup	25	<1.0	4.0	230	na	1.0	(mq)
COUNTRY								
(Heinz) 'Homestyle' jar	2 oz	25	0.0	4.0	210	na	1.0	na
CREAM *(Franco-American)* canned	2 oz	35	0.0	4.0	220	na	2.0	na
HERB *(McCormick/Schilling)* mix, prepared	1/4 cup	20	0.5	3.0	312	na	0.5	na
MUSHROOM								
Canned or in jars								
(Franco-American)	2 oz	25	0.0	3.0	290	na	1.0	na
(Heinz) 'HomeStyle'	1/4 cup	25	1.0	3.0	340	na	1.0	na
Prepared from mix								
(French's)	1/4 cup	20	1.0	3.0	250	na	1.0	na
(McCormick/Schilling)	1/4 cup	19	0.5	3.0	270	na	0.5	na
ONION								
(French's) mix, prepared	1/4 cup	25	1.0	4.0	270	na	1.0	na
(McCormick/Schilling) mix, prepared	1/4 cup	22	0.6	3.6	na	na	0.6	337
PORK								
Canned or in jars								
(Franco-American)	1/4 cup	40	0.0	3.0	330	na	3.0	na
(Heinz) 'HomeStyle'	1/4 cup	25	1.0	3.0	310	na	1.0	na
(Hormel) 'Great Beginnings' w/chunky pork	5 oz	140	14.0	5.0	567	na	8.0	(mq)
Prepared from mix								
(French's)	1/4 cup	20	1.0	4.0	250	na	1.0	na
(McCormick/Schilling)	1/4 cup	20	0.6	4.0	297	na	0.6	na
TURKEY								
Canned or in jars								
(Franco-American)	2 oz	30	0.0	3.0	290	na	2.0	na
(Heinz) 'HomeStyle'	1/4 cup	25	1.0	3.0	370	na	1.0	(mq)
(Hormel) 'Great Beginnings' w/chunky turkey	5 oz	138	11.0	7.0	585	na	8.0	(mq)
Prepared from mix								
(Lawry's)	1 cup	102	2.6	13.4	1400	>.1 c	4.1	na
(McCormick/Schilling)	1/4 cup	22	0.5	4.0	353	na	0.5	na
GREAT NORTHERN BEAN								
boiled	4 oz	134	9.4	23.9	2	6.1	0.5	0
boiled, mature seeds	1/2 cup	104	7.3	18.6	2	>2.6 c	0.4	0
raw	1/2 cup	308	19.9	56.8	13	36.4	1.0	0
raw	1 oz	96	6.2	17.7	4	11.3	0.3	0
Canned								
(A&P)	1 cup	210	14.0	38.0	0	(mq)	1.0	0

Food Name	Serv. Size	Total Cal.	Prot. GMS	Carbs GMS	Sod. MGS	Fiber GMS	Fat GMS	Chol. MGS
(Allens)	1/2 cup	105	5.0	17.0	440	(mq)	<1.0	0
(Allens) w/pork	1/2 cup	100	5.0	19.0	320	(mq)	1.0	(mq)
(Bush's Best)	1/2 cup	70	5.0	16.0	380	5.0	0.0	na
(Eden Foods) organically grown, w/liquid	1/2 cup	110	6.0	20.0	15	6.4	<1.0	0
(Green Giant)	1/2 cup	80	6.0	18.0	290	5.0	1.0	0
(Joan of Arc)	1/2 cup	80	6.0	18.0	290	5.0	1.0	0
(Luck's) w/pork	7.25 oz	220	12.0	32.0	645	13.0	5.0	(mq)

GREEK SALAD, w/feta cheese and pitted Kalamata olives, refrigerated

(Trader Joe's)	1 salad	310	6.0	10.0	530	1.0	28.0	20

GREEN BEAN/string bean

boiled, drained	4 oz	40	2.1	8.9	3	2.0	0.3	0
boiled, drained	1/2 cup	22	1.2	4.9	2	1.1	0.2	0
raw, trimmed	1/2 cup	17	1.0	3.9	3	1.2	0.1	0
raw, trimmed	1 oz	9	0.5	2.0	2	.6	<.1	0
raw, untrimmed	1 lb	123	7.3	28.5	23	8.4	0.5	0

GREEN BEAN, CANNED

Cut

(A&P)	1/2 cup	20	1.0	4.0	350	(mq)	<1.0	0
(A&P) 'No Salt Added'	1/2 cup	20	1.0	4.0	10	(mq)	<1.0	0
(Allens)	1/2 cup	20	1.0	4.0	350	(mq)	<1.0	0
(Bush's Best)	1/2 cup	20	1.0	5.0	360	2.0	0.0	na
(Del Monte) w/liquid	1/2 cup	20	1.0	4.0	355	(mq)	0.0	0
(Del Monte) w/liquid 'No Salt Added'	1/2 cup	20	1.0	4.0	10	(mq)	0.0	0
(Bush's Best) 'Blue Lake'	1/2 cup	20	1.0	5.0	360	2.0	0.0	na
(Bush's Best) w/Shelly beans	1/2 cup	35	3.0	8.0	290	4.0	0.0	na
(Featherweight)	1/2 cup	25	1.0	5.0	10	(mq)	0.0	0
(Finast)	1/2 cup	20	1.0	4.0	400	(mq)	0.0	0
(Finast) 'No Salt Added'	1/2 cup	20	1.0	4.0	10	(mq)	0.0	0
(Finast) 'Veri-Green'	1/2 cup	20	1.0	4.0	320	(mq)	0.0	0
(Freshlike)	1/2 cup	20	1.0	4.0	340	na	0.0	na
(Freshlike) no salt added	1/2 cup	20	1.0	4.0	5	na	0.0	na
(Freshlike) no sugar or salt, in water	1/2 cup	20	1.0	4.0	5	na	0.0	na
(Freshlike) wax, water packed, w/o salt	1/2 cup	18	1.0	4.0	5	na	0.0	na
(Freshlike) wax, water packed, w/o sugar or salt	1/2 cup	18	1.0	4.0	5	na	0.0	na
(Green Giant)	1/2 cup	16	1.0	4.0	300	1.0	0.0	0
(Green Giant) 50% less salt	1/2 cup	16	<1.0	4.0	195	1.0	0.0	0
(Green Giant) kitchen sliced	1/2 cup	16	<1.0	4.0	390	1.0	0.0	0
(Green Giant) 'Pantry Express'	1/2 cup	12	<1.0	3.0	20	1.0	0.0	0
(IGA)	1/2 cup	20	1.0	5.0	10	(mq)	0.0	0
(Pathmark)	1/2 cup	20	1.0	4.0	430	(mq)	0.0	0
(Pathmark) 'Blue Lake'	1/2 cup	20	1.0	4.0	430	(mq)	0.0	0

Food Name	Serv. Size	Total Cal.	Prot. GMS	Carbs GMS	Sod. MGS	Fiber GMS	Fat GMS	Chol. MGS
(Pathmark) 'No Frills'	1 cup	35	2.0	8.0	640	(mq)	0.0	0
(Pathmark) 'No Salt Added'	1/2 cup	20	1.0	5.0	10	(mq)	0.0	0
(Quincy's)	4.3 oz	40	2.0	7.0	500	(mq)	1.0	0
(S&W) 'Premium Blue Lake'	1/2 cup	20	1.0	4.0	385	(mq)	0.0	0
(S&W) 'Premium Gold'	1/2 cup	20	1.0	5.0	385	(mq)	0.0	0
(S&W) stringless, w/liquid	1/2 cup	20	1.0	4.0	3850	(mq)	0.0	0
(S&W Nutradiet)	1/2 cup	20	1.0	4.0	5	(mq)	0.0	0
(Stokely)	1/2 cup	20	1.0	4.0	360	(mq)	0.0	0
(Stokely) 'No Salt or Sugar'	1/2 cup	20	1.0	4.0	5	(mq)	0.0	0
(Veg•All)	1/2 cup	20	1.0	4.0	340	na	0.0	na
French style								
(A&P)	1/2 cup	20	1.0	4.0	350	(mq)	<1.0	0
(A&P) 'No Salt Added'	1/2 cup	20	1.0	4.0	10	(mq)	<1.0	0
(Allens)	1/2 cup	20	1.0	4.0	350	(mq)	<1.0	0
(Bush's Best)	1/2 cup	20	1.0	5.0	360	2.0	0.0	na
(Del Monte) seasoned, w/liquid	1/2 cup	20	1.0	4.0	355	(mq)	0.0	0
(Finast)	1/2 cup	20	1.0	4.0	400	(mq)	0.0	0.
(Freshlike)	1/2 cup	20	1.0	4.0	340	na	0.0	na
(Freshlike) in water, w/o salt	1/2 cup	20	1.0	4.0	5	na	0.0	na
(Green Giant)	1/2 cup	16	<1.0	4.0	390	1.0	0.0	0
(Pathmark) 'Blue Lake'	1/2 cup	20	1.0	4.0	430	(mq)	0.0	0
(Pathmark) 'No Frills'	1 cup	35	2.0	8.0	640	(mq)	0.0	0
(Pathmark) 'No Salt Added'	1/2 cup	20	1.0	5.0	10	(mq)	0.0	0
(S&W) 'Premium Blue Lake'	1/2 cup	20	1.0	4.0	385	(mq)	0.0	0
(S&W) stringless, w/liquid	1/2 cup	20	1.0	4.0	3850	(mq)	0.0	0
(Veg•All)	1/2 cup	20	1.0	4.0	340	na	0.0	na
Italian								
(Allens)	1/2 cup	18	1.0	3.0	260	(mq)	<1.0	0
(Del Monte) cut	1/2 cup	25	1.0	6.0	355	(mq)	0.0	0
Whole								
(A&P)	1/2 cup	20	1.0	4.0	350	(mq)	<1.0	0
(Allens) Shelly beans	1/2 cup	35	2.0	6.0	395	(mq)	<1.0	0
(Bush's Best)	1/2 cup	20	1.0	5.0	360	2.0	0.0	na
(Del Monte) w/liquid	1/2 cup	20	1.0	4.0	355	(mq)	0.0	0
(Finast)	1/2 cup	25	1.0	4.0	400	(mq)	0.0	0
(Freshlike)	1/2 cup	20	1.0	4.0	340	na	0.0	na
(Green Giant) amandine	1/2 cup	45	2.0	5.0	300	2.0	3.0	0
(IGA)	1 cup	45	2.0	8.0	640	(mq)	0.0	0
(Pathmark)	1/2 cup	20	1.0	4.0	430	(mq)	0.0	0
(S&W) dilled	1/2 cup	60	1.0	15.0	3850	(mq)	0.0	0
(S&W) stringless, w/liquid	1/2 cup	20	1.0	4.0	3850	(mq)	0.0	0
(S&W) 'Vertical Pak'	1/2 cup	20	1.0	4.0	385	(mq)	0.0	0

Food Name	Serv. Size	Total Cal.	Prot. GMS	Carbs GMS	Sod. MGS	Fiber GMS	Fat GMS	Chol. MGS
GREEN BEAN, FREEZE-DRIED								
(Mountain House) diluted as directed	1/2 cup	35	1.0	6.0	tr	(mq)	0.0	0
GREEN BEAN, FROZEN								
Cut								
(A&P)	3 oz	25	1.0	6.0	140	(mq)	<1.0	0
(Birds Eye)	3 oz	25	1.0	6.0	0	2.0	0.0	0
(Birds Eye) 'Portion Pack'	3 oz	25	1.0	6.0	0	2.0	0.0	0
(Finast)	3 oz	25	1.0	6.0	5	(mq)	0.0	0
(Freshlike)	3 oz	25	1.0	6.0	5	na	0.0	na
(Frosty Acres)	3 oz	25	1.0	6.0	3	2.0	0.0	0
(Green Giant) 'Harvest Fresh'	1/2 cup	16	1.0	4.0	95	1.0	0.0	0
(Green Giant) in butter sauce	1/2 cup	30	1.0	4.0	230	1.5	1.0	5
(Seabrook)	3 oz	25	1.0	6.0	3	2.0	0.0	0
(Stokely) 'Singles'	3 oz	30	2.0	6.0	5	(mq)	1.0	0
French style								
(A&P)	3 oz	25	1.0	6.0	0	(mq)	<1.0	0
(Birds Eye)	3 oz	25	1.0	6.0	0	2.0	0.0	0
(Bird's Eye) w/almonds								
'Combination Vegetables'	3 oz	50	3.0	8.0	340	2.0	2.0	0
(Finast)	3 oz	25	1.0	6.0	5	(mq)	0.0	0
(Freshlike)	3 oz	25	1.0	6.0	5	na	0.0	na
(Frosty Acres)	3 oz	25	1.0	6.0	3	2.0	0.0	0
(Seabrook)	3 oz	25	1.0	6.0	3	2.0	0.0	0
(Southern)	3.5 oz	34	1.6	6.9	20	(mq)	0.1	0
(Veg•All)	3 oz	25	1.0	6.0	5	na	0.0	na
Italian								
(Birds Eye)	3 oz	30	2.0	7.0	0	3.0	0.0	0
(Finast) cut	3 oz	30	2.0	7.0	5	(mq)	0.0	0
(Freshlike)	3 oz	30	2.0	7.0	5	na	0.0	na
(Frosty Acres)	3 oz	30	2.0	7.0	3	2.0	0.0	0
(Seabrook)	3 oz	30	2.0	7.0	3	2.0	0.0	0
(Veg•All)	3 oz	30	2.0	7.0	5	na	0.0	na
Whole								
(Bird's Eye) Bavarian style, w/spaetzle	3.3 oz	100	2.0	11.0	350	2.0	5.0	10
(Birds Eye) 'Deluxe'	3 oz	25	1.0	5.0	0	2.0	0.0	0
(Bird's Eye) 'Farm Fresh Whole Vegetables'	4 oz	30	2.0	7.0	0	2.0	0.0	0
(Bird's Eye) petite 'Deluxe'	2.6 oz	20	1.0	5.0	0	2.0	0.0	0
(Freshlike)	3 oz	25	1.0	5.0	5	na	0.0	na
(Green Giant)	1/2 cup	14	1.0	4.0	10	1.5	0.0	0
(Green Giant) and creamy mushroom								
'Garden Gourmet'	1 pkg	220	6.0	29.0	860	4.0	11.0	25
(Green Giant) in butter sauce								
'One Serving'	5.5 oz	60	2.0	8.0	370	3.0	2.0	5

Food Name	Serv. Size	Total Cal.	Prot. GMS	Carbs GMS	Sod. MGS	Fiber GMS	Fat GMS	Chol. MGS
(Green Giant) 'Plain Polybag'	1/2 cup	14	1.0	4.0	10	1.0	0.0	0
(Seabrook)	3 oz	25	1.0	5.0	1	2.0	0.0	0
(Southern)	3.5 oz	33	1.6	6.8	20	(mq)	0.1	0
(Stouffer's) mushroom casserole	4.75 oz	160	3.0	13.0	680	(mq)	11.0	na
(Veg·All)	3 oz	25	1.0	5.0	5	na	0.0	na

GREEN ONION. See ONION, GREEN.

GRENADINE. See ALCOHOLIC BEVERAGES.

GRITS

Dry

white *(Arrowhead Mills)*	2 oz	200	5.0	43.0	1	1.5	1.0	0
white, enriched	1 cup	579	13.7	124.2	2	2.5	1.9	0
white, enriched	1 tbsp	36	0.9	7.7	0	.2	0.1	0
white, enriched 'Regular/Quick'								
(Aunt Jemima)	3 tbsp	101	2.4	22.4	1	1.4	0.2	0
white, unenriched	1 cup	579	13.7	124.2	2	2.5	1.9	0
white, unenriched	1 tbsp	36	0.9	7.7	0	.2	0.1	0
yellow *(Arrowhead Mills)*	2 oz	200	5.0	44.0	1	1.5	1.0	0
yelllow, enriched	1 cup	579	13.7	124.2	2	2.5	1.9	0
yellow, enriched	1 tbsp	36	0.9	7.7	0	.2	0.1	0
yellow, enriched *(Quick)*	3 tbsp	101	2.4	22.4	1	1.2	0.2	0
yellow, unenriched	1 cup	579	13.7	124.2	2	2.5	1.9	0
yellow, unenriched	1 tbsp	36	0.9	7.7	0	.2	0.1	0

Prepared

white, enriched, cooked w/water	1 cup	145	3.4	31.5	0	.5	0.5	0
white, unenriched, cooked w/water	1 cup	145	3.4	31.5	0	.5	0.5	0
yellow, enriched, cooked w/water	1 cup	145	3.4	31.5	0	.5	0.5	0
yellow, unenriched, cooked w/water	1 cup	145	3.4	31.5	0	.5	0.5	0

GRITS, CANNED

golden *(Allens)*	1/2 cup	80	2.0	16.0	370	(mq)	<1.0	0
golden *(Bush's Best)*	1/2 cup	45	1.0	11.0	390	na	0.0	na
golden *(Van Camp's)*	1 cup	128	2.7	27.9	701	>.8 c	0.6	0
golden, w/red and green peppers								
(Van Camp's)	1 cup	129	2.6	28.5	685	>.7 c	0.5	0
Mexican *(Allens)*	1/2 cup	80	2.0	16.0	330	(mq)	<1.0	0
white	1 cup	115	2.4	22.8	336	>.7 c	1.4	0
white	4 oz	82	1.7	16.2	238	>.5 c	1.0	0
white *(Allens)*	1/2 cup	70	2.0	16.0	430	(mq)	<1.0	0
white *(Bush's Best)*	1/2 cup	45	<1.0	11.0	450	na	0.0	na
white *(Van Camp's)*	1 cup	138	3.0	30.0	708	>.8 c	0.7	0
yellow	1 cup	115	2.4	22.8	336	>.7 c	1.4	0
yellow	4 oz	82	1.7	16.2	238	>.5 c	1.0	0

Food Name	Serv. Size	Total Cal.	Prot. GMS	Carbs GMS	Sod. MGS	Fiber GMS	Fat GMS	Chol. MGS
GRITS, INSTANT								
white, hominy product, dry, one packet								
(Quaker)	.8 oz	79	1.9	17.7	440	1.2	0.1	0
w/imitation bacon bits, dry, one packet								
(Quaker)	1 oz	101	2.7	21.6	590	1.5	0.4	0
w/imitation ham bits, dry, one packet								
(Quaker)	1 oz	99	2.7	21.3	800	1.7	0.3	0
w/real cheddar cheese flavor, dry, one								
packet *(Quaker)*	1 oz	104	2.2	21.6	497	1.3	1.0	na
GRITS, QUICK-COOKING								
Dry								
white, enriched	1 cup	579	13.7	124.2	2	2.5	1.9	0
white, enriched	1 tbsp	36	0.9	7.7	0	.2	0.1	0
white, unenriched	1 cup	579	13.7	124.2	2	2.5	1.9	0
white, unenriched	1 tbsp	36	0.9	7.7	0	.2	0.1	0
yellow, enriched	1 cup	579	13.7	124.2	2	2.5	1.9	0
yellow, enriched	1 tbsp	36	0.9	7.7	0	.2	0.1	0
yellow, enriched 'Quick' *(Quaker)*	3 tbsp	101	2.4	22.4	1	1.2	0.2	na
yellow, unenriched	1 cup	579	13.7	124.2	2	2.5	1.9	0
yellow, unenriched	1 tbsp	36	0.9	7.7	0	.2	0.1	0
Prepared								
white, enriched, cooked w/water	1 cup	145	3.4	31.5	0	.5	0.5	0
white, unenriched, cooked w/water	1 cup	145	3.4	31.5	0	.5	0.5	0
yellow, enriched, cooked w/water	1 cup	145	3.4	31.5	0	.5	0.5	0
yellow, unenriched, cooked w/water	1 cup	145	3.4	31.5	0	.5	0.5	0
GROUND CHERRY. See CAPE GOOSEBERRY.								
GROUND HUSK TOMATO. See TOMATILLO.								
GROUPER, MIXED SPECIES								
broiled	4 oz	134	28.2	0.0	60	0	1.5	53
dry-heat cooked	4 oz	134	28.2	0.0	60	0	1.5	53
dry-heat cooked	3 oz	100	21.1	0.0	45	0	1.1	40
microwaved	4 oz	134	28.2	0.0	60	0	1.5	53
raw	1 lb	417	87.9	0.0	239	0	4.6	166
raw	3 oz	78	16.5	0.0	45	0	0.9	31
raw	1 oz	26	5.5	0.0	15	0	0.3	10
GUACAMOLE. See DIP, AVOCADO.								
GUACAMOLE SEASONING								
(Lawry's) 'Seasoning Blend' dry mix	1 pkg	60	1.7	12.6	1495	>.8 c	0.4	0
(Old El Paso) dry mix	1/7 pkg	7	0.0	2.0	240	0	0.0	0
GUANABANA/soursop								
raw, approx 2.1 lb	1 med	416	6.3	105.3	87	>6.9 c	1.9	0
trimmed	1 oz	19	0.3	4.8	4	>.3 c	0.1	0
trimmed	1/2 cup	75	1.1	18.9	16	>1.2 c	0.3	0

Food Name	Serv. Size	Total Cal.	Prot. GMS	Carbs GMS	Sod. MGS	Fiber GMS	Fat GMS	Chol. MGS
untrimmed	1 lb	202	3.0	51.2	42	>3.3 c	0.9	0
GUANABANA NECTAR *(Libby's)*	6 oz	110	0.0	26.0	15	na	0.0	na
GUANABANA PUNCH, 'Rain Forest'								
(Knudsen & Sons)	8 oz	125	<1.0	29.0	na	na	0.0	na
GUAVA								
trimmed	1 cup	84	1.4	19.6	5	8.9	1.0	0
trimmed	1 fruit	46	0.7	10.7	3	4.9	0.5	0
trimmed	1 oz	15	0.2	3.4	1	>1.6 c	0.2	0
untrimmed	1 lb	183	3.0	43.1	9	>20.3 c	2.2	0
w/edible seeds *(Sunfresh)*	3.5 oz	70	0.0	18.0	15	6.0	0.0	7
GUAVA, STRAWBERRY								
trimmed	1 cup	168	1.4	42.4	90	>15.6 c	1.5	0
trimmed	1 oz	20	0.2	4.9	11	>1.8 c	0.2	0
trimmed	1 fruit	4	0.0	1.0	2	>.4 c	0.0	0
untrimmed	1 lb	268	2.2	66.9	141	>24.7 c	2.3	0
GUAVA CRANBERRY JUICE								
organic 'Cruz' *(Santa Cruz Natural)*	8 oz	130	1.0	30.0	na	na	<1.0	na
GUAVA FRUIT DRINK								
Hawaiian 'Mauna La'i' *(Ocean Spray)*	6 oz	100	0.0	24.0	15	(tr)	0.0	0
GUAVA JUICE								
'Orchard Tropicals' bottled, diluted *(Welch's)*	6 oz	100	0.0	25.0	20	0	0.0	0
'Orchard Tropicals' frozen, diluted *(Welch's)*	6 oz	100	0.0	25.0	20	0	0.0	0
GUAVA NECTAR								
(Kern's)	6 oz	110	0.0	28.0	0	na	0.0	na
(Libby's)	6 oz	110	0.0	26.0	15	(mq)	0.0	0
GUAVA PASSION DRINK								
Hawaiian 'Hawaii' *(Pathmark)*	6 oz	100	0.0	25.0	10	(tr)	0.0	0
Hawaiian 'Mauna La'i' *(Ocean Spray)*	6 oz	100	0.0	25.0	10	(tr)	0.0	0
GUAVA STRAWBERRY DRINK 'Refresher'								
(Veryfine)	8 oz	120	0.3	30.0	25	(tr)	0.0	0
GUINEA HEN								
giblets, raw	100 gm	157	20.8	1.2	70	0	7.0	350
meat and skin, raw	1 lb	567	84.0	0.0	241	0	23.2	266
meat only, raw	1 oz	31	5.9	0.0	(mq)	0	0.7	18
GUMBO. See OKRA.								
GUMBO FILE POWDER *(Tone's)*	1 tsp	8	0.2	1.7	<1	.6	0.2	0

H

Food Name	Serv. Size	Total Cal.	Prot. GMS	Carbs GMS	Sod. MGS	Fiber GMS	Fat GMS	Chol. MGS
HADDOCK								
baked	4 oz	127	27.5	0.0	99	0	1.1	84

Food Name	Serv. Size	Total Cal.	Prot. GMS	Carbs GMS	Sod. MGS	Fiber GMS	Fat GMS	Chol. MGS
broiled	4 oz	127	27.5	0.0	99	0	1.1	84
dry-heat cooked	3 oz	95	20.6	0.0	74	0	0.8	63
microwaved	4 oz	127	27.5	0.0	99	0	1.1	84
raw	1 lb	396	85.8	0.0	310	0	3.3	261
raw	3 oz	74	16.1	0.0	58	0	0.6	48
smoked	3 oz	99	21.5	0.0	649	0	0.8	65
HADDOCK FILLET, FROZEN								
(SeaPak)	4 oz	90	18.0	0.0	120	0	1.0	(mq)
battered (Van de Kamp's)	2 pieces	250	12.0	19.0	580	na	15.0	30
battered, 'Crunchy' (Mrs. Paul's)	2 pieces	190	14.0	22.0	580	(mq)	5.0	25
breaded (Van de Kamp's)	2 pieces	270	12.0	19.0	290	na	16.0	25
breaded, in lemon butter, 'Microwave' (Gorton's)	1 pkg	360	23.0	19.0	730	(mq)	21.0	100
breaded, 'Light' (Mrs. Paul's)	1 piece	220	17.0	15.0	350	(mq)	9.0	45
breaded, 'Light' (Van de Kamp's)	1 piece	240	15.0	21.0	380	(mq)	11.0	35
'Fishmarket Fresh' (Gorton's)	5 oz	110	25.0	0.0	120	0	1.0	(mq)
natural (Van de Kamp's)	4 oz	90	21.0	0.0	125	0	1.0	20
HALIBUT								
ATLANTIC								
broiled	4 oz	159	30.3	0.0	78	0	3.3	46
dry-heat cooked	4 oz	159	30.3	0.0	78	0	3.3	46
dry-heat cooked	3 oz	119	22.7	0.0	59	0	2.5	35
microwaved	4 oz	159	30.3	0.0	78	0	3.3	46
raw	1 lb	497	94.4	0.0	245	0	10.4	146
raw	3 oz	94	17.7	0.0	46	0	2.0	27
raw	1 oz	31	5.9	0.0	15	0	0.6	9
GREENLAND								
dry-heat cooked	3 oz	203	15.7	0.0	88	0	15.1	50
raw	1 lb	845	65.2	0.0	363	0	62.8	209
raw	3 oz	158	12.2	0.0	68	0	11.8	39
raw	1 oz	53	4.1	0.0	23	0	3.9	13
PACIFIC								
broiled	4 oz	159	30.3	0.0	78	0	3.3	46
dry-heat cooked	4 oz	159	30.3	0.0	78	0	3.3	46
dry-heat cooked	3 oz	119	22.7	0.0	59	0	2.5	35
microwaved	4 oz	159	30.3	0.0	78	0	3.3	46
raw	1 lb	497	94.4	0.0	245	0	10.4	146
raw	3 oz	94	17.7	0.0	46	0	2.0	27
raw	1 oz	31	5.9	0.0	15	0	0.6	9
raw, fillet portions, skinless (Peter Pan Seafoods)	3.5 oz	110	20.8	na	54	na	2.3	32
HALIBUT, FROZEN								
fillet, battered (Van de Kamp's)	2 pieces	150	8.0	16.0	400	na	6.0	10

Food Name	Serv. Size	Total Cal.	Prot. GMS	Carbs GMS	Sod. MGS	Fiber GMS	Fat GMS	Chol. MGS
steaks, w/o seasoning mix *(SeaPak)* ..	6-oz pkg	160	36.0	0.0	120	0	1.0	(mq)

HAM. See HAM, ALTERNATIVE; HAM, CANNED; HAM, CURED; HAM, FRESH; HAM, MINCED; HAM PATTY.

HAM, ALTERNATIVE

Food Name	Serv. Size	Total Cal.	Prot. GMS	Carbs GMS	Sod. MGS	Fiber GMS	Fat GMS	Chol. MGS
(Worthington) frozen, roll 'Wham' approx .9-oz slices	3 slices	120	11.0	3.0	940	(mq)	7.0	0

HAM, CANNED

Food Name	Serv. Size	Total Cal.	Prot. GMS	Carbs GMS	Sod. MGS	Fiber GMS	Fat GMS	Chol. MGS
chopped	1 oz	68	4.6	0.1	387	0	5.3	14
chopped	.75-oz slice	50	3.4	0.1	287	0	4.0	10
cured, extra lean, approx 4% fat, baked ..	3 oz	116	18.0	0.4	965	0	4.2	25
cured, extra lean, approx 4% fat, unheated	1 oz	34	5.2	0.0	356	0	1.3	11
cured, extra lean and regular, baked	3 oz	142	17.8	0.4	908	0	7.2	35
cured, extra lean and regular, unheated ...	1 oz	41	5.1	0.0	362	0	2.1	11
cured, regular, approx 13% fat, baked	3 oz	192	17.5	0.4	800	0	12.9	53
cured, regular, approx 13% fat, unheated ..	1 oz	54	4.8	0.0	352	0	3.7	11
(Armour) chopped	3 oz	190	13.0	1.0	1260	na	14.0	na
(Black Label)								
'5-lb can'	4 oz	140	20.0	0.0	1245	0	7.0	(mq)
'3-lb can'	4 oz	140	20.0	0.0	1315	0	7.0	(mq)
'1 1/2-lb can'	4 oz	150	21.0	0.0	1324	0	7.0	(mq)
(Chi-Chi's) 'Black Label'	1 oz	37	5.0	2.0	303	na	1.0	15
(EXL) 'Deli Ham' 10-lb can	4 oz	130	20.0	0.0	1368	0	6.0	(mq)
(Holiday Glaze) '3-lb can'	4 oz	130	21.0	2.0	(mq)	0	4.0	(mq)
(Hormel)								
'Bone-In'	4 oz	210	17.0	1.0	(mq)	0	15.0	(mq)
chopped, '8-lb can'	3 oz	240	12.0	1.0	1062	0	21.0	(mq)
chopped, '12-oz can'	2 oz	120	10.0	0.0	703	0	9.0	(mq)
chunk	6.75 oz	310	32.0	0.0	2241	0	20.0	(mq)
chunk	2.5 oz	110	11.0	1.0	780	na	7.0	35
'Cure/81'	4 oz	160	22.0	0.0	1322	0	8.0	(mq)
'Cure/81'	1 oz	31	5.0	2.0	291	na	1.0	15
'Curemaster'	4 oz	140	22.0	1.0	1361	0	5.0	(mq)
'Curemaster'	2 oz	60	10.0	1.0	627	na	2.0	26
'Light and Lean 97'	2 oz	60	10.0	1.0	450	na	2.0	26
roll	4 oz	170	21.0	0.0	1338	0	10.0	(mq)
spiced	3 oz	240	13.0	1.0	1093	0	21.0	(mq)
(JM) '95% Fat-free'	2 oz	60	10.0	1.0	680	0	2.0	(mq)
(Light & Lean) 'Boneless'	2 oz	60	10.0	1.0	574	0	2.0	(mq)
(Oscar Mayer) 'Jubilee'	1 oz	29	5.0	0.1	287	0	0.9	14
(Rath) hickory smoked, 'Black Hawk'	2 oz	60	10.0	1.0	720	0	2.0	(mq)

Food Name	Serv. Size	Total Cal.	Prot. GMS	Carbs GMS	Sod. MGS	Fiber GMS	Fat GMS	Chol. MGS
HAM, CURED								
(NOTE: TRIMMED = Lean; separable fat removed. UNTRIMMED = Separable fat not removed.)								
BONELESS								
center slice, country-style, trimmed,								
unheated	1 oz	55	7.9	0.1	764	0	2.4	20
center slice, untrimmed, unheated	1 oz	58	5.7	0.0	393	0	3.7	15
extra lean, approx 5% fat, baked	3 oz	123	17.8	1.3	1023	0	4.7	45
extra lean, approx 5% fat, unheated	1 oz	37	5.5	0.3	405	0	1.4	13
extra lean and regular, baked	3 oz	140	18.7	0.4	1177	0	6.5	48
extra lean and regular, unheated	1 oz	46	5.2	0.7	362	0	2.4	15
extra lean and regular, unheated,								
4 x 6 1/4 inch slice	1 slice	46	5.2	0.7	362	0	2.4	15
mini *(JM)*	3 oz	90	17.0	0.0	40	0	3.0	(mq)
regular, approx 11% fat, baked	3 oz	151	19.2	0.0	1275	0	7.7	50
regular, approx 11% fat, unheated	1 oz	52	5.0	0.9	373	0	3.0	16
steak, 'Jubilee' *(Oscar Mayer)*	2 oz	57	9.7	0.2	754	0	1.9	31
steak, unheated	2 oz	69	11.1	0.0	720	0	2.4	26
w/natural juices, 'EZ Cut' *(JM)*	2 oz	70	11.0	1.0	660	0	3.0	(mq)
WHOLE								
trimmed, fully cooked, baked	3 oz	133	21.3	0.0	1128	0	4.7	47
trimmed, fully cooked, unheated	1 oz	42	6.3	0.0	430	0	1.6	15
trimmed *(JM)*	3 oz	140	17.0	0.0	40	0	8.0	na
untrimmed, fully cooked, baked	3 oz	207	18.3	0.0	1009	0	14.2	53
untrimmed, fully cooked, unheated	1 oz	70	5.2	0.0	364	0	5.3	16
HAM, FRESH. See also PORK.								
(NOTE: TRIMMED = Lean; separable fat removed. UNTRIMMED = Separable fat not removed.)								
LEG, RUMP HALF								
Trimmed								
raw	1 lb	621	96.3	0.0	313	0	23.5	277
raw	1 oz	39	6.0	0.0	20	0	1.5	17
roasted	3 oz	175	26.3	0.0	55	0	6.9	82
roasted, diced	1 cup	278	41.8	0.0	88	0	11.0	130
Untrimmed								
raw	1 lb	1007	85.0	0.0	277	0	71.2	299
raw	1 oz	63	5.3	0.0	17	0	4.4	19
roasted	3 oz	214	24.5	0.0	53	0	12.1	82
roasted	1.5 oz	117	11.3	0.0	26	0	7.6	40
roasted, diced	1 cup	340	39.0	0.0	84	0	19.3	130
LEG, SHANK HALF								
Trimmed								
raw	1 lb	631	93.5	0.0	304	0	25.5	272
raw	1 oz	39	5.8	0.0	19	0	1.6	17
roasted	3 oz	183	24.0	0.0	54	0	8.9	78

Food Name	Serv. Size	Total Cal.	Prot. GMS	Carbs GMS	Sod. MGS	Fiber GMS	Fat GMS	Chol. MGS
roasted, diced	1 cup	290	38.1	0.0	86	0	14.2	124
Untrimmed								
raw	1 lb	1193	77.5	0.0	249	0	95.4	308
raw	1 oz	75	4.8	0.0	16	0	6.0	19
roasted	3 oz	246	21.5	0.0	50	0	17.0	78
roasted	1.5 oz	129	10.3	0.0	25	0	9.4	39
roasted, diced	1 cup	390	34.2	0.0	80	0	27.1	124
LEG, WHOLE								
Trimmed								
raw	1 lb	617	92.9	0.0	249	0	24.5	308
raw	1 oz	39	5.8	0.0	16	0	1.5	19
roasted	3 oz	179	25.0	0.0	54	0	8.0	80
roasted	1.5 oz	94	12.0	0.0	27	0	4.7	40
roasted	1 cup	285	39.7	0.0	86	0	12.7	127
Untrimmed								
raw	1 lb	1111	79.1	0.0	213	0	85.6	331
raw	1 oz	69	4.9	0.0	13	0	5.3	21
roasted	3 oz	232	22.8	0.0	51	0	15.0	80
roasted	1.5 oz	125	10.6	0.0	25	0	8.8	40
roasted, diced	1 cup	369	36.2	0.0	81	0	23.8	127
HAM, MINCED	1 oz	75	4.6	0.5	353	0	5.9	20
HAM ENTRÉE, FROZEN								
and asparagus bake *(Stouffer's)*	9.5 oz	520	18.0	32.0	1100	na	35.0	na
and cheese casserole, 'Microwave Classic'								
(Pillsbury)	1 pkg	470	18.0	34.0	1300	na	29.0	(mq)
dinner *(Morton)*	10 oz	290	15.0	49.0	1400	(mq)	4.0	45
'Platters' *(Banquet)*	10 oz	400	20.0	43.0	1180	(mq)	17.0	50
steak *(Le Menu)*	10 oz	300	19.0	31.0	1500	(mq)	11.0	(mq)
steak 'Classics' *(Armour)*	10.75 oz	270	15.0	36.0	1320	(mq)	7.0	50
w/scalloped potatoes 'Homestyle Recipe'								
(Swanson)	9 oz	300	19.0	26.0	1080	(mq)	13.0	(mq)
HAM LUNCHEON MEAT. See LUNCHEON MEAT.								
HAM PATTY								
canned *(Hormel)*	1 patty	180	7.0	0.0	456	0	16.0	(mq)
canned, w/cheese *(Hormel)*	1 patty	190	7.0	0.0	468	0	18.0	(mq)
cured, boneless steak, extra lean,								
unheated	2-oz slice	69	11.1	0.0	720	0	2.4	26
cured, unheated	1 oz	89	3.6	0.5	308	0	8.0	20
grilled	4 oz	388	15.1	1.9	1205	0	35.0	82
'Premium Brown 'N Serve' *(Swift)*	1 patty	130	3.0	1.0	260	0	13.0	(mq)
HAM SPREAD								
deviled	1 cup	790	31.3	0.0	2776	0	72.7	146
deviled	4.5-oz can	449	17.8	0.0	1580	0	41.3	83

Food Name	Serv. Size	Total Cal.	Prot. GMS	Carbs GMS	Sod. MGS	Fiber GMS	Fat GMS	Chol. MGS
deviled *(Hormel)*	1 oz	76	4.0	1.0	214	na	6.0	19
deviled *(Hormel)*	1 tbsp	35	2.0	0.0	108	0	3.0	(mq)
deviled *(Underwood)*	2 1/8 oz	220	8.0	<1.0	430	na	19.0	50
deviled *(Underwood)* 'Light'	2 1/8 oz	120	11.0	1.0	250	na	8.0	35
deviled *(Underwood)* 'Smoked'	2 1/8 oz	190	9.0	<1.0	260	na	18.0	65
ham and cheese	1 oz	69	4.6	0.6	339	0	5.3	17
ham and cheese	1 tbsp	37	2.4	0.3	179	0	2.8	9
ham salad	1 oz	61	2.5	3.0	259	0	4.4	10
ham salad	1 tbsp	32	1.3	1.6	137	0	2.3	6
ham salad 'Spreadables' *(Libby's)*	1.9 oz	70	5.0	6.0	380	1.1	3.0	10
HAM TACO, refrigerated, 'Border Breakfasts' *(Owens)*	2.17 oz	90	7.0	13.0	430	(mq)	6.0	50

HAMBURG PARSLEY. See PARSLEY ROOT.

HAMBURGER. See BEEF, GROUND.

HAMBURGER BUN. See BUN, HAMBURGER.

HAMBURGER ENTRÉE MIX

(Betty Crocker) 'Hamburger Helper'

Food Name	Serv. Size	Total Cal.	Prot. GMS	Carbs GMS	Sod. MGS	Fiber GMS	Fat GMS	Chol. MGS
beef noodle, dry	1/5 pkg	140	5.0	26.0	1000	(mq)	2.0	na
beef noodle, prepared	1 cup	320	20.0	26.0	1050	(mq)	15.0	(mq)
beef Romanoff, dry	1/5 pkg	180	7.0	31.0	1030	(mq)	3.0	na
beef Romanoff, prepared	1 cup	350	22.0	31.0	1070	(mq)	16.0	(mq)
beef taco, dry	1/5 pkg	160	4.0	33.0	930	na	1.0	na
beef taco, prepared	1 cup	330	19.0	33.0	970	na	14.0	na
beef teriyaki, dry	1/5 pkg	180	4.0	38.0	1110	na	1.0	na
beef teriyaki, prepared	1 cup	360	20.0	38.0	1160	na	14.0	na
cheddar and bacon, dry	1/5 pkg	190	7.0	28.0	950	na	6.0	na
cheddar and bacon, prepared	1 cup	400	24.0	30.0	1020	na	20.0	na
cheeseburger macaroni, dry	1/5 pkg	190	6.0	26.0	980	(mq)	6.0	na
cheeseburger macaroni, prepared	1 cup	370	21.0	28.0	1030	(mq)	19.0	(mq)
cheesy Italian, dry	1/5 pkg	160	5.0	27.0	970	(mq)	3.0	na
cheesy Italian, prepared w/2% milk	1 cup	360	22.0	30.0	1040	(mq)	17.0	(mq)
chili macaroni, dry	1/5 pkg	150	4.0	32.0	920	na	1.0	na
chili macaroni, prepared	1 cup	330	19.0	32.0	960	na	14.0	na
chili tomato, dry	1/5 pkg	150	5.0	31.0	1360	(mq)	1.0	na
chili tomato, prepared	1 cup	330	20.0	31.0	1410	(mq)	14.0	(mq)
chili w/beans, dry	1/4 pkg	130	5.0	25.0	1680	(mq)	1.0	na
chili w/beans, prepared	1 1/4 cup	350	24.0	25.0	1740	(mq)	17.0	(mq)
creamy Stroganoff, dry	1/5 pkg	190	5.0	30.0	800	(mq)	5.0	na
creamy Stroganoff, prepared w/whole milk	1 cup	390	22.0	30.0	870	(mq)	20.0	(mq)
hamburger hash, dry	1/5 pkg	140	3.0	27.0	970	(mq)	2.0	na
hamburger hash, prepared	1 cup	320	18.0	27.0	1020	(mq)	15.0	(mq)
hamburger stew, dry	1/5 pkg	120	3.0	25.0	960	(mq)	1.0	na

Food Name	Serv. Size	Total Cal.	Prot. GMS	Carbs GMS	Sod. MGS	Fiber GMS	Fat GMS	Chol. MGS
hamburger stew, prepared	1 cup	300	18.0	25.0	1010	(mq)	14.0	(mq)
lasagna, dry	1/5 pkg	160	5.0	33.0	1000	(mq)	1.0	na
lasagna, prepared	1 cup	340	21.0	33.0	1050	(mq)	14.0	(mq)
meat loaf, dry	1/5 pkg	70	2.0	13.0	620	(mq)	1.0	na
meat loaf, prepared	1 cup	360	27.0	14.0	710	(mq)	22.0	(mq)
mushroom and wild rice, dry	1/5 pkg	180	4.0	34.0	880	na	3.0	na
mushroom and wild rice, prepared	1 cup	380	21.0	37.0	950	na	16.0	na
nacho cheese, dry	1/5 pkg	160	4.0	32.0	980	na	2.0	na
nacho cheese, prepared	1 cup	360	21.0	35.0	1050	na	15.0	na
pizza dish, dry	1/5 pkg	180	6.0	37.0	960	(mq)	1.0	na
pizza dish, prepared	1 cup	360	21.0	37.0	1010	(mq)	14.0	(mq)
'Pizzabake' dry	1/6 pkg	150	4.0	29.0	800	(mq)	2.0	na
'Pizzabake' prepared	4.5 oz	320	19.0	29.0	840	(mq)	14.0	(mq)
potato au gratin, dry	1/5 pkg	150	4.0	28.0	860	(mq)	2.0	na
potato au gratin, prepared	1 cup	320	19.0	28.0	910	(mq)	15.0	(mq)
potato Stroganoff, dry	1/5 pkg	140	3.0	28.0	900	(mq)	2.0	na
potato Stroganoff, prepared	1 cup	320	18.0	28.0	950	(mq)	15.0	(mq)
rice Oriental, dry	1/5 pkg	180	4.0	38.0	1070	(mq)	1.0	na
rice Oriental, prepared	1 cup	340	19.0	38.0	1120	(mq)	14.0	(mq)
'Sloppy Joe Bake' dry	1/6 pkg	180	5.0	33.0	1060	(mq)	3.0	na
'Sloppy Joe Bake' prepared	5 oz	340	18.0	33.0	1100	(mq)	15.0	(mq)
spaghetti, dry	1/5 pkg	170	5.0	32.0	1060	(mq)	2.0	na
spaghetti, prepared	1 cup	340	20.0	32.0	1110	(mq)	15.0	(mq)
'Tacobake' dry	1/6 pkg	170	4.0	31.0	920	(mq)	4.0	na
'Tacobake' prepared	5.75 oz	320	17.0	31.0	940	(mq)	15.0	(mq)
tamale pie, dry	1/5 pkg	200	4.0	39.0	890	(mq)	3.0	na
tamale pie, prepared	1 cup	380	19.0	39.0	940	(mq)	16.0	(mq)
three cheese, dry	1/5 pkg	210	7.0	30.0	910	na	7.0	na
three cheese, prepared	1/5 pkg	400	24.0	32.0	980	na	20.0	na
zesty Italian, dry	1/5 pkg	170	6.0	35.0	940	(mq)	1.0	na
zesty Italian, prepared	1 cup	340	21.0	35.0	980	(mq)	13.0	(mq)
HAWAIIAN YAM. See YAM, MOUNTAIN.								
HAWS/hawthorn tree fruit								
scarlet, flesh and skin, raw	100 gm	87	2.0	20.8	0	>2.1 c	0.7	0
HAZELNUT, SHELLED/cobnut/filbert								
blanched	1 oz	191	3.6	4.5	1	>.5 c	19.1	0
dry-roasted, unblanched	1 oz	188	2.8	5.1	1	1.7	18.8	0
dry-roasted, unblanched, w/salt	1 oz	188	2.8	5.1	221	1.7	18.8	0
oil-roasted, unblanched	1 oz	187	4.1	5.4	1	1.8	18.1	0
oil-roasted, unblanched, w/salt	1 oz	187	4.1	5.4	223	1.8	18.1	0
unblanched	1 oz	179	3.7	4.4	1	1.7	17.8	0
unblanched, chopped	1 cup	727	15.0	17.6	3	7.0	72.0	0
HAZELNUT BUTTER, gourmet *(Roaster Fresh)*	1 oz	188	4.0	5.0	1	na	18.9	na

Food Name	Serv. Size	Total Cal.	Prot. GMS	Carbs GMS	Sod. MGS	Fiber GMS	Fat GMS	Chol. MGS
HAZELNUT OIL								
....	1 cup	1927	0.0	0.0	0	0	218.0	0
....	1 oz	251	0.0	0.0	0	0	28.4	0
....	1 tbsp	120	0.0	0.0	0	0	13.6	0
HAZELNUT SPREAD, Nutella, with milk								
and cocoa *(Ferrero)*	1 tbsp	80	1.0	9.0	10	na	5.0	0
HEART NUT. See CASHEW.								
HERB AND GARLIC MARINADE, w/lemon								
(Lawry's)	2 tbsp	36	3.6	3.8	3688	.4	<1.0	0
HERB SEASONING MIX								
Italian, 'Bag 'n Season' *(Schilling)*	1 pkg	94	2.0	21.0	1367	(mq)	0.2	na
mixed, 'Pinch of Herbs' *(Lawry's)*	1 tsp	9	0.3	0.9	259	>.2 c	0.5	0
HERBAL TEA. See TEA.								
HERRING								
ATLANTIC								
broiled	4 oz	230	26.1	0.0	130	0	13.1	87
dry-heat cooked	4 oz	230	26.1	0.0	130	0	13.1	87
dry-heat cooked	3 oz	173	19.6	0.0	98	0	9.9	65
kippered	4 oz	246	27.9	0.0	1041	0	14.0	93
kippered snacks, w/smoke flavoring,								
drained *(Beach Cliff)*	3.3 oz	220	17.0	1.0	350	na	17.0	na
microwaved	4 oz	230	26.1	0.0	130	0	13.1	87
pickled	4 oz	297	16.1	10.9	987	0	20.4	15
raw	1 lb	718	81.5	0.0	407	0	41.0	272
raw	3 oz	134	15.3	0.0	77	0	7.7	51
raw	1 oz	45	5.1	0.0	26	0	2.6	17
steaks, in soybean oil, drained *(Beach Cliff)*	3 oz	240	16.0	0.0	350	na	20.0	na
steaks, in water, drained *(Beach Cliff)*	3 oz	230	17.0	1.0	350	na	18.0	na
steaks, w/mustard, drained *(Beach Cliff)* ..	3 oz	227	13.0	4.0	350	na	18.0	na
steaks, w/tomato, drained *(Beach Cliff)* ...	3 oz	210	15.0	0.0	350	na	17.0	na
LAKE								
raw	1 lb	446	86.1	0.0	249	0	8.7	(mq)
raw	2.8-oz fillet	78	15.0	0.0	47	0	1.5	(mq)
raw	1 oz	28	5.4	0.0	16	0	0.5	(mq)
smoked	4 oz	201	18.6	0.0	545	0	13.5	36
PACIFIC								
dry-heat cooked	3 oz	213	17.9	0.0	81	0	15.1	84
raw	1 lb	885	74.4	0.0	335	0	63.0	348
raw	3 oz	166	13.9	0.0	63	0	11.8	65
raw	1 oz	55	4.6	0.0	21	0	3.9	22
HIBISCUS COOLER *(Knudsen & Sons)* ...	8 oz	95	<1.0	24.0	na	na	0.0	na
HIBISCUS CRANBERRY JUICE								
(Knudsen & Sons)	8 oz	110	<1.0	28.0	na	na	0.0	na

Food Name	Serv. Size	Total Cal.	Prot. GMS	Carbs GMS	Sod. MGS	Fiber GMS	Fat GMS	Chol. MGS
HICKORY NUT								
in shell	1 lb	954	18.5	26.5	1	>4.7 c	93.4	0
shelled	1 oz	187	3.6	5.2	0	1.9	18.3	0
HOG PLUM. See JOBO.								
HOMINY GRITS. See GRITS.								
HONEY								
extracted	1 cup	1031	1.0	279.0	17	0	0.0	0
extracted	1 tbsp	64	0.1	17.3	1	0	0.0	0
strained	1 cup	1031	1.0	279.0	17	0	0.0	0
strained	1 tbsp	64	0.1	17.3	1	0	0.0	0
(Golden Blossom)	1 tbsp	60	0.0	16.0	na	0	0.0	0
(Knott's Berry Farm)	1 oz	90	0.0	23.0	0	na	0.0	na
(Knott's Berry Farm)	1 tbsp	60	0.0	17.0	0	na	0.0	na
(Knott's Berry Farm)	.5 oz	30	0.0	17.0	0	na	0.0	na
(Sioux)	1 tbsp	60	0.0	16.0	na	0	0.0	0
HONEY BUTTER	1 tbsp	50	<1.0	11.0	5	0	1.0	na
HONEY ROLL SAUSAGE								
	1 oz	52	5.3	0.6	375	0	3.0	14
4 inch diam	1/8-inch slice	42	4.3	0.5	304	0	2.4	11
HONEYDEW MELON								
pulp	1 oz	10	0.1	2.6	3	>.2 c	<.1	0
raw, cubed	1 cup	59	0.8	15.6	17	1.0	0.2	0
raw, wedge	7 x 2 inches	45	0.6	11.8	13	.8	0.1	0
untrimmed	1 lb	74	1.0	19.2	21	>1.3 c	0.2	0
untrimmed (Dole)	7 x 2 inches	50	1.0	12.0	50	>1.0 c	0.0	na
HORSE								
roasted	3 oz	149	23.9	0.0	47	na	5.1	58
roasted, diced	1 cup	245	39.4	0.0	77	0	8.5	95
raw	1 lb	603	97.0	0.0	240	na	20.9	236
raw	1 oz	37	6.0	0.0	15	na	1.3	15
HORSE BEAN. See FAVA BEAN.								
HORSERADISH								
Prepared								
	1 tbsp	6	0.2	1.4	14	>.1 c	0.0	0
	1 tsp	2	0.1	0.5	5	>.1 c	0.0	0
(Crowley)	1 oz	10	<1.0	2.0	25	(mq)	<1.0	0
(Kraft)	1 tbsp	10	0.0	1.0	140	(mq)	0.0	0
(Kraft) cream style	1 tbsp	12	0.0	1.0	85	(mq)	0.0	0
(Gold's) hot	1 tsp	4	<1.0	<1.0	60	(mq)	<1.0	0
(Gold's) red	1 tsp	4	<1.0	<1.0	75	(mq)	<1.0	0
(Gold's) white	1 tsp	4	<1.0	<1.0	55	(mq)	<1.0	0
(Silver Spring) cream style	1 tsp	0	0.0	0.0	10	na	0.0	na
Raw	1 lb	288	10.6	65.3	27	>7.9 c	1.0	0

Food Name	Serv. Size	Total Cal.	Prot. GMS	Carbs GMS	Sod. MGS	Fiber GMS	Fat GMS	Chol. MGS
HORSERADISH, JAPANESE. See WASABI.								
HORSERADISH TREE								
Leafy tips								
boiled, drained	4 oz	68	6.0	12.6	10	>2.0 c	1.1	0
boiled, drained, chopped	1 cup	25	2.2	4.7	4	.8	0.4	0
raw, chopped	1 cup	13	2.0	1.7	2	.4	0.3	0
raw, trimmed	1 oz	18	2.7	2.3	3	>.4 c	0.4	0
raw, untrimmed	1 lb	181	26.4	23.3	26	>4.2 c	3.9	0
Pods								
boiled, drained	4 oz	41	2.4	9.3	49	5.0	0.2	0
boiled, drained, sliced	1 cup	42	2.5	9.6	51	5.0	0.2	0
boiled, drained, sliced	1/2 cup	21	1.2	4.8	25	2.5	0.1	0
raw, sliced	1 cup	37	2.1	8.5	42	3.2	0.2	0
raw, trimmed	1 oz	10	0.6	2.4	12	1.2	0.1	0
raw, untrimmed	1 lb	88	5.0	20.1	99	>3.1 c	0.5	0
raw, whole, approx 15 1/3 inches long	1 pod	4	0.2	0.9	5	.3	0.0	0
HOT CHOCOLATE. See COCOA MIX.								
HOT DOG. See FRANKFURTER.								
HOT DOG BUN. See BUN, FRANKFURTER.								
HUBBARD SQUASH. See SQUASH, HUBBARD.								
HUMMUS								
mix, dry (Casbah)	1 oz	110	5.0	10.0	na	(mq)	5.0	0
prepared	1/2 cup	210	6.0	24.8	300	>1.7 c	10.4	0
prepared	1 oz	48	1.4	5.7	69	>.4 c	2.4	0
HUSHPUPPY, FROZEN, 'Regular' (SeaPak)	4 oz	330	6.0	56.0	690	(mq)	9.0	na
HUSHPUPPY MIX								
deluxe, dry (Golden Dipt)	1.25 oz	120	3.0	26.0	520	(mq)	0.0	0
jalapeño, dry (Golden Dipt)	1.25 oz	120	3.0	27.0	570	(mq)	0.0	0
w/onion, dry (Golden Dipt)	1.25 oz	120	3.0	27.0	520	(mq)	0.0	0
HYACINTH BEAN								
boiled, drained	4 oz	57	3.3	10.4	2	>2.0 c	0.3	0
immature, boiled, drained	1/2 cup	22	1.3	4.1	1	>.8 c	0.1	0
immature, raw	1/2 cup	18	0.8	3.7	1	>.5 c	0.1	0
mature, boiled	1/2 cup	113	7.9	20.1	7	>2.4 c	0.6	0
mature, raw	1/2 cup	361	25.1	63.8	22	>7.5 c	1.8	0
raw, trimmed	1 oz	13	0.6	2.6	<1	>.4 c	0.1	0
raw, untrimmed	1 lb	196	8.9	38.8	8	>5.5 c	0.8	0
HYACINTH BEAN, DRIED								
mature, boiled	1/2 cup	114	7.9	20.1	7	>2.4 c	0.6	0
mature, boiled	4 oz	133	9.2	23.5	8	>2.8 c	0.7	0
mature, raw	1/2 cup	362	25.1	63.8	22	>7.5 c	1.8	0
mature, raw	1 oz	98	6.8	17.2	6	>2.0 c	0.5	0

I

Food Name	Serv. Size	Total Cal.	Prot. GMS	Carbs GMS	Sod. MGS	Fiber GMS	Fat GMS	Chol. MGS
ICE BARS AND DESSERTS. See also FRUIT BAR, FROZEN; SHERBET; SORBET.								
BAR								
'All Natural' all flavors (Popsicle)	1 bar	60	0.0	14.0	0	(tr)	0.0	0
'Ice Stripes' 1.5 oz, all flavors								
(Good Humor)	1 bar	35	0.0	8.6	0	(tr)	0.0	0
'Twin Pop' all flavors (Gold Bond)	1 bar	60	0.0	14.0	0	(tr)	0.0	0
'Water Ice' all flavors except cherry and								
wildberry (Popsicle)	1 bar	50	0.0	12.0	10	(tr)	0.0	0
Cherry								
'Calippo' 4.5 oz (Good Humor)	1 bar	138	0.1	34.9	5	(tr)	0.1	0
'Jumbo Jet Star' 4.5 oz (Good Humor)	1 bar	85	0.0	19.5	0	na	0.7	0
'Water Ice' (Popsicle)	1 bar	70	0.0	17.0	15	(tr)	0.0	0
Fruit								
and juice, 3 oz	1 bar	75	1.1	18.6	4	0	0.1	0
and water, aspartame-sweetened	1 bar	12	0.3	3.2	3	na	0.1	0
Lemon								
'Calippo' 4.5 oz (Good Humor)	1 bar	112	0.0	27.6	0	(tr)	0.1	0
'Great White Shark' 3 oz (Good Humor)	1 bar	68	0.0	17.0	7	na	0.1	(mq)
Orange								
'Calippo' 4.5 oz (Good Humor)	1 bar	111	0.0	27.2	0	(tr)	0.2	0
Wildberry, 'Water Ice' (Popsicle)	1 bar	40	0.0	10.0	10	(tr)	0.0	0
DESSERT								
cherry, Italian (Good Humor)	6 oz	138	0.0	34.2	0	(tr)	0.1	0
daiquiri (Baskin-Robbins)	1 scoop	140	0.0	35.0	15	na	0.0	0
lime	4 oz	75	0.4	31.3	21	0	0.0	0
pineapple-coconut	4 oz	108	0.0	22.9	34	na	2.5	0
ICE CREAM. See also ICE CREAM, ALTERNATIVE; ICE CREAM BAR; ICE CREAM BAR, ALTERNATI*								
ICE CREAM CAKE; ICE CREAM CONE; ICE CREAM MIX; ICE CREAM SNACKS AND SANDWICHE								
ICE MILK; ICE MILK BAR.								
ALMOND FUDGE (Baskin-Robbins)								
'Jamoca'	1 scoop	270	5.0	30.0	115	na	14.0	32
BANANA								
(Baskin-Robbins) sugar-free								
'Chunky Banana'	4 oz	100	3.0	20.0	50	na	1.0	3
(Ben & Jerry's) 'Chunky Monkey'	1/2 cup	280	4.0	29.0	50	1.0	19.0	70
BORDEAUX CHERRY (Healthy Choice)								
'Dairy Dessert'	4 oz	120	3.0	23.0	50	na	2.0	5
BORDEAUX CHERRY CHOCOLATE CHIP								
(Healthy Choice) 'Dairy Dessert'	4 oz	120	3.0	23.0	50	na	2.0	5
BOYSENBERRY (Good Humor) 'King Cone'	5 oz	340	3.9	51.6	151	(mq)	13.1	(mq)

Food Name	Serv. Size	Total Cal.	Prot. GMS	Carbs GMS	Sod. MGS	Fiber GMS	Fat GMS	Chol. MGS
BROWNIES 'N CREME *(Weight Watchers)*								
'ONE-ders'	4 oz	130	4.0	20.0	115	na	4.0	10
BUTTER ALMOND *(Breyers)*	4 oz	170	4.0	15.0	125	(mq)	10.0	25
BUTTER CRUNCH *(Sealtest)*	4 oz	150	2.0	18.0	90	(tr)	7.0	25
BUTTER PECAN								
(Ben & Jerry's)	1/2 cup	310	4.0	20.0	160	1.0	26.0	100
(Breyers)	4 oz	180	3.0	15.0	125	(mq)	12.0	25
(Frusen Glädjé)	4 oz	280	5.0	16.0	160	(mq)	21.0	85
(Häagen-Dazs)	4 oz	390	5.0	29.0	100	(mq)	24.0	110
(Lady Borden)	4 oz	180	3.0	16.0	65	(mq)	12.0	(mq)
(Sealtest)	4 oz	160	3.0	16.0	125	(mq)	9.0	15
BUTTER PECAN CRUNCH *(Healthy Choice)*								
'Dairy Dessert'	4 oz	140	3.0	26.0	80	na	2.0	5
CHERRY								
(Ben & Jerry's) 'Cherry Garcia'	1/2 cup	240	4.0	25.0	60	0	16.0	80
(Breyers) vanilla	4 oz	150	3.0	17.0	45	(tr)	7.0	20
CHOCOLATE								
(Baskin-Robbins)	1 scoop	270	5.0	32.0	160	na	14.0	37
(Baskin-Robbins) 'World Class'	1 scoop	280	5.0	35.0	145	na	14.0	36
(Ben & Jerry's) deep dark chocolate	1/2 cup	260	4.0	32.0	55	2.0	15.0	55
(Breyers)	4 oz	160	3.0	20.0	30	(tr)	8.0	20
(Darigold)	4 oz	140	2.0	17.0	70	(tr)	7.0	(mq)
(Darigold) 'Alpine'	4 oz	140	2.0	17.0	70	(tr)	7.0	(mq)
(Darigold) 'Classic'	4 oz	180	3.0	16.0	30	(tr)	13.0	(mq)
(Frusen Glädjé)	4 oz	240	5.0	17.0	65	(tr)	17.0	75
(Häagen-Dazs)	4 oz	270	5.0	24.0	50	(tr)	17.0	120
(Häagen-Dazs) deep	4 oz	290	5.0	26.0	70	(tr)	14.0	(mq)
(Healthy Choice) 'Dairy Dessert'	4 oz	130	3.0	24.0	70	na	2.0	5
(Sealtest)	4 oz	140	2.0	18.0	50	(tr)	6.0	20
CHOCOLATE, DUTCH *(Borden)*								
'Olde Fashioned Recipe'	4 oz	130	2.0	16.0	65	(tr)	6.0	(mq)
CHOCOLATE CARAMEL NUT								
(Baskin-Robbins) light	4 oz	130	3.0	19.0	8	na	5.0	0
CHOCOLATE CHIP								
(Baskin-Robbins)	1 scoop	260	4.0	27.0	110	na	15.0	40
(Breyers)	4 oz	170	3.0	18.0	45	na	10.0	35
(Dreyer's)	4 oz	150	3.0	16.0	40	(tr)	9.0	30
(Eskimo Pie) cone 'Cookie Dough'	1 cone	280	4.0	33.0	103	na	14.0	14
(Healthy Choice) 'Dairy Dessert'	4 oz	130	3.0	24.0	70	na	2.0	5
(Sealtest)	4 oz	150	2.0	17.0	50	(tr)	8.0	15
(Weight Watchers) 'ONE-ders'	4 oz	120	3.0	19.0	80	na	4.0	10
CHOCOLATE CHIP CHOCOLATE								
(Häagen-Dazs)	4 oz	290	5.0	28.0	40	(tr)	20.0	105

Food Name	Serv. Size	Total Cal.	Prot. GMS	Carbs GMS	Sod. MGS	Fiber GMS	Fat GMS	Chol. MGS
CHOCOLATE CHIP COOKIE DOUGH								
(Ben & Jerry's) .... 1/2 cup	270	4.0	30.0	92	0	17.0	80	
CHOCOLATE CHOCOLATE CHIP								
(Frusen Glädjé) .... 4 oz	270	5.0	21.0	60	(tr)	18.0	55	
CHOCOLATE CHUNK								
(Ben & Jerry's) 'New York Super Fudge								
Chunk' .... 1/2 cup	290	5.0	28.0	55	2.0	20.0	50	
CHOCOLATE FUDGE								
(Ben & Jerry's) 'Chocolate Fudge								
Brownie' .... 1/2 cup	250	4.0	31.0	100	2.0	14.0	50	
(Ben & Jerry's) double chocolate fudge 1/2 cup	280	5.0	35.0	60	3.0	16.0	55	
(Häagen-Dazs) deep .... 4 oz	290	5.0	26.0	70	(tr)	14.0	(mq)	
CHOCOLATE MINT (Häagen-Dazs) ..... 4 oz	300	5.0	26.0	50	(tr)	20.0	(mq)	
CHOCOLATE PEANUT BUTTER COOKIE DOUGH								
(Ben & Jerry's) .... 1/2 cup	300	6.0	32.0	85	2.0	20.0	55	
CHOCOLATE RASPBERRY TRUFFLE								
(Baskin-Robbins) 'International								
Creams' .... 1 scoop	310	4.0	35.0	115	na	17.0	45	
CHOCOLATE SWIRL (Borden) .... 4 oz	130	2.0	18.0	65	(tr)	6.0	(mq)	
CHOCOLATE TRIPLE STRIPES (Sealtest) .. 4 oz	140	2.0	17.0	50	(tr)	7.0	(mq)	
CHOCOLATE-PEANUT BUTTER, DEEP								
(Häagen-Dazs) .... 4 oz	330	7.0	25.0	90	(tr)	19.0	(mq)	
COCONUT ALMOND FUDGE CHIP								
(Ben & Jerry's) .... 1/2 cup	320	6.0	24.0	82	2.0	28.0	75	
COFFEE								
(Baskin-Robbins) light 'Espresso and Cream' 4 oz	120	3.0	15.0	0	na	5.0	12	
(Ben & Jerry's) Aztec harvest coffee ... 1/2 cup	230	4.0	22.0	55	0	16.0	90	
(Breyers) .... 4 oz	150	3.0	16.0	50	0	8.0	30	
(Häagen-Dazs) .... 4 oz	270	5.0	23.0	120	0	17.0	55	
(Sealtest) .... 4 oz	140	2.0	16.0	50	0	7.0	15	
COFFEE ALMOND FUDGE								
(Ben & Jerry's) .... 1/2 cup	290	6.0	24.0	85	2.0	20.0	75	
COFFEE TOFFEE								
(Ben & Jerry's) 'Coffee Toffee Crunch' .. 1/2 cup	280	4.0	28.0	120	0	19.0	80	
(Healthy Choice) 'Dairy Dessert' .... 4 oz	130	3.0	25.0	80	na	2.0	5	
COOKIE DOUGH DYNAMO (Häagen-Dazs) 4 oz	300	4.0	31.0	110	na	18.0	na	
COOKIES 'N' CREAM								
(Breyers) .... 4 oz	170	3.0	19.0	60	(tr)	9.0	20	
(Dreyer's) .... 4 oz	160	3.0	18.0	80	(tr)	9.0	28	
(Healthy Choice) 'Dairy Dessert' .... 4 oz	130	4.0	24.0	80	na	2.0	5	
FUDGE, MARBLE (Dreyer's) .... 4 oz	150	3.0	18.0	50	(tr)	8.0	28	
FUDGE BROWNIE (Healthy Choice)								
'Dairy Dessert' .... 4 oz	130	3.0	27.0	70	na	2.0	5	

Food Name	Serv. Size	Total Cal.	Prot. GMS	Carbs GMS	Sod. MGS	Fiber GMS	Fat GMS	Chol. MGS
FUDGE ROYALE *(Sealtest)*	4 oz	140	3.0	19.0	55	(tr)	7.0	15
FUDGE SWIRL, DOUBLE *(Healthy Choice)*								
'Dairy Dessert'	4 oz	130	3.0	24.0	70	na	2.0	5
HEAVENLY HASH								
(Sealtest)	4 oz	150	2.0	19.0	50	(tr)	7.0	15
(Weight Watchers) 'ONE-ders'	4 oz	130	4.0	22.0	90	na	3.0	10
MACADAMIA BRITTLE *(Häagen-Dazs)*	4 oz	280	4.0	25.0	60	(mq)	18.0	(mq)
MAPLE WALNUT *(Sealtest)*	4 oz	160	3.0	17.0	40	(mq)	9.0	20
MINT CHOCOLATE *(Breyers)*	4 oz	170	3.0	18.0	45	(tr)	10.0	25
MINT CHOCOLATE CHIP *(Healthy Choice)*								
'Dairy Dessert'	4 oz	140	3.0	25.0	80	na	2.0	5
MINT WITH CHOCOLATE COOKIE								
(Ben & Jerry's)	1/2 cup	260	4.0	27.0	120	1.0	17.0	80
MOCHA ALMOND FUDGE *(Breyers)*	4 oz	190	4.0	20.0	60	na	10.0	na
MOCHA FUDGE *(Ben & Jerry's)*	1/2 cup	270	5.0	30.0	65	1.0	18.0	85
NEAPOLITAN *(Healthy Choice)*								
'Dairy Dessert'	4 oz	120	3.0	22.0	60	na	2.0	5
PEACH								
(Baskin-Robbins) fat-free 'Just Peachy' ...	4 oz	100	3.0	22.0	60	na	0.0	0
(Breyers) natural	4 oz	130	2.0	18.0	35	(tr)	6.0	15
PEANUT BUTTER CUP *(Ben & Jerry's)* ..	1/2 cup	370	8.0	30.0	140	2.0	26.0	75
PRALINE								
(Baskin-Robbins) light 'Praline Dream'	4 oz	130	3.0	17.0	85	na	6.0	11
(Baskin-Robbins) pralines 'n cream ...	1 scoop	280	4.0	35.0	180	na	14.0	36
(Healthy Choice) and caramel								
'Dairy Dessert'	4 oz	130	3.0	26.0	70	na	2.0	5
(Weight Watchers) pralines 'n creme								
'ONE-ders'	4 oz	120	3.0	19.0	110	na	4.0	10
RASPBERRY SWIRL *(Healthy Choice)*								
'Dairy Dessert'	4 oz	120	3.0	23.0	60	na	2.0	5
ROCKY ROAD								
(Baskin-Robbins)	1 scoop	300	5.0	39.0	135	na	14.0	32
(Dreyer's)	4 oz	170	3.0	18.0	30	(tr)	10.0	30
(Healthy Choice) 'Dairy Dessert'	4 oz	160	3.0	32.0	70	na	2.0	5
RUM RAISIN *(Häagen-Dazs)*	4 oz	250	4.0	21.0	45	(tr)	17.0	110
STRAWBERRY								
(Baskin-Robbins) light 'Strawberry Royale'	4 oz	110	2.0	19.0	120	na	3.0	9
(Baskin-Robbins) 'Very Berry'	1 scoop	220	3.0	30.0	95	na	10.0	30
(Borden)	4 oz	130	2.0	18.0	55	(tr)	6.0	(mq)
(Borden) cream 'Olde Fashioned Recipe' .	4 oz	130	2.0	19.0	55	(tr)	5.0	(mq)
(Breyers)	4 oz	130	2.0	16.0	40	(tr)	6.0	20
(Frusen Glädjé)	4 oz	230	4.0	20.0	60	(tr)	15.0	65
(Häagen-Dazs)	4 oz	250	4.0	23.0	40	(tr)	15.0	95

Food Name	Serv. Size	Total Cal.	Prot. GMS	Carbs GMS	Sod. MGS	Fiber GMS	Fat GMS	Chol. MGS
(Healthy Choice) 'Dairy Dessert'	4 oz	120	2.0	23.0	50	na	2.0	5
(Sealtest)	4 oz	130	2.0	18.0	40	(tr)	5.0	15
SUNDAE								
(Häagen-Dazs) caramel nut	4 oz	310	5.0	26.0	100	(mq)	21.0	(mq)
(Sealtest) chocolate-marshmallow	4 oz	150	2.0	21.0	40	(tr)	6.0	20
(Sealtest) peanut fudge	4 oz	140	3.0	17.0	50	(mq)	7.0	20
(Weight Watchers) hot caramel fudge	4.5 oz	160	5.0	27.0	140	na	4.0	15
(Weight Watchers) hot chocolate fudge	4.5 oz	160	6.0	26.0	115	na	4.0	15
(Weight Watchers) hot mocha fudge	4.5 oz	160	5.0	24.0	120	na	5.0	15
SWISS CHOCOLATE CANDY ALMOND								
(Frusen Glädjé)	4 oz	270	6.0	18.0	60	(mq)	19.0	55
TOFFEE (Ben & Jerry's) 'English Toffee								
Crunch'	1/2 cup	310	4.0	30.0	130	0	21.0	90
VANILLA								
regular, 10% fat, hardened	1 oz	57	1.0	6.8	25	0	3.1	13
rich, 16% fat, hardened	1 oz	67	0.8	6.1	21	0	4.5	17
(Baskin-Robbins)	1 scoop	240	4.0	24.0	115	0	14.0	52
(Ben & Jerry's)	1/2 cup	230	4.0	21.0	55	0	17.0	95
(Ben & Jerry's) vanilla bean	1/2 cup	230	4.0	21.0	55	0	17.0	95
(Borden) 'Olde Fashioned Recipe'	4 oz	130	2.0	15.0	55	0	7.0	(mq)
(Breyers)	4 oz	150	3.0	15.0	50	0	8.0	25
(Darigold)	4 oz	130	2.0	15.0	50	0	7.0	(mq)
(Darigold) 'Alpine'	4 oz	130	2.0	15.0	50	0	7.0	(mq)
(Darigold) 'Classic'	4 oz	180	2.0	16.0	40	0	12.0	(mq)
(Dreyer's)	4 oz	160	2.0	14.0	30	0	10.0	40
(Eagle Brand) 'Homestyle'	4 oz	150	3.0	16.0	55	0	9.0	(mq)
(Frusen Glädjé)	4 oz	230	5.0	16.0	70	0	17.0	65
(Good Humor) 'Cup'	3 oz	98	1.5	11.6	35	0	5.1	(mq)
(Häagen-Dazs)	4 oz	260	5.0	23.0	55	0	17.0	120
(Healthy Choice) 'Dairy Dessert'	4 oz	120	4.0	21.0	60	na	2.0	5
(Sealtest)	4 oz	140	2.0	16.0	50	0	7.0	20
VANILLA, FRENCH								
(Baskin-Robbins)	1 scoop	280	4.0	25.0	90	0	18.0	90
(Sealtest)	4 oz	140	2.0	16.0	50	0	7.0	35
VANILLA CARAMEL FUDGE								
(Ben & Jerry's)	1/2 cup	280	4.0	33.0	75	1.0	17.0	95
VANILLA CRUNCH								
(Ben & Jerry's) 'Rainforest Crunch'	1/2 cup	300	5.0	24.0	140	0	23.0	85
(Ben & Jerry's) 'Wavy Gravy'	1/2 cup	330	6.0	29.0	95	2.0	24.0	80
VANILLA FUDGE (Häagen-Dazs)	4 oz	270	5.0	26.0	100	(tr)	17.0	(mq)
VANILLA FUDGE TWIRL (Breyers)	4 oz	160	3.0	19.0	55	(tr)	8.0	20
VANILLA HONEY (Häagen-Dazs)	4 oz	250	5.0	22.0	55	0	16.0	135

Food Name	Serv. Size	Total Cal.	Prot. GMS	Carbs GMS	Sod. MGS	Fiber GMS	Fat GMS	Chol. MGS
VANILLA SWISS ALMOND								
(Frusen Glädjé)	4 oz	270	6.0	18.0	65	(mq)	19.0	65
(Häagen-Dazs)	4 oz	290	5.0	24.0	55	(mq)	19.0	(mq)
VANILLA TOFFEE CHUNK (Frusen Glädjé)	4 oz	270	5.0	22.0	160	0	17.0	85
VANILLA-CHOCOLATE								
(Baskin-Robbins) fat-free 'Just Chocolate								
Vanilla'	4 oz	100	4.0	21.0	60	na	0.0	0
(Breyers)	4 oz	160	3.0	17.0	40	(tr)	8.0	25
(Good Humor) cup 'Combo'	6 oz	201	3.8	25.6	80	(mq)	9.2	(mq)
VANILLA-CHOCOLATE-STRAWBERRY								
(Breyers)	4 oz	150	3.0	17.0	40	(tr)	8.0	20
(Sealtest)	4 oz	140	2.0	18.0	50	(tr)	6.0	20
(Sealtest) 'Cubic Scoops'	4 oz	130	2.0	17.0	50	(tr)	6.0	20
VANILLA-PEANUT BUTTER SWIRL								
(Häagen-Dazs)	4 oz	280	5.0	19.0	120	(tr)	21.0	110
WHITE RUSSIAN (Ben & Jerry's)	1/2 cup	240	4.0	23.0	55	0	16.0	90
ICE CREAM, ALTERNATIVE								
ALL FLAVORS (Lite Lite Tofutti)	4 oz	90	2.0	20.0	80	na	<1.0	0
BLACK CHERRY (Sealtest) 'Free'	4 oz	100	2.0	25.0	45	(tr)	0.0	0
CAPPUCCINO								
(Rice Dream)	4 oz	130	1.0	17.0	80	na	5.0	0
(Tofutti) 'Love Drops'	4 oz	230	3.0	26.0	120	na	12.0	0
CAROB (Rice Dream)	4 oz	130	1.0	20.0	80	na	5.0	0
CAROB ALMOND (Rice Dream)	4 oz	140	1.0	20.0	80	na	6.0	0
CAROB CHIP (Rice Dream)	4 oz	140	1.0	20.0	80	na	6.0	0
CHOCOLATE								
(Lite Lite Tofutti) soft-serve	4 oz	90	2.0	20.0	80	(tr)	<1.0	0
(Rice Dream) 'Dream Pie'	1 pie	380	3.0	47.0	225	na	19.0	0
(Sealtest) 'Free'	4 oz	100	3.0	23.0	50	(tr)	0.0	0
(Simple Pleasures)	4 oz	140	9.0	25.0	15	0	<1.0	na
(Tofutti) 'Love Drops'	4 oz	230	3.0	26.0	100	(tr)	13.0	0
(Tofutti) supreme	4 oz	210	3.0	20.0	130	(tr)	13.0	0
(Weight Watchers)	4 oz	80	3.0	19.0	75	(tr)	0.0	5
CHOCOLATE CHIP (Low, Lite 'n Luscious)	4 oz	100	3.0	19.0	80	(tr)	2.0	4
CHOCOLATE SWIRL (Weight Watchers)	4 oz	90	3.0	22.0	75	(tr)	0.0	5
COCOA MARBLE FUDGE (Rice Dream)	4 oz	140	1.0	19.0	80	na	6.0	0
COFFEE (Simple Pleasures)	4 oz	120	8.0	22.0	15	0	<1.0	na
COOKIES N' DREAM (Rice Dream)	4 oz	130	1.0	21.0	80	na	5.0	0
JAMOCA SWISS ALMOND (Low, Lite 'n								
Luscious)	4 oz	90	3.0	19.0	100	(tr)	2.0	4
LEMON (Rice Dream)	4 oz	130	1.0	17.0	80	na	5.0	0
MINT (Rice Dream) 'Dream Pie'	1 pie	380	3.0	47.0	225	na	19.0	0
MINT CAROB CHIP (Rice Dream)	4 oz	140	1.0	20.0	80	na	6.0	0

Food Name	Serv. Size	Total Cal.	Prot. GMS	Carbs GMS	Sod. MGS	Fiber GMS	Fat GMS	Chol. MGS
MOCHA *(Rice Dream)* 'Dream Pie'	1 pie	380	3.0	47.0	225	na	19.0	0
NEAPOLITAN								
(Rice Dream)	4 oz	130	1.0	21.0	80	na	5.0	0
(Weight Watchers)	4 oz	80	3.0	19.0	75	(tr)	0.0	5
PEACH								
(Sealtest) 'Free'	4 oz	100	2.0	23.0	45	(tr)	0.0	0
(Simple Pleasures)	4 oz	135	9.0	24.0	5	0	<1.0	na
PEANUT BUTTER FUDGE *(Rice Dream)* ..	4 oz	160	3.0	19.0	100	na	7.0	0
PINEAPPLE COCONUT *(Low, Lite 'n Luscious)*	4 oz	90	3.0	19.0	70	(tr)	1.0	3
RUM RAISIN *(Simple Pleasures)*	4 oz	130	7.0	25.0	10	0	<1.0	na
STRAWBERRY								
(Low, Lite 'n Luscious)	4 oz	80	3.0	17.0	70	(tr)	1.0	3
(Rice Dream)	4 oz	130	1.0	17.0	80	na	5.0	0
(Sealtest) 'Free'	4 oz	100	2.0	23.0	40	(tr)	0.0	0
(Simple Pleasures)	4 oz	120	8.0	22.0	55	0	<1.0	11
VANILLA								
(Lite Lite Tofutti) soft-serve	4 oz	90	2.0	20.0	80	na	<1.0	0
(Rice Dream)	4 oz	130	1.0	17.0	80	na	5.0	0
(Rice Dream) 'Dream Pie'	1 pie	380	3.0	47.0	225	na	19.0	0
(Sealtest) 'Free'	4 oz	100	3.0	24.0	45	0	0.0	0
(Tofutti) ...,....................	4 oz	200	2.0	21.0	90	na	11.0	0
(Tofutti) 'Love Drops'	4 oz	220	3.0	26.0	100	na	12.0	0
(Weight Watchers)	4 oz	80	3.0	20.0	75	0	0.0	5
VANILLA ALMOND BARK *(Tofutti)*	4 oz	230	3.0	23.0	950	na	14.0	0
VANILLA CHOCOLATE *(Tofutti)* dipped 'O's'	1 piece	40	1.0	4.0	20	na	2.0	0
VANILLA SWISS ALMOND *(Rice Dream)* ...	4 oz	140	1.0	20.0	80	na	6.0	0
VANILLA-CHOCOLATE-STRAWBERRY *(Sealtest)* 'Free'	4 oz	100	3.0	23.0	40	(tr)	0.0	0
VANILLA-FUDGE *(Rice Dream)*	4 oz	140	1.0	21.0	80	na	6.0	0
VANILLA-FUDGE ROYALE *(Sealtest)* 'Free'	4 oz	100	3.0	24.0	50	(tr)	0.0	0
VANILLA-STRAWBERRY ROYALE *(Sealtest)* 'Free'	4 oz	100	3.0	25.0	35	(tr)	0.0	0
WILDBERRY								
(Rice Dream)	4 oz	130	1.0	17.0	80	na	5.0	0
(Tofutti)	4 oz	210	2.0	22.0	100	(tr)	12.0	0
ICE CREAM BAR								
ALMOND *(Good Humor)* toasted, 3 oz	1 bar	212	1.8	24.3	34	(mq)	11.8	(mq)
CARAMEL ALMOND *(Häagen-Dazs)* 'Crunch Bar'	1 bar	240	3.0	17.0	65	(mq)	18.0	40
CHIP CANDY CRUNCH *(Good Humor)* 3 oz	1 bar	255	2.2	21.2	40	na	17.9	(mq)

Food Name	Serv. Size	Total Cal.	Prot. GMS	Carbs GMS	Sod. MGS	Fiber GMS	Fat GMS	Chol. MGS
CHOCOLATE								
(Häagen-Dazs) w/dark chocolate coating	1 bar	390	5.0	32.0	60	0	27.0	(mq)
(Klondike) 5 oz	1 bar	270	4.0	23.0	60	na	19.0	(mq)
(Nestlé) w/milk chocolate coating 'Quik' 3 oz	1 bar	210	3.0	19.0	40	na	14.0	(mq)
(Weight Watchers) 'Treat Bars' 2.75 oz	1 bar	100	4.0	18.0	75	(tr)	1.0	0
CHOCOLATE DIP (Weight Watchers) 1.7 oz	1 bar	110	2.0	10.0	35	(tr)	7.0	5
CHOCOLATE ECLAIR (Good Humor) 3 oz	1 bar	188	2.1	22.6	54	na	9.9	(mq)
CHOCOLATE FUDGE								
(Baker's) sundae, crunchy 'Fudgetastic' 4 oz	1 bar	230	3.0	24.0	40	na	14.0	20
(Baker's) sundae 'Fudgetastic' 4 oz	1 bar	220	3.0	23.0	45	na	15.0	20
(Good Humor) cake, 6.3 oz	1 bar	214	1.7	18.1	50	na	15.0	(mq)
(Weight Watchers) double, 1.75 oz	1.75 oz	60	3.0	12.0	50	(tr)	1.0	5
CHOCOLATE MOUSSE								
(Weight Watchers) sugar-free, 1.75 oz	1 bar	35	2.0	9.0	30	(tr)	<1.0	5
MILK CHOCOLATE (Nestlé) w/almonds, milk chocolate coating, 3.7 oz	3.7 oz	350	6.0	28.0	45	na	23.0	5
ORANGE-VANILLA								
(Weight Watchers) 'Sugar-free Treat Bars'	1 bar	30	2.0	8.0	40	(tr)	<1.0	5
PEANUT BUTTER (Häagen-Dazs) 'Crunch Bar'	4 oz	270	6.0	16.0	55	(mq)	21.0	35
STRAWBERRY SHORTCAKE								
(Good Humor) 3 oz	1 bar	176	1.7	23.8	88	na	8.2	(mq)
VANILLA								
(Eskimo Pie) w/dark chocolate coating	1 bar	180	2.0	16.0	35	na	12.0	na
(Eskimo Pie) w/dark chocolate coating 'Sugar-freedom'	1 bar	140	2.0	13.0	30	na	11.0	na
(Eskimo Pie) w/milk chocolate coating	1 bar	190	5.0	18.0	16	na	12.0	na
(Eskimo Pie) w/milk chocolate coating and almonds 'Sugar-freedom'	1 bar	140	3.0	12.0	35	na	13.0	na
(Eskimo Pie) w/milk chocolate coating and crisp rice 'Sugar-freedom'	1 bar	150	4.0	12.0	40	na	11.0	na
(Good Humor) w/chocolate flavor coating, 3 oz	1 bar	198	1.9	16.8	44	na	13.7	(mq)
(Häagen-Dazs) 'Crunch Bar' 4 oz	1 bar	220	3.0	16.0	55	(mq)	16.0	40
(Häagen-Dazs) w/dark chocolate coating, 4 oz	1 bar	390	5.0	32.0	60	na	27.0	(mq)
(Häagen-Dazs) w/milk chocolate coating, 4 oz	1 bar	360	4.0	26.0	55	na	27.0	(mq)
(Häagen-Dazs) w/milk chocolate-almond coating, 4 oz	1 bar	370	5.0	27.0	55	(mq)	27.0	(mq)
(Häagen-Dazs) w/milk chocolate-brittle coating, 4 oz	1 bar	370	5.0	32.0	160	(tr)	25.0	(mq)
(Klondike) w/chocolate flavor coating 'Lite'	1 bar	110	3.0	14.0	50	na	6.0	5

Food Name	Serv. Size	Total Cal.	Prot. GMS	Carbs GMS	Sod. MGS	Fiber GMS	Fat GMS	Chol. MGS
(Nestlé) w/chocolate coating and crisp rice 'Crunch' 3 oz	1 bar	180	2.0	15.0	(mq)	(mq)	13.0	(mq)
(Nestlé) w/chocolate coating and crisp rice 'Crunch Lite'	1 bar	120	2.0	16.0	50	na	5.0	na
(Nestlé) w/white chocolate coating 'Alpine Premium' 3.7 oz	1 bar	350	6.0	25.0	5	na	25.0	50
(Oh Henry!) w/caramel peanut, milk chocolate coating, 3 oz	1 bar	320	1.0	34.0	75	(mq)	20.0	(mq)
ICE CREAM BAR, ALTERNATIVE								
(Rice Dream) chocolate	1 bar	270	1.0	33.0	115	na	16.0	0
(Rice Dream) chocolate nutty bar	1 bar	330	5.0	29.0	110	na	23.0	0
(Rice Dream) strawberry	1 bar	260	1.0	31.0	110	na	14.8	0
(Rice Dream) vanilla	1 bar	275	1.0	33.0	120	na	15.8	0
(Rice Dream) vanilla nutty bar	1 bar	330	5.0	29.0	100	na	23.0	0
ICE CREAM CAKE *(Breyers)* 'Viennetta'	1 slice	190	3.0	18.0	40	0	12.0	25
ICE CREAM CONE								
Cup style, wafer								
(Bozo) cake	1 cone	16	1.0	3.0	13	0	0.0	0
(Keebler)	1 cone	15	1.0	4.0	20	na	1.0	0
(Keebler) assorted colors	1 cone	15	1.0	4.0	20	na	1.0	0
(Little Debbie)	1 cone	15	0.4	3.0	15	(mq)	0.1	<1
(Nabisco) 'Comet'	1 cone	18	<1.0	4.0	5	na	<1.0	0
Sugar								
(Baskin-Robbins)	1 cone	60	1.0	11.0	45	(mq)	1.0	0
(Bozo)	1 cone	53	1.0	11.0	29	.2	1.0	na
(Keebler)	1 cone	45	1.0	11.0	35	na	1.0	0
(Nabisco)	1 cone	50	1.0	11.0	40	na	<1.0	0
(Nabisco) 'Comet'	1 cone	50	1.0	11.0	40	na	<1.0	0
Waffle, Baskin-Robbins	1 cone	140	3.0	28.0	5	(mq)	2.0	0
ICE CREAM MIX								
Dutch chocolate, prepared *(Salada)*	8 oz	310	4.0	31.0	75	(tr)	19.0	(mq)
peach, prepared *(Salada)*	8 oz	310	4.0	32.0	60	(tr)	18.0	(mq)
vanilla, prepared *(Salada)*	8 oz	310	4.0	32.0	60	(tr)	18.0	(mq)
wild strawberry, prepared *(Salada)*	8 oz	310	4.0	32.0	60	(tr)	18.0	(mq)
ICE CREAM SNACKS AND SANDWICHES								
Nuggets								
vanilla, dark chocolate coated 'Bon Bons' *(Carnation)*	5 pieces	170	2.0	15.0	50	(tr)	11.0	14
vanilla, milk chocolate coated 'Bon Bons' *(Carnation)*	5 pieces	165	2.0	14.0	50	(tr)	11.0	16
Round novelties								
mocha, 4 oz *(Natural Nectar)*	1 bar	300	4.0	40.0	135	na	14.0	10
nectar, 4 oz *(Natural Nectar)*	1 bar	300	4.0	38.0	120	na	15.0	15

Food Name	Serv. Size	Total Cal.	Prot. GMS	Carbs GMS	Sod. MGS	Fiber GMS	Fat GMS	Chol. MGS
Sandwich								
chocolate chip cookie, 4 oz								
(Good Humor)	1 sandwich	246	2.9	35.1	181	(mq)	10.5	(mq)
chocolate chip cookie, 2.7 oz								
(Good Humor)	1 sandwich	204	2.2	30.1	166	(mq)	8.3	(mq)
vanilla (Weight Watchers)	1 sandwich	150	3.0	28.0	170	(tr)	3.0	5
vanilla, 5 oz (Klondike)	1 sandwich	230	5.0	33.0	220	(mq)	9.0	(mq)
vanilla 'Lite' (Klondike)	1 sandwich	100	2.0	18.0	110	na	2.0	5
vanilla, 1.5 oz snacks								
(Weight Watchers)	1 sandwich	90	2.0	17.0	120	na	2.0	0
vanilla, 3 oz (Good Humor)	1 sandwich	191	3.7	31.1	155	(mq)	5.7	(mq)
vanilla, 2.5 oz (Good Humor)	1 sandwich	165	3.2	26.9	134	(mq)	4.9	(mq)
vanilla 'Sugar-freedom'								
(Eskimo Pie)	1 sandwich	170	4.0	26.0	142	na	6.0	na
Stick novelties								
banana cream (Natural Nectar)	1 bar	170	3.0	22.0	70	na	8.0	20
cocoa-fudge 'n' cream (Natural Nectar)	1 bar	170	3.0	22.0	70	na	8.0	20
strawberries 'n' cream (Natural Nectar)	1 bar	120	2.0	18.0	40	na	5.0	15
wildberry cream (Natural Nectar)	1 bar	120	2.0	22.0	50	na	3.0	15
ICE CREAM TOPPING. See individual toppings.								
ICE MILK								
CARAMEL NUT (Light n' Lively)	4 oz	120	3.0	18.0	85	(tr)	4.0	10
CHOCOLATE								
(Breyers) 'Light'	4 oz	120	3.0	18.0	55	(tr)	4.0	15
(Borden)	4 oz	100	3.0	18.0	80	0	2.0	(mq)
(Darigold) 'Lite'	4 oz	110	3.0	19.0	65	(tr)	3.0	(mq)
(Weight Watchers) 'Grand Collection'	4 oz	110	4.0	18.0	75	(tr)	3.0	10
CHOCOLATE CHIP								
(Light n' Lively)	4 oz	120	3.0	18.0	35	0	4.0	10
(Weight Watchers) 'Grand Collection'	4 oz	120	3.0	19.0	75	(tr)	4.0	10
CHOCOLATE CHOCOLATE CHIP (Breyers)								
'Light'	4 oz	140	4.0	20.0	55	na	5.0	25
CHOCOLATE FUDGE TWIRL (Breyers)								
'Light'	4 oz	130	4.0	21.0	60	(tr)	4.0	10
CHOCOLATE SWIRL (Weight Watchers)								
'Grand Collection'	4 oz	120	3.0	19.0	75	(tr)	3.0	5
COFFEE (Light n' Lively)	4 oz	100	3.0	16.0	40	0	3.0	10
COOKIES N' CREAM (Light n' Lively)	4 oz	110	3.0	18.0	65	0	3.0	10
HEAVENLY HASH								
(Breyers) 'Light'	4 oz	150	3.0	21.0	55	(tr)	5.0	10
(Light n' Lively)	4 oz	120	3.0	20.0	35	(tr)	4.0	10
NEAPOLITAN (Weight Watchers)								
'Grand Collection'	4 oz	110	3.0	18.0	75	(tr)	3.0	10

Food Name	Serv. Size	Total Cal.	Prot. GMS	Carbs GMS	Sod. MGS	Fiber GMS	Fat GMS	Chol. MGS
PECAN PRALINES 'N CREME								
(Weight Watchers) 'Grand Collection' ...	4 oz	120	3.0	20.0	80	(tr)	4.0	10
PRALINE ALMOND (Breyers) 'Light'	4 oz	130	3.0	19.0	70	(tr)	5.0	10
STRAWBERRY								
(Borden)	4 oz	90	2.0	17.0	65	0	2.0	(mq)
(Breyers) 'Light'	4 oz	110	3.0	18.0	50	(tr)	3.0	15
SWISS ALMOND FUDGE TWIRL (Breyers)	4 oz	150	4.0	21.0	65	na	6.0	na
TOFFEE FUDGE PARFAIT (Breyers) 'Light'	4 oz	140	3.0	22.0	90	(tr)	5.0	10
VANILLA								
(Borden)	4 oz	90	2.0	17.0	60	0	2.0	(mq)
(Breyers) 'Light'	4 oz	120	3.0	18.0	60	0	4.0	10
(Darigold)	4 oz	110	2.0	18.0	66	0	3.0	(mq)
(Light n' Lively)	4 oz	100	3.0	16.0	40	0	3.0	10
(Light n' Lively) w/chocolate covered								
almonds	4 oz	120	3.0	17.0	45	(tr)	4.0	10
(Weight Watchers) 'Grand Collection'	4 oz	100	3.0	16.0	75	0	3.0	10
VANILLA-CHOCOLATE-STRAWBERRY								
(Breyers) 'Light'	4 oz	120	3.0	18.0	55	(tr)	4.0	15
(Light n' Lively)	4 oz	100	2.0	17.0	35	(tr)	3.0	10
VANILLA-FUDGE TWIRL (Light n' Lively) ...	4 oz	110	3.0	18.0	45	0	3.0	10
VANILLA-RASPBERRY								
(Breyers) parfait 'Light'	4 oz	130	3.0	23.0	50	(tr)	3.0	15
(Light n' Lively) swirl	4 oz	110	3.0	19.0	35	0	3.0	10
ICE MILK BAR								
CHOCOLATE ALMOND CRUNCH								
(Weight Watchers)	1 bar	120	2.0	12.0	45	na	7.0	5
CHOCOLATE FUDGE, DOUBLE								
(Light n' Lively) nonfat	1 bar	50	2.0	11.0	45	na	0.0	0
CHOCOLATE MOUSSE (Light n' Lively)								
nonfat	1 bar	50	2.0	12.0	45	na	0.0	0
CHOCOLATE W/FUDGE SWIRL (Sealtest)								
nonfat 'Free'	1 bar	80	3.0	19.0	55	na	0.0	0
ORANGE VANILLA (Light n' Lively) nonfat ..	1 bar	40	1.0	10.0	15	na	0.0	0
PRALINE (Weight Watchers) 'Crispy Praline								
'N Creme'	1 bar	120	2.0	13.0	45	na	6.0	5
STRAWBERRY (Light n' Lively) nonfat	1 bar	80	2.0	12.0	25	na	0.0	0
TOFFEE (Weight Watchers) 'English Toffee								
Crunch'	1 bar	120	2.0	11.0	60	na	8.0	5
VANILLA								
(Light n' Lively) chocolate dipped	1 bar	110	2.0	14.0	35	na	6.0	5
(Sealtest) w/fudge swirl, nonfat 'Free'	1 bar	80	2.0	18.0	55	na	0.0	0
(Sealtest) w/strawberry swirl, nonfat 'Free'	1 bar	70	2.0	17.0	60	na	0.0	0
ICED TEA. See TEA, ICED.								

Food Name	Serv. Size	Total Cal.	Prot. GMS	Carbs GMS	Sod. MGS	Fiber GMS	Fat GMS	Chol. MGS
IMBU. See JOBO.								
INDIAN DATE. See TAMARIND.								
INDIAN FRY BREAD. See BREAD.								
INFANT FORMULA. See BABY FOOD.								
IRISH MOSS. See SEAWEED.								
ITALIAN SEASONING *(Schilling)*								
'Spice Blends'	1/4 tsp	1	<.1	0.1	<1	na	na	0
ITALIAN STONE PINE NUT. See PINE NUT.								

J

Food Name	Serv. Size	Total Cal.	Prot. GMS	Carbs GMS	Sod. MGS	Fiber GMS	Fat GMS	Chol. MGS
JACK BEAN. See FAVA BEAN.								
JACKFRUIT								
trimmed	1 oz	27	0.4	6.8	1	>.3 c	0.1	0
untrimmed	1 lb	119	1.9	30.5	3	>1.3 c	0.4	0
JALAPEÑO. See PEPPER, JALAPEÑO.								
JAM. See also FRUIT SPREAD; JELLY; PRESERVES.								
(Bama) all flavors	2 tsp	30	0.0	8.0	5	(mq)	0.0	0
(Estee) all flavors	1 tsp	2	0.0	0.0	10	(mq)	0.0	0
(Featherweight) all flavors	1 tsp	4	0.0	1.0	0	(mq)	0.0	0
(Kraft) all flavors	1 tsp	17	0.0	4.0	0	(mq)	0.0	0
(S&W Nutradiet) all flavors	1 tsp	4	0.0	1.0	0	(mq)	0.0	0
APRICOT								
(Finast)	2 tsp	35	0.0	9.0	1	(mq)	0.0	0
(Smucker's) natural ingredients	1 tsp	18	0.0	4.0	0	na	0.0	na
APRICOT-PINEAPPLE *(Smucker's)* natural								
ingredients	1 tsp	18	0.0	4.0	0	na	0.0	na
BLACK RASPBERRY *(Smucker's)* natural								
ingredients	1 tsp	18	0.0	4.0	0	na	0.0	na
BLACKBERRY								
(Finast)	2 tsp	16	0.0	4.0	5	(mq)	0.0	0
(Smucker's) natural ingredients	1 tsp	18	0.0	4.0	0	na	0.0	na
BLUEBERRY								
(Finast)	2 tsp	16	0.0	4.0	5	(mq)	0.0	0
(Smucker's) natural ingredients	1 tsp	18	0.0	4.0	0	na	0.0	na
BOYSENBERRY *(Smucker's)* natural								
ingredients	1 tsp	18	0.0	4.0	0	na	0.0	na
CHERRY								
(Finast)	2 tsp	25	0.0	9.0	5	(mq)	0.0	0
(Smucker's) natural ingredients	1 tsp	18	0.0	4.0	0	na	0.0	na

Food Name	Serv. Size	Total Cal.	Prot. GMS	Carbs GMS	Sod. MGS	Fiber GMS	Fat GMS	Chol. MGS
GRAPE								
(Finast) Concord or regular	2 tsp	35	0.0	9.0	5	(tr)	0.0	0
(Polaner)	2 tsp	35	0.0	9.0	5	na	0.0	na
(Smucker's) Concord, natural ingredients	1 tsp	18	0.0	4.0	0	na	0.0	na
(Welch's)	2 tsp	35	0.0	9.0	5	0	0.0	0
ORANGE MARMALADE (Polaner)	2 tsp	35	0.0	9.0	5	na	0.0	na
PEACH								
(Finast)	2 tsp	35	0.0	9.0	1	(mq)	0.0	0
(Smucker's) natural ingredients	1 tsp	18	0.0	4.0	0	na	0.0	na
PINEAPPLE								
(Finast)	2 tsp	35	0.0	9.0	1	(mq)	0.0	0
(Smucker's) natural ingredients	1 tsp	18	0.0	4.0	0	na	0.0	na
PLUM (Smucker's) natural ingredients	1 tsp	18	0.0	4.0	0	na	0.0	na
RASPBERRY								
(Finast)	2 tsp	35	0.0	9.0	3	(mq)	0.0	0
(Smucker's) natural ingredients, seedless	1 tsp	18	0.0	4.0	0	na	0.0	na
RASPBERRY-APPLE (Welch's)	2 tsp	35	0.0	9.0	5	0	0.0	0
STRAWBERRY								
(Finast)	2 tsp	35	0.0	9.0	3	(mq)	0.0	0
(Kraft) 'Reduced Calorie'	1 tsp	6	0.0	2.0	5	(mq)	0.0	0
(Piedmont)	2 tsp	35	0.0	9.0	10	na	0.0	na
(Smucker's) natural ingredients, seedless	1 tsp	18	0.0	4.0	0	na	0.0	na
(Welch's)	2 tsp	35	0.0	9.0	5	0	0.0	0
TOMATO (Smucker's) natural ingredients . .	1 tsp	18	0.0	4.0	0	na	0.0	na
JAMAICAN BREADNUT. See BREADNUT TREE SEEDS.								
JAMBERRY, fresh (Frieda's)	3.5 oz	25	1.4	4.2	na	(mq)	0.5	0
JAMBOLAN. See JAVA PLUM.								
JAPANESE MEDLAR. See LOQUAT.								
JAPANESE WHITE RADISH. See RADISH, ORIENTAL.								
JAVA PLUM/jambolan								
raw	1 cup	81	1.0	21.0	19	>.4 c	0.3	0
raw	3 fruits	5	0.1	1.4	1	(mq)	0.0	0
w/seeds	1 lb	222	2.7	57.2	50	>1.0 c	0.9	0
w/o seeds	1 oz	17	0.2	4.4	4	>.1 c	0.1	0
JELLY. See also JAM; FRUIT SPREAD; PRESERVES.								
(Bama) and peanut butter, spread,								
all flavors	2 tbsp	150	3.0	20.0	75	(mq)	7.0	0
(Estee) all flavors	1 tsp	2	0.0	0.0	10	0	0.0	0
(Featherweight) all flavors, except grape . .	1 tsp	4	0.0	1.0	0	0	0.0	0
(Kraft) all flavors	1 tsp	17	0.0	4.0	0	0	0.0	0
(Smucker's) 'Slenderella' all flavors	1 tsp	7	0.0	2.0	0	0	0.0	0
APPLE								
(Bama)	2 tsp	30	0.0	8.0	5	0	0.0	0

Food Name	Serv. Size	Total Cal.	Prot. GMS	Carbs GMS	Sod. MGS	Fiber GMS	Fat GMS	Chol. MGS
(Finast)	2 tsp	35	0.0	9.0	2	0	0.0	0
(Lucky Leaf)	1 oz	80	0.0	20.0	5	0	0.0	0
(Musselman's)	1 oz	80	0.0	20.0	5	0	0.0	0
(Polaner)	2 tsp	35	0.0	9.0	5	na	0.0	na
(Smucker's) cinnamon-flavored, natural ingredients	1 tsp	18	0.0	4.0	0	na	0.0	na
(Smucker's) mint-flavored, natural ingredients	1 tsp	18	0.0	4.0	0	na	0.0	na
(Smucker's) natural ingredients	1 tsp	18	0.0	4.0	0	na	0.0	na
APPLE-BLACKBERRY *(Musselman's)*	1 oz	80	0.0	19.0	0	0	0.0	0
APPLE-CHERRY *(Musselman's)*	1 oz	80	0.0	19.0	5	0	0.0	0
APPLE-GRAPE								
(Musselman's)	1 oz	80	0.0	20.0	5	0	0.0	0
(Welch's)	2 tsp	35	0.0	9.0	5	0	0.0	0
APPLE-RASPBERRY *(Musselman's)*	1 oz	80	0.0	19.0	0	0	0.0	0
APPLE-STRAWBERRY *(Musselman's)*	1 oz	80	0.0	20.0	5	0	0.0	0
APRICOT-PINEAPPLE								
(Knott's Berry Farm) 'Light' w/NutraSweet	1 tsp	8	0.0	2.0	0	na	0.0	na
BLACK RASPBERRY *(Smucker's)* natural ingredients	1 tsp	18	0.0	4.0	0	na	0.0	na
BLACKBERRY								
(Bama)	2 tsp	30	0.0	8.0	5	0	0.0	0
(Knott's Berry Farm) 'Light' w/NutraSweet	1 tsp	8	0.0	2.0	0	na	0.0	na
(Smucker's) natural ingredients	1 tsp	18	0.0	4.0	0	na	0.0	na
BOYSENBERRY *(Knott's Berry Farm)* 'Light' w/NutraSweet	1 tsp	8	0.0	2.0	0	na	0.0	na
CHERRY *(Smucker's)* natural ingredients	1 tsp	18	0.0	4.0	0	na	0.0	na
CRABAPPLE *(Smucker's)* natural ingredients	1 tsp	18	0.0	4.0	0	na	0.0	na
CURRANT								
(Finast)	2 tsp	35	0.0	9.0	2	0	0.0	0
(Polaner)	2 tsp	35	0.0	9.0	5	na	0.0	na
(Smucker's) natural ingredients	1 tsp	18	0.0	4.0	0	na	0.0	na
ELDERBERRY *(Smucker's)* natural ingredients	1 tsp	18	0.0	4.0	0	na	0.0	na
GRAPE								
(Bama)	2 tsp	30	0.0	8.0	5	0	0.0	0
(Featherweight)	1 tsp	4	0.0	1.0	5	0	0.0	0
(Finast)	2 tsp	35	0.0	9.0	5	0	0.0	0
(Kraft) 'Reduced Calorie'	1 tsp	6	0.0	2.0	5	0	0.0	0
(Musselman's)	1 oz	80	0.0	20.0	0	0	0.0	0
(Polaner)	2 tsp	35	0.0	9.0	5	na	0.0	na
(Smucker's) Concord, natural ingredients	1 tsp	18	0.0	4.0	0	na	0.0	na
(Welch's)	2 tsp	35	0.0	9.0	5	0	0.0	0

Food Name	Serv. Size	Total Cal.	Prot. GMS	Carbs GMS	Sod. MGS	Fiber GMS	Fat GMS	Chol. MGS
GREEN PEPPER *(Great Impressions)*	1 tbsp	50	0.0	12.6	<1	na	0.0	0
GUAVA *(Smucker's)* natural ingredients	1 tsp	18	0.0	4.0	0	na	0.0	na
JALAPEÑO								
(Great Impressions)	1 tbsp	58	0.0	14.6	51	na	0.0	0
(Knott's Berry Farm)	1 oz	70	0.0	18.0	0	na	0.0	na
(Knott's Berry Farm)	1 tsp	18	0.0	4.0	0	na	0.0	na
MINT								
(Finast)	2 tsp	35	0.0	9.0	2	0	0.0	0
(Polaner)	2 tsp	35	0.0	9.0	5	na	0.0	na
MIXED FRUIT *(Smucker's)* natural ingredients	1 tsp	18	0.0	4.0	0	na	0.0	na
PLUM *(Smucker's)* natural ingredients	1 tsp	18	0.0	4.0	0	na	0.0	na
QUINCE *(Smucker's)* natural ingredients ..	1 tsp	18	0.0	4.0	0	na	0.0	na
RASPBERRY								
(Knott's Berry Farm) 'Light' w/NutraSweet	1 tsp	8	0.0	2.0	0	na	0.0	na
(Polaner)	2 tsp	35	0.0	9.0	5	na	0.0	na
(Smucker's) natural ingredients	1 tsp	18	0.0	4.0	0	na	0.0	na
RED PEPPER *(Great Impressions)*	1 tbsp	50	0.0	12.6	9	na	0.0	0
STRAWBERRY								
(Finast)	2 tsp	35	0.0	9.0	2	0	0.0	0
(Knott's Berry Farm) 'Light' w/NutraSweet	1 tsp	8	0.0	2.0	0	na	0.0	na
(Polaner)	2 tsp	35	0.0	9.0	5	na	0.0	na
(Smucker's) natural ingredients	1 tsp	18	0.0	4.0	0	na	0.0	na
STRAWBERRY-APPLE *(Polaner)*	2 tsp	35	0.0	9.0	5	na	0.0	na

JERKY. See BEEF JERKY.

JERUSALEM ARTICHOKE. See ARTICHOKES, JERUSALEM.

JEW'S EAR. See CHINESE FUNGUS.

JICAMA/Chinese yam/fon goot yam/Mexican potato/sicama/yambean tuber

boiled, drained	4 oz	52	1.3	11.8	7	>1.3 c	0.1	0
raw, trimmed	1 oz	12	0.4	2.5	2	>.2 c	0.1	0
raw, trimmed, sliced	1/2 cup	25	0.8	5.3	4	>.4 c	0.1	0
raw, untrimmed	1 lb	170	5.8	36.5	26	>2.9 c	0.3	0

JOBO/hog plum/imbu/yellow mombin

seeded	1 oz	20	0.2	3.9	na	>.3 c	0.6	0

JUICE. See individual listings.

JUJUBE, CHINESE

dried	100 gm	287	3.7	73.6	9	>3.0 c	1.1	0
dried	1 oz	81	1.0	20.1	3	>.9 c	0.3	0
raw	100 gm	79	1.2	20.2	3	>1.4 c	0.2	0
raw	1 oz	22	0.3	5.7	1	>.4 c	0.1	0
raw, w/seeds	1 lb	331	5.1	85.3	11	>5.9 c	0.8	0

Food Name	Serv. Size	Total Cal.	Prot. GMS	Carbs GMS	Sod. MGS	Fiber GMS	Fat GMS	Chol. MGS
JUNKET MIX								
CHOCOLATE								
mix only, dry	2-oz pkg	207	1.4	52.2	40	>.5 c	1.9	0
mix only, dry	1 tbsp	33	0.2	8.2	6	>.1 c	0.3	0
prepared *(Junket)*	1/2 cup	120	5.0	15.0	65	na	4.0	(mq)
prepared w/2% milk	1/2 cup	110	4.3	18.4	71	>.1 c	2.9	10
prepared w/whole milk	1/2 cup	125	4.3	18.1	69	>.1 c	4.5	16
STRAWBERRY OR RASPBERRY								
mix only, dry	1.5-oz pkg	165	0.0	42.6	3	0	0.0	0
mix only, dry	1 tbsp	38	0.0	9.9	1	0	0.0	0
prepared *(Junket)*	1/2 cup	120	4.0	16.0	60	na	4.0	(mq)
prepared w/whole milk	1 cup	238	8.0	32.0	115	0	9.0	33
VANILLA								
mix only, dry	1.5-oz pkg	165	0.0	42.6	3	0	0.0	0
mix only, dry	1 tbsp	41	0.0	10.7	1	0	0.0	0
prepared *(Junket)*	1/2 cup	120	4.0	16.0	60	na	4.0	(mq)
prepared w/2% milk	1/2 cup	101	4.1	16.4	61	0	2.4	9
prepared w/whole milk	1/2 cup	116	4.0	16.2	61	0	4.1	17
JUTE POTHERB								
boiled, drained	4 oz	42	4.2	8.3	12	>2.2 c	0.2	0
raw, trimmed	1 oz	10	1.3	1.6	2	>.3 c	0.1	0
raw, untrimmed	1 lb	96	13.1	16.3	23	>3.4 c	0.7	0

K

Food Name	Serv. Size	Total Cal.	Prot. GMS	Carbs GMS	Sod. MGS	Fiber GMS	Fat GMS	Chol. MGS
KALE/borecole/cole/colewort								
boiled, drained	4 oz	36	2.2	6.4	26	>.9 c	0.5	0
boiled, drained, chopped	1 cup	42	2.5	7.3	30	2.6	0.5	0
chopped *(Dole)*	1/2 cup	17	1.0	3.0	15	1.3	0.5	na
raw, chopped	1 cup	33	2.2	6.7	29	1.3	0.5	0
raw, trimmed	1 oz	14	0.9	2.8	12	>.4 c	0.2	0
raw, untrimmed	1 lb	137	9.1	27.7	119	>4.2 c	1.9	0
Canned, chopped *(Allen's)*	1/2 cup	25	2.0	3.0	15	(mq)	<1.0	0
Frozen								
boiled, drained	4 oz	34	3.2	5.9	17	>1.1 c	0.6	0
boiled, drained, chopped	1 cup	39	3.7	6.8	20	>1.2 c	0.6	0
chopped *(Frosty Acres)*	3.3 oz	25	3.0	5.0	15	>1.0 c	0.0	0
chopped *(Seabrook)*	3.3 oz	25	3.0	5.0	14	>1.0 c	0.0	0
chopped *(Southern)*	3.5 oz	30	2.6	4.8	30	(mq)	0.5	0
unprepared, 10-oz pkg	3.3 oz	26	2.5	4.6	14	1.88	0.4	0

Food Name	Serv. Size	Total Cal.	Prot. GMS	Carbs GMS	Sod. MGS	Fiber GMS	Fat GMS	Chol. MGS
KALE, SCOTCH								
boiled, drained	4 oz	32	2.2	6.4	51	>1.0 c	0.5	0
boiled, drained, chopped	1 cup	36	2.5	7.3	58	>1.1 c	0.5	0
raw, chopped	1 cup	28	1.9	5.6	47	>.8 c	0.4	0
raw, trimmed	1 oz	12	0.8	2.4	20	>.3 c	0.2	0
raw, untrimmed	1 lb	115	7.8	23.0	194	>3.4 c	1.7	0
KANPYO/dried gourd strips								
	1 lb	1169	38.9	295.0	68	0	2.5	0
	1 oz	73	2.4	18.4	4	0	0.2	0
	1/2 cup	70	2.3	17.6	4	>2.5 c	0.2	0
KANTEN								
raw	1 lb	116	2.5	30.6	40	>2.0 c	0.1	0
raw	1 oz	7	0.2	1.9	3	>.1 c	tr	0
KASHA. See BUCKWHEAT GROATS.								
KATSUO. See TUNA, SKIPJACK.								
KATURAY/sesbania flower								
raw, approx .1 oz	1 flower	1	<.1	0.2	tr	>.1 c	tr	0
raw, trimmed	1 cup	5	0.3	1.4	3	>.3 c	<.1	0
raw, trimmed	1 oz	8	0.4	1.9	4	>.4 c	<.1	0
raw, untrimmed	1 lb	106	4.9	25.9	59	>5.8 c	0.2	0
steamed	4 oz	25	1.3	5.9	12	>1.8 c	0.1	0
KAUAI PUNCH, organic *(Santa Cruz Natural)*	8 oz	120	<1.0	28.0	na	na	1.0	na
KEFIR, CULTURED								
black cherry *(Alta•Dena)*	1 cup	200	9.0	24.0	120	na	9.0	na
boysenberry *(Alta•Dena)*	1 cup	200	9.0	24.0	120	na	9.0	na
peach *(Alta•Dena)*	1 cup	200	9.0	24.0	120	na	9.0	na
red raspberry *(Alta•Dena)*	1 cup	200	9.0	24.0	120	na	9.0	na
KELP. See SEAWEED.								
KETCHUP. See CATSUP.								
KIDNEY BEAN								
California red, mature								
boiled	4 oz	141	10.4	25.4	5	>2.7 c	0.1	0
boiled	1/2 cup	109	8.0	19.7	4	>2.1 c	0.1	0
raw	1/2 cup	304	22.4	55.0	10	22.91	0.2	0
raw	1 oz	94	6.9	17.0	3	>1.8 c	0.1	0
Red, mature								
boiled	1/2 cup	112	7.6	20.1	2	6.51	0.4	0
boiled	4 oz	144	9.8	25.9	2	4.1	0.6	0
boiled *(A&P)*	1 cup	230	17.0	41.0	5	(mq)	1.0	0
raw	1/2 cup	310	20.7	56.4	11	14.0	1.0	0
raw	1 oz	96	6.4	17.4	3	2.9	0.1	0
raw *(Arrowhead Mills)*	2 oz	190	13.0	35.0	3	11.7	1.0	0

Food Name	Serv. Size	Total Cal.	Prot. GMS	Carbs GMS	Sod. MGS	Fiber GMS	Fat GMS	Chol. MGS
Royal red, mature								
boiled	4 oz	139	10.8	24.8	6	>2.6 c	0.2	0
boiled	1/2 cup	108	8.4	19.2	4	>2.0 c	0.2	0
raw	1/2 cup	303	23.3	53.7	12	>5.7 c	0.4	0
raw	1 oz	93	7.2	16.5	4	>1.7 c	0.1	0
Sprouted, mature								
boiled, drained	4 oz	37	5.5	5.4	(mq)	(mq)	0.7	0
raw	1 lb	132	19.1	18.6	(mq)	(mq)	2.3	0
raw	1 cup	53	7.7	7.5	11	>1.4 c	0.9	0
raw	1 oz	8	1.2	1.2	(mq)	(mq)	0.1	0
KIDNEY BEAN, CANNED								
Dark red								
(Allens)	1/2 cup	105	5.0	20.0	290	(mq)	<1.0	0
(Bush's Best)	1/2 cup	70	6.0	17.0	300	6.0	0.0	na
(Finast)	1/2 cup	110	6.0	20.0	350	(mq)	2.0	0
(Green Giant)	1/2 cup	90	7.0	20.0	330	5.0	<1.0	0
(Green Giant) 50% less salt	1/2 cup	90	7.0	20.0	165	5.0	<1.0	0
(Joan of Arc)	1/2 cup	90	7.0	20.0	330	5.0	<1.0	0
(Joan of Arc) 50% less salt	1/2 cup	90	7.0	20.0	165	5.0	<1.0	0
(Pathmark)	1/2 cup	110	8.0	18.0	370	(mq)	0.0	0
(S&W) 50% less salt 'Lite'	1/2 cup	120	7.0	22.0	355	(mq)	1.0	0
(S&W) 'Premium'	1/2 cup	120	6.0	22.0	596	(mq)	1.0	0
(Stokely)	1/2 cup	110	7.0	20.0	360	(mq)	1.0	0
(Van Camp's)	1 cup	182	11.7	35.0	830	(mq)	0.5	0
Light red								
(Allens)	1/2 cup	105	5.0	2.0	290	(mq)	<1.0	0
(Bush's Best)	1/2 cup	70	6.0	17.0	300	6.0	0.0	na
(Finast)	1/2 cup	110	6.0	20.0	350	(mq)	2.0	0
(Green Giant)	1/2 cup	90	7.0	20.0	330	5.0	<1.0	0
(Green Giant) 50% less salt	1/2 cup	90	7.0	20.0	165	5.0	<1.0	0
(Joan of Arc)	1/2 cup	90	7.0	20.0	330	5.0	<1.0	0
(Joan of Arc) 50% less salt	1/2 cup	90	7.0	20.0	165	5.0	<1.0	0
(Stokely)	1/2 cup	110	7.0	20.0	360	(mq)	1.0	0
(Van Camp's)	1 cup	184	11.5	36.0	650	(mq)	0.5	0
Red								
(A&P)	1/2 cup	110	7.0	20.0	440	(mq)	<1.0	0
(B&M) baked	8 oz	250	15.0	42.0	640	11.0	7.0	5
(Eden Foods) organic, very low sodium, no salt added	1/2 cup	60	8.0	18.0	20	10.0	<1.0	0
(Friends) baked	8 oz	340	17.0	57.0	1060	11.0	4.0	4
(Friends) baked, w/pork	8 oz	270	14.0	55.0	990	11.0	4.0	4
(Green Giant)	1/2 cup	90	7.0	20.0	250	5.9	0.0	0
(Hunt's)	4 oz	120	7.0	21.0	400	(mq)	0.0	0

Food Name	Serv. Size	Total Cal.	Prot. GMS	Carbs GMS	Sod. MGS	Fiber GMS	Fat GMS	Chol. MGS
(Joan of Arc)	1/2 cup	90	7.0	20.0	250	5.9	0.0	0
(Pathmark)	1/2 cup	110	8.0	18.0	370	(mq)	0.0	0
(Progresso)	1/2 cup	100	9.0	21.0	210	7.0	<1.0	0
(S&W) 50% less salt 'Lite'	1/2 cup	120	7.0	22.0	355	(mq)	1.0	0
(S&W) 'Premium'	1/2 cup	120	6.0	22.0	596	(mq)	1.0	0
(S&W Nutradiet)	1/2 cup	90	7.0	16.0	1	(mq)	1.0	0
(Stokely)	1/2 cup	110	7.0	20.0	360	(mq)	1.0	0
(Van Camp's)	1 cup	184	11.5	36.0	650	(mq)	0.5	0
(Van Camp's) 'New Orleans Style'	1 cup	178	12.1	34.0	940	(mq)	0.6	na
KIELBASA/kolbassy								
'Bun Size' *(Hillshire Farm)*	2 oz	180	8.0	2.0	570	0	16.0	(mq)
'Kolbase' *(Hormel)*	3 oz	220	12.0	1.0	904	0	19.0	(mq)
'Lean Supreme Polska' *(Eckrich)*	1 oz	72	4.0	1.0	224	0	6.0	(mq)
'Polska Flavorseal' *(Hillshire Farm)*	2 oz	190	8.0	2.0	540	0	17.0	(mq)
'Polska Flavorseal' beef *(Hillshire Farm)*	2 oz	190	7.0	1.0	550	0	17.0	(mq)
'Polska Flavorseal Lite' *(Hillshire Farm)*	2 oz	160	8.0	2.0	(mq)	0	13.0	(mq)
'Polska Flavorseal' mild *(Hillshire Farm)*	2 oz	190	7.0	2.0	530	0	17.0	(mq)
'Polska Links' *(Hillshire Farm)*	2 oz	190	7.0	2.0	530	0	17.0	(mq)
'Polska' skinless *(Eckrich)*	1 link	180	7.0	2.0	420	0	16.0	(mq)
skinless *(Hormel)*	1/2 link	180	12.0	1.0	826	0	14.0	(mq)
KIWI FRUIT/Chinese gooseberry								
fresh, raw, w/o skin	1 large	56	0.9	13.5	5	3.1	0.4	0
fresh, raw, w/o skin	1 med	46	0.8	11.3	4	2.6	0.3	0
trimmed	1 oz	17	0.3	4.2	1	1.0	0.1	0
untrimmed *(Dole)*	2 fruit	90	1.0	18.0	0	4.0	1.0	na
w/skin	1 lb	237	3.9	58.1	18	13.3	1.7	0
KIWI NECTAR *(Knudsen & Sons)*	8 oz	60	<1.0	14.0	na	na	0.0	na
KNACKWURST								
	4-inch link	209	8.1	1.2	687	0	18.9	39
	1 oz	87	3.4	0.5	286	0	7.9	16
beef *(Hebrew National)*	3-oz link	263	10.2	<1.0	877	0	25.0	26
'Links' *(Hillshire Farm)*	2 oz	180	7.0	1.0	460	0	16.0	(mq)
KOHLRABI/cabbage turnip								
boiled, drained	4 oz	33	2.0	7.6	24	>1.2 c	0.1	0
boiled, drained, sliced	1/2 cup	24	1.5	5.5	17	.9	0.1	0
raw, sliced	1/2 cup	19	1.2	4.3	14	2.52	0.1	0
raw, trimmed	1 oz	8	0.5	1.8	6	.3	<1	0
raw, untrimmed	1 lb	57	3.6	12.9	42	2.3	0.2	0
KOLBASSY. See KIELBASA								
KOOL-AID. See individual flavors.								
KOYADOFU. See TOFU.								
KUMQUAT								
raw, trimmed	1 fruit	12	0.2	3.1	1	>.7 c	0.0	0

Food Name	Serv. Size	Total Cal.	Prot. GMS	Carbs GMS	Sod. MGS	Fiber GMS	Fat GMS	Chol. MGS
w/seeds	1 lb	266	3.8	69.3	25	>15.6 c	0.4	0

L

Food Name	Serv. Size	Total Cal.	Prot. GMS	Carbs GMS	Sod. MGS	Fiber GMS	Fat GMS	Chol. MGS

LAMB, DOMESTIC

(NOTE: All USDA choice grade. TRIMMED = Lean; separable fat removed. UNTRIMMED = Separable fat not removed.)

BRAINS

Food Name	Serv. Size	Total Cal.	Prot. GMS	Carbs GMS	Sod. MGS	Fiber GMS	Fat GMS	Chol. MGS
braised	3 oz	123	10.7	0.0	114	0	8.6	1737
braised, yield from 1 lb raw	12.25 oz	503	43.5	0.0	465	0	35.3	7089
pan-fried	3 oz	232	14.4	0.0	133	0	18.9	2128
raw	4 oz	138	11.8	0.0	127	0	9.7	1533

COMPOSITE CUTS/LEG AND SHOULDER
Trimmed

Food Name	Serv. Size	Total Cal.	Prot. GMS	Carbs GMS	Sod. MGS	Fiber GMS	Fat GMS	Chol. MGS
braised, cubes	3 oz	190	28.6	0.0	59	0	7.5	92
broiled, cubes	3 oz	158	23.9	0.0	65	0	6.2	77
broiled, ground	3 oz	241	21.0	0.0	69	na	16.7	82
raw, cubes	1 lb	608	91.7	0.0	295	0	24.0	295
raw, cubes	1 oz	38	5.7	0.0	18	0	1.5	18
raw, ground	1 lb	1279	75.1	0.0	268	na	106.2	331
raw, ground	1 oz	79	4.6	0.0	17	na	6.6	20
stewed, cubes	4 oz	253	38.2	0.0	79	0	10.0	122

HEART

Food Name	Serv. Size	Total Cal.	Prot. GMS	Carbs GMS	Sod. MGS	Fiber GMS	Fat GMS	Chol. MGS
braised	3 oz	157	21.2	1.6	54	0	6.7	212
raw	4 oz	138	18.7	0.2	101	0	6.4	153
simmered	4 oz	210	28.3	2.2	71	0	9.0	282

KIDNEYS

Food Name	Serv. Size	Total Cal.	Prot. GMS	Carbs GMS	Sod. MGS	Fiber GMS	Fat GMS	Chol. MGS
braised	3 oz	116	20.1	0.8	128	0	3.1	480
raw	4 oz	110	17.8	0.9	177	0	3.3	382

LEG/FORESHANK
Trimmed

Food Name	Serv. Size	Total Cal.	Prot. GMS	Carbs GMS	Sod. MGS	Fiber GMS	Fat GMS	Chol. MGS
braised	3 oz	159	26.4	0.0	63	0	5.1	88
braised	1 oz	53	8.8	0.0	21	0	1.7	29
braised, diced	1 cup	262	43.4	0.0	104	0	8.4	146
broiled, ground	1 cup	328	28.7	0.0	94	0	23.1	113
broiled, ground	4 oz	321	28.1	0.0	92	0	22.3	110
raw	1 lb	544	95.6	0.0	358	0	14.9	313
raw	1 oz	34	5.9	0.0	22	0	0.9	19
raw, ground	1 cup	637	37.4	0.0	133	0	52.9	165
stewed	4 oz	212	35.2	0.0	84	0	6.8	118
stewed	1 oz	53	8.8	0.0	21	0	1.7	29

Food Name	Serv. Size	Total Cal.	Prot. GMS	Carbs GMS	Sod. MGS	Fiber GMS	Fat GMS	Chol. MGS
stewed, diced	1 cup	262	43.4	0.0	104	0	8.4	146
Untrimmed								
braised	3 oz	207	24.1	0.0	61	0	11.4	90
braised	1 oz	69	8.0	0.0	20	0	3.8	30
braised, diced	1 cup	340	39.7	0.0	101	0	18.8	148
raw	1 lb	912	85.8	0.0	327	0	60.7	327
raw	1 oz	56	5.3	0.0	20	0	3.8	20
stewed	1 oz	69	8.0	0.0	20	0	3.8	30
stewed, diced	1 cup	340	39.7	0.0	101	0	18.8	148
LEG/SHANK								
Trimmed								
raw	1 lb	567	93.1	0.0	277	0	19.0	290
raw	1 oz	35	5.8	0.0	17	0	1.2	18
roasted	3 oz	153	23.9	0.0	56	0	5.7	74
roasted	1 oz	51	8.0	0.0	19	0	1.9	25
roasted, diced	1 cup	252	39.4	0.0	92	0	9.3	122
Untrimmed								
raw	1 lb	912	84.3	0.0	259	0	61.2	304
raw	1 oz	56	5.2	0.0	16	0	3.8	19
roasted	3 oz	191	22.5	0.0	55	0	10.6	77
roasted	1 oz	64	7.5	0.0	18	0	3.5	26
roasted, diced	1 cup	315	37.0	0.0	91	0	17.4	126
LEG/SIRLOIN								
Trimmed								
raw	1 lb	608	93.2	0.0	290	0	23.0	299
raw	1 oz	38	5.8	0.0	18	0	1.4	18
roasted	3 oz	173	24.1	0.0	60	0	7.8	78
roasted	1 oz	58	8.0	0.0	20	0	2.6	26
roasted, diced	1 cup	286	39.7	0.0	99	0	12.8	129
Untrimmed								
raw	1 lb	1234	76.8	0.0	254	0	100.3	327
raw	1 oz	76	4.7	0.0	16	0	6.2	20
roasted	3 oz	248	20.9	0.0	58	0	17.6	82
roasted	1 oz	83	7.0	0.0	19	0	5.9	27
roasted, diced	1 cup	409	34.5	0.0	95	0	28.9	136
LEG/WHOLE								
Trimmed								
raw	1 lb	581	93.3	0.0	281	0	20.5	290
raw	1 oz	36	5.8	0.0	17	0	1.3	18
roasted	3 oz	162	24.1	0.0	58	0	6.6	76
roasted	1 oz	54	8.0	0.0	19	0	2.2	25
roasted, diced	1 cup	267	39.6	0.0	95	0	10.8	125

Food Name	Serv. Size	Total Cal.	Prot. GMS	Carbs GMS	Sod. MGS	Fiber GMS	Fat GMS	Chol. MGS
Untrimmed								
raw	1 lb	1043	81.2	0.0	254	0	77.4	313
raw	1 oz	64	5.0	0.0	16	0	4.8	19
roasted	3 oz	219	21.7	0.0	56	0	14.0	79
roasted	1 oz	73	7.2	0.0	19	0	4.7	26
roasted, diced	1 cup	361	35.8	0.0	92	0	23.0	130
LIVER								
braised	3 oz	187	26.0	2.2	48	na	7.5	426
pan-fried	3 oz	202	21.7	3.2	105	na	10.8	419
raw	4 oz	158	23.1	2.0	79	na	5.7	421
LOIN								
Trimmed								
broiled	3 oz	184	25.5	0.0	71	0	8.3	81
raw	1 oz	40	5.8	0.0	19	0	1.7	18
roasted	3 oz	172	22.6	0.0	56	0	8.3	74
Untrimmed								
broiled	3 oz	269	21.4	0.0	65	0	19.6	85
roasted	3 oz	263	19.2	0.0	54	0	20.0	81
LUNGS								
braised	3 oz	96	16.9	0.0	71	0	2.6	241
raw	4 oz	108	18.9	0.0	178	0	3.0	na
PANCREAS								
braised	3 oz	199	19.4	0.0	44	0	12.8	340
raw	4 oz	172	16.8	0.0	85	0	11.1	295
RIB								
Trimmed								
broiled	3 oz	200	23.6	0.0	72	0	11.0	77
raw	1 lb	767	90.6	0.0	327	0	41.9	299
raw	1 oz	47	5.6	0.0	20	0	2.6	18
roasted	3 oz	197	22.2	0.0	69	0	11.3	75
Untrimmed								
broiled	3 oz	307	18.8	0.0	65	0	25.1	84
raw	1 lb	1687	65.9	0.0	254	0	156.0	345
raw	1 oz	104	4.1	0.0	16	0	9.6	21
roasted	3 oz	305	18.0	0.0	62	0	25.3	82
SHOULDER/ARM								
Trimmed								
braised	3 oz	237	30.2	0.0	65	0	12.0	103
broiled	3 oz	170	23.5	0.0	70	0	7.7	78
raw	1 oz	37	5.6	0.0	19	0	1.5	18
roasted	3 oz	163	21.6	0.0	57	0	7.9	73
Untrimmed								
braised	3 oz	294	25.8	0.0	61	0	20.4	102

Food Name	Serv. Size	Total Cal.	Prot. GMS	Carbs GMS	Sod. MGS	Fiber GMS	Fat GMS	Chol. MGS
broiled	3 oz	239	20.8	0.0	65	0	16.6	82
raw	1 oz	73	4.7	0.0	17	0	5.8	20
roasted	3 oz	237	19.1	0.0	55	0	17.2	78
SHOULDER/BLADE								
Trimmed								
braised	1 oz	81	9.1	0.0	22	0	4.7	33
broiled	3 oz	179	21.7	0.0	75	0	9.6	77
raw	3 oz	128	16.4	0.0	59	0	6.5	57
roasted	3 oz	178	20.9	0.0	58	0	9.8	74
Untrimmed								
braised	3 oz	293	24.2	0.0	64	0	21.0	99
broiled	3 oz	236	19.6	0.0	70	0	17.0	81
raw	1 lb	1175	75.4	0.0	281	0	94.6	327
raw	1 oz	73	4.7	0.0	17	0	5.8	20
roasted	3 oz	239	18.9	0.0	56	0	17.5	78
SHOULDER/WHOLE								
Trimmed								
braised	4 oz	321	37.2	0.0	90	0	10.0	133
braised, diced	1 cup	396	45.9	0.0	111	0	22.2	164
broiled	4 oz	238	30.8	0.0	94	0	11.9	105
roasted	4 oz	231	28.3	0.0	77	0	12.2	99
roasted, diced	1 cup	286	34.9	0.0	95	0	15.1	122
stewed	4 oz	321	37.2	0.0	90	0	10.0	133
stewed, diced	1 cup	396	45.9	0.0	111	0	22.2	164
Untrimmed								
braised, diced	1 cup	482	40.2	0.0	105	0	34.4	162
broiled	4 oz	315	27.7	0.0	88	0	21.8	110
broiled, diced	1 cup	389	34.2	0.0	109	0	27.0	136
roasted	4 oz	313	25.5	0.0	75	0	22.6	104
roasted, diced	1 cup	386	31.5	0.0	92	0	28.0	129
stewed	4 oz	390	32.5	0.0	85	0	27.8	132
stewed, diced	1 cup	482	40.2	0.0	105	0	34.4	162
SPLEEN								
braised	3 oz	133	22.5	0.0	49	0	4.1	327
raw	4 oz	115	19.5	0.0	95	0	3.5	283
TONGUE								
braised	3 oz	234	18.3	0.0	57	0	17.2	161
raw	4 oz	252	17.8	0.0	88	0	19.5	177
LAMB, NEW ZEALAND, FROZEN								
COMPOSITE CUTS								
Trimmed								
cooked	4 oz	234	33.6	0.0	57	0	10.0	124
raw	1 oz	36	5.9	0.0	13	0	1.3	21

Food Name	Serv. Size	Total Cal.	Prot. GMS	Carbs GMS	Sod. MGS	Fiber GMS	Fat GMS	Chol. MGS
Untrimmed								
raw	1 oz	182	2.0	0.0	6	0	19.2	25
LEG/FORESHANK								
Trimmed								
braised	3 oz	158	26.1	0.0	42	0	5.1	86
braised, diced	1 cup	260	43.1	0.0	69	0	8.5	141
raw	1 lb	535	94.4	0.0	227	0	14.9	304
raw	1 oz	33	5.8	0.0	14	0	0.9	19
stewed	4 oz	211	34.9	0.0	56	0	6.8	115
stewed, diced	1 cup	260	43.1	0.0	69	0	8.5	141
Untrimmed								
braised	3 oz	219	22.9	0.0	40	0	13.5	87
braised, diced	1 cup	361	37.8	0.0	66	0	22.2	143
raw	1 lb	1012	81.8	0.0	204	0	73.3	322
raw	1 oz	62	5.1	0.0	13	0	4.5	20
stewed	4 oz	293	30.6	0.0	53	0	18.0	116
stewed, diced	1 cup	361	37.8	0.0	66	0	22.2	143
LEG/WHOLE								
Trimmed								
raw	1 lb	558	94.6	0.0	200	0	17.2	331
raw	1 oz	34	5.8	0.0	12	0	1.1	20
roasted	3 oz	154	23.5	0.0	38	0	6.0	85
roasted, diced	1 cup	253	38.8	0.0	63	0	9.8	140
Untrimmed								
raw	1 lb	980	83.2	0.0	181	0	69.4	345
raw	1 oz	60	5.1	0.0	11	0	4.3	21
roasted	3 oz	209	21.1	0.0	37	0	13.2	86
roasted, diced	1 cup	344	34.7	0.0	60	0	21.8	141
LOIN								
Trimmed								
broiled	4 oz	226	33.2	0.0	62	0	9.3	129
raw	1 oz	36	5.9	0.0	13	0	1.2	22
roasted	3 oz	169	24.9	0.0	47	0	7.0	97
Untrimmed								
broiled	3 oz	268	19.9	0.0	42	0	20.3	95
raw	1 oz	85	4.6	0.0	10	0	7.3	23
RIB								
Trimmed								
raw	1 lb	644	92.9	0.0	236	0	27.5	345
raw	1 oz	40	5.7	0.0	15	0	1.7	21
roasted	3 oz	167	20.8	0.0	41	0	8.6	80
Untrimmed								
raw	1 lb	1569	67.7	0.0	181	0	142.0	367

Food Name	Serv. Size	Total Cal.	Prot. GMS	Carbs GMS	Sod. MGS	Fiber GMS	Fat GMS	Chol. MGS
raw	1 oz	97	4.2	0.0	11	0	8.8	23
roasted	3 oz	289	16.1	0.0	37	0	24.4	85
SHOULDER/WHOLE								
Trimmed								
braised	3 oz	242	29.0	0.0	48	0	13.2	108
braised, diced	1 cup	399	47.7	0.0	78	0	21.7	178
raw	1 lb	612	91.8	0.0	213	0	24.6	322
raw	1 oz	38	5.8	0.0	13	0	1.5	20
stewed	6.5 oz	522	62.3	0.0	103	0	28.3	232
stewed, diced	1 cup	399	47.7	0.0	78	0	21.7	178
Untrimmed								
braised	3 oz	303	24.0	0.0	43	0	22.3	105
braised, diced	1 cup	491	40.2	0.0	73	0	35.5	172
raw	1 lb	1234	75.5	0.0	186	0	100.8	340
stewed	4 oz	398	32.5	0.0	59	0	28.8	139
stewed, diced	1 cup	491	40.2	0.0	73	0	35.5	172
LAMB'S QUARTERS								
boiled, drained	4 oz	36	3.6	5.7	(mq)	>2.0 c	0.8	0
boiled, drained, chopped	1 cup	58	5.8	9.0	52	>3.2 c	1.3	0
raw	100 gm	43	4.2	7.3	43	>4.0	0.8	0
raw, trimmed	1 lb	195	19.1	33.1	(mq)	>9.5 c	3.6	0
raw, trimmed	1 oz	12	1.2	2.1	(mq)	>.6 c	0.2	0
LARD								
pork, fresh	1 cup	1849	0.0	0.0	0	0	205.0	195
pork, fresh	1 tbsp	115	0.0	0.0	0	0	12.8	12
pork leaf, fresh	1 oz	243	0.5	0.0	1	0	26.7	31
LASAGNA ENTRÉE, FROZEN								
(Banquet) 'Extra Helping'	16.5 oz	645	24.0	88.0	1582	(mq)	23.0	38
(Celentano)	10 oz	460	24.0	40.0	870	(mq)	24.0	(mq)
(Celentano)	8 oz	370	19.0	32.0	700	(mq)	19.0	(mq)
(Celentano)	6.25 oz	230	13.0	22.0	600	(mq)	14.0	(mq)
(Chef Boyardee)	5.97 oz	280	15.0	42.0	900	(mq)	8.0	(mq)
(Green Giant) 'Entrées'	12 oz	490	33.0	44.0	1660	(mq)	20.0	(mq)
(Stouffer's) 96-oz tray	9.75 oz	400	30.0	37.0	940	na	14.0	na
(Stouffer's) 21-oz pkg	10.5 oz	360	28.0	33.0	1020	na	13.0	na
(Stouffer's) 10-oz pkg	10 oz	340	18.0	40.0	840	na	12.0	na
(Tyson) 'Gourmet Selection'	11.5 oz	380	20.0	47.0	840	(mq)	14.0	(mq)
(Weight Watchers)	10.25 oz	270	24.0	29.0	510	na	6.0	5
CHEESE								
(Budget Gourmet) three cheese	10 oz	400	22.0	38.0	760	(mq)	17.0	65
(Dining Lite)	9 oz	260	14.0	36.0	800	(mq)	6.0	30
(Lean Cuisine) casserole 'Lunch Express'	9.5 oz	290	17.0	42.0	560	na	6.0	10
(Weight Watchers) Italian	11 oz	290	28.0	29.0	510	na	7.0	20

Food Name	Serv. Size	Total Cal.	Prot. GMS	Carbs GMS	Sod. MGS	Fiber GMS	Fat GMS	Chol. MGS
FLORENTINE *(Smart Ones)* w/spinach								
cheese	11 oz	220	18.0	34.0	460	na	1.0	10
IN SAUCE *(Buitoni)* 'Family Style'	7.3 oz	370	13.0	30.0	940	(mq)	13.0	55
LOW FAT *(Celentano)* 'Great Choice'	10 oz	260	18.0	42.0	650	na	2.0	na
MEAT *(Buitoni)* 'Single Serving'	9 oz	580	23.0	57.0	820	(mq)	19.0	110
PRIMAVERA *(Celentano)*	11 oz	330	18.0	34.0	470	(mq)	14.0	na
SAUSAGE *(Budget Gourmet)* Italian	10 oz	420	20.0	38.0	950	(mq)	20.0	80
SEAFOOD *(Mrs. Paul's)* seafood 'Light'	9.5 oz	290	14.0	39.0	750	(mq)	8.0	57
TOFU								
(Amy's Kitchen) vegetable, organic	9.5 oz	310	14.0	36.0	500	4.0	10.0	0
(Legume) and sauce 'Classic'	8 oz	210	15.0	20.0	410	8.2	8.0	0
TUNA *(Lean Cuisine)* w/spinach noodles	9.75 oz	240	16.0	29.0	520	na	7.0	20
VEGETABLE								
(Amy's Kitchen) organic	9.5 oz	310	20.0	36.0	470	3.0	8.5	26
(Le Menu) garden 'Light Style'	10.5 oz	260	11.0	35.0	500	(mq)	8.0	25
(Legume) w/tofu and sauce	12 oz	240	14.0	26.0	520	5.8	8.0	0
(Stouffer's)	10.5 oz	430	20.0	35.0	820	na	23.0	na
(Stouffer's) 96-oz tray	9.5 oz	400	23.0	33.0	760	na	20.0	na
(Weight Watchers) garden 'Lowfat'	11 oz	260	19.0	30.0	430	na	7.0	15
W/MEAT SAUCE								
(Banquet) 'Family Entrees'	7 oz	270	15.0	30.0	(mq)	(mq)	10.0	(mq)
(Dining Lite)	9 oz	240	13.0	36.0	800	(mq)	5.0	25
(Freezer Queen) 'Deluxe Family Suppers'	7 oz	200	8.0	28.0	730	(mq)	6.0	(mq)
(Healthy Choice)	10 oz	260	18.0	37.0	420	na	5.0	20
(Le Menu) 'LightStyle'	10 oz	290	19.0	36.0	510	(mq)	8.0	30
(Lean Cuisine)	10.25 oz	280	20.0	36.0	560	na	6.0	25
(Swanson) 'Homestyle Recipe'	10.5 oz	400	26.0	39.0	1070	(mq)	15.0	(mq)
ZUCCHINI								
(Healthy Choice)	11.5 oz	250	14.0	41.0	400	na	3.0	15
(Lean Cuisine)	11 oz	260	17.0	34.0	520	na	6.0	20
LASAGNA ENTRÉE, MICROWAVE								
(Chef Boyardee)	7.5 oz	230	7.0	31.0	1080	(mq)	9.0	18
(Chef Boyardee) hearty 'Main Meals'	10.5 oz	290	13.0	41.0	na	na	8.0	na
(Chef Boyardee) in garden vegetable sauce	7.5 oz	170	5.0	14.0	940	(mq)	1.0	3
(Hormel)	7.5 oz	250	8.0	25.0	949	na	13.0	23
(Libby's) w/meat sauce 'Diner'	7.75 oz	200	9.0	29.0	790	2.4	5.0	15
(Lunch Bucket) w/meat sauce	7.5 oz	220	8.0	38.0	870	na	4.0	30
LASAGNA ENTRÉE, PACKAGED								
(Dinty Moore) w/meat sauce								
'American Classics'	10 oz	320	16.0	33.0	870	na	14.0	35
(Top Shelf) Italian	10 oz	350	23.0	30.0	840	na	16.0	60
(Top Shelf) vegetable	10.6 oz	275	18.0	34.0	1024	(mq)	8.0	35
(Ultra Slim Fast) vegetable	12 oz	240	17.0	39.0	730	na	4.0	15

Food Name	Serv. Size	Total Cal.	Prot. GMS	Carbs GMS	Sod. MGS	Fiber GMS	Fat GMS	Chol. MGS
(Ultra Slim Fast) w/meat sauce .... 12 oz		330	28.0	38.0	980	na	9.0	55
LASAGNA NOODLE. See PASTA.								
LAVER. See SEAWEED.								
LEEK								
boiled, drained .... 4 oz		35	0.9	8.6	11	>.9 c	0.2	0
boiled, drained, chopped .... 1/4 cup		8	0.2	2.0	3	>.2 c	0.1	0
raw, chopped .... 1/2 cup		32	0.8	7.4	10	.6	0.2	0
raw, trimmed .... 1 oz		17	0.4	4.0	6	.3	0.1	0
raw, untrimmed .... 1 lb		122	3.0	28.2	40	2.4	0.6	0
LEEK, FREEZE-DRIED								
bulb-lower leaf portion .... 1 oz		91	4.3	21.2	10	>2.5 c	0.6	0
bulb-lower leaf portion .... 1/4 cup		3	0.1	0.6	0	>.1 c	0.0	0
bulb-lower leaf portion .... 1 tbsp		1	0.0	0.2	0	0	0.0	0
LEMON								
w/peel, approx 3.9 oz .... 1 med		22	1.3	11.6	3	na	0.3	0
w/peel, whole .... 1 lb		89	5.3	47.6	13	(mq)	1.3	0
w/o peel, approx 3.9 oz .... 1 med		17	0.6	5.4	1	1.6	0.2	0
w/o peel, approx 5.6 oz .... 1 large		24	0.9	7.8	2	2.3	0.3	0
w/o peel, trimmed .... 1-oz wedge		5	0.3	2.9	1	na	0.1	0
LEMON AND HERB SEASONING								
(Schilling) 'Spice Blends' .... 1/4 tsp		1	0.1	0.2	154	na	0.1	0
LEMON DILL SEASONING MIX								
(Schilling) 'Bag 'n Season' .... 1 pkg		161	3.0	15.0	2035	(mq)	11.0	0
LEMON DRINK. See also LEMONADE.								
(Crowley) chilled .... 8 oz		130	0.0	32.0	15	(tr)	0.0	0
(Gatorade) 'Thirst Quencher' .... 8 oz		50	0.0	14.0	110	na	0.0	na
(Pathmark) 'No Frills' mix, prepared ...... 8 oz		90	0.0	20.0	55	(tr)	0.0	0
LEMON GINGER JUICE								
(Santa Cruz Natural) organic 'Cruz' ...... 8 oz		125	1.0	29.0	na	na	<1.0	na
LEMON HERB MARINADE *(Golden Dipt)* .. 1 oz		130	0.0	2.0	210	na	14.0	0
LEMON JUICE								
.... 1 cup		61	0.9	21.1	2	0	0.0	0
.... 1 oz		8	0.1	2.6	<1	(tr)	0.0	0
.... 1 tbsp		4	0.1	1.3	0	0	0.0	0
Canned or bottled								
(A&P) reconstituted, natural strength ..... 1 oz		6	<1.0	2.0	0	(tr)	<1.0	0
(Lucky Leaf) .... 6 oz		30	1.0	6.0	35	(tr)	0.0	0
(ReaLemon) reconstituted, natural strength,								
refrigerated .... 1 oz		6	0.0	2.0	10	(tr)	0.0	0
(ReaLemon) reconstituted, '100%' .... 1 oz		6	0.0	2.0	5	(tr)	0.0	0
Frozen								
single strength .... 1/2 cup		27	0.6	7.9	1	(tr)	0.4	0
single strength .... 1 tbsp		3	0.1	1.0	tr	(tr)	0.1	0

Food Name	Serv. Size	Total Cal.	Prot. GMS	Carbs GMS	Sod. MGS	Fiber GMS	Fat GMS	Chol. MGS
(Minute Maid) concentrate	6 oz	8	0.0	2.0	0	na	0.0	na
(Sunkist)	1 oz	7	0.1	2.0	<1	(tr)	0.1	0
LEMON PEEL								
candied	1 oz	88	0.1	22.6	0	>.6 c	0.1	0
raw	1 tbsp	na	0.1	1.0	0	.6	0.0	0
raw	1 tsp	na	0.0	0.3	0	na	0.0	0
LEMON PEPPER								
Dry seasoning								
(Lawry's)	1 tsp	6	0.2	1.2	340	>.1 c	0.1	0
(Schilling) 'Parsley Patch'	1 tsp	13	0.4	1.0	2	(mq)	0.6	0
(Schilling) 'Spice Blends'	1 tsp	7	0.2	0.8	618	(mq)	0.0	0
Marinade *(Lawry's)*	1 oz	20	0.3	2.1	800	na	1.1	na
LEMONADE								
Can, bottle, or box								
(Fruitopia) 'Lemonade, Love & Hope' real fruit	8 oz	110	0.0	28.0	25	na	0.0	na
(Fruitopia) 'Pink Lemonade Euphoria' real fruit	8 oz	120	0.0	29.0	25	na	0.0	na
(Hi-C)	8.45 oz	109	0.1	27.2	73	(tr)	0.1	0
(J. Hungerford) pink, 20% plus juice	9.03 oz	41	0.1	10.7	39	0	0.0	0
(Knudsen & Sons) 'Natural'	8 oz	100	<1.0	26.0	na	na	0.0	na
(Minute Maid)	6 oz	80	0.0	21.0	20	na	0.0	na
(Minute Maid) country style	6 oz	80	0.0	21.0	20	na	0.0	na
(Minute Maid) cranberry	6 oz	90	0.0	23.0	20	na	0.0	na
(Minute Maid) pink	6 oz	80	0.0	21.0	20	na	0.0	na
(Minute Maid) raspberry	6 oz	90	0.0	23.0	20	na	0.0	na
(Santa Cruz Natural) organic	8 oz	60	<1.0	21.0	na	na	<1.0	na
(Santa Cruz Natural) organic 'Sparkling'	8 oz	85	<1.0	20.0	na	na	<1.0	na
(Shasta)	12 oz	146	0.0	39.0	106	(tr)	0.0	0
(Sunkist)	8 oz	141	0.0	36.0	0	(tr)	0.0	0
(10-K) pink	8 oz	60	0.0	15.0	55	na	0.0	na
(Tropicana)	6 oz	100	<1.0	22.0	35	na	<1.0	na
(Tropicana) 'Single Serve'	8 oz	120	(tr)	30.0	3	(tr)	0.0	0
(Veryfine)	8 oz	120	0.2	30.0	25	(tr)	0.0	0
(Wyler's)	6 oz	64	0.0	16.5	33	(tr)	0.0	0
(Wyler's) pink 'Fruit Slush'	4 oz	157	0.0	39.3	10	(tr)	0.0	0
LEMONADE DRINK MIX								
Prepared from dry mix								
(Country Time)	8 oz	80	0.0	20.0	20	0	0.0	0
(Country Time) pink	8 oz	80	0.0	20.0	20	0	0.0	0
(Country Time) pink, 'Sugar Free'	8 oz	4	0.0	0.0	0	0	0.0	0
(Country Time) pink, sugar sweetened	8 oz	80	0.0	20.0	20	na	0.0	0

Food Name	Serv. Size	Total Cal.	Prot. GMS	Carbs GMS	Sod. MGS	Fiber GMS	Fat GMS	Chol. MGS
(Country Time) pink, sugar-free, w/NutraSweet	8 oz	4	0.0	0.0	0	na	0.0	0
(Country Time) 'Sugar-free'	8 oz	4	0.0	0.0	0	0	0.0	0
(Crystal Light) 'Sugar-free'	8 oz	4	0.0	0.0	0	0	0.0	0
(Crystal Light) sugar-free, w/NutraSweet	8 oz	4	0.0	0.0	0	na	0.0	0
(Finast)	8 oz	80	0.0	20.0	15	0	0.0	0
(Gatorade) instant 'Thirst Quencher'	8 oz	60	0.0	15.0	110	na	0.0	na
(Kool-Aid) pink, unsweetened, prepared w/sugar	8 oz	100	0.0	25.0	0	na	0.0	0
(Kool-Aid) pink, unsweetened, prepared w/o sugar	8 oz	2	0.0	0.0	0	na	0.0	0
(Kool-Aid) sugar free, w/NutraSweet	8 oz	4	0.0	0.0	0	na	0.0	0
(Kool-Aid) sugar sweetened	8 oz	80	0.0	20.0	0	na	0.0	0
(Wyler's) 'Crystals' 32-serving pkg	8 oz	78	0.0	19.4	39	0	0.0	0
Prepared from frozen concentrate								
(A&P)	8 oz	110	<1.0	28.0	0	(tr)	<1.0	0
(A&P) pink	8 oz	110	<1.0	28.0	0	(tr)	<1.0	0
(Minute Maid)	6 oz	90	0.0	22.0	0	na	0.0	na
(Minute Maid) country style	6 oz	90	0.0	22.0	0	na	0.0	na
(Minute Maid) cranberry	6 oz	90	0.0	22.0	0	na	0.0	na
(Minute Maid) pink	6 oz	90	0.0	22.0	0	na	0.0	na
(Minute Maid) raspberry	6 oz	90	0.0	22.0	0	na	0.0	na
(Sunkist)	8 oz	92	0.1	24.2	1	(tr)	0.0	0
LEMONADE PUNCH MIX *(Country Time)*								
sugar sweetened	8 oz	80	0.0	20.0	15	na	0.0	0
LEMON-LIME DRINK								
Can, bottle, or box								
(All-Sports) thirst quencher, caffeine-free	8 oz	70	0.0	19.0	55	na	0.0	na
(Gatorade) 'Thirst Quencher'	8 oz	50	0.0	14.0	110	na	0.0	na
(Gatorade) 'Thirst Quencher Light'	8 oz	25	0.0	7.0	80	na	0.0	na
(PowerAde) thirst quencher, high energy	8 oz	70	0.0	19.0	70	na	0.0	na
(10-K)	8 oz	60	0.0	15.0	55	na	0.0	na
(Veryfine)	8 oz	120	0.1	30.0	10	(tr)	0.0	0
Prepared from dry mix								
(Crystal Light) w/NutraSweet	8 oz	4	0.0	0.0	0	na	0.0	0
(GatorAde) instant 'Thirst Quencher'	8 oz	60	0.0	15.0	110	na	0.0	na
(Kool-Aid) unsweetened, prepared w/sugar	8 oz	100	0.0	25.0	0	na	0.0	0
(Kool-Aid) unsweetened, prepared w/o sugar	8 oz	2	0.0	0.0	0	na	0.0	0
LENTIL								
boiled	1/2 cup	115	8.9	19.9	2	4.0	0.4	0
boiled	4 oz	132	10.2	22.8	2	4.5	0.4	0
boiled *(A&P)*	1 cup	210	16.0	39.0	0	(mq)	1.0	0
raw	1/2 cup	324	26.9	54.8	9	10.9	0.9	0

Food Name	Serv. Size	Total Cal.	Prot. GMS	Carbs GMS	Sod. MGS	Fiber GMS	Fat GMS	Chol. MGS
raw	1 oz	96	8.0	16.2	3	3.2	0.3	0
raw, green *(Arrowhead Mills)*	2 oz	190	13.0	35.0	9	8.8	1.0	0
raw, red *(Arrowhead Mills)*	2 oz	195	14.0	34.0	10	8.8	1.0	0
raw, sprouted	1 oz	30	2.5	6.3	3	>.9 c	0.2	0
LENTIL DINNER, CANNED								
hearty, w/garden vegetables 'Fast Menu' fat-free *(Health Valley)*	7.5 oz	160	13.0	18.0	204	15.5	4.0	0
hearty, w/garden vegetables 'Fast Menu' fat-free *(Health Valley)*	5 oz	80	9.0	12.0	140	10.3	0.0	0
LETTUCE								
BIBB, BOSTON, OR BUTTERHEAD								
raw, approx 7.75 oz, 5-inch diam	1 head	21	2.1	3.8	8	1.6	0.4	0
trimmed	1 oz	4	0.4	0.7	1	.3	0.1	0
untrimmed	1 lb	45	4.3	7.8	18	3.4	0.7	0
COS								
raw, shredded	1/2 cup	4	0.5	0.7	2	.5	0.1	0
trimmed	1 oz	5	0.5	0.7	2	.5	0.1	0
untrimmed	1 lb	68	6.9	10.1	32	7.2	0.9	0
ICEBERG								
raw, 6 inch diam	1 head	70	5.4	11.3	49	5.4	1.0	0
trimmed	1 oz	4	0.3	0.6	3	.3	0.1	0
untrimmed	1 lb	55	4.3	9.0	39	4.3	0.8	0
LEAF, shredded *(Dole)*	1.5 cups	12	1.0	1.0	40	1.0	0.0	na
LOOSELEAF								
raw, shredded	1/2 cup	5	0.4	1.0	3	.53	0.1	0
trimmed	1 oz	5	0.4	1.0	3	>.2 c	0.1	0
untrimmed	1 lb	52	3.8	10.2	26	>2.0 c	0.9	0
ROMAINE								
raw, shredded	1/2 cup	4	0.5	0.7	2	.5	0.1	0
trimmed	1 oz	5	0.5	0.7	2	.5	0.1	0
untrimmed	1 lb	68	6.9	10.1	32	7.2	0.9	0
LIMA BEAN /butterbean								
boiled, drained	4 oz	139	7.7	26.8	19	4.8	0.4	0
raw, trimmed	1 oz	32	1.9	5.7	2	1.0	0.2	0
raw, untrimmed	1 lb	226	13.7	40.2	16	7.4	1.7	0
MATURE, DRY								
Baby								
boiled	4 oz	143	9.1	26.4	3	4.9	0.4	0
boiled *(A&P)*	1 cup	230	16.0	40.0	15	(mq)	1.0	0
boiled, thin-seeded	1/2 cup	115	7.3	21.2	3	7.01	0.4	0
raw	1 oz	95	5.8	17.8	4	2.8	0.3	0
raw, thin-seeded	1/2 cup	338	20.8	63.5	13	>5.8 c	0.9	0

Food Name	Serv. Size	Total Cal.	Prot. GMS	Carbs GMS	Sod. MGS	Fiber GMS	Fat GMS	Chol. MGS
Large								
boiled	4 oz	130	8.8	23.7	2	8.2	0.4	0
boiled	1/2 cup	108	7.3	19.6	2	6.8	0.4	0
boiled (A&P)	1 cup	230	15.0	35.0	0	(mq)	1.0	0
raw	1/2 cup	301	19.1	56.4	16	16.9	0.6	0
raw	1 oz	96	6.1	18.0	5	5.4	0.2	0
LIMA BEAN, CANNED								
(A&P)	1/2 cup	110	7.0	20.0	380	(mq)	<1.0	0
(Allens) large	1/2 cup	110	5.0	18.0	370	(mq)	<1.0	0
(Featherweight)	1/2 cup	80	5.0	16.0	25	(mq)	0.0	0
(Freshlike)	1/2 cup	80	5.0	16.0	320	na	0.0	na
(Freshlike) water packed, w/o salt	1/2 cup	80	5.0	16.0	5	na	0.0	na
(Green Giant)	1/2 cup	80	6.0	16.0	420	3.7	0.0	0
(Joan of Arc)	1/2 cup	80	6.0	16.0	420	3.7	0.0	0
(S&W)	1/2 cup	100	5.0	19.0	440	(mq)	1.0	0
(Stokely)	1/2 cup	80	5.0	16.0	390	(mq)	0.0	0
(Stokely) 'No Salt or Sugar Added'	1/2 cup	80	5.0	16.0	5	(mq)	0.0	0
(Van Camp's)	1 cup	162	11.0	30.0	710	(mq)	0.5	0
(Veg•All)	1/2 cup	80	5.0	16.0	320	na	0.0	na
FORDHOOK (Stokely)	1/2 cup	80	5.0	14.0	300	(mq)	0.0	0
GREEN								
(A&P)	1/2 cup	80	5.0	15.0	320	(mq)	<1.0	0
(Allens) medium	1/2 cup	90	5.0	15.0	350	(mq)	<1.0	0
(Allens) tiny, small	1/2 cup	90	5.0	15.0	350	(mq)	<1.0	0
(Bush's Best)	1/2 cup	90	4.0	17.0	400	4.0	0.0	na
(Del Monte) w/liquid	1/2 cup	70	4.0	14.0	355	(mq)	0.0	0
(Luck's) small, w/pork	7.5 oz	220	10.0	33.0	640	8.0	7.0	(mq)
(S&W) small 'Fancy'	1/2 cup	80	6.0	16.0	390	(mq)	0.0	0
GREEN AND WHITE								
(Allens)	1/2 cup	90	5.0	15.0	370	(mq)	<1.0	0
(Bush's Best) gem	1/2 cup	80	5.0	17.0	300	4.0	0.0	na
W/HAM (Dennison's)	7.5 oz	250	14.0	33.0	935	9.0	7.0	(mq)
W/PORK (Luck's)	7.5 oz	230	12.0	34.0	720	9.0	7.0	(mq)
LIMA BEAN, FROZEN								
(Green Giant)	1/2 cup	100	6.0	19.0	30	5.0	0.0	0
(Green Giant) 'Harvest Fresh'	1/2 cup	80	6.0	18.0	170	4.0	0.0	0
(Green Giant) in butter sauce	1/2 cup	100	6.0	17.0	310	2.0	2.0	5
(Health Valley)	1/2 cup	94	6.0	18.0	26	3.4	0.0	0
BABY								
boiled, drained	10-oz pkg	376	21.6	71.4	147	>6.2 c	1.3	0
boiled, drained	4 oz	119	7.5	22.1	33	(mq)	0.3	0
boiled, drained, immature seeds	10-oz pkg	327	20.7	60.5	90	>5.4 c	0.9	0
boiled, drained, immature seeds	1/2 cup	94	6.0	17.5	26	>1.6 c	0.3	0

Food Name	Serv. Size	Total Cal.	Prot. GMS	Carbs GMS	Sod. MGS	Fiber GMS	Fat GMS	Chol. MGS
unprepared, immature seeds	10-oz pkg	375	21.6	71.4	148	>6.2 c	1.3	0
unprepared, immature seeds	1/2 cup	108	6.2	20.6	43	>1.8 c	0.4	0
(A&P) green	3.3 oz	130	7.0	24.0	130	(mq)	<1.0	0
(Birds Eye)	3.3 oz	130	7.0	24.0	115	(mq)	0.0	0
(Freshlike)	3.3 oz	130	7.0	24.0	100	na	1.0	na
(Frosty Acres)	3.3 oz	130	7.0	24.0	125	>2.0 c	0.0	0
(Seabrook)	3.3 oz	130	7.0	24.0	125	>2.0 c	0.0	0
(Seabrook) butter	3.3 oz	140	7.0	26.0	213	>2.0 c	1.0	0
(Southern)	3.5 oz	135	7.3	25.2	125	(mq)	0.5	0
(Stokely) in butter sauce 'Singles'	4 oz	140	7.0	25.0	450	(mq)	2.0	5
(Veg•All)	3.3 oz	130	7.0	24.0	100	na	1.0	na
FORDHOOK								
boiled, drained	10-oz pkg	301	18.2	56.3	166	>5.6 c	1.0	0
boiled, drained	4 oz	113	6.9	21.3	60	>2.1 c	0.4	0
boiled, drained, immature seeds	10-oz pkg	311	18.9	58.5	165	22.4	1.1	0
boiled, drained, immature seeds	1/2 cup	85	5.2	16.0	45	6.1	0.3	0
unprepared, immature seeds	1/2 cup	85	5.1	15.9	46	1.6	0.3	0
(A&P)	3.3 oz	100	6.0	19.0	70	(mq)	<1.0	0
(Birds Eye)	3.3 oz	100	6.0	19.0	100	(mq)	0.0	0
(Frosty Acres)	3.3 oz	100	6.0	19.0	71	>2.0 c	0.0	0
(Seabrook)	3.3 oz	100	6.0	19.0	71	>2.0 c	0.0	0
(Southern)	3.5 oz	105	6.4	19.1	100	(mq)	0.3	0
SPECKLED								
(Seabrook)	3.3 oz	120	7.0	23.0	19	>2.0 c	0.0	0
(Southern)	3.5 oz	135	7.8	25.0	30	(mq)	0.4	0
TINY (Seabrook)	3.3 oz	110	6.0	21.0	144	>2.0 c	1.0	0
LIME								
peeled and seeded	1 oz	9	0.2	3.0	1	>.1 c	0.1	0
raw, 2 inch diam	1 med	20	0.5	7.1	1	1.9	0.1	0
untrimmed	1 lb	115	2.7	40.2	8	>1.9 c	0.8	0
LIME JUICE								
fresh	1 cup	66	1.1	22.2	2	0	0.3	0
fresh	1 oz	8	0.1	2.8	<1	(tr)	<.1	0
fresh	1 tbsp	4	0.1	1.4	0	0	0.0	0
Canned or bottled								
	1/2 cup	26	0.3	8.2	20	(tr)	0.3	0
	1 tbsp	3	<.1	1.0	2	(tr)	<.1	0
unsweetened	1 cup	52	0.6	16.5	39	0	0.6	0
unsweetened	1 tbsp	3	0.0	1.0	2	0	0.0	0
(ReaLime) reconstituted, natural strength	1 oz	6	0.0	2.0	10	(tr)	0.0	0
(Roses)	1 oz	48	0.0	12.0	6	(tr)	0.0	0
(Santa Cruz Natural) organic, 'Cruz'	8 oz	120	1.0	27.0	na	na	<1.0	na

Food Name	Serv. Size	Total Cal.	Prot. GMS	Carbs GMS	Sod. MGS	Fiber GMS	Fat GMS	Chol. MGS
LIMEADE								
(Minute Maid) frozen concentrate, diluted	6 oz	70	0.0	19.0	0	na	0.0	na
(Santa Cruz Natural) organic, 'Sparkling'	8 oz	60	<1.0	23.0	na	na	<1.0	na
LING								
dry-heat cooked	3 oz	94	20.7	0.0	147	0	0.7	43
raw	1 lb	394	86.1	0.0	612	0	2.9	(mq)
raw	3 oz	74	16.1	0.0	115	0	0.5	34
raw	1 oz	25	5.4	0.0	38	0	0.2	(mq)
LINGCOD								
dry-heat cooked	3 oz	93	19.2	0.0	65	0	1.2	57
raw	1 lb	385	80.1	0.0	266	0	4.8	236
raw	3 oz	72	15.0	0.0	50	0	0.9	44
raw	1 oz	24	5.0	0.0	17	0	0.3	15
LINGUINE ENTRÉE								
Frozen								
(Banquet) w/meat sauce 'Healthy Balance'	11.5 oz	290	11.0	49.0	560	na	6.0	25
(Budget Gourmet) w/shrimp	10 oz	330	15.0	33.0	1250	(mq)	15.0	75
(Healthy Choice) w/shrimp	9.5 oz	230	13.0	40.0	420	na	2.0	60
(Lean Cuisine) w/clam sauce	9 5/8 oz	280	17.0	36.0	560	na	8.0	30
Packaged (Top Shelf) w/clam sauce	1 serving	330	12.0	30.0	1420	(mq)	18.0	85
Refrigerated								
(Contadina) egg, angel hair 'Fresh'	3 oz	260	12.0	45.0	30	na	3.0	75
(DiGiorno) herb, approx 1 1/3 cups cooked	3 oz	250	11.0	46.0	135	na	3.0	0
LINGUINE NOODLE. See PASTA.								
LINSEED OIL								
edible	1/2 cup	964	0.0	0.0	0	0	109.0	0
edible	1 oz	251	0.0	0.0	0	0	28.4	0
edible	1 tbsp	120	0.0	0.0	0	0	13.6	0
LIQUEUR. See ALCOHOLIC BEVERAGES.								
LIQUOR. See ALCOHOLIC BEVERAGES.								
LITCHI/lychee								
Dried								
	100 gm	277	3.8	70.7	3	>1.4 c	1.2	0
	1 oz	79	1.1	20.0	1	4.6	0.3	0
Raw								
approx .6 oz	1 med	6	0.1	1.6	tr	<.1	<.1	0
shelled and seeded	1/2 cup	63	0.8	15.7	1	>.2 c	0.4	0
shelled and seeded	1 oz	19	0.2	4.7	<1	>.1 c	0.1	0
untrimmed	1 lb	179	2.3	45.0	2	>.6 c	1.2	0
LIVER. See individual animal listings.								
LIVERWURST. See LUNCHEON MEATS.								
LIVERWURST SPREAD								
(Hormel) canned	.5 oz	35	2.0	0.0	(mq)	0	3.0	(mq)

Food Name	Serv. Size	Total Cal.	Prot. GMS	Carbs GMS	Sod. MGS	Fiber GMS	Fat GMS	Chol. MGS
(Underwood) canned	2 1/8 oz	180	8.0	4.0	470	na	15.0	90
LOBSTER, NORTHERN								
boiled	1 cup	142	29.7	1.9	551	0	0.9	104
boiled	4 oz	111	23.2	1.5	431	0	0.7	82
moist-heat cooked	1 cup	142	29.7	1.9	551	0	0.9	104
moist-heat cooked	3 oz	83	17.4	1.1	323	0	0.5	61
poached	1 cup	142	29.7	1.9	551	0	0.9	104
poached	4 oz	111	23.2	1.5	431	0	0.7	82
raw	1 lb	410	85.3	2.3	(mq)	0	4.1	432
raw	3 oz	77	16.0	0.4	252	0	0.8	81
raw	1 oz	26	5.3	0.1	(mq)	0	0.3	27
steamed	1 cup	142	29.7	1.9	551	0	0.9	104
steamed	4 oz	111	23.2	1.5	431	0	0.7	82
LOBSTER, SPINY, MIXED SPECIES								
moist-heat cooked	3 oz	122	22.5	2.7	193	0	1.6	77
raw	1 lb	506	93.4	11.0	803	0	6.9	318
raw	3 oz	95	17.5	2.1	150	0	1.3	59
raw	1 oz	32	5.8	0.7	50	0	0.4	20
LOBSTER PASTE, canned	1 tsp	13	1.5	0.1	10	0	0.7	12
LOGANBERRY								
fresh, trimmed	1 lb	281	4.5	67.6	5	(mq)	2.7	0
fresh, trimmed	1 cup	89	1.4	21.5	1	>4.3 c	0.9	0
fresh, untrimmed	1 lb	267	4.3	64.2	4	(mq)	2.6	0
frozen	1 cup	81	2.2	19.1	1	7.2	0.5	0
frozen	4 oz	62	1.7	14.8	1	(mq)	0.4	0
LONGAN/dragon's eye								
raw, approx .2 oz	1 med	2	<.1	0.5	tr	<.1	tr	0
raw, shelled and seeded	1 oz	17	0.4	4.3	tr	>.1 c	<.1	0
raw, untrimmed	1 lb	144	3.2	36.4	1	>1.0 c	0.2	0
LONGAN, DRIED								
	100 gm	286	4.9	74.0	48	>2.0 c	0.4	0
	1 oz	81	1.4	21.0	14	>.6 c	0.1	0
LONGBEAN								
boiled, drained	4 oz	53	2.9	10.4	5	>1.7 c	0.1	0
boiled, drained, sliced	1/2 cup	25	1.3	4.8	2	>.8 c	0.1	0
boiled, drained, 13 1/4 inches long x 1/4 inch diam	1 pod	7	0.4	1.3	1	>.2 c	<.1	0
raw, sliced	1/2 cup	22	1.3	3.8	2	(mq)	0.2	0
raw, 13 1/4 inches long x 1/4 inch diam	1 pod	6	0.3	1.0	tr	(mq)	0.1	0
raw, trimmed	1 oz	13	0.8	2.4	1	(mq)	0.1	0
raw, untrimmed	1 lb	203	12.1	36.0	17	(mq)	1.7	0
LONGBEAN, DRIED								
boiled	1/2 cup	102	7.1	18.1	4	>1.4 c	0.4	0

Food Name	Serv. Size	Total Cal.	Prot. GMS	Carbs GMS	Sod. MGS	Fiber GMS	Fat GMS	Chol. MGS
boiled	4 oz	134	9.4	23.9	6	>1.8 c	0.5	0
raw	1/2 cup	292	20.4	52.0	14	>4.0 c	1.1	0
raw	1 oz	98	6.9	17.6	5	>1.4 c	0.4	0

LOOFAH GOURD. See GOURD, DISHCLOTH.

LOQUAT/Japanese medlar

peeled and seeded	1 oz	13	0.1	3.4	<1	>.1 c	0.1	0
trimmed, .6 oz	1 med	5	0.0	1.2	0	.2	0.0	0
untrimmed	1 lb	132	1.2	34.1	3	>1.4 c	0.6	0

LOTTE. See MONKFISH.

LOTUS ROOT

boiled, drained	4 oz	75	1.8	18.2	51	>1.0 c	0.1	0
boiled, drained, 2.5-inch diam	10 slices	59	1.4	14.3	40	2.8	0.1	0
raw, 2.5-inch diam	10 slices	45	2.1	14.0	32	4.0	0.1	0
raw, 9.5 inches long	1 root	64	3.0	19.8	46	5.6	0.1	0
raw, trimmed	1 oz	16	0.7	4.9	11	>.2 c	<.1	0
raw, untrimmed	1 lb	201	9.3	61.8	145	>2.9 c	0.4	0

LOTUS SEED

dried	1 cup	106	4.9	20.6	2	>.8 c	0.6	0
dried, approx 42 medium seeds	1 oz	94	4.4	18.3	1	>.7 c	0.6	0
raw	1 oz	25	1.2	4.9	0	>.2 c	0.2	0
raw, in shell	1 lb	214	9.9	41.5	3	>1.6 c	1.3	0

LOX. See SALMON, CHINOOK.

LUNCHEON MEAT

BARBECUE LOAF (Oscar Mayer)	1 oz	46	4.5	1.7	333	0	2.3	14

BOLOGNA

(Eckrich)	1 oz	100	3.0	1.0	240	0	9.0	(mq)
(Eckrich) 'German Brand'	1 oz	80	4.0	1.0	300	0	7.0	(mq)
(Eckrich) 'Lean Supreme'	1 oz	70	4.0	1.0	240	0	6.0	(mq)
(Eckrich) 'Sandwich'	1 oz	100	3.0	1.0	240	0	9.0	(mq)
(Eckrich) 'Smorgas Pac'	1 oz	100	3.0	1.0	240	0	9.0	(mq)
(Eckrich) 'Thick Sliced, 1-lb pkg'	1.8 oz	170	5.0	2.0	430	0	15.0	(mq)
(Hillshire Farm) 'Large'	1 oz	90	3.0	<1.0	(mq)	0	8.0	(mq)
(Hillshire Farm) 'Ring'	1 oz	89	3.0	<1.0	(mq)	0	8.0	(mq)
(Hormel) 'Fine Ground, 1-lb'	2 oz	170	7.0	1.0	596	0	16.0	(mq)
(Hormel) 'Perma-Fresh'	2 slices	180	7.0	0.0	599	0	16.0	(mq)
(JM)	1 oz	90	3.0	1.0	350	0	8.0	(mq)
(JM) 'German Brand'	1 oz	70	4.0	1.0	270	0	6.0	(mq)
(Kahn's)	1 slice	90	3.0	1.0	330	0	8.0	(mq)
(Kahn's) 'Deluxe Club'	1 slice	90	3.0	1.0	290	0	8.0	na
(Kahn's) 'Deluxe Club Family Pack'	1 slice	70	2.0	1.0	220	0	6.0	(mq)
(Kahn's) 'Giant Deluxe'	1 slice	90	3.0	1.0	290	0	8.0	(mq)
(Kahn's) 'Giant Thick Deluxe'	1 slice	110	4.0	1.0	330	0	10.0	(mq)
(Kahn's) 'Thick Deluxe'	1 slice	140	5.0	1.0	450	0	13.0	(mq)

Food Name	Serv. Size	Total Cal.	Prot. GMS	Carbs GMS	Sod. MGS	Fiber GMS	Fat GMS	Chol. MGS
(Kahn's) 'Thin Sliced Deluxe'	1 slice	60	2.0	1.0	190	0	5.0	(mq)
(Light & Lean)	2 slices	140	6.0	2.0	(mq)	0	12.0	(mq)
(Light & Lean) 'Thin Sliced'	2 slices	70	3.0	1.0	(mq)	0	6.0	(mq)
(OHSE)	1 oz	75	3.0	3.0	280	0	6.0	(mq)
(Oscar Mayer)	1.6 oz	144	5.0	1.1	500	0	13.3	30
(Oscar Mayer)	1 oz	90	3.1	0.7	311	0	8.3	19
(Oscar Mayer)	.53 oz	48	1.7	0.4	167	0	4.4	10
(Oscar Mayer) 'Light'	1 oz	64	3.2	0.7	310	0	5.4	11
(Oscar Mayer) Wisconsin made, ring	1 oz	90	3.0	<1.0	230	na	8.0	15
(Oscar Mayer) w/cheese	.8 oz	74	2.7	0.6	232	0	6.8	15
(Pilgrim's Pride)	1 oz	59	3.9	0.6	228	0	4.4	16
Beef								
(Boar's Head)	1 oz	74	4.0	<1.0	270	0	7.0	17
(Boar's Head) 'Premium' low cholesterol	1 oz	70	4.0	1.0	270	na	7.0	15
(Eckrich)	1 oz	90	3.0	1.0	230	0	8.0	(mq)
(Eckrich) 'Thick Sliced'	1.5 oz	130	4.0	2.0	340	0	12.0	(mq)
(Hebrew National) 'Original Deli Style'	1 oz	90	3.0	<1.0	330	0	3.0	15
(Hormel) 'Coarse Ground, 1 lb'	2 oz	160	8.0	1.0	576	0	14.0	(mq)
(Hormel) 'Perma-Fresh'	2 slices	170	6.0	1.0	592	0	16.0	(mq)
(JM)	1 oz	90	3.0	1.0	350	0	8.0	(mq)
(Kahn's)	1 slice	90	3.0	1.0	300	0	8.0	(mq)
(Kahn's) 'Family Pack'	1 slice	70	2.0	1.0	230	0	6.0	(mq)
(Kahn's) 'Giant'	1 slice	90	3.0	1.0	300	0	8.0	(mq)
(Kahn's) 'Pounder'	1 slice	90	3.0	1.0	300	0	8.0	(mq)
(OHSE)	1 oz	85	3.0	1.0	310	0	8.0	(mq)
(Oscar Mayer)	1.6 oz	143	5.0	1.0	489	0	13.3	31
(Oscar Mayer)	1 oz	89	3.1	0.6	304	0	8.2	19
(Oscar Mayer)	.53 oz	48	1.7	0.3	163	0	4.4	10
(Oscar Mayer) 'Light'	1 oz	64	3.5	0.9	316	0	5.3	10
Beef and cheddar *(Kahn's)*	1 slice	90	4.0	1.0	320	0	8.0	(mq)
Beef and pork								
(Boar's Head)	1 oz	80	4.0	<1.0	250	0	7.0	15
(Boar's Head) 'Premium' low cholesterol	1 oz	80	4.0	1.0	250	na	7.0	15
(Healthy Deli)	1 oz	41	4.4	1.1	200	0	2.0	9
Chicken								
(Health Valley)	1 slice	85	4.0	1.0	329	0	8.0	13
(OHSE) '15% Chicken'	1 oz	90	3.0	1.0	320	0	8.0	(mq)
(Tyson)	1 slice	44	2.2	3.7	185	na	0.5	na
Garlic								
(Eckrich)	1 oz	90	3.0	1.0	230	0	9.0	(mq)
(Eckrich) w/cheese	1 oz	90	3.0	1.0	250	0	9.0	(mq)
(JM)	1 oz	90	3.0	1.0	350	0	8.0	(mq)
(Kahn's)	1 slice	90	3.0	1.0	290	0	8.0	(mq)

Food Name	Serv. Size	Total Cal.	Prot. GMS	Carbs GMS	Sod. MGS	Fiber GMS	Fat GMS	Chol. MGS
Ham								
(Boar's Head)	1 oz	40	5.0	1.0	(mq)	0	2.0	15
(Oscar Mayer)	1 oz	90	3.1	0.7	301	0	8.3	18
Lebanon (Oscar Mayer)	.8 oz	46	4.7	0.4	302	0	2.9	16
Turkey								
(Butterball) 'Cold Cuts'	1 oz	70	4.0	2.0	370	0	6.0	(mq)
(Butterball) 'Deli/Slice 'n Serve'	1 oz	70	4.0	2.0	370	0	6.0	(mq)
(Butterball) 'Turkey Variety Pak'	.75 oz	50	3.0	1.0	280	0	4.0	(mq)
(Healthy Choice) beef and pork	.75-oz slice	25	3.0	1.0	240	na	1.0	10
(Longacre) sliced	1 oz	61	4.0	0.0	270	0	5.0	25
(Louis Rich)	1 oz	61	3.4	0.6	244	0	5.0	22
(Louis Rich) mild	1 oz	59	3.8	0.7	298	0	4.5	18
(Norbest) 'Blue Label' 2-2.5 lb	1 oz	68	3.5	0.5	331	0	5.6	(mq)
(Norbest) 'Blue Label' 5-lb	1 oz	57	3.8	0.3	339	0	4.4	(mq)
(OHSE)	1 oz	70	3.0	2.0	300	0	6.0	(mq)
CHICKEN								
Breast								
(Healthy Choice) deli-thin, 97% fat-free	1 slice	10	2.0	<1.0	90	na	<1.0	5
(Healthy Choice) oven roasted, 97% fat-free	1 slice	30	6.0	1.0	300	na	<1.0	15
(Healthy Favorites) oven roasted	.4-oz slice	12	2.0	<1.0	110	na	<1.0	5
(Hillshire Farm) smoked 'Deli Select'	1 oz	31	6.0	<1.0	290	0	0.2	(mq)
(Longacre) 'Premium'	1 oz	45	4.0	1.0	280	0	3.0	20
(Louis Rich) hickory smoked	1 oz	30	5.1	0.6	356	0	0.8	14
(Louis Rich) oven roasted 'Deluxe'	1 oz	30	4.9	0.6	332	0	0.8	14
(Louis Rich) oven roasted 'Thin Sliced'	.4-oz slice	12	1.9	0.2	130	0	0.3	6
(Louis Rich) oven roasted, white meat	1-oz slice	35	4.9	0.1	301	0	1.7	16
(Mr. Turkey)	1 oz	32	4.8	0.6	242	0	1.1	9
(Oscar Mayer) oven roasted	1 oz	29	5.2	0.6	414	0	0.7	15
(Oscar Mayer) smoked	1 oz	25	5.3	0.2	397	0	0.4	15
(Oscar Mayer) 'Thin Sliced'	.4-oz slice	13	2.1	0.3	151	0	0.4	5
(Tyson) hickory smoked	1 slice	25	4.0	0.8	195	na	1.0	na
(Tyson) honey flavored	1 slice	25	4.0	0.8	na	na	1.0	na
(Tyson) mesquite, oven roasted	1 slice	25	4.0	0.8	na	na	1.0	na
(Tyson) oven roasted	1 slice	25	3.7	0.8	185	na	0.5	na
Roll								
(Longacre)	1 oz	60	4.0	1.0	210	0	5.0	25
(Pilgrim's Pride)	1-oz slice	35	5.2	0.4	260	0	1.2	15
(Tyson)	1 slice	26	3.2	1.4	153	na	0.5	na

Food Name	Serv. Size	Total Cal.	Prot. GMS	Carbs GMS	Sod. MGS	Fiber GMS	Fat GMS	Chol. MGS
CHICKEN HAM								
(Healthy Favorites) smoked, w/natural								
juices	.4-oz slice	13	2.2	0.2	116	0	0.4	7
(Pilgrim's Pride)	1-oz slice	35	4.0	0.8	430	0	1.8	18
CORNED BEEF LOAF, jellied	1 oz	43	6.5	0.0	270	0	1.7	13
DUTCH BRAND LOAF								
....	1-oz slice	68	3.8	1.6	354	0	5.1	13
(Eckrich)	1-oz slice	70	3.0	2.0	300	0	6.0	(mq)
(Eckrich) 'Lean Supreme'	1-oz slice	60	4.0	2.0	250	0	4.0	(mq)
(Eckrich) 'Smorgas Pac'	1-oz slice	70	3.0	2.0	300	0	6.0	(mq)
(Kahn's)	1 slice	80	3.0	1.0	280	0	7.0	(mq)
HAM								
(Boar's Head) boiled 'Deluxe'	1 oz	28	5.0	1.0	275	0	<1.0	15
(Boar's Head) deluxe 'Deli-trition' low								
cholesterol	1 oz	30	5.0	1.0	280	na	1.0	15
(Boar's Head) 'Lower Salt'	1 oz	28	5.0	<1.0	250	0	<1.0	15
(Healthy Deli)	1 oz	33	5.9	0.2	120	0	0.8	13
(Healthy Deli) 'Deluxe'	1 oz	31	4.7	1.1	245	0	0.9	12
(Healthy Deli) 'Lessalt'	1 oz	32	4.7	1.4	190	0	0.9	13
(Healthy Deli) 'Light AM'	1 oz	27	3.9	1.4	200	0	0.6	11
(Healthy Deli) 'Taverne'	1 oz	31	5.4	0.3	210	0	0.8	15
(Healthy Favorites) boiled	.4-oz slice	12	2.0	<1.0	115	na	<1.0	5
(Hormel)	1 oz	29	4.0	1.0	344	na	1.0	11
(JM)	1 oz	30	4.0	1.0	360	0	1.0	(mq)
(JM) 'Slice 'n Eat' 93% fat-free	2 oz	70	10.0	1.0	630	0	3.0	24
(JM) 'Slice 'n Eat' 95% fat-free, presliced	2 slices	60	9.0	1.0	620	0	2.0	30
(Jones Dairy Farm) 'Farm'	1 slice	50	8.8	tr	381	0	1.1	21
(Jones Dairy Farm) 'Four Family Ham' ...	1 oz	35	5.8	tr	298	0	1.2	14
(Kahn's)	1 slice	30	5.0	1.0	360	0	1.0	(mq)
(Kahn's) 'Low Salt'	1 slice	30	5.0	1.0	290	0	1.0	(mq)
(Light & Lean)	2 slices	50	9.0	0.0	(mq)	0	2.0	(mq)
(OHSE)	1 oz	30	5.0	1.0	260	0	1.0	(mq)
(Oscar Mayer) boiled	.75-oz slice	23	3.9	0.3	275	0	0.7	12
(Oscar Mayer) boiled 'Thin Sliced'	.4 oz	13	2.2	0.2	157	0	0.4	7
(Oscar Mayer) 'Breakfast Ham'	1.5-oz slice	47	7.2	1.2	582	0	1.5	21
(Oscar Mayer) 'Jubilee'	1 oz	43	5.3	0.1	365	0	2.4	15
(Oscar Mayer) 'Lower Salt'	.7 oz	23	3.6	0.6	174	0	0.7	10
(Swift) 'Premium Hostess'	1 oz	30	5.0	0.0	330	0	1.0	(mq)
(Swift) 'Premium Sugar Plum'	1 oz	30	5.0	1.0	280	0	1.0	(mq)
Baked								
(Healthy Deli) Virginia	1 oz	34	4.8	1.6	245	0	0.9	12
(Healthy Deli) Virginia 'Lessalt'	1 oz	32	4.7	1.4	19	0	0.9	13

Food Name	Serv. Size	Total Cal.	Prot. GMS	Carbs GMS	Sod. MGS	Fiber GMS	Fat GMS	Chol. MGS
(Louis Rich) 'Carving Board' cooked								
w/natural juices .... 22 grams		22	4.0	0.5	248	0	0.4	12
(Oscar Mayer) .... .75-oz slice		21	3.9	0.4	238	0	0.5	11
Barbecue *(Light & Lean)* .... 2 slices		50	8.0	0.0	(mq)	0	2.0	(mq)
Black Forest *(Healthy Deli)* .... 1 oz		32	5.9	0.4	220	0	0.6	16
Cajun *(Hillshire Farm)* 'Deli Select' ..... 1 oz		31	6.0	<1.0	350	(tr)	0.9	(mq)
Capocollo *(Hormel)* .... 1 oz		80	5.0	0.0	273	0	6.0	(mq)
Chopped								
(Eckrich) .... 1-oz slice		45	5.0	<1.0	350	0	2.0	(mq)
(Eckrich) 'Lean Supreme' .... 1-oz slice		35	10.0	<1.0	350	0	2.0	(mq)
(Hormel) 'Black Label' .... 1 oz		70	4.0	1.0	326	na	6.0	16
(Hormel) 'Perma-Fresh' .... 2 slices		88	11.0	0.0	685	0	5.0	(mq)
(JM) .... 1-oz slice		80	4.0	1.0	370	0	7.0	(mq)
(Kahn's) .... 1 slice		50	5.0	1.0	360	0	3.0	(mq)
(Light & Lean) .... 2 slices		70	8.0	0.0	(mq)	0	4.0	(mq)
(OHSE) .... 1 oz		65	4.0	1.0	260	0	5.0	(mq)
(Oscar Mayer) .... 1-oz slice		41	4.4	0.7	303	0	2.3	14
Glazed *(Light & Lean)* .... 2 slices		50	9.0	0.0	(mq)	0	2.0	(mq)
Honey								
(Boar's Head) 'Premium' low cholesterol .. 1 oz		35	5.0	2.0	310	na	1.0	15
(Carl Buddig) 'Lean' smoked, chopped ... 1 oz		50	5.0	1.0	na	na	3.0	na
(Healthy Choice) 'Deli-Thin' .... 1 slice		10	2.0	<1.0	90	na	<1.0	5
(Healthy Deli) 'Honey Valley' .... 1 oz		31	4.8	1.2	26	0	0.8	10
(Healthy Favorites) .... 1 slice		14	2.0	<1.0	115	na	<1.0	5
(Healthy Favorites) 'Breakfast' water added 1 oz		30	4.7	0.7	346	0	0.9	14
(Hillshire Farm) 'Deli Select' .... 1 oz		31	6.0	<1.0	270	0	0.9	(mq)
(Louis Rich) 'Carving Board'								
w/natural juices .... 2.1 oz		68	10.9	1.8	761	0	1.9	33
(Oscar Mayer) .... .75-oz slice		23	3.8	0.5	268	0	0.6	12
(Oscar Mayer) 'Thin Sliced' .... .4-oz slice		13	2.2	0.3	153	0	0.4	7
Jalapeño *(Healthy Deli)* .... 1 oz		25	3.7	0.8	260	(tr)	0.6	11
Peppered								
(Light & Lean) black pepper .... 2 slices		50	9.0	0.0	(mq)	(tr)	2.0	(mq)
(Light & Lean) red pepper .... 2 slices		50	9.0	0.0	(mq)	(tr)	2.0	(mq)
(Oscar Mayer) cracked black pepper .75-oz slice		22	3.8	0.2	284	(tr)	0.8	11
Prosciutto *(Hormel)* .... 1 oz		90	7.0	0.0	502	0	7.0	(mq)
Smoked								
(Carl Buddig) 'Lean' chopped .... 1 oz		50	5.0	1.0	na	na	3.0	na
(Eckrich) 'Slender Sliced' .... 1 oz		40	5.0	1.0	360	0	2.0	(mq)
(Healthy Favorites) .... .4-oz slice		14	2.0	<1.0	115	na	<1.0	5
(Hillshire Farm) 'Deli Select' .... 1 oz		31	6.0	<1.0	300	0	0.9	(mq)
(JM) golden .... 2 oz		80	8.0	1.0	630	0	5.0	(mq)
(JM) golden, water added .... 2 oz		70	8.0	4.0	810	0	2.0	23

Food Name	Serv. Size	Total Cal.	Prot. GMS	Carbs GMS	Sod. MGS	Fiber GMS	Fat GMS	Chol. MGS
(Light & Lean)	2 slices	50	9.0	0.0	(mq)	0	2.0	(mq)
(Louis Rich) 'Carving Board' w/natural juices	10 grams	11	1.8	0.0	124	0	0.4	5
(OHSE) '95% Fat-Free'	1 oz	30	5.0	1.0	310	0	1.0	(mq)
(Oscar Mayer)	.75-oz slice	22	3.8	0.1	266	0	0.7	12
HAM AND CHEESE LOAF								
(Eckrich)	1-oz slice	50	4.0	1.0	300	0	4.0	(mq)
(Hormel) '8 lb' canned	3 oz	260	13.0	1.0	1135	0	22.0	(mq)
(Hormel) 'Perma-Fresh'	2 slices	110	11.0	0.0	668	0	7.0	(mq)
(Kahn's)	1 slice	70	4.0	1.0	310	0	6.0	(mq)
(Light & Lean)	2 slices	90	8.0	0.0	(mq)	0	6.0	(mq)
(OHSE)	1 oz	65	4.0	2.0	190	0	5.0	(mq)
(Oscar Mayer)	1-oz slice	66	4.2	1.0	358	0	5.0	19
HEAD CHEESE (Oscar Mayer)	1-oz slice	55	4.5	0.1	347	0	4.0	25
HONEY LOAF								
(Eckrich)	1-oz slice	35	4.0	2.0	280	0	1.0	(mq)
(Eckrich) 'Smorgas Pac'	1-oz slice	35	4.0	2.0	280	0	1.0	(mq)
(Hormel) 'Perma-Fresh'	2 slices	90	1.0	0.0	584	0	5.0	(mq)
(Kahn's)	1 slice	40	4.0	1.0	320	0	2.0	(mq)
(Oscar Mayer)	1-oz slice	34	5.2	1.0	378	0	1.0	16
IOWA BRAND LOAF (Hormel) 'Perma-Fresh'	2 slices	90	10.0	0.0	607	0	6.0	(mq)
JALAPEÑO LOAF (Kahn's)	1 slice	70	3.0	2.0	340	na	6.0	(mq)
LIVER CHEESE								
(JM)	1-oz slice	70	4.0	1.0	(mq)	0	6.0	(mq)
(Oscar Mayer)	1.34-oz slice	116	5.8	0.5	418	0	10.0	80
LIVER LOAF								
(Hormel) 'Perma-Fresh'	2 slices	160	9.0	1.0	704	0	13.0	(mq)
(Kahn's)	1 slice	170	6.0	3.0	370	0	15.0	(mq)
LIVERWURST/liver sausage								
(Hickory Farms)	1 oz	97	4.0	1.0	249	0	9.0	74
(Jones Dairy Farm) 'Farm Club'	1 oz	80	4.5	tr	254	0	6.3	43
(Jones Dairy Farm) 'Farm Slices'	1 slice	75	3.5	tr	186	0	6.6	43
LOAF								
(Hormel) spiced, canned	3 oz	280	11.0	2.0	1110	0	26.0	(mq)
(JM) 'P&B'	1-oz slice	70	3.0	2.0	330	0	5.0	(mq)
(Kahn's) 'P&B'	1 slice	40	5.0	1.0	270	0	2.0	(mq)
(OHSE)	1 oz	75	3.0	1.0	320	0	6.0	(mq)
MACARONI AND CHEESE LOAF								
(Eckrich)	1-oz slice	75	3.0	3.0	320	(mq)	6.0	(mq)
(OHSE)	1 oz	60	4.0	4.0	310	(mq)	3.0	(mq)
OLD-FASHIONED LOAF (Oscar Mayer)	1-oz slice	62	4.0	2.4	337	(tr)	4.0	16

Food Name	Serv. Size	Total Cal.	Prot. GMS	Carbs GMS	Sod. MGS	Fiber GMS	Fat GMS	Chol. MGS
OLIVE LOAF								
(Eckrich)	1-oz slice	80	3.0	2.0	320	(tr)	6.0	(mq)
(Hormel) 'Perma-Fresh'	2 slices	110	7.0	5.0	810	(tr)	7.0	(mq)
(Oscar Mayer)	1-oz slice	63	2.9	3.2	392	(tr)	4.3	8
PASTRAMI. See also TURKEY PASTRAMI.								
(Boar's Head) 'Round'	1 oz	40	6.0	<1.0	270	0	1.5	16
(Carl Buddig) 'Lean' smoked, chopped, sliced	1 oz	40	5.0	1.0	na	na	2.0	na
(Healthy Deli) 'Deli Round'	1 oz	34	5.3	0.8	195	0	1.1	14
(Hillshire Farm) 'Deli Select'	1 oz	31	6.0	<1.0	290	0	0.4	(mq)
(Oscar Mayer)	.6-oz slice	16	3.4	0.1	217	0	0.3	7
PEPPERED BEEF								
(Carl Buddig) 'Lean' smoked, chopped, sliced	1 oz	40	5.0	1.0	na	na	2.0	na
(Eckrich)	1-oz slice	35	5.0	2.0	340	(tr)	1.0	(mq)
(Kahn's)	1 slice	40	5.0	1.0	340	(tr)	2.0	(mq)
(Oscar Mayer)	1-oz slice	39	5.1	1.2	367	(tr)	1.5	14
PICKLE LOAF								
(Eckrich)	1-oz slice	80	3.0	2.0	270	(tr)	6.0	(mq)
(Eckrich) 'Smorgas-Pac'	1-oz slice	80	3.0	2.0	270	(tr)	6.0	(mq)
(Hormel) 'Perma-Fresh'	2 slices	102	8.0	3.0	752	(tr)	7.0	(mq)
(Kahn's)	1 slice	80	3.0	2.0	280	(tr)	7.0	(mq)
(Kahn's) 'Family-Pack'	1 slice	70	3.0	2.0	220	(tr)	6.0	(mq)
(Light & Lean)	2 slices	100	8.0	3.0	(mq)	(tr)	6.0	(mq)
(OHSE)	1 oz	60	3.0	2.0	330	(tr)	4.0	(mq)
PICKLE-PIMIENTO LOAF (Oscar Mayer)	1-oz slice	66	3.1	4.1	370	(mq)	4.1	13
PORK LOAF (Eckrich) 'Slender Sliced'	1 oz	45	5.0	1.0	320	0	2.0	(mq)
ROAST BEEF								
(Healthy Deli)	1 oz	30	6.4	0.2	130	0	0.4	13
(Healthy Deli) Italian	1 oz	31	6.2	0.1	140	0	0.6	16
(Hillshire Farm) 'Deli Select' oven roasted, cured, w/o added ingredients	1 oz	31	6.0	<1.0	270	0	0.5	(mq)
(Oscar Mayer) 'Thin Sliced'	.4-oz slice	14	2.4	0.2	55	0	0.4	5
SALAMI. See also TURKEY SALAMI.								
Beef								
(Boar's Head)	1 oz	60	5.0	<1.0	288	0	4.0	20
(Hebrew National) 'Original Deli-Style'	1 oz	80	7.0	<1.0	230	0	7.0	15
(Hormel) 'Party'	1 oz	90	5.0	0.0	399	0	8.0	(mq)
(Hormel) 'Perma-Fresh'	2 slices	50	3.0	0.0	219	0	5.0	(mq)
(Kahn's)	1 slice	70	3.0	1.0	250	0	6.0	(mq)
(Kahn's) 'Family-Pack'	1 slice	60	2.0	1.0	190	0	5.0	(mq)
(Oscar Mayer) 'Machiaeh Brand'	.8-oz slice	60	3.0	0.0	265	0	5.0	15
Beer								
(Eckrich)	1-oz slice	70	4.0	1.0	330	0	6.0	(mq)

Food Name	Serv. Size	Total Cal.	Prot. GMS	Carbs GMS	Sod. MGS	Fiber GMS	Fat GMS	Chol. MGS
(Oscar Mayer) 'Salami for Beer'	.8-oz slice	50	3.2	0.4	286	0	4.0	15
(Oscar Mayer) 'Salami for Beer' beef	.8-oz slice	63	2.9	0.4	280	0	5.6	16
Cooked								
(Kahn's)	1 slice	60	4.0	1.0	300	0	4.0	(mq)
(OHSE)	1 oz	65	4.0	1.0	330	0	5.0	(mq)
Cotto								
(Eckrich)	1-oz slice	70	4.0	1.0	380	0	6.0	(mq)
(Eckrich) beef	1.3 oz	100	5.0	2.0	460	0	8.0	(mq)
(Hormel) 'Club'	1 oz	100	5.0	0.0	385	0	5.0	(mq)
(Hormel) 'Perma-Fresh'	2 slices	105	9.0	1.0	750	0	7.0	(mq)
(JM)	1-oz slice	80	4.0	2.0	270	0	6.0	(mq)
(Kahn's) 'Family Pack'	1 slice	45	3.0	1.0	230	0	3.0	(mq)
(Light & Lean)	2 slices	80	6.0	0.0	(mq)	0	6.0	(mq)
(Oscar Mayer) beef	.8-oz slice	45	3.3	0.4	296	0	3.4	19
(Oscar Mayer) beef	.5-oz slice	29	2.1	0.3	193	0	2.2	12
Dry or hard								
(Hickory Farms)	1 oz	120	6.0	0.0	535	0	10.0	30
(Hormel)	1 oz	110	7.0	0.0	468	0	10.0	(mq)
(Hormel) 'Homeland'	1 oz	117	6.0	2.0	448	na	10.0	29
(Hormel) 'National Brand'	1 oz	120	6.0	2.0	463	0	11.0	(mq)
(Hormel) 'Perma-Fresh'	2 slices	80	4.0	0.0	339	0	7.0	(mq)
(Hormel) 'Sliced'	1 oz	110	6.0	0.0	483	0	10.0	(mq)
(JM)	1-oz slice	110	6.0	1.0	580	0	9.0	(mq)
(Oscar Mayer)	.8-oz slice	52	3.1	0.4	287	0	4.2	19
(Oscar Mayer) 'Hard'	.3-oz slice	33	2.0	0.1	169	0	2.8	8
Genoa								
(Hickory Farms)	1 oz	110	6.0	0.0	540	0	10.0	20
(Hormel)	1 oz	110	6.0	0.0	456	0	10.0	(mq)
(Hormel) 'DiLusso'	1 oz	100	6.0	0.0	443	0	8.0	(mq)
(Hormel) 'Gran Valore'	1 oz	110	6.0	0.0	453	0	10.0	(mq)
(Hormel) 'San Remo Brand'	1 oz	118	7.0	0.0	541	0	10.0	(mq)
(JM)	1-oz slice	100	6.0	1.0	540	0	8.0	(mq)
(Oscar Mayer)	.3-oz slice	34	1.9	0.1	162	0	2.8	9
Piccolo *(Hormel)* 'Stick'	1 oz	120	6.0	0.0	512	0	11.0	(mq)
SOUSE LOAF *(Kahn's)*	1 slice	90	4.0	1.0	190	0	7.0	(mq)
SPICE LOAF								
(Hormel) canned	3 oz	280	11.0	2.0	1110	0	26.0	(mq)
(Hormel) 'Perma-Fresh'	2 slices	118	9.0	1.0	702	0	9.0	(mq)
(JM)	1-oz slice	70	4.0	1.0	370	0	6.0	(mq)
(Kahn's) 'Family Pack'	1 slice	70	3.0	1.0	180	0	6.0	(mq)
(Kahn's) 'Family Pack' beef	1 slice	60	2.0	1.0	200	0	5.0	(mq)
(Kahn's) 'Luncheon Loaf'	1 slice	80	3.0	1.0	240	0	7.0	(mq)

Food Name	Serv. Size	Total Cal.	Prot. GMS	Carbs GMS	Sod. MGS	Fiber GMS	Fat GMS	Chol. MGS
TURKEY. See also TURKEY LOAF/ROLL.								
(Boar's Head) 'Premium' skin on, low cholesterol	1 oz	35	6.0	1.0	200	na	1.0	20
(Butterball) 'Cold Cuts'	1 oz	30	5.0	1.0	230	0	1.0	(mq)
(Butterball) 'Deli No Salt Added'	1 oz	45	7.0	0.0	15	0	2.0	(mq)
(Healthy Choice) 97% fat-free	1 slice	30	6.0	<1.0	240	na	1.0	10
(Healthy Deli) 'Gourmet'	1 oz	28	4.9	0.5	170	0	0.6	9
(Healthy Deli) 'Lessalt'	1 oz	25	4.5	0.4	140	0	0.5	9
(Hormel) 'Perma-Fresh'	2 slices	60	9.0	0.0	484	0	2.0	(mq)
(Light & Lean)	2 slices	60	8.0	0.0	(mq)	0	2.0	(mq)
(Longacre) 'Catering'	1 oz	35	6.0	<1.0	280	0	1.0	15
(Norbest) white meat, diced	1 oz	31	4.4	1.0	318	0	0.9	(mq)
(Tyson)	1 slice	20	4.0	0.3	136	na	0.4	na
Honey roasted (Healthy Deli)	1 oz	28	4.9	0.5	170	0	0.5	9
Honey roasted and smoked								
(Healthy Choice)	1-oz slice	35	6.0	1.0	230	na	1.0	15
(Healthy Choice) deli thin	1 slice	10	2.0	<1.0	70	na	<1.0	5
Oven roasted								
(Healthy Choice) deli thin	1 slice	10	2.0	<1.0	85	na	<1.0	5
(Healthy Choice) 97% fat-free	1-oz slice	30	6.0	<1.0	290	na	1.0	10
(Healthy Deli)	1 oz	26	4.7	0.4	180	0	0.2	8
(Healthy Favorites)	.4-oz slice	12	2.0	<1.0	100	na	<1.0	5
(Hillshire Farm) 'Deli Select'	1 oz	31	6.0	<1.0	340	0	0.2	(mq)
(Longacre)	1 oz	30	5.0	1.0	280	0	1.0	10
(Louis Rich)	1 oz	31	4.8	1.1	323	0	0.8	11
(Louis Rich) 'Thin Sliced'	.4-oz slice	12	1.9	0.4	127	0	0.3	4
(Oscar Mayer)	.75-oz slice	23	4.2	0.5	290	0	0.5	9
(Oscar Mayer) 'Thin Sliced'	.4-oz slice	12	2.2	0.3	151	0	0.2	5
Smoked								
(Butterball) 'Cold Cuts'	1 oz	35	5.0	0.0	190	0	1.0	(mq)
(Butterball) 'Turkey Variety Pak'	.75 oz	25	4.0	1.0	160	0	1.0	(mq)
(Carl Buttig) 'Lean' chopped, sliced	1 oz	50	5.0	1.0	na	na	3.0	na
(Healthy Choice) deli thin	1 slice	10	2.0	<1.0	70	na	<1.0	5
(Healthy Deli) '3 lb'	1 oz	29	4.8	0.5	180	0	0.5	8
(Healthy Favorites)	1 slice	12	2.0	<1.0	80	na	<1.0	5
(Hillshire Farm) 'Deli Select'	1 oz	31	6.0	<1.0	290	0	0.2	(mq)
(Longacre)	1 oz	26	5.0	1.0	260	0	<1.0	10
(Louis Rich)	.74-oz slice	21	4.5	0.2	211	0	0.3	9
(Louis Rich) 'Thin Sliced'	.4-oz slice	11	2.3	0.1	111	0	0.1	5
(Mr. Turkey)	1 oz	31	5.9	0.3	332	0	0.7	10
(Oscar Mayer)	.75-oz slice	20	4.3	0.2	300	0	0.2	9
TURKEY HAM								
(Butterball) 'Cold Cuts'	1 oz	35	5.0	1.0	390	0	1.0	(mq)

Food Name	Serv. Size	Total Cal.	Prot. GMS	Carbs GMS	Sod. MGS	Fiber GMS	Fat GMS	Chol. MGS
(Butterball) 'Deli Thin'	1 oz	35	5.0	1.0	390	0	1.0	(mq)
(Butterball) 'Slice 'n Serve'	1 oz	35	5.0	1.0	340	0	2.0	(mq)
(Longacre)	1 oz	33	6.0	0.0	310	0	1.0	20
(Longacre) lean lite 'Deli'	1 oz	37	6.0	0.0	150	0	2.0	25
(Louis Rich) cured	1 oz	25	4.2	0.6	217	0	0.7	14
Chopped								
(Louis Rich)	1 oz	46	5.2	0.2	289	0	2.8	19
(Louis Rich) 92% fat-free, water added	1 oz	45	5.0	<1.0	285	na	2.0	25
(Mr. Turkey)	1 oz	37	5.4	0.3	301	0	1.6	17
Chunk (Longacre)	1 oz	37	5.0	0.0	360	0	2.0	25
Honey cured								
(Butterball) 'Cold Cuts'	1 oz	35	5.0	1.0	380	0	1.0	(mq)
(Butterball) 'Cold Cuts' chopped	1 oz	35	5.0	2.0	290	0	1.0	(mq)
(Butterball) 'Slice 'n Serve'	1 oz	40	5.0	1.0	370	0	2.0	(mq)
(Louis Rich) 96% fat-free	1 oz	25	4.0	<1.0	215	na	<1.0	15
(Mr. Turkey)	1 oz	32	5.4	0.3	286	0	1.0	18
(Mr. Turkey) breakfast	1 oz	33	5.0	0.4	306	0	1.3	16
(Mr. Turkey) buffet style	1 oz	32	4.7	0.4	340	0	1.3	17
(Mr. Turkey) 'Chub'	1 oz	32	4.7	0.4	340	0	1.3	17
Smoked								
(Louis Rich) 'Deli Thin' 96% fat-free	1 slice	15	2.0	<1.0	110	na	<1.0	5
(Louis Rich) 94% fat-free, water added	1 oz	35	5.0	<1.0	300	na	2.0	20
(Louis Rich) 'Round'	1 oz	34	5.4	0.4	300	0	1.2	19
(Louis Rich) 'Round' 95% fat-free, water added	1-oz slice	30	5.0	<1.0	325	na	1.0	20
(Louis Rich) 'Square'	.75-oz slice	24	4.1	0.3	213	0	0.7	14
(Louis Rich) 'Square' 96% fat free	1-oz slice	25	4.0	<1.0	215	na	<1.0	15
(Louis Rich) 'Thin Sliced'	.4-oz slice	12	2.2	0.1	111	0	0.4	7
(Louis Rich) 'Water Added'	1 oz	33	4.9	0.4	294	0	1.4	19
(Norbest) roll	1 oz	31	4.6	0.5	346	0	1.1	(mq)
(Norbest) thigh meat, Canadian style	1 oz	35	5.1	0.3	331	0	1.4	(mq)
(Norbest) thigh meat 'Gold Label'	1 oz	27	6.1	0.3	297	0	0.7	(mq)
(Norbest) thigh meat 'Tavern' 5-6 lb, whole	1 oz	27	5.4	0.3	311	0	0.8	(mq)
(Norbest) thigh meat 'Tavern' 2-2.5 lb, half	1 oz	29	4.7	0.6	312	0	0.8	(mq)
(OHSE)	1 oz	30	4.0	2.0	370	0	1.0	(mq)
TURKEY LOAF/ROLL								
(Louis Rich)	1 oz	45	4.6	0.4	270	0	2.8	16
(Louis Rich) 89% fat free	1 oz	45	5.0	<1.0	270	na	3.0	15
(Mr. Turkey) spiced	1 oz	51	4.2	0.5	292	0	3.6	11
TURKEY PASTRAMI								
(Butterball) 'Cold Cuts'	1 oz	30	5.0	1.0	290	0	1.0	(mq)
(Butterball) 'Slice 'n Serve'	1 oz	35	5.0	1.0	320	0	1.0	(mq)
(Longacre)	1 oz	32	5.0	0.0	260	0	1.0	20

Food Name	Serv. Size	Total Cal.	Prot. GMS	Carbs GMS	Sod. MGS	Fiber GMS	Fat GMS	Chol. MGS
(Louis Rich) 'Deli Thin' 96% fat-free	1 oz	10	2.0	<1.0	125	na	<1.0	5
(Louis Rich) 'Round'	1 oz	32	5.2	0.3	288	0	1.1	18
(Louis Rich) 'Round' 96% fat-free	1 oz	35	5.0	<1.0	290	na	1.0	20
(Louis Rich) 'Square'	1 oz	24	4.2	0.1	262	0	0.7	14
(Louis Rich) 'Square' 96% fat-free	1 oz	25	4.0	<1.0	260	na	<1.0	15
(Louis Rich) Thin Sliced	1 oz	11	2.0	0.1	125	0	0.4	7
(Mr. Turkey)	1 oz	28	4.8	0.1	383	0	0.9	17
(Norbest) '5-6 lb Slab'	1 oz	29	5.1	0.5	305	0	0.6	(mq)
(Norbest) '3 lb'	1 oz	29	4.8	0.3	302	0	0.8	(mq)
TURKEY SALAMI								
(Butterball) 'Cold Cuts'	1 oz	50	4.0	1.0	350	0	4.0	(mq)
(Butterball) 'Deli/Slice 'n Serve'	1 oz	50	4.0	1.0	350	0	4.0	(mq)
(Butterball) 'Turkey Variety Pak'	.75 oz	40	3.0	1.0	260	0	3.0	(mq)
(Longacre)	1 oz	52	4.4	0.2	290	0	4.0	20
(Louis Rich)	1 oz	54	4.4	0.2	263	0	4.0	20
(Louis Rich) cotto	1 oz	53	4.4	0.3	271	0	3.8	21
(Louis Rich) cotto, 85% fat-free	1-oz slice	55	4.0	<1.0	275	na	4.0	25
(Louis Rich) 85% fat-free	1-oz slice	55	4.0	<1.0	265	na	4.0	20
(Mr. Turkey) cotto	1 oz	45	4.3	0.4	369	0	2.9	16
(Norbest) 'Blue Label' 5 lb	1 oz	46	4.3	0.5	270	0	2.9	(mq)
(Norbest) 'Blue Label' 2-2.5 lb	1 oz	45	4.2	0.9	314	0	2.6	(mq)
(OHSE)	1 oz	50	4.0	1.0	260	0	3.0	(mq)
LUNCHEON MEAT, ALTERNATIVE								
(Worthington) canned 'Numete' 1/2-inch slice	2.4 oz	160	8.0	6.0	570	(mq)	11.0	0
(Worthington) canned 'Protose' 1/2-inch slice	2.7 oz	180	17.0	9.0	470	(mq)	8.0	0
BOLOGNA TYPE								
(Worthington) frozen 'Bolono' approx .65-oz slices	2 slices	60	7.0	2.0	390	(mq)	2.0	0
SALAMI TYPE								
(Worthington) frozen, roll, approx 1.5-oz slices	2 slices	90	8.0	3.0	760	(mq)	5.0	0
(Worthington) frozen, sliced, approx 1.3-oz slices	2 slices	80	7.0	3.0	675	(mq)	4.0	0
LUNCHEON MEAT, CANNED. See also POTTED MEAT SPREAD; SANDWICH SPREAD.								
(Armour) 'Treet'	2 oz	200	6.0	3.0	840	na	17.0	na
(Armour) 'Treet' low salt	2 oz	190	6.0	3.0	610	na	16.0	na
(Spam)	1 oz	86	4.0	<2.0	376	na	8.0	20
(Spam) less salt	2 oz	176	8.0	1.0	550	na	15.0	38
(Spam) lite	2 oz	140	8.0	1.0	560	na	12.0	43
(Spam) smoke flavored	2 oz	170	8.0	0.0	774	0	15.0	(mq)
(Spam) w/cheese chunks	2 oz	170	8.0	0.0	811	0	16.0	(mq)

Food Name	Serv. Size	Total Cal.	Prot. GMS	Carbs GMS	Sod. MGS	Fiber GMS	Fat GMS	Chol. MGS
LUNCHEON MEAT COMBINATIONS, PACKAGED								
(Eckrich) 'Lunch Makers'								
ham/Swiss cheese/crackers	1 pc each	40	2.0	2.0	170	na	2.0	5
turkey/cheddar cheese/crackers	1 pc each	40	2.0	2.0	160	na	2.0	5
(Hillshire Farms) 'Lunch 'n Munch'								
bologna/American cheese/crackers/								
Snickers	4.25 oz	490	15.0	31.0	1110	na	34.0	na
bologna/American cheese/crackers/								
Snickers/6-oz drink	4.25 oz	590	15.0	55.0	1130	na	34.0	na
chicken/Monterey jack cheese/crackers/								
Snickers	4.25 oz	400	19.0	31.0	1080	na	23.0	na
ham/cheddar cheese/crackers/Snickers	4.25 oz	400	17.0	32.0	1010	na	23.0	na
ham/cheddar cheese/crackers/								
Snickers/6-oz drink	4.25 oz	500	17.0	56.0	1030	na	23.0	na
ham/Swiss cheese/crackers/Oreo	4.1 oz	370	16.0	30.0	1160	na	21.0	na
turkey/cheddar cheese/crackers/brownie	4.5 oz	400	17.0	34.0	1240	na	22.0	na
(Louis Rich) 'Lunch Breaks'								
turkey/cheddar cheese	1 pkg	410	22.0	23.0	1715	na	26.0	70
turkey/Monterey jack cheese	1 pkg	400	21.0	27.0	1665	na	25.0	75
turkey ham/Swiss cheese	1 pkg	380	24.0	25.0	1875	na	22.0	75
turkey salami/cheddar cheese	1 pkg	430	22.0	25.0	1595	na	29.0	85
(Oscar Mayer) 'Lunchables'								
bologna/American cheese/crackers	4.5 oz	480	18.0	20.0	1520	na	38.0	80
chicken/Monterey jack cheese/crackers/								
pudding	6.2 oz	380	19.0	32.0	1200	na	21.0	45
ham/American cheese/crackers/pudding	6.2 oz	410	19.0	33.0	1380	na	23.0	45
ham/cheddar cheese/crackers	4.5 oz	370	21.0	18.0	1680	na	25.0	70
ham/Swiss cheese/crackers	4.5 oz	340	22.0	18.0	1660	na	21.0	65
ham/Swiss cheese/crackers/cookie	4.2 oz	380	18.0	29.0	1370	na	23.0	50
turkey/cheddar cheese/crackers	4.5 oz	360	22.0	19.0	1600	na	22.0	70
turkey/cheddar cheese/crackers/trail mix	5 oz	460	20.0	41.0	1230	na	26.0	40
turkey/ham, deluxe variety pak	5.1 oz	370	23.0	23.0	1760	na	20.0	60
turkey/Monterey jack cheese/wheat crackers	4.5 oz	360	21.0	18.0	1600	na	22.0	75
LUPIN, mature seeds								
boiled	4 oz	135	17.7	11.2	5	>.8 c	3.3	0
boiled	1/2 cup	99	12.9	8.2	3	2.3	2.4	0
raw	1/2 cup	334	32.5	36.3	14	>12.4 c	8.8	0
raw	1 oz	105	10.3	11.4	4	>3.9 c	2.8	0
LYCHEE. See LITCHI.								

M

Food Name	Serv. Size	Total Cal.	Prot. GMS	Carbs GMS	Sod. MGS	Fiber GMS	Fat GMS	Chol. MGS
MACADAMIA NUT/bushnut								
in shell	1 lb	987	11.7	19.3	6	>7.4 c	103.7	0
shelled	1 cup	941	11.1	18.4	7	12.5	98.8	0
shelled	1 oz	199	2.4	3.9	1	2.6	20.9	0
shelled, oil roasted, chopped	1 cup	790	8.0	14.2	8	>1.9 c	84.2	0
shelled, oil roasted, kernels, 10-12	1 oz	204	2.1	3.7	2	>.5 c	21.7	0
shelled, oil roasted, whole or halves	1 cup	962	9.7	17.3	9	>2.3 c	102.5	0
shelled, w/salt *(Maunu Loa)*	1 oz	210	2.0	4.0	75	(mq)	21.0	0
MACADAMIA NUT BUTTER, roasted								
(Maranatha Natural)	2 tbsp	200	2.0	6.0	5	na	19.0	na
MACARONI. See PASTA.								
MACARONI ENTRÉE, CANNED								
(Chef Boyardee) shells	7.5 oz	150	6.0	31.0	930	na	1.0	na
(Heinz)	7.5 oz	190	5.0	26.0	1105	(mq)	8.0	(mq)
W/BEEF, IN TOMATO SAUCE								
(Heinz)	7.5 oz	200	8.0	23.0	850	(mq)	8.0	(mq)
(Pathmark) 'No Frills'	7.5 oz	200	9.0	22.0	880	(mq)	8.0	(mq)
W/CHEESE								
(Chef Boyardee)	7.5 oz	170	7.0	33.0	970	2.0	2.0	25
(Franco-American)	7 3/8 oz	170	6.0	24.0	870	(mq)	6.0	(mq)
Shells w/cheddar *(Lipton)* 'Hearty Ones'	11 oz	367	15.4	60.0	1406	(mq)	7.4	14
MACARONI ENTRÉE, FROZEN								
W/BEEF								
(Swanson)	12 oz	370	12.0	48.0	930	(mq)	15.0	(mq)
(Weight Watchers)	9 oz	220	14.0	31.0	510	na	4.0	10
In tomato sauce *(Lean Cuisine)*	10 oz	250	14.0	35.0	540	na	6.0	25
W/tomatoes *(Stouffer's)*	11.5-oz pkg	340	21.0	38.0	1440	na	12.0	na
W/CHEESE								
(Banquet)	10 oz	420	14.0	46.0	450	(mq)	20.0	30
(Banquet) 'Casserole'	8 oz	350	11.0	36.0	930	(mq)	17.0	(mq)
(Banquet) 'Family Entrees'	8 oz	290	12.0	32.0	(mq)	(mq)	13.0	(mq)
(Budget Gourmet) 'Side Dish'	5.3 oz	210	9.0	23.0	370	(mq)	8.0	25
(Freezer Queen) 'Family Side Dish'	4 oz	110	3.0	19.0	420	(mq)	2.0	(mq)
(Green Giant)	5.7 oz	220	10.0	27.0	480	1.5	8.0	25
(Green Giant) 'One Serving'	5.7 oz	230	9.0	28.0	590	(mq)	9.0	25
(Healthy Choice)	9 oz	280	12.0	45.0	520	na	6.0	20
(Healthy Choice)	8.5 oz	260	11.0	42.0	490	na	5.0	15
(Kid Cuisine) 'Mega Meal'	12.45 oz	470	14.0	75.0	1270	na	13.0	na
(Lean Cuisine)	9 oz	290	15.0	37.0	550	na	9.0	30
(Myers)	3.5 oz	168	7.0	16.0	516	(mq)	9.0	(mq)
(Stouffer's) 76-oz pkg	9.5 oz	440	18.0	39.0	1150	na	24.0	na

Food Name	Serv. Size	Total Cal.	Prot. GMS	Carbs GMS	Sod. MGS	Fiber GMS	Fat GMS	Chol. MGS
(Stouffer's) 12-oz pkg	6 oz	250	11.0	23.0	640	na	13.0	na
(Swanson)	12.25 oz	370	13.0	43.0	1070	(mq)	15.0	(mq)
(Swanson) 'Homestyle Recipe'	10 oz	390	17.0	37.0	1150	(mq)	19.0	(mq)
Casserole *(Morton)*	6.5 oz	290	8.0	30.0	760	na	14.0	na
Organic *(Amy's Kitchen)*	9 oz	452	22.0	58.0	434	na	18.0	na
Pot pie *(Swanson)*	7 oz	200	7.0	24.0	740	(mq)	8.0	(mq)
W/broccoli *(Lean Cuisine)*								
'Lunch Express'	9.75 oz	240	12.0	32.0	560	na	7.0	25
W/cheddar and parmesan cheese								
(Budget Gourmet) 'Light & Healthy'	10.5 oz	330	19.0	49.0	760	na	8.0	30
W/mini franks *(Kid Cuisine)*	9 oz	380	9.0	55.0	1000	(mq)	14.0	40
W/soy cheese, organic *(Amy's Kitchen)*	9 oz	380	17.0	42.0	500	na	14.0	0
W/three cheeses *(Weight Watchers)*	9 oz	280	15.0	43.0	550	na	6.0	20
MACARONI ENTRÉE, MICROWAVE								
W/BEEF								
(Chef Boyardee) 'Beefaroni'	7.5 oz	220	7.0	31.0	1145	2.0	7.0	18
(Chef Boyardee) elbows in sauce	7.5 oz	210	8.0	29.0	1000	(mq)	7.0	15
(Kid's Kitchen) microwave cup	7.5 oz	200	11.0	25.0	780	na	6.0	25
(Nalley's)	7.5 oz	180	9.0	29.0	900	(mq)	3.0	(mq)
W/CHEESE								
(Chef Boyardee)	7.5 oz	180	7.0	27.0	970	1.0	5.0	20
(Hormel) micro cup	7.5 oz	189	7.0	26.0	874	(mq)	6.0	17
(Kid's Kitchen) microwave cup	7.5 oz	260	12.0	28.0	650	na	11.0	45
(Libby's) 'Diner' microwave cup	7.5 oz	360	14.0	27.0	1020	2.0	22.0	35
(Lunch Bucket) microwave cup	7.5 oz	210	9.0	24.0	990	na	9.0	na
MACARONI ENTRÉE, PACKAGED								
(Ultra Slim Fast) w/cheese sauce,								
prepared	1 cup	230	9.0	46.0	700	4.0	3.0	na
MACARONI ENTRÉE MIX								
(Kraft) 'Dinner' spirals, prepared	3/4 cup	340	9.0	36.0	600	(mq)	18.0	10
MEXICAN STYLE								
(Velveeta) 'Touch of Mexico' shells,								
prepared	1/2 cup	210	10.0	27.0	630	(mq)	8.0	20
W/CHEDDAR								
(Fantastic Foods) 'Traditional' prepared	1/2 cup	112	5.0	19.0	205	(mq)	2.0	(mq)
(Golden Grain) dry mix	1.81 oz	190	7.4	35.6	466	1.4	2.1	4
(Golden Grain) prepared	1 serving	310	8.0	36.0	620	(mq)	15.0	(mq)
W/CHEESE								
(Kraft) 'Deluxe Dinner' prepared	3/4 cup	260	11.0	36.0	590	(mq)	8.0	20
(Kraft) 'Dinner' prepared	3/4 cup	290	9.0	34.0	530	(mq)	13.0	5
(Kraft) 'Dinomac Dinner' prepared	3/4 cup	310	9.0	36.0	560	(mq)	14.0	10
(Kraft) 'Family Size Dinner' prepared	3/4 cup	290	9.0	34.0	490	(mq)	13.0	5
(Kraft) 'Teddy Bears Dinner' prepared	3/4 cup	310	9.0	36.0	560	(mq)	14.0	10

Food Name	Serv. Size	Total Cal.	Prot. GMS	Carbs GMS	Sod. MGS	Fiber GMS	Fat GMS	Chol. MGS
(Kraft) 'Wild Wheels Dinner' prepared	3/4 cup	310	9.0	36.0	560	(mq)	14.0	10
(Velveeta) 'Bits of Bacon' shells, w/bacon, prepared	1/2 cup	240	11.0	27.0	690	(mq)	10.0	25
(Velveeta) shells, prepared	1/2 cup	210	10.0	25.0	570	(mq)	8.0	20
W/CURRY								
(Tofu Classics) 'Shells 'n Curry' prepared w/tofu	1/2 cup	103	8.0	15.0	275	(mq)	3.0	na
(Tofu Classics) 'Shells 'n Curry' prepared w/tofu and salted butter	1/2 cup	143	8.0	15.0	330	(mq)	7.0	(mq)
W/PARMESAN AND HERBS *(Fantastic Foods)* prepared w/whole milk	1/2 cup	109	5.0	19.0	264	(mq)	2.0	(mq)
MACE								
ground	1 oz	135	1.9	14.3	23	5.9	9.2	0
ground	1 tbsp	25	0.4	2.7	4	1.1	1.7	0
ground	1 tsp	8	0.1	0.9	1	.3	0.6	0
ground *(Durkee)*	1 tsp	10	0.0	0.0	0	0	<0.1	na
ground *(Laurel Leaf)*	1 tsp	10	0.0	0.0	0	0	<0.1	na
ground *(Spice Islands)*	1 tsp	10	0.1	0.8	1	>.1 c	0.7	0
MACKEREL								
ATLANTIC								
baked	4 oz	297	27.0	0.0	94	0	20.2	85
broiled	4 oz	297	27.0	0.0	94	0	20.2	85
dry-heat cooked	3 oz	223	20.3	0.0	71	0	15.1	64
microwaved	4 oz	297	27.0	0.0	94	0	20.2	85
raw	1 lb	929	84.4	0.0	408	0	63.0	318
raw	3 oz	174	15.8	0.0	77	0	11.8	59
raw	1 oz	58	5.3	0.0	26	0	3.9	20
JACK, mixed species								
canned, drained	1 cup	296	44.1	0.0	720	0	12.0	150
canned, drained	4 oz	177	26.3	0.0	430	0	7.1	90
dry-heat cooked	3 oz	171	21.9	0.0	94	0	8.6	51
raw	1 lb	712	91.0	0.0	391	0	35.8	213
raw	3 oz	134	17.1	0.0	73	0	6.7	40
raw	1 oz	45	5.7	0.0	24	0	2.2	13
KING								
dry-heat cooked	3 oz	114	22.1	0.0	173	0	2.2	58
raw	1 lb	475	92.0	0.0	717	0	9.1	242
raw	3 oz	89	17.2	0.0	134	0	1.7	45
raw	1 oz	30	5.7	0.0	45	0	0.6	15
PACIFIC, mixed species								
dry-heat cooked	3 oz	171	21.9	0.0	94	0	8.6	51
raw	1 lb	712	91.0	0.0	391	0	35.8	213
raw	3 oz	134	17.1	0.0	73	0	6.7	40

Food Name	Serv. Size	Total Cal.	Prot. GMS	Carbs GMS	Sod. MGS	Fiber GMS	Fat GMS	Chol. MGS
raw	1 oz	45	5.7	0.0	24	0	2.2	13
SPANISH								
baked	5.1-oz fillet	230	34.4	0.0	96	0	9.2	107
baked	4 oz	179	26.8	0.0	75	0	7.2	83
broiled	5.1-oz fillet	230	34.4	0.0	96	0	9.2	107
broiled	4 oz	179	26.8	0.0	75	0	7.2	83
dry-heat cooked	3 oz	134	20.0	0.0	56	0	5.4	62
microwaved	5.1-oz fillet	230	34.4	0.0	96	0	9.2	107
microwaved	4 oz	179	26.8	0.0	75	0	7.2	83
raw	1 lb	631	87.5	0.0	266	0	28.6	345
raw	3 oz	118	16.4	0.0	50	0	5.3	65
raw	1 oz	39	5.5	0.0	17	0	1.8	22
MAHI MAHI/dolphin fish								
dry-heat cooked	3 oz	93	20.2	0.0	96	0	0.8	80
raw	1 lb	387	83.9	0.0	397	0	3.2	331
raw	3 oz	72	15.7	0.0	75	0	0.6	62
raw	1 oz	24	5.2	0.0	25	0	0.2	21
Fillet portions *(Peter Pan Seafoods)* raw	3.5 oz	85	18.5	na	88	na	0.7	73
MALACCA APPLE, w/o seeds	1 oz	9	0.2	2.3	na	>.2 c	<.1	0
MALT, DRY	1 oz	103	3.7	21.7	22	>1.6 c	0.5	0
MALT EXTRACT, DRIED	1 oz	103	1.7	25.0	22	0	0.0	0
MALT LIQUOR. See ALCOHOLIC BEVERAGES.								
MALT SYRUP								
	1 cup	1221	23.8	273.8	134	0	0.0	0
	1 tbsp	76	1.5	17.1	8	0	0.0	0
MALTED MILK DRINK MIX. See also BREAKFAST DRINK MIX, INSTANT.								
CHOCOLATE FLAVOR								
	1 oz	106	1.4	24.9	71	<.1	1.1	1
w/added nutrients	1 oz	101	1.4	23.9	168	tr	1.0	na
w/added nutrients	4-5 heap tsp	75	1.0	17.7	125	0	0.7	1
(Carnation)	3 heap tsp	80	1.0	18.0	55	na	0.8	0
(Kraft) 'Instant'	3 tsp	90	1.0	18.0	45	na	1.0	na
NATURAL FLAVOR								
	1 oz	117	3.2	21.5	140	tr	2.2	6
w/added nutrients	1 oz	109	2.5	23.0	115	<.1	0.8	na
w/added nutrients	4-5 heap tsp	80	1.9	17.0	85	0	0.6	4
w/o added nutrients	3/4 oz	87	2.3	15.9	104	0	1.7	4
(Carnation) 'Original'	3 heap tsp	90	3.0	15.0	100	na	1.8	0
(Kraft) 'Instant'	3 tsp	90	3.0	16.0	100	na	2.0	na
MAMMY APPLE								
peeled, w/o seeds	1 oz	14	0.1	3.5	4	.9	0.1	0
raw	3 1/2 oz	51	0.5	12.5	15	3.0	0.5	0
raw, trimmed, approx 3.1 lb	1 med	431	4.2	105.8	127	25.4	4.2	0

Food Name	Serv. Size	Total Cal.	Prot. GMS	Carbs GMS	Sod. MGS	Fiber GMS	Fat GMS	Chol. MGS
raw, untrimmed .... 1 lb		139	1.4	34.0	41	>2.7 c	1.4	0
MANDARIN ORANGE								
fresh, whole, approx 2 3/8-inch diam,								
4.1 oz .... 1 med		37	0.5	9.4	1	1.9	0.2	0
peeled, w/o seeds .... 1 oz		12	0.2	3.2	<1	.6	0.1	0
sections, w/o membrane .... 1/2 cup		43	0.6	10.9	2	2.3	0.2	0
untrimmed .... 1 lb		144	2.1	36.6	4	7.4	0.6	0
MANDARIN ORANGE, CANNED *(Dole)*								
sections .... 1/2 cup		70	0.0	19.0	10	na	<1.0	na
MANDARIN ORANGE DRINK								
w/papaya *(Tropicana)* 'Twister' .... 6 oz		90	<1.0	21.0	30	na	<1.0	na
MANGO								
peeled, w/o seed .... 1 oz		18	0.1	4.8	1	.3	0.1	0
raw, sliced .... 1 cup		107	0.8	28.1	3	3.0	0.5	0
raw, trimmed, approx 10.6 oz ...... 1 med		135	1.1	35.2	4	3.7	0.6	0
raw, untrimmed .... 1 lb		204	1.6	53.2	6	3.4	0.9	0
sliced, chilled, in jar *(Sun Fresh)* ...... 3.5 oz		89	0.5	21.0	11	1.9	0.3	1
MANGO DRINK								
(Arizona) 'Mucho Mango Cowboy Cocktail' 8 oz		100	0.0	27.0	20	na	0.0	na
(Kern's) nectar, canned or bottled .... 6 oz		100	0.0	28.0	0	na	0.0	na
(Libby's) nectar, canned or bottled ...... 6 oz		110	0.0	26.0	0	na	0.0	na
MANGO FLAVOR DRINK MIX *(Tang)*								
prepared .... 6 oz		80	0.0	20.0	0	na	0.0	0
MANGO-PEACH JUICE *(Knudsen & Sons)* 8 oz		110	<1.0	29.0	na	na	0.0	na
MANHATTAN. See ALCOHOLIC BEVERAGES.								
MANICOTTI ENTRÉE, FROZEN								
(Budget Gourmet) cheese, w/meat sauce 10 oz		450	20.0	33.0	920	(mq)	26.0	50
(Buitoni) 'Single Serving' .... 9 oz		470	18.0	45.0	830	(mq)	14.0	130
(Celentano) .... 8 oz		300	16.0	36.0	690	(mq)	11.0	(mq)
(Celentano) cheese, w/sauce .... 10 oz		380	20.0	45.0	860	(mq)	14.0	(mq)
(Celentano) cheese, w/sauce .... 7 oz		360	21.0	35.0	580	(mq)	16.0	(mq)
(Celentano) low-fat, 'Great Choice' ..... 10 oz		250	16.0	41.0	675	na	3.0	na
(Healthy Choice) cheese .... 9.25 oz		220	15.0	34.0	310	na	3.0	30
(Le Menu) three cheese .... 11.75 oz		390	19.0	44.0	870	(mq)	15.0	(mq)
(Legume) cheese, w/spinach, tofu, and								
sauce .... 11 oz		260	18.0	30.0	650	8.7	7.0	0
(Legume) cheese, w/tofu and sauce, 'Classic' 8 oz		220	17.0	24.0	370	7.0	11.0	0
(Weight Watchers) cheese .... 9.25 oz		260	17.0	31.0	510	na	8.0	25
MANICOTTI NOODLE. See PASTA.								
MAPLE SYRUP. See also PANCAKE SYRUP.								
.... 1 cup		825	0.0	211.7	28	0	0.6	0
.... 1 tbsp		52	0.0	13.4	2	0	0.0	0
(Knudsen & Sons) 'Fruit 'N Maple' .... 1 oz		105	<1.0	26.0	na	na	<1.0	na

Food Name	Serv. Size	Total Cal.	Prot. GMS	Carbs GMS	Sod. MGS	Fiber GMS	Fat GMS	Chol. MGS
(Maple House) 100% pure	1 oz	100	0.0	61.0	4	na	0.0	0
MARGARINE								
hydrogenated and regular corn oil	1 stick	815	1.0	1.0	1070	0	91.3	0
hydrogenated and regular corn oil	1 tsp	34	0.0	0.0	44	0	3.8	0
hydrogenated and regular soybean oil	1 stick	815	1.0	1.0	1070	0	91.3	0
hydrogenated and regular soybean oil	1 tsp	34	0.0	0.0	44	0	3.8	0
hydrogenated safflower and soybean oil	1 stick	815	1.0	1.0	1070	0	91.3	0
hydrogenated safflower and soybean oil	1 tsp	34	0.0	0.0	44	0	3.8	0
hydrogenated soybean and cottonseed oil	1 stick	815	1.0	1.0	1070	0	91.3	0
hydrogenated soybean and cottonseed oil	1 tsp	34	0.0	0.0	44	0	3.8	0
(A&P)								
'Corn Oil Quarters'	1 tbsp	100	<1.0	<1.0	105	0	11.0	0
'Premium'	1 tbsp	100	<1.0	<1.0	110	0	11.0	0
(Ann Page) 'Quarters'	1 tbsp	100	<1.0	<1.0	110	0	11.0	0
(Blue Bonnet) stick	1 tbsp	100	0.0	0.0	95	na	11.0	0
(Canoleo) 100% canola oil, all natural, dairy-free	1 tbsp	100	0.0	0.0	120	0	11.0	0
(Fleischmann's)								
reduced calorie, 'Diet'	1 tbsp	50	0.0	0.0	50	na	6.0	0
stick	1 tbsp	100	0.0	0.0	95	na	11.0	0
unsalted, stick	1 tbsp	100	0.0	0.0	0	na	11.0	0
(Hain)								
safflower oil	1 tbsp	100	0.0	0.0	170	0	11.0	0
safflower oil, unsalted	1 tbsp	100	0.0	0.0	5	0	11.0	0
(Hollywood)								
safflower oil	1 tbsp	100	0.0	0.0	130	0	11.0	0
safflower oil, unsalted	1 tbsp	100	0.0	0.0	2	0	11.0	0
(Imperial) reduced calorie, 'Diet'	1 tbsp	50	0.0	0.0	140	na	6.0	0
(Land O'Lakes)								
premium, corn oil, stick	1 tsp	35	0.0	0.0	35	na	4.0	0
regular, soy oil, stick	1 tsp	35	0.0	0.0	35	na	4.0	0
tub	1 tsp	35	0.0	0.0	35	0	4.0	0
(Mazola)								
reduced calorie, 'Diet'	1 tbsp	50	0.0	0.0	130	0	6.0	0
regular	1 tbsp	100	0.0	0.0	100	0	11.0	0
unsalted	1 tbsp	100	0.0	0.0	0	0	11.0	0
(Nucoa)	1 tbsp	100	0.0	0.0	160	0	11.0	0
(Parkay)	1 tbsp	100	0.0	0.0	105	0	11.0	0
(Quincy's)	1 oz	204	<1.0	<1.0	268	0	22.0	0
(Spectrum Naturals) non-hydrogenated canola oil, 100% dairy-free	1 tbsp	94	0.0	0.0	84	na	11.0	0
MARGARINE, ALTERNATIVE								
hydrogenated and regular corn oil	1 cup	801	1.2	0.9	2226	0	90.0	0

Food Name	Serv. Size	Total Cal.	Prot. GMS	Carbs GMS	Sod. MGS	Fiber GMS	Fat GMS	Chol. MGS
hydrogenated and regular corn oil	1 tsp	17	0.0	0.0	46	0	1.9	0
hydrogenated soybean and cottonseed oil	1 cup	801	1.2	0.9	2226	0	90.0	0
hydrogenated soybean and cottonseed oil	1 tsp	17	0.0	0.0	46	0	1.9	0
hydrogenated soybean oil	1 cup	801	1.2	0.9	2226	0	90.0	0
hydrogenated soybean oil	1 tsp	17	0.0	0.0	46	0	1.9	0
MARGARINE, SOFT								
(A&P) bowl	1 tbsp	100	<1.0	<1.0	105	0	11.0	0
(Blue Bonnet)	1 tbsp	100	0.0	0.0	95	na	11.0	0
(Chiffon)								
cup	1 tbsp	90	0.0	0.0	95	0	10.0	0
stick	1 tbsp	100	0.0	0.0	105	0	11.0	0
unsalted	1 tbsp	90	0.0	0.0	0	0	10.0	0
(Fleischmann's)								
lightly salted	1 tbsp	100	0.0	0.0	95	na	11.0	0
unsalted	1 tbsp	100	0.0	0.0	0	na	11.0	0
(Imperial)	1 tbsp	100	0.0	0.0	95	na	11.0	0
(Nucoa)	1 tbsp	90	0.0	0.0	150	0	10.0	0
(Parkay)								
reduced calorie, 'Diet'	1 tbsp	50	0.0	0.0	110	0	6.0	0
regular	1 tbsp	100	0.0	0.0	105	0	11.0	0
'Squeezable'	1 tbsp	90	0.0	0.0	110	0	10.0	0
MARGARINE, WHIPPED								
(Blue Bonnet) stick	1 tbsp	70	0.0	0.0	70	na	7.0	0
(Chiffon)	1 tbsp	70	0.0	0.0	80	0	8.0	0
(Fleischmann's)								
lightly salted	1 tbsp	70	0.0	0.0	60	na	7.0	0
unsalted	1 tbsp	70	0.0	0.0	0	na	7.0	0
(Miracle Brand)								
cup	1 tbsp	60	0.0	0.0	70	0	7.0	0
stick	1 tbsp	70	0.0	0.0	65	0	7.0	0
(Parkay)								
cup	1 tbsp	70	0.0	0.0	70	0	7.0	0
stick	1 tbsp	70	0.0	0.0	65	0	7.0	0
MARGARINE SPREAD								
hydrogenated soybean and cottonseed oil, tub	1 cup	1236	1.4	0.0	2276	0	139.2	0
hydrogenated soybean and cottonseed oil, tub	1 tsp	26	0.0	0.0	48	0	2.9	0
hydrogenated soybean and hydrogenated and regular palm oils	1 tsp	26	0.0	0.0	48	0	2.9	0
hydrogenated soybean and hydrogenated and regular palm oils, tub	1 cup	1236	1.4	0.0	2276	0	139.2	0
hydrogenated soybean and palm oil, stick	1 cup	1236	1.4	0.0	2276	0	139.2	0

Food Name	Serv. Size	Total Cal.	Prot. GMS	Carbs GMS	Sod. MGS	Fiber GMS	Fat GMS	Chol. MGS
hydrogenated soybean and palm oil, stick	1 tsp	26	0.0	0.0	48	0	2.9	0
60% corn oil margarine, 40% butter	1 stick	811	1.0	0.7	1014	na	91.2	99
60% corn oil margarine, 40% butter	1 tsp	36	0.0	0.0	45	na	4.0	4
(Blue Bonnet)								
48% vegetable oil	1 tbsp	60	<1.0	<1.0	115	na	6.0	5
75% vegetable oil	1 tbsp	90	0.0	0.0	95	na	11.0	0
whipped, 60% vegetable oil	1 tbsp	80	0.0	0.0	100	na	8.0	0
(Blue Bonnet) 'Better Blend'								
soft	1 tbsp	90	0.0	0.0	95	na	11.0	0
stick	1 tbsp	90	0.0	0.0	95	na	11.0	na
unsalted	1 tbsp	90	0.0	0.0	0	na	11.0	5
(Country Crock)								
'Churn Style' stick	1 tbsp	80	0.0	0.0	55	na	9.0	0
regular	1 tbsp	60	0.0	0.0	110	na	7.0	0
(Fleischmann's) 'Move Over Butter'	1 tbsp	90	0.0	0.0	100	na	10.0	0
(Hollywood) soft	1 tbsp	90	0.0	1.0	135	0	10.0	0
(Imperial) 'Light'	1 tbsp	60	0.0	0.0	110	na	6.0	0
(Kraft) 'Touch of Butter'								
bowl	1 tbsp	50	0.0	0.0	110	na	6.0	0
stick	1 tbsp	90	0.0	0.0	110	0	10.0	0
(Land O'Lakes) 'Country Morning Blend'								
stick	1 tsp	35	0.0	0.0	35	0	4.0	5
tub	1 tsp	30	0.0	0.0	25	0	3.0	5
unsalted, stick	1 tsp	35	0.0	0.0	0	0	4.0	4
unsalted, tub	1 tsp	30	0.0	0.0	0	0	3.0	5
(Land O'Lakes) 'Country Morning Light'								
stick	1 tsp	20	0.0	0.0	30	0	2.0	3
tub	1 tsp	20	0.0	0.0	25	0	2.0	3
(Land O'Lakes) w/sweet cream								
stick	1 tsp	30	0.0	0.0	35	0	4.0	0
tub	1 tsp	25	0.0	0.0	25	0	3.0	0
unsalted	1 tsp	30	0.0	0.0	0	0	4.0	0
(Mazola) 'Corn Oil Light'	1 tbsp	50	0.0	0.0	100	0	6.0	0
(Nucoa) 'Heart Beat'								
regular	1 tbsp	25	0.0	0.0	110	0	3.0	0
unsalted	1 tbsp	24	0.0	0.0	0	0	3.0	0
(P&Q) 60% vegetable oil, stick	1 tbsp	80	<1.0	<1.0	105	0	8.0	0
(Parkay) 50% vegetable oil	1 tbsp	60	0.0	0.0	110	0	7.0	0
(Promise)								
'Extra Light'	1 tbsp	50	0.0	0.0	50	na	6.0	0
regular	1 tbsp	90	0.0	0.0	90	na	10.0	0
'Ultra' fat-free	1 tbsp	5	0.0	0.0	90	na	0.0	0
'Ultra' w/canola oil	1 tbsp	35	0.0	0.0	50	na	4.0	0

Food Name	Serv. Size	Total Cal.	Prot. GMS	Carbs GMS	Sod. MGS	Fiber GMS	Fat GMS	Chol. MGS
(Shedd's Spread) 52% vegetable oil	1 tbsp	60	0.0	0.0	110	na	7.0	0
(Van Den Bergh Foods) 'I Can't Believe It's Not Butter'								
light	1 tbsp	60	0.0	0.0	110	na	7.0	0
regular	1 tbsp	90	0.0	0.0	0	0	10.0	0
(Weight Watchers)								
'Country Cottage Farms' extra light, sweet,								
unsalted	1 tbsp	50	0.0	0.0	0	na	6.0	0
'Country Cottage Farms' extra light, tub	1 tbsp	45	0.0	2.0	75	na	4.0	0
'Country Cottage Farms' light	1 tbsp	50	0.0	0.0	130	0	6.0	0
light, stick	1 tbsp	60	0.0	0.0	130	0	7.0	0
MARGARITA. See ALCOHOLIC BEVERAGES.								
MARINADE. See individual listings.								
MARJORAM								
dried	1 oz	77	3.6	17.2	22	5.1	2.0	0
dried	1 tbsp	5	0.2	1.0	1	.3	0.1	0
dried	1 tsp	2	0.1	0.4	0	.1	0.0	0
dried (Durkee)	1 tsp	2	0.0	0.0	0	0	tr	na
dried (Laurel Leaf)	1 tsp	2	0.0	0.0	0	0	tr	na
dried (Spice Islands)	1 tsp	4	0.2	0.7	1	.2	0.1	0
MARMALADE, ORANGE								
(Finast)	2 tsp	35	0.0	9.0	0	(mq)	0.0	2
(Knott's Berry Farm) light, w/NutraSweet	1 tsp	8	0.0	2.0	0	na	0.0	na
(Knudsen & Sons)	2 tsp	35	<1.0	8.0	na	na	<1.0	na
(Smucker's)	1 tsp	18	0.0	4.0	0	(mq)	0.0	0
(Smucker's) low-sugar	1 tsp	8	0.0	2.0	0	na	0.0	na
(Smucker's) 'Simply Fruit'	1 tsp	16	0.0	4.0	0	na	0.0	na
(Smucker's) sweet, natural ingredients	1 tsp	18	0.0	4.0	0	na	0.0	na
MARMALADE PLUM. See SAPOTE.								
MARROW BEAN								
boiled	4 oz	158	11.0	28.5	7	7.2	0.4	0
boiled	1/2 cup	125	8.6	22.5	6	5.7	0.3	0
raw	1/2 cup	337	23.6	60.9	16	15.4	0.9	0
raw	1 oz	94	6.6	17.1	5	4.3	0.2	0
small, boiled	4 oz	161	10.2	29.3	2	5.0	0.7	0
small, boiled	1/2 cup	127	8.1	23.2	2	3.7	0.6	0
small, raw	1/2 cup	363	22.8	67.2	13	11.1	1.3	0
small, raw	1 oz	95	6.0	17.6	3	2.9	0.3	0
MARROW SQUASH. See SQUASH, MARROW.								
MARSHMALLOW								
(Campfire) large	2 pieces	40	0.0	10.0	10	0	0.0	0
(FunMallows)	1 piece	30	0.0	7.0	15	0	0.0	0
(FunMallows) miniature	10 pieces	18	0.0	5.0	5	0	0.0	0
(Kraft) 'Jet Puffed'	1 piece	25	0.0	6.0	5	0	0.0	0

Food Name	Serv. Size	Total Cal.	Prot. GMS	Carbs GMS	Sod. MGS	Fiber GMS	Fat GMS	Chol. MGS
(Kraft) miniature	10 pieces	18	0.0	5.0	5	0	0.0	0
MARSHMALLOW CREME TOPPING								
(Finast)	1 oz	95	0.0	23.0	45	0	0.0	0
(Kraft)	1 oz	90	0.0	23.0	20	0	0.0	0
(Marshmallow Fluff)	1 tsp	59	0.0	15.0	12	0	0.0	0
(Smucker's)	2 tbsp	120	0.0	29.0	0	na	0.0	na
MARTINI. See ALCOHOLIC BEVERAGES.								
MASA HARINA. See CORN FLOUR.								
MATAI. See WATER CHESTNUT, CHINESE.								
MATZO. See cracker.								
MAYONNAISE								
(Bama)	1 tbsp	100	0.0	0.0	65	0	11.0	(mq)
(Bennett's) 'Real'	1 tbsp	110	0.0	1.0	65	0	12.0	(mq)
(Best Foods)	1 tbsp	100	0.0	0.0	80	0	11.0	5
(Cains)	1 tbsp	100	0.0	0.0	80	0	11.0	10
(Finast)	1 tbsp	100	0.0	0.0	80	0	11.0	10
(Hain) cold processed	1 tbsp	110	0.0	0.0	70	0	12.0	5
(Hellmann's)	1 tbsp	100	0.0	0.0	80	0	11.0	5
(Hollywood)	1 tbsp	110	0.0	0.0	80	0	12.0	5
(Kraft) 'Real'	1 tbsp	100	0.0	0.0	70	0	12.0	5
(Pathmark)	1 tbsp	100	0.0	0.0	70	0	11.0	5
(Pathmark) 'No Frills'	1 tbsp	100	0.0	0.0	75	0	11.0	10
(Rokeach)	1 tbsp	100	0.0	0.0	70	0	11.0	10
(Westbrae)	1 tbsp	100	0.0	0.0	75	na	11.0	5
CANOLA								
(Hain)	1 tbsp	100	0.0	<1.0	100	0	11.0	5
(Hollywood)	1 tbsp	100	0.0	<1.0	100	0	11.0	5
(Spectrum Naturals)	1 tbsp	100	0.0	0.0	80	(tr)	12.0	4
(Spectrum Naturals) 'Lite Mayo'	1 tbsp	35	0.0	1.0	60	0.0	3.0	0
(Westbrae)	1 tbsp	100	0.0	0.0	75	na	11.0	5
LOW-SODIUM								
(Hain) 'Real No Salt Added'	1 tbsp	110	0.0	0.0	0	0	12.0	5
(Weight Watchers) 'Low Sodium'	1 tbsp	50	0.0	1.0	45	0	5.0	5
REDUCED CALORIE								
(Best Foods) 'Light'	1 tbsp	50	0.0	1.0	115	0	5.0	5
(Estee)	1 tbsp	50	0.0	1.0	80	na	5.0	0
(Featherweight)	1 tbsp	30	0.0	3.0	40	0	2.0	10
(Finast) 'Lite'	1 tbsp	40	0.0	1.0	100	0	4.0	5
(Hain) 'Light Low Sodium'	1 tbsp	60	0.0	2.0	95	0	6.0	10
(Hellmann's) 'Light'	1 tbsp	50	0.0	1.0	115	0	5.0	5
(Janet Lee) 'Light'	1 tbsp	50	0.0	1.0	115	na	5.0	5
(Kraft) 'Light'	1 tbsp	50	0.0	1.0	110	0	5.0	0
(Pathmark)	1 tbsp	40	0.0	1.0	100	0	4.0	5

Food Name	Serv. Size	Total Cal.	Prot. GMS	Carbs GMS	Sod. MGS	Fiber GMS	Fat GMS	Chol. MGS
(Smart Beat) 'Golden Corn Light'	1 tbsp	40	0.0	1.0	110	na	4.0	0
(Weight Watchers) 'Light'	1 tbsp	50	0.0	1.0	100	na	5.0	5
SAFFLOWER								
(Hain)	1 tbsp	110	0.0	0.0	70	0	12.0	5
(Hollywood)	1 tbsp	100	0.0	0.0	75	0	12.0	5
SAFFLOWER AND SOYBEAN	1 tbsp	99	0.2	0.4	78	0	11.0	(mq)
SOYBEAN								
	1 tbsp	99	0.2	0.4	78	0	11.0	8
(Featherweight) 'Soyamaise'	1 tbsp	100	0.0	0.0	3	0	11.0	5
MAYONNAISE, ALTERNATIVE								
(Best Foods) 'Cholesterol Free'	1 tbsp	50	0.0	1.0	80	na	5.0	0
(Hain) 'Eggless No Salt Added'	1 tbsp	110	0.0	0.0	5	0	12.0	0
(Hellman's) 'Cholesterol Free'	1 tbsp	50	0.0	1.0	80	0	5.0	na
(Kraft) 'Free'	1 tbsp	8	0.0	3.0	125	na	0.0	0
(Nucoa) 'Heart Beat'	1 tbsp	40	0.0	1.0	110	0	4.0	0
(Weight Watchers) 'Cholesterol Free'	1 tbsp	50	0.0	1.0	90	0	5.0	0
CANOLA *(Hain)* reduced calorie	1 tbsp	60	0.0	2.0	160	0	5.0	0
MILK CREAM	1 tbsp	15	0.3	1.7	76	0	0.8	6
SOYBEAN	1 tbsp	35	tr	2.4	75	0	2.9	4
SUNFLOWER *(Life)* 'All Natural'	1 tbsp	71	<1.0	1.0	3	0	8.0	0
TOFU *(Nasoya)* 'Nayonaise'	1 tbsp	40	1.0	1.0	50	(tr)	4.0	0
MEAT. See individual listings.								
MEAT, ALTERNATIVE. See also individual listings.								
chops *(Worthington)* 'Choplets' canned	2 slices	100	17.0	5.0	350	(mq)	2.0	0
cutlet *(Worthington)* 'Multigrain' canned	2 slices	90	14.0	6.0	260	(mq)	1.0	0
unflavored *(Heartline)* lite	.5 oz	22	5.0	1.0	135	3.0	0.0	0
MEAT EXTENDER								
soybean	1 cup	275	33.5	33.7	8	>1.5 c	2.6	0
soybean	1 oz	88	10.7	10.7	3	>.5 c	0.8	0
MEAT LOAF ENTRÉE, FROZEN								
(Armour) 'Classics'	11.25 oz	360	20.0	32.0	1170	(mq)	17.0	65
(Banquet)	11 oz	440	26.0	27.0	770	(mq)	27.0	85
(Banquet) 'Cookin' Bags'	4 oz	200	10.0	8.0	(mq)	(mq)	14.0	(mq)
(Freezer Queen)	10 oz	350	19.0	26.0	910	(mq)	19.0	(mq)
(Freezer Queen) 'Family Suppers'								
w/tomato sauce	7 oz	230	12.0	15.0	850	(mq)	13.0	(mq)
(Healthy Choice) low-fat, low-cholesterol	12 oz	340	17.0	48.0	560	na	8.0	40
(Lean Cuisine) w/macaroni and cheese	9 3/8 oz	280	26.0	26.0	540	na	8.0	55
(Morton)	10 oz	310	11.0	26.0	1520	na	17.0	50
(Stouffer's) homestyle, in gravy,								
w/whipped potatoes	9 7/8 oz	370	22.0	25.0	860	na	20.0	na
(Swanson)	10.75 oz	360	15.0	41.0	960	(mq)	15.0	(mq)

Food Name	Serv. Size	Total Cal.	Prot. GMS	Carbs GMS	Sod. MGS	Fiber GMS	Fat GMS	Chol. MGS
MEAT LOAF ENTRÉE, PACKAGED								
(Dinty Moore) 'American Classics' w/mashed								
potatoes and gravy	10 oz	262	18.0	26.0	na	na	9.0	na
(Ultra Slim Fast) w/tomato sauce	10.5 oz	340	19.0	52.0	780	na	9.0	35
MEAT LOAF MIX								
(Hunt's) 'Meatloaf Fixins'	2.222 oz	23	1.5	3.9	600	.7	0.4	0
(Lipton) 'Microeasy' homestyle	1/4 pkg	90	4.0	15.0	630	(mq)	1.0	na
MEAT LOAF MIX, ALTERNATIVE								
(Natural) 'Touch Loaf Mix' vegetarian	4 oz	180	21.0	7.0	25	(mq)	7.0	0
MEAT LOAF SEASONING								
(French's)	1/8 pkg	20	1.0	5.0	620	na	0.0	0
(Lawry's) 'Seasoning Blends'	1 pkg	355	15.5	64.5	6547	>1.8 c	1.2	na
(Schilling) 'Bag 'n Season'	1 pkg	111	0.6	26.0	3090	na	0.7	1
MEAT MARINADE MIX *(French's)*	1/8 pkg	10	0.0	2.0	540	na	0.0	0
MEAT STICKS								
smoked	1 oz	156	6.1	1.5	420	na	14.1	38
smoked	1 stick	109	4.3	1.1	293	na	9.8	26
MEAT TENDERIZER								
(Tone's) seasoned	1 tsp	7	<.1	1.2	1650	<.1	0.2	0
(Tone's) unseasoned	1 tsp	7	0.0	1.2	1760	tr	0.2	0
MEATBALL, ALTERNATIVE								
vegetarian *(Worthington)* 'Non-Meat Balls'	3 pieces	100	7.0	4.0	220	(mq)	6.0	0
MEATBALL ENTRÉE								
Canned, stew								
(Chef Boyardee)	8 oz	350	9.0	24.0	1315	(mq)	24.0	(mq)
(Dinty Moore)	8 oz	240	11.0	14.0	980	na	16.0	30
Frozen, BBQ homestyle *(Banquet)*								
'Healthy Balance'	10.25 oz	270	14.0	43.0	680	na	5.0	25
Microwave *(Dinty Moore)* microwave cup	7.5 oz	240	11.0	14.0	980	na	16.0	30
MEATBALL SEASONING *(French's)*								
dry mix	1/4 pkg	35	1.0	7.0	830	na	0.0	0
MELBA TOAST. See CRACKER.								
MELON. See individual listings.								
MELON, BITTER. See BALSAM PEAR.								
MELON BALLS, FROZEN								
cantaloupe and honeydew	1 lb	144	3.8	36.0	139	(mq)	1.1	0
cantaloupe and honeydew	1 cup	57	1.5	13.7	54	1.2	0.4	0
cantaloupe and honeydew	1 oz	9	0.2	2.3	9	(mq)	0.1	0
MENUDO MIX								
(Gebhardt)	1 tsp	5	<1.0	1.0	310	<1.0	<1.0	0
(Gebhardt) spice	.0141 oz	1	0.0	0.1	45	.1	0.0	0
MESQUITE MARINADE *(Lawry's)*	2 tbsp	24	3.0	3.0	4142	tr	0.4	0
MESQUITE SEASONING *(Tone's)*	1 tsp	13	0.1	3.2	467	na	<.1	0

Food Name	Serv. Size	Total Cal.	Prot. GMS	Carbs GMS	Sod. MGS	Fiber GMS	Fat GMS	Chol. MGS
MEXICAN FOODS. See individual listings.								
MEXICAN POTATO. See JICAMA.								
MEXICAN SEASONING (Tone's)	1 tsp	6	0.3	1.3	4185	.4	0.1	tr
MEXICAN STYLE DINNER, FROZEN. See also individual listings.								
(Banquet)	12 oz	490	18.0	62.0	2000	(mq)	18.0	(mq)
(Banquet) combination	12 oz	520	20.0	72.0	1980	(mq)	17.0	(mq)
(Morton)	10 oz	300	9.0	44.0	1390	(mq)	10.0	20
(Patio)	13.25 oz	540	15.0	64.0	1940	(mq)	25.0	45
(Patio) 'Fiesta'	12.25 oz	470	16.0	55.0	2040	(mq)	20.0	30
(Swanson) combination	14.25 oz	490	19.0	62.0	1760	(mq)	18.0	(mq)
(Swanson) 'Hungry Man'	20.25 oz	820	25.0	88.0	2080	(mq)	41.0	(mq)
(Van de Kamp's)	1/2 pkg	220	7.0	25.0	640	(mq)	10.0	(mq)
MILK, ALTERNATIVE. See RICE BEVERAGE; SOY BEVERAGE.								
MILK, COW'S, CANNED								
CONDENSED, SWEETENED								
	1 cup	982	24.2	166.5	389	0	26.6	104
(Borden)	1/3 cup	320	7.0	54.0	115	0	8.0	(mq)
(Carnation)	1/3 cup	320	7.0	56.0	110	0	8.0	(mq)
(Diehl) 'Jerzee'	1/3 cup	320	7.0	52.0	120	0	9.0	(mq)
(Eagle)	1/2 cup	320	7.0	52.0	120	0	9.0	(mq)
EVAPORATED								
	1/2 cup	169	8.6	12.6	133	0	9.5	37
(Carnation)	1/2 cup	170	8.0	12.0	135	0	10.0	(mq)
(Diehl)	1/2 cup	170	8.0	12.0	135	0	10.0	(mq)
(Finast)	1/2 cup	170	8.0	12.0	135	0	10.0	(mq)
(IGA)	1/2 cup	170	8.0	12.0	140	0	10.0	(mq)
(Pathmark)	1/2 cup	170	8.0	12.0	140	0	10.9	(mq)
(Pet)	1/2 cup	170	8.0	12.0	140	0	10.0	36
Filled (Pet)	1/2 cup	150	8.0	12.0	140	0	8.0	5
Low-fat (Carnation)	1/2 cup	110	8.0	12.0	140	0	3.0	10
Skim								
	1/2 cup	100	9.7	14.5	147	0	0.3	5
(Carnation) 'Lite'	1/2 cup	100	9.0	14.0	150	0	<1.0	5
(Diehl)	1/2 cup	100	9.0	14.0	150	0	<1.0	(mq)
(Finast)	1/2 cup	100	9.0	14.0	150	0	<1.0	(mq)
(Pathmark)	1/2 cup	100	9.0	14.0	15	0	0.0	(mq)
(Pet) 'Lite'	1/2 cup	100	9.0	14.0	150	0	<1.0	10
MILK, COW'S, DRY								
LOW-FAT								
(Milkman)	1/4 pkg	90	9.0	12.0	125	na	1.0	na
(Milkman) reconstituted	1 quart	380	35.0	48.0	500	na	5.0	na
SKIM								
(Alba) reconstituted	8 oz	80	8.0	13.0	190	na	0.0	na

Food Name	Serv. Size	Total Cal.	Prot. GMS	Carbs GMS	Sod. MGS	Fiber GMS	Fat GMS	Chol. MGS
(Carnation)	1/3 cup	80	8.0	12.0	125	na	0.0	na
(Lucerne)	1/3 cup	80	8.0	12.0	125	na	0.0	na
(Saco Foods)	5 tbsp	80	8.0	12.0	125	na	<1.0	5
(Sanalac) 'Dairy Fresh' reconstituted	8 oz	80	8.0	12.0	85	0	0.1	5
(Sanalac) reconstituted	9.03 oz	80	7.5	12.3	110	0	0.1	5
(Weight Watchers) 'Dairy Creamer'	1 pkt	10	1.0	1.0	15	0	0.0	na

MILK, COW'S, FLUID
WHOLE

Food Name	Serv. Size	Total Cal.	Prot. GMS	Carbs GMS	Sod. MGS	Fiber GMS	Fat GMS	Chol. MGS
(A&P)	1 cup	150	8.0	11.0	120	0	8.0	(mq)
(Borden)	1 cup	150	8.0	11.0	130	0	8.0	(mq)
(Borden) 'Hi-Calcium'	1 cup	150	8.0	11.0	130	0	8.0	(mq)
(Carnation)	1 cup	150	8.0	12.0	120	0	8.0	33
(Crowley)	1 cup	150	8.0	11.0	125	0	8.0	30
(Darigold)	1 cup	150	8.0	11.0	125	0	8.0	33
(Knudsen)	1 cup	160	9.0	12.0	180	0	8.0	(mq)
Low-sodium	1 cup	149	7.6	10.9	6	0	8.4	33
3.7% fat	1 cup	157	8.0	11.4	119	0	8.9	35
3.3% fat	1 cup	150	8.0	11.4	120	0	8.1	33

2% FAT

Food Name	Serv. Size	Total Cal.	Prot. GMS	Carbs GMS	Sod. MGS	Fiber GMS	Fat GMS	Chol. MGS
	1 cup	121	8.1	11.7	122	0	4.7	18

Protein-fortified

Food Name	Serv. Size	Total Cal.	Prot. GMS	Carbs GMS	Sod. MGS	Fiber GMS	Fat GMS	Chol. MGS
	1 cup	137	9.7	13.5	145	0	4.9	19
(A&P)	1 cup	120	8.0	12.0	120	0	5.0	(mq)
(Borden) 'Hi-Protein'	1 cup	140	10.0	13.0	150	0	5.0	(mq)
(Crowley) 'Tone Acidophilus'	1 cup	120	8.0	11.0	125	0	5.0	15
(Darigold) 'Nutrish Acidophilus'	1 cup	120	8.0	11.0	130	0	5.0	18
(Finast)	1 cup	130	9.0	12.0	130	0	5.0	(mq)
(Knudsen) 'Sweet Acidophilus'	1 cup	140	10.0	13.0	150	0	5.0	(mq)
(Viva)	1 cup	120	8.0	11.0	125	0	5.0	(mq)
W/non-fat milk solids added	1 cup	125	8.5	12.2	128	0	4.7	18

1% FAT

Food Name	Serv. Size	Total Cal.	Prot. GMS	Carbs GMS	Sod. MGS	Fiber GMS	Fat GMS	Chol. MGS
	1 cup	102	8.0	11.7	123	0	2.6	10
(Crowley)	1 cup	100	8.0	11.0	130	0	2.0	10

Protein-fortified

Food Name	Serv. Size	Total Cal.	Prot. GMS	Carbs GMS	Sod. MGS	Fiber GMS	Fat GMS	Chol. MGS
	1 cup	119	9.7	13.6	143	0	2.9	10
(A&P)	1 cup	100	8.0	12.0	120	0	3.0	(mq)
(Borden)	1 cup	100	8.0	11.0	130	0	2.0	(mq)
(Crowley)	1 cup	120	10.0	14.0	150	0	2.0	10
(Crowley) 'Lactaid'	1 cup	100	8.0	11.0	125	0	2.0	10
(Darigold)	1 cup	100	8.0	13.0	130	0	2.0	10
(Knudsen) 'Nice n' Light'	1 cup	130	10.0	15.0	153	0	3.0	(mq)
W/calcium added *(Darigold)*	1 cup	100	8.0	11.0	130	0	2.0	10
W/non-fat milk solids added	1 cup	104	8.5	12.2	128	0	2.4	10

Food Name	Serv. Size	Total Cal.	Prot. GMS	Carbs GMS	Sod. MGS	Fiber GMS	Fat GMS	Chol. MGS
SKIM								
....	1 cup	86	8.4	11.9	126	0	0.4	4
Protein-fortified								
(A&P)	1 cup	90	8.0	12.0	125	0	<1.0	(mq)
(Borden)	1 cup	90	8.0	12.0	130	0	1.0	(mq)
(Borden) 'Skim-Line'	1 cup	100	10.0	13.0	150	0	1.0	(mq)
(Crowley)	1 cup	90	9.0	12.0	130	0	<1.0	<1
(Darigold) 'Trim'	1 cup	80	8.0	11.0	130	0	1.0	4
(Knudsen)	1 cup	80	9.0	12.0	130	0	(mq)	(mq)
(Weight Watchers)	1 cup	90	9.0	13.0	140	0	<1.0	(mq)
W/non-fat milk solids added	1 cup	90	8.8	12.3	130	0	0.6	5
W/vitamin A added	1 cup	86	8.4	11.9	126	0	0.4	4
MILK, GOAT'S								
evaporated (Meyenberg) canned, undiluted	4 oz	143	7.9	10.0	86	na	7.9	na
fluid, whole	1 cup	168	8.7	10.9	122	0	10.1	28
fluid, whole	1 oz	20	1.0	1.3	14	0	1.2	3
MILK, HUMAN								
fluid, whole	1 cup	171	2.5	17.0	42	0	10.8	34
fluid, whole	1 oz	21	0.3	2.1	5	0	1.4	4
fluid, whole	1 tbsp	11	0.2	1.1	3	0	0.7	2
MILK, INDIA BUFFALO								
fluid, whole	1 cup	236	9.1	12.6	127	0	16.8	46
fluid, whole	1 oz	27	1.1	1.5	15	0	2.0	5
MILK, LACTOSE-REDUCED								
2% FAT								
(Lactaid) 70% lactose reduced, w/vitamins								
A and D	1 cup	130	8.0	12.0	125	0	5.0	20
(Lucerne) 70% lactose reduced, w/vitamins								
A and D	1 cup	120	9.0	12.0	110	0	5.0	25
1% FAT								
(First Alternative) lactose free	1 cup	80	8.0	6.0	180	0	2.0	0
SKIM								
(Lactaid) 70% lactose reduced, w/calcium								
and vitamins A and D	1 cup	80	8.0	13.0	125	0	0.0	5
(Lactaid) 70% lactose reduced, w/vitamins								
A and D	1 cup	80	8.0	13.0	125	0	0.0	5
(Lactaid 100) lactose free, w/vitamins								
A and D	1 cup	80	8.0	13.0	125	0	0.0	5
(Lucerne) 70% lactose reduced, w/vitamins								
A and D	1 cup	80	9.0	12.0	115	0	0.0	5
MILK, REINDEER	1 cup	580	26.8	10.2	389	0	48.6	35
MILK, SHEEP'S								
fluid, whole	1 cup	264	14.7	13.1	108	0	17.2	66

Food Name	Serv. Size	Total Cal.	Prot. GMS	Carbs GMS	Sod. MGS	Fiber GMS	Fat GMS	Chol. MGS
fluid, whole	1 oz	31	1.7	1.5	12	0	2.0	(mq)
MILKFISH. See AWA.								
MILKSHAKE								
chocolate, thick	10.6 oz	356	9.1	63.5	333	.9	8.1	32
vanilla, thick	11 oz	350	12.1	55.6	299	0	9.5	37
(MicroMagic) chocolate, frozen	11.5 oz	340	5.0	55.0	120	(tr)	8.0	40
(MicroMagic) chocolate, frozen	7 oz	200	2.0	32.0	70	(tr)	4.0	25
(MicroMagic) strawberry, frozen	11.5 oz	340	5.0	54.0	120	(tr)	9.0	40
(MicroMagic) vanilla, frozen	11.5 oz	380	8.0	60.0	150	0	13.0	45
MILKSHAKE MIX								
(Alba '77) chocolate, 'Fit'N' prepared	6 oz	346	26.1	56.0	709	>1.0 c	2.5	na
(Alba '77) chocolate marshmallow, 'Fit'N' prepared	6 oz	346	27.5	51.5	690	>.8 c	3.6	na
(Alba '77) double fudge, frosty, 'Fit'N' prepared	6 oz	346	28.0	52.2	728	>1.0 c	3.3	na
(Alba '77) strawberry, 'Fit'N' prepared	6 oz	333	24.6	55.0	805	>.2 c	1.7	na
(Alba '77) vanilla, 'Fit'N' prepared	6 oz	333	26.0	54.5	810	>.4 c	1.4	na
(Weight Watchers) chocolate fudge	1 pkt	70	6.0	11.0	170	(tr)	1.0	na
(Weight Watchers) orange sherbet	1 pkt	70	6.0	11.0	210	(tr)	0.0	0
MILLET								
pearl, cooked	1/2 cup	143	4.2	28.4	2	1.6	1.2	0
pearl, cooked	4 oz	135	4.0	26.8	2	1.5	1.1	0
pearl, raw	1/2 cup	378	11.0	72.9	5	8.5	4.2	0
pearl, raw	1 oz	107	3.1	20.7	1	2.4	1.2	0
pearl, raw, hulled *(Arrowhead Mills)*	1 oz	90	3.0	21.0	1	1.8	1.0	0
Proso/hog millet, whole grain	3 1/2 oz	327	9.9	72.9	1	>3.2 c	2.9	0
MILLET FLOUR, whole grain								
(Arrowhead Mills)	2 oz	185	6.0	41.0	1	3.7	2.0	0
MISO								
....	1/2 cup	284	16.3	38.6	5033	7.4	8.4	0
....	1 oz	58	3.3	7.9	1034	1.5	1.7	0
w/barley malt/mugi-koji	1 oz	56	2.7	8.0	1191	(mq)	1.2	0
w/rice malt, dark yellow/kome-koji	1 oz	53	3.7	5.4	1446	(mq)	1.6	0
w/rice malt, sweet/kome-koji	1 oz	62	2.7	10.4	680	(mq)	0.9	0
w/soybean malt/mame-koji	1 oz	62	4.9	3.2	1219	(mq)	3.9	0
(Eden Foods) barley/mugi, organic	1 tbsp	25	2.0	3.0	760	na	<1.0	na
(Eden Foods) brown rice/genmai, organic	1 tbsp	25	2.0	3.0	810	na	1.0	na
(Eden Foods) rice/shiro, organic	1 tbsp	35	2.0	5.0	410	na	1.0	na
(Eden Foods) soybean and rice/kome, organic	1 tbsp	25	2.0	3.0	850	na	1.0	na
(Eden Foods) soybean/hacho, organic ..	1 tbsp	35	3.0	2.0	600	na	2.0	na
(Westbrae) barley, pasteurized	1 tsp	12	<1.0	2.0	310	na	0.0	0
(Westbrae) brown rice, pasteurized	1 tsp	10	1.0	2.0	360	na	0.0	0

Food Name	Serv. Size	Total Cal.	Prot. GMS	Carbs GMS	Sod. MGS	Fiber GMS	Fat GMS	Chol. MGS
(Westbrae) red, instant	.35 oz	35	3.0	3.0	750	na	1.0	na
(Westbrae) red, pasteurized	1 tsp	10	1.0	1.0	375	na	0.0	0
(Westbrae) soybean, pasteurized	1 tsp	12	1.0	1.0	265	na	0.0	0
(Westbrae) soybean/hacho	1 tsp	14	1.0	1.0	240	na	0.0	0
(Westbrae) white, instant	.35 oz	35	2.0	4.0	740	na	1.0	na
MOLASSES								
....	1 cup	872	0.0	225.7	121	0	0.3	0
....	1 tbsp	53	0.0	13.8	7	0	0.0	0
Barbados	1 cup	889	0.0	229.6	49	0	0.0	0
Barbados	1 oz	111	0.0	28.7	6	0	0.0	0
1st extraction/light	1 cup	827	0.0	213.2	49	0	0.0	0
1st extraction/light	1 oz	103	0.0	26.7	6	0	0.0	0
2nd extraction/medium	1 cup	761	0.0	196.8	121	0	0.0	0
2nd extraction/medium	1 oz	95	0.0	24.6	15	0	0.0	0
3rd extraction/blackstrap	1 cup	771	0.0	199.4	180	0	0.0	0
3rd extraction/blackstrap	1 tbsp	47	0.0	12.2	11	0	0.0	0
(Br'er Rabbit) dark	1 oz	110	0.0	28.0	20	na	0.0	0
(Br'er Rabbit) light	1 oz	110	0.0	29.0	15	na	0.0	0
(Grandma's) mild flavor, gold	1 tbsp	70	0.0	17.0	28	0	0.0	0
(Grandma's) robust flavor, green	1 tbsp	70	0.0	16.0	57	0	0.0	0
(LaChoy) bead	.7055 oz	52	0.4	12.5	48	0	0.0	0
(LaChoy) bead	1/2 tsp	7	<1.0	2.0	1	0	0.0	0
MONKFISH/angler fish/bellyfish/frogfish/goosefish/lotte/sea devil								
dry-heat cooked	3 oz	82	15.8	0.0	20	0	1.7	27
raw	1 lb	343	65.7	0.0	84	0	6.9	115
raw	3 oz	65	12.3	0.0	15	0	1.3	21
raw	1 oz	22	4.1	0.0	5	0	0.4	7
MONOSODIUM GLUTAMATE/MSG								
flavor enhancer *(Tone's)* 'MSG'	1 tsp	0	0.0	0.0	638	0	0.0	0
MOOSE								
raw	1 lb	463	100.9	0.0	295	na	3.4	268
raw	1 oz	29	6.2	0.0	18	na	0.2	17
roasted	3 oz	114	24.9	0.0	59	na	0.8	66
roasted, diced	1 cup	188	41.0	0.0	97	0	1.4	109
MOSTACCIOLI. See PASTA.								
MOSTACCIOLI ENTRÉE								
(Banquet) frozen, w/meat sauce 'Family Entrees'	7 oz	170	7.0	28.0	(mq)	(mq)	3.0	(mq)
MOTH BEAN								
boiled	4 oz	133	8.9	23.8	11	>1.5 c	0.6	0
boiled	1/2 cup	103	6.9	18.4	9	>1.2 c	0.5	0
raw	1/2 cup	336	22.5	60.3	29	>3.9 c	1.6	0
raw	1 oz	97	6.5	17.4	9	>1.1 c	0.5	0

Food Name	Serv. Size	Total Cal.	Prot. GMS	Carbs GMS	Sod. MGS	Fiber GMS	Fat GMS	Chol. MGS
MOUNTAIN YAM. See YAM.								
MOUSSE *(Estee)* orange chocolate	1/2 cup	70	3.0	9.0	50	na	3.0	0
MOUSSE, FROZEN								
(Weight Watchers) 'Sweet Celebrations' chocolate	2.5 oz	170	6.0	24.0	190	na	6.0	5
(Weight Watchers) 'Sweet Celebrations' praline pecan	2.75 oz	190	5.0	27.0	180	na	7.0	5
(Weight Watchers) 'Sweet Celebrations' triple chocolate caramel	2.75 oz	170	4.0	31.0	120	na	4.0	5
MOUSSE MIX								
(Jell-O) 'Rich & Luscious' chocolate, dry mix	1 pkg	110	3.0	18.0	45	na	3.0	0
(Jell-O) 'Rich & Luscious' chocolate, prepared	1/2 cup	150	5.0	21.0	75	na	6.0	10
(Jell-O) 'Rich & Luscious' chocolate fudge, dry mix	1 pkg	110	3.0	18.0	45	na	4.0	0
(Jell-O) 'Rich & Luscious' chocolate fudge, prepared	1/2 cup	140	5.0	20.0	75	na	6.0	10
(Weight Watchers) chocolate, prepared w/skim milk	1/2 cup	60	3.0	9.0	45	na	3.0	(mq)
(Weight Watchers) chocolate cheesecake, prepared w/skim milk	1/2 cup	60	4.0	12.0	75	na	2.0	(mq)
(Weight Watchers) chocolate raspberry, prepared w/skim milk	1/2 cup	60	3.0	12.0	75	na	3.0	(mq)
(Weight Watchers) white chocolate almond, prepared w/skim milk	1/2 cup	60	3.0	6.0	50	na	3.0	(mq)
MSG. See MONOSODIUM GLUTAMATE.								
MUFFIN. See also ENGLISH MUFFIN.								
APPLE								
(Awrey's) 1.5-oz muffin	1 muffin	130	2.0	17.0	210	0	6.0	20
(Awrey's) 2.5-oz muffin	1 muffin	220	3.0	30.0	350	1.0	10.0	35
(Awrey's) w/banana nut 'Grande' 4.2-oz muffin	1 muffin	260	3.0	27.0	160	.6	16.0	40
(Hostess) w/banana walnut, mini muffin	5 muffins	160	2.0	17.0	90	(mq)	9.0	0
APPLE SPICE								
(Dunkin' Donuts) 3.5-oz muffin	1 muffin	300	6.0	52.0	360	na	8.0	25
(Health Valley) fat-free	1 muffin	130	4.0	30.0	110	5.1	0.0	0
APPLE STREUSEL *(Awrey's)* 'Grande' 4.2-oz muffin	1 muffin	340	6.0	50.0	540	1.0	13.0	35
BANANA *(Health Valley)* fat-free	1 muffin	130	4.0	29.0	110	4.5	0.0	0
BANANA NUT								
(Break Cake) .5-oz muffin	1 muffin	60	1.0	7.0	45	na	3.0	10
(Dunkin' Donuts) 3.6-oz muffin	1 muffin	310	7.0	49.0	410	3.0	10.0	30

Food Name	Serv. Size	Total Cal.	Prot. GMS	Carbs GMS	Sod. MGS	Fiber GMS	Fat GMS	Chol. MGS
BLUEBERRY								
(Awrey's) 1.5-oz muffin	1 muffin	130	2.0	18.0	180	1.0	5.0	10
(Awrey's) 2.5-oz muffin	1 muffin	210	3.0	31.0	280	1.0	8.0	20
(Awrey's) 'Grande' 4.2-oz muffin	1 muffin	360	5.0	52.0	480	2.0	14.0	35
(Break Cake)	1 muffin	60	1.0	8.0	50	na	3.0	10
(Dunkin' Donuts) 3.6-oz muffin	1 muffin	280	6.0	46.0	340	na	8.0	30
(Entenmann's)	1 muffin	200	3.0	29.0	250	na	8.0	na
(Hostess) mini muffin	5 muffins	240	3.0	29.0	180	.7	13.0	40
BLUEBERRY-APPLE (Health Valley) fat-free, twin pack	1 muffin	140	4.0	32.0	100	5.0	0.0	0
BRAN (Dunkin' Donuts) w/raisins, 3.7-oz muffin	1 muffin	310	6.0	51.0	560	4.0	9.0	15
CARROT (Health Valley) fat-free, twin pack	1 muffin	130	4.0	30.0	110	5.0	0.0	0
CINNAMON APPLE (Hostess) mini muffin	5 muffins	260	3.0	27.0	180	.6	16.0	45
CORN								
(Awrey's) 1.5-oz muffin	1 muffin	130	2.0	20.0	270	0	5.0	15
(Awrey's) 2.5-oz muffin	1 muffin	220	4.0	33.0	430	1.0	8.0	25
(Dunkin' Donuts) 3.4-oz muffin	1 muffin	340	7.0	51.0	560	na	12.0	40
CRANBERRY (Awrey's) 1.5-oz muffin	1 muffin	120	2.0	20.0	210	0	4.0	10
CRANBERRY NUT (Dunkin' Donuts) 3.5-oz muffin	1 muffin	290	6.0	44.0	360	2.0	9.0	25
OAT BRAN								
(Awrey's) 2.75-oz muffin	1 muffin	180	5.0	27.0	330	2.0	7.0	0
(Awrey's) pineapple raisin, 2.75-oz muffin	1 muffin	180	5.0	26.0	320	2.0	6.0	0
(Dunkin' Donuts) 3.4-oz muffin	1 muffin	330	7.0	50.0	450	3.0	11.0	0
(Hostess)	1 muffin	160	2.0	21.0	150	1.5	7.0	0
(Hostess) banana nut	1 muffin	140	2.0	20.0	160	1.0	5.0	0
(Health Valley) almond and date	1 muffin	180	4.0	31.0	81	8.2	4.0	0
(Health Valley) blueberry	1 muffin	180	4.0	32.0	99	7.5	4.0	0
(Health Valley) 'Fancy Fruit Muffins' raisin	1 muffin	180	4.0	31.0	90	7.8	5.0	0
RAISIN								
(Dunkin' Donuts)	1 muffin	310	6.0	51.0	560	na	9.0	15
(Wonder) 'Raisin Rounds'	1 muffin	140	4.0	27.0	280	1.2	2.0	0
RAISIN BRAN								
(Awrey's) 1.5-oz muffin	1 muffin	110	2.0	18.0	170	1.0	4.0	15
(Awrey's) 2.5-oz muffin	1 muffin	190	3.0	30.0	280	2.0	7.0	20
(Awrey's) 'Grande' 4.2-oz muffin	1 muffin	320	5.0	50.0	470	3.0	12.0	35
RAISIN SPICE (Health Valley) fat-free	1 muffin	140	4.0	32.0	100	5.1	0.0	0

Food Name	Serv. Size	Total Cal.	Prot. GMS	Carbs GMS	Sod. MGS	Fiber GMS	Fat GMS	Chol. MGS
RASPBERRY *(Health Valley)* fat-free, twin pack	1 muffin	130	4.0	30.0	110	5.0	0.0	0
RICE BRAN-RAISIN *(Health Valley)*	1 muffin	215	5.0	35.0	124	5.5	7.0	0
SOURDOUGH *(Wonder)*	1 muffin	130	4.0	27.0	250	1.2	1.0	0
MUFFIN, FROZEN								
APPLE SPICE								
(Healthy Choice) 2.5-oz muffin	1 muffin	190	3.0	40.0	90	na	4.0	0
(Sara Lee) 2.5-oz muffin	1 muffin	220	4.0	36.0	280	(mq)	8.0	0
(Weight Watchers) 'Microwave' 2.5-oz muffin	1 muffin	160	3.0	29.0	260	(mq)	5.0	na
BANANA NUT								
(Healthy Choice) 2.5-oz muffin	1 muffin	180	3.0	32.0	80	na	6.0	0
(Weight Watchers) 'Microwave' 2.5-oz muffin	1 muffin	170	3.0	32.0	250	(mq)	5.0	10
BLUEBERRY								
(Healthy Choice) 2.5-oz muffin	1 muffin	190	3.0	39.0	110	na	4.0	0
(Pepperidge Farm) 'Old Fashioned'	1 muffin	170	2.0	27.0	250	1.0	7.0	25
(Sara Lee) 2.5-oz muffin	1 muffin	200	3.0	34.0	290	(mq)	8.0	0
(Sara Lee) 'Free & Light'	1 muffin	120	3.0	28.0	140	(mq)	0.0	0
(Weight Watchers) 'Microwave' 2.5-oz muffin	1 muffin	170	3.0	32.0	220	(mq)	5.0	10
CHEESE STREUSEL *(Sara Lee)* 2.1-oz muffin	1 muffin	220	4.0	27.0	170	(mq)	11.0	na
CHOCOLATE CHUNK *(Sara Lee)* 2.1-oz muffin	1 muffin	220	3.0	33.0	210	(mq)	8.0	na
CINNAMON SWIRL *(Pepperidge Farm)* 'Old Fashioned'	1 muffin	190	2.0	30.0	170	1.0	6.0	35
CORN *(Pepperidge Farm)* 'Old Fashioned'	1 muffin	180	3.0	27.0	260	2.0	7.0	30
HONEY BRAN								
(Sara Lee) golden, 2.5-oz muffin	1 muffin	250	4.0	31.0	310	(mq)	13.0	0
(Weight Watchers) 2.5-oz muffin	1 muffin	160	3.0	32.0	150	na	4.0	5
OAT BRAN								
(Pepperidge Farm) apple 'Old Fashioned Cholesterol Free'	1 muffin	190	3.0	29.0	200	2.0	7.0	0
(Sara Lee) 2.5-oz muffin	1 muffin	210	4.0	35.0	320	(mq)	8.0	0
(Sara Lee) apple, 2.5-oz muffin	1 muffin	210	4.0	35.0	320	(mq)	8.0	0
RAISIN BRAN								
(Pepperidge Farm) 'Old Fashioned Cholesterol Free'	1 muffin	170	4.0	30.0	280	3.0	6.0	0
(Sara Lee) 2.5-oz muffin	1 muffin	220	4.0	37.0	400	(mq)	7.0	0

Food Name	Serv. Size	Total Cal.	Prot. GMS	Carbs GMS	Sod. MGS	Fiber GMS	Fat GMS	Chol. MGS
MUFFIN MIX								
ALMOND *(Krusteaz)* w/poppy seed,								
prepared	1 muffin	160	3.0	29.0	230	2.0	4.0	27
APPLE CINNAMON								
(Betty Crocker) prepared w/egg,								
2% milk	1/12 recipe	120	2.0	18.0	140	(mq)	4.0	25
(Betty Crocker) prepared w/egg white,								
skim milk	1/12 recipe	110	2.0	18.0	140	(mq)	3.0	0
(General Mills) prepared	1 muffin	100	1.0	17.0	130	na	3.0	0
(General Mills) prepared w/egg,								
1/2 cup 2% milk	1 muffin	120	2.0	18.0	140	na	4.0	25
(General Mills) prepared w/egg white,								
skim milk	1 muffin	110	2.0	18.0	140	na	3.0	0
(Krusteaz) prepared	1 muffin	180	3.0	36.0	340	na	3.0	4
(Martha White) prepared	1/16 recipe	140	2.0	25.0	250	(mq)	3.0	3
(Martha White) prepared w/2% milk	1 muffin	140	2.0	25.0	250	na	3.0	2
APPLE STREUSEL								
(Betty Crocker) Dutch, prepared w/egg,								
whole milk	1/12 recipe	200	3.0	32.0	240	(mq)	7.0	(mq)
APPLESAUCE								
(Gold Medal) 'Pouch Mix' prepared								
w/egg, whole milk	1/6 recipe	160	3.0	26.0	240	(mq)	5.0	(mq)
(Robin Hood) 'Pouch Mix' prepared								
w/egg, whole milk	1/6 recipe	160	3.0	26.0	240	(mq)	5.0	(mq)
BANANA								
(Gold Medal) 'Pouch Mix' prepared								
w/egg, whole milk	1/12 recipe	150	3.0	24.0	240	(mq)	5.0	(mq)
(Robin Hood) 'Pouch Mix' prepared								
w/egg, whole milk	1/12 recipe	150	3.0	24.0	240	(mq)	5.0	(mq)
BANANA NUT								
(Betty Crocker) prepared w/egg,								
2% milk	1/12 recipe	120	2.0	17.0	140	(mq)	5.0	25
(Betty Crocker) prepared w/egg white,								
skim milk	1/12 recipe	110	2.0	17.0	140	(mq)	4.0	0
(General Mills) prepared	1 muffin	110	1.0	17.0	140	na	4.0	0
(General Mills) prepared w/egg,								
1/3 cup 2% milk	1 muffin	120	2.0	18.0	150	na	4.0	20
(General Mills) prepared w/egg white,								
skim milk	1 muffin	120	2.0	18.0	150	na	4.0	0
(Martha White) prepared w/2% milk	1 muffin	180	3.0	23.0	240	na	8.0	35
BLACKBERRY								
(Martha White) prepared	1/6 recipe	140	2.0	25.0	250	(mq)	3.0	3
(Martha White) prepared w/2% milk	1 muffin	140	2.0	25.0	250	na	3.0	2

Food Name	Serv. Size	Total Cal.	Prot. GMS	Carbs GMS	Sod. MGS	Fiber GMS	Fat GMS	Chol. MGS
BLUEBERRY								
(Betty Crocker) streusel 'Bake Shop' prepared	1/12 recipe	210	3.0	31.0	230	(mq)	8.0	(mq)
(Betty Crocker) wild blueberries, prepared w/egg, 2% milk	1/12 recipe	120	2.0	18.0	150	(mq)	4.0	25
(Betty Crocker) wild blueberries, prepared w/egg white, skim milk	1/12 recipe	110	2.0	18.0	150	(mq)	3.0	0
(Duncan Hines) 'Bakery Style' prepared	1 muffin	190	2.0	32.0	250	na	6.0	na
(Duncan Hines) prepared	1 muffin	120	2.0	21.0	185	na	3.0	na
(General Mills) 'Twice the Blueberries' prepared	1 muffin	100	1.0	17.0	130	na	3.0	0
(General Mills) 'Twice the Blueberries' prepared, no cholesterol recipe	1 muffin	110	2.0	18.0	140	na	3.0	0
(General Mills) 'Twice the Blueberries' prepared w/egg, 1/2 cup 2% milk	1 muffin	120	2.0	18.0	140	na	4.0	20
(Gold Medal) 'Pouch Mix' prepared w/egg, whole milk	1/6 recipe	170	3.0	26.0	240	(mq)	6.0	(mq)
(Krusteaz) prepared	1 muffin	150	3.0	27.0	260	1.0	4.0	27
(Lovin' Lites) dry mix	1/12 pkg	100	2.0	21.0	150	na	1.0	0
(Lovin' Lites) prepared w/egg, water	1/12 recipe	100	2.0	21.0	160	na	1.0	20
(Lovin' Lites) prepared w/2 egg whites, water	1/12 recipe	100	3.0	21.0	160	na	1.0	0
(Martha White) prepared	1/6 recipe	140	2.0	25.0	260	(mq)	3.0	3
(Martha White) prepared w/2% milk	1 muffin	140	2.0	25.0	260	na	3.0	2
(Robin Hood) 'Pouch Mix' prepared w/egg, whole milk	1/6 recipe	170	3.0	26.0	240	(mq)	6.0	(mq)
BRAN								
(Duncan Hines) w/honey 'Bakery Style' prepared	1 muffin	200	2.0	32.0	220	(mq)	7.0	na
(Martha White) prepared	1/6 recipe	150	3.0	24.0	330	(mq)	5.0	14
(Martha White) prepared w/2% milk	1 muffin	150	3.0	24.0	330	na	5.0	35
CARAMEL								
(Gold Medal) 'Pouch Mix' prepared w/egg, whole milk	1/6 recipe	150	3.0	23.0	250	(mq)	5.0	(mq)
(Robin Hood) 'Pouch Mix' prepared w/egg, whole milk	1/6 recipe	150	3.0	23.0	250	(mq)	5.0	(mq)
CARROT NUT								
(Betty Crocker) prepared w/egg, 2% milk	1/12 recipe	150	3.0	22.0	160	(mq)	5.0	25
(Betty Crocker) prepared w/egg white, skim milk	1/12 recipe	150	3.0	22.0	160	(mq)	5.0	0
CHOCOLATE CHIP								
(Betty Crocker) prepared	1/12 recipe	140	2.0	22.0	180	(mq)	5.0	0

Food Name	Serv. Size	Total Cal.	Prot. GMS	Carbs GMS	Sod. MGS	Fiber GMS	Fat GMS	Chol. MGS
(Betty Crocker) prepared w/egg, 2% milk	1/12 recipe	150	2.0	22.0	180	(mq)	6.0	20
(Krusteaz) prepared	1 muffin	200	3.0	35.0	340	na	5.0	11
CINNAMON								
(Betty Crocker) streusel, prepared w/egg, 2% milk	1/12 recipe	200	3.0	27.0	240	(mq)	9.0	30
(Duncan Hines) swirl 'Bakery Style' prepared	1 muffin	200	2.0	32.0	245	na	7.0	na
(General Mills) streusel, prepared	1 muffin	190	2.0	27.0	220	na	8.0	0
CORN								
(Arrowhead Mills) blue, prepared	1 muffin	110	4.0	15.0	na	2.6	4.0	na
(Dromedary) dry mix	3 1/2 tbsp	110	1.0	20.0	250	(mq)	3.0	na
(Dromedary) prepared	1 muffin	120	3.0	20.0	270	(mq)	4.0	na
(Flako) prepared	1 muffin	116	1.8	19.8	351	.7	3.3	na
(Gold Medal) prepared w/egg, whole milk	1/6 pkg	130	3.0	24.0	250	(mq)	2.0	(mq)
(Krusteaz) prepared	1 muffin	220	4.0	36.0	450	2.0	7.0	5
(Martha White) yellow, prepared w/water	1 muffin	160	2.0	30.0	230	na	3.0	<1
(Robin Hood) prepared w/egg, whole milk	1/6 pkg	130	3.0	24.0	250	(mq)	2.0	(mq)
CRANBERRY-ORANGE NUT								
(Duncan Hines) 'Bakery Style' prepared	1 muffin	200	2.0	30.0	215	(mq)	8.0	na
HONEY BRAN								
(Gold Medal) 'Pouch Mix' prepared w/egg, whole milk	1/6 recipe	170	5.0	25.0	240	(mq)	6.0	(mq)
(Krusteaz) prepared	1 muffin	140	3.0	23.0	290	3.0	4.0	0
(Martha White) w/poppy seed, prepared w/2% milk	1 muffin	200	2.0	30.0	260	na	9.0	35
(Robin Hood) 'Pouch Mix' prepared w/egg, whole milk	1/6 recipe	170	5.0	25.0	240	(mq)	6.0	(mq)
OAT								
(Gold Medal) 'Pouch Mix' prepared w/egg, 2% milk	1/6 recipe	150	4.0	23.0	220	(mq)	5.0	45
(Robin Hood) 'Pouch Mix' prepared w/egg, 2% milk	1/6 recipe	150	4.0	23.0	220	(mq)	5.0	45
OAT BRAN								
(Arrowhead Mills) apple spice, prepared	1 muffin	120	6.0	15.0	(mq)	5.4	4.0	na
(General Mills) prepared	1 muffin	170	3.0	26.0	230	na	6.0	0
(Krusteaz) prepared	1 muffin	190	3.0	33.0	310	4.0	5.0	0
(Hain) apple cinnamon, prepared	1 muffin	140	4.0	28.0	200	5.0	3.0	0
(Hain) banana nut, prepared	1 muffin	140	4.0	26.0	190	4.0	4.0	0

Food Name	Serv. Size	Total Cal.	Prot. GMS	Carbs GMS	Sod. MGS	Fiber GMS	Fat GMS	Chol. MGS
(Hain) raspberry spice, prepared ..... 1 muffin		140	5.0	27.0	190	4.0	3.0	0
OATMEAL RAISIN								
(Arrowhead Mills) wheat-free, prepared	1 muffin	100	5.0	11.0	na	4.5	5.0	(mq)
(Betty Crocker) prepared w/egg,								
2% milk .... 1/8 recipe		190	4.0	25.0	240	(mq)	8.0	35
(Betty Crocker) prepared w/egg white,								
skim milk .... 1/8 recipe		180	4.0	25.0	240	(mq)	7.0	0
(General Mills) prepared w/egg,								
1/2 cup 2% milk .... 1 muffin		180	4.0	26.0	250	na	7.0	35
(General Mills) prepared w/egg white,								
skim milk .... 1 muffin		170	4.0	26.0	260	na	6.0	0
ORANGEBERRY								
(Martha White) prepared .... 1/6 recipe		140	2.0	25.0	220	(mq)	3.0	2
(Martha White) prepared w/2% milk ... 1 muffin		140	2.0	25.0	220	na	3.0	2
PECAN CRUNCH (Duncan Hines)								
'Bakery Style' prepared .... 1 muffin		220	3.0	27.0	250	(mq)	11.0	na
RASPBERRY								
(Martha White) prepared .... 1/6 recipe		140	2.0	25.0	184	(mq)	3.0	3
(Martha White) prepared w/2% milk ... 1 muffin		140	2.0	25.0	180	na	3.0	2
STRAWBERRY								
(Arrowhead Mills) wheat bran,								
prepared .... 2 muffins		270	10.0	43.0	(mq)	10.5	7.0	na
(Betty Crocker) prepared w/egg,								
2% milk .... 1/10 recipe		150	2.0	24.0	170	(mq)	5.0	25
(Betty Crocker) prepared w/egg white,								
skim milk .... 1/10 recipe		140	2.0	24.0	170	(mq)	4.0	0
(Martha White) prepared .... 1/6 recipe		140	2.0	25.0	270	(mq)	3.0	3
(Martha White) prepared w/2% milk ... 1 muffin		140	2.0	25.0	270	na	3.0	2
WILD BERRY								
(General Mills) 'Light' prepared ...... 1 muffin		90	1.0	20.0	140	na	<1.0	0
(General Mills) 'Light' prepared w/egg .. 1 muffin		90	2.0	20.0	140	na	1.0	20
(General Mills) prepared .... 1 muffin		100	1.0	18.0	140	na	3.0	0
(General Mills) prepared w/egg, 1/2 cup								
2% milk .... 1 muffin		120	2.0	19.0	150	na	4.0	20
(General Mills) prepared w/egg white,								
skim milk .... 1 muffin		110	2.0	19.0	150	na	3.0	0
MUFFIN/PASTRY, TOASTER								
APPLE								
(Kellogg's) Dutch, 'Frosted Pop-Tarts'								
1.8 oz each .... 1 pastry		210	2.0	37.0	200	0	6.0	0
(Pastry Poppers) fruit juice sweetened,								
low-sodium, 2 oz each .... 1 pastry		212	2.9	38.0	115	na	5.4	na
(Pillsbury) 'Toaster Strudel' .... 1/6 pkg		200	3.0	26.0	190	na	9.0	5

Food Name	Serv. Size	Total Cal.	Prot. GMS	Carbs GMS	Sod. MGS	Fiber GMS	Fat GMS	Chol. MGS
(Toastettes) 'Frosted Tarts' 1.5 oz each	1 pastry	190	2.0	35.0	170	1.0	5.0	0
(Toastettes) 'Tarts' 1.5 oz each	1 pastry	190	2.0	36.0	170	1.0	5.0	0
APPLE SPICE, *(Toaster)* 'Muffins'	1 muffin	130	2.0	21.0	100	(mq)	5.0	na
APPLE-CINNAMON								
(Pepperidge Farm) 'Croissant Toaster Tarts'	1 pastry	170	3.0	25.0	120	(mq)	7.0	0
BANANA NUT								
(Pastry Poppers) fruit juice sweetened, low-sodium, 2 oz each	1 pastry	212	2.5	38.0	115	na	4.5	na
(Thomas') 'Toast-r-Cakes'	1 muffin	111	1.7	16.7	192	.6	4.4	10
(Toaster) 'Muffins'	1 muffin	130	2.0	19.0	85	(mq)	6.0	na
(Toaster) 'Strudel Breakfast Pastries'	1 pastry	190	2.0	28.0	190	(mq)	8.0	na
BLUEBERRY								
(Kellogg's) 'Frosted Pop-Tarts' 1.8 oz each	1 pastry	210	2.0	37.0	210	0	6.0	0
(Kellogg's) 'Pop-Tarts' 1.8 oz each	1 pastry	210	2.0	37.0	210	0	6.0	0
(Pillsbury) 'Toaster Strudel'	1/6 pkg	190	3.0	26.0	210	na	9.0	5
(Thomas') 'Toast-r-Cakes'	1 muffin	108	1.6	18.0	158	(mq)	3.3	na
(Toaster) 'Strudel Breakfast Pastries'	1 pastry	190	2.0	28.0	200	(mq)	8.0	na
(Toaster) wild, Maine	1 muffin	120	2.0	23.0	135	(mq)	3.0	na
(Toastettes) 'Frosted Tarts' 1.5 oz each	1 pastry	190	2.0	35.0	200	1.0	5.0	0
(Toastettes) 'Tarts' 1.5 oz each	1 pastry	190	2.0	35.0	200	1.0	5.0	0
BRAN *(Thomas')* 'Toast-r-Cakes'	1 muffin	103	1.7	17.6	163	(mq)	2.9	na
BROWN SUGAR-CINNAMON								
(Kellogg's) 'Frosted Pop-Tarts'	1 pastry	210	3.0	34.0	180	0	7.0	0
(Toastettes) 'Frosted Tarts' 1.5 oz each	1 pastry	190	2.0	35.0	180	1.0	5.0	0
(Kellogg's) 'Pop-Tarts' 1.8 oz each	1 pastry	210	3.0	33.0	210	0	8.0	0
CHEESE *(Pepperidge Farm)* 'Croissant Toaster Tarts'	1 pastry	190	5.0	22.0	180	(mq)	10.0	10
CHERRY								
(Kellogg's) 'Frosted Pop-Tarts' 1.8 oz each	1 pastry	200	2.0	37.0	220	0	5.0	0
(Kellogg's) 'Pop-Tarts' 1.8 oz each	1 pastry	210	2.0	37.0	220	0	6.0	0
(Pastry Poppers) fruit juice sweetened, low-sodium, 2 oz each	1 pastry	212	2.5	38.0	115	na	4.5	na
(Toaster) 'Strudel Breakfast Pastries'	1 pastry	190	2.0	26.0	200	(mq)	9.0	na
(Toastettes) 'Frosted Tarts' 1.5 oz each	1 pastry	190	2.0	35.0	200	1.0	5.0	0
(Toastettes) 'Tarts' 1.5 oz each	1 pastry	190	2.0	35.0	200	1.0	5.0	0
CHOCOLATE FUDGE								
(Kellogg's) 'Frosted Pop-Tarts' 1.8 oz each	1 pastry	200	3.0	37.0	220	0	5.0	0

Food Name	Serv. Size	Total Cal.	Prot. GMS	Carbs GMS	Sod. MGS	Fiber GMS	Fat GMS	Chol. MGS
CHOCOLATE-VANILLA CREME								
(Kellogg's) 'Frosted Pop-Tarts'								
1.8 oz each .... 1 pastry		200	3.0	37.0	230	0	5.0	0
CINNAMON								
(Pillsbury) 'Toaster Strudel' .... 1/6 pkg		200	5.0	23.0	200	na	10.0	5
(Toaster) 'Strudel Breakfast Pastries' .. 1 pastry		190	2.0	26.0	200	(mq)	8.0	na
CORN								
(Thomas') 'Toast-r-Cakes' .... 1 muffin		120	1.8	19.2	142	(mq)	4.0	na
(Toaster) 'Old Fashioned Muffins' ..... 1 muffin		120	2.0	17.0	200	(mq)	5.0	na
FRUIT PUNCH *(Toastettes)* 'Frosted Tarts'								
1.5 oz each .... 1 pastry		190	2.0	35.0	200	1.0	5.0	0
FUDGE *(Toastettes)* 'Frosted Tarts'								
1.5 oz each .... 1 pastry		200	2.0	34.0	280	1.0	5.0	0
GRAPE *(Kellogg's)* 'Frosted Pop-Tarts'								
1.8 oz each .... 1 pastry		200	2.0	37.0	200	0	5.0	200
OAT BRAN *(Awrey's)* 'Toastums'								
w/raisins .... 1 muffin		130	3.0	17.0	310	1.0	5.0	0
PEACH-APRICOT *(Pastry Poppers)* fruit juice								
sweetened, low-sodium, 2 oz each ... 1 pastry		212	2.5	38.0	115	na	4.5	na
RAISIN BRAN *(Toaster)* 'Muffins' ...... 1 muffin		120	3.0	16.0	220	(mq)	5.0	na
RASPBERRY								
(Kellogg's) 'Frosted Pop-Tarts'								
1.8 oz each .... 1 pastry		200	2.0	37.0	210	0	5.0	0
(Pastry Poppers) fruit juice sweetened,								
low-sodium, 2 oz each .... 1 pastry		212	2.5	38.0	115	na	4.5	na
(Toaster) 'Strudel Breakfast Pastries' .. 1 pastry		190	2.0	27.0	200	(mq)	8.0	na
STRAWBERRY								
(Kellogg's) 'Frosted Pop-Tarts'								
1.8 oz each .... 1 pastry		200	2.0	37.0	190	0	5.0	0
(Kellogg's) 'Pop-Tarts' 1.8 oz each ..... 1 pastry		210	2.0	37.0	200	0	6.0	0
(Pastry Poppers) fruit juice sweetened,								
low-sodium, 2 oz each .... 1 pastry		212	2.5	38.0	115	na	4.5	na
(Pepperidge Farm) 'Croissant Toaster								
Tarts' .... 1 pastry		190	3.0	28.0	120	(mq)	7.0	0
(Pillsbury) 'Toaster Strudel' .... 1/6 pkg		190	3.0	26.0	200	na	9.0	5
(Toaster) 'Strudel Breakfast Pastries' .. 1 pastry		190	2.0	27.0	200	(mq)	8.0	na
(Toastettes) 'Frosted Tarts' 1.5 oz each	1 pastry	190	2.0	35.0	200	1.0	5.0	0
(Toastettes) 'Tarts' 1.5 oz each ...... 1 pastry		190	2.0	35.0	200	1.0	5.0	0
MULBERRY								
raw .... 1 lb		197	6.5	44.5	46	>4.4 c	1.8	0
raw .... 1 cup		60	2.0	13.7	14	2.4	0.6	0
raw .... 1/2 cup		31	1.0	6.9	7	1.2	0.3	0
raw .... 1 oz		12	0.4	2.8	3	>.3 c	0.1	0

Food Name	Serv. Size	Total Cal.	Prot. GMS	Carbs GMS	Sod. MGS	Fiber GMS	Fat GMS	Chol. MGS
MULLANGI. See DAIKON.								
MULLET, STRIPED								
baked	4 oz	170	28.1	0.0	81	0	5.5	71
broiled	4 oz	170	28.1	0.0	81	0	5.5	71
dry-heat cooked	3 oz	127	21.1	0.0	60	0	4.1	54
microwaved	4 oz	170	28.1	0.0	81	0	5.5	71
raw	1 lb	530	87.8	0.0	294	0	17.2	224
raw	3 oz	99	16.5	0.0	55	0	3.2	42
raw	1 oz	33	5.5	0.0	18	0	1.1	14
MUNG BEAN								
boiled	4 oz	119	8.0	21.7	2	2.8	0.4	0
boiled	1/2 cup	106	7.1	19.3	2	7.7	0.4	0
raw	1/2 cup	361	24.8	65.1	16	17.0	1.2	0
raw	1 oz	98	6.8	17.8	4	2.7	0.3	0
sprouted, boiled, drained	4 oz	24	2.3	4.8	11	>.6 c	0.1	0
sprouted, boiled, drained	1/2 cup	13	1.3	2.6	6	.5	0.1	0
sprouted, raw	1 lb	136	13.8	26.9	26	5.0	0.8	0
sprouted, raw	1/2 cup	16	1.6	3.1	3	.9	0.1	0
sprouted, raw	1 oz	9	0.9	1.7	2	.3	0.1	0
sprouted, stir-fried	4 oz	57	4.9	12.0	(mq)	>.8 c	0.2	0
sprouted, stir-fried	1/2 cup	31	2.7	6.6	6	>.4 c	0.1	0
MUNG BEAN, CANNED								
drained	4 oz	14	1.6	2.4	(mq)	>.3 c	0.1	0
sprouted (LaChoy)	2 oz	8	0.8	1.0	20	.7	0.1	0
sprouted, drained	1/2 cup	7	0.9	1.3	87	.5	0.0	0
MUNG BEAN LONG RICE								
dehydrated	1/2 cup	246	0.1	60.3	7	.4	0.0	0
dehydrated	1 oz	99	<.1	24.4	3	tr	tr	0
MUNGO BEAN								
boiled	1/2 cup	94	6.8	16.5	6	5.8	0.5	0
raw	1/2 cup	365	26.1	63.5	27	>4.6 c	1.9	0
MUSHROOM, ENOKI								
raw	1 large	2	0.1	0.4	0	na	0.0	0
raw	1 med	1	0.1	0.2	0	na	0.0	0
MUSHROOM, JAPANESE HONEY/hon shimeji								
trimmed	1 lb	136	9.5	20.0	(mq)	(mq)	1.4	0
trimmed	1 oz	9	0.6	1.2	(mq)	(mq)	<.1	0
MUSHROOM, OYSTER/abalone/hiritake/shimeji/tree mushroom								
(Frieda's)	1 lb	113	9.5	20.9	18	3.6	1.8	0
(Frieda's)	1 oz	7	0.6	1.3	1	.2	0.1	0
MUSHROOM, SHIITAKE								
cooked	4 oz	62	1.8	16.2	5	>2.2 c	0.2	0
cooked, pieces	1 cup	80	2.3	20.7	6	3.0	0.3	0

Food Name	Serv. Size	Total Cal.	Prot. GMS	Carbs GMS	Sod. MGS	Fiber GMS	Fat GMS	Chol. MGS
dried	1 lb	1343	43.5	341.9	60	>52.2 c	4.5	0
dried	1 oz	84	2.7	21.4	4	>3.3 c	0.3	0
MUSHROOM, STRAW								
(Green Giant) canned	2 oz	12	1.0	2.0	290	1.0	0.0	0
(Green Giant) canned, whole	1/4 cup	12	1.0	2.0	290	1.0	0.0	0
MUSHROOM, WHITE								
boiled, drained	4 oz	31	2.5	5.8	2	2.5	0.5	0
boiled, drained, pieces	1/2 cup	21	1.7	4.0	2	1.7	0.4	0
raw, pieces	1/2 cup	9	0.7	1.6	1	.5	0.2	0
raw, trimmed	1 oz	7	0.6	1.3	1	.4	0.1	0
raw, untrimmed	1 lb	111	9.2	20.5	16	5.7	1.9	0
Canned								
drained	4 oz	27	2.1	5.6	(mq)	(mq)	0.3	0
pieces, drained	1/2 cup	19	1.5	3.9	331	1.9	0.2	0
(Allens) pieces and stems	1/2 cup	20	2.0	3.0	450	(mq)	<1.0	0
(B In B)	1/4 cup	12	1.0	2.0	240	1.0	0.0	0
(B In B) w/garlic	1/4 cup	12	1.0	2.0	200	1.0	0.0	0
(Empress) pieces and stems	2 oz	14	1.0	2.0	260	(mq)	na	0
(Green Giant) in butter sauce	1/2 cup	30	2.0	4.0	330	.6	1.0	na
(Green Giant) whole, pieces, and stems	1/4 cup	12	1.0	2.0	220	1.0	0.0	0
Frozen								
(Birds Eye) whole 'Deluxe'	2.6 oz	20	2.0	4.0	0	2.0	0.0	0
(Freshlike)	3.5 oz	30	3.0	4.0	15	na	0.0	na
(Green Giant) creamy 'Right for Lunch'	9.5-oz pkg	220	6.0	29.0	860	4.0	11.0	25
(Stilwell) battered 'Quick Krisp'	2 oz	140	2.0	15.0	280	(mq)	8.0	5
(Veg•All)	3.5 oz	30	3.0	4.0	15	na	0.0	na
MUSKMELON. See CANTALOUPE.								
MUSKRAT								
raw	1 lb	735	94.2	0.0	372	na	36.7	na
raw	1 oz	45	5.8	0.0	23	na	2.3	na
roasted	3 oz	199	25.6	0.0	81	0	10.0	103
roasted, diced	1 cup	258	33.0	0.0	105	0	12.9	(mq)
MUSSEL, BLUE								
moist-heat cooked	4 oz	195	27.0	8.4	418	0	5.1	64
moist-heat cooked	3 oz	146	20.2	6.3	314	0	3.8	48
raw	1 lb	391	54.0	16.8	1296	0	10.2	127
raw	1 cup	129	17.8	5.5	429	0	3.4	42
raw	3 oz	73	10.1	3.1	243	0	1.9	24
MUSTARD, DRY. See MUSTARD POWDER.								
MUSTARD, PREPARED								
(Featherweight)	1 tsp	5	0.0	0.0	0	0	0.0	0
(French's) 'Medford'	1 tbsp	16	1.0	1.0	240	na	1.0	0

Food Name	Serv. Size	Total Cal.	Prot. GMS	Carbs GMS	Sod. MGS	Fiber GMS	Fat GMS	Chol. MGS
(Grey Poupon) 'Parisian'	1 tsp	6	0.0	0.0	55	0	0.0	0
(Kraft) 'Pure'	1 tbsp	11	0.0	1.0	160	0	1.0	0
(Life) 'English All Natural'	1 tbsp	22	2.0	<1.0	2	na	2.0	0
(Westbrae) 'Mt. Fuji'	1 tbsp	16	1.0	1.0	195	na	1.0	0
DIJON								
(French's)	1 tsp	8	0.0	0.0	140	0	1.0	0
(Grey Poupon)	1 tbsp	18	0.0	0.0	450	0	1.0	0
(Grey Poupon) 'Country Style'	1 tsp	6	0.0	0.0	120	0	0.0	0
(Westbrae)	1 tbsp	16	1.0	1.0	195	na	1.0	0
HORSERADISH								
(French's)	1 tbsp	16	1.0	1.0	265	na	1.0	0
(Kraft)	1 tbsp	14	1.0	1.0	135	0	1.0	0
JALAPEÑO (Great Impressions)	2 tsp	7	0.4	0.7	173	na	0.3	0
ONION (French's)	1 tsp	8	0.0	2.0	70	na	0.0	0
SPICY								
(French's) 'Bold 'n Spicy'	1 tsp	6	0.0	0.0	50	na	0.0	0
(Gulden's) hot, 'Diablo'	.25 oz	8	0.0	0.0	55	0	0.0	0
(Gulden's) 'Spicy Brown'	.25 oz	8	0.0	0.0	45	0	0.0	0
(Heinz) 'Brown'	1 tbsp	14	<1.0	1.0	115	na	1.0	0
STONE GROUND								
(Hain)	1 tbsp	14	1.0	1.0	185	na	1.0	0
(Hain) no salt added	1 tbsp	14	1.0	1.0	10	na	1.0	0
(Westbrae)	1 tbsp	16	1.0	1.0	195	na	1.0	0
(Westbrae) no salt added	1 tbsp	16	1.0	1.0	195	na	1.0	0
YELLOW								
(French's)	1 tbsp	10	1.0	1.0	180	na	1.0	0
(Gulden's) 'Creamy Mild'	.25 oz	6	0.0	0.0	60	0	0.0	0
(Heinz)	1 tsp	3	0.2	0.2	55	na	0.2	0
(Heinz) 'Mild'	1 tbsp	8	1.0	1.0	175	na	1.0	0
(Westbrae)	1 tbsp	16	1.0	1.0	195	na	1.0	0
MUSTARD BLEND (Best Foods)								
'Dijonnaise'	1 tsp	12	0.0	1.0	70	na	1.0	0
MUSTARD GREENS								
boiled, drained	4 oz	17	2.6	2.4	18	>.8 c	0.3	0
boiled, drained, chopped	1/2 cup	10	1.6	1.5	11	1.4	0.2	0
raw, chopped	1/2 cup	7	0.8	1.4	7	.6	0.1	0
raw, untrimmed	1 lb	109	11.4	20.7	107	2.5	0.8	0
Canned (Allens) chopped	1/2 cup	20	1.0	2.0	35	(mq)	<1.0	0
Frozen								
boiled, drained	10-oz pkg	40	4.8	6.6	53	>1.5 c	0.5	0
boiled, drained	4 oz	22	2.6	3.5	28	>.8 c	0.3	0
boiled, drained, chopped	1/2 cup	14	1.7	2.3	19	>.6 c	0.2	0
chopped	1/2 cup	15	1.8	2.5	21	1.5	0.2	0

Food Name	Serv. Size	Total Cal.	Prot. GMS	Carbs GMS	Sod. MGS	Fiber GMS	Fat GMS	Chol. MGS
unprepared	10-oz pkg	57	7.1	9.7	82	>2.3 c	0.8	0
(Frosty Acres)	3.3 oz	20	2.0	3.0	20	>1.0 c	0.0	0
(Seabrook) chopped	3.3 oz	20	2.0	3.0	20	>1.0 c	0.0	0
(Southern) chopped	3.5 oz	25	2.5	3.6	40	(mq)	0.3	0
MUSTARD OIL								
	1 cup	1927	0.0	0.0	0	0	218.0	na
	1 oz	251	0.0	0.0	0	0	28.4	0
	1 tbsp	124	0.0	0.0	0	0	14.0	na
MUSTARD POWDER								
ground *(Durkee)*	1 tsp	19	0.0	0.0	0	0	<0.1	na
ground *(Laurel Leaf)*	1 tsp	19	0.0	0.0	0	0	<0.1	na
ground *(Spice Islands)*	1 tsp	9	0.5	0.3	<1	<.1	0.6	0
MUSTARD SEED, YELLOW								
whole	1 oz	133	7.1	9.9	1	>1.9 c	8.2	0
whole	1 tbsp	53	2.8	3.9	1	>.7 c	3.2	0
whole	1 tsp	15	0.8	1.1	0	>.2 c	1.0	0
MUSTARD SPINACH/tendergreen								
boiled, drained	4 oz	18	1.9	3.2	(mq)	>.9 c	0.2	0
boiled, drained, chopped	1/2 cup	14	1.5	2.5	13	>.7 c	0.2	0
raw, chopped	1/2 cup	16	1.6	2.9	16	>.8 c	0.2	0
raw, trimmed	1 oz	6	0.6	1.1	(mq)	>.3 c	0.1	0
raw, untrimmed	1 lb	93	9.3	16.5	(mq)	>4.2 c	1.3	0
MUSTARD TALLOW	1 oz	256	0.0	0.0	0	0	28.4	29
MUTTON TALLOW								
	1 cup	1849	0.0	0.0	0	0	205.0	209
	1 tbsp	115	0.0	0.0	0	0	12.8	13

MUTTONFISH. See OCEAN POUT.

N

Food Name	Serv. Size	Total Cal.	Prot. GMS	Carbs GMS	Sod. MGS	Fiber GMS	Fat GMS	Chol. MGS
NACHO CHIPS. See CORN CHIPS AND SNACKS.								
NACHO SEASONING *(Lawry's)*								
'Seasoning Blends'	1 pkg	141	6.7	15.0	2168	>1.6 c	6.8	na
NAPA CABBAGE. See CABBAGE, NAPA.								
NATAL PLUM. See CARISSA.								
NATTO. See SOYBEAN, FERMENTED.								
NAVY BEAN								
boiled	4 oz	161	9.9	29.8	1	4.1	0.6	0
boiled	1/2 cup	129	7.9	23.9	1	>2.9 c	0.5	0
cooked 'Michigan #1' *(A&P)*	1 cup	220	15.0	40.0	15	(mq)	1.0	0
raw	1/2 cup	348	23.2	63.1	15	25.0	1.3	0

Food Name	Serv. Size	Total Cal.	Prot. GMS	Carbs GMS	Sod. MGS	Fiber GMS	Fat GMS	Chol. MGS
raw	1 oz	95	6.3	17.2	4	2.7	0.4	0
NAVY BEAN, CANNED								
(Allens)	1/2 cup	160	8.0	24.0	440	(mq)	<1.0	0
(Bush's Best)	1/2 cup	60	5.0	17.0	370	7.0	0.0	na
(Eden Foods) organic, very low sodium	1/2 cup	70	6.0	18.0	15	7.0	<1.0	0
(Hunt's) w/ham 'Homestyle'	9.03 oz	239	16.2	37.6	737	10.0	2.7	10
NAVY BEAN, SPROUTED								
boiled, drained	4 oz	88	8.0	17.0	(mq)	>3.3 c	0.9	0
raw	1 lb	306	27.9	59.2	(mq)	>11.3 c	3.2	0
raw	1/2 cup	35	3.2	6.8	7	>1.3 c	0.4	0
raw	1 oz	19	1.7	3.7	(mq)	>.7 c	0.2	0
NECTAR. See individual flavors.								
NECTARINE								
pitted	1 oz	14	0.3	3.3	tr	.5	0.1	0
sliced	1 cup	68	1.3	16.3	0	2.2	0.6	0
trimmed, approx 2.5-inch diam	1 med	67	1.3	16.0	0	2.2	0.6	0
untrimmed (Dole)	1 med	70	1.0	16.0	0	3.0	1.0	na
whole	1 lb	204	3.9	48.6	1	6.6	1.9	0
NEW ZEALAND SPINACH. See SPINACH, NEW ZEALAND.								
NOODLE. See NOODLE, CHINESE; NOODLE, EGG; NOODLE, JAPANESE; PASTA.								
NOODLE, CHINESE								
cellophane, dehydrated	1 lb	1594	0.7	390.6	44	>.3 c	0.3	0
cellophane, dehydrated	2 oz	199	0.1	48.8	6	<.1	<.1	0
chow mein	1 cup	237	3.8	25.9	198	1.8	13.8	0
chow mein	1.5 oz	227	3.6	24.7	189	1.7	13.2	0
long rice, dehydrated	1 lb	1594	0.7	390.6	44	>.3 c	0.3	0
long rice, dehydrated	2 oz	199	0.1	48.8	6	<.1	<.1	0
NOODLE, EGG								
(NOTE: All of the following egg noodles are dry unless otherwise noted.)								
DUMPLING (Creamette) w/pasteurized eggs	2 oz	220	8.0	40.0	20	na	3.0	70
ENRICHED								
	2 oz	217	8.0	40.5	12	1.8	2.4	54
cooked	1 cup	213	7.6	39.7	11	1.5	2.3	53
EXTRA WIDE (American Beauty) enriched	2 oz	220	8.0	42.0	15	na	3.0	55
FINE								
(American Beauty) enriched	2 oz	220	8.0	42.0	15	na	3.0	55
(Herb's)	2 oz	230	10.0	40.0	5	na	2.0	60
JERUSALEM ARTICHOKE								
(De Boles)	2 oz	210	9.0	41.0	0	na	1.0	0
(De Boles) w/garlic and parsley	2 oz	210	9.0	41.0	15	na	1.0	0
MEDIUM (American Beauty) enriched	2 oz	220	8.0	42.0	15	na	3.0	55
PLAIN								
cooked	4 oz	151	5.4	28.2	8	2.5	1.7	37

Food Name	Serv. Size	Total Cal.	Prot. GMS	Carbs GMS	Sod. MGS	Fiber GMS	Fat GMS	Chol. MGS
(Creamette) enriched	2 oz	221	8.0	40.0	3	.8	2.5	70
(Gioia)	2 oz	220	8.0	40.0	(mq)	(mq)	3.0	(mq)
(Golden Grain)	2 oz	210	8.2	39.3	10	1.8	2.2	65
(Goodman's) 'Country Style'	2 oz	220	8.0	40.0	15	(mq)	3.0	(mq)
(Mrs. Grass)	2 oz	220	8.0	40.0	200	(mq)	3.0	(mq)
(Mueller's)	2 oz	220	8.0	40.0	10	(mq)	3.0	55
(P&R)	2 oz	220	8.0	42.0	15	(mq)	3.0	(mq)
(Prince)	2 oz	210	8.0	40.0	35	(mq)	2.0	65
(San Giorgio)	2 oz	220	8.0	42.0	15	(mq)	3.0	(mq)
SPINACH								
cooked	4 oz	150	5.7	27.5	14	(mq)	1.8	37
enriched	1 cup	145	5.6	26.7	27	2.6	1.7	36
enriched	2 oz	218	8.3	40.1	41	3.9	2.6	54
enriched, cooked	1 cup	211	8.1	38.8	19	3.7	2.5	53
SUBSTITUTE *(No Yolks)* broad	2 oz	200	8.0	40.0	25	na	1.0	0
UNENRICHED								
	2 oz	74	1.5	16.1	218	.2	0.2	0
cooked	1 cup	213	7.6	39.7	11	1.8	2.3	53
VERY LOW SODIUM *(Ronzoni)*								
'Egg Pastina'	2 oz	220	8.0	42.0	15	na	3.0	65
WIDE								
(American Beauty) enriched	2 oz	220	8.0	42.0	15	na	3.0	55
(Creamette) w/pasteurized eggs 'Fancy'	2 oz	220	8.0	40.0	20	na	3.0	70
(Hospitality) enriched 'Valu Pack'	1 1/4 cup	235	9.0	43.0	5	2.0	2.5	80
(Ronzoni) enriched 'Country Kitchen Style'	2 oz	220	8.0	42.0	15	na	3.0	65
NOODLE, JAPANESE								
GENMAI, dry *(Westbrae)*	2 oz	200	5.0	41.0	411	na	1.0	0
SOBA/BUCKWHEAT								
cooked	1 cup	113	5.8	24.4	68	>.4 c	0.1	0
dry	1 lb	1526	65.2	338.5	3593	(mq)	3.2	0
dry	2 oz	192	8.2	42.5	451	>.7 c	0.4	0
dry *(Westbrae)*	2 oz	190	7.0	40.0	5	na	2.0	0
SOMEN/WHEAT								
cooked	1 cup	231	7.0	48.5	283	>.4 c	0.3	0
cooked	4 oz	149	4.5	31.2	183	>.3 c	0.2	0
dry	2 oz	203	6.5	42.2	1049	2.5	0.5	0
whole wheat, dry *(Westbrae)*	2 oz	200	7.0	41.0	375	na	1.0	0
TRADITIONAL, dry *(Westbrae)*	2 oz	190	7.0	41.0	198	na	2.0	0
UDON/WHEAT								
cooked	4 oz	115	2.8	23.0	51	(mq)	0.6	0
dry	2 oz	159	3.9	32.3	340	(mq)	0.7	0
whole wheat, organic, dry *(Westbrae)*	2 oz	200	7.0	41.0	375	na	1.0	0

Food Name	Serv. Size	Total Cal.	Prot. GMS	Carbs GMS	Sod. MGS	Fiber GMS	Fat GMS	Chol. MGS
NOODLE ENTRÉE/DISH								
(Dinty Moore)								
and chicken 'American Classics'	10 oz	230	17.0	24.0	1020	na	7.0	65
tuna casserole 'American Classics'	10 oz	240	16.0	28.0	1280	na	7.0	65
(LaChoy)								
and beef	9.03 oz	156	7.4	26.8	1332	2.9	3.5	6
and chicken	8.995 oz	163	10.2	24.4	859	1.4	3.3	19
and vegetables	9.383 oz	131	4.8	26.6	1311	2.9	1.3	0
chow mein	2 tbsp	140	4.5	17.0	209	1.9	6.1	0
chow mein, narrow	1/2 cup	150	3.0	16.0	230	<1.0	8.0	0
chow mein, wide	1/2 cup	150	3.0	16.0	300	<1.0	8.0	0
crispy, wide	2 tbsp	148	2.3	17.1	258	1.1	7.8	0
rice	1/2 cup	130	2.0	21.0	420	<1.0	5.0	0
rice	2 tbsp	122	2.1	21.9	362	.4	3.1	0
(Westbrae)								
brown rice, steamed 'Ramen'	1 oz	100	3.0	21.0	500	na	1.0	0
buckwheat, steamed 'Ramen'	1 oz	100	3.0	20.0	500	na	0.0	0
carrot, steamed 'Ramen'	1 oz	100	3.0	20.0	460	na	1.0	0
curry, steamed 'Ramen'	1 oz	100	3.0	20.0	420	na	1.0	0
five-spice, steamed 'Ramen'	1 oz	100	3.0	20.0	420	na	1.0	0
miso, steamed 'Ramen'	1 oz	100	3.0	20.0	540	na	1.0	0
mushroom, steamed 'Ramen'	1 oz	100	3.0	20.0	340	na	1.0	0
onion, steamed 'Ramen'	1 oz	100	3.0	20.0	460	na	1.0	0
seaweed, steamed 'Ramen'	1 oz	100	3.0	20.0	460	na	1.0	0
spinach, steamed 'Ramen'	1 oz	100	3.0	20.0	460	na	1.0	0
tofu, steamed 'Ramen'	1 oz	100	3.0	20.0	460	na	1.0	0
whole wheat, steamed 'Ramen'	1 oz	110	3.0	22.0	480	na	1.0	0
NOODLE ENTRÉE/DISH, CANNED								
(Heinz)								
and chicken	7.5 oz	160	6.0	19.0	930	(mq)	7.0	(mq)
w/beef, in sauce	7.5 oz	170	8.0	17.0	825	(mq)	8.0	(mq)
w/tuna	7.5 oz	170	11.0	20.0	950	(mq)	5.0	(mq)
(Nalley's)								
and chicken	7 3/8 oz	150	9.0	17.0	1000	(mq)	5.0	(mq)
and chicken w/vegetables	7 3/8 oz	160	10.0	18.0	1450	(mq)	5.0	(mq)
(Van Camp's) w/franks 'Noodle Weenee'	1 cup	245	9.3	32.9	1245	>5.0 c	8.5	(mq)
NOODLE ENTRÉE/DISH, FREEZE-DRIED								
(Mountain House) w/chicken, prepared	1 cup	270	10.0	34.0	201	(mq)	10.0	(mq)
NOODLE ENTRÉE/DISH, FROZEN								
(Banquet)								
and beef w/gravy 'Family Entrées'	8 oz	200	13.0	22.0	(mq)	(mq)	7.0	(mq)
and julienne beef w/sauce 'Family Entrées'	7 oz	170	12.0	22.0	(mq)	(mq)	3.0	(mq)
w/chicken	10 oz	350	10.0	42.0	460	(mq)	15.0	45

Food Name	Serv. Size	Total Cal.	Prot. GMS	Carbs GMS	Sod. MGS	Fiber GMS	Fat GMS	Chol. MGS
w/chicken 'Family Favorites'	10 oz	340	11.0	42.0	455	(mq)	15.0	45
(Stouffer's) Romanoff	6 oz	260	11.0	23.0	1260	na	14.0	na
(Swanson) w/chicken	10.5 oz	280	7.0	45.0	740	(mq)	8.0	(mq)
NOODLE ENTRÉE/DISH, MICROWAVE								
(Hormel) and chicken 'Micro-Cup'	7.5 oz	180	7.0	18.0	1000	(mq)	8.0	20
(Kid's Kitchen) rings and chicken	7.5 oz	150	11.0	17.0	840	na	4.0	25
(Minute)								
Alfredo, family size, prepared w/salted butter	1/2 cup	170	7.0	23.0	670	(mq)	6.0	45
Alfredo, single size, prepared w/salted butter	1/2 cup	160	7.0	23.0	660	(mq)	5.0	40
chicken or chicken flavor, family size, prepared	1/2 cup	160	6.0	23.0	570	(mq)	5.0	35
chicken or chicken flavor, single size, prepared	1/2 cup	160	6.0	25.0	610	(mq)	4.0	35
Parmesan, family size, prepared w/salted butter	1/2 cup	170	6.0	23.0	470	(mq)	6.0	45
Parmesan, single size, prepared w/salted butter	1/2 cup	160	6.0	23.0	460	(mq)	5.0	40
w/cheddar cheese, family size, prepared w/salted butter	1/2 cup	160	6.0	20.0	530	na	7.0	15
w/cheddar cheese, single size, prepared w/salted butter	1/2 cup	160	6.0	20.0	520	na	6.0	15
NOODLE ENTRÉE/DISH, MIX								
(Kraft)								
cheese 'Dinner' prepared	3/4 cup	340	10.0	37.0	670	(mq)	17.0	50
chicken flavor 'Dinner' prepared	3/4 cup	240	8.0	32.0	1050	(mq)	9.0	45
(LaChoy)								
beef flavor 'Ramen' prepared	1 cup	225	6.0	33.0	865	4.0	8.0	0
chicken flavor 'Ramen' prepared	1 cup	200	6.0	29.0	740	4.0	7.0	0
(Lipton)								
Alfredo 'Noodles and Sauce' dry mix ...	1/4 pkg	150	6.0	22.0	510	(mq)	4.0	(mq)
beef 'Noodles and Sauce' dry mix	1/4 pkg	120	5.0	23.0	640	(mq)	2.0	(mq)
broccoli 'Noodles and Sauce' dry mix ...	1/4 pkg	130	5.0	22.0	430	(mq)	2.0	(mq)
butter 'Noodles and Sauce' dry mix	1/4 pkg	150	6.0	23.0	450	(mq)	4.0	(mq)
butter and herb 'Noodles and Sauce' dry mix	1/4 pkg	140	5.0	23.0	460	(mq)	3.0	(mq)
carbonara Alfredo 'Noodles and Sauce' dry mix	1/4 pkg	140	5.0	20.0	460	(mq)	4.0	(mq)
cheese 'Noodles and Sauce' dry mix ...	1/4 pkg	140	5.0	25.0	470	(mq)	2.0	(mq)
chicken flavor 'Noodles and Sauce' dry mix	1/4 pkg	130	5.0	23.0	390	(mq)	2.0	(mq)
Parmesan 'Noodles and Sauce' dry mix	1/4 pkg	140	6.0	21.0	410	(mq)	4.0	(mq)

Food Name	Serv. Size	Total Cal.	Prot. GMS	Carbs GMS	Sod. MGS	Fiber GMS	Fat GMS	Chol. MGS
sour cream and chives 'Noodles and								
Sauce' dry mix	1/4 pkg	150	5.0	24.0	440	(mq)	3.0	(mq)
Stroganoff 'Noodles and Sauce' dry mix	1/4 pkg	130	6.0	22.0	330	(mq)	3.0	(mq)
(Mueller's)								
Alfredo 'Chef's Series' prepared	1/2 cup	190	5.0	23.0	580	(mq)	9.0	(mq)
chicken flavor 'Chef's Series' prepared	1/2 cup	160	3.0	21.0	550	(mq)	8.0	(mq)
garlic and butter 'Chef's Series' prepared	1/2 cup	170	3.0	21.0	480	(mq)	7.0	(mq)
sour cream and chives 'Chef's Series'								
prepared	1/2 cup	190	4.0	22.0	470	(mq)	8.0	(mq)
Stroganoff 'Chef's Series' prepared	1/2 cup	190	5.0	22.0	620	(mq)	9.0	(mq)
(Noodle Roni)								
angel hair pasta, w/Parmesan cheese,								
prepared	1/2 cup	210	6.0	26.0	580	na	9.0	na
fettuccini, prepared	1/2 cup	300	7.0	29.0	560	(mq)	18.0	(mq)
garlic, creamy, prepared	1/2 cup	300	7.0	29.0	630	(mq)	17.0	(mq)
herb and butter, prepared	1/2 cup	160	5.0	19.0	290	(mq)	7.0	(mq)
mushroom, prepared	1/2 cup	160	6.0	25.0	550	(mq)	4.0	(mq)
Parmesan, prepared	1/2 cup	240	7.0	23.0	470	(mq)	13.0	(mq)
Parmesano 'Less Fat' prepared	1/2 cup	190	6.0	24.0	460	na	8.0	na
Romanoff, prepared	1/2 cup	240	8.0	28.0	730	(mq)	11.0	(mq)
Stroganoff, prepared	1/2 cup	350	11.0	37.0	1190	(mq)	17.0	(mq)
(Ultra Slim Fast) w/Alfredo sauce,								
prepared	8 oz	240	9.0	47.0	1110	4.0	4.0	na
NORI. See SEAWEED.								
NORWAY HADDOCK. See OCEAN PERCH, ATLANTIC.								
NUT TOPPING								
(Fisher) fancy	1 oz	170	5.0	7.0	60	na	15.0	0
(Fisher) oil-roasted, w/peanuts	1 oz	160	6.0	7.0	115	na	14.0	0
(Planters)	1 oz	180	5.0	6.0	0	(mq)	16.0	0
(Smucker's) pecan, in syrup	2 tbsp	130	2.0	28.0	0	(mq)	1.0	0
(Smucker's) walnut, in syrup	2 tbsp	130	2.0	27.0	0	(mq)	1.0	0
NUTMEG								
ground	1 oz	149	1.7	14.0	5	>1.1 c	10.3	0
ground	1 tbsp	37	0.4	3.5	1	1.5	2.5	0
ground	1 tsp	12	0.1	1.1	0	.5	0.8	0
ground *(Durkee)*	1 tsp	12	0.0	0.0	0	0	<0.1	na
ground *(Laurel Leaf)*	1 tsp	12	0.0	0.0	0	0	<0.1	na
ground *(Spice Islands)*	1 tsp	11	0.1	0.9	<1	>.1 c	0.7	0
NUTMEG BUTTER OIL								
	1 cup	1927	0.0	0.0	0	0	218.0	0
	1 oz	251	0.0	0.0	0	0	28.4	0
	1 tbsp	120	0.0	0.0	0	0	13.6	0
NUTRASWEET. See SUGAR, ALTERNATIVE.								

Food Name	Serv. Size	Total Cal.	Prot. GMS	Carbs GMS	Sod. MGS	Fiber GMS	Fat GMS	Chol. MGS
NUTS, MIXED								
(Guy's) w/peanuts	1 oz	170	8.0	3.0	140	(mq)	14.0	0
(Planters) 'Select Mix' cashews, almonds, and peanuts	1 oz	170	5.0	7.0	100	na	14.0	0
(Planters) 'Select Mix' cashews, almonds, and pecans	1 oz	180	4.0	6.0	85	na	16.0	0
(Planters) 'Select Mix' cashews, pecans, and peanuts	1 oz	180	4.0	6.0	80	na	16.0	0
Dry-roasted								
(Finast) 'No Frills' w/peanuts, salted	1 oz	180	5.0	7.0	150	(mq)	14.0	0
(Fisher) lightly salted	1 oz	170	6.0	7.0	na	na	15.0	0
(Fisher) salted	1 oz	170	6.0	7.0	125	na	15.0	0
(Pathmark) 'No Frills' w/peanuts, salted	1 oz	180	6.0	7.0	220	(mq)	14.0	0
(Planters)	1 oz	160	5.0	7.0	250	(mq)	14.0	0
(Planters) sesame nut mix	1 oz	160	5.0	8.0	330	(mq)	12.0	0
(Planters) 'Unsalted'	1 oz	170	6.0	7.0	0	(mq)	15.0	0
w/peanuts	1 cup	814	23.7	34.7	16	12.3	70.5	0
w/peanuts	1 oz	169	4.9	7.2	3	2.6	14.6	0
w/peanuts, salted	1 cup	814	23.7	34.7	917	12.3	70.5	0
w/peanuts, salted	1 oz	169	4.9	7.2	190	2.6	14.6	0
Honey-roasted								
(Fisher) peanuts and cashews	1 oz	150	5.0	6.0	105	na	13.0	0
(Planters)	1 oz	170	5.0	9.0	140	na	13.0	0
(Planters) cashews and peanuts	1 oz	170	5.0	9.0	170	(mq)	12.0	0
Oil-roasted								
(Fisher) lightly salted	1 oz	170	6.0	6.0	50	na	16.0	0
(Fisher) salted	1 oz	170	6.0	6.0	110	na	16.0	0
(Flavor House)	1 oz	180	5.0	6.0	125	(mq)	18.0	0
(Pathmark) 'No Frills' salted	1 oz	180	4.0	7.0	150	(mq)	15.0	0
(Pathmark) 'No Frills' w/peanuts, salted	1 oz	180	6.0	5.0	150	(mq)	15.0	0
(Pathmark) 'No Frills Fancy' salted	1 oz	180	4.0	7.0	150	(mq)	15.0	0
(Planters)	1 oz	180	5.0	6.0	110	na	16.0	0
(Planters) 'Deluxe'	1 oz	180	4.0	6.0	110	na	17.0	0
(Planters) lightly salted	1 oz	180	5.0	6.0	80	na	16.0	0
(Planters) sesame nut mix	1 oz	160	5.0	8.0	200	na	13.0	0
salted	1 cup	886	22.4	32.1	1008	7.9	80.9	0
salted	1 oz	175	4.4	6.3	199	1.6	15.9	0
w/peanuts	1 cup	876	23.8	30.4	16	14.1	80.0	0
w/peanuts	1 oz	175	4.8	6.1	3	2.8	16.0	0
w/peanuts, salted	1 cup	876	23.8	30.4	926	12.8	80.0	0
w/peanuts, salted	1 oz	175	4.8	6.1	185	2.6	16.0	0

O

Food Name	Serv. Size	Total Cal.	Prot. GMS	Carbs GMS	Sod. MGS	Fiber GMS	Fat GMS	Chol. MGS
OAT. See also CEREAL, HOT.								
cooked	1 cup	87	7.0	25.1	2	3.5	1.9	0
cooked	4 oz	45	3.6	13.0	1	>.4 c	1.0	0
raw	1 cup	231	16.3	62.2	4	14.9	6.6	0
raw	1 oz	70	4.9	18.8	1	4.5	2.0	0
steel-cut *(Arrowhead Mills)*	2 oz	220	10.0	37.0	1	2.8	4.0	0
whole grain	1 cup	607	26.3	103.4	3	(mq)	10.8	0
whole grain	1 oz	110	4.8	18.8	1	(mq)	2.0	0
OAT BRAN. See CEREAL, HOT.								
OAT FLOUR								
(Arrowhead Mills) whole grain	2 oz	200	7.0	43.0	1	8.3	1.0	0
(Gold Medal) blend	1 cup	390	14.0	81.0	0	4.0	3.0	0
OAT GROATS *(Arrowhead Mills)*	2 oz	220	8.0	38.0	1	5.6	4.0	0
OAT VEGETABLE OIL								
	1 cup	1927	0.0	0.0	0	0	218.0	0
	1 tbsp	120	0.0	0.0	0	0	13.6	0
OATMEAL. See CEREAL, HOT.								
OCEAN CATFISH. See WOLF FISH.								
OCEAN PERCH, ATLANTIC/Norway haddock/red perch/redfish/rosefish/sea perch								
baked	4 oz	137	27.1	0.0	109	0	2.4	61
broiled	4 oz	137	27.1	0.0	109	0	2.4	61
dry-heat cooked	3 oz	103	20.3	0.0	82	0	1.8	46
microwaved	4 oz	137	27.1	0.0	109	0	2.4	61
raw	1 lb	427	84.5	0.0	339	0	7.4	191
raw	1 oz	27	5.3	0.0	21	0	0.5	12
OCEAN PERCH, FROZEN								
(Booth)	4 oz	100	20.0	0.0	250	0	1.0	(mq)
(Gorton's) 'Fishmarket Fresh'	5 oz	140	25.0	2.0	100	0	3.0	(mq)
(Van de Kamp's) breaded 'Light'	1 piece	280	17.0	21.0	450	(mq)	14.0	35
(Van de Kamp's) 'Natural'	4 oz	130	20.0	0.0	65	0	5.0	40
OCEAN POUT/muttonfish								
dry-heat cooked	3 oz	87	18.1	0.0	66	0	1.0	57
raw	1 lb	360	75.5	0.0	277	0	4.1	236
raw	1 oz	22	4.7	0.0	17	0	0.3	15
OCEANIC BONITO. See TUNA, SKIPJACK.								
OCTOBER BEAN, CANNED, w/pork *(Luck's)*	7.25 oz	230	12.0	32.0	550	10.0	6.0	(mq)
OCTOPUS								
moist-heat cooked	3 oz	139	25.3	3.7	391	0	1.8	82
raw	1 lb	372	67.6	10.0	(mq)	0	4.7	219
raw	1 oz	23	4.2	0.6	(mq)	0	0.3	14

Food Name	Serv. Size	Total Cal.	Prot. GMS	Carbs GMS	Sod. MGS	Fiber GMS	Fat GMS	Chol. MGS
OHELOBERRY								
raw	1 lb	126	1.7	31.0	6	>6.0 c	1.0	0
raw	1 cup	39	0.5	9.6	1	>1.9 c	0.3	0
raw	1 oz	8	0.1	1.9	<1	>.4 c	0.1	0
raw, approx .4 oz	10 fruits	3	0.0	0.8	0	>.2 c	0.0	0
OIL. See individual listings.								
OKRA/gumbo								
boiled, drained	4 oz	36	2.1	8.2	6	>1.0 c	0.2	0
boiled, drained, approx 3 inches long	8 pods	27	1.6	6.1	4	2.1	0.1	0
boiled, drained, sliced	1/2 cup	26	1.5	5.8	4	2.0	0.1	0
raw, approx 3 inches long	8 pods	36	1.9	7.3	8	2.5	0.1	0
raw, sliced	1/2 cup	19	1.0	3.8	4	1.3	0.1	0
raw, trimmed	1 oz	11	0.6	2.2	2	>.3 c	<.1	0
raw, untrimmed	1 lb	148	7.8	29.8	32	>3.7 c	0.4	0
OKRA, FROZEN								
boiled, drained	10 oz	94	5.3	20.8	8	7.1	0.8	0
boiled, drained, sliced	1/2 cup	34	1.9	7.5	3	2.6	0.3	0
cut (Freshlike)	3.3 oz	25	1.0	6.0	5	na	0.0	na
cut (Seabrook)	3.3 oz	25	1.0	6.0	3	>1.0 c	0.0	0
cut (Southern)	3.5 oz	31	1.6	6.5	20	(mq)	0.2	0
cut (Veg·All)	3.3 oz	25	1.0	6.0	5	na	0.0	na
whole (Freshlike)	3.3 oz	30	2.0	7.0	5	na	0.0	na
whole (Seabrook)	3.3 oz	30	2.0	7.0	2	>1.0 c	0.0	0
whole (Southern)	3.5 oz	35	1.9	7.4	20	(mq)	0.2	0
whole (Veg·All)	3.3 oz	30	2.0	7.0	5	na	0.0	na
whole, baby (Frosty Acres)	3.3 oz	30	2.0	7.0	2	>1.0 c	0.0	0
OLD FASHIONED. See ALCOHOLIC BEVERAGES.								
OLIVE								
all varieties, all sizes, pickled (S&W)	1 oz	46	0.0	0.0	215	(mq)	5.1	0
black, jumbo, canned	1 olive	7	0.1	0.5	75	.3	0.6	0
black, large, canned	1 olive	5	0.0	0.3	38	.1	0.5	0
black, small, canned	1 olive	4	0.0	0.2	28	.1	0.3	0
black, super colossal, canned	1 olive	12	0.2	0.9	136	.5	1.0	0
mixed varieties, chopped, pickled (Lindsay)	1 oz	29	0.2	1.7	249	.8	2.7	0
mixed varieties, pitted, pickled (Vlasic)	1 oz	37	0.3	0.7	230	>.4 c	3.9	0
mixed varieties, sliced, pickled (Lindsay)	1/2 cup	70	0.6	4.1	598	2.0	6.5	0
mixed varieties, sliced, pickled (Lindsay)	1 oz	29	0.2	1.7	249	.8	2.7	0
salad, pickled (Progresso)	1/2 cup	120	1.0	1.0	2400	4.0	15.0	0
OLIVE, ASCOLANO								
all sizes, pitted, pickled	1 oz	23	0.3	1.6	255	.9	1.9	0
all sizes, pitted, pickled (Lindsay)	1 oz	23	0.3	1.6	255	.7	1.9	0
colossal, pitted, pickled (Lindsay)	10 olives	90	1.1	6.3	1010	2.8	7.7	0
jumbo, pitted, pickled	10 olives	67	0.8	4.7	745	2.5	5.7	0

Food Name	Serv. Size	Total Cal.	Prot. GMS	Carbs GMS	Sod. MGS	Fiber GMS	Fat GMS	Chol. MGS
jumbo, pitted, pickled *(Lindsay)*	10 olives	66	0.8	4.7	745	2.1	5.7	0
super colossal, pitted, pickled	10 olives	123	1.5	8.5	1365	4.6	10.4	0
super colossal, pitted, pickled								
(Lindsay)	10 olives	122	1.5	8.5	1365	3.8	10.4	0
OLIVE, GREEK								
all sizes, pitted, salt-cured, oil-coated,								
pickled	1 oz	96	0.6	2.5	932	(mq)	10.2	0
extra large, w/pits, salt-cured, oil-coated,								
pickled	10 olives	89	0.6	2.3	868	(mq)	9.5	0
extra large, w/pits, salt-cured, pickled	10 olives	89	0.6	2.3	868	(mq)	9.5	0
medium, w/pits, salt-cured, oil-coated,								
pickled	10 olives	65	0.4	1.7	631	(mq)	6.9	0
medium, w/pits, salt-cured, pickled ...	10 olives	65	0.4	1.7	631	(mq)	6.9	0
OLIVE, GREEN								
all sizes, pitted, pickled	1 oz	33	0.4	0.4	680	.7	3.6	0
giant, w/pits, pickled	10 olives	76	0.9	0.9	1572	1.7	8.3	0
large, w/pits, pickled	10 olives	45	0.5	0.5	926	1.0	4.9	0
small, select, w/pits, pickled	10 olives	33	0.4	0.4	686	.7	3.6	0
small, standard, w/pits, pickled	10 olives	33	0.4	0.4	686	.7	3.6	0
OLIVE, MANZANILLA								
all sizes, pitted, pickled	1 oz	33	0.2	1.8	247	.9	3.0	0
all sizes, pitted, pickled *(Lindsay)*	1 oz	32	0.2	1.8	247	.9	3.0	0
extra large, pitted, pickled *(Lindsay)* ..	10 olives	63	0.5	3.5	484	1.8	5.9	0
large, pitted, pickled	10 olives	51	0.5	2.8	384	1.3	4.7	0
large, pitted, pickled *(Lindsay)*	10 olives	50	0.4	2.8	388	1.4	4.8	0
medium, pitted, pickled *(Lindsay)*	10 olives	44	0.3	2.4	336	1.2	4.1	0
small, pitted, pickled	10 olives	37	0.3	2.0	279	1.0	3.4	0
small, pitted, pickled *(Lindsay)*	10 olives	37	0.3	2.0	283	1.0	3.5	0
OLIVE, MISSION								
all sizes, pitted, pickled	1 oz	33	0.2	1.8	247	.9	3.0	0
all sizes, pitted, pickled *(Lindsay)*	1 oz	32	0.2	1.8	247	.9	3.0	0
extra large, pitted, pickled *(Lindsay)* ..	10 olives	63	0.5	3.5	484	1.8	5.9	0
large, pitted, pickled	10 olives	51	0.5	2.8	384	1.3	4.7	0
large, pitted, pickled *(Lindsay)*	10 olives	50	0.4	2.8	388	1.4	4.8	0
medium, pitted, pickled *(Lindsay)*	10 olives	44	0.3	2.4	336	1.2	4.1	0
small, pitted, pickled	10 olives	37	0.3	2.0	279	1.0	3.4	0
small, pitted, pickled *(Lindsay)*	10 olives	37	0.3	2.0	283	1.0	3.5	0
OLIVE, SEVILLANO								
all sizes, pitted, pickled	1 oz	23	0.3	1.6	255	.9	1.9	0
all sizes, pitted, pickled *(Lindsay)*	1 oz	23	0.3	1.6	255	.7	1.9	0
colossal, pitted, pickled *(Lindsay)*	10 olives	90	1.1	6.3	1010	2.8	7.7	0
jumbo, pitted, pickled	10 olives	67	0.8	4.7	745	2.5	5.7	0
jumbo, pitted, pickled *(Lindsay)*	10 olives	66	0.8	4.7	745	2.1	5.7	0

Food Name	Serv. Size	Total Cal.	Prot. GMS	Carbs GMS	Sod. MGS	Fiber GMS	Fat GMS	Chol. MGS
super colossal, pitted, pickled .... 10 olives		123	1.5	8.5	1365	4.6	10.4	0
super colossal, pitted, pickled								
(Lindsay) .... 10 olives		122	1.5	8.5	1365	3.8	10.4	0
OLIVE APPETIZER								
(Progresso) .... 1/2 cup		180	1.0	6.0	1600	2.5	21.0	0
(Progresso) 'Condite' .... 1/2 cup		130	<1.0	5.0	870	2.0	14.0	0
OLIVE OIL								
.... 1/2 cup		955	0.0	0.0	tr	0	108.0	0
.... 1 oz		251	0.0	0.0	tr	0	28.4	0
(Amore) 'Extra Virgin' .... 1 tbsp		130	0.0	0.0	0	0	14.0	0
(Amore) 'Pure' .... 1 tbsp		130	0.0	0.0	0	0	14.0	0
(Bertolli) .... 1 tbsp		120	0.0	0.0	(tr)	0	14.0	0
(Filippo Berio) .... 1 tbsp		120	0.0	0.0	(tr)	0	14.0	0
(Hain) .... 1 tbsp		120	0.0	0.0	0	0	14.0	0
(Pope) 100% Italian cold press, no salt . 1 tbsp		120	0.0	0.0	0	na	14.0	0
(Progresso) all varieties .... 1 tbsp		119	0.0	0.0	0	0	14.0	0
(Spectrum Naturals) .... 1 tbsp		120	0.0	0.0	0	(tr)	14.0	(tr)
(Spectrum Naturals) organic .... 1 tbsp		120	0.0	0.0	0	(tr)	14.0	(tr)
(Wesson) .... 1 tbsp		120	0.0	0.0	0	0	14.0	0
OMELET, FROZEN								
(Healthy Choice) turkey sausage, on								
English muffin .... 1 serving		210	16.0	30.0	470	na	4.0	20
(Healthy Choice) western style, on								
English muffin .... 1 serving		200	16.0	29.0	480	na	3.0	15
(Weight Watchers) ham and cheese								
'Handy' .... 4 oz		180	14.0	18.0	420	na	5.0	10
ONION								
Mature								
boiled, drained .... 4 oz		50	1.5	11.5	3	>.8 c	0.2	0
chopped, boiled, drained .... 1/2 cup		46	1.4	10.7	3	1.7	0.2	0
chopped, boiled, drained .... 1 tbsp		7	0.2	1.5	0	.2	0.0	0
raw (Dole) .... 1 med		60	1.0	14.0	10	3.0	0.0	na
raw, chopped .... 1/2 cup		30	0.9	6.9	2	1.3	0.1	0
raw, chopped .... 1 tbsp		4	0.1	0.9	tr	.2	<.1	0
raw, trimmed .... 1 oz		11	0.3	2.4	1	5	<.1	0
raw, untrimmed .... 1 lb		154	4.7	35.2	12	6.5	0.7	0
ONION, CANNED								
sweet (Heinz) .... 1 oz		40	0.0	9.0	165	(mq)	0.0	0
whole, small (Pathmark) .... 1/2 cup		35	2.0	7.0	280	(mq)	0.0	0
whole, small (S&W) .... 1/2 cup		35	1.0	9.0	345	(mq)	0.0	0
w/liquid .... 4 oz		22	1.0	4.5	421	1.2	0.1	0
w/liquid, chopped .... 1/2 cup		21	1.0	4.5	416	1.5	0.1	0
ONION, COCKTAIL, lightly spiced (Vlasic) .. 1 oz		4	0.0	1.0	365	(mq)	0.0	0

Food Name	Serv. Size	Total Cal.	Prot. GMS	Carbs GMS	Sod. MGS	Fiber GMS	Fat GMS	Chol. MGS
ONION, DRIED								
flakes	1 oz	92	2.5	23.6	6	>1.3 c	0.1	0
flakes	1/4 cup	45	1.3	11.7	3	1.3	0.1	0
flakes	1 tbsp	16	0.5	4.2	1	.5	0.0	0
w/green onion, minced (Lawry's)	1 tsp	7	0.4	1.6	1	>.6 c	0.2	0
ONION, FROZEN								
Chopped								
boiled, drained	1/2 cup	29	0.8	6.9	13	1.7	0.1	0
boiled, drained	4 oz	32	0.9	7.5	14	>5.0 c	0.1	0
boiled, drained	1 tbsp	4	0.1	1.0	2	.2	0.0	0
unprepared	10 oz	82	2.2	19.3	34	4.5	0.3	0
(Ore-Ida)	2 oz	20	0.0	4.0	10	(mq)	<1.0	0
(Seabrook)	1 oz	8	0.0	2.0	2	0	0.0	0
Diced								
(Freshlike)	3.3 oz	8	0.0	2.0	0	na	0.0	na
(Veg·All)	3.3 oz	8	0.0	2.0	0	na	0.0	na
Whole								
boiled, drained	4 oz	32	0.8	7.6	9	>.6 c	0.1	0
(Birds Eye) small	4 oz	40	1.0	10.0	10	2.0	0.0	0
(Birds Eye) small, w/cream sauce								
'Combination Vegetables'	5 oz	140	2.0	12.0	400	1.0	10.0	0
(Freshlike)	3.3 oz	35	1.0	8.0	10	na	0.0	na
(Seabrook) small	3.3 oz	35	1.0	8.0	9	>1.0 c	0.0	0
(Veg·All)	3.3 oz	35	1.0	8.0	10	na	0.0	na
ONION, GREEN/scallion/spring onion								
chopped (Dole)	1 tbsp	2	0.1	0.3	0	tr	0.1	na
trimmed, w/top	1 oz	19	0.5	2.1	5	.7	<.1	0
trimmed, w/top, chopped	1/2 cup	16	0.9	3.7	8	1.2	0.1	0
trimmed, w/top, chopped	1 tbsp	2	0.1	0.4	1	.1	<.1	0
untrimmed	1 lb	140	8.0	32.0	71	10.5	0.8	0
ONION, SPRING. See ONION, GREEN.								
ONION, WELSH								
trimmed	1 lb	160	8.0	28.8	na	>4.8 c	1.6	0
trimmed	1 oz	10	0.5	1.8	na	>.3 c	0.1	0
ONION POWDER								
ground	1 tbsp	23	0.7	5.2	3	>.4 c	0.1	0
ground	1 tsp	7	0.2	1.7	1	>.1 c	0.0	0
ground (Durkee)	1 tsp	8	0.0	0.0	0	0	tr	na
ground (Laurel Leaf)	1 tsp	8	0.0	0.0	0	0	tr	na
ground (Spice Islands)	1 tsp	8	0.2	1.7	1	>.1 c	<.1	0
ONION RINGS, FROZEN								
breaded, partially fried in vegetable oil,								
prepared in oven	4 oz	462	6.1	43.3	425	>.5 c	30.3	0

Food Name	Serv. Size	Total Cal.	Prot. GMS	Carbs GMS	Sod. MGS	Fiber GMS	Fat GMS	Chol. MGS
breaded, partially fried in vegetable oil, prepared in oven	2 rings	81	1.1	7.6	75	>.1 c	5.3	0
breaded, partially fried in vegetable oil, unprepared	16 oz	1171	14.3	138.6	1117	5.9	64.0	0
breaded, partially fried in vegetable oil, unprepared	9 oz	658	8.0	77.8	627	3.3	36.0	0
(Farm Rich) battered, precooked 'Batter Dipt'	4 oz	260	3.0	32.0	580	(mq)	13.0	na
(Farm Rich) crispy 'Onion O's'	5 rings	190	3.0	26.0	480	(mq)	9.0	0
(Mrs. Paul's) crispy	2.5 oz	190	2.0	19.0	230	(mq)	12.0	na
(Ore-Ida) 'Onion Ringers'	2 oz	140	2.0	18.0	190	(mq)	7.0	0
(Stilwell) battered	3 oz	250	2.0	22.0	300	(mq)	16.0	<1
ONION SALT (Tone's)	1 tsp	1	0.1	0.4	1599	<.1	tr	0
OPOSSUM								
roasted	4 oz	251	34.2	0.0	(mq)	0	11.6	(mq)
roasted	3 oz	188	25.7	0.0	na	na	8.7	na
roasted, diced	1 cup	309	42.3	0.0	(mq)	0	14.3	(mq)
ORANGE								
All commercial varieties								
approx 2 5/8-inch diam	1 med	62	1.2	15.4	0	3.1	0.2	0
peeled and seeded	1 oz	13	0.3	3.3	0	.7	<.1	0
sections, w/o membrane	1 cup	85	1.7	21.1	0	4.3	0.2	0
untrimmed	1 lb	156	3.1	38.9	0	7.9	0.4	0
California navel								
approx 2 7/8-inch diam	1 med	64	1.4	16.3	1	>.6 c	0.1	0
peeled and seeded	1 oz	13	0.3	3.3	<1	>.1 c	<.1	0
sections, w/o membrane	1 cup	76	1.7	19.2	2	>.8 c	0.2	0
untrimmed	1 lb	142	3.2	35.9	2	>1.4 c	0.3	0
California Valencia								
approx 2 5/8 inch diam	1 med	59	1.3	14.4	0	>.6 c	0.4	0
peeled and seeded	1 oz	14	0.3	3.4	0	>.1 c	0.1	0
sections, w/o membrane	1 cup	88	1.9	21.4	0	>.9 c	0.5	0
untrimmed	1 lb	167	3.5	40.5	0	>1.7 c	1.0	0
Florida								
approx 2 5/8 inch diam	1 med	69	1.1	17.4	0	3.6	0.3	0
peeled and seeded	1 oz	13	0.2	3.3	tr	>.1 c	0.1	0
sections, w/o membrane	1 cup	85	1.3	21.4	0	4.4	0.4	0
untrimmed	1 lb	153	2.4	38.7	2	>1.2 c	0.7	0
ORANGE APRICOT DRINK (Tropicana)								
'Twister'	8 oz	115	(mq)	30.0	2	(mq)	0.0	0
ORANGE APRICOT JUICE								
(Musselman's) 'Breakfast Cocktail'	6 oz	90	0.0	21.0	20	(tr)	0.0	0
ORANGE APRICOT JUICE DRINK	1 oz	16	0.1	4.0	1	na	0.0	0

Food Name	Serv. Size	Total Cal.	Prot. GMS	Carbs GMS	Sod. MGS	Fiber GMS	Fat GMS	Chol. MGS
ORANGE BANANA NECTAR *(Kern's)*	6 oz	110	1.0	25.0	0	na	0.0	na
ORANGE CRANBERRY JUICE								
(Santa Cruz Natural) organic 'Cruz'	8 oz	125	1.0	29.0	na	na	<1.0	na
ORANGE CRANBERRY JUICE DRINK								
(Ocean Spray) 'Refreshers'	6 oz	100	0.0	26.0	15	na	0.0	na
(Tropicana) 'Single Serve'	10 oz	175	(mq)	43.0	3	(mq)	0.0	0
(Tropicana) 'Twister'	8 oz	115	(mq)	30.0	1	(mq)	0.0	0
(Tropicana) 'Twister'	6 oz	100	<1.0	23.0	25	na	<1.0	na
(Tropicana) 'Twister Light' w/NutraSweet	6 oz	18	<1.0	5.0	27	na	<1.0	na
ORANGE DRINK								
Can, bottle, or box								
....	8 oz	128	0.0	32.0	40	(tr)	tr	0
(Bama)	8.45 oz	120	0.0	29.0	60	(tr)	0.0	0
(Crowley)	8 oz	130	0.0	32.0	15	(tr)	0.0	0
(Hawaiian Punch)	6 oz	100	0.0	24.0	20	(tr)	0.0	0
(Hi-C)	8.45 oz	134	0.2	32.9	24	(tr)	<.1	0
(Hi-C)	6 oz	95	0.1	23.3	17	(tr)	<.1	0
(Hi-C) aseptic box	6 oz	90	0.0	23.0	20	na	0.0	na
(J. Hungerford) 20% plus juice	9.03 oz	41	0.1	10.8	23	0	0.0	0
(Pathmark) 'No Frills Sodium Free'	6 oz	80	0.0	22.0	0	(tr)	0.0	0
(Squeezit) 'Smarty Arty Orange'	6.75 oz	100	0.0	26.0	50	na	0.0	na
(Sunny Delight) California style	8 oz	130	0.0	31.0	130	na	0.0	na
(Tropicana)	6 oz	90	<1.0	22.0	35	na	<1.0	na
(Tropicana) 'Single Serve'	10 oz	132	(tr)	33.0	3	(tr)	0.0	0
(Veryfine)	8 oz	130	<1.0	33.0	70	(tr)	0.0	0
(Wyler's) 'Fruit Slush'	4 oz	157	0.0	39.3	10	(tr)	0.0	0
Chilled *(Hi-C)*	6 oz	90	0.0	23.0	20	na	0.0	na
Frozen, w/juice and pulp, diluted	6 oz	85	0.2	21.2	19	>.2 c	0.0	0
Mix								
(Finast) breakfast, prepared	8 oz	80	0.0	20.0	15	(tr)	0.0	0
(Kool-Aid) sugar-free, w/NutraSweet, prepared	8 oz	4	0.0	0.0	0	0	0.0	0
(Kool-Aid) sugar-sweetened, prepared	8 oz	80	0.0	20.0	0	na	0.0	0
(Kool-Aid) unsweetened, prepared w/sugar	8 oz	100	0.0	25.0	0	na	0.0	0
(Kool-Aid) unsweetened, prepared w/o sugar	8 oz	2	0.0	0.0	0	na	0.0	0
(Pathmark) breakfast 'No Frills' prepared	4 oz	60	0.0	15.0	0	(tr)	0.0	0
ORANGE FLAVOR DRINK								
Can, bottle, or box	12 oz	729	0.3	182.0	103	.4	2.2	0
Chilled *(Bright & Early)* diluted	6 oz	90	0.1	20.8	18	(mq)	0.2	0
Frozen								
(Bright & Early) diluted	6 oz	90	0.1	20.8	18	(mq)	0.2	0
w/orange pulp, diluted	1 oz	15	tr	3.8	3	(mq)	tr	0
Mix								
powder, unprepared	1 oz	109	<.1	28.0	5	(tr)	<.1	0

Food Name	Serv. Size	Total Cal.	Prot. GMS	Carbs GMS	Sod. MGS	Fiber GMS	Fat GMS	Chol. MGS
powder, unprepared .... 3 rounded tsp		93	tr	23.7	4	(tr)	tr	0
(Tang) crystals, prepared .... 6 oz		90	0.0	22.0	0	(tr)	0.0	0
(Tang) crystals 'Sugar-free' prepared ..... 6 oz		6	0.0	1.0	0	(tr)	0.0	0
ORANGE FRUIT JUICE BLEND								
(Mott's) .... 10 oz		144	1.0	35.0	6	(tr)	0.0	0
(Mott's) .... 9.5 oz		139	1.0	34.0	6	(tr)	0.0	0
ORANGE GRAPEFRUIT JUICE								
canned .... 8 oz		106	1.5	25.4	7	>.3 c	0.3	0
canned .... 1 oz		13	0.2	3.2	1	0	0.0	0
(Kraft) chilled 'Pure 100%' .... 6 oz		80	1.0	19.0	0	(mq)	0.0	0
ORANGE JUICE								
fresh squeezed .... 8 oz		112	1.7	25.8	2	.5	0.5	0
Can, bottle, or box								
.... 6 oz		78	1.1	18.4	5	.4	0.3	0
(Del Monte) 'Unsweetened' .... 6 oz		80	1.0	19.0	10	(mq)	0.0	0
(J. Hungerford) .... 9.03 oz		112	0.5	27.8	1	0	0.0	0
(Minute Maid) blend 'Juices to Go' .... 6 oz		90	1.0	22.0	20	na	0.0	na
(Minute Maid) 'Juices to Go' .... 6 oz		80	1.0	20.0	20	na	0.0	na
(Ocean Spray) .... 6 oz		80	0.0	19.0	15	(mq)	0.0	0
(S&W) .... 6 oz		83	2.0	18.0	2	(mq)	0.0	0
(Sippin' Pak) .... 8.45 oz		110	1.0	26.0	25	(mq)	0.0	0
(Snapple) .... 8 oz		130	0.0	29.0	55	na	0.0	0
(Stokely) 'Unsweetened' .... 6 oz		89	1.0	21.0	5	(mq)	1.0	0
(Sunkist) .... 6 oz		84	1.3	20.0	2	(mq)	0.1	0
(Tree Top) .... 6 oz		90	1.0	22.0	5	(mq)	0.0	0
(TreeSweet) .... 6 oz		78	1.0	18.0	15	(mq)	0.0	0
(Tropicana) '100% Pure' .... 8 oz		109	(mq)	24.9	3	(mq)	0.0	0
(Tropicana) 'Pure Premium' 100% pure ... 6 oz		80	1.0	19.0	0	na	<1.0	na
(Tropicana) reconstituted, 100% pure .... 6 oz		80	1.0	16.0	20	na	<1.0	na
(Veryfine) blend '100%' .... 8 oz		120	<1.0	30.0	35	(mq)	0.0	0
(Veryfine) '100%' .... 8 oz		121	1.5	24.0	10	(mq)	0.0	0
Chilled								
.... 8 oz		110	2.0	25.0	2	.5	0.7	0
(Citrus Hill) 'Plus Calcium' .... 6 oz		90	<1.0	20.0	10	(mq)	<1.0	0
(Citrus Hill) 'Select' .... 6 oz		90	<1.0	20.0	10	(mq)	<1.0	0
(Crowley) .... 8 oz		110	2.0	26.0	5	(mq)	0.0	0
(Kraft) 'Pure 100% Unsweetened' .... 6 oz		80	1.0	19.0	0	(mq)	0.0	0
(Minute Maid) calcium fortified .... 6 oz		80	1.0	20.0	20	na	0.0	na
(Minute Maid) country style .... 6 oz		80	1.0	20.0	20	na	0.0	na
(Minute Maid) country style, premium choice 6 oz		90	1.0	21.0	0	na	0.0	na
(Minute Maid) premium choice .... 6 oz		90	1.0	21.0	0	na	0.0	na
(Minute Maid) regular .... 6 oz		80	1.0	20.0	20	na	0.0	na
(Sunkist) .... 6 oz		84	1.3	20.0	2	(mq)	0.1	0

Food Name	Serv. Size	Total Cal.	Prot. GMS	Carbs GMS	Sod. MGS	Fiber GMS	Fat GMS	Chol. MGS
(Sunkist) 'Fresh Squeezed'	6 oz	77	1.2	17.7	2	(mq)	0.3	0
Frozen								
(A&P) diluted	6 oz	80	1.0	19.0	0	(mq)	<1.0	0
(Minute Maid) calcium fortified	6 oz	80	1.0	20.0	0	na	0.0	na
(Minute Maid) country style	6 oz	80	1.0	20.0	0	na	0.0	na
(Minute Maid) reduced acid	6 oz	80	1.0	20.0	0	na	0.0	na
(Minute Maid) regular	6 oz	80	1.0	20.0	0	na	0.0	na
(Sunkist) '8-16 servings per pkg' diluted	6 oz	112	1.7	26.8	3	(mq)	0.1	0
(TreeSweet) diluted	6 oz	84	1.0	20.0	15	(mq)	0.0	0
ORANGE JUICE COCKTAIL								
(Musselman's) w/grapefruit juice								
'Breakfast Cocktail'	6 oz	90	1.0	22.0	20	(tr)	0.0	0
(Ocean Spray)	6 oz	100	0.0	25.0	15	na	0.0	na
(Welch's) 'Orchard'	10 oz	150	0.0	37.0	0	0	0.0	0
ORANGE JUICE DRINK								
(Citrus Hill) 'Lite Premium'	6 oz	60	<1.0	14.0	10	(tr)	<1.0	0
(Kool-Aid) 'Koolers'	8.45 oz	110	0.0	30.0	10	(tr)	0.0	0
(Tang) 'Fruit Box'	8.45 oz	130	0.0	32.0	10	na	0.0	0
(Tropicana) tropical 'Juice Sparkler'	8 oz	110	(mq)	26.0	50	(tr)	0.0	0
ORANGE JUICE FLOAT *(Knudsen & Sons)*	8 oz	120	2.0	27.0	na	na	0.0	na
ORANGE KIWI PASSION JUICE								
(Tropicana) 100% pure	6 oz	80	1.0	17.0	35	na	<1.0	na
ORANGE MANGO DRINK *(Tropicana)*								
'Twister'	6 oz	90	<1.0	21.0	45	na	<1.0	na
ORANGE MANGO JUICE								
(Knudsen & Sons)	8 oz	110	<1.0	24.0	na	na	0.0	na
ORANGE PASSION DRINK								
(Tropicana) 'Twister'	8 oz	90	(mq)	22.0	1	(mq)	0.0	0
(Tropicana) 'Twister'	6 oz	80	<1.0	19.0	35	na	<1.0	na
ORANGE PEACH DRINK								
(Tropicana) 'Twister'	8 oz	115	(mq)	30.0	2	(mq)	0.0	0
(Tropicana) 'Twister'	6 oz	90	<1.0	21.0	35	na	<1.0	na
ORANGE PEACH MANGO JUICE								
(Tropicana) 100% pure	6 oz	80	1.0	19.0	20	na	<1.0	na
ORANGE PEEL								
candied	1 oz	88	0.1	22.6	0	>.6 c	0.1	0
fresh	1 oz	na	0.4	7.1	1	(mq)	0.1	0
fresh	1 tbsp	na	0.1	1.5	tr	.2	<.1	0
fresh	1 tsp	na	<.1	0.5	tr	.1	tr	0
ORANGE PINEAPPLE JUICE								
(Kraft) 'Pure 100%'	6 oz	80	1.0	19.0	0	(mq)	0.0	0
(Musselman's) 'Breakfast Cocktail'	6 oz	90	1.0	23.0	15	(tr)	0.0	0
(Tropicana) 100% pure	6 oz	80	1.0	19.0	15	na	<1.0	na

Food Name	Serv. Size	Total Cal.	Prot. GMS	Carbs GMS	Sod. MGS	Fiber GMS	Fat GMS	Chol. MGS
ORANGE PUNCH *(Minute Maid)* aseptic box	6 oz	80	0.0	20.0	20	na	0.0	na
ORANGE RASPBERRY DRINK								
(Tropicana) 'Twister'	6 oz	80	<1.0	20.0	30	na	<1.0	na
(Tropicana) 'Twister Light'	6 oz	30	<1.0	6.0	30	na	<1.0	na
ORANGE ROUGHY/slimehead								
dry-heat cooked	3 oz	76	16.0	0.0	69	0	0.8	22
raw	1 lb	571	66.7	0.0	286	0	31.8	91
raw	1 oz	36	4.2	0.0	18	0	2.0	6
ORANGE STRAWBERRY BANANA JUICE								
(Tropicana) 100% pure	6 oz	80	1.0	18.0	25	na	<1.0	na
ORANGE STRAWBERRY DRINK								
(Tropicana) w/banana 'Twister'	6 oz	80	<1.0	20.0	45	na	<1.0	na
(Tropicana) w/banana 'Twister Light'	6 oz	25	<1.0	6.0	20	na	<1.0	na
(Tropicana) w/guava 'Twister'	6 oz	80	<1.0	20.0	40	na	<1.0	na
ORANGEADE								
(Santa Cruz Natural) organic	8 oz	90	1.0	22.0	na	na	<1.0	na
(Santa Cruz Natural) organic 'Sparkling'	8 oz	90	<1.0	24.0	na	na	<1.0	na
OREGANO								
dried *(Golden Dipt)*	2 grams	6	0.0	0.0	88	na	0.0	0
dried *(Spice Islands)*	1 tsp	6	0.2	1.0	<1	>.2 c	0.1	0
ground	1 tbsp	14	0.5	2.9	1	>.7 c	0.5	0
ground	1 tsp	5	0.2	1.0	0	>.2 c	0.2	0
ground *(Durkee)*	1 tsp	5	0.0	0.0	0	0	tr	na
ground *(Laurel Leaf)*	1 tsp	5	0.0	0.0	0	0	tr	na
ORIENTAL SEASONING MIX *(Schilling)*								
'Bag 'n Season'	1 pkg	152	5.0	31.0	1912	na	8.0	na
OYSTER, CANNED								
Eastern	1 cup	171	17.5	9.7	278	0	6.1	136
Eastern	3 oz	59	6.0	3.3	95	0	2.1	47
Eastern, w/liquid	4 oz	78	8.0	4.4	127	0	2.8	62
(Bumble Bee)	1 cup	218	25.4	15.4	185	0	5.3	(mq)
(S&W) mole 'Fancy'	2 oz	95	12.0	4.0	(mq)	0	3.0	(mq)
OYSTER, EASTERN								
Farmed								
dry-heat cooked	3 oz	67	5.9	6.2	139	0	1.8	32
dry-heat cooked	6 med	47	4.1	4.3	96	0	1.3	22
raw, approx 3 oz	6 med	50	4.4	4.7	150	0	1.3	21
Wild								
dry-heat cooked	3 oz	61	7.0	4.1	207	0	1.6	42
dry-heat cooked	6 med	42	4.9	2.8	144	0	1.1	29
moist-heat cooked	4 oz	155	16.0	8.9	254	0	5.6	124
moist-heat cooked	3 oz	116	12.0	6.7	359	0	4.2	89
moist-heat cooked, approx 1.5 oz	6 med	58	5.9	3.3	177	0	2.1	44

Food Name	Serv. Size	Total Cal.	Prot. GMS	Carbs GMS	Sod. MGS	Fiber GMS	Fat GMS	Chol. MGS
raw	1 cup	169	17.5	9.7	523	0	6.1	131
raw	1 oz	20	2.0	1.1	32	0	0.7	16
raw, approx 3 oz	6 med	57	5.9	3.3	177	0	2.1	45
OYSTER, PACIFIC								
moist-heat cooked	3 oz	139	16.1	8.4	180	0	3.9	85
moist-heat cooked	1 med	41	4.7	2.5	53	0	1.1	25
raw	1 lb	370	42.9	22.5	481	0	10.4	(mq)
raw	3 oz	69	8.0	4.2	90	0	2.0	43
raw	1 oz	23	2.7	1.4	30	0	0.7	(mq)
raw, approx 1.75 oz	1 med	41	4.7	2.5	53	0	1.1	25
OYSTER PLANT. See SALSIFY.								
OYSTER STEW. See SOUP.								

P

Food Name	Serv. Size	Total Cal.	Prot. GMS	Carbs GMS	Sod. MGS	Fiber GMS	Fat GMS	Chol. MGS
PALM KERNEL OIL/babassu oil								
	1 cup	1927	0.0	0.0	0	0	218.0	0
	1/2 cup	964	0.0	0.0	0	0	109.0	0
	1 oz	251	0.0	0.0	0	0	28.4	0
	1 tbsp	120	0.0	0.0	0	0	13.6	0
PALM OIL								
	1 oz	251	0.0	0.0	0	0	28.4	0
	1 tbsp	120	0.0	0.0	0	0	13.6	0
PAM COOKING SPRAY. See COOKING SPRAY.								
PANANG CURRY BASE (A Taste of Thai)	1 tbsp	25	0.0	2.0	180	0	2.0	0
PANCAKE, FROZEN								
(Aunt Jemima) blueberry	3.5 oz	220	6.2	42.3	826	1.7	3.7	21
(Aunt Jemima) buttermilk 'Lite Microwave'	3.5 oz	140	7.0	28.0	660	(mq)	3.0	na
(Aunt Jemima) buttermilk 'Microwave'	3.5 oz	210	6.4	41.3	860	1.8	3.0	20
(Aunt Jemima) 'Original Microwave'	3.5 oz	211	6.2	40.3	801	1.8	3.6	44
(Downyflake)	3 pancakes	280	5.0	45.0	920	(mq)	9.0	na
(Downyflake) blueberry	3 pancakes	290	5.0	48.0	920	(mq)	9.0	na
(Downyflake) buttermilk	3 pancakes	280	5.0	45.0	920	(mq)	9.0	na
(Krusteaz) blueberry, 4.5 oz	3 pancakes	280	8.0	49.0	710	na	5.0	14
(Krusteaz) buttermilk, 4.75 oz	3 pancakes	290	8.0	53.0	900	na	5.0	14
(Krusteaz) mini, microwave	6 pancakes	120	3.0	21.0	280	na	2.0	4
(Krusteaz) whole wheat honey, 4.75 oz	3 pancakes	250	8.0	45.0	990	.7	4.0	12
(Pillsbury) blueberry 'Microwave'	3 pancakes	250	5.0	49.0	540	(mq)	4.0	na
(Pillsbury) buttermilk 'Microwave'	3 pancakes	260	6.0	51.0	590	(mq)	4.0	na

Food Name	Serv. Size	Total Cal.	Prot. GMS	Carbs GMS	Sod. MGS	Fiber GMS	Fat GMS	Chol. MGS
(Pillsbury) harvest wheat								
'Microwave'	3 pancakes	240	6.0	48.0	420	(mq)	4.0	na
(Pillsbury) 'Original Microwave'	3 pancakes	240	6.0	47.0	550	(mq)	4.0	na
(Weight Watchers) buttermilk								
'Microwave' approx 2.5 oz	1/2 pkg	140	5.0	22.0	270	(mq)	3.0	10
PANCAKE BATTER, FROZEN								
(Aunt Jemima) blueberry	3.6 oz	204	5.0	38.7	688	1.8	4.0	27
(Aunt Jemima) buttermilk	3.6 oz	180	5.5	36.0	778	1.8	2.3	27
(Aunt Jemima) 'Original'	3.6 oz	183	5.7	36.5	763	1.8	2.4	19
PANCAKE ENTRÉE, FROZEN								
(Aunt Jemima) and sausages 'Homestyle'	6 oz	420	12.0	57.0	1140	(mq)	16.0	(mq)
(Aunt Jemima) lite, w/lite links 'Homestyle'	6 oz	310	14.0	43.0	970	(mq)	10.0	(mq)
(Aunt Jemima) lite, w/lite syrup 'Homestyle'	6 oz	260	10.0	53.0	860	(mq)	3.0	na
(Downyflake) and sausages	5.5 oz	430	11.0	47.0	1170	(mq)	23.0	(mq)
(Swanson) and sausages 'Great Starts'	6 oz	460	15.0	52.0	920	(mq)	22.0	(mq)
(Swanson) silver dollar, and sausage								
'Great Starts'	3.75 oz	310	10.0	37.0	680	(mq)	14.0	(mq)
(Swanson) whole wheat, w/lite links								
'Great Starts'	5.5 oz	350	15.0	39.0	600	(mq)	16.0	(mq)
(Swanson) w/bacon 'Great Starts'	4.5 oz	400	11.0	47.0	1000	(mq)	20.0	(mq)
PANCAKE MIX. See also PANCAKE/WAFFLE MIX.								
(NOTE: Unless otherwise stated, all pancakes are 4 inches in diameter.)								
(Hungry Jack) dry	1/14 pkg	180	4.0	33.0	650	na	3.0	0
(Hungry Jack) prepared w/water	3 pancakes	180	4.0	33.0	650	na	3.0	0
BLUEBERRY *(Krusteaz)* imitation,								
prepared	3 pancakes	205	5.0	39.0	660	na	4.0	14
BLUEBERRY, WILD								
(Hungry Jack) dry	1/5 pkg	170	3.0	38.0	780	na	1.0	0
(Hungry Jack) prepared w/milk/								
oil/egg	3 pancakes	320	6.0	41.0	820	na	14.0	45
BUCKWHEAT *(Krusteaz)* prepared	3 pancakes	215	8.0	40.0	770	6.0	3.0	9
BUTTERMILK								
(Health Valley) 'Biscuit & Pancake'	1 oz	100	4.0	20.0	170	3.3	1.0	0
(Hungry Jack) 'Complete' dry	1/17 pkg	180	5.0	38.0	720	1.0	1.0	5
(Hungry Jack) 'Complete' prepared								
w/water	3 pancakes	180	5.0	38.0	720	1.0	1.0	5
(Hungry Jack) dry	1/25 pkg	120	3.0	26.0	530	.5	0.0	0
(Hungry Jack) prepared w/skim milk/								
oil/egg whites	3 pancakes	200	6.0	28.0	570	.5	7.0	0
(Hungry Jack) prepared w/2% milk/								
oil/egg	3 pancakes	210	6.0	28.0	560	.5	9.0	55
(Krusteaz) prepared	3 pancakes	200	5.0	39.0	770	na	3.0	10

Food Name	Serv. Size	Total Cal.	Prot. GMS	Carbs GMS	Sod. MGS	Fiber GMS	Fat GMS	Chol. MGS
EXTRA LIGHT								
(Hungry Jack) 'Complete' dry	1/17 pkg	180	4.0	38.0	730	1.0	3.0	0
(Hungry Jack) dry	1/17 pkg	180	4.0	38.0	730	1.0	3.0	0
(Hungry Jack) dry	1/26 pkg	120	2.0	26.0	450	.5	0.0	0
(Hungry Jack) prepared w/skim milk/ oil/egg whites	3 pancakes	170	6.0	28.0	500	.5	4.0	0
(Hungry Jack) prepared w/2% milk/ oil/egg	3 pancakes	190	5.0	28.0	490	.5	6.0	55
OAT BRAN *(Krusteaz)* 'Lite'	3 pancakes	130	5.0	36.0	370	10.0	1.0	0
WHOLE WHEAT *(Krusteaz)* honey	3 pancakes	215	8.0	42.0	630	5.0	1.0	9
PANCAKE MIX, MICROWAVE								
(Hungry Jack) blueberry, dry	3/4 pkg	230	5.0	47.0	550	1.0	4.0	10
(Hungry Jack) buttermilk, dry	3/4 pkg	260	5.0	51.0	590	1.0	4.0	10
(Hungry Jack) harvest wheat, dry	3/4 pkg	230	6.0	46.0	560	3.0	4.0	10
(Hungry Jack) oat bran, dry	3/4 pkg	230	6.0	45.0	580	3.0	4.0	10
(Hungry Jack) original, dry	3/4 pkg	240	5.0	49.0	570	2.0	4.0	10
PANCAKE SYRUP. See also MAPLE SYRUP.								
15% maple	1 cup	879	0.3	236.9	328	na	0.3	0
15% maple	1 tbsp	56	0.0	15.0	21	na	0.0	0
2% maple	1 cup	762	2.2	202.9	126	na	0.6	0
2% maple	1 tbsp	48	0.1	12.9	8	na	0.0	0
reduced calorie	100 gm	164	0.0	44.3	200	na	0.0	0
(Aunt Jemima)								
'ButterLite'	1 oz	50	0.0	13.0	65	(tr)	0.0	0
'Lite'	1 oz	54	0.1	13.1	92	.3	0.1	0
'Original' rich maple taste	1 oz	100	0.0	26.0	60	na	0.0	na
(Br'er Rabbit)								
dark	1 oz	120	0.0	31.0	0	na	0.0	0
light	1 oz	120	0.0	31.0	0	na	0.0	0
(Estee)								
	1 tbsp	4	0.0	1.0	25	(tr)	0.0	0
'Breakfast'	1 tbsp	12	0.0	3.0	35	na	0.0	0
(Featherweight)	1 tbsp	16	0.0	4.0	25	(tr)	0.0	0
(Hungry Jack)								
'Lite'	2 tbsp	50	0.0	14.0	105	0	0.0	0
regular	2 tbsp	100	0.0	26.0	25	0	0.0	0
(Knott's Berry Farm)								
	1 oz	110	0.0	28.0	0	na	0.0	na
'Country'	1 oz	110	0.0	27.0	0	na	0.0	na
'Light' microwavable	1 oz	45	0.0	11.0	70	na	0.0	na
w/30% real maple syrup, microwavable	1 oz	110	0.0	28.0	90	na	0.0	na
(Log Cabin)								
'Country Kitchen'	1 oz	100	0.0	26.0	20	(tr)	0.0	0

Food Name	Serv. Size	Total Cal.	Prot. GMS	Carbs GMS	Sod. MGS	Fiber GMS	Fat GMS	Chol. MGS
'Country Kitchen' butter flavor	1 oz	100	0.0	27.0	100	na	0.0	0
'Country Kitchen Lite'	1 oz	50	0.0	13.0	85	na	0.0	0
'Lite,' reduced calorie	1 oz	50	0.0	13.0	90	na	0.0	0
'Pancake and Waffle'	1 oz	100	0.0	26.0	35	(tr)	0.0	0
(Maple Valley)								
maple syrup substitute	2 tbsp	110	0.0	27.0	50	na	0.0	na
maple syrup substitute, 'Lite'	2 tbsp	60	0.0	16.0	60	na	0.0	na
(Mrs. Butterworth's) thick 'n rich, 'Lite'	2 tbsp	60	0.0	15.0	65	na	0.0	na
(Mrs. Richardson's)								
'Lite'	1 oz	50	0.0	13.0	90	na	0.0	na
original recipe	1 oz	100	0.0	25.0	60	na	0.0	na
(S&W) maple flavor, saccharin sweetened	1 tsp	4	0.0	1.0	25	(tr)	0.0	0
(Vermont Maid)	1 tbsp	50	0.0	13.0	5	(tr)	0.0	0
(Weight Watchers) 'Reduced Calorie'	1 tbsp	25	0.0	7.0	40	0	0.0	0

PANCAKE/WAFFLE MIX. See also PANCAKE MIX.

(NOTE: Unless otherwise stated, all pancakes are 4 inches in diameter.)

Food Name	Serv. Size	Total Cal.	Prot. GMS	Carbs GMS	Sod. MGS	Fiber GMS	Fat GMS	Chol. MGS
(Arrowhead Mills) 'Griddle Lite' prepared	1/2 cup	260	8.0	50.0	(mq)	(mq)	3.0	0
(Aunt Jemima) 'Original' prepared	3 pancakes	116	3.4	25.4	609	1.4	0.8	0
(Aunt Jemima) 'Original Complete' prepared	3 pancakes	253	7.0	50.2	1024	2.1	3.6	16
(Bisquick) 'Shake 'n Pour' prepared	3 pancakes	260	6.0	48.0	850	(mq)	5.0	0
(Estee) prepared, 3 inches each	3 pancakes	100	3.0	21.0	130	na	0.0	0
(Featherweight) prepared	3 pancakes	140	6.0	24.0	90	(mq)	2.0	5
(Gold Medal) 'Pouch Mix' prepared w/egg	1/8 pouch	100	3.0	17.0	280	(mq)	2.0	na
(Hungry Jack) 'Panshakes' prepared	3 pancakes	250	7.0	43.0	880	(mq)	6.0	na
(Krusteaz) Belgian waffle, prepared, 4-inch square	1 waffle	170	5.0	22.0	350	na	7.0	45
(Martha White) 'FlapStax' 1/4-cup batter per pancake	1 pancake	80	3.0	17.0	320	na	1.0	tr
(Martha White) 'Light Crust' dry	2 oz	120	4.0	20.0	290	(mq)	3.0	25
(Robin Hood) 'Pouch Mix' prepared w/egg	1/8 pouch	100	3.0	17.0	280	(mq)	2.0	na
APPLE CINNAMON *(Bisquick)* 'Shake 'n Pour' prepared	3 pancakes	270	6.0	49.0	870	(mq)	5.0	0
BLUE CORN *(Arrowhead Mills)* prepared	1/2 cup	330	10.0	36.0	295	1.2	5.0	0
BLUEBERRY								
(Bisquick) 'Shake 'n Pour' prepared	3 pancakes	280	6.0	53.0	860	(mq)	5.0	0
(Hungry Jack) prepared	3 pancakes	320	6.0	41.0	820	(mq)	15.0	na
BUCKWHEAT								
(Arrowhead Mills) prepared	1/2 cup	270	11.0	53.0	(mq)	(mq)	2.0	na
(Aunt Jemima) prepared	3 pancakes	143	5.5	31.7	773	5.0	1.6	na

Food Name	Serv. Size	Total Cal.	Prot. GMS	Carbs GMS	Sod. MGS	Fiber GMS	Fat GMS	Chol. MGS
BUTTERMILK								
(Aunt Jemima) 'Complete' prepared	3 pancakes	231	7.2	46.4	950	2.0	2.8	9
(Aunt Jemima) 'Lite Complete' prepared	3 pancakes	130	7.0	25.0	570	(mq)	2.0	na
(Aunt Jemima) prepared	3 pancakes	122	4.2	26.1	698	1.3	0.7	1
(Betty Crocker) complete, dry	1/2 cup	210	5.0	41.0	500	na	3.0	na
(Betty Crocker) complete, prepared	3 pancakes	210	5.0	41.0	500	na	3.0	na
(Betty Crocker) dry	1/2 cup	170	4.0	36.0	760	na	1.0	na
(Betty Crocker) prepared w/milk/oil/egg	3 pancakes	280	8.0	39.0	810	na	10.0	na
(Bisquick) 'Shake 'n Pour' prepared	3 pancakes	260	7.0	47.0	860	(mq)	5.0	0
(Hungry Jack) 'Complete' prepared	3 pancakes	180	4.0	39.0	710	(mq)	1.0	na
(Hungry Jack) 'Complete Packets' prepared	3 pancakes	180	4.0	35.0	680	(mq)	3.0	na
(Hungry Jack) prepared	3 pancakes	240	7.0	29.0	570	(mq)	11.0	na
EXTRA LIGHT (Hungry Jack) 'Complete' prepared w/water	3 pancakes	180	4.0	38.0	730	1.0	3.0	0
MULTIGRAIN (Arrowhead Mills) prepared	1/2 cup	350	12.0	70.0	(mq)	.8	2.0	na
OAT BRAN								
(Arrowhead Mills) prepared	1/2 cup	200	9.0	64.0	230	1.8	2.0	na
(Bisquick) 'Shake 'n Pour' prepared	3 pancakes	240	7.0	45.0	580	1.0	4.0	0
WHOLE WHEAT (Aunt Jemima) prepared	3 pancakes	161	7.0	34.5	892	3.6	1.0	0
PAPAYA								
peeled and seeded	1 oz	11	0.2	2.8	1	.3	<.1	0
raw (Calavo Growers)	1/2 med	80	0.0	19.0	15	2.7	0.0	0
raw (Del Monte)	1/3 med	60	0.0	15.0	5	(mq)	0.0	0
raw, approx 3 1/2-inch diam	1 med	119	1.9	29.8	9	5.5	0.4	0
raw, cubed	1 cup	55	0.9	13.7	4	2.5	0.2	0
raw, slices in light syrup (Sunfresh)	2/3 cup	80	<1.0	19.0	10	<1.0	0.0	0
PAPAYA DRINK (Knudsen & Sons) concentrate	1.5 oz	90	<1.0	22.0	37	na	0.0	na
PAPAYA JUICE (Knudsen & Sons) cream	2 oz	25	<1.0	6.0	na	na	0.0	na
PAPAYA LIME JUICE (Knudsen & Sons)	8 oz	115	1.0	29.0	na	na	0.0	na
PAPAYA NECTAR								
canned	1 cup	142	0.4	36.3	13	1.5	0.4	0
canned	1 oz	18	0.1	4.5	2	.2	0.1	0
(Kern's)	6 oz	110	0.0	27.0	5	na	0.0	na
(Knudsen & Sons)	8 oz	100	<1.0	26.0	na	na	0.0	na
(Knudsen & Sons) concentrate	1.5 oz	90	<1.0	22.0	na	na	0.0	na
(Libby's)	6 oz	110	0.0	28.0	10	(mq)	0.0	0

Food Name	Serv. Size	Total Cal.	Prot. GMS	Carbs GMS	Sod. MGS	Fiber GMS	Fat GMS	Chol. MGS
PAPAYA PUNCH *(Veryfine)*	8 oz	120	<1.0	30.0	10	(mq)	0.0	0
PAPRIKA								
ground	1 oz	82	4.2	15.8	10	>5.9 c	3.7	0
ground	1 tbsp	20	1.0	3.8	2	1.4	0.9	0
ground	1 tsp	6	0.3	1.2	1	.4	0.3	0
ground *(Durkee)*	1 tsp	8	0.0	0.0	0	0	tr	na
ground *(Laurel Leaf)*	1 tsp	8	0.0	0.0	0	0	tr	na
ground *(Spice Islands)*	1 tsp	7	0.3	1.1	<1	>.4 c	0.2	0
PARANUT. See BRAZIL NUT.								
PARFAIT								
chocolate *(Pearson)*	1 oz	120	1.0	23.0	70	na	3.0	na
chocolate *(Swiss Miss)*	4 oz	170	3.0	27.0	200	0	6.0	1
chocolate vanilla, fat-free *(Swiss Miss)*	4 oz	104	1.9	23.3	171	0	0.3	1
peanut butter *(Pearson)*	1 oz	120	1.0	23.0	70	na	3.0	na
vanilla *(Swiss Miss)*	4 oz	180	2.0	29.0	150	0	6.0	1
vanilla chocolate *(Swiss Miss)*	4 oz	164	2.9	24.5	196	0	6.0	1
vanilla chocolate 'Light' *(Swiss Miss)*	4 oz	100	2.0	20.0	110	0	1.0	0
PARROT FISH/pollyfish								
raw	1 lb	390	87.5	0.0	(mq)	0	1.8	(mq)
raw	1 oz	24	5.5	0.0	(mq)	0	0.1	(mq)
PARSLEY								
dried	1 oz	78	6.4	14.6	128	>2.9 c	1.3	0
dried	1 tbsp	4	0.3	0.7	6	.1	0.1	0
dried	1 tsp	1	0.1	.2	1	0	tr	0
dried *(Durkee)*	1 tsp	1	0.0	0.0	0	0	tr	na
dried *(Laurel Leaf)*	1 tsp	1	0.0	0.0	0	0	tr	na
dried flakes *(Spice Islands)*	1 tsp	4	0.2	0.6	6	>.1 c	0.1	0
freeze-dried	1 oz	77	8.9	12.0	111	>2.9 c	1.5	0
freeze-dried	1/4 cup	4	0.4	0.6	5	>.1 c	0.1	0
freeze-dried	1 tbsp	1	0.1	0.2	2	0	tr	0
raw	10 sprigs	4	0.3	0.6	6	na	0.1	0
raw, chopped	1/2 cup	11	0.9	1.9	17	na	0.2	0
raw, trimmed	1 oz	9	0.6	2.0	11	1.2	0.1	0
raw, untrimmed	1 lb	140	9.5	29.8	169	19.0	1.3	0
PARSLEY ROOT/hamburg parsley/turnip-rooted parsley								
fresh	1 lb	50	12.7	10.4	454	5.9	2.7	0
fresh	1 oz	3	0.8	0.7	28	.4	0.2	0
PARSLEY SEASONING								
(Schilling) all-purpose 'Parsley Patch'	1 tsp	6	0.3	1.0	3	(mq)	0.0	0
PARSNIP								
boiled, drained	4 oz	92	1.5	22.1	11	3.1	0.3	0
boiled, drained, 9 inches long	1 parsnip	130	2.1	31.3	16	6.4	0.5	0
boiled, drained, slices	1/2 cup	63	1.0	15.2	8	3.1	0.2	0

Food Name	Serv. Size	Total Cal.	Prot. GMS	Carbs GMS	Sod. MGS	Fiber GMS	Fat GMS	Chol. MGS
raw, slices	1/2 cup	50	0.8	12.0	7	3.3	0.2	0
raw, trimmed	1 oz	21	0.3	5.1	3	>.6 c	0.1	0
raw, untrimmed	1 lb	289	4.6	69.4	39	>7.7 c	1.2	0
PASSION FRUIT/granadilla								
purple, trimmed	1 oz	27	0.6	6.6	na	>3.1 c	0.2	0
purple, trimmed, approx 1.2 oz	1 med	17	0.4	4.2	5	1.9	0.1	0
purple, untrimmed	1 lb	230	5.2	55.1	na	>25.8 c	1.7	0
PASSION FRUIT BEVERAGES								
COCKTAIL								
fresh, purple	1 cup	126	1.0	33.6	15	.5	0.1	0
fresh, purple	1 oz	16	0.1	4.2	2	tr	0.0	0
fresh, yellow	1 cup	148	1.6	35.7	15	.5	0.4	0
(Welch's) bottled 'Orchard Tropicals" diluted	6 oz	100	0.0	25.0	20	0	0.0	0
(Welch's) frozen 'Orchard Tropicals' diluted	6 oz	100	0.0	25.0	20	0	0.0	0
(Welch's) 'Orchard Tropicals Cocktails-In-A-Box'	8.45 oz	140	0.0	34.0	20	0	0.0	0
JUICE								
fresh, yellow	1 oz	19	0.2	4.5	2	.1	0.1	0
(Knudsen & Sons) raspberry	8 oz	130	<1.0	32.0	na	na	0.0	na
(Snapple) passion juice 'Passion Supreme'	8 oz	160	0.0	39.0	20	na	0.0	0
(Veryfine) refresher, w/orange, tropical	8 oz	110	<1.0	26.0	25	na	0.0	0
PASTA/macaroni. See also NOODLE, CHINESE; NOODLE, EGG; NOODLE, JAPANESE; TORTELLINI PASTA.								
(NOTE: 2 ounces uncooked pasta = approximately 1 cup cooked.)								
ACINI PEPE *(Ronzoni)* dry	2 oz	210	7.0	42.0	0	na	1.0	0
AGNOLOTTI, refrigerated, 'Fresh' *(Contadina)*	3 oz	270	13.0	38.0	230	na	7.0	40
ANGEL HAIR								
Dry								
corn *(Westbrae)*	2 oz	210	4.0	46.0	10	na	2.0	10
Jerusalem artichoke *(De Boles)*	2 oz	210	9.0	41.0	0	na	1.0	0
Jerusalem artichoke, garlic and parsley *(De Boles)*	2 oz	210	9.0	41.0	15	na	1.0	0
Jerusalem artichoke, tomato and basil *(De Boles)*	2 oz	210	9.0	41.0	10	na	1.0	0
100% durum wheat semolina *(American Beauty)*	2 oz	210	7.0	42.0	0	na	1.0	0
wheat *(Creamette)*	2 oz	210	7.0	42.0	0	2.0	1.0	0
wheat *(DiGiorno)*	3 oz	250	11.0	47.0	140	na	3.0	0
whole wheat *(De Boles)*	2 oz	210	9.0	40.0	0	na	2.0	0
Refrigerated, fresh								
'Fresh' *(Contadina)*	3 oz	260	12.0	45.0	30	na	3.0	75
BOW TIE. See FARFELLE.								

Food Name	Serv. Size	Total Cal.	Prot. GMS	Carbs GMS	Sod. MGS	Fiber GMS	Fat GMS	Chol. MGS
CAPELLINI								
100% durum wheat semolina								
(American Beauty) dry	2 oz	210	7.0	42.0	0	na	1.0	0
CURLY								
100% durum wheat semolina 'Curly-Roni'								
(American Beauty) dry	2 oz	210	7.0	42.0	0	na	1.0	0
ELBOW								
Dry								
corn (Westbrae)	2 oz	210	4.0	46.0	10	na	2.0	0
corn, wheat-free (De Boles)	2 oz	210	5.0	45.0	0	na	1.0	na
Jerusalem artichoke (De Boles)	2 oz	210	9.0	41.0	0	na	1.0	0
100% durum wheat semolina								
(American Beauty)	2 oz	210	7.0	42.0	0	na	1.0	0
'Primavera' (De Boles)	2 oz	210	9.0	41.0	0	na	<1.0	0
quinoa 'Supergrain Wheat Free'								
(Ancient Harvest)	2 oz	180	5.0	36.0	5	2.5	2.0	0
quinoa 'Supergrain Wheat Free' (Quinoa)	2 oz	180	5.0	36.0	5	2.5	2.0	0
'Valu Pack' (Hospitality)	1/2 cup	240	8.0	48.0	0	2.0	0.5	0
wheat (Creamette)	2 oz	210	7.0	42.0	0	.1	1.0	0
whole wheat	1 cup	365	15.4	78.8	8	12.4	1.5	0
whole wheat (De Boles)	2 oz	210	9.0	40.0	0	na	2.0	0
FARFELLE/bow tie								
Dry								
wheat (De Cecco)	2 oz	210	7.0	41.0	0	na	1.0	0
wheat (Ronzoni)	2 oz	210	7.0	42.0	0	na	1.0	0
FETTUCCINE								
Dry								
basil (Al Dente)	2 oz	220	8.0	40.0	20	(mq)	2.0	(mq)
curry (Al Dente)	2 oz	220	8.0	40.0	20	(mq)	2.0	(mq)
dill (Al Dente)	2 oz	220	8.0	40.0	20	(mq)	2.0	(mq)
egg noodle (Antoine's)	2 oz	210	7.0	41.0	0	na	1.0	0
egg noodle, extra long (Ronzoni)	2 oz	220	8.0	42.0	15	na	3.0	65
egg noodle 'Home-Style' (De Cecco)	2 oz	210	8.0	40.0	35	na	3.0	0
Jerusalem artichoke (De Boles)	2 oz	210	9.0	41.0	0	na	1.0	0
spinach (Al Dente)	2 oz	220	8.0	40.0	20	(mq)	2.0	(mq)
spinach (DiGiorno)	3 oz	250	12.0	46.0	140	na	3.0	0
spinach, Jerusalem artichoke (De Boles)	2 oz	210	9.0	41.0	5	na	<1.0	0
spinach and egg 'Florentine'								
(American Beauty)	2 oz	220	8.0	42.0	35	na	3.0	65
tarragon (Al Dente)	2 oz	220	8.0	40.0	20	(mq)	2.0	(mq)
wheat (DiGiorno)	3 oz	250	11.0	47.0	140	na	3.0	0
wheat, bell pepper/basil, organic (Herb's)	2 oz	220	10.0	40.0	5	na	2.0	60
whole wheat (Al Dente)	2 oz	210	8.0	42.0	10	(mq)	1.0	0

Food Name	Serv. Size	Total Cal.	Prot. GMS	Carbs GMS	Sod. MGS	Fiber GMS	Fat GMS	Chol. MGS
Refrigerated, fresh								
spinach 'Fresh' *(Contadina)*	3 oz	260	12.0	45.0	70	na	4.0	80
FUSILLI								
Dry								
rainbow *(Antoine's)*	2 oz	210	7.0	41.0	20	(mq)	1.0	0
spinach *(De Cecco)*	2 oz	210	7.0	41.0	5	na	1.0	0
tricolor *(Antoine's)*	2 oz	210	7.0	41.0	20	(mq)	1.0	0
tricolor, vegetable *(Antoine's)*	2 oz	210	7.0	41.0	25	2.0	1.0	0
vegetable *(Antoine's)*	2 oz	210	7.0	41.0	20	(mq)	1.0	0
wheat *(De Cecco)*	2 oz	210	7.0	41.0	0	na	1.0	0
GEMELLI *(Antoine's)* dry	2 oz	210	7.0	41.0	0	na	1.0	0
LASAGNA								
Dry								
curly edge *(Ronzoni)*	2 oz	210	7.0	42.0	0	na	1.0	0
Jerusalem artichoke *(De Boles)*	2 oz	210	9.0	41.0	0	na	1.0	0
100% durum wheat semolina *(American Beauty)*	2 oz	210	7.0	42.0	0	na	1.0	0
100% semolina *(Creamette)*	2 oz	210	7.0	42.0	0	na	1.0	0
100% semolina *(De Cecco)*	2 oz	210	7.0	41.0	0	na	1.0	0
spinach, whole wheat, no egg *(Westbrae)*	2 oz	210	8.0	40.0	0	6.0	2.0	0
whole wheat *(De Boles)*	2 oz	210	9.0	40.0	0	na	2.0	0
whole wheat *(Health Valley)*	2 oz	170	9.0	40.0	10	7.2	1.0	0
whole wheat, no egg *(Westbrae)*	2 oz	210	8.0	40.0	0	7.0	2.0	0
whole wheat, spinach *(Health Valley)*	2 oz	170	9.0	40.0	15	7.2	1.0	0
LINGUINE								
Dry								
Jerusalem artichoke *(De Boles)*	2 oz	210	9.0	41.0	0	na	1.0	0
quinoa 'Supergrain Wheat Free' *(Ancient Harvest)*	2 oz	180	5.0	35.0	5	2.5	2.0	0
quinoa 'Supergrain Wheat Free' *(Quinoa)*	2 oz	180	5.0	35.0	5	2.5	2.0	0
wheat *(Creamette)*	2 oz	210	7.0	42.0	0	na	1.0	0
wheat *(De Cecco)*	2 oz	210	7.0	41.0	0	na	1.0	0
wheat *(DiGiorno)*	3 oz	250	11.0	46.0	135	na	3.0	0
wheat *(Ronzoni)*	2 oz	210	7.0	42.0	0	na	1.0	0
Refrigerated, fresh								
(DiGiorno)	3 oz	250	11.0	47.0	140	na	3.0	0
MANICOTTI, extra fancy *(Ronzoni)* dry	2 oz	210	7.0	42.0	0	na	1.0	0
MOSTACCIOLI								
Dry								
100% durum wheat semolina *(American Beauty)*	2 oz	210	7.0	42.0	0	na	1.0	0
wheat *(Creamette)*	2 oz	210	7.0	42.0	0	2.0	1.0	0
wheat *(Ronzoni)*	2 oz	210	9.0	40.0	0	2.0	1.0	0

Food Name	Serv. Size	Total Cal.	Prot. GMS	Carbs GMS	Sod. MGS	Fiber GMS	Fat GMS	Chol. MGS
ORZO *(Ronzoni)* dry	2 oz	210	7.0	42.0	0	na	3.0	0
PENNE RIGATI								
Dry								
(Antoine's)	2 oz	210	7.0	41.0	0	(mq)	1.0	0
(De Cecco)	2 oz	210	7.0	41.0	0	na	1.0	0
PENNONI *(De Cecco)* dry	2 oz	210	7.0	41.0	0	na	1.0	0
QUINOA								
Dry								
garden pagodas 'Supergrain Wheat Free'								
(Ancient Harvest)	2 oz	180	5.0	35.0	5	2.5	2.0	0
veggie curls 'Supergrain Wheat Free'								
(Ancient Harvest)	2 oz	180	5.0	35.0	5	2.5	2.0	0
veggie curls 'Supergrain Wheat Free'								
(Quinoa)	2 oz	180	5.0	35.0	5	2.5	2.0	0
RADIATORE								
Dry								
tomato and spinach, tri-color *(Ronzoni)* . . .	2 oz	210	7.0	42.0	30	na	1.0	0
wheat *(Antoine's)*	2 oz	210	7.0	41.0	0	na	1.0	na
RAINBOW								
100% durum wheat semolina 'Rainbo Twirl'								
(American Beauty) dry	2 oz	210	7.0	42.0	30	na	1.0	0
RIBBON								
Dry								
spinach *(Creamette)*	2 oz	210	7.0	42.0	70	na	1.0	na
wheat, mixed vegetable, organic *(Herb's)*	2 oz	220	10.0	40.0	5	na	2.0	60
wheat, paella, w/saffron, organic								
(Eden Foods)	2 oz	228	8.0	44.0	0	na	<1.0	0
wheat, parsley garlic, organic *(Eden Foods)*	2 oz	228	8.0	44.0	0	na	<1.0	0
whole wheat *(De Boles)*	2 oz	210	9.0	40.0	0	na	2.0	0
yolk-free 'Pennsylvania Dutch' *(Creamette)*	2 oz	210	7.0	42.0	0	na	1.0	0
RIGATONI								
Dry								
(Creamette)	2 oz	210	7.0	42.0	0	na	1.0	0
(De Cecco)	2 oz	210	7.0	41.0	0	na	1.0	0
(Ronzoni)	2 oz	210	7.0	42.0	0	na	1.0	0
Refrigerated, fresh								
'Fresh' *(Contadina)*	2.3 oz	200	9.0	34.0	25	na	3.0	85
Jerusalem artichoke *(De Boles)*	2 oz	210	9.0	41.0	0	na	1.0	0
ROTELLE								
Dry								
100% durum wheat semolina								
(American Beauty)	2 oz	210	7.0	42.0	30	na	1.0	0

Food Name	Serv. Size	Total Cal.	Prot. GMS	Carbs GMS	Sod. MGS	Fiber GMS	Fat GMS	Chol. MGS
quinoa 'Supergrain Wheat Free'								
(Ancient Harvest)	2 oz	180	5.0	35.0	5	2.5	2.0	0
quinoa 'Supergrain Wheat Free' (Quinoa)	2 oz	180	5.0	35.0	5	2.5	2.0	0
wheat (Creamette)	2 oz	210	7.0	42.0	0	na	1.0	0
wheat (De Cecco)	2 oz	210	7.0	41.0	0	na	1.0	0
wheat (Ronzoni)	2 oz	210	9.0	40.0	0	2.0	1.0	0
ROTINI								
Dry								
garlic and parsley (De Boles)	2 oz	210	9.0	41.0	15	na	1.0	0
Jerusalem artichoke (De Boles)	2 oz	210	9.0	41.0	0	na	1.0	0
100% durum wheat semolina								
(American Beauty)	2 oz	210	7.0	42.0	0	na	1.0	0
quinoa 'Supergrain' (Ancient Harvest)	2 oz	210	10.0	40.0	11	8.0	1.0	0
vegetable 'Primavera' (De Boles)	2 oz	210	9.0	41.0	0	na	<1.0	0
vegetable, tomato, and basil (De Boles)	2 oz	210	9.0	41.0	10	na	1.0	0
SALAD PASTA								
100% durum wheat semolina 'Salad-Roni'								
(American Beauty) dry	2 oz	210	7.0	42.0	0	na	1.0	0
SEA SHELL								
durum wheat semolina (American Beauty)								
dry	2 oz	210	7.0	42.0	0	na	1.0	0
SHELL								
Dry								
corn (Westbrae)	2 oz	210	4.0	46.0	10	na	2.0	0
corn, wheat-free (De Boles)	2 oz	210	5.0	45.0	0	na	1.0	na
extra fancy (Ronzoni)	2 oz	210	7.0	42.0	0	na	1.0	0
jumbo (Ronzoni)	2 oz	210	7.0	42.0	0	na	1.0	0
medium (Creamette)	2 oz	210	7.0	42.0	0	na	1.0	0
medium, 100% durum wheat semolina								
(American Beauty)	2 oz	210	7.0	42.0	0	na	1.0	0
100% durum wheat semolina 'Shel-Roni'								
(American Beauty) dry	2 oz	210	7.0	42.0	0	na	1.0	0
quinoa 'Supergrain Wheat Free'								
(Ancient Harvest)	2 oz	180	5.0	35.0	5	2.5	2.0	0
quinoa 'Supergrain Wheat Free' (Quinoa)	2 oz	180	5.0	35.0	5	2.5	2.0	0
'Primavera' (De Boles)	2 oz	210	9.0	41.0	0	na	<1.0	0
wheat (Ronzoni)	2 oz	210	7.0	42.0	0	na	1.0	0
wheat, vegetable, no eggs, organic								
(Eden Foods)	2 oz	228	8.0	44.0	0	na	<1.0	0
whole wheat (De Boles)	2 oz	210	9.0	40.0	0	na	2.0	0
SPAGHETTI								
Dry								
amaranth (Health Valley)	2 oz	170	7.0	40.0	10	8.8	1.0	0

Food Name	Serv. Size	Total Cal.	Prot. GMS	Carbs GMS	Sod. MGS	Fiber GMS	Fat GMS	Chol. MGS
corn *(Westbrae)*	2 oz	210	4.0	46.0	10	na	2.0	0
corn, wheat-free *(De Boles)*	2 oz	210	5.0	45.0	0	na	1.0	na
Jerusalem artichoke *(De Boles)*	2 oz	210	9.0	41.0	0	na	1.0	0
oat bran *(Health Valley)*	2 oz	120	4.0	23.0	2	3.8	1.0	0
100% durum wheat semolina *(American Beauty)*	2 oz	210	7.0	42.0	0	na	1.0	0
100% semolina *(Hospitality)*	2 oz	210	7.0	42.0	0	2.0	0.5	0
pepper 'Three Pepper Pasta' *(Al Dente)*	2 oz	220	8.0	40.0	20	(mq)	2.0	(mq)
protein-fortified	2 oz	213	12.4	37.4	5	>.5 c	1.3	0
quinoa 'Supergrain' *(Ancient Harvest)*	2 oz	210	10.0	40.0	11	8.0	1.0	0
quinoa 'Supergrain' *(Quinoa)*	2 oz	210	10.0	40.0	11	8.0	1.0	0
quinoa 'Supergrain Wheat Free' *(Ancient Harvest)*	2 oz	180	5.0	35.0	5	2.5	2.0	0
quinoa 'Supergrain Wheat Free' *(Quinoa)*	2 oz	180	5.0	35.0	5	2.5	2.0	0
spinach	2 oz	212	7.6	42.6	21	>1.8 c	0.9	0
spinach, Jerusalem artichoke *(De Boles)*	2 oz	210	9.0	41.0	5	na	<1.0	0
spinach, whole wheat, no egg *(Westbrae)*	2 oz	210	8.0	40.0	0	6.0	2.0	0
thin *(Creamette)*	2 oz	210	7.0	42.0	0	na	1.0	0
thin *(Ronzoni)*	2 oz	210	7.0	42.0	0	na	1.0	0
thin, 100% durum wheat semolina *(American Beauty)*	2 oz	210	7.0	42.0	0	na	1.0	0
unenriched	2 oz	211	7.3	42.6	4	>.2 c	0.9	0
wheat *(DiGiorno)*	3 oz	250	11.0	47.0	140	na	3.0	0
wheat *(Rummo)*	2 oz	210	7.0	41.0	10	na	1.0	na
whole wheat	2 oz	198	8.3	42.8	5	>1.7 c	0.8	0
whole wheat *(De Boles)*	2 oz	210	9.0	40.0	0	na	2.0	0
whole wheat *(Health Valley)*	2 oz	170	9.0	40.0	10	7.2	1.0	0
whole wheat, no egg *(Westbrae)*	2 oz	210	8.0	40.0	0	7.0	2.0	0
whole wheat, spinach *(Health Valley)*	2 oz	170	9.0	40.0	10	7.2	1.0	0
SPAGHETTINI *(De Cecco)* dry	2 oz	210	7.0	41.0	0	na	1.0	0
SPIRAL								
Dry								
spicy *(Antoine's)*	2 oz	210	7.0	41.0	40	(mq)	1.0	0
vegetable	1 cup	308	11.0	62.9	36	3.6	0.9	0
wheat, sesame rice, organic *(Eden Foods)*	2 oz	212	10.0	40.0	0	na	1.0	0
wheat, vegetable, no eggs, organic *(Eden Foods)*	2 oz	228	8.0	44.0	0	na	<1.0	0
TRICOLOR								
Dry								
'Primavera' *(De Boles)*	2 oz	200	8.0	41.0	8	(mq)	1.0	0
spirals	1 cup	308	11.0	62.9	36	3.6	0.9	0
wheat *(Creamette)*	2 oz	210	8.0	42.0	5	1.3	1.0	0

Food Name	Serv. Size	Total Cal.	Prot. GMS	Carbs GMS	Sod. MGS	Fiber GMS	Fat GMS	Chol. MGS
TRIO ITALIANO								
rotini, mostaccioli, shells								
(American Beauty) dry	2 oz	210	7.0	42.0	0	na	1.0	0
VERMICELLI								
Dry								
extra thin (Creamette)	2 oz	210	7.0	42.0	0	na	1.0	0
100% durum wheat semolina								
(American Beauty)	2 oz	210	7.0	42.0	0	na	1.0	0
wheat (Ronzoni)	2 oz	210	7.0	42.0	0	na	1.0	0
ZITI Jerusalem artichoke (De Boles) dry	2 oz	210	9.0	41.0	0	na	1.0	0
ZITI RIGATI (Ronzoni) dry	2 oz	210	7.0	42.0	0	na	1.0	0
PASTA DINNER, FROZEN								
penne, w/tomato sauce, Italian sausage								
(Budget Gourmet)	10 oz	320	12.0	53.0	520	na	9.0	5
primavera (Healthy Choice)	11 oz	280	11.0	51.0	360	na	3.0	15
stuffed, shells, 3-cheese 'LightStyle'								
(Le Menu)	10 oz	280	17.0	34.0	690	(mq)	8.0	25
w/chicken and herb tomato sauce								
(Lean Cuisine)	9.5 oz	270	17.0	38.0	460	na	6.0	35
zesty tomato sauce over ziti 'Classics'								
(Healthy Choice)	12 oz	350	16.0	59.0	530	na	5.0	30
PASTA DINNER MIX								
artichoke elbow 'Mac & Cheese' dry								
(De Boles)	2 oz	210	9.0	40.0	160	na	2.0	na
artichoke elbow 'Mac & Cheese' prepared								
(De Boles)	3/4 cup	220	8.0	31.0	140	na	7.0	na
artichoke shells and cheddar, dry								
(De Boles)	2 oz	210	9.0	40.0	160	na	2.0	na
artichoke shells and cheddar, prepared								
(De Boles)	3/4 cup	220	8.0	31.0	140	na	7.0	na
wheat elbow 'Mac & Cheese' dry								
(De Boles)	2 oz	210	9.0	39.0	150	na	3.0	na
wheat elbow 'Mac & Cheese' prepared								
(De Boles)	3/4 cup	200	7.0	27.0	120	na	8.0	na
w/beef flavored sauce, prepared								
(Ultra Slim Fast)	8 oz	230	8.0	45.0	1070	4.0	3.0	na
w/chicken flavored sauce, prepared								
(Ultra Slim Fast)	8 oz	220	8.0	45.0	980	4.0	3.0	na
w/tomato herb sauce, prepared								
(Ultra Slim Fast)	8 oz	220	8.0	46.0	1090	5.0	3.0	na
w/zesty cheese sauce, prepared								
(Ultra Slim Fast)	8 oz	230	9.0	44.0	770	4.0	4.0	na

Food Name	Serv. Size	Total Cal.	Prot. GMS	Carbs GMS	Sod. MGS	Fiber GMS	Fat GMS	Chol. MGS
PASTA DISH MIX. See also NOODLE ENTRÉE/DISH MIX; ROTINI ENTRÉE MIX; SPAGHETTI ENTRÉE MIX.								
Alfredo 'Pasta For One' (Villa Lorenzo)	2.3 oz	270	9.0	39.0	910	na	8.0	na
butter and herbs 'Pasta For One' (Villa Lorenzo)	2.3 oz	270	8.0	43.0	800	na	7.0	na
cream sauce and mushrooms 'Pasta For One' (Villa Lorenzo)	2.3 oz	260	8.0	42.0	800	na	6.0	na
cream sauce and spinach 'Pasta For One' (Villa Lorenzo)	2.3 oz	270	9.0	43.0	900	na	6.0	na
pesto and herbs 'Pasta For One' (Villa Lorenzo)	2.3 oz	260	9.0	41.0	850	na	6.0	na
three cheese and broccoli 'Pasta For One' (Villa Lorenzo)	2.3 oz	260	9.0	43.0	910	na	5.0	na
zesty tomato 'Pasta For One' (Villa Lorenzo)	2.3 oz	250	8.0	47.0	680	na	3.0	na
PASTA ENTRÉE, CANNED. See also NOODLE ENTRÉE/DISH, CANNED; RAVIOLI ENTRÉE; SPAGHETTI ENTRÉE, CANNED.								
(Chef Boyardee)								
and chicken	7.5 oz	180	10.0	30.0	850	1.0	2.0	15
in cheese sauce 'ABC's & 123's'	8.6 oz	200	6.0	42.0	1020	na	1.0	2
in cheese sauce 'Dinosaurs'	8.6 oz	200	6.0	42.0	1060	na	1.0	2
in cheese sauce 'Dinosaurs'	7.5 oz	160	4.0	33.0	790	3.0	1.0	1
in cheese sauce 'Sharks'	7.5 oz	170	5.0	34.0	780	na	1.0	2
in cheese sauce 'Smurfs'	7.5 oz	150	6.0	29.0	830	3.0	1.0	2
in cheese sauce 'Tic Tac Toes'	8.6 oz	190	5.0	41.0	1080	na	1.0	na
in cheese sauce 'Tic Tac Toes'	7.5 oz	160	5.0	31.0	870	3.0	1.0	1
in chicken sauce 'Pac Man'	7.5 oz	170	6.0	22.0	905	na	7.0	na
in meat sauce, shells	7.5 oz	190	7.0	31.0	810	4.0	6.0	5
in pizza sauce, spirals	7.5 oz	180	5.0	35.0	1080	3.0	3.0	5
in sauce 'ABC's & 123's'	7.5 oz	160	5.0	31.0	830	3.0	1.0	2
in sauce 'Turtles'	7.5 oz	150	4.0	31.0	830	na	1.0	0
in tomato sauce 'Pac Man'	7.5 oz	150	6.0	30.0	830	na	1.0	2
mini bites	7.5 oz	260	8.0	30.0	1020	1.0	12.0	17
'Roller Coasters'	7.5 oz	230	7.0	28.0	1070	3.0	10.0	19
w/meatballs 'ABC's & 123's'	8.6 oz	280	9.0	35.0	1090	na	11.0	23
w/meatballs 'Dinosaurs'	8.6 oz	280	9.0	36.0	1131	na	11.0	21
w/meatballs 'Pac Man'	7.5 oz	230	7.0	32.0	880	5.0	9.0	17
w/meatballs 'Sharks'	7.5 oz	230	8.0	31.0	900	na	8.0	15
w/meatballs 'Smurfs'	7.5 oz	240	8.0	31.0	900	2.0	9.0	19
w/meatballs 'Tic Tac Toes'	8.6 oz	290	8.0	39.0	1045	na	11.0	na
w/meatballs 'Tic Tac Toes'	7.5 oz	240	8.0	31.0	1000	na	9.0	18
w/meatballs 'Turtles'	7.5 oz	220	7.0	30.0	940	na	8.0	20
w/meatballs in sauce 'Zooroni'	7.5 oz	240	8.0	33.0	970	na	8.0	17

Food Name	Serv. Size	Total Cal.	Prot. GMS	Carbs GMS	Sod. MGS	Fiber GMS	Fat GMS	Chol. MGS
w/mini meatballs 'ABC's & 123's'	7.5 oz	240	8.0	33.0	920	na	9.0	18
w/mini meatballs 'Dinosaurs'	7.5 oz	230	7.0	32.0	960	na	8.0	19

PASTA ENTRÉE, FROZEN. See also NOODLE ENTRÉE/DISH, FROZEN; RAVIOLI ENTRÉE; ROTINI ENTRÉE, FROZEN; SPAGHETTI ENTRÉE, FROZEN; TORTELLINI PASTA DISH/ENTRÉE, FROZEN; ZITI ENTRÉE, FROZEN.

Food Name	Serv. Size	Total Cal.	Prot. GMS	Carbs GMS	Sod. MGS	Fiber GMS	Fat GMS	Chol. MGS
angel hair (Smart Ones)	8.55 oz	120	8.0	18.0	290	na	<1.0	0
angel hair pasta (Lean Cuisine)	10 oz	240	10.0	38.0	410	na	5.0	10
baked, and cheese (Celentano)	6 oz	290	12.0	29.0	350	(mq)	13.0	(mq)
broccoli stuffed shells, low fat 'Great Choice' (Celentano)	10 oz	190	12.0	31.0	520	na	4.0	na
creamy cheddar 'Pasta Accents' (Green Giant)	1/2 cup	90	4.0	14.0	280	2.0	3.0	5
Dijon 'Microwave Garden Gourmet' (Green Giant)	1 pkg	300	7.0	24.0	560	3.0	20.0	na
garden herb seasoning 'Pasta Accents' (Green Giant)	1/2 cup	80	3.0	12.0	290	3.0	3.0	5
garlic seasoning 'Pasta Accents' (Green Giant)	1/2 cup	100	3.0	14.0	260	2.0	4.0	5
Italiano (Ultimate 200)	8 oz	190	17.0	19.0	450	na	4.0	5
'Looney Tunes Bugs Bunny & Tazmanian Devil' (Tyson)	8 oz	290	13.0	41.0	420	na	8.0	na
'Looney Tunes Daffy Duck' spaghetti & meatballs (Tyson)	8.65 oz	340	11.0	49.0	570	na	10.0	20
'Looney Tunes Daffy Duck & Elmer Fudd' (Tyson)	8 oz	270	11.0	40.0	430	na	7.0	na
'Looney Tunes Foghorn Leghorn & Henry Hawk' (Tyson)	8 oz	230	9.0	39.0	320	na	4.0	na
'Looney Tunes Sylvester & Tweety' (Tyson)	8 oz	250	13.0	41.0	380	na	4.0	na
'Looney Tunes Tweety' macaroni and cheese (Tyson)	8 oz	340	12.0	49.0	650	na	10.0	28
Parmesan, w/sweet peas 'One Serving' (Green Giant)	5.5 oz	160	9.0	21.0	420	2.5	5.0	10
Portafino, in wine sauce (Smart Ones)	9.5 oz	160	8.0	30.0	220	na	1.0	0
primavera 'Pasta Accents' (Green Giant)	1/2 cup	110	5.0	15.0	190	2.5	4.0	5
Romanoff supreme (Weight Watchers)	9 oz	230	12.0	29.0	540	na	7.0	20
shells, cheese, w/tomato sauce (Stouffer's)	9.25 oz	300	17.0	28.0	820	na	13.0	na
shells, stuffed (Celentano)	8 oz	330	18.0	41.0	680	(mq)	11.0	(mq)
shells, stuffed, in tomato sauce 'Classics' (Healthy Choice)	12 oz	330	24.0	53.0	470	na	3.0	35
shells, stuffed, low fat 'Great Choice' (Celentano)	10 oz	250	16.0	41.0	675	na	2.0	na
shells, stuffed 'Single Serving' (Buitoni)	9 oz	460	18.0	46.0	840	(mq)	13.0	80

Food Name	Serv. Size	Total Cal.	Prot. GMS	Carbs GMS	Sod. MGS	Fiber GMS	Fat GMS	Chol. MGS
shells, stuffed, w/sauce *(Celentano)*	10 oz	410	23.0	51.0	850	(mq)	14.0	(mq)
shells, stuffed, w/sauce *(Celentano)*	6.25 oz	340	17.0	31.0	420	(mq)	16.0	(mq)
shells, stuffed, w/vegetables, tofu, sauce *(Legume)*	11 oz	240	15.0	26.0	660	6.2	12.0	0
shells and beef *(Budget Gourmet)*	10 oz	340	20.0	34.0	985	(mq)	14.0	35
teriyaki pasta, w/chicken 'Classics' *(Healthy Choice)*	12.6 oz	350	24.0	58.0	370	na	3.0	45
trio 'Gourmet Selection' *(Tyson)*	11 oz	450	21.0	53.0	890	(mq)	17.0	na
w/shrimp 'Classics' *(Healthy Choice)* ...	12.5 oz	270	16.0	44.0	490	na	4.0	50
w/turkey, Dijon sauce 'Lunch Express' *(Lean Cuisine)*	9 7/8 oz	290	18.0	39.0	540	na	7.0	35

PASTA ENTRÉE, MICROWAVE. See also NOODLE ENTRÉE/DISH, MICROWAVE; RAVIOLI ENTRÉE SPAGHETTI ENTRÉE, MICROWAVE.

(Chef Boyardee)

Food Name	Serv. Size	Total Cal.	Prot. GMS	Carbs GMS	Sod. MGS	Fiber GMS	Fat GMS	Chol. MGS
in cheese sauce 'ABC's & 123's'	7.5 oz	180	5.0	37.0	940	3.0	1.0	3
in cheese sauce 'Dinosaurs'	7.5 oz	180	6.0	36.0	880	3.0	1.0	3
in cheese sauce 'Tic Tac Toes'	7.5 oz	170	5.0	36.0	930	2.0	1.0	2
in sauce 'Turtles'	7.5 oz	160	5.0	33.0	870	2.0	1.0	3
rings and franks	7.5 oz	190	7.0	31.0	980	3.0	5.0	20
rings and meatballs	7.5 oz	220	8.0	33.0	990	4.0	8.0	25
shells, in meat sauce	7.5 oz	210	8.0	32.0	1090	na	6.0	15
shells, in mushroom sauce	7.5 oz	170	6.0	35.0	1080	na	1.0	2
w/meatballs 'Dinosaurs'	7.5 oz	240	8.0	32.0	900	4.0	9.0	17
w/meatballs 'Tic Tac Toes'	7.5 oz	250	7.0	32.0	1035	3.0	10.0	16
w/meatballs 'Turtles'	7.5 oz	210	7.0	30.0	990	2.0	8.0	20
w/mini meatballs 'ABC's & 123's'	7.5 oz	260	7.0	32.0	1005	2.0	11.0	17

(Lunch Bucket)

Food Name	Serv. Size	Total Cal.	Prot. GMS	Carbs GMS	Sod. MGS	Fiber GMS	Fat GMS	Chol. MGS
and garden vegetables 'Light 'n Healthy'	7.5 oz	150	4.0	30.0	630	na	1.0	0
elbows, in tomato sauce	7.5 oz	190	4.0	38.0	860	na	2.0	na
in wine sauce, beef 'Light 'n Healthy'	7.5 oz	130	5.0	21.0	600	na	3.0	10
Italian style chicken 'Light 'n Healthy'	7.5 oz	130	7.0	23.0	630	na	1.0	10
'Pasta 'n Chicken'	7.5 oz	180	9.0	22.0	860	na	6.0	45

PASTA SALAD MIX

Food Name	Serv. Size	Total Cal.	Prot. GMS	Carbs GMS	Sod. MGS	Fiber GMS	Fat GMS	Chol. MGS
Caesar, dry *(Suddenly Salad)*	1/6 pkg	110	4.0	20.0	450	na	1.0	na
Caesar, prepared *(Suddenly Salad)* ...	1/2 cup	170	4.0	20.0	450	(mq)	8.0	na
creamy macaroni, dry *(Suddenly Salad)*	1/6 pkg	100	4.0	20.0	210	na	1.0	na
creamy macaroni, prepared *(Suddenly Salad)*	1/2 cup	200	4.0	21.0	280	(mq)	10.0	na
garden primavera, dry *(Kraft)*	1/6 box	170	5.0	21.0	490	na	7.0	0
Italian 'Light' dry *(Kraft)*	1/6 box	120	5.0	22.0	480	na	1.0	0
pasta, classic, dry *(Suddenly Salad)* ...	1/6 pkg	120	4.0	23.0	530	na	1.0	na
pasta, classic, prepared *(Suddenly Salad)*	1/2 cup	160	4.0	23.0	530	(mq)	6.0	na

Food Name	Serv. Size	Total Cal.	Prot. GMS	Carbs GMS	Sod. MGS	Fiber GMS	Fat GMS	Chol. MGS
pasta primavera, dry *(Suddenly Salad)*	1/6 pkg	90	3.0	19.0	270	na	1.0	na
pasta primavera, prepared *(Suddenly Salad)*	1/2 cup	190	4.0	20.0	340	(mq)	10.0	na
ranch and bacon, dry *(Suddenly Salad)*	1/6 pkg	110	5.0	21.0	250	na	1.0	na
ranch and bacon, prepared *(Suddenly Salad)*	1/2 cup	210	6.0	22.0	320	(mq)	11.0	na
tortellini, Italiano, dry *(Suddenly Salad)*	1/5 pkg	120	4.0	21.0	450	na	2.0	na
tortellini, Italiano, prepared *(Suddenly Salad)*	1/2 cup	160	4.0	21.0	450	(mq)	7.0	na

PASTA SAUCE. See SAUCE.

PASTRAMI. See LUNCHEON MEAT.

PASTRY. See also BREAD, SWEET; BUN, SWEET; CAKE; DANISH PASTRY; MUFFIN; PIE; ROLL, SWEET; TURNOVER.

Food Name	Serv. Size	Total Cal.	Prot. GMS	Carbs GMS	Sod. MGS	Fiber GMS	Fat GMS	Chol. MGS
(Charlotte Russe) w/lady fingers, whipped cream filling	1 serving	326	6.7	38.2	49	0	16.6	225
(Pillsbury) pocket, refrigerated	1 piece	240	4.0	25.0	520	(mq)	13.0	0

PASTRY, BAVARIAN CREAM

Food Name	Serv. Size	Total Cal.	Prot. GMS	Carbs GMS	Sod. MGS	Fiber GMS	Fat GMS	Chol. MGS
(Entenmann's)	1.3 oz	80	2.0	20.0	90	na	0.0	0
(Rich's) puff, frozen	1 piece	150	2.0	17.0	70	(mq)	8.0	25

PASTRY, CINNAMON *(Entenmann's)*

Food Name	Serv. Size	Total Cal.	Prot. GMS	Carbs GMS	Sod. MGS	Fiber GMS	Fat GMS	Chol. MGS
filbert ring	1.5 oz	190	3.0	19.0	160	na	12.0	na

PASTRY, DATE NUT *(Awrey's)* 1 piece | 1.6 oz | 230 | 2.0 | 35.0 | 150 | 1.0 | 10.0 | 15 |

PASTRY, ÉCLAIR

Food Name	Serv. Size	Total Cal.	Prot. GMS	Carbs GMS	Sod. MGS	Fiber GMS	Fat GMS	Chol. MGS
(Rich's) frozen, chocolate, 2 oz	1 piece	210	2.0	27.0	110	(mq)	10.0	35
(Weight Watchers) frozen, chocolate 'Sweet Celebrations'	2.1 oz	150	3.0	26.0	110	na	4.0	15

PATÉ, CANNED

Food Name	Serv. Size	Total Cal.	Prot. GMS	Carbs GMS	Sod. MGS	Fiber GMS	Fat GMS	Chol. MGS
chicken liver	1 oz	57	3.8	1.9	109	0	3.7	111
chicken liver	1 tbsp	26	1.8	0.9	50	0	1.7	51
foie gras, goose liver, smoked	1 oz	131	3.2	1.3	198	0	12.4	43
foie gras, goose liver, smoked	1 tbsp	60	1.5	0.6	91	0	5.7	20
liver *(Sells)*	2 1/8 oz	190	8.0	4.0	470	0	16.0	90

PATTYPAN SQUASH. See SQUASH, SCALLOP.

PEACH

Food Name	Serv. Size	Total Cal.	Prot. GMS	Carbs GMS	Sod. MGS	Fiber GMS	Fat GMS	Chol. MGS
peeled, pitted	1 oz	12	0.2	3.1	tr	.5	<.1	0
peeled, sliced	1/2 cup	37	0.6	9.4	1	1.4	0.1	0
raw, approx 4 oz	1 med	37	0.6	9.7	0	1.4	0.1	0
raw, slices	1 cup	73	1.2	18.9	0	2.7	0.2	0
untrimmed	1 lb	148	2.4	38.2	2	5.5	0.3	0
untrimmed *(Dole)*	2 pieces	70	1.0	19.0	0	1.0	0.0	na

PEACH, CANNED

Food Name	Serv. Size	Total Cal.	Prot. GMS	Carbs GMS	Sod. MGS	Fiber GMS	Fat GMS	Chol. MGS
'Fruit Pak' *(Mott's)*	3.75 oz	75	0.0	18.0	7	(mq)	0.0	0
halves *(Hunt's)*	4 oz	90	<1.0	23.0	7	<1.0	<1.0	0

Food Name	Serv. Size	Total Cal.	Prot. GMS	Carbs GMS	Sod. MGS	Fiber GMS	Fat GMS	Chol. MGS
slices *(Hunt's)*	4 oz	90	<1.0	23.0	7	<1.0	<1.0	0
FREESTONE								
halves *(Del Monte)*	1/2 cup	90	0.0	23.0	10	(mq)	0.0	0
halves *(S&W Nutradiet)*	1/2 cup	30	0.0	7.0	10	(mq)	0.0	0
halves 'Lite' *(Del Monte)*	1/2 cup	60	0.0	13.0	10	(mq)	0.0	0
in heavy syrup, halves *(S&W)*	1/2 cup	100	0.0	26.0	10	(mq)	0.0	0
in heavy syrup, slices *(S&W)*	1/2 cup	100	0.0	26.0	10	(mq)	0.0	0
slices *(Del Monte)*	1/2 cup	90	0.0	23.0	10	(mq)	0.0	0
slices *(S&W Nutradiet)*	1/2 cup	30	0.0	7.0	10	(mq)	0.0	0
slices 'Lite' *(Del Monte)*	1/2 cup	60	0.0	13.0	10	(mq)	0.0	0
YELLOW CLING								
diced 'Fruit Cup' *(Del Monte)*	5 oz	110	0.0	28.0	10	(mq)	0.0	0
halves *(Del Monte)*	1/2 cup	80	0.0	22.0	10	(mq)	0.0	0
halves *(S&W Nutradiet)*	1/2 cup	30	0.0	8.0	5	(mq)	0.0	0
halves 'Lite' *(Del Monte)*	1/2 cup	50	0.0	13.0	10	(mq)	0.0	0
halves 'Lite' *(Finast)*	1/2 cup	50	0.0	14.0	10	(mq)	0.0	0
in heavy syrup, halves *(A&P)*	1/2 cup	100	<1.0	25.0	10	(mq)	<1.0	0
in heavy syrup, halves *(S&W)*	1/2 cup	100	0.0	25.0	10	(mq)	0.0	0
in heavy syrup, slices *(A&P)*	1/2 cup	100	<1.0	25.0	10	(mq)	<1.0	0
in heavy syrup, slices *(Finast)*	1/2 cup	100	0.0	25.0	6	(mq)	0.0	0
in heavy syrup, slices *(Pathmark)*	1/2 cup	100	0.0	25.0	10	(mq)	0.0	0
in heavy syrup, slices *(S&W)*	1/2 cup	100	0.0	25.0	10	(mq)	0.0	0
in heavy syrup, whole, spiced *(S&W)*	1/2 cup	90	0.0	23.0	10	(mq)	0.0	0
in juice *(A&P)*	1/2 cup	50	<1.0	12.0	10	(mq)	<1.0	0
in juice, halves *(A&P)*	1/2 cup	50	<1.0	12.0	10	(mq)	<1.0	0
in juice, halves *(Featherweight)*	1/2 cup	50	0.0	14.0	10	(mq)	0.0	0
in juice, halves 'Lite' *(Libby's)*	1/2 cup	50	0.0	13.0	0	(mq)	0.0	10
in juice, slices *(Featherweight)*	1/2 cup	50	0.0	14.0	10	(mq)	0.0	0
in juice, slices *(IGA)*	1/2 cup	50	1.0	14.0	10	(mq)	0.0	0
in juice, slices *(Pathmark)*	1/2 cup	50	0.0	14.0	10	(mq)	0.0	0
in juice, slices 'Lite' *(Libby's)*	1/2 cup	50	0.0	13.0	0	(mq)	0.0	10
in juice, slices, sweetened *(S&W)*	1/2 cup	90	0.0	20.0	10	(mq)	0.0	0
in light syrup, slices 'No Frills' *(Pathmark)*	1/2 cup	140	1.0	36.0	15	(mq)	0.0	0
slices *(Del Monte)*	1/2 cup	80	0.0	22.0	10	(mq)	0.0	0
slices 'Lite' *(Del Monte)*	1/2 cup	50	0.0	13.0	10	(mq)	0.0	0
slices 'Lite' *(Finast)*	1/2 cup	50	0.0	14.0	10	(mq)	0.0	0
slices, unsweetened *(S&W Nutradiet)*	1/2 cup	30	0.0	8.0	5	(mq)	0.0	0
spiced, w/pits *(Del Monte)*	3.5 oz	80	0.0	20.0	10	(mq)	0.0	0
PEACH, DRIED								
sulfured, cooked, sweetened	4 oz	117	1.2	30.2	2	>1.0 c	0.2	0
sulfured, cooked, sweetened, halves	1/2 cup	139	1.4	35.9	3	3.2	0.3	0
sulfured, cooked, unsweetened	4 oz	87	1.3	22.3	2	>1.1 c	0.3	0

Food Name	Serv. Size	Total Cal.	Prot. GMS	Carbs GMS	Sod. MGS	Fiber GMS	Fat GMS	Chol. MGS
sulfured, cooked, unsweetened, halves	1/2 cup	91	1.5	25.4	3	3.5	0.3	0
sulfured, uncooked	4 oz	271	4.1	69.5	8	9.3	0.9	0
sulfured, uncooked, approx 4.6 oz . . .	10 halves	311	4.7	79.7	9	10.7	1.0	0
sulfured, uncooked, halves	1/2 cup	192	2.9	49.1	6	6.6	0.6	0
(Del Monte) uncooked	2 oz	140	2.0	35.0	10	(mq)	0.0	0
(Mountain House) freeze-dried, prepared	1/4 cup	50	1.0	12.0	<1	(mq)	0.0	0
(Sun•Maid)	2 oz	140	2.0	38.0	10	(mq)	0.0	0
(SunSweet)	2 oz	140	2.0	38.0	10	(mq)	0.0	0
PEACH, FROZEN								
slices, sweetened	10-oz pkg	267	1.8	68.1	17	4.0	0.4	0
slices, sweetened	1/2 cup	118	0.8	30.0	8	1.8	0.2	0
slices, sweetened	4 oz	107	0.7	27.2	7	>.5 c	0.1	0
PEACH BUTTER (Smucker's)	1 tsp	15	0.0	4.0	0	(mq)	0.0	0
PEACH DRINK								
(Hi-C)	6 oz	101	0.1	24.8	18	(tr)	<.1	0
(Ocean Spray) citrus 'Refreshers'	6 oz	90	0.0	23.0	15	na	0.0	na
PEACH JUICE								
(Dole) orchard blend 'Pure & Light'	6 oz	90	0.0	24.0	10	(mq)	0.0	0
(Smucker's) 'Naturally 100%'	8 oz	120	1.0	30.0	10	(mq)	0.0	0
(Snapple) 'Dixie Peach'	8 oz	160	0.0	39.0	20	na	0.0	0
PEACH NECTAR								
w/added ascorbic acid	1 cup	134	0.7	34.7	17	>.4 c	0.1	0
w/added ascorbic acid	1 oz	17	0.1	4.3	2	0	0.0	0
w/o added ascorbic acid	1 cup	134	0.7	34.7	17	1.5	0.1	0
w/o added ascorbic acid	1 oz	17	0.1	4.3	2	0	0.0	0
(Kern's)	6 oz	110	1.0	26.0	0	na	0.0	na
(Knudsen & Sons)	8 oz	107	<1.0	32.0	na	na	0.0	na
(Libby's)	6 oz	100	0.0	24.0	5	na	0.0	na
PEANUT, SHELLED								
(Beer Nuts)	1 oz	180	7.0	7.0	60	(mq)	14.0	0
(Frito Lay) salted	1 oz	170	6.0	6.0	170	na	15.0	0
(Little Debbie) salted	1.25 oz	230	10.0	5.0	90	(mq)	18.0	<1
(Pathmark) 'Sweet and Crunchy'	1 oz	140	4.0	15.0	30	(mq)	8.0	0
(Planters)								
hot spicy 'Heat'	1 oz	170	7.0	5.0	190	na	14.0	0
mild spicy 'Heat'	1 oz	170	7.0	5.0	130	na	14.0	0
'Sweet-N-Crunchy'	1 oz	140	4.0	15.0	20	na	8.0	0
(Weight Watchers)	1 pouch	100	8.0	4.0	50	(mq)	7.0	0
BOILED								
salted	1/2 cup	102	4.3	6.8	240	2.82	7.0	0
salted	1 oz	90	3.8	6.0	213	>.6 c	6.2	0

Food Name	Serv. Size	Total Cal.	Prot. GMS	Carbs GMS	Sod. MGS	Fiber GMS	Fat GMS	Chol. MGS
DRY-ROASTED								
(Finast)								
lightly salted	1 oz	160	7.0	5.0	15	(mq)	14.0	0
salted	1 oz	160	8.0	6.0	120	(mq)	14.0	0
(Flavor House)								
salted	1 oz	180	8.0	5.0	200	(mq)	14.0	0
unsalted	1 oz	180	8.0	5.0	0	(mq)	14.0	0
(Frito Lay) salted	1 1/8 oz	190	7.0	7.0	300	(mq)	16.0	0
(Guy's) salted	1 oz	170	8.0	3.0	310	(mq)	14.0	0
(Pathmark)								
'No Frills' salted	1 oz	170	7.0	5.0	150	(mq)	14.0	0
'No Frills' unsalted	1 oz	180	8.0	5.0	0	(mq)	14.0	0
(Planters)								
lightly salted	1 oz	170	7.0	5.0	110	na	15.0	0
salted	1 oz	160	7.0	6.0	250	(mq)	14.0	0
unsalted	1 oz	170	7.0	5.0	0	na	15.0	0
HONEY-ROASTED								
(Eagle) 'Honey Roast'	1 oz	170	7.0	7.0	140	(mq)	13.0	0
(Fisher)								
lightly salted	1 oz	150	6.0	5.0	0	na	13.0	na
salted	1 oz	150	6.0	5.0	115	na	13.0	0
(Flavor House)	1 oz	160	6.0	9.0	120	(mq)	11.0	0
(Little Debbie)	1.13 oz	190	8.0	9.0	15	(mq)	13.0	<1
(Pathmark)	1 oz	170	6.0	8.0	75	(mq)	13.0	0
(Planters)	1 oz	170	6.0	8.0	180	(mq)	13.0	0
(Weight Watchers)	1 pouch	100	8.0	4.0	50	(mq)	7.0	0
OIL-ROASTED								
(Fisher) salted	1 oz	160	7.0	6.0	130	na	14.0	0
(Flavor House) salted	1 oz	170	7.0	5.0	125	(mq)	15.0	0
(Pathmark) salted	1 oz	180	8.0	5.0	150	(mq)	14.0	0
(Planters)								
cocktail	1 oz	170	7.0	5.0	160	(mq)	15.0	0
cocktail, unsalted	1 oz	170	7.0	5.0	0	(mq)	15.0	0
lightly salted	1 oz	170	7.0	5.0	80	na	14.0	0
redskin	1 oz	170	7.0	5.0	150	(mq)	15.0	0
salted	1 oz	170	7.0	5.0	160	(mq)	15.0	0
unsalted	1 oz	170	7.0	5.0	0	na	14.0	0
PEANUT, SPANISH								
DRY-ROASTED *(Planters)*	1 oz	160	7.0	6.0	200	(mq)	14.0	0
OIL-ROASTED								
salted	1/2 cup	426	20.6	12.8	319	>3.7 c	36.0	0
salted	1 oz	162	7.8	4.9	121	>1.4 c	13.7	0
salted *(Flavor House)*	1 oz	170	7.0	5.0	125	(mq)	15.0	0

Food Name	Serv. Size	Total Cal.	Prot. GMS	Carbs GMS	Sod. MGS	Fiber GMS	Fat GMS	Chol. MGS
salted *(Planters)*	1 oz	170	7.0	5.0	100	na	15.0	0
shelled, salted *(Flavor House)*	1 oz	170	7.0	5.0	125	(mq)	15.0	0
shelled, salted *(Guy's)*	1 oz	170	8.0	3.0	170	(mq)	14.0	0
unsalted	1/2 cup	426	20.6	12.8	4	>3.7 c	36.0	0
unsalted	1 oz	162	7.8	4.9	2	>1.4 c	13.7	0
RAW								
	1 cup	832	38.2	23.1	32	13.9	72.4	0
	1 oz	160	7.3	4.4	6	2.7	13.9	0
(Planters)	1 oz	160	7.0	5.0	5	na	14.0	0
PEANUT, VALENCIA								
oil-roasted	1 cup	848	38.9	23.5	9	>3.3 c	73.8	0
oil-roasted	1/2 cup	424	19.5	11.7	4	>1.6 c	36.9	0
oil-roasted	1 oz	165	7.6	4.6	2	>.6 c	14.4	0
raw	1/2 cup	417	18.3	15.3	<1	>1.6 c	34.7	0
raw	1 oz	160	7.0	5.8	0	>.6 c	13.3	0
PEANUT, VIRGINIA								
oil-roasted, unsalted	1 cup	827	37.0	28.4	9	>7.7 c	69.5	0
oil-roasted, unsalted	1 oz	162	7.2	5.6	2	>1.5 c	13.6	0
raw	1 cup	822	36.8	24.2	15	>7.1 c	71.2	0
raw	1 oz	158	7.1	4.6	3	>1.4 c	13.6	0
PEANUT BUTTER								
(Hollywood) 'Unsalted'	1 tbsp	35	2.0	1.0	0	1.0	3.0	0
(Pathmark) 'Natural'	2 tbsp	200	9.0	5.0	130	(mq)	17.0	0
(Roaster Fresh) gourmet	1 oz	166	8.0	5.0	2	na	14.0	na
(S&W Nutradiet)	1 tbsp	93	3.0	2.0	10	(mq)	8.0	0
(Smucker's)								
honey sweetened	2 tbsp	200	7.0	7.0	150	na	16.0	0
no salt added 'Natural'	2 tbsp	200	8.0	6.0	10	na	16.0	0
CHUNKY								
(Arrowhead Mills)	2 tbsp	190	9.0	6.0	<1	4.5	16.0	0
(Bama)	2 tbsp	200	7.0	6.0	115	(mq)	17.0	0
(Estee)	2 tbsp	200	8.0	6.0	0	na	18.0	0
(Featherweight)	1 tbsp	90	4.0	2.0	5	(mq)	7.0	0
(Finast) 'Crunchy'	2 tbsp	195	9.0	6.0	175	(mq)	17.0	0
(Health Valley) 'No Salt Added'	2 tbsp	180	8.0	6.0	2	2.6	14.0	0
(Hollywood)	1 tbsp	35	2.1	1.0	25	1.0	3.0	0
(Jif)								
regular	2 tbsp	190	9.0	6.0	155	(mq)	16.0	0
'Simply Jif'	2 tbsp	180	9.0	5.0	50	na	16.0	0
(Maranatha Natural) crunchy	2 tbsp	190	8.0	7.0	•5	na	15.0	na
(Pathmark) 'Super Chunky'	2 tbsp	200	7.0	6.0	140	(mq)	17.0	0
(Peter Pan)								
'Extra Crunchy'	2 tbsp	190	9.1	5.1	122	(mq)	16.3	0

Food Name	Serv. Size	Total Cal.	Prot. GMS	Carbs GMS	Sod. MGS	Fiber GMS	Fat GMS	Chol. MGS
regular	2 tbsp	190	9.0	5.0	120	2.0	16.0	0
'Salt Free'	2 tbsp	190	9.0	5.0	0	2.0	17.0	0
(Skippy) 'Super Chunk'	2 tbsp	190	9.0	4.0	130	.6	17.0	0
(Smucker's) 'Chunky Natural'	2 tbsp	200	8.0	6.0	120	(mq)	16.0	0
(Westbrae)								
'Natural' w/salt	2 tbsp	190	8.0	7.0	5	na	16.0	0
'Natural' w/o salt	2 tbsp	190	8.0	7.0	0	na	16.0	0
SMOOTH								
(Arrowhead Mills)	2 tbsp	190	9.0	6.0	<1	4.5	16.0	0
(Bama)	2 tbsp	200	7.0	6.0	140	(mq)	17.0	0
(Estee)	1 tbsp	100	4.0	3.0	2	(mq)	8.0	0
(Featherweight)	1 tbsp	90	4.0	2.0	3	(mq)	7.0	0
(Finast)	2 tbsp	195	9.0	6.0	175	(mq)	17.0	0
(Health Valley) 'No Salt Added'	2 tbsp	180	8.0	6.0	2	2.6	14.0	0
(Hollywood)	1 tbsp	35	2.1	1.0	25	1.0	3.0	0
(Jif)								
regular	2 tbsp	190	9.0	6.0	155	(mq)	16.0	0
'Simply Jif'	2 tbsp	180	9.0	5.0	65	na	16.0	0
(Pathmark) 'No Frills Creamy'	2 tbsp	200	7.0	6.0	170	(mq)	17.0	0
(Peter Pan)								
'Creamy'	2 tbsp	190	8.6	5.7	150	(mq)	16.4	0
'Creamy Salt Free'	2 tbsp	195	8.7	5.3	1	(mq)	17.1	0
(Skippy) 'Creamy'	2 tbsp	190	9.0	4.0	150	.6	17.0	0
(Smucker's)								
'Natural'	2 tbsp	200	8.0	6.0	120	(mq)	16.0	0
'No Salt Added Natural'	2 tbsp	200	8.0	6.0	10	(mq)	17.0	0
(Westbrae) 'Natural' no salt	2 tbsp	190	8.0	7.0	0	na	16.0	0
(Woodstock) 'Old Fashioned Unsalted'	2 tbsp	200	9.0	6.0	3	(mq)	16.0	0
W/JELLY								
(Bama)	2 tbsp	150	3.0	20.0	75	(mq)	7.0	0
(Smucker's)								
'Goober Grape'	2 tbsp	180	5.0	18.0	120	na	10.0	0
'Goober Strawberry'	2 tbsp	180	5.0	18.0	120	na	10.0	0
PEANUT BUTTER CHIPS (Hershey's)								
'Reese's'	1.5 oz	230	9.0	19.0	90	na	13.0	5
PEANUT BUTTER TOPPING (Smucker's)								
caramel	2 tbsp	150	3.0	29.0	120	(mq)	2.0	0
PEANUT FLOUR								
defatted	1 cup	196	31.3	20.8	108	>2.4 c	0.3	0
defatted	1 oz	92	14.6	9.7	50	>1.1 c	0.2	0
low-fat	1 cup	257	20.3	18.8	1	>4.6 c	13.1	0
low-fat	1 oz	120	9.5	8.8	0	>2.2 c	6.1	0

Food Name	Serv. Size	Total Cal.	Prot. GMS	Carbs GMS	Sod. MGS	Fiber GMS	Fat GMS	Chol. MGS
PEANUT OIL								
....	1/2 cup	955	0.0	0.0	0	0	108.0	0
....	1 oz	251	0.0	0.0	0	0	28.4	0
(Hain)	1 tbsp	120	0.0	0.0	0	0	14.0	0
(Planters)	1 tbsp	120	0.0	0.0	0	0	14.0	0
(Spectrum Naturals)	1 tbsp	120	0.0	0.0	0	(tr)	14.0	(tr)
(Wesson)	1 tbsp	122	0.0	0.0	0	0	13.6	0
PEAR								
Asian, raw	1 fruit	51	0.6	13.0	0	na	0.3	0
raw, slices	1 cup	97	0.6	24.9	0	4.3	0.7	0
trimmed, w/skin	1 oz	17	0.1	4.3	tr	.7	0.1	0
untrimmed	1 lb	247	1.6	63.1	2	10.9	1.7	0
untrimmed *(Dole)*	1 fruit	100	1.0	25.0	1	4.0	1.0	na
w/skin, sliced	1/2 cup	49	0.3	12.5	1	2.1	0.3	0
PEAR, CANNED								
in extra heavy syrup	4 oz	110	0.2	28.6	6	>.7 c	0.1	0
in extra heavy syrup, halves	1/2 cup	127	0.3	33.0	7	>.8 c	0.2	0
in extra heavy syrup, solid and liquid, halves	1 cup	253	0.5	65.9	13	>1.5 c	0.3	0
in extra light syrup	4 oz	53	0.3	13.8	2	>.7 c	0.1	0
in extra light syrup, halves	1/2 cup	58	0.4	15.1	3	>.7 c	0.1	0
in extra light syrup, solid and liquid, halves	1 cup	116	0.7	30.1	5	>.3 c	0.3	0
in heavy syrup	4 oz	84	0.2	21.7	6	>.7 c	0.1	0
in heavy syrup, halves	1/2 cup	94	0.3	24.4	7	>.7 c	0.2	0
in heavy syrup, solid and liquid, halves ...	1 cup	189	0.5	48.9	13	5.1	0.3	0
in juice	4 oz	57	0.4	14.7	5	1.0	0.1	0
in juice, halves	1/2 cup	62	0.4	16.0	5	1.1	0.1	0
in juice, solid and liquid, halves	1 cup	124	0.8	32.1	10	5.0	0.2	0
in light syrup	4 oz	65	0.2	17.2	6	>.7 c	<.1	0
in light syrup, halves	1/2 cup	72	0.2	19.0	7	>.7 c	<.1	0
in light syrup, solid and liquid, halves	1 cup	143	0.5	38.1	13	5.0	0.1	0
in water	4 oz	33	0.2	8.9	2	>.7 c	<.1	0
in water, halves	1/2 cup	36	0.2	9.5	3	>.7 c	<.1	0
in water, solid and liquid, halves	1 cup	71	0.5	19.1	5	4.9	0.1	0
(A&P)								
in heavy syrup, halves or slices	1/2 cup	95	<1.0	25.0	10	(mq)	<1.0	0
in juice, halves or slices	1/2 cup	60	<1.0	15.0	10	(mq)	<1.0	0
in light syrup, halves or slices	1/2 cup	70	<1.0	20.0	10	(mq)	<1.0	0
(Del Monte)								
Bartlett, halves 'Lite'	1/2 cup	50	0.0	14.0	10	(mq)	0.0	0
Bartlett, halves or slices	1/2 cup	80	0.0	22.0	10	(mq)	0.0	0
Bartlett, slices 'Lite'	1/2 cup	50	0.0	14.0	10	(mq)	0.0	0

Food Name	Serv. Size	Total Cal.	Prot. GMS	Carbs GMS	Sod. MGS	Fiber GMS	Fat GMS	Chol. MGS
(Featherweight) in juice, halves	1/2 cup	60	0.0	15.0	10	(mq)	0.0	0
(Finast)								
Bartlett, halves or slices, in heavy syrup	1/2 cup	100	0.0	25.0	10	(mq)	0.0	0
Bartlett, halves or slices, 'Lite No Sugar Added'	1/2 cup	60	0.0	15.0	10	(mq)	0.0	0
(Hunt's) halves	4 oz	90	1.0	23.0	6	<1.0	1.0	0
(IGA) Bartlett, halves, unsweetened	1/2 cup	60	0.0	15.0	10	(mq)	0.0	0
(Libby's) in juice, halves or slices, 'Lite' ..	1/2 cup	60	0.0	19.0	10	(mq)	0.0	0
(Pathmark)								
Bartlett, halves, in heavy syrup	1/2 cup	90	0.0	23.0	10	(mq)	0.0	0
Bartlett, halves, in juice	1/2 cup	60	0.0	15.0	10	(mq)	0.0	0
Bartlett, in light syrup 'No Frills'	1 cup	140	0.0	38.0	10	(mq)	0.0	0
Bartlett, slices, in heavy syrup	1 cup	180	0.0	46.0	20	(mq)	0.0	0
(S&W Nutradiet)								
Bartlett, peeled, unsweetened	1/2 cup	35	0.0	10.0	10	(mq)	0.0	0
in heavy syrup, halves	1/2 cup	100	0.0	25.0	10	(mq)	0.0	0
in juice, slices, sweetened 'Natural Style'	1/2 cup	80	0.0	20.0	10	(mq)	0.0	0
peeled, quarters	1/2 cup	35	0.0	10.0	10	(mq)	0.0	0
PEAR, DRIED								
Sulfured								
cooked, sweetened	4 oz	159	1.0	42.1	3	>3.0 c	0.3	0
cooked, unsweetened	4 oz	144	1.0	38.3	3	>3.1 c	0.4	0
stewed, w/added sugar, halves	1/2 cup	196	1.2	52.0	4	8.1	0.4	0
stewed, w/o added sugar, halves	1/2 cup	163	1.2	43.3	4	8.2	0.4	0
uncooked	10 halves	458	3.3	122.0	10	13.1	1.1	0
uncooked	4 oz	297	2.1	79.0	7	>6.5 c	0.7	0
PEAR JUICE								
(Knudsen & Sons)	8 oz	110	<1.0	28.0	na	na	0.0	na
(Santa Cruz Natural) organic 'Cruz'	8 oz	135	1.0	32.0	na	na	<1.0	na
PEAR NECTAR								
(Kern's)	6 oz	120	0.0	28.0	0	na	0.0	na
(Libby's)	6 oz	110	0.0	28.0	0	na	0.0	na
PEAS, CROWDER								
(Allens) canned, 'Fresh'	1/2 cup	80	5.0	15.0	370	(mq)	<1.0	0
(Seabrook) frozen	3 oz	130	8.0	23.0	na	>1.0 c	1.0	0
PEAS, GREEN								
(NOTE: All peas are shelled unless otherwise noted.)								
boiled, drained	4 oz	95	6.1	17.7	3	4.2	0.2	0
boiled, drained	1/2 cup	67	4.3	12.5	2	>1.9 c	0.2	0
boiled, drained, in pod	4 oz	48	3.7	8.0	5	3.2	0.3	0
boiled, drained, in pod	1/2 cup	34	2.6	5.6	3	2.2	0.2	0
raw	1/2 cup	58	3.9	10.4	4	>1.6 c	0.3	0
raw	1 oz	23	1.5	4.1	1	1.0	0.1	0

Food Name	Serv. Size	Total Cal.	Prot. GMS	Carbs GMS	Sod. MGS	Fiber GMS	Fat GMS	Chol. MGS
raw, in pod	1 lb	140	9.3	24.9	8	5.9	0.7	0
raw, trimmed	1/2 cup	30	2.0	5.4	3	1.9	0.1	0
raw, trimmed	1 oz	12	0.8	2.1	1	.7	0.1	0
raw, untrimmed	1 lb	180	11.9	32.2	18	11.1	0.9	0
CANNED								
dietary pack, drained solids	1/2 cup	59	3.8	10.7	2	>1.7 c	0.3	0
dietary pack, solids and liquid	1/2 cup	61	3.7	11.1	2	>1.8 c	0.4	0
drained, low-sodium	4 oz	78	5.0	14.3	2	3.9	0.4	0
regular pack, drained solids	1/2 cup	59	3.8	10.7	186	2.9	0.3	0
regular pack, solids and liquid	1/2 cup	61	3.7	11.1	340	2.5	0.4	0
Early/June								
(A&P)	1/2 cup	70	4.0	15.0	350	(mq)	<1.0	0
(Allens) dry	1/2 cup	80	5.0	15.0	320	(mq)	<1.0	0
(Del Monte) small, w/liquid	1/2 cup	50	3.0	9.0	355	(mq)	0.0	0
(Green Giant)	1/2 cup	50	3.0	12.0	330	3.0	0.0	0
(Green Giant) very young, small	1/2 cup	50	3.0	12.0	390	3.0	0.0	0
(S&W) 'Petit Pois'	1/2 cup	70	4.0	12.0	330	(mq)	0.0	0
(Stokely)	1/2 cup	60	4.0	12.0	320	(mq)	0.0	0
Mixed sizes								
(A&P)	1/2 cup	60	4.0	12.0	350	(mq)	<1.0	0
(IGA) 'No Salt or Sugar Added'	1/2 cup	50	4.0	10.0	10	(mq)	0.0	0
Sweet								
wrinkled, dietary pack, drained, low-sodium	1 lb	82	5.9	15.4	14	0	0.0	0
wrinkled, dietary pack, drained, low-sodium	1 oz	5	0.4	1.0	1	0	0.0	0
wrinkled, regular pack, drained	1 lb	100	5.9	19.5	1071	0	0.0	0
wrinkled, regular pack, drained	1 oz	6	0.4	1.2	66	0	0.0	0
(Featherweight)	1/2 cup	70	5.0	12.0	10	(mq)	0.0	0
(Finast)	1/2 cup	70	4.0	13.0	300	(mq)	1.0	0
(Finast) 'No Salt Added'	1/2 cup	60	4.0	12.0	10	(mq)	0.0	0
(Green Giant)	1/2 cup	50	4.0	11.0	320	4.0	0.0	0
(Green Giant) 50% less salt	1/2 cup	50	4.0	11.0	195	3.0	0.0	0
(Green Giant) mini	1/2 cup	50	4.0	12.0	340	4.0	0.0	0
(Green Giant) mini, in brine	1/2 cup	60	4.0	12.0	240	4.0	<1.0	0
(Green Giant) very young, small	1/2 cup	50	4.0	12.0	390	4.0	0.0	0
(Green Giant) very young, tender	1/2 cup	50	4.0	11.0	390	4.0	0.0	0
(IGA) tiny, early/June	1/2 cup	70	4.0	12.0	340	(mq)	0.0	0
(Pathmark) garden, fancy	1/2 cup	70	4.0	12.0	350	(mq)	1.0	0
(Pathmark) large, tender	1/2 cup	70	4.0	12.0	350	(mq)	1.0	0
(Pathmark) 'Little Gem'	1/2 cup	70	4.0	12.0	350	(mq)	1.0	0
(Pathmark) mixed sizes 'No Salt Added'	1/2 cup	50	4.0	10.0	10	(mq)	0.0	0
(Pathmark) 'No Frills'	1 cup	120	8.0	25.0	640	(mq)	1.0	0
(Pathmark) small	1/2 cup	70	4.0	12.0	350	(mq)	1.0	0
(S&W) 'Perfection'	1/2 cup	70	4.0	12.0	330	(mq)	0.0	0

Food Name	Serv. Size	Total Cal.	Prot. GMS	Carbs GMS	Sod. MGS	Fiber GMS	Fat GMS	Chol. MGS
(S&W Nutradiet)	1/2 cup	40	3.0	8.0	5	(mq)	0.0	0
(Stokely)	1/2 cup	60	4.0	10.0	320	(mq)	0.0	0
W/liquid								
low-sodium	4 oz	56	3.4	10.2	2	2.3	0.3	0
(Del Monte)	1/2 cup	60	3.0	10.0	355	(mq)	0.0	0
(Del Monte) 'No Salt Added'	1/2 cup	60	3.0	11.0	10	(mq)	0.0	0
FREEZE-DRIED (Mountain House)								
prepared	1/2 cup	70	4.0	12.0	21	(mq)	1.0	0
FROZEN								
boiled, drained	4 oz	88	5.8	16.2	99	4.3	0.3	0
boiled, drained	1/2 cup	62	4.1	11.4	70	>1.7 c	0.2	0
unprepared	1/2 cup	55	3.8	9.9	81	>1.5 c	0.3	0
(Birds Eye)	3.3 oz	80	5.0	13.0	130	4.0	0.0	0
(Birds Eye) 'Portion Pack'	3 oz	70	5.0	12.0	120	4.0	0.0	0
(Freshlike)	3.3 oz	80	5.0	13.0	75	na	0.0	na
(Frosty Acres)	3.3 oz	80	5.0	13.0	91	>2.0 c	0.0	0
(Health Valley)	1/2 cup	65	4.0	11.0	70	3.0	0.0	0
(Seabrook)	3.3 oz	80	5.0	13.0	91	>2.0 c	0.0	0
(Southern)	3.5 oz	79	5.5	14.0	130	(mq)	0.5	0
(Stokely) 'Singles'	3 oz	65	4.0	12.0	95	(mq)	1.0	0
(Veg•All)	3.3 oz	80	5.0	13.0	75	na	0.0	na
Chinese								
(Chun King)	1.5 oz	20	1.0	3.0	10	(mq)	0.0	0
(Seabrook)	2 oz	20	2.0	4.0	na	(mq)	0.0	0
Combinations								
(Bird's Eye) w/cream sauce 'Combination Vegetables'	5 oz	180	5.0	16.0	480	3.0	11.0	0
(Bird's Eye) w/pearl onions 'Combination Vegetables'	3.3 oz	70	5.0	13.0	440	3.0	0.0	0
(Bird's Eye) w/potatoes, cream sauce 'Combination Vegetables'	5 oz	190	4.0	17.0	490	2.0	12.0	0
(Budget Gourmet) and cauliflower, in cream sauce	5.75 oz	170	6.0	16.0	280	(mq)	7.0	20
(Budget Gourmet) Oriental, and water chestnuts 'Side Dish'	5 oz	120	5.0	15.0	240	(mq)	3.0	5
(Green Giant) 'LeSueur Valley'	1/2 cup	70	4.0	12.0	400	2.1	2.0	0
(Green Giant) mini, pea pods, water chestnut, butter 'LeSueur Valley'	1/2 cup	80	4.0	10.0	410	3.0	2.0	na
(Green Giant) w/onions and carrots in butter sauce 'LeSueur Valley'	1/2 cup	80	4.0	11.0	470	3.0	3.0	na
Early/June								
(Finast) in butter sauce	1/2 cup	80	8.0	15.0	400	(mq)	4.0	0
(Green Giant) 'Harvest Fresh'	1/2 cup	60	4.0	12.0	140	3.0	1.0	0

Food Name	Serv. Size	Total Cal.	Prot. GMS	Carbs GMS	Sod. MGS	Fiber GMS	Fat GMS	Chol. MGS
(Green Giant) in butter sauce								
'One Serving'	4.5 oz	90	6.0	16.0	500	5.0	2.0	5
(Green Giant) in butter sauce								
'Select LeSueur'	1/2 cup	80	5.0	14.0	440	3.0	2.0	5
(Southern) petite	3.5 oz	64	4.7	11.0	50	(mq)	0.4	0
Sweet								
(Finast)	3.3 oz	80	5.0	13.0	125	(mq)	0.0	0
(Green Giant)	1/2 cup	50	4.0	11.0	95	4.0	0.0	0
(Green Giant) 'Harvest Fresh'	1/2 cup	50	4.0	12.0	135	3.0	0.0	0
(Green Giant) in butter sauce	1/2 cup	80	5.0	14.0	410	4.0	2.0	5
(Stokely) in butter sauce 'Singles'	4 oz	90	5.0	16.0	335	(mq)	1.0	5
Tiny								
(Birds Eye) tender, 'Deluxe'	3.3 oz	60	4.0	11.0	120	4.0	0.0	0
(Freshlike)	3.3 oz	60	4.0	11.0	75	na	0.0	na
(Frosty Acres)	3.3 oz	60	4.0	11.0	127	>2.0 c	0.0	0
(Seabrook)	3.3 oz	60	4.0	11.0	127	>2.0 c	0.0	0
(Veg•All)	3.3 oz	60	4.0	11.0	75	na	0.0	na
PEAS, PIGEON								
immature seeds, boiled, drained	1/2 cup	85	4.6	15.0	4	na	1.0	0
immature seeds, raw	10 seeds	5	0.3	1.0	0	.2	0.1	0
raw, in pods	1 lb	296	15.7	52.0	11	>5.8 c	3.6	0
red gram, mature seeds, boiled	1/2 cup	102	5.7	19.5	4	>.9 c	0.3	0
red gram, mature seeds, raw	1/2 cup	350	22.1	64.0	17	15.3	1.5	0
shelled, boiled, drained	4 oz	126	6.8	22.1	5	>3.3 c	1.5	0
shelled, raw	1 oz	39	2.0	6.8	1	>.8 c	0.5	0
shelled, raw, approx .1 oz	10 peas	5	0.3	1.0	tr	>.1 c	0.1	0
Dried								
shelled, mature, boiled	4 oz	137	7.8	26.4	6	5.3	0.4	0
shelled, mature, boiled	1/2 cup	102	5.7	19.5	5	3.9	0.3	0
shelled, mature, raw	1/2 cup	350	22.1	64.0	17	13.8	1.5	0
shelled, mature, raw	1 oz	97	6.2	17.8	5	3.8	0.4	0
PEAS, PURPLE HULL								
(Allens) canned 'Fresh'	1/2 cup	100	6.0	16.0	370	(mq)	<1.0	0
(Frosty Acres) frozen	3.3 oz	130	9.0	23.0	6	(mq)	0.0	0
PEAS, SNAP								
(Birds Eye) carrots, water chestnuts	3.2 oz	50	2.0	11.0	20	4.0	0.0	0
(Birds Eye) 'Deluxe'	2.6 oz	45	2.0	9.0	5	4.0	0.0	0
(Green Giant) 'Harvest Fresh'	1/2 cup	30	2.0	8.0	100	2.0	0.0	0
(Green Giant) 'Sugar Snap' frozen	1/2 cup	30	2.0	8.0	0	2.0	0.0	0
PEAS, SNOW, 'Deluxe' *(Birds Eye)*	3 oz	35	2.0	6.0	0	3.0	0.0	0
PEAS, WHITE ACRE, canned *(Allens)*	1/2 cup	90	7.0	14.0	440	(mq)	<1.0	0
PEAS AND CARROTS, CANNED								
regular pack, solid and liquid	1/2 cup	49	2.8	10.9	333	4.2	0.4	0

Food Name	Serv. Size	Total Cal.	Prot. GMS	Carbs GMS	Sod. MGS	Fiber GMS	Fat GMS	Chol. MGS
special dietary pack, solid and liquid	1/2 cup	49	2.8	10.9	5	4.2	0.4	0
w/liquid	4 oz	43	2.5	9.6	295	>1.3 c	0.3	0
w/liquid, low-sodium	4 oz	43	2.5	9.6	5	>1.3 c	0.3	0
(A&P) early/June 'No Salt Added'	1/2 cup	60	4.0	12.0	10	(mq)	<1.0	0
(A&P) mixed sizes	1/2 cup	60	4.0	12.0	10	(mq)	<1.0	0
(Del Monte) w/liquid	1/2 cup	50	2.0	10.0	355	(mq)	0.0	0
(Finast)	1/2 cup	55	3.0	9.0	315	(mq)	0.0	0
(Freshlike)	1/2 cup	50	3.0	12.0	340	na	0.0	na
(Freshlike) water pack, w/o salt	1/2 cup	50	3.0	12.0	30	na	0.0	na
(Freshlike) water pack, w/o sugar, salt	1/2 cup	50	3.0	12.0	30	na	0.0	na
(Kohl's)	1/2 cup	50	3.0	20.0	330	(mq)	<1.0	0
(Pathmark)	1/2 cup	60	3.0	18.0	330	(mq)	1.0	0
(S&W)	1/2 cup	50	3.0	9.0	310	(mq)	0.0	0
(S&W Nutradiet)	1/2 cup	35	2.0	7.0	5	(mq)	0.0	0
(Stokely)	1/2 cup	50	3.0	9.0	320	(mq)	0.0	0
(Stokely) 'No Salt or Sugar Added'	1/2 cup	45	3.0	8.0	20	(mq)	0.0	0
(Veg•All)	1/2 cup	50	3.0	12.0	340	na	0.0	na
PEAS AND CARROTS, FROZEN								
boiled, drained	10-oz pkg	133	8.6	28.1	189	10.0	1.2	0
boiled, drained	4 oz	54	3.5	11.5	77	>1.6 c	0.5	0
boiled, drained	1/2 cup	38	2.5	8.1	54	2.9	0.3	0
unprepared	10-oz pkg	151	9.7	31.7	224	9.9	1.3	0
unprepared	1/2 cup	37	2.4	7.8	55	2.5	0.3	0
(A&P)	3.3 oz	60	3.0	11.0	75	(mq)	<1.0	0
(A&P) sweet peas	1/2 cup	80	5.0	13.0	90	(mq)	<1.0	0
(Freshlike)	3.3 oz	60	3.0	11.0	60	na	0.0	na
(Frosty Acres)	3.3 oz	60	3.0	11.0	75	>1.0 c	0.0	0
(Seabrook)	3.3 oz	60	3.0	11.0	75	>1.0 c	0.0	0
(Southern)	3.5 oz	64	3.2	11.7	80	(mq)	0.0	0
(Veg•All)	3.3 oz	60	3.0	11.0	60	na	0.0	na
PEAS AND ONIONS, CANNED								
solid and liquid	1/2 cup	31	2.0	5.1	265	>.7 c	0.2	0
w/liquid	4 oz	58	3.7	9.7	501	>1.4 c	0.4	0
(Freshlike) sweet peas, tiny onions	1/2 cup	60	4.0	12.0	440	na	0.0	na
(Green Giant) pearl onions, w/liquid	1/2 cup	50	4.0	11.0	510	4.0	0.0	0
(S&W) tiny pearl onions, w/liquid	1/2 cup	60	3.0	10.0	490	(mq)	1.0	0
PEAS AND ONIONS, FROZEN								
boiled, drained	4 oz	51	2.9	9.8	na	(mq)	0.2	0
boiled, drained	1/2 cup	41	2.3	7.8	33	2.7	0.2	0
unprepared	10-oz pkg	199	11.3	38.4	173	9.1	0.9	0
unprepared	1/2 cup	48	2.8	9.3	42	2.2	0.2	0
(Birds Eye) pearl onions 'Cheese Sauce Combinations'	5 oz	140	6.0	17.0	470	3.0	5.0	5

Food Name	Serv. Size	Total Cal.	Prot. GMS	Carbs GMS	Sod. MGS	Fiber GMS	Fat GMS	Chol. MGS
(Birds Eye) pearl onions 'Combination								
Vegetables'	3.3 oz	70	5.0	13.0	440	3.0	0.0	0
(Freshlike)	3.3 oz	70	4.0	13.0	100	na	0.0	na
(Frosty Acres) pearl onions	3.3 oz	70	4.0	13.0	80	(mq)	0.0	0
(Seabrook)	3.3 oz	70	4.0	13.0	na	(mq)	0.0	0
(Veg•All)	3.3 oz	70	4.0	13.0	100	na	0.0	na
PECAN, SHELLED								
chopped *(Fisher)*	1 oz	190	2.0	5.0	0	na	19.0	0
dried, chopped	1 cup	794	9.2	21.7	1	7.7	80.5	0
dried, ground	1 cup	634	7.4	17.3	1	6.2	64.3	0
dried, halves	1 cup	721	8.4	19.7	1	7.0	73.1	0
dried, halves, pieces, or chips *(Planters)*	1 oz	190	2.0	5.0	0	(mq)	20.0	0
dried, 31 large or 20 medium halves	1 oz	190	2.2	5.2	tr	1.8	19.2	0
dry-roasted	1 oz	187	2.3	6.3	0	>.5 c	18.4	0
ground *(Fisher)*	1 oz	190	2.0	5.0	0	na	19.0	0
honey-roasted *(Planters)*	1 oz	200	2.0	8.0	0	na	18.0	80
oil-roasted	1 cup	753	7.6	17.6	1	>1.8 c	78.3	0
oil-roasted, 15 halves	1 oz	195	2.0	4.6	0	>.5 c	20.2	0
raw *(Fisher)*	1 oz	190	2.0	5.0	0	na	19.0	0
raw, chips *(Planters)*	1 oz	190	2.0	5.0	0	na	20.0	0
raw, halves *(Planters)*	1 oz	190	2.0	5.0	0	(mq)	20.0	0
raw, pieces *(Planters)*	1 oz	190	2.0	5.0	0	na	20.0	0
PECAN FLOUR	1 oz	93	9.1	14.4	0	>.4 c	0.4	0
PECTIN, unsweetened, dry mix	.5 oz	39	0.0	10.9	24	0	0.0	0
PEPITAS								
In shell								
dried	1 lb	1817	82.4	59.8	59	>7.5 c	153.9	0
roasted, whole	1 cup	285	11.9	34.4	12	>23.0 c	12.4	0
roasted, whole, approx 85 seeds	1 oz	127	5.3	15.3	5	>10.2 c	5.5	0
Shelled								
dried	1 cup	747	33.9	24.6	24	>3.1 c	63.3	0
dried, approx 142 kernels	1 oz	154	7.0	5.1	5	>.6 c	13.0	0
roasted	1 cup	1184	74.8	30.5	40	>4.1 c	95.6	0
roasted	1 oz	148	9.4	3.8	5	>.5 c	12.0	0
salted	1 lb	2021	84.1	243.8	2608	>162.8 c	88.0	0
salted	1 cup	285	11.9	34.4	368	>23.0 c	12.4	0
salted	1 oz	127	5.3	15.3	163	>10.2 c	5.5	0
PEPPER, BANANA, hot rings *(Vlasic)*	1 oz	4	0.0	1.0	465	(mq)	0.0	0
PEPPER, BELL. See PEPPER, SWEET.								
PEPPER, CHERRY								
hot *(Progresso)*	1/2 cup	190	0.0	3.0	130	1.0	20.0	0
hot *(Vlasic)*	1 oz	10	0.0	2.0	425	(mq)	0.0	0
hot, pickled *(Progresso)*	1/2 cup	130	0.0	3.0	110	1.0	12.0	0

Food Name	Serv. Size	Total Cal.	Prot. GMS	Carbs GMS	Sod. MGS	Fiber GMS	Fat GMS	Chol. MGS
mild (Vlasic)	1 oz	8	0.0	2.0	410	(mq)	0.0	0

PEPPER, CHILI

Food Name	Serv. Size	Total Cal.	Prot. GMS	Carbs GMS	Sod. MGS	Fiber GMS	Fat GMS	Chol. MGS
green, raw, approx 1.6 oz	1 med	18	0.9	4.3	3	.7	0.1	0
green, raw, chopped	1/2 cup	30	1.5	7.1.	5	1.1	0.2	0
green, raw, trimmed	1 oz	11	0.6	2.7	2	.5	0.1	0
green, raw, untrimmed	1 lb	134	6.6	31.3	23	6.0	0.7	0
red, raw, approx 1.6 oz	1 med	18	0.9	4.3	3	.7	0.1	0
red, raw, chopped	1/2 cup	30	1.5	7.1	5	1.1	0.2	0
red, raw, trimmed	1 oz	11	0.6	2.7	2	.5	0.1	0
red, raw, untrimmed	1 lb	134	6.6	31.3	23	6.0	0.7	0
Canned								
green, chopped (Old El Paso)	2 tbsp	8	<1.0	2.0	70	(mq)	<1.0	0
green, diced (Rosarita)	1.058 oz	6	0.1	1.4	85	.5	0.1	0
green, diced, w/liquid (Del Monte)	1/2 cup	20	0.0	5.0	690	(mq)	0.0	0
green, whole (Old El Paso)	1 pepper	8	<1.0	1.0	105	(mq)	<1.0	0
green, whole (Rosarita)	1.235 oz	4	0.2	1.1	74	.5	0.1	0
green, whole, diced, sliced, or strips (Ortega)	1 oz	10	0.0	3.0	20	(mq)	0.0	0
green, whole, w/liquid (Del Monte)	1/2 cup	20	0.0	5.0	690	(mq)	0.0	0
green and red, seeded, chopped, w/liquid	1/2 cup	17	0.6	4.2	(mq)	>.8 c	0.1	0
green and red, seeded, w/liquid	4 oz	28	1.0	6.9	(mq)	>1.4 c	0.1	0
hot, green, pods, w/o seeds, solid and liquid, chopped	1/2 cup	17	0.6	4.2	798	>.8 c	0.1	0
hot, green and red, seeded, w/liquid, approx 2.6 oz	1 med	18	0.7	4.5	(mq)	1.0	0.1	0

PEPPER, GREEN. See PEPPER, SWEET.

PEPPER, GROUND

Food Name	Serv. Size	Total Cal.	Prot. GMS	Carbs GMS	Sod. MGS	Fiber GMS	Fat GMS	Chol. MGS
black	1 oz	72	3.1	18.4	12	>3.7 c	0.9	0
black	1 tbsp	16	0.7	4.2	3	1.7	0.2	0
black	1 tsp	5	0.2	1.4	1	.6	0.1	0
black (Durkee)	1 tsp	8	0.0	0.0	0	0	tr	na
black (Laurel Leaf)	1 tsp	8	0.0	0.0	0	0	tr	na
black (Spice Islands)	1 tsp	9	0.2	1.5	<1	>.2 c	0.2	0
cayenne/red	1 oz	90	3.4	16.1	9	>7.1 c	4.9	0
cayenne/red	1 tbsp	17	0.6	3.0	2	>1.3 c	0.9	0
cayenne/red	1 tsp	6	0.2	1.0	1	>.5 c	0.3	0
cayenne/red (Durkee)	1 tsp	8	0.0	0.0	0	0	<0.1	na
cayenne/red (Laurel Leaf)	1 tsp	8	0.0	0.0	0	0	<0.1	na
cayenne/red (Spice Islands)	1 tsp	9	0.3	1.1	<1	>.5 c	0.3	0
chili (Spice Islands)	1 tsp	9	0.3	1.2	<1	>.3 c	0.3	0
pizza (Lawry's)	1 tsp	2	1.5	3.2	11	na	0.2	0
seasoned (Lawry's)	1 tsp	9	0.3	1.8	5	>.2 c	0.1	0

Food Name	Serv. Size	Total Cal.	Prot. GMS	Carbs GMS	Sod. MGS	Fiber GMS	Fat GMS	Chol. MGS
seasoned 'All Pepper' (Schilling)	1/4 tsp	1	<.1	0.3	106	(mq)	0.0	0
white	1 oz	84	2.9	19.5	1	>1.2 c	0.6	0
white	1 tbsp	21	0.7	4.9	0	>.3 c	0.2	0
white	1 tsp	7	0.3	1.6	0	>.1 c	0.1	0
white (Durkee)	1 tsp	9	0.0	0.0	0	0	tr	na
white (Laurel Leaf)	1 tsp	9	0.0	0.0	0	0	tr	na
white (Spice Islands)	1 tsp	9	0.3	1.5	<1	>.1 c	0.2	0

PEPPER, JALAPEÑO

Food Name	Serv. Size	Total Cal.	Prot. GMS	Carbs GMS	Sod. MGS	Fiber GMS	Fat GMS	Chol. MGS
diced (Ortega)	1 oz	10	0.0	3.0	20	(mq)	0.0	0
diced (Rosarita)	1.058 oz	5	0.4	0.8	121	.6	0.2	0
for nachos (La Victoria)	14 pieces	5	0.0	1.0	330	na	0.0	na
for nachos (La Victoria)	1 tbsp	2	<1.0	1.0	335	(mq)	<1.0	0
hot, diced (Ortega)	1 oz	8	0.0	2.0	(mq)	(mq)	0.0	0
hot 'Mexican' (Vlasic)	1 oz	8	0.0	2.0	380	(mq)	0.0	0
hot, tiny, Mexican (Vlasic)	1 oz	6	0.0	2.0	430	(mq)	0.0	0
hot, whole (Ortega)	1 oz	8	0.0	2.0	(mq)	(mq)	0.0	0
marinated (La Victoria)	1.5 pieces	10	0.0	2.0	300	na	0.0	na
marinated (La Victoria)	1 tbsp	4	<1.0	1.0	251	(mq)	<1.0	0
nacho sliced (Rosarita)	1.058 oz	4	0.1	1.0	448	.6	0.1	0
sliced, w/liquid (Del Monte)	1/2 cup	30	1.0	6.0	1690	(mq)	1.0	0
whole (Old El Paso)	2 peppers	14	0.0	1.0	480	(mq)	1.0	0
whole (Ortega)	1 oz	10	0.0	3.0	20	(mq)	0.0	0
whole (Rosarita)	1.34 oz	6	0.2	1.3	568	.7	0.2	0
whole, w/escabeche (Rosarita)	1.164 oz	8	0.6	1.4	430	.9	0.2	0
whole, w/liquid (Del Monte)	1/2 cup	30	1.0	6.0	1690	(mq)	1.0	0

PEPPER, PEPPERONCINI

Food Name	Serv. Size	Total Cal.	Prot. GMS	Carbs GMS	Sod. MGS	Fiber GMS	Fat GMS	Chol. MGS
mild, Greek, salad (Vlasic)	1 oz	4	0.0	1.0	450	(mq)	0.0	0
Tuscan (Progresso)	1/2 cup	20	0.0	7.0	5	1.0	0.0	0
PEPPER, PICCALILLI (Progresso)	1/2 cup	190	<1.0	4.0	220	1.0	20.0	0

PEPPER, SWEET/bell pepper/green pepper/red pepper/yellow pepper

Food Name	Serv. Size	Total Cal.	Prot. GMS	Carbs GMS	Sod. MGS	Fiber GMS	Fat GMS	Chol. MGS
boiled, drained	4 oz	32	1.0	7.6	2	>.5 c	0.2	0
boiled, drained, approx 2.6 oz	1 med	20	0.7	4.9	1	>.3 c	0.2	0
boiled, drained, chopped	1/2 cup	19	0.6	4.6	1	.9	0.1	0
raw, approx 3.2 oz	1 med	20	0.7	4.8	1	1.5	0.1	0
raw, chopped	1/2 cup	14	0.4	3.2	1	.8	0.1	0
raw (Dole)	1 med	25	1.0	5.0	0	2.0	1.0	na
raw, trimmed	1 oz	8	0.3	1.8	<1	.5	0.1	0
raw, untrimmed	1 lb	99	3.3	23.9	7	6.0	0.7	0
Canned								
roasted (Progresso)	1/2 cup	20	<1.0	5.0	2	1.7	<1.0	0
solid and liquid, halves	1/2 cup	13	0.6	2.7	958	>.6 c	0.2	0
'Sweet Pepper Mementos' (Heinz)	1 oz	6	0.0	1.0	320	(mq)	0.0	0
w/liquid	4 oz	20	0.9	4.4	1552	>.9 c	0.3	0

Food Name	Serv. Size	Total Cal.	Prot. GMS	Carbs GMS	Sod. MGS	Fiber GMS	Fat GMS	Chol. MGS
Freeze-dried								
....	1 oz	89	5.1	19.5	55	>4.6 c	0.9	0
....	1/4 cup	5	0.3	1.1	3	>.3 c	0.1	0
Frozen								
boiled, drained, chopped	4 oz	20	1.1	4.4	5	>1.0 c	0.2	0
chopped, unprepared	10-oz pkg	57	3.1	12.6	14	4.5	0.6	0
chopped, unprepared	1 oz	6	0.3	1.3	1	.5	0.1	0
green *(Seabrook)*	1 oz	6	0.0	1.0	1	(mq)	0.0	0
red *(Seabrook)*	1 oz	8	0.0	1.0	na	(mq)	0.0	0
PEPPER DILL SEASONING								
(Golden Dipt)	2 grams	8	0.0	1.0	96	na	0.0	0
PEPPER STEAK DINNER								
(Armour) frozen, beef 'Classics Lite' ...	11.25 oz	220	17.0	29.0	970	(mq)	4.0	35
(Healthy Choice) frozen	11 oz	260	20.0	40.0	500	na	5.0	40
(LaChoy)	3.81 oz	36	1.9	7.4	942	1.4	0.2	0
(Le Menu) frozen	11.5 oz	370	26.0	36.0	1020	(mq)	13.0	(mq)
PEPPER STEAK DINNER MIX								
(LaChoy) 'Dinner Classics'	1/5 pkg	35	2.0	9.0	720	1.0	<1.0	0
(LaChoy) 'Dinner Classics' prepared ...	3/4 cup	180	17.0	9.0	760	1.0	9.0	60
PEPPER STEAK ENTRÉE								
pork and beef	1 oz	141	6.0	0.8	578	0	12.5	(mq)
pork and beef, approx .2 oz	1 slice	27	1.2	0.2	112	0	2.4	(mq)
(Budget Gourmet) frozen, w/rice	10 oz	300	15.0	39.0	800	(mq)	9.0	25
(Dining Lite) frozen	9 oz	260	18.0	33.0	1050	(mq)	6.0	40
(Healthy Choice) frozen	9.5 oz	250	18.0	36.0	560	na	4.0	40
(LaChoy) frozen, w/rice & vegetables								
'Fresh & Lite'	10 oz	280	21.0	33.0	1082	2.0	8.0	36
(Stouffer's) frozen, green, w/rice, 1 pkg	10.5 oz	310	20.0	35.0	700	na	10.0	na
(Top Shelf) Oriental, microwave bowl	1 serving	290	25.0	25.0	1700	(mq)	10.0	45
(Tyson) frozen 'Gourmet Selection' ...	11.25 oz	330	20.0	38.0	1130	(mq)	11.0	(mq)
(Ultra Slim Fast) beef, and parsley rice ...	12 oz	270	22.0	36.0	690	na	4.0	45
PEPPERONI								
(Hickory Farms)	1 oz	140	6.0	1.0	578	0	13.0	23
(Hormel)								
'Chunk'	1 oz	140	6.0	0.0	423	0	12.0	(mq)
'Leoni Brand'	1 oz	130	6.0	0.0	508	0	12.0	(mq)
'Perma-Fresh'	2 slices	80	3.0	0.0	281	0	7.0	(mq)
'Rosa'	1 oz	140	6.0	0.0	626	0	13.0	(mq)
'Rosa Grande'	1 oz	140	6.0	0.0	512	0	13.0	(mq)
(JM) approx .5 oz	8 slices	70	3.0	1.0	290	0	6.0	(mq)
PEPPERS AND ONIONS *(Quincy's)*	4 oz	80	1.0	8.0	11	(mq)	5.0	na
PERCH								
frozen *(Booth)*	4 oz	100	20.0	0.0	90	0	1.0	(mq)

Food Name	Serv. Size	Total Cal.	Prot. GMS	Carbs GMS	Sod. MGS	Fiber GMS	Fat GMS	Chol. MGS
frozen *(SeaPak)*	4 oz	100	19.0	0.0	80	0	2.0	(mq)
frozen, fillet, battered *(Van de Kamp's)*	2 pieces	310	12.0	18.0	500	na	21.0	30
mixed species, dry-heat cooked	4 oz	133	28.2	0.0	90	0	1.3	130
mixed species, dry-heat cooked	3 oz	99	21.1	0.0	67	0	1.0	98
mixed species, raw	1 lb	413	87.9	0.0	280	0	4.2	407
mixed species, raw	3 oz	77	16.5	0.0	53	0	0.8	77
mixed species, raw	1 oz	26	5.5	0.0	18	0	0.3	26
PERSIMMON								
Japanese, dried	1 oz	78	0.4	20.8	1	>1.0 c	0.2	0
Japanese, fresh, trimmed	1 oz	20	0.2	5.3	<1	>.4 c	0.1	0
Japanese, fresh, untrimmed	1 lb	268	2.2	70.8	6	>5.6 c	0.7	0
Japanese, raw, 2.5-inch diam	1 med	118	1.0	31.2	2	6.1	0.3	0
native, fresh, trimmed	1 oz	36	0.2	9.5	<1	>.4 c	0.1	0
native, fresh, untrimmed	1 lb	472	3.0	124.6	4	>5.6 c	1.5	0
native, raw, trimmed, approx 1.1 oz	1 med	32	0.2	8.4	0	>.4 c	0.1	0
PE-TSAI. See CABBAGE, NAPA.								
PHEASANT								
breast meat only, raw	1 oz	38	6.9	0.0	9	0	0.9	(mq)
leg meat only, raw	1 oz	38	6.3	0.0	13	0	1.2	(mq)
meat and skin, raw	1 oz	51	6.4	0.0	11	0	2.6	(mq)
meat only, raw	1 oz	38	6.7	0.0	10	0	1.0	(mq)
PHYLLO DOUGH								
1 sheet	1 oz	85	2.0	14.9	137	na	1.7	0
1 sheet *(Apollo)*	1 oz	80	3.0	18.0	200	na	.4	0
PICKLES								
BREAD AND BUTTER								
chunks 'Old-Fashion' *(Vlasic)*	1 oz	25	0.0	6.0	120	(mq)	0.0	0
'Deli' *(Vlasic)*	1 oz	25	0.0	6.0	120	(mq)	0.0	0
fresh	2 slices	11	0.1	2.7	101	>.1 c	0.0	0
one slice *(Claussen)*	.4 oz	7	0.1	1.7	61	(mq)	tr	0
slices	1 cup	124	1.5	30.4	1144	>.9 c	0.3	0
slices *(Claussen)*	1 oz	20	0.2	4.7	172	(mq)	0.1	0
slices, approx 2/3 oz *(Mrs. Fanning's)*	2 slices	16	0.0	3.0	140	(mq)	0.0	0
slices 'Cucumber Slices' *(Heinz)*	1 oz	25	0.0	6.0	170	(mq)	0.0	0
'Sweet Butter Chips' *(Vlasic)*	1 oz	30	0.0	7.0	160	(mq)	0.0	0
'Sweet Butter Stix' *(Vlasic)*	1 oz	18	0.0	5.0	110	(mq)	0.0	0
DILL								
	1 lb	81	2.8	18.7	5813	5.4	0.9	0
	1 oz	5	0.2	1.2	363	.3	0.1	0
baby *(Heinz)*	1 oz	4	0.0	1.0	285	(mq)	0.0	0
baby *(Vlasic)*	1 oz	4	0.0	1.0	210	(mq)	0.0	0
chips *(Heinz)*	1 oz	4	0.0	1.0	275	(mq)	0.0	0
chunks, snack *(Vlasic)*	1 oz	4	0.0	1.0	220	(mq)	0.0	0

Food Name	Serv. Size	Total Cal.	Prot. GMS	Carbs GMS	Sod. MGS	Fiber GMS	Fat GMS	Chol. MGS
chunks, zesty, snacks (Vlasic)	1 oz	4	0.0	1.0	290	(mq)	0.0	0
crunchy (Vlasic)	1 oz	4	0.0	1.0	210	(mq)	0.0	0
crunchy, half salt (Vlasic)	1 oz	4	0.0	1.0	125	(mq)	0.0	0
crunchy, zesty (Vlasic)	1 oz	4	0.0	1.0	250	(mq)	0.0	0
gherkins (Vlasic)	1 oz	4	0.0	1.0	210	(mq)	0.0	0
halves 'Deli' (Vlasic)	1 oz	4	0.0	1.0	290	(mq)	0.0	0
halves 'Deli Style' (Heinz)	1 oz	4	0.0	1.0	280	(mq)	0.0	0
hamburger chips, half salt (Vlasic)	1 oz	2	0.0	1.0	175	(mq)	0.0	0
hamburger slices (Heinz)	1 oz	2	0.0	0.0	405	(mq)	0.0	0
low sodium	1 lb	81	2.8	18.7	82	5.4	0.9	0
low sodium	1 oz	5	0.2	1.2	5	.3	0.1	0
no garlic (Claussen)	1 oz	6	0.2	1.0	313	(mq)	0.1	0
no garlic, 1 piece (Claussen)	2.9 oz	17	0.6	2.8	895	(mq)	0.3	0
'Original' (Vlasic)	1 oz	4	0.0	1.0	375	(mq)	0.0	0
'Polish Snack Chunks' (Vlasic)	1 oz	4	0.0	1.0	300	(mq)	0.0	0
spears (Claussen)	1 oz	4	0.1	0.5	330	(mq)	0.1	0
spears, half salt (Vlasic)	1 oz	4	0.0	1.0	120	(mq)	0.0	0
spears, kosher (Heinz)	1 oz	4	0.0	1.0	295	(mq)	0.0	0
spears, kosher (Vlasic)	1 oz	4	0.0	1.0	175	(mq)	0.0	0
spears, no garlic (Vlasic)	1 oz	4	0.0	1.0	210	(mq)	0.0	0
spears, 1 piece (Claussen)	1.1 oz	4	0.2	0.6	373	(mq)	0.1	0
spears, Polish style (Heinz)	1 oz	4	0.0	1.0	285	(mq)	0.0	0
spears, zesty (Vlasic)	1 oz	4	0.0	1.0	230	(mq)	0.0	0
whole (Featherweight)	1 piece	4	0.0	1.0	5	(mq)	0.0	0
whole 'Genuine' (Heinz)	1 oz	2	0.0	1.0	420	(mq)	0.0	0
whole, kosher (Heinz)	1 oz	4	0.0	1.0	295	(mq)	0.0	0
whole, Polish style (Heinz)	1 oz	4	0.0	1.0	285	(mq)	0.0	0
whole, processed (Heinz)	1 oz	2	0.0	0.0	435	(mq)	0.0	0
HOT AND SPICY, garden, mixed (Vlasic)	1 oz	4	0.0	1.0	380	(mq)	0.0	0
KOSHER. See also DILL.								
chips, 'Old Fashioned' (Heinz)	1 oz	4	0.0	1.0	270	(mq)	0.0	0
halves (Claussen)	1 oz	4	0.1	0.5	330	(mq)	0.1	0
halves 'Old Fashioned Deli Halves' (Heinz)	1 oz	4	0.0	1.0	275	(mq)	0.0	0
halves, 2.3 oz (Claussen)	1 piece	9	0.3	1.3	769	(mq)	0.2	0
slices (Claussen)	1 oz	3	0.1	0.5	319	(mq)	0.1	0
slices, .3 oz (Claussen)	1 piece	1	tr	0.2	107	(mq)	tr	0
SOUR								
	1 lb	48	1.5	10.2	5477	>2.8 c	0.9	0
	1 oz	3	0.1	0.6	342	>.2 c	0.1	0
low sodium	1 lb	48	1.5	10.2	82	>2.8 c	0.9	0
low sodium	1 oz	3	0.1	0.6	5	>.2 c	0.1	0
whole (Claussen)	1 oz	3	0.2	0.5	332	(mq)	0.1	0
whole 'Old Fashioned' (Heinz)	1 oz	4	0.0	1.0	280	(mq)	0.0	0

Food Name	Serv. Size	Total Cal.	Prot. GMS	Carbs GMS	Sod. MGS	Fiber GMS	Fat GMS	Chol. MGS
whole, 1 piece *(Claussen)*	2.5 oz	9	0.4	1.3	832	(mq)	0.2	0
SWEET								
....	1 lb	529	1.7	144.3	4257	5.0	1.2	0
....	1 oz	33	0.1	9.0	266	.3	0.1	0
cubes, salad *(Heinz)*	1 oz	30	0.0	7.0	270	(mq)	0.0	0
'Cucumber Stix' *(Heinz)*	1 oz	25	0.0	6.0	145	(mq)	0.0	0
gherkins *(Heinz)*	1 oz	35	0.0	8.0	210	(mq)	0.0	0
gherkins, midget *(Heinz)*	1 oz	35	0.0	8.0	205	(mq)	0.0	0
half salt 'Sweet Butter Chips' *(Vlasic)*	1 oz	30	0.0	7.0	80	(mq)	0.0	0
low sodium	1 lb	529	1.7	144.3	82	5.0	1.2	0
low sodium	1 med	41	0.1	11.1	6	>.2 c	0.1	0
low sodium	1 oz	33	0.1	9.0	5	.3	0.1	0
low sodium	1 slice	7	0.0	1.9	1	0.0	0.0	0
low sodium, mixed *(Heinz)*	1 oz	40	0.0	9.0	200	(mq)	0.0	0
low sodium, 3 inches long, approx 1.2 oz	1 large	41	0.1	11.1	6	.4	0.1	0
sliced *(Featherweight)*	3-4 slices	24	0.0	6.0	5	(mq)	0.0	0
sliced *(Heinz)*	1 oz	35	0.0	8.0	205	(mq)	0.0	0
sliced 'Cucumber Slices' *(Heinz)*	1 oz	20	0.0	5.0	195	(mq)	0.0	0
whole, 3 inches long, approx 1.2 oz	1 large	41	0.1	11.1	328	.4	0.1	0
PICKLING SPICE *(Tone's)*	1 tsp	10	0.3	1.2	1	.3	0.6	0
PIE								
APPLE								
Fresh								
(Entenmann's) homestyle	2.1 oz	140	1.0	21.0	150	na	7.0	na
(McMillin's)	4 oz	430	4.0	51.0	340	na	23.0	na
Frozen								
(Amy's Kitchen)	8 oz	282	4.0	42.0	180	na	12.0	na
(Banquet) 'Family Size' 3 1/3 oz	1/6 pie	250	2.0	37.0	290	(mq)	11.0	na
(Mrs. Smith's) 'Pie In Minutes' 8-inch pie	1/8 pie	210	2.0	29.0	250	(mq)	9.0	0
(Pet-Ritz)	1/16 pie	330	2.0	53.0	385	(mq)	12.0	0
(Sara Lee) apple streusel 'Free & Light'	1/8 pie	170	1.0	36.0	140	(mq)	2.0	0
(Sara Lee) Dutch apple 'Homestyle'								
9-inch pie	1/10 pie	300	2.0	45.0	310	(mq)	12.0	0
(Sara Lee) 'Homestyle' 9-inch pie	1/10 pie	280	2.0	42.0	220	(mq)	12.0	0
(Sara Lee) 'Homestyle High' 10-inch pie	1/10 pie	400	3.0	46.0	450	(mq)	23.0	0
(Weight Watchers) 3.5 oz	1/2 pkg	200	2.0	39.0	280	(mq)	5.0	5
BANANA CREAM								
Frozen								
(Banquet) 2 1/3 oz	1/6 pie	180	2.0	21.0	150	(mq)	10.0	na
(Pet-Ritz) 2 1/3 oz	1/6 pie	170	2.0	22.0	155	(mq)	9.0	na
BERRY, fresh *(McMillin's)*	4 oz	430	3.0	52.0	410	na	23.0	na
BLACKBERRY, frozen *(Banquet)*								
'Family Size' 3 1/3 oz	1/6 pie	270	3.0	40.0	350	(mq)	11.0	na

Food Name	Serv. Size	Total Cal.	Prot. GMS	Carbs GMS	Sod. MGS	Fiber GMS	Fat GMS	Chol. MGS
BLUEBERRY								
Frozen								
(Banquet) 'Family Size' 3 1/3 oz	1/6 pie	270	3.0	40:0	350	(mq)	11.0	na
(Mrs. Smith's) 'Pie In Minutes' 8-inch pie	1/8 pie	220	2.0	32.0	240	(mq)	9.0	0
(Pet-Ritz)	1/6 pie	370	3.0	50.0	330	(mq)	12.0	na
(Sara Lee) 'Homestyle' 9-inch pie	1/10 pie	300	2.0	45.0	210	(mq)	12.0	0
BOSTON CREAM, frozen (Weight Watchers)	3 oz	160	3.0	34.0	260	(mq)	4.0	5
CHERRY								
Fresh (McMillin's)	4 oz	430	3.0	51.0	350	na	24.0	na
Frozen								
(Banquet) 'Family Size' 3 1/3 oz	1/6 pie	250	3.0	36.0	260	(mq)	11.0	na
(Mrs. Smith's) 'Pie In Minutes' 8-inch pie	1/8 pie	220	2.0	32.0	200	(mq)	9.0	0
(Pet-Ritz)	1/6 pie	300	3.0	48.0	330	(mq)	12.0	na
(Sara Lee) cherry streusel 'Free & Light'	1/10 pie	160	2.0	34.0	140	(mq)	2.0	0
(Sara Lee) 'Homestyle' 9-inch pie	1/10 pie	270	2.0	37.0	270	(mq)	13.0	0
CHOCOLATE								
Fresh (McMillin's) chocolate pudding	4 oz	420	3.0	54.0	350	na	21.0	na
Frozen								
(Banquet) chocolate cream, 2 1/3 oz	1/6 pie	190	2.0	24.0	110	(mq)	10.0	na
(Pet Ritz) chocolate cream, 2 1/3 oz	1/6 pie	190	1.0	27.0	145	(mq)	8.0	na
(Weight Watchers) chocolate mocha 'Sweet Celebrations' 2.75 oz	1/2 pkg	160	5.0	23.0	150	(mq)	5.0	5
COCONUT								
Fresh (McMillin's) coconut pudding	4 oz	450	4.0	50.0	420	na	26.0	na
Frozen								
(Banquet) cream, 2 1/3 oz	1/6 pie	190	2.0	22.0	120	(mq)	11.0	na
(Pet Ritz) cream, 2 1/3 oz	1/6 pie	190	2.0	27.0	145	(mq)	8.0	na
COCONUT CUSTARD, fresh								
(Entenmann's)	1.8 oz	140	3.0	16.0	160	na	8.0	na
EGG CUSTARD, frozen (Pet-Ritz)	1/6 pie	200	5.0	28.0	(mq)	(mq)	8.0	(mq)
LEMON								
Fresh (McMillin's)	4 oz	450	4.0	52.0	330	na	25.0	na
Frozen								
(Banquet) cream, 2 1/3 oz	1/6 pie	170	2.0	23.0	120	(mq)	9.0	na
(Mrs. Smith's) meringue, 8-inch pie	1/8 pie	210	2.0	38.0	130	(mq)	5.0	na
(Pet Ritz) cream, 2 1/3 oz	1/6 pie	190	2.0	26.0	150	(mq)	9.0	na
MINCE								
Frozen								
(Banquet) mincemeat 'Family Size' 3 1/3 oz	1/6 pie	260	3.0	38.0	370	(mq)	11.0	na
(Pet-Ritz)	1/6 pie	280	2.0	48.0	(mq)	(mq)	9.0	na
(Sara Lee) 'Homestyle' 9-inch pie	1/10 pie	300	3.0	43.0	340	(mq)	13.0	0

Food Name	Serv. Size	Total Cal.	Prot. GMS	Carbs GMS	Sod. MGS	Fiber GMS	Fat GMS	Chol. MGS
NEAPOLITAN CREAM, frozen,								
(Pet Ritz) 2 1/3 oz	1/6 pie	180	1.0	17.0	185	(mq)	10.0	na
PEACH								
Fresh (McMillin's)	4 oz	430	4.0	52.0	370	na	24.0	na
Frozen								
(Banquet) 'Family Size' 3 1/3 oz	1/6 pie	245	3.0	35.0	280	(mq)	11.0	na
(Mrs. Smith's) 'Pie In Minutes' 8-inch pie	1/8 pie	210	2.0	29.0	190	(mq)	9.0	0
(Pet-Ritz)	1/6 pie	320	2.0	51.0	320	(mq)	12.0	na
(Sara Lee) 'Homestyle' 9-inch pie	1/10 pie	280	2.0	41.0	170	(mq)	12.0	0
PECAN								
Frozen								
(Mrs. Smith's) 'Pie In Minutes' 8-inch pie	1/8 pie	330	3.0	51.0	200	(mq)	13.0	35
(Sara Lee) 'Homestyle' 9-inch pie	1/10 pie	400	4.0	56.0	290	(mq)	18.0	55
PUMPKIN								
Frozen								
(Banquet) 'Family Size' 3 1/3 oz	1/6 pie	200	3.0	29.0	350	(mq)	8.0	na
(Mrs. Smith's) 'Pie In Minutes' 8-inch pie	1/8 pie	190	3.0	30.0	230	(mq)	6.0	35
(Pet Ritz) pumpkin custard	1/6 pie	250	4.0	39.0	(mq)	(mq)	9.0	na
(Sara Lee) 'Homestyle' 9-inch pie	1/10 pie	240	4.0	34.0	250	(mq)	10.0	40
RASPBERRY, frozen (Sara Lee)								
'Homestyle' 9-inch pie	1/10 pie	280	2.0	39.0	150	(mq)	13.0	0
STRAWBERRY								
Fresh (McMillin's)	4 oz	400	3.0	50.0	370	na	20.0	na
Frozen								
(Banquet) strawberry cream, 2 1/3 oz ..	1/6 pie	170	2.0	22.0	120	(mq)	9.0	na
(Pet Ritz) strawberry cream, 2 1/3 oz ...	1/6 pie	170	2.0	20.0	145	(mq)	9.0	na
SWEET POTATO, frozen (Pet-Ritz)	1/6 pie	150	2.0	21.0	110	(mq)	7.0	na
PIE, SNACK								
APPLE								
(Break Cake) 'Fried Pie' 4.5 oz	2 pies	430	5.0	63.0	370	na	18.0	0
(Drake's) approx 2 oz	1 piece	210	2.0	29.0	135	(mq)	10.0	0
(Hostess)	1 piece	430	3.0	60.0	390	2.0	20.0	15
(Hostess) French apple	1 piece	430	3.0	60.0	390	2.0	20.0	15
(Little Debbie) Dutch apple, 2.17 oz ...	1 piece	230	2.0	42.0	150	(mq)	8.0	<1
(Little Debbie) Dutch apple, 2.5 oz	1 piece	270	2.0	48.0	170	(mq)	8.0	<1
(Tastykake) 4 oz	1 piece	296	3.0	46.0	339	2.5	12.3	0
(Tastycake) French apple, 4.2 oz	1 piece	353	3.0	63.0	225	1.9	10.7	0
BANANA CREAM (Tastycake) 4.2 oz ...	1 piece	382	5.2	53.9	428	1.7	16.1	26
BLACKBERRY (Hostess)	1 piece	420	4.0	59.0	360	2.4	18.0	15
BLUEBERRY								
(Hostess)	1 piece	420	4.0	59.0	360	2.4	18.0	15
(Tastykake) 4 oz	1 piece	308	2.8	55.0	410	2.1	9.4	0
BLUEBERRY APPLE (Drake's) approx 2 oz	1 piece	210	2.0	30.0	135	(mq)	10.0	0

Food Name	Serv. Size	Total Cal.	Prot. GMS	Carbs GMS	Sod. MGS	Fiber GMS	Fat GMS	Chol. MGS
CHERRY								
(Break Cake) 'Fried Pie' 4.5 oz	2 pies	410	5.0	64.0	370	na	16.0	0
(Hostess)	1 piece	460	4.0	65.0	380	2.4	20.0	15
(Tastykake) 4 oz	1 piece	298	3.0	48.8	306	2.0	9.7	0
CHERRY APPLE (Drake's) approx 2 oz	1 piece	220	2.0	30.0	135	(mq)	10.0	0
CHOCOLATE PUDDING								
(Hostess) chocolate pudding	1 piece	490	5.0	76.0	439	(mq)	19.0	21
(Tastycake) chocolate pudding, 4.2 oz	1 piece	443	6.0	68.3	(mq)	(mq)	16.2	na
COCONUT CREME (Tastykake) 4 oz	1 piece	377	4.9	46.0	416	2.3	20.2	65
LEMON								
(Break Cake) 'Fried Pie' 4.5 oz	2 pies	490	5.0	66.0	370	na	23.0	0
(Drake's) approx 2 oz	1 piece	210	2.0	27.0	115	(mq)	11.0	0
(Hostess)	1 piece	440	4.0	60.0	370	1.4	20.0	30
(Tastykake) 4 oz	1 piece	319	3.6	48.1	375	1.7	13.2	39
LEMON-LIME (Tastykake) 4 oz	1 piece	310	3.3	54.1	329	.2	8.8	55
MARSHMALLOW BANANA								
(Little Debbie) 3 oz	1 piece	360	3.0	60.0	180	(mq)	12.0	<1
(Little Debbie) 1.4 oz	1 piece	170	1.0	28.0	85	(mq)	6.0	<1
MARSHMALLOW CHOCOLATE								
(Little Debbie) 3 oz	1 piece	370	3.0	59.0	170	(mq)	13.0	<1
(Little Debbie) 1.4 oz	1 piece	170	1.0	28.0	85	(mq)	6.0	<1
MISSISSIPPI MUD (Pepperidge Farm) frozen 'American Collection'	1 ramekin	310	3.0	23.0	60	(mq)	23.0	45
OATMEAL CREME								
(Little Debbie) 1.33 oz	1 piece	160	2.0	25.0	125	(mq)	6.0	<1
(Little Debbie) 2.75 oz	1 piece	350	4.0	51.0	260	(mq)	14.0	<1
PEACH								
(Hostess)	1 piece	420	4.0	60.0	360	2.0	19.0	15
(Tastykake) 4 oz	1 piece	310	3.3	54.1	329	.2	8.8	55
PECAN								
(Little Debbie) 1.83 oz	1 piece	170	2.0	37.0	200	(mq)	2.0	<1
(Little Debbie) 3 oz	1 piece	280	3.0	60.0	340	(mq)	3.0	<1
PINEAPPLE CHEESE (Tastykake) 4.2 oz	1 piece	343	4.5	53.9	405	2.2	13.2	19
PUMPKIN (Tastykake) 4 oz	1 piece	324	4.5	46.5	520	1.9	14.2	28
RAISIN CREME								
(Little Debbie) 2.5 oz	1 piece	290	2.0	47.0	190	(mq)	10.0	<1
(Little Debbie) 1.17 oz	1 piece	140	1.0	21.0	90	(mq)	6.0	<1
STRAWBERRY								
(Hostess)	1 piece	410	4.0	56.0	360	2.2	19.0	15
(Tastykake) 4 oz	1 piece	342	3.1	57.4	303	.6	11.4	0
PIE CRUST								
Mix								
(Betty Crocker) dry	1/16 pkg	120	1.0	10.0	140	(mq)	8.0	0

Food Name	Serv. Size	Total Cal.	Prot. GMS	Carbs GMS	Sod. MGS	Fiber GMS	Fat GMS	Chol. MGS
(Flako) prepared	1 serving	247	3.7	24.4	393	1.2	15.0	9
(General Mills) dry	1/16 pkg	120	1.0	10.0	150	na	8.0	0
(Krusteaz) 9-inch pie	1/8 shell	90	1.0	10.0	120	.1	5.0	0
(Nabisco) chocolate cookie crumbs								
'Oreo' dry	2 tbsp	80	1.0	13.0	140	na	3.0	0
(Nabisco) graham crumbs								
'Honey Maid' dry	2 1/2 tbsp	70	1.0	13.0	90	na	2.0	0
(Nabisco) wafer crumbs 'Nilla' dry	2 tbsp	70	1.0	12.0	55	na	2.0	5
(Pillsbury) dry	1/8 pkg	200	3.0	20.0	300	na	13.0	0
Shell								
(Mrs. Smith's) 8-inch pie	1/8 shell	80	1.0	8.0	105	(mq)	5.0	0
(Mrs. Smith's) '9-inch pie'	1/8 shell	90	1.0	10.0	125	(mq)	5.0	0
(Mrs. Smith's) '9 5/8-inch pie'	1/8 shell	120	2.0	12.0	160	(mq)	7.0	0
(Oronoque) deep dish, 9-inch pie	1/6 shell	130	2.0	11.0	130	na	9.0	0
(Oronoque) regular, 9-inch pie	1/6 shell	120	2.0	9.0	115	na	8.0	0
(Pet-Ritz)	1/6 shell	110	1.0	11.0	110	(mq)	7.0	7
(Pet-Ritz) all vegetable shortening	1/6 shell	110	2.0	10.0	60	(mq)	8.0	0
(Pet-Ritz) deep dish, 1 oz	1/6 shell	130	1.0	12.0	120	(mq)	8.0	7
(Pet-Ritz) deep dish, whole-grain	1/6 shell	130	1.0	14.0	125	(mq)	8.0	na
(Pet-Ritz) graham cracker	1/6 shell	110	1.0	8.0	80	(mq)	6.0	7
(Pet-Ritz) 9 5/8-inch pie	1/6 shell	170	2.0	15.0	180	(mq)	11.0	7
(Pet-Ritz) tart	3-inch shell	150	3.0	12.0	150	(mq)	10.0	7
(Pet-Ritz) vegetable shortening,								
deep dish	1/6 shell	140	2.0	12.0	75	(mq)	9.0	0
(Pillsbury) 'All Ready' 2-crust pie	1/8 shell	240	2.0	24.0	210	(mq)	15.0	15
Stick *(Betty Crocker)*	1/8 stick	120	1.0	10.0	140	(mq)	8.0	0

PIE FILLING

(NOTE: All pie fillings are canned unless otherwise noted.)

APPLE

Food Name	Serv. Size	Total Cal.	Prot. GMS	Carbs GMS	Sod. MGS	Fiber GMS	Fat GMS	Chol. MGS
(Comstock)	3.5 oz	120	0.0	30.0	15	.4	0.0	0
(Comstock) 'Lite'	3.5 oz	80	0.0	20.0	10	.4	0.0	0
(Lucky Leaf)	4 oz	120	0.0	30.0	60	(mq)	0.0	0
(Lucky Leaf) apple turnover, diced	4 oz	120	0.0	30.0	60	(mq)	0.0	0
(Lucky Leaf) 'Deluxe'	4 oz	120	0.0	35.0	40	(mq)	0.0	0
(Lucky Leaf) 'Plus'	4 oz	121	0.3	30.2	24	(mq)	0.0	0
(Musselman's)	4 oz	120	0.0	30.0	60	(mq)	0.0	0
(Musselman's) apple turnover, diced	4 oz	120	0.0	30.0	60	(mq)	0.0	0
(Musselman's) 'Deluxe'	4 oz	120	0.0	35.0	40	(mq)	0.0	0
(Musselman's) 'Plus'	4 oz	121	0.3	30.2	24	(mq)	0.0	0
(Pathmark) 'No Frills'	4 oz	130	0.0	33.0	60	(mq)	0.0	0
(White House)	3.5 oz	121	0.0	29.0	44	(mq)	1.0	0

APRICOT

Food Name	Serv. Size	Total Cal.	Prot. GMS	Carbs GMS	Sod. MGS	Fiber GMS	Fat GMS	Chol. MGS
(Comstock)	3.5 oz	110	0.0	29.0	100	.4	0.0	0

Food Name	Serv. Size	Total Cal.	Prot. GMS	Carbs GMS	Sod. MGS	Fiber GMS	Fat GMS	Chol. MGS
(Lucky Leaf)	4 oz	150	0.0	39.0	90	(mq)	0.0	0
(Musselman's)	4 oz	150	0.0	39.0	90	(mq)	0.0	0
BANANA *(Comstock)*	3.5 oz	110	1.0	22.0	300	.5	2.0	0
BLACKBERRY								
(Lucky Leaf)	4 oz	120	1.0	31.0	140	(mq)	0.0	0
(Lucky Leaf) 'Plus'	4 oz	121	0.9	30.1	20	(mq)	0.0	0
(Musselman's)	4 oz	120	1.0	31.0	140	(mq)	0.0	0
(Musselman's) 'Plus'	4 oz	121	0.9	30.1	20	(mq)	0.0	0
BLUEBERRY								
(Comstock)	3.5 oz	110	0.0	28.0	15	.5	0.0	0
(Comstock) 'Lite'	3.5 oz	75	0.0	17.0	15	.6	0.0	0
(Lucky Leaf) cultivated	4 oz	120	1.0	31.0	150	(mq)	0.0	0
(Lucky Leaf) 'Plus'	4 oz	145	0.3	35.2	17	(mq)	0.0	0
(Musselman's) cultivated	4 oz	120	1.0	31.0	150	(mq)	0.0	0
(Musselman's) 'Plus'	4 oz	145	0.3	35.2	17	(mq)	0.0	0
(White House)	3.5 oz	118	0.0	28.0	48	(mq)	1.0	0
BOYSENBERRY								
(Lucky Leaf)	4 oz	120	1.0	31.0	140	(mq)	0.0	0
(Musselman's)	4 oz	120	1.0	31.0	140	(mq)	0.0	0
CHERRY								
(Comstock)	3.5 oz	110	0.0	28.0	15	.3	0.0	0
(Comstock) 'Lite'	3.5 oz	75	0.0	19.0	15	.3	0.0	0
(Lucky Leaf)	4 oz	120	1.0	29.0	50	(mq)	0.0	0
(Musselman's)	4 oz	120	1.0	29.0	50	(mq)	0.0	0
(Musselman's) 'Plus'	4 oz	108	0.8	26.0	10	(mq)	0.2	0
(Pathmark) 'No Frills'	4 oz	130	0.0	33.0	60	(mq)	0.0	0
(White House)	3.5 oz	141	0.0	33.0	54	(mq)	1.0	0
CHOCOLATE *(Comstock)*	3.5 oz	130	1.0	26.0	240	.2	3.0	0
COCONUT *(Comstock)*	3.5 oz	120	1.0	22.0	290	.2	3.0	0
GOOSEBERRY								
(Lucky Leaf)	4 oz	180	0.0	45.0	30	(mq)	0.0	0
(Musselman's)	4 oz	180	0.0	45.0	30	(mq)	0.0	0
LEMON								
(Comstock)	3.5 oz	140	0.0	34.0	110	.1	1.0	0
(Lucky Leaf)	4 oz	200	0.0	48.0	235	(mq)	2.0	na
(Lucky Leaf) 'French'	4 oz	180	0.0	42.0	140	(mq)	1.0	na
(Musselman's)	4 oz	200	0.0	48.0	235	(mq)	2.0	na
(Musselman's) 'French'	4 oz	180	0.0	42.0	140	(mq)	1.0	na
MINCEMEAT								
(Comstock)	3.5 oz	150	0.0	39.0	180	.7	1.0	0
(Lucky Leaf)	4 oz	190	0.0	48.0	145	(mq)	1.0	na
(Musselman's)	4 oz	190	0.0	48.0	145	(mq)	1.0	na
(None Such)	1/3 cup	200	1.0	48.0	280	(mq)	1.0	na

Food Name	Serv. Size	Total Cal.	Prot. GMS	Carbs GMS	Sod. MGS	Fiber GMS	Fat GMS	Chol. MGS
(None Such) condensed	1/4 pkg	220	1.0	50.0	310	(mq)	2.0	na
(None Such) w/brandy and rum	1/3 cup	220	1.0	48.0	260	(mq)	2.0	na
(S&W) w/brandy, 'Old Fashioned'	4 oz	234	1.1	55.6	234	(mq)	2.3	na
PEACH								
(Comstock)	3.5 oz	110	0.0	26.0	20	.2	0.0	0
(Lucky Leaf)	4 oz	150	0.0	37.0	65	(mq)	0.0	0
(Lucky Leaf) 'Plus'	4 oz	113	0.7	27.4	16	(mq)	0.0	0
(Musselman's)	4 oz	150	0.0	37.0	65	(mq)	0.0	0
(Musselman's) 'Plus'	4 oz	113	0.7	27.4	16	(mq)	0.0	0
(White House)	3.5 oz	117	0.0	28.0	30	(mq)	1.0	0
PINEAPPLE								
(Comstock)	3.5 oz	100	0.0	28.0	65	.4	0.0	0
(Lucky Leaf)	4 oz	110	0.0	30.0	65	(mq)	0.0	0
(Musselman's)	4 oz	110	0.0	30.0	65	(mq)	0.0	0
PUMPKIN								
(Comstock)	3.5 oz	100	0.0	24.0	180	(mq)	0.0	0
(Libby's)	1 cup	260	2.0	64.0	0	(mq)	0.3	440
(Lucky Leaf)	4 oz	170	1.0	33.0	200	(mq)	4.0	na
(Musselman's)	4 oz	170	1.0	33.0	200	(mq)	4.0	na
(Stokely)	1/2 cup	170	1.0	44.0	420	(mq)	0.0	0
RAISIN								
(Comstock)	3.5 oz	120	0.0	32.0	80	(mq)	0.0	0
(Lucky Leaf)	4 oz	130	1.0	34.0	120	(mq)	1.0	na
(Musselman's)	4 oz	130	1.0	34.0	120	(mq)	1.0	na
RASPBERRY, BLACK								
(Lucky Leaf)	4 oz	190	0.0	43.0	50	(mq)	0.0	0
(Musselman's)	4 oz	190	0.0	43.0	50	(mq)	0.0	0
RASPBERRY, RED								
(Lucky Leaf)	4 oz	190	0.0	46.0	80	(mq)	0.0	0
(Musselman's)	4 oz	190	0.0	46.0	80	(mq)	0.0	0
STRAWBERRY								
(Comstock)	3.5 oz	100	0.0	25.0	20	.6	0.0	0
(Lucky Leaf)	4 oz	120	0.0	30.0	75	(mq)	0.0	0
(Lucky Leaf) 'Plus'	4 oz	138	0.9	33.5	17	(mq)	0.0	0
(Musselman's)	4 oz	120	0.0	30.0	75	(mq)	0.0	0
(Musselman's) 'Plus'	4 oz	138	0.9	33.5	17	(mq)	0.0	0
STRAWBERRY-RHUBARB								
(Lucky Leaf) strawberry-rhubarb	4 oz	120	0.0	31.0	95	(mq)	0.0	0
(Musselman's) strawberry-rhubarb	4 oz	120	0.0	31.0	95	(mq)	0.0	0
PIE MIX								
BANANA CREAM								
(Jell-O) 'No Bake' dry	1 pkg	140	1.0	25.0	190	na	5.0	0
(Jell-O) 'No Bake' prepared	1/8 pie	240	3.0	27.0	300	(mq)	14.0	30

Food Name	Serv. Size	Total Cal.	Prot. GMS	Carbs GMS	Sod. MGS	Fiber GMS	Fat GMS	Chol. MGS
BOSTON CREAM								
(Betty Crocker) 'Classic' dry	1/8 pkg	230	1.0	48.0	370	na	4.0	0
(Betty Crocker) 'Classic' prepared w/egg and 2% milk	1/8 pkg	270	4.0	50.0	390	na	6.0	30
(Jell-O) mousse 'No Bake' dry	1 pkg	160	2.0	22.0	320	na	7.0	0
(Jell-O) mousse 'No Bake' prepared	1/8 pie	260	4.0	25.0	430	(mq)	17.0	30
CHOCOLATE								
(Royal) chocolate mint 'No-Bake' prepared	1/8 pie	260	5.0	25.0	280	(mq)	15.0	na
(Royal) mousse 'No Bake' prepared	1/8 pie	230	4.0	27.0	260	(mq)	12.0	na
COCONUT CREAM								
(Jell-O) 'No Bake' dry	1 pkg	160	1.0	25.0	200	na	7.0	0
(Jell-O) 'No Bake' prepared	1/8 pie	260	3.0	27.0	300	(mq)	16.0	30
KEY LIME *(Royal)* dry	1 serving	50	0.0	13.0	120	na	0.0	0
LEMON								
(Royal) dry	1 serving	50	0.0	13.0	120	0	0.0	0
(Royal) lemon meringue 'No Bake' prepared	1/8 pie	310	3.0	50.0	250	(mq)	11.0	na
PUMPKIN								
(Jell-O) 'No Bake' dry	1 pkg	140	1.0	28.0	330	na	3.0	0
(Jell-O) 'No Bake' prepared	1/8 pie	250	4.0	31.0	450	(mq)	13.0	30
(Libby's) prepared	1/6 pie	390	7.0	53.0	70	(mq)	17.0	380
VANILLA CREME								
(Lucky Leaf) prepared	4 oz	150	0.0	32.0	145	(mq)	3.0	na
(Musselman's) prepared	4 oz	150	0.0	32.0	145	(mq)	3.0	na
PIROGIES, FROZEN								
pasta pocket, potato and American cheese filled *(Mrs. T's)*	1 pocket	70	3.0	10.0	180	na	2.0	5
pasta pocket, potato and cheddar cheese filled *(Mrs. T's)*	1 pocket	60	2.0	11.0	170	8.0	<1.0	2
pasta pocket, potato and onion filled *(Mrs. T's)*	1 pocket	50	2.0	10.0	140	na	<1.0	2
pasta pocket, sauerkraut filled *(Mrs. T's)*	1 pocket	50	2.0	9.0	220	na	<1.0	0
PIGEON. See SQUAB.								
PIGNOLIA. See PINE NUT.								
PIG'S EAR								
frozen, raw	1 oz	66	6.4	0.0	54	0	4.3	23
frozen, simmered	4 oz	188	18.1	0.0	189	0	12.2	102
PIG'S FEET								
pickled *(Penrose)*	6 oz	220	19.0	2.0	2890	0	15.0	(mq)
pickled, cured	1 lb	921	61.3	0.1	4187	0	73.2	417
pickled, cured	1 oz	58	3.8	0.0	262	0	4.6	26

Food Name	Serv. Size	Total Cal.	Prot. GMS	Carbs GMS	Sod. MGS	Fiber GMS	Fat GMS	Chol. MGS
raw	1 oz	75	6.3	0.0	18	0	5.3	30
simmered	5 oz	275	27.3	0.0	43	0	17.6	142
PIG'S HEART								
braised	1 cup	215	34.2	0.6	51	0	7.3	320
braised	4 oz	168	26.8	0.5	40	0	5.7	251
raw	1 oz	33	4.9	0.4	16	0	1.2	37
PIG'S JOWL, raw	1 oz	186	1.8	0.0	7	0	19.7	26
PIG'S KNUCKLES, pickled *(Penrose)*	6 oz	290	23.0	1.0	2380	0	21.0	(mq)
PIG'S TAIL								
raw	1 oz	107	5.0	0.0	18	0	9.5	28
simmered	3 oz	337	14.4	0.0	21	0	30.4	110
PIG'S TONGUE								
braised	3 oz	230	20.5	0.0	93	0	15.8	124
cured, '8-lb can' *(Hormel)*	3 oz	190	17.0	0.0	966	0	13.0	(mq)
raw	1 oz	64	4.6	0.0	31	0	4.9	29
PIKE, NORTHERN								
dry-heat cooked	3 oz	96	21.0	0.0	42	0	0.8	43
raw	1 lb	401	87.3	0.0	177	0	3.1	177
raw	3 oz	75	16.4	0.0	33	0	0.6	33
raw	1 oz	25	5.5	0.0	11	0	0.2	11
PIKE, WALLEYE								
dry-heat cooked	3 oz	101	20.9	0.0	55	0	1.3	94
raw	1 lb	420	86.8	0.0	230	0	5.5	390
raw	3 oz	79	16.3	0.0	43	0	1.0	73
raw	1 oz	26	5.4	0.0	14	0	0.3	24
PILAF DINNER, CANNED								
oat bran, w/garden vegetables 'Fast Menu' *(Health Valley)*	7.5 oz	210	8.0	31.0	445	5.8	7.0	0
PILAF MIX								
lentil, approx 1/2 cup cooked or 1 oz dry *(Casbah)*	1 serving	100	5.0	20.0	(mq)	(mq)	0.0	0
three-grain, w/herbs, prepared w/salted butter *(Quick Pilaf)*	1/2 cup	142	3.0	24.0	324	(mq)	4.0	(mq)
three-grain, w/herbs, prepared w/o butter *(Quick Pilaf)*	1/2 cup	110	3.0	24.0	278	(mq)	0.6	0
PILI NUT, CANARY TREE								
dried	1 cup	863	13.0	4.8	4	>3.4 c	95.5	0
dried, 15 kernels	1 oz	204	3.1	1.1	1	>.8 c	22.6	0
dried, in shell	1 lb	619	9.3	3.4	3	>2.4 c	68.5	0
PIMIENTO, CAN OR JAR								
	2 oz	13	0.6	2.9	8	>.6 c	0.2	0
	1 tbsp	3	0.1	0.6	2	>.1 c	<.1	0
all varieties, drained *(Dromedary)*	1 oz	10	0.0	2.0	5	(mq)	0.0	0

Food Name	Serv. Size	Total Cal.	Prot. GMS	Carbs GMS	Sod. MGS	Fiber GMS	Fat GMS	Chol. MGS
PIMIENTO SPREAD (Price's)	1 oz	80	3.0	2.0	na	na	6.0	(mq)
PINE NUT/Colorado pinyon pine nut/Italian stone pine nut/pignolia/pinocchio/piñon								
whole	1 oz	161	3.3	5.5	20	3.0	17.3	0
whole	1 tbsp	52	2.4	1.4	0	.4	5.1	0
whole	10 kernels	6	0.1	0.2	1	.1	0.6	0
PINEAPPLE								
candied, approx 1/2 cup	4-oz pkg	357	0.9	90.4	7	>.9 c	0.5	0
raw, diced pieces	1 cup	76	0.6	19.2	2	1.9	0.7	0
raw, 3 1/2-inch diam	1 slice	41	0.3	10.4	1	1.0	0.4	0
raw, 3 1/2-inch diam, 3/4 inch thick								
(Del Monte)	2 slices	90	1.0	24.0	5	(mq)	0.0	0
trimmed	1 oz	14	0.1	3.5	<1	.3	0.1	0
untrimmed	1 lb	117	0.9	29.2	2	2.8	1.0	0
untrimmed (Dole)	2 slices	90	1.0	21.0	10	2.0	1.0	na
PINEAPPLE, CANNED								
chunks	1/2 cup	75	0.5	19.6	2	.9	0.1	0
chunks (A&P)	1/2 cup	70	<1.0	18.0	10	(mq)	<1.0	0
chunks, unsweetened 'Hawaiian'								
(Pathmark)	1/2 cup	70	0.0	18.0	10	(mq)	0.0	0
crushed (A&P)	1/2 cup	70	<1.0	18.0	10	(mq)	<1.0	0
crushed (Empress)	1/2 cup	70	0.0	18.0	10	(mq)	0.0	0
crushed, unsweetened 'Hawaiian'								
(Pathmark)	1/2 cup	70	0.0	18.0	10	(mq)	0.0	0
'Fruit Pak' (Mott's)	3.75 oz	86	0.0	21.0	2	(mq)	0.0	0
in extra heavy syrup	4 oz	94	0.4	24.4	1	>.5 c	0.1	0
in extra heavy syrup, chunks	1/2 cup	109	0.4	28.0	2	>.6 c	0.1	0
in extra heavy syrup, chunks, w/liquid ...	1 cup	216	0.9	55.9	3	>1.1 c	0.3	0
in extra heavy syrup, crushed	1/2 cup	109	0.4	28.0	2	>.6 c	0.1	0
in extra heavy syrup, w/1.25 tbsp liquid ..	1 slice	48	0.2	12.5	1	>.3 c	0.1	0
in heavy syrup	4 oz	88	0.4	22.9	1	>.5 c	0.1	0
in heavy syrup, chunks (A&P)	1/2 cup	90	<1.0	23.0	10	(mq)	<1.0	0
in heavy syrup, chunks 'Hawaiian'								
(Pathmark)	1/2 cup	90	0.0	23.0	10	(mq)	0.0	0
in heavy syrup, chunks, tidbits, or								
crushed	1/2 cup	100	0.5	25.8	2	>.6 c	0.1	0
in heavy syrup, chunks or crushed,								
w/liquid	1 cup	199	0.9	51.5	3	1.8	0.3	0
in heavy syrup, crushed (A&P)	1/2 cup	90	<1.0	23.0	10	(mq)	<1.0	0
in heavy syrup, slices (A&P)	2 slices	90	<1.0	23.0	10	(mq)	<1.0	0
in heavy syrup, slices 'Hawaiian'								
(Pathmark)	1/2 cup	90	0.0	23.0	10	(mq)	0.0	0
in heavy syrup, slices '100% Hawaiian'								
(S&W)	2 slices	90	0.0	23.0	0	(mq)	0.0	0

Food Name	Serv. Size	Total Cal.	Prot. GMS	Carbs GMS	Sod. MGS	Fiber GMS	Fat GMS	Chol. MGS
in heavy syrup, w/1.25 tbsp liquid	1 slice	45	0.2	11.7	1	.4	0.1	0
in juice	4 oz	68	0.5	17.8	1	.9	0.1	0
in juice, all cuts (Dole)	1/2 cup	70	0.5	17.5	1	(mq)	0.5	0
in juice, chunks (Del Monte)	1/2 cup	70	0.0	18.0	10	(mq)	0.0	0
in juice, chunks or tidbits, w/liquid	1 cup	150	1.0	39.2	3	1.8	0.2	0
in juice, crushed (Del Monte)	1/2 cup	70	0.0	18.0	10	(mq)	0.0	0
in juice, slices (A&P)	2 slices	70	<1.0	18.0	10	(mq)	<1.0	0
in juice, slices (Del Monte)	1/2 cup	70	0.0	18.0	10	(mq)	0.0	0
in juice, slices (Featherweight)	1/2 cup	70	0.0	18.0	10	(mq)	0.0	0
in juice, slices '100% Hawaiian' (S&W)	1/2 cup	70	0.0	17.0	10	(mq)	0.0	0
in juice, tidbits (Del Monte)	1/2 cup	70	0.0	18.0	10	(mq)	0.0	0
in juice, w/1.25 tbsp liquid	1 slice	35	0.2	9.1	1	.4	0.1	0
in light syrup	1/2 cup	66	0.5	16.9	2	>.6 c	0.1	0
in light syrup	4 oz	59	0.4	15.3	1	>.5 c	0.1	0
in light syrup, w/liquid	1 cup	131	0.9	33.9	3	1.8	0.3	0
in light syrup, w/1.75 tbsp liquid	1 slice	30	0.2	7.8	1	.4	0.1	0
in pineapple juice (Dole)	1/2 cup	70	0.0	18.0	10	na	<1.0	na
in pineapple syrup (Dole)	1/2 cup	90	0.0	23.0	10	na	0.0	na
in syrup, all cuts (Del Monte)	1/2 cup	90	0.0	23.0	10	(mq)	0.0	0
in syrup, all cuts (Dole)	1/2 cup	95	0.4	24.8	2	(mq)	0.2	0
in water	4 oz	36	0.5	9.4	1	>.5 c	0.1	0
in water, tidbits	1/2 cup	40	0.5	10.2	2	>.6 c	0.1	0
in water, tidbits, w/liquid	1 cup	79	1.1	20.4	2	1.7	0.2	0
in water, w/1.25 tbsp liquid	1 slice	19	0.3	4.8	1	.4	0.1	0
spears, approx 3.1 oz (Del Monte)	2 spears	50	0.0	14.0	10	(mq)	0.0	0
spears or slices, unsweetened 'Hawaiian' (Pathmark)	1/2 cup	70	0.0	18.0	10	(mq)	0.0	0
tidbits	1/2 cup	75	0.5	19.6	2	.9	0.1	0
unsweetened, slices (S&W Nutradiet)	1/2 cup	60	0.0	15.0	10	(mq)	0.0	0
PINEAPPLE, FROZEN								
sweetened, chunks	1/2 cup	104	0.5	27.1	2	1.3	0.1	0
sweetened, chunks	4 oz	96	0.5	25.2	2	>.3 c	0.1	0
PINEAPPLE CITRUS DRINK								
'Thirst Quencher Light' (Gatorade)	8 oz	25	0.0	7.0	80	na	0.0	na
PINEAPPLE COCKTAIL JUICE								
w/banana 'Orchard Tropicals' (Welch's) bottled	6 oz	100	0.0	24.0	20	0	0.0	0
w/banana 'Orchard Tropicals' (Welch's) boxed	8.45 oz	140	0.0	34.0	20	0	0.0	0
w/banana 'Orchard Tropicals' (Welch's) frozen	6 oz	100	0.0	24.0	20	0	0.0	0
w/grapefruit juice (Ocean Spray)	6 oz	110	0.0	26.0	5	(mq)	0.0	0

Food Name	Serv. Size	Total Cal.	Prot. GMS	Carbs GMS	Sod. MGS	Fiber GMS	Fat GMS	Chol. MGS
PINEAPPLE COCONUT JUICE								
(Knudsen & Sons)	8 oz	110	<1.0	24.0	na	na	0.0	na
PINEAPPLE DRINK								
frozen 'Bright & Early Pineapple' prepared								
(Bright & Early)	6 oz	90	0.0	23.0	0	na	0.0	na
w/grapefruit juice	6 oz	90	0.6	21.6	24	tr	0.2	0
w/grapefruit juice (Del Monte)	6 oz	90	0.0	24.0	50	(mq)	0.0	0
w/grapefruit juice (Pathmark)	6 oz	80	0.0	21.0	0	(mq)	0.0	0
w/grapefruit juice (Tropicana)	6 oz	100	<1.0	24.0	10	na	<1.0	na
w/grapefruit juice 'Single Serve'								
(Tropicana)	10 oz	159	(tr)	39.0	3	(mq)	0.0	0
w/grapefruit juice 'Twister' (Tropicana)	8 oz	125	(tr)	32.0	2	(mq)	0.0	0
w/pink grapefruit juice (Del Monte)	6 oz	90	0.0	24.0	50	(mq)	0.0	0
PINEAPPLE GRAPEFRUIT JUICE								
canned	1 cup	117	0.5	29.0	35	.3	0.3	0
canned	1 oz	15	0.1	3.6	4	tr	0.0	0
PINEAPPLE JUICE								
Can, bottle, or box								
....	6 oz	104	0.6	25.8	2	>.2 c	0.2	0
(Dole)	6 oz	103	0.8	25.4	2	(mq)	0.2	0
(Knudsen & Sons)	8 oz	110	<1.0	25.0	na	na	0.0	na
(Minute Maid)	6 oz	90	1.0	23.0	20	na	0.0	na
(Mott's)	9.5 oz	169	0.0	42.0	0	(mq)	0.0	0
50% juice (J. Hungerford)	9.03 oz	123	0.4	30.8	0	0	0.0	0
float (Knudsen & Sons)	8 oz	130	2.0	31.0	na	na	0.0	na
'Hawaiian' (Pathmark)	6 oz	100	0.0	25.0	10	(mq)	0.0	0
'No Frills Unsweetened' (Pathmark)	6 oz	100	0.0	25.0	0	(mq)	0.0	0
'100%' (Veryfine)	8 oz	125	0.7	31.0	10	(mq)	0.0	0
100% juice (J. Hungerford)	9.03 oz	124	0.6	31.3	9	.3	0.0	0
regular (J. Hungerford)	9.03 oz	114	0.4	28.6	0	0	0.0	0
'Unsweetened' (Del Monte)	6 oz	100	0.0	25.0	10	(mq)	0.0	0
'Unsweetened' (IGA)	6 oz	100	0.0	25.0	10	(mq)	0.0	0
'Unsweetened' (S&W)	6 oz	100	0.0	25.0	0	(mq)	0.0	0
unsweetened, w/added ascorbic acid ...	1 cup	140	0.8	34.4	3	.3	0.2	0
unsweetened, w/added ascorbic acid	1 oz	18	0.1	4.3	0	0	0.0	0
unsweetened, w/o added ascorbic acid ..	1 cup	140	0.8	34.4	3	.3	0.2	0
unsweetened, w/o added ascorbic acid ...	1 oz	18	0.1	4.3	0	0	0.0	0
Frozen or chilled								
(Dole)	6 oz	90	0.0	22.0	5	na	0.0	na
(Minute Maid)	6 oz	90	1.0	23.0	0	na	0.0	na
concentrate (Dole) diluted	6 oz	100	0.0	25.0	7	(mq)	na	0
unsweetened concentrate, diluted	1 cup	130	1.0	31.9	3	.3	0.1	0
unsweetened concentrate, diluted	1 oz	16	0.1	4.0	0	0	0.0	0

Food Name	Serv. Size	Total Cal.	Prot. GMS	Carbs GMS	Sod. MGS	Fiber GMS	Fat GMS	Chol. MGS
unsweetened concentrate, undiluted	6 oz	387	2.8	95.7	6	.7	0.2	0
w/grapefruit juice (Dole)	6 oz	90	1.0	23.0	8	(mq)	na	0
w/grapefruit juice '100% Pure' (Tropicana)	8 oz	120	(mq)	29.3	3	(mq)	0.0	0
w/pink grapefruit juice (Dole)	6 oz	101	0.4	25.4	tr	(mq)	0.1	0
PINEAPPLE NECTAR (Libby's)	6 oz	110	0.0	27.0	na	na	0.0	30
PINEAPPLE ORANGE DRINK								
	6 oz	96	2.4	22.2	6	0	0.0	0
(Del Monte)	6 oz	90	0.0	24.0	20	0	0.0	0
(Veryfine)	8 oz	130	0.0	32.0	10	(mq)	0.0	0
PINEAPPLE ORANGE JUICE								
(Dole)	6 oz	100	1.0	23.0	8	(mq)	na	0
chilled, carton (Dole)	6 oz	90	0.0	22.0	10	na	0.0	na
chilled, w/banana, carton (Dole)	6 oz	100	0.0	23.0	10	na	0.0	na
chilled, w/guava, carton (Dole)	6 oz	100	<1.0	21.0	10	na	0.0	na
frozen, can (Dole)	6 oz	90	1.0	22.0	10	na	0.0	na
frozen, w/banana, can (Dole)	6 oz	90	1.0	21.0	5	na	0.0	na
frozen, w/guava, can (Dole)	6 oz	100	<1.0	22.0	10	na	0.0	na
frozen or chilled (Minute Maid)	6 oz	90	1.0	23.0	0	na	0.0	na
w/banana (Dole)	6 oz	90	0.8	23.0	5	(mq)	0.1	0
PINEAPPLE PASSION JUICE								
frozen, can, w/banana (Dole)	6 oz	100	<1.0	21.0	10	na	0.0	na
frozen, carton, w/banana (Dole)	6 oz	100	<1.0	21.0	10	na	0.0	na
PINEAPPLE TOPPING								
	1 cup	860	0.3	225.8	214	3.4	0.3	0
	2 tbsp	106	0.0	27.9	26	.4	0.0	0
(Kraft)	1 tbsp	50	0.0	13.0	0	(mq)	0.0	0
(Smucker's)	2 tbsp	130	0.0	32.0	0	(mq)	0.0	0
PINK BEAN								
boiled	4 oz	169	10.3	31.6	2	5.0	0.6	0
mature seeds, boiled	1/2 cup	125	7.6	23.4	2	4.5	0.4	0
mature seeds, raw	1/2 cup	360	22.0	67.4	8	13.3	1.2	0
raw	1 oz	97	5.9	18.2	2	2.5	0.3	0
PINOCCHIO. See PINE NUT.								
PIÑON. See PINE NUT.								
PINTO BEAN								
(Allens)	1/2 cup	105	5.0	18.0	480	(mq)	<1.0	0
boiled	4 oz	155	9.3	29.1	2	4.5	0.6	0
boiled (A&P)	1 cup	230	17.0	42.0	5	na	1.0	0
mature seeds, boiled	1/2 cup	116	7.0	21.8	2	7.3	0.4	0
mature seeds, raw	1/2 cup	326	20.0	60.9	10	23.4	1.1	0
raw	1 oz	96	5.9	18.0	3	3.4	0.3	0
raw (Arrowhead Mills)	2 oz	200	13.0	36.0	3	11.2	1.0	0
raw, dry (Evans)	1 cup	660	43.0	121.0	19	na	2.0	na

Food Name	Serv. Size	Total Cal.	Prot. GMS	Carbs GMS	Sod. MGS	Fiber GMS	Fat GMS	Chol. MGS
sprouted, mature seeds, boiled, drained	4 oz	25	2.1	4.6	58	>1.1 c	0.4	0
sprouted, mature seeds, raw	1 lb	280	23.8	52.6	694	>12.3 c	4.1	0
sprouted, mature seeds, raw	1 oz	18	1.5	3.3	43	>.8 c	0.3	0
Canned								
(Bush's Best)	1/2 cup	60	5.0	15.0	350	5.0	0.0	na
(Gebhardt)	4 oz	197	12.8	35.7	608	(mq)	0.5	0
(Green Giant)	1/2 cup	90	6.0	20.0	280	5.0	1.0	0
(Joan of Arc)	1/2 cup	90	6.0	20.0	280	5.2	1.0	0
(Old El Paso)	1/2 cup	100	6.0	19.0	320	8.0	0.0	0
(Progresso)	1/2 cup	110	8.0	21.0	410	6.5	<1.0	0
baked style, and Great Northern, w/pork (Luck's)	7.25 oz	200	12.0	29.0	822	(mq)	5.0	(mq)
baked style, w/pork, 15-oz can (Luck's)	7.5 oz	220	12.0	30.0	787	7.0	6.0	(mq)
baked style, w/pork, 29-oz can (Luck's)	7.25 oz	220	11.0	30.0	520	11.0	6.0	(mq)
mature seeds	1/2 cup	94	5.5	17.5	499	4.2	0.4	0
organic, very low sodium, no salt added (Eden Foods)	1/2 cup	70	6.0	17.0	15	6.0	<1.0	0
organic, w/liquid (Eden Foods)	1/2 cup	110	6.0	20.0	20	6.4	<1.0	0
picante style (Green Giant)	1/2 cup	100	7.0	21.0	580	6.6	1.0	0
picante style (Joan of Arc)	1/2 cup	100	7.0	21.0	580	6.6	1.0	0
w/liquid	4 oz	88	5.2	16.5	472	>1.4 c	0.4	0
Frozen								
	10-oz pkg	484	27.8	92.3	na	(mq)	1.4	0
(Seabrook)	3.2 oz	160	9.0	29.0	na	(mq)	0.0	0
boiled, drained	4 oz	184	10.6	35.0	na	(mq)	0.5	0
immature seeds, boiled, drained, 10-oz pkg	1/3 pkg	152	8.8	29.0	78	>2.8 c	0.5	0
immature seeds, unprepared, 10-oz pkg	1/3 pkg	160	9.2	30.6	86	5.4	0.5	0
PISTACHIO BUTTER, roasted								
(Maranatha Natural)	2 tbsp	170	6.0	7.0	5	na	13.0	na
PISTACHIO NUT								
In shell								
dried	1 lb	1309	46.7	56.3	13	24.5	109.7	0
dried (Dole)	1 oz	90	3.0	3.0	250	na	7.0	na
dried (Fisher)	1 oz	170	5.0	7.0	85	na	14.0	0
dried (Fisher) red tint	1 oz	170	5.0	7.0	85	na	14.0	0
dry-roasted	1 lb	1429	35.2	64.9	14	>4.3 c	124.5	0
dry-roasted, salted	1 lb	1429	35.2	64.9	1840	>4.3 c	124.5	0
Shelled								
dried	1 cup	739	26.3	31.8	8	13.8	61.9	0
dried, approx 47 kernels	1 oz	164	5.8	7.1	2	3.1	13.7	0
dry-roasted	1 cup	776	19.1	35.2	8	13.8	67.6	0
dry-roasted	1 oz	172	4.2	7.8	2	3.1	15.0	0

Food Name	Serv. Size	Total Cal.	Prot. GMS	Carbs GMS	Sod. MGS	Fiber GMS	Fat GMS	Chol. MGS
dry-roasted *(Dole)*	1 oz	163	6.0	7.0	2	(mq)	14.0	0
dry-roasted *(Planters)*	1 oz	170	5.0	6.0	250	(mq)	15.0	0
dry-roasted, natural *(Planters)*	1 oz	170	6.0	6.0	250	na	14.0	0
dry-roasted, red tint *(Planters)*	1 oz	170	6.0	6.0	250	na	14.0	0
PITA BREAD. See BREAD.								
PITANGA/Surinam cherry								
raw	1 cup	57	1.4	13.0	5	>1.0 c	0.7	0
raw, trimmed	1/2 cup	29	0.7	6.5	3	>.5 c	0.3	0
raw, trimmed	1 oz	9	0.2	2.1	1	>.2 c	0.1	0
raw, trimmed, approx .3 oz	1 med	2	0.1	0.5	0	tr	0.0	0
raw, untrimmed	1 lb	132	3.2	29.9	11	>2.4 c	1.6	0
PIZZA, FRENCH BREAD, FROZEN								
Canadian style bacon, 1 pkg *(Stouffer's)*	5.5 oz	370	18.0	40.0	1070	na	15.0	na
cheese *(Healthy Choice)*	5.6 oz	300	21.0	48.0	500	na	3.0	20
cheese *(Lean Cuisine)*	5 1/8 oz	300	17.0	38.0	310	na	9.0	15
cheese *(Pappalo's)*	1 piece	360	16.0	40.0	830	(mq)	15.0	(mq)
cheese, microwave *(Oven Lovin')*	1 serving	350	17.0	40.0	700	na	14.0	15
cheese 'Microwave' *(Pillsbury)*	1 piece	370	18.0	41.0	680	(mq)	15.0	(mq)
cheese, 1 pkg *(Stouffer's)*	5 1/8 oz	350	16.0	40.0	630	na	14.0	na
cheese 'Zap' *(Banquet)*	4.5 oz	310	14.0	41.0	800	(mq)	10.0	35
combination *(Pappalo's)*	1 piece	430	19.0	41.0	1120	(mq)	21.0	(mq)
combination, microwave *(Oven Lovin')*	1 serving	420	18.0	41.0	910	na	21.0	30
deluxe *(Healthy Choice)*	6.25 oz	330	23.0	41.0	490	na	8.0	35
deluxe *(Lean Cuisine)*	6 1/8 oz	350	22.0	40.0	580	na	11.0	30
deluxe, 1 pkg *(Stouffer's)*	6 1/8 oz	420	21.0	40.0	950	na	19.0	na
deluxe 'Zap' *(Banquet)*	4.8 oz	330	14.0	39.0	890	(mq)	13.0	25
double cheese, 1 pkg *(Stouffer's)*	5 7/8 oz	420	22.0	43.0	850	na	18.0	na
hamburger, 1 pkg *(Stouffer's)*	6 oz	410	23.0	39.0	650	na	18.0	na
Italian turkey sausage *(Healthy Choice)*	6.45 oz	320	23.0	42.0	440	na	7.0	30
pepperoni *(Healthy Choice)*	6.25 oz	320	22.0	41.0	490	na	8.0	30
pepperoni *(Lean Cuisine)*	5 1/4 oz	340	19.0	41.0	580	na	11.0	25
pepperoni *(Pappalo's)*	1 piece	410	16.0	41.0	1130	(mq)	20.0	(mq)
pepperoni, microwave *(Oven Lovin')*	1 serving	410	18.0	40.0	980	na	21.0	35
pepperoni 'Microwave' *(Pillsbury)*	1 piece	430	19.0	45.0	940	(mq)	19.0	(mq)
pepperoni, 1 pkg *(Stouffer's)*	5 3/4 oz	400	19.0	39.0	880	na	19.0	na
pepperoni 'Zap' *(Banquet)*	4.5 oz	350	15.0	36.0	1060	(mq)	16.0	40
pepperoni and mushroom *(Stouffer's)*	6 oz	410	19.0	40.0	920	na	19.0	na
sausage *(Lean Cuisine)*	6 oz	350	22.0	42.0	600	na	10.0	35
sausage *(Pappalo's)*	1 piece	410	18.0	41.0	1000	(mq)	18.0	(mq)
sausage *(Stouffer's)*	6 oz	430	20.0	40.0	840	na	21.0	na
sausage, microwave *(Oven Lovin')*	1 serving	400	18.0	41.0	830	na	20.0	25
sausage 'Microwave' *(Pillsbury)*	1 piece	410	18.0	48.0	860	(mq)	16.0	(mq)
sausage and pepperoni *(Stouffer's)*	6.25 oz	460	23.0	41.0	920	na	23.0	na

Food Name	Serv. Size	Total Cal.	Prot. GMS	Carbs GMS	Sod. MGS	Fiber GMS	Fat GMS	Chol. MGS
sausage combo, and pepperoni								
'Microwave' (Pillsbury)	1 piece	450	19.0	47.0	950	(mq)	21.0	(mq)
three cheese (Lean Cuisine)	5.5 oz	330	23.0	38.0	350	na	10.0	20
vegetable deluxe (Stouffer's)	6.5 oz	420	18.0	41.0	830	na	20.0	na
PIZZA, FROZEN								
(Banquet)								
pepperoni 'Pizza Pie'	6-oz pie	470	11.0	45.0	970	na	27.0	35
sausage 'Pizza Pie'	6-oz pie	500	11.0	48.0	860	na	29.0	35
sausage and pepperoni 'Pizza Pie'	6-oz pie	470	12.0	43.0	930	na	27.0	40
(Celeste)								
cheese	1/4 pie	315	14.0	28.0	690	2.2	17.0	20
cheese 'Pizza for One'	1 pie	500	21.0	48.0	1070	3.6	25.0	40
deluxe	1/4 pie	380	16.0	29.0	870	3.1	22.0	20
deluxe 'Pizza for One'	1 pie	580	23.0	51.0	1290	4.4	32.0	20
four cheese, original 'Pizza for One'	1 pie	540	25.0	47.0	1500	na	30.0	50
four cheese, zesty 'Pizza for One'	1 pie	550	24.0	45.0	1500	na	31.0	50
pepperoni	1/4 pie	370	15.0	29.0	940	2.4	21.0	15
pepperoni 'Pizza for One'	1 pie	545	20.0	50.0	1290	3.9	30.0	20
sausage	1/4 pie	375	16.0	30.0	900	3.3	22.0	15
sausage 'Pizza for One'	1 pie	570	23.0	49.0	1300	4.2	32.0	20
suprema	1/4 pie	380	17.0	29.0	970	3.0	24.0	15
suprema 'Pizza for One'	1 pie	680	27.0	54.0	1590	4.5	39.0	20
vegetable 'Pizza for One'	1 pie	490	20.0	44.0	1200	na	26.0	na
(Jeno's)								
combination 'Crisp 'N Tasty'	1/2 pizza	280	10.0	27.0	680	1.0	15.0	15
pepperoni 'Crisp 'N Tasty'	1/2 pizza	280	10.0	28.0	710	1.0	15.0	15
pepperoni 'Pizza Pocket'	1 serving	370	12.0	35.0	790	na	20.0	25
sausage 'Crisp 'N Tasty'	1/2 pizza	280	10.0	27.0	640	1.0	15.0	10
sausage 'Pizza Pocket'	1 serving	360	11.0	35.0	660	na	19.0	15
sausage and pepperoni 'Pizza Pocket'	1 serving	360	12.0	35.0	710	na	20.0	20
supreme 'Pizza Pocket'	1 serving	370	12.0	36.0	720	na	19.0	20
(Oven Lovin')								
cheese, microwave	1/2 pie	250	11.0	24.0	430	na	12.0	10
combination, microwave	1/2 pie	310	13.0	26.0	580	na	18.0	20
pepperoni, microwave	1/2 pie	300	13.0	25.0	620	na	17.0	25
sausage, microwave	1/2 pie	290	12.0	26.0	510	na	16.0	15
supreme, microwave	1/2 pie	310	13.0	27.0	570	na	18.0	20
(Pappalo's)								
pepperoni, 9 inch, traditional crust	1/2 pie	390	23.0	47.0	870	4.0	14.0	45
pepperoni, 12 inch, traditional crust	1/4 pie	350	22.0	40.0	700	4.0	11.0	45
pepperoni, pan pizza	1/6 pie	350	22.0	40.0	720	3.0	11.0	50
sausage, 9 inch, traditional crust	1/2 pie	380	22.0	47.0	680	4.0	13.0	40
sausage, 12 inch, traditional crust	1/4 pie	350	22.0	39.0	600	4.0	12.0	40

Food Name	Serv. Size	Total Cal.	Prot. GMS	Carbs GMS	Sod. MGS	Fiber GMS	Fat GMS	Chol. MGS
sausage, pan pizza	1/5 pie	350	22.0	39.0	530	3.0	11.0	40
sausage and pepperoni, 9 inch, traditional crust	1/2 pie	390	23.0	45.0	650	4.0	15.0	45
sausage and pepperoni, 12 inch, traditional crust	1/4 pie	360	23.0	40.0	730	4.0	12.0	45
sausage and pepperoni, pan pizza	1/5 pie	360	22.0	40.0	630	3.0	12.0	45
supreme, 9 inch, traditional crust	1/2 pie	400	25.0	46.0	700	4.0	16.0	45
supreme, 12 inch, traditional crust	1/4 pie	350	22.0	38.0	640	4.0	12.0	45
supreme, pan pizza	1/5 pie	340	22.0	37.0	610	3.0	12.0	45
three cheese, 9 inch, traditional crust	1/2 pie	350	21.0	47.0	640	4.0	11.0	30
three cheese, 12 inch, traditional crust	1/4 pie	310	20.0	41.0	440	4.0	7.0	30
three cheese, pan pizza	1/5 pie	310	20.0	39.0	490	3.0	8.0	30
(Pepperidge Farm)								
cheese, croissant pastry	1 pie	430	15.0	41.0	640	(mq)	23.0	(mq)
deluxe, croissant pastry	1 pie	440	16.0	43.0	790	(mq)	23.0	(mq)
pepperoni, croissant pastry	1 pie	420	14.0	43.0	690	(mq)	22.0	(mq)
(Tombstone)								
bacon, Canadian style, 'Original' 12 inch	3.6 oz	230	12.0	23.0	580	na	10.0	25
bacon cheeseburger, 'Special Order' 12 inch	4.7 oz	330	17.0	29.0	730	na	16.0	40
cheese, microwave, 7 inch	7.7 oz	500	25.0	45.0	940	na	24.0	40
cheese, 'Original' 9 inch	5.6 oz	380	18.0	40.0	730	na	17.0	35
cheese, 'Original' 12 inch	3.4 oz	230	11.0	23.0	460	na	10.0	25
cheese, w/hamburger, 'Original' 12 inch	3.7 oz	250	13.0	23.0	570	na	12.0	30
cheese, w/Italian sausage 'Italian Style Thincrust'	3.2 oz	220	11.0	15.0	490	na	13.0	30
cheese, w/pepperoni 'Italian Style Thincrust'	3 oz	230	11.0	15.0	540	na	14.0	25
cheese, w/pepperoni, 'Original' 12 inch	3.6 oz	260	12.0	23.0	620	na	14.0	30
cheese, w/sausage, mushrooms, 'Original' 12 inch	3.8 oz	240	13.0	23.0	570	na	11.0	30
cheese, w/sausage, 'Original' 12 inch	3.7 oz	240	13.0	23.0	590	na	11.0	30
cheese and hamburger, 'Original' 9 inch	6.3 oz	440	22.0	41.0	960	na	21.0	50
cheese and pepperoni, microwave, 7 inch	7.5 oz	550	27.0	38.0	1240	na	32.0	55
cheese and pepperoni, 'Original' 9 inch	6.3 oz	480	21.0	40.0	1100	na	26.0	50
cheese and sausage, 'Original' 9 inch	6.3 oz	420	22.0	41.0	1000	na	19.0	50
chicken, 'Light' 8 inch	4.5 oz	240	17.0	28.0	450	na	8.0	25
chicken deluxe 'Light' approx 1/2 pizza	3.7 oz	180	13.0	23.0	440	2.0	4.0	15
deluxe, 'Original' 9 inch	7.0 oz	440	24.0	41.0	1010	na	20.0	55
deluxe, 'Original' 12 inch	3.9 oz	240	13.0	23.0	570	na	11.0	30
four cheese 'Special Order'	4.3 oz	300	15.0	28.0	630	na	14.0	35
four meat 'Special Order'	4.6 oz	320	17.0	28.0	810	na	15.0	40
four meat, 'Special Order' 9 inch	3.9 oz	280	14.0	24.0	670	na	14.0	35

Food Name	Serv. Size	Total Cal.	Prot. GMS	Carbs GMS	Sod. MGS	Fiber GMS	Fat GMS	Chol. MGS
Italian sausage, microwave, 7 inch	8.0 oz	550	28.0	38.0	1210	na	32.0	65
Italian sausage 'Special Order'	4.5 oz	300	17.0	28.0	740	na	13.0	40
pepperoni, 'Double Top' w/double cheese, 12 inch	4.8 oz	360	20.0	24.0	920	na	20.0	50
pepperoni 'Light' 8 inch	4.0 oz	250	16.0	27.0	630	na	10.0	20
pepperoni 'Special Order'	4.4 oz	320	16.0	28.0	780	na	16.0	40
pepperoni 'Special Order' 9 inch	3.7 oz	280	13.0	24.0	650	na	14.0	30
pepperoni and sausage, 'Original' 9 inch	6.6 oz	490	24.0	40.0	1230	na	26.0	60
ranchero deluxe 'Mexican Style Thincrust'	3.4 oz	230	11.0	16.0	530	na	13.0	40
sausage, 'Double Top' w/double cheese, 12 inch	4.8 oz	330	21.0	24.0	860	na	16.0	50
sausage, w/pepperoni, 'Original' 12 inch	3.7 oz	260	13.0	23.0	640	na	13.0	30
sausage and pepperoni, 'Double Top' w/double cheese, 12 inch	4.8 oz	340	21.0	24.0	910	na	18.0	50
sausage and pepperoni, microwave, 7 inch	8 oz	570	32.0	39.0	1430	na	32.0	70
supreme 'Italian Style Thincrust'	3.38 oz	230	11.0	16.0	520	na	14.0	30
supreme, 'Light' 8 inch	4.6 oz	250	17.0	26.0	660	na	9.0	20
supreme, 'Light' 12 inch	4.5 oz	250	15.0	29.0	630	na	9.0	35
supreme, microwave, 7 inch	8.5 oz	550	27.0	40.0	1260	na	31.0	55
supreme, 'Original' 12 inch	3.8 oz	270	12.0	24.0	630	na	14.0	30
supreme 'Special Order'	4.4 oz	320	17.0	29.0	800	na	15.0	40
supreme, 'Special Order' 9 inch	4.0 oz	280	13.0	24.0	640	na	14.0	35
taco, microwave, 7 inch	8.4 oz	590	28.0	41.0	1460	na	34.0	100
three sausage, 'Special Order' 9 inch	3.8 oz	260	14.0	24.0	600	na	12.0	35
vegetable, 'Light' 8 inch	4.4 oz	240	14.0	30.0	500	na	8.0	10
vegetable, 'Light' 12 inch	4.3 oz	230	12.0	30.0	420	na	7.0	10
(Totino's)								
Canadian bacon 'Party Pizza'	1/2 pie	330	15.0	42.0	860	3.0	13.0	10
cheese 'Pan Pizza'	1/6 pie	290	15.0	35.0	440	na	10.0	10
cheese 'Party Pizza'	1/2 pie	290	13.0	40.0	530	2.0	10.0	15
cheese 'Party Pizza Family Size'	1/3 pie	320	14.0	43.0	580	2.0	11.0	15
combination 'Party Pizza'	1/2 pie	370	15.0	43.0	920	3.0	17.0	20
combination 'Party Pizza Family Size'	1/3 pie	400	17.0	47.0	990	3.0	18.0	20
hamburger 'Party Pizza'	1/2 pie	350	16.0	37.0	780	3.0	17.0	15
pepperoni 'Pan Pizza'	1/6 pie	330	16.0	35.0	620	na	15.0	30
pepperoni 'Party Pizza'	1/2 pie	380	14.0	41.0	980	3.0	19.0	15
pepperoni 'Party Pizza Family Size'	1/3 pie	410	16.0	44.0	1060	3.0	20.0	20
sausage 'Pan Pizza'	1/6 pie	320	16.0	35.0	500	na	13.0	20
sausage 'Party Pizza'	1/2 pie	370	15.0	44.0	800	3.0	17.0	10
sausage 'Party Pizza Family Size'	1/3 pie	410	16.0	48.0	870	4.0	18.0	15
sausage and pepperoni 'Pan Pizza'	1/6 pie	330	16.0	35.0	560	na	15.0	25

Food Name	Serv. Size	Total Cal.	Prot. GMS	Carbs GMS	Sod. MGS	Fiber GMS	Fat GMS	Chol. MGS
PIZZA CRUST, 'All Ready' *(Pillsbury)* ..	1/8 crust	90	3.0	16.0	170	(mq)	1.0	0
PIZZA CRUST MIX								
deep dish, prepared w/water, crust only								
(Martha White)	1 slice	110	3.0	23.0	110	na	<1.0	0
'Pouch Mix' *(Gold Medal)*	1/6 pkg	110	3.0	22.0	220	(mq)	1.0	na
'Pouch Mix' *(Robin Hood)*	1/6 pkg	110	3.0	22.0	220	(mq)	1.0	na
'Quick & Easy' *(Chef Boyardee)*	1/6 pkg	150	6.0	26.0	300	(mq)	2.0	na
regular, prepared w/water, crust only								
(Martha White)	1 slice	100	2.0	19.0	125	na	2.0	0
PIZZA DINNER, FROZEN								
cheese *(Kid Cuisine)*	6.85 oz	380	11.0	57.0	390	na	12.0	25
cheese 'Mega Meal' *(Kid Cuisine)*	9.7 oz	430	17.0	75.0	700	na	7.0	na
hamburger *(Kid Cuisine)*	6.85 oz	330	11.0	50.0	700	na	10.0	15
PIZZA ENTRÉE, FROZEN								
cheese *(Weight Watchers)*	6.03 oz	300	24.0	36.0	310	na	7.0	10
deluxe combination 'Lowfat'								
(Weight Watchers)	7.32 oz	320	25.0	36.0	370	na	9.0	10
hamburger 'Looney Tunes Wile E.								
Coyote' *(Tyson)*	6 oz	310	12.0	40.0	630	na	11.0	13
pepperoni 'Looney Tunes Foghorn								
Leghorn' *(Tyson)*	6.35 oz	400	13.0	57.0	610	na	13.0	18
pepperoni 'Lowfat' *(Weight Watchers)* ..	6.08 oz	320	25.0	36.0	550	na	8.0	15
supreme, hand held 'Aussie Pie'								
(Mrs. Paterson's)	5.5 oz	470	12.0	44.0	880	na	27.0	75
PIZZA MIX								
cheese 'Complete' *(Chef Boyardee)*	1/4 pkg	230	9.0	36.0	740	(mq)	6.0	na
cheese, kit *(Contadina)*	4.94 oz	320	16.0	41.0	850	na	10.0	20
cheese '2 Complete' *(Chef Boyardee)* ..	1/8 pkg	210	10.0	31.0	650	(mq)	5.0	(mq)
pepperoni 'Complete' *(Chef Boyardee)* .	1/4 pkg	250	13.0	31.0	870	(mq)	9.0	(mq)
pepperoni, kit *(Contadina)*	4.94 oz	370	18.0	38.0	980	na	16.0	30
pepperoni '2 Complete' *(Chef Boyardee)*	1/8 pkg	210	10.0	31.0	595	(mq)	7.0	(mq)
plain *(Chef Boyardee)*	1/4 pkg	180	6.0	32.0	640	(mq)	3.0	na
sausage *(Chef Boyardee)*	1/4 pkg	270	14.0	34.0	930	(mq)	10.0	(mq)
PIZZA ROLL, FROZEN								
cheese, approx 6 rolls *(Jeno's)*	3 oz	240	8.0	23.0	350	(mq)	12.0	(mq)
combination *(Jeno's)*	3 oz	220	10.0	26.0	230	1.9	9.0	15
hamburger, approx 6 rolls *(Jeno's)*	3 oz	240	9.0	21.0	280	(mq)	13.0	(mq)
pepperoni, approx 6 rolls *(Jeno's)*	3 oz	220	9.0	26.0	350	1.8	9.0	20
pepperoni and cheese, approx 6 rolls								
(Jeno's)	3 oz	230	7.0	22.0	390	(mq)	13.0	(mq)
pepperoni and cheese 'Microwave' 6 rolls								
(Jeno's)	3 oz	240	7.0	23.0	440	(mq)	13.0	(mq)
sausage *(Jeno's)*	3 oz	210	9.0	26.0	340	1.6	7.0	15

Food Name	Serv. Size	Total Cal.	Prot. GMS	Carbs GMS	Sod. MGS	Fiber GMS	Fat GMS	Chol. MGS
sausage and cheese 'Microwave'								
approx 6 rolls (Jeno's)	3 oz	250	8.0	24.0	440	(mq)	13.0	(mq)
sausage and pepperoni, approx 6 rolls								
(Jeno's)	3 oz	230	7.0	22.0	380	(mq)	13.0	(mq)
PLANTAIN								
cooked	4 oz	132	0.9	35.3	6	(mq)	0.2	0
cooked, sliced	1 cup	179	1.2	48.0	8	3.5	0.3	0
raw, approx 9.7 oz	1 med	218	2.3	57.1	7	>.9 c	0.7	0
raw, sliced	1 cup	181	1.9	47.2	6	3.4	0.6	0
raw, trimmed	1 oz	35	0.4	9.0	1	>.1 c	0.1	0
raw, trimmed, approx 9.7 oz	1 med	218	2.3	57.1	7	4.1	0.7	0
raw, untrimmed	1 lb	360	3.8	94.0	12	>1.5 c	1.1	0
PLUM								
pitted	1 oz	16	0.2	3.7	tr	>.2 c	0.2	0
raw, sliced	1 cup	91	1.3	21.5	0	2.5	1.0	0
raw, 2 1/8-inch diam	1 med	36	0.5	8.6	0	1.0	0.4	0
untrimmed (Dole)	2 pieces	70	1.0	17.0	0	1.0	1.0	na
w/pits	1 lb	235	3.4	55.5	2	>2.6 c	2.6	0
PLUM, JAPANESE								
peeled and seeded	1 oz	13	0.1	3.4	<1	>.1 c	0.1	0
raw, approx .6 oz	1 med	5	<.1	1.2	tr	>.1 c	<.1	0
untrimmed	1 lb	132	1.2	34.1	3	>1.4 c	0.6	0
PLUM, PURPLE, CANNED								
halves or whole, unpeeled								
(S&W Nutradiet)	1/2 cup	52	0.0	13.0	0	(mq)	0.0	0
in extra heavy syrup	1/2 cup	133	0.5	34.3	25	>.4 c	0.1	0
in extra heavy syrup, pitted	4 oz	115	0.4	29.8	22	>.4 c	0.1	0
in extra heavy syrup, unpeeled, halves								
(S&W)	1/2 cup	135	0.0	35.0	25	(mq)	0.0	0
in extra heavy syrup, unpeeled, whole								
(S&W)	1/2 cup	135	0.0	35.0	25	(mq)	0.0	0
in extra heavy syrup, w/liquid	1 cup	264	0.9	68.7	50	>.8 c	0.3	0
in extra heavy syrup, w/2.75 tbsp liquid	3 plums	134	0.5	35.0	25	>.4 c	0.1	0
in heavy syrup	1/2 cup	115	0.5	30.0	25	>.4 c	0.1	0
in heavy syrup (Stokely)	1/2 cup	130	0.0	30.0	25	(mq)	0.0	0
in heavy syrup, pitted	4 oz	101	0.4	26.4	22	>.4 c	0.1	0
in heavy syrup, w/liquid	1 cup	230	0.9	60.0	49	2.6	0.3	0
in heavy syrup, w/2.75 tbsp liquid	3 plums	118	0.5	30.9	25	1.3	0.1	0
in juice	1/2 cup	73	0.7	19.1	2	.5	<.1	0
in juice, pitted	4 oz	66	0.6	17.2	1	.4	<.1	0
in juice, whole (Featherweight)	1/2 cup	80	1.0	18.0	10	(mq)	0.0	0
in light syrup	1/2 cup	79	0.5	20.5	25	>.4 c	0.1	0
in light syrup (Stokely)	1/2 cup	100	0.0	16.0	20	(mq)	0.0	0

Food Name	Serv. Size	Total Cal.	Prot. GMS	Carbs GMS	Sod. MGS	Fiber GMS	Fat GMS	Chol. MGS
in light syrup, pitted	4 oz	71	0.4	18.5	23	>.4 c	0.1	0
in water	1/2 cup	51	0.5	13.7	1	>.3 c	<.1	0
in water, pitted	4 oz	46	0.4	12.5	1	>.3 c	<.1	0

POHA. See CAPE GOOSEBERRY.

POI

fresh	1/2 cup	134	0.5	32.7	14	.5	0.2	0
fresh	1 oz	32	0.1	7.7	3	.1	<.1	0

POKEBERRY SHOOTS

boiled, drained	4 oz	23	2.6	3.5	na	(mq)	0.5	0
boiled, drained	1/2 cup	16	1.9	2.5	15	1.2	0.3	0
raw	1/2 cup	18	2.1	3.0	18	1.4	0.3	0
raw, trimmed	4 oz	26	2.9	4.2	na	(mq)	0.5	0

POLENTA MIX, prepared

(Fantastic Foods)	1/2 cup	106	3.0	18.0	246	(mq)	2.0	na

POLISH SAUSAGE

	1 oz	92	4.0	0.5	248	0	8.1	20
link, 10 inches long x 1 1/4 inch diam, 8 oz	1 large	739	32.0	3.7	1989	0	65.2	158
(Hillshire Farm) 'Links'	2 oz	190	7.0	2.0	520	0	17.0	(mq)
(Hormel)	2 links	170	9.0	0.0	574	0	14.0	(mq)
(OHSE)	1 oz	80	4.0	1.0	290	0	7.0	(mq)
(OHSE) hot	1 oz	70	4.0	3.0	270	0	5.0	(mq)
(Pilgrim's Pride)	3 oz	131	13.2	2.3	780	0	7.7	72

POLLACK, ALASKAN

baked	4 oz	128	26.7	0.0	132	0	1.3	109
broiled	4 oz	128	26.7	0.0	132	0	1.3	109
microwaved	4 oz	128	26.7	0.0	132	0	1.3	109
raw	1 lb	365	77.9	0.0	449	0	3.6	323
raw	1 oz	23	4.9	0.0	28	0	0.2	20

POLLACK, ATLANTIC

raw	1 lb	416	88.2	0.0	391	0	4.4	320
raw	3 oz	78	16.5	0.0	73	0	0.8	60
raw	1 oz	26	5.5	0.0	24	0	0.3	20

POLLACK, WALLEYE

baked	4 oz	128	26.7	0.0	132	0	1.3	109
broiled	4 oz	128	26.7	0.0	132	0	1.3	109
dry-heat cooked	3 oz	96	20.0	0.0	99	0	1.0	82
microwaved	4 oz	128	26.7	0.0	132	0	1.3	109
raw	1 lb	365	77.9	0.0	449	0	3.6	323
raw	3 oz	69	14.6	0.0	84	0	0.7	60
raw	1 oz	23	4.9	0.0	28	0	0.2	20

POLLYFISH. See PARROTFISH.

Food Name	Serv. Size	Total Cal.	Prot. GMS	Carbs GMS	Sod. MGS	Fiber GMS	Fat GMS	Chol. MGS
POMEGRANATE/Chinese apple								
raw, approx 3 3/8-inch diam	1 med	105	1.5	26.4	5	.9	0.5	0
trimmed	1 oz	19	0.3	4.9	1	>.1 c	0.1	0
untrimmed	1 lb	172	2.4	43.6	8	>.5 c	0.8	0
POMEGRANATE JUICE (Knudsen & Sons)	8 oz	85	<1.0	21.0	na	na	0.0	na
POMELO/pumelo								
raw, approx 5 1/2-inch diam, 2.4 lbs	1 med	228	4.6	58.6	7	6.1	0.2	0
sections	1/2 cup	36	0.7	9.1	1	1.0	<.1	0
trimmed	1 oz	11	0.2	2.7	1	>.1 c	<.1	0
untrimmed	1 lb	95	1.9	24.4	3	>.5 c	0.1	0
POMFRET								
raw	1 lb	663	78.4	0.0	401	0	36.4	295
raw	1 oz	41	4.9	0.0	25	0	2.3	18
POMPANO, FLORIDA								
baked	4 oz	239	26.4	0.0	86	0	13.8	73
broiled	4 oz	239	26.4	0.0	86	0	13.8	73
dry-heat cooked	3 oz	179	20.1	0.0	65	0	10.3	54
microwaved	4 oz	239	26.4	0.0	86	0	13.8	73
raw	1 lb	745	83.8	0.0	294	0	42.9	227
raw	1 oz	46	5.2	0.0	18	0	2.7	14
POPCORN								
(NOTE: All popcorn is popped unless otherwise noted.)								
(Bachman)								
cheese flavor	.5 oz	90	1.0	7.0	165	(mq)	6.0	na
'Lite'	.5 oz	50	1.0	10.0	35	2.0	1.0	0
regular	.5 oz	80	1.0	7.0	160	(mq)	6.0	0
white cheddar cheese flavor	.5 oz	70	1.0	7.0	150	(mq)	4.0	na
(Bearitos)								
cheese flavor 'Organic'	1 oz	137	3.1	13.2	122	2.0	8.0	na
'Organic 50% Less Oil'	.5 oz	70	2.0	9.0	70	na	3.0	0
'Organic Lite'	1 oz	132	2.8	14.7	39	2.7	6.9	0
'Organic No Salt'	1 oz	108	3.6	21.7	1	.7	0.8	0
'Organic Traditional'	1 oz	140	2.4	12.0	85	3.0	9.2	0
(Bonnie Lee)								
w/oil and salt	1 oz	172	3.0	20.0	230	(mq)	8.0	na
w/o oil and salt	1 oz	109	3.0	20.0	<1	(mq)	1.0	0
(Cape Cod) white cheddar cheese flavor	.5 oz	80	2.0	6.0	150	(mq)	5.0	na
(Clover Club) white cheddar cheese flavor	.5 oz	70	1.0	6.0	140	(mq)	5.0	na
(Cracker Jack) caramel coated, w/peanuts	1 oz	120	2.0	22.0	85	(mq)	3.0	80
(Estee) caramel coated	1 oz	140	3.0	25.0	55	(mq)	3.0	5
(Frito Lay)								
cheese flavor	.5 oz	80	1.0	7.0	180	(mq)	5.0	0
regular	.5 oz	70	1.0	9.0	200	(mq)	3.0	0

Food Name	Serv. Size	Total Cal.	Prot. GMS	Carbs GMS	Sod. MGS	Fiber GMS	Fat GMS	Chol. MGS
(Jiffy Pop)								
butter flavor 'Pan Popcorn'	4 cups	130	3.0	16.0	270	2.0	6.0	0
'Pan Popcorn'	4 cups	130	3.0	16.0	270	2.0	6.0	0
(Jolly Time)								
white, air-popped	3 cups	60	2.0	15.0	2	4.0	<1.0	0
white, w/o salt	4 cups	75	3.0	20.0	2	5.0	1.0	0
yellow, air-popped	3 cups	60	2.0	14.0	2	4.0	<1.0	0
yellow, w/o salt	4 cups	75	3.0	19.0	2	5.0	1.0	0
(Keebler)								
honey caramel 'Pop Deluxe'	1 oz	120	<1.0	22.0	180	(mq)	3.0	0
white cheddar cheese flavor	1 oz	140	1.0	13.0	270	(mq)	10.0	5
(Kettle Poppins)								
lightly salted	.5 oz	70	2.0	9.0	40	1.0	2.5	0
white cheddar	.5 oz	70	2.0	9.0	120	1.0	2.5	1
(Laura Scudder)								
'Tender Baby White Corn'	.5 oz	80	1.0	6.0	140	(mq)	6.0	0
white cheddar cheese flavor	.5 oz	70	1.0	6.0	140	(mq)	5.0	na
(Nature's Choice)								
caramel, original	1 oz	108	1.0	25.0	na	na	1.0	0
caramel, w/peanuts	1 oz	114	1.0	23.0	na	na	1.0	0
(Orville Redenbacher)								
caramel 'Ready-to-Eat'	1 oz	112	0.9	22.4	65	3.2	3.5	1
hot air 'Gourmet' prepared	3 cups	40	1.0	10.0	0	3.0	<1.0	0
original 'Gourmet' prepared	3 cups	80	1.0	10.0	0	3.0	4.0	0
white 'Gourmet'	3 cups	80	1.0	10.0	0	3.0	4.0	0
white cheddar cheese 'Ready-to-Eat'	1.058 oz	139	3.4	16.5	285	4.4	8.6	1
(Pops-Rite)								
white, w/o salt, air popped	1 oz	100	3.0	20.0	na	.6	2.0	0
white, w/o salt, oil popped	1 oz	220	3.0	20.0	na	.6	15.0	0
yellow, w/o salt, air popped	1 oz	100	2.0	21.0	na	.6	2.0	0
yellow, w/o salt, oil popped	1 oz	220	2.0	21.0	na	.6	15.0	0
(Smartfood) white cheddar cheese flavor	.5 oz	80	2.0	7.0	150	(mq)	5.0	na
(Ultra Slim Fast) butter flavor 'Lite 'N Tasty'	.5 oz	60	2.0	10.0	150	2.0	2.0	0
(Vic's)								
caramel, lite 'Gourmet'	1/2 cup	60	1.0	10.0	50	na	2.0	0
white, lite 'Gourmet'	1 cup	35	1.0	6.0	15	na	2.0	0
white cheddar cheese, lite 'Gourmet'	2/3 cup	40	1.0	4.0	50	na	2.0	1
yellow cheddar cheese, lite 'Gourmet'	2/3 cup	40	1.0	4.0	60	na	2.0	1
(Weight Watchers)								
butter	.66-oz pkg	90	2.0	13.0	100	na	3.0	na
caramel	.9-oz pkg	100	1.0	23.0	45	na	1.0	0
'Lightly Salted'	.66-oz pkg	80	2.0	12.0	65	(mq)	4.0	0
white cheddar cheese flavor	.66-oz pkg	100	2.0	10.0	85	(mq)	6.0	na

Food Name	Serv. Size	Total Cal.	Prot. GMS	Carbs GMS	Sod. MGS	Fiber GMS	Fat GMS	Chol. MGS
(Wise)								
butter flavor, 1 cup	.5 oz	80	1.0	7.0	140	(mq)	5.0	0
'Tender Baby White Corn'	.5 oz	80	1.0	6.0	140	(mq)	6.0	0
'Tender Eating Baby Popcorn'	.5 oz	70	1.0	4.0	120	(mq)	6.0	0
white cheddar cheese flavor	.5 oz	70	1.0	6.0	140	(mq)	5.0	na
POPCORN, FROZEN								
(Orville Redenbacher)								
butter flavor 'Gourmet' microwave	3 cups	100	2.0	11.0	240	3.0	6.0	0
natural 'Gourmet' microwave	3 cups	100	2.0	11.0	200	3.0	6.0	0
(Pillsbury)								
butter flavor	3 cups	210	3.0	20.0	480	(mq)	13.0	na
'Original'	3 cups	210	3.0	20.0	420	(mq)	13.0	na
'Salt-Free'	3 cups	170	3.0	23.0	na	(mq)	7.0	0
POPCORN, MICROWAVE								
(NOTE: All microwave popcorn is popped unless otherwise noted.)								
(Betty Crocker)								
butter flavor 'Pop•Secret'	1/4 bag	120	2.0	13.0	250	2.0	8.0	0
butter flavor 'Pop•Secret By Request'	1/3 bag	60	2.0	12.0	160	na	1.0	0
butter flavor 'Pop•Secret Light'	1/4 bag	90	2.0	13.0	160	2.0	4.0	0
butter flavor 'Pop•Secret Pop Qwiz'	1 bag	110	2.0	11.0	210	2.0	7.0	0
butter flavor, salt-free 'Pop•Secret'	1/4 bag	120	2.0	13.0	5	2.0	7.0	0
butter flavor, singles 'Pop•Secret'	1 bag	250	4.0	27.0	460	4.0	16.0	0
butter flavor, singles 'Pop•Secret Light'	1 bag	180	4.0	28.0	310	4.0	8.0	0
cheese flavor 'Pop•Secret'	1/3 bag	170	3.0	15.0	260	2.0	11.0	0
natural 'Pop•Secret'	1/4 bag	120	2.0	13.0	250	2.0	8.0	0
natural 'Pop•Secret By Request'	1/3 bag	60	2.0	12.0	170	na	1.0	0
natural 'Pop•Secret Light'	1/4 bag	90	2.0	13.0	200	2.0	4.0	0
natural 'Pop•Secret Pop Qwiz'	1 bag	110	2.0	11.0	220	2.0	7.0	0
natural, singles 'Pop•Secret Light'	1 bag	170	4.0	26.0	440	4.0	7.0	0
(Featherweight)								
butter flavor 'Low Salt'	3 cups	100	3.0	14.0	70	(mq)	3.0	0
'Natural Low Salt'	3 cups	80	3.0	14.0	0	(mq)	1.0	0
(Jiffy Pop)								
butter flavor	4 cups	140	3.0	17.0	270	3.0	7.0	0
natural	4 cups	140	3.0	17.0	270	3.0	7.0	0
(Jolly Time)								
butter flavor	3 cups	90	2.0	13.0	95	3.0	5.0	0
butter flavor, light	3 cups	60	2.0	12.0	105	3.0	2.0	0
cheddar flavor	3 cups	155	3.0	17.0	220	4.0	10.0	0
natural	3 cups	120	2.0	15.0	125	3.0	7.0	0
natural, light	3 cups	70	2.0	13.0	110	3.0	2.0	0
(Orville Redenbacher)								
butter flavor 'Gourmet'	3 cups	100	2.0	11.0	240	3.0	6.0	0

Food Name	Serv. Size	Total Cal.	Prot. GMS	Carbs GMS	Sod. MGS	Fiber GMS	Fat GMS	Chol. MGS
butter flavor, light 'Gourmet'	3 cups	70	2.0	8.0	110	3.0	3.0	0
butter flavor, light, snack size	3 cups	70	2.0	11.0	90	na	3.0	0
butter flavor, salt-free 'Gourmet'	3 cups	100	2.0	11.0	0	3.0	6.0	0
butter flavor 'Smart•Pop'	3 cups	50	2.0	11.0	100	na	1.0	0
butter flavor, snack size	3 cups	100	2.0	11.0	140	na	6.0	0
butter toffee flavor 'Gourmet'	2 1/2 cups	210	2.0	26.0	85	2.0	12.0	<1
caramel flavor 'Gourmet'	2 1/2 cups	240	2.0	29.0	90	2.0	14.0	<1
cheddar cheese flavor 'Gourmet'	3 cups	130	2.0	14.0	280	3.0	8.0	2
natural 'Gourmet'	3 cups	100	2.0	11.0	200	3.0	6.0	0
natural, light 'Gourmet'	3 cups	70	2.0	8.0	115	3.0	3.0	0
natural, salt-free 'Gourmet'	3 cups	100	2.0	11.0	0	3.0	6.0	0
red herb and garlic flavor, 2 tbsp unpopped	1.27 oz	150	1.9	15.4	366	4.0	10.7	0
sour cream 'n onion flavor 'Gourmet'	3 cups	160	2.0	12.0	270	3.0	12.0	0
zesty butter flavor 'Reddenbutter' 2 tbsp unpopped	1.27 oz	148	2.1	15.9	259	4.0	10.2	0
(Pillsbury)								
butter flavor	3 cups	210	3.0	20.0	410	(mq)	13.0	na
'Original'	3 cups	210	3.0	20.0	410	(mq)	13.0	0
(Planters)								
butter flavor	3 cups	140	2.0	13.0	0	(mq)	10.0	560
natural	3 cups	140	2.0	14.0	0	(mq)	9.0	560
(Pop Weavers)								
butter flavor	4 cups	140	3.0	20.0	230	4.0	8.0	0
'Natural'	4 cups	140	3.0	20.0	230	4.0	8.0	0
(Pops-Rite)								
butter flavor	3 cups	90	2.0	13.0	140	(mq)	5.0	0
'Natural'	3 cups	90	2.0	13.0	190	(mq)	5.0	0
(Weight Watchers)	1-oz pkg	100	4.0	22.0	5	(mq)	1.0	0
POPCORN OIL								
(Orville Redenbacher) popping	1 tbsp	120	0.0	0.0	0	0	14.0	0
(Planters)	1 tbsp	120	0.0	0.0	0	na	14.0	0
(Wesson) buttery flavor popping oil	1 tbsp	120	0.0	0.0	0	0	13.5	0
(Wesson) popping and topping oil 'Food Service'	1 tbsp	122	0.0	0.0	0	0	13.5	0
POPCORN SEASONING								
(McCormick/Schilling) 'Parsley Patch'	1 tsp	10	0.6	3.0	4	na	0.1	0
POPPY SEED								
whole	1 oz	151	5.1	6.7	6	>1.8 c	12.6	0
whole	1 tbsp	47	1.6	2.1	2	2.6	3.9	0
whole	1 tsp	15	0.5	0.7	1	.8	1.3	0
whole *(Durkee)*	1 tsp	15	0.0	0.0	0	0	<0.1	na
whole *(Laurel Leaf)*	1 tsp	15	0.0	0.0	0	0	<0.1	na

Food Name	Serv. Size	Total Cal.	Prot. GMS	Carbs GMS	Sod. MGS	Fiber GMS	Fat GMS	Chol. MGS
whole *(Spice Islands)*	1 tsp	13	0.6	0.8	<1	>.2 c	0.9	0
POPPY SEED OIL								
	1 cup	1927	0.0	0.0	0	0	218.0	0
	1 oz	251	0.0	0.0	0	0	28.4	0
	1 tbsp	120	0.0	0.0	0	0	13.6	0

PORK. See also HAM, CANNED; HAM, CURED; HAM, FRESH; HAM PATTY.

(NOTE: TRIMMED = Lean; separable fat removed. UNTRIMMED = Separable fat not removed.)

BACKFAT

Food Name	Serv. Size	Total Cal.	Prot. GMS	Carbs GMS	Sod. MGS	Fiber GMS	Fat GMS	Chol. MGS
wholesale cuts, raw	1 lb	3683	13.3	0.0	50	0	402.3	259
wholesale cuts, raw	1 oz	230	0.8	0.0	3	0	25.1	16
BACKRIB								
Untrimmed								
raw	1 lb	1279	73.1	0.0	340	0	107.0	367
raw	1 oz	80	4.6	0.0	21	0	6.7	23
raw 'Gourmet' *(JM)*	5.5 oz	220	15.0	0.0	50	0	18.0	(mq)
roasted	3 oz	315	20.6	0.0	86	0	25.1	100
BELLY								
wholesale cuts, raw	1 lb	2350	42.4	0.0	145	0	240.5	327
wholesale cuts, raw	1 oz	147	2.7	0.0	9	0	15.0	20
BOSTON BUTT								
Trimmed								
cured, medium fat, chopped, roasted	1 cup	340	38.9	0.0	1393	0	19.3	123
cured, medium fat, roasted	9.8 oz	678	77.6	0.0	2777	0	38.5	246
BRAINS								
braised	3 oz	117	10.3	0.0	77	0	8.1	2169
in milk gravy *(Armour)*	2.75 oz	110	7.0	1.0	400	na	8.0	na
raw	1 oz	36	2.9	0.0	34	0	2.6	622
CENTER LOIN								
Trimmed								
braised	3 oz	172	25.3	0.0	53	0	7.1	72
broiled	3 oz	172	25.7	0.0	51	0	6.9	70
chopped, braised	1 cup	381	48.7	0.0	77	0	19.2	155
chopped, broiled	1 cup	323	44.8	0.0	109	0	14.7	137
chopped, roasted	1 cup	336	39.9	0.0	97	0	18.3	127
pan-fried	3 oz	197	27.4	0.0	73	0	8.9	78
pan-fried in vegetable oil	4 oz	302	32.6	0.0	96	0	14.0	121
raw	1 oz	45	6.2	0.0	19	0	2.0	18
roasted	3 oz	169	23.4	0.0	56	0	7.7	67
Untrimmed								
braised	3 oz	210	23.8	0.0	50	0	12.0	73
broiled	3 oz	204	24.4	0.0	49	0	11.1	70
chopped, braised	1 cup	496	41.2	0.0	71	0	35.5	150
chopped, broiled	1 cup	442	38.4	0.0	98	0	30.9	136

Food Name	Serv. Size	Total Cal.	Prot. GMS	Carbs GMS	Sod. MGS	Fiber GMS	Fat GMS	Chol. MGS
chopped, pan-fried in vegetable oil	1 cup	372	40.3	0.0	119	0	22.3	150
chopped, roasted	1 cup	427	35.6	0.0	90	0	30.5	127
pan-fried	3 oz	235	25.4	0.0	68	0	14.1	78
pan-fried in vegetable oil	4 oz	425	26.4	0.0	82	0	34.6	117
raw	1 oz	80	5.2	0.0	16	0	6.2	20
roasted	3 oz	199	22.4	0.0	54	0	11.4	68
CENTER RIB								
Trimmed								
braised	3 oz	175	24.1	0.0	35	0	8.0	60
broiled	3 oz	186	26.1	0.0	55	0	8.3	69
chopped, braised	1 cup	388	48.2	0.0	73	0	20.2	136
chopped, broiled	1 cup	361	40.3	0.0	94	0	20.9	132
chopped, pan-fried in vegetable oil	1 cup	360	39.1	0.0	70	0	21.4	113
chopped, roasted	1 cup	343	39.5	0.0	64	0	19.3	111
pan-fried	3 oz	185	23.9	0.0	44	0	9.2	59
pan-fried in vegetable oil	4 oz	291	31.7	0.0	57	0'	17.4	92
raw	1 lb	676	100.3	0.0	204	0	27.3	249
roasted	3 oz	190	24.4	0.0	40	0	9.5	60
Untrimmed								
braised	3 oz	213	22.7	0.0	34	0	12.8	62
broiled	3 oz	224	24.5	0.0	53	0	13.2	70
chopped, braised	1 cup	514	40.0	0.0	67	0	38.0	133
chopped, broiled	1 cup	480	34.4	0.0	85	0	36.9	130
chopped, pan-fried in vegetable oil	1 cup	546	30.3	0.0	63	0	46.2	118
chopped, roasted	1 cup	445	34.6	0.0	62	0	33.0	113
pan-fried	3 oz	225	22.3	0.0	43	0	14.4	62
pan-fried in vegetable oil	4 oz	442	24.5	0.0	51	0	37.4	95
raw	1 oz	82	5.1	0.0	11	0	6.6	18
roasted	3 oz	217	23.3	0.0	39	0	13.0	62
CHITTERLINGS								
raw	1 oz	71	2.8	0.1	10	0	6.5	45
simmered	3 oz	258	8.7	0.0	33	0	24.4	122
CHOP, BONELESS, 'America's Cut' *(JM)*	6 oz	330	38.0	0.0	90	0	20.0	(mq)
COMPOSITE CUTS								
Trimmed								
loin and shoulder, cooked	3 oz	179	25.0	0.0	48	0	8.0	72
loin and shoulder, raw	1 lb	653	96.3	0.0	245	0	26.7	272
loin and shoulder, raw	1 oz	41	6.0	0.0	15	0	1.7	17
retail cuts, cooked	3 oz	232	23.4	0.0	53	0	14.6	77
retail cuts, raw	1 lb	980	86.0	0.0	249	0	67.8	304
retail cuts, raw	1 oz	61	5.4	0.0	16	0	4.2	19
roasted	3 oz	180	24.9	0.0	50	0	8.2	73

Food Name	Serv. Size	Total Cal.	Prot. GMS	Carbs GMS	Sod. MGS	Fiber GMS	Fat GMS	Chol. MGS
Untrimmed								
loin and shoulder, cooked	3 oz	214	23.6	0.0	48	0	12.6	73
loin and shoulder, raw	1 lb	907	88.6	0.0	231	0	58.5	290
loin and shoulder, raw	1 oz	57	5.5	0.0	14	0	3.7	18
raw	1 lb	1030	82.8	0.0	245	0	74.8	313
raw	1 oz	64	5.2	0.0	15	0	4.7	20
KIDNEYS								
braised	1 cup	211	35.6	0.0	112	0	6.6	672
braised	3 oz	128	21.6	0.0	68	0	4.0	408
raw	1 oz	28	4.7	0.0	34	0	0.9	90
LIVER								
braised	3 oz	140	22.1	3.2	42	0	3.7	302
fried	3 oz	205	25.4	2.1	94	0	9.8	372
raw	1 oz	38	6.1	0.7	25	0	1.0	85
LOIN								
Trimmed								
blade, braised	3 oz	191	21.3	0.0	53	0	11.1	71
blade, broiled	3 oz	199	21.6	0.0	68	0	11.8	71
blade, chopped, braised	1 cup	438	41.6	0.0	113	0	28.8	158
blade, chopped, broiled	1 cup	420	34.9	0.0	108	0	30.1	140
blade, chopped, roasted	1 cup	391	34.6	0.0	95	0	27.0	125
blade, pan-fried	3 oz	205	21.0	0.0	66	0	12.8	70
blade, pan-fried in vegetable oil	4 oz	321	27.6	0.0	84	0	22.5	110
blade, raw	1 lb	712	87.4	0.0	304	0	37.4	290
blade, roasted	3 oz	210	22.6	0.0	25	0	12.6	79
country-style ribs, braised	3 oz	199	22.1	0.0	54	0	11.6	73
country-style ribs, raw	1 lb	712	87.4	0.0	304	0	37.4	290
country-style ribs, raw	1 oz	45	5.5	0.0	19	0	2.3	18
country-style ribs, roasted	3 oz	210	22.6	0.0	25	0	12.6	79
whole, braised	3 oz	173	24.3	0.0	43	0	7.8	67
whole, broiled	3 oz	178	24.3	0.0	54	0	8.3	67
whole, chopped, braised	1 cup	382	46.2	0.0	105	0	20.4	147
whole, chopped, broiled	1 cup	360	39.0	0.0	105	0	21.4	133
whole, chopped, roasted	1 cup	336	37.7	0.0	97	0	19.5	126
whole, raw	1 oz	44	5.9	0.0	18	0	2.1	17
whole, roasted	3 oz	178	24.3	0.0	49	0	8.2	69
whole or half, center cut, boneless *(JM)*	3 oz	190	16.0	0.0	50	0	13.0	(mq)
Untrimmed								
blade, braised	3 oz	275	18.6	0.0	47	0	21.6	72
blade, broiled	3 oz	272	19.1	0.0	59	0	21.1	73
blade, chopped, braised	1 cup	574	33.5	0.0	97	0	47.7	151
blade, chopped, broiled	1 cup	550	28.9	0.0	94	0	47.4	137
blade, chopped, roasted	1 cup	510	29.5	0.0	85	0	42.6	126

Food Name	Serv. Size	Total Cal.	Prot. GMS	Carbs GMS	Sod. MGS	Fiber GMS	Fat GMS	Chol. MGS
blade, pan-fried	3 oz	291	18.3	0.0	57	0	23.6	72
blade, pan-fried in vegetable oil	4 oz	469	21.3	0.0	69	0	41.9	108
blade, raw	1 lb	1293	71.8	0.0	245	0	109.4	327
blade, roasted	3 oz	275	20.2	0.0	25	0	20.9	79
country-style ribs, braised	3 oz	252	20.3	0.0	50	0	18.3	74
country-style ribs, raw	1 lb	1093	77.1	0.0	263	0	84.9	313
country-style ribs, raw	1 oz	68	4.8	0.0	16	0	5.3	20
country-style ribs, roasted	3 oz	279	19.9	0.0	44	0	21.5	78
whole, braised	4 oz	417	30.8	0.0	74	0	31.6	116
whole, broiled	3 oz	206	23.2	0.0	53	0	11.8	68
whole, chopped, braised	1 cup	515	38.0	0.0	91	0	39.1	143
whole, chopped, broiled	1 cup	484	33.0	0.0	92	0	38.1	132
whole, chopped, roasted	1 cup	447	32.8	0.0	88	0	34.0	126
whole, raw	1 lb	898	89.5	0.0	227	0	57.1	286
whole, roasted	3 oz	211	23.0	0.0	50	0	12.4	70
LUNGS								
braised	3 oz	84	14.1	0.0	69	0	2.6	329
raw	1 oz	24	4.0	0.0	43	0	0.8	91
PANCREAS								
braised	3 oz	186	24.2	0.0	36	0	9.2	268
raw	1 oz	56	5.3	0.0	12	0	3.8	55
SHOULDER								
Trimmed								
arm picnic, braised	3 oz	211	27.4	0.0	87	0	10.4	97
arm picnic, chopped, braised	1 cup	347	45.2	0.0	143	0	17.1	160
arm picnic, chopped, roasted	1 cup	319	37.4	0.0	112	0	17.7	133
arm picnic, raw	1 lb	635	89.6	0.0	372	0	27.9	295
arm picnic, raw	1 oz	40	5.6	0.0	23	0	1.8	18
arm picnic, roasted	3 oz	194	22.7	0.0	68	0	10.7	81
Boston blade, braised	3 oz	232	26.4	0.0	64	0	13.2	99
Boston blade, broiled	3 oz	193	22.7	0.0	63	0	10.7	80
Boston blade, chopped, braised	1 cup	412	43.6	0.0	105	0	24.6	162
Boston blade, chopped, broiled	1 cup	384	35.2	0.0	118	0	25.8	147
Boston blade, chopped, roasted	1 cup	358	34.1	0.0	102	0	23.6	137
Boston blade, raw	1 oz	47	5.4	0.0	20	0	2.6	19
Boston blade, roasted	3 oz	197	20.6	0.0	75	0	12.2	72
whole, chopped, roasted	1 cup	341	35.5	0.0	107	0	21.0	135
whole, raw	1 lb	671	88.7	0.0	345	0	32.4	304
whole, raw	1 oz	42	5.5	0.0	22	0	2.0	19
whole, roasted	3 oz	195	21.5	0.0	64	0	11.5	77
whole, roasted, diced	1 cup	310	34.2	0.0	101	0	18.3	122
Untrimmed								
arm picnic, roasted	3 oz	269	20.0	0.0	59	0	20.4	80

Food Name	Serv. Size	Total Cal.	Prot. GMS	Carbs GMS	Sod. MGS	Fiber GMS	Fat GMS	Chol. MGS
Boston blade, braised	3 oz	271	24.4	0.0	59	0	18.5	96
Boston blade, broiled	3 oz	220	21.7	0.0	59	0	14.1	81
Boston blade, chopped, braised	1 cup	519	37.0	0.0	94	0	40.1	155
Boston blade, chopped, broiled	1 cup	490	30.6	0.0	105	0	39.8	144
Boston blade, raw	1 lb	989	80.1	0.0	286	0	71.8	322
Boston blade, roasted	3 oz	229	19.6	0.0	57	0	16.0	73
whole, chopped, roasted	1 cup	456	30.8	0.0	96	0	36.0	134
whole, diced, roasted	1 cup	394	31.4	0.0	92	0	28.9	122
whole, raw	1 lb	1070	77.9	0.0	295	0	81.6	322
whole, raw	1 oz	67	4.9	0.0	18	0	5.1	20
whole, roasted	3 oz	248	19.8	0.0	58	0	18.2	77
SIRLOIN								
Trimmed								
boneless, braised	3 ogz	149	23.0	0.0	39	0	5.6	69
boneless, broiled	3 oz	164	26.5	0.0	48	0	5.7	78
boneless, raw	1 lb	581	95.5	0.0	231	0	19.1	286
boneless, roasted	3 oz	168	24.5	0.0	48	0	7.0	73
braised	3 oz	167	23.0	0.0	45	0	7.7	69
broiled	3 oz	181	24.2	0.0	61	0	8.6	72
chopped, braised	1 cup	365	46.9	0.0	83	0	18.2	154
chopped, broiled	1 cup	340	39.6	0.0	84	0	19.0	137
chopped, roasted	1 cup	330	38.5	0.0	87	0	18.4	126
raw	1 oz	43	6.0	0.0	14	0	1.9	18
raw, approx 3.1 oz	1 chop	133	19.8	0.0	48	0	5.4	59
roasted	3 oz	184	24.5	0.0	54	0	8.8	73
Untrimmed								
boneless, braised	3 oz	161	22.6	0.0	39	0	7.1	69
boneless, broiled	3 oz	177	25.9	0.0	48	0	7.3	77
boneless, raw	1 lb	658	93.3	0.0	227	0	28.6	290
boneless, roasted	3 oz	176	24.2	0.0	48	0	8.0	73
braised	3 oz	208	21.6	0.0	43	0	12.8	70
broiled	3 oz	220	22.6	0.0	58	0	13.7	73
chopped, braised	1 cup	493	39.2	0.0	76	0	36.0	148
chopped, broiled	1 cup	463	33.8	0.0	77	0	35.4	136
chopped, roasted	1 cup	407	35.1	0.0	83	0	28.6	127
raw	1 oz	78	4.9	0.0	12	0	6.3	20
roasted	3 oz	222	23.1	0.0	51	0	13.6	74
SPARERIBS								
Untrimmed								
braised	3 oz	337	24.7	0.0	79	0	25.8	103
raw	1 lb	1297	77.5	0.0	345	0	107.0	354
raw	1 oz	81	4.8	0.0	22	0	6.7	22
raw 'Gourmet' *(JM)*	4.5 oz	250	14.0	0.0	70	0	22.0	(mq)

Food Name	Serv. Size	Total Cal.	Prot. GMS	Carbs GMS	Sod. MGS	Fiber GMS	Fat GMS	Chol. MGS
SPLEEN								
braised	3 oz	127	24.0	0.0	91	0	2.7	428
raw	1 oz	28	5.1	0.0	28	0	0.7	103
STOMACH, raw	1 oz	45	4.7	0.0	15	0	2.7	55
TENDERLOIN								
Trimmed								
boneless *(JM)*	3 oz	120	17.0	0.0	40	0	5.0	(mq)
broiled	3 oz	159	25.9	0.0	55	0	5.4	80
chopped or diced, roasted	1 cup	232	40.3	0.0	94	0	6.7	130
raw	1 lb	544	95.2	0.0	227	0	15.5	295
raw	1 oz	34	5.9	0.0	14	0	1.0	18
roasted	3 oz	139	23.9	0.0	48	0	4.1	67
Untrimmed								
broiled	3 oz	171	25.4	0.0	54	0	6.9	80
raw	1 lb	617	93.2	0.0	222	0	24.5	299
raw	1 oz	39	5.8	0.0	14	0	1.5	19
roasted	3 oz	147	23.6	0.0	47	0	5.1	67
TOP LOIN								
Trimmed								
braised	3 oz	172	24.7	0.0	36	0	7.3	62
broiled	3 oz	173	26.5	0.0	55	0	6.6	68
chopped, braised	1 cup	388	48.2	0.0	73	0	20.2	136
chopped, broiled	1 cup	361	40.3	0.0	94	0	20.9	132
chopped, pan-fried in vegetable oil	1 cup	360	39.1	0.0	70	0	21.4	113
chopped, roasted	1 cup	343	39.5	0.0	64	0	19.3	111
pan-fried	3 oz	191	25.9	0.0	48	0	8.9	65
pan-fried in vegetable oil	4 oz	291	31.7	0.0	57	0	17.4	92
raw	1 oz	46	6.2	0.0	13	0	2.1	16
roast, boneless, raw	1 lb	640	98.9	0.0	204	0	24.0	249
roast, boneless, raw	1 oz	40	6.2	0.0	13	0	1.5	16
roasted	3 oz	165	25.7	0.0	38	0	6.1	66
Untrimmed								
braised	3 oz	198	23.6	0.0	36	0	10.8	64
broiled	3 oz	195	25.5	0.0	54	0	9.6	69
chopped, braised	1 cup	533	38.7	0.0	66	0	40.8	133
chopped, broiled	1 cup	504	33.2	0.0	83	0	40.1	130
chopped, pan-fried in vegetable oil	1 cup	549	30.1	0.0	63	0	46.5	118
chopped, roasted	1 cup	462	33.9	0.0	62	0	35.2	115
pan-fried	3 oz	218	24.7	0.0	47	0	12.6	66
pan-fried in vegetable oil	3 oz	337	18.5	0.0	39	0	28.6	72
raw	1 oz	86	4.9	0.0	11	0	7.3	18
roast, boneless, raw	1 lb	866	91.8	0.0	195	0	52.7	268
roast, boneless, raw	1 oz	54	5.7	0.0	12	0	3.3	17

Food Name	Serv. Size	Total Cal.	Prot. GMS	Carbs GMS	Sod. MGS	Fiber GMS	Fat GMS	Chol. MGS
roasted	3 oz	192	24.5	0.0	37	0	9.7	66
PORK, CANNED								
	1 oz	95	3.5	0.6	365	0	8.6	18
approx .75 oz	1 slice	70	2.6	0.4	271	0	6.4	13
(Hormel)	3 oz	240	11.0	2.0	1056	0	21.0	(mq)
(Hormel) chopped	3 oz	200	12.0	2.0	1073	0	16.0	(mq)
PORK, CURED								
blade roll, untrimmed, diced, roasted	1 cup	402	24.2	0.5	1362	0	32.9	94
blade roll, untrimmed, diced, unheated	1 cup	377	23.1	0.0	1750	0	30.8	74
blade roll, untrimmed, roasted	4 oz	325	19.6	0.4	1103	0	26.6	76
blade roll, untrimmed, unheated	1 oz	76	4.7	0.0	354	0	6.2	15
boneless, blade roll, untrimmed, roasted	3 oz	244	14.7	0.3	827	0	20.0	57
boneless, blade roll, untrimmed, unheated	1 oz	76	4.7	0.0	354	0	6.2	15
PORK, GROUND								
cooked	3 oz	252	21.8	0.0	62	0	17.6	80
raw	1 oz	75	4.8	0.0	16	0	6.0	20
(JM)	3 oz	190	15.0	0.0	40	0	14.0	(mq)
PORK, SALT, cured, raw	1 oz	212	1.4	0.0	404	0	22.8	24
PORK DINNER, FROZEN, chow mein								
'Bi-Pack' *(LaChoy)*	8.642 oz	87	5.6	10.3	1218	2.9	3.2	10
PORK ENTRÉE								
Canned								
chow mein 'Bi-Pack' *(LaChoy)*	3/4 cup	80	6.0	7.0	970	2.0	3.0	14
sweet and sour *(LaChoy)*	3/4 cup	250	6.0	48.0	1540	1.0	4.0	18
Frozen								
barbecued back ribs 'Pork Classics'								
(John Morrell)	4.75 oz	240	12.0	8.0	480	0	17.0	62
barbecued chops, center cut								
'Pork Classics' *(John Morrell)*	4.5 oz	230	29.0	7.0	410	0	9.0	90
barbecued loin, thin sliced 'Pork Classics'								
(John Morrell)	3 oz	150	17.0	5.0	440	0	6.0	52
barbecued spare ribs 'Pork Classics'								
(John Morrell)	4.5 oz	250	12.0	7.0	470	0	18.0	51
barbecued tenderloin 'Pork Classics'								
(John Morrell)	3 oz	130	18.0	3.0	220	0	5.0	53
breaded, steak *(Hormel)*	3 oz	220	12.0	11.0	(mq)	(mq)	15.0	(mq)
patty deluxe 'Looney Tunes Porky Pig'								
(Tyson)	6.5 oz	370	14.0	48.0	490	na	14.0	35
sweet and sour *(Chun King)*	13 oz	400	11.0	78.0	1460	na	5.0	(mq)
PORK FAT								
separable fat from fully cooked ham,								
roasted	1 oz	167	2.2	0.0	177	0	17.5	24

Food Name	Serv. Size	Total Cal.	Prot. GMS	Carbs GMS	Sod. MGS	Fiber GMS	Fat GMS	Chol. MGS
separable fat from fully cooked ham, unheated	1 oz	164	1.6	<.1	143	0	17.4	19
separable fat from ham and arm picnic, roasted	3 oz	502	6.5	0.0	530	0	52.6	73
separable fat from ham and arm picnic, roasted	1 oz	168	2.2	.0.0	177	0	17.5	24
separable fat from ham and arm picnic, unheated	1 oz	164	1.6	0.0	143	0	17.4	19
PORK RIND SNACK								
(Baken-ets)	1 oz	160	12.0	2.0	850	na	10.0	25
(Baken-ets) hot 'n spicy	1 oz	150	17.0	1.0	750	na	9.0	25
PORK SEASONING AND COATING MIX								
'Bag 'n Season' *(Schilling)*	1 pkg	103	1.1	23.6	3126	(mq)	0.4	0
POT ROAST DINNER/ENTRÉE, FROZEN								
homestyle *(Right Course)*	9.25 oz	220	17.0	22.0	550	(mq)	7.0	35
homestyle, w/browned potatoes *(Stouffer's)*	8 7/8 oz	280	20.0	24.0	690	na	11.0	na
Yankee *(Budget Gourmet)*	11 oz	380	27.0	22.0	690	(mq)	21.0	70
Yankee *(Healthy Choice)*	11 oz	260	19.0	36.0	400	na	4.0	55
Yankee *(Le Menu)*	10 oz	330	26.0	27.0	700	(mq)	13.0	(mq)
Yankee 'Classics' *(Armour)*	10 oz	310	25.0	26.0	670	(mq)	12.0	85
POT ROAST SEASONING MIX								
'Bag 'n Season' *(Schilling)*	1 pkg	55	3.9	8.5	3030	na	0.6	0
'Seasoning Blends' *(Lawry's)*	1 pkg	122	3.7	25.0	4008	>.5 c	0.7	0
POTATO								
Baked								
in skin	4 oz	124	2.6	28.6	9	>.7 c	0.1	0
in skin, pulp only	4 oz	105	2.2	24.4	6	1.7	0.1	0
in skin, skin only	2 oz	112	2.4	26.1	12	2.3	0.1	0
pulp	1/2 cup	57	1.2	13.1	3	.9	0.1	0
Boiled								
in skin	2 oz	44	1.6	9.8	8	>2.1 c	0.1	0
in skin, pulp only	4 oz	99	2.1	22.8	5	1.7	0.1	0
in skin, pulp only	1/2 cup	68	1.5	15.7	3	1.4	0.1	0
in skin, pulp only, approx 2.5 inch diam	1 potato	118	2.5	27.4	5	2.5	0.1	0
pulp only	4 oz	98	1.9	22.7	6	>.4 c	0.1	0
pulp only	1/2 cup	67	1.3	15.6	4	1.4	0.1	0
pulp only, approx 2.5 inch diam	1 potato	116	2.3	27.0	7	2.4	0.1	0
Hash brown, cooked in vegetable oil	4 oz	237	2.7	24.2	27	>.5 c	15.8	0
Microwaved								
in skin	4 oz	119	2.8	27.4	9	>.9 c	0.1	0
in skin, pulp only	4 oz	113	2.4	26.4	8	>.5 c	0.1	0
in skin, pulp only	1/2 cup	78	1.6	18.2	5	>.3 c	0.1	0

Food Name	Serv. Size	Total Cal.	Prot. GMS	Carbs GMS	Sod. MGS	Fiber GMS	Fat GMS	Chol. MGS
in skin, skin only	2 oz	75	2.5	16.8	9	>1.8 c	0.1	0
Raw								
peeled	1 oz	22	0.6	5.1	2	.5	<.1	0
pulp only, diced	1/2 cup	59	1.5	13.5	5	1.2	0.1	0
skin only	2 oz	33	1.5	7.1	6	>1.0 c	0.1	0
unpeeled	1 lb	269	7.1	61.2	21	5.4	0.3	0
POTATO, CANNED								
(Stokely)	1/2 cup	50	2.0	11.0	360	(mq)	0.0	0
(Veg•All)	1/2 cup	60	1.0	13.0	260	na	0.0	na
approx 1.2 oz	1 potato	21	0.5	4.8	(mq)	>.1 c	0.1	0
diced (Bush's Best)	1/2 cup	40	1.0	8.0	340	na	0.0	na
diced (Taylor's Brand)	1 cup	90	3.0	25.0	292	(mq)	0.0	0
drained	4 oz	68	1.6	15.4	(mq)	>.3 c	0.2	0
drained	1/2 cup	54	1.3	12.3	234	>.2 c	0.2	0
drained, approx 1-inch diam	1 potato	21	0.5	4.8	91	>.1 c	0.1	0
new, extra small, whole (S&W)	1/2 cup	45	2.0	9.0	310	na	0.0	0
new, small, whole (IGA)	1/2 cup	45	2.0	9.0	300	na	0.0	0
new, whole, drained (Hunt's)	4 oz	70	2.0	15.0	230	<1.0	<1.0	0
sliced (Bush's Best)	1/2 cup	40	1.0	8.0	340	na	0.0	na
sliced (Taylor's Brand)	1 cup	90	3.0	25.0	292	(mq)	0.0	0
sliced, w/liquid (Del Monte)	1/2 cup	45	1.0	10.0	355	(mq)	0.0	0
white, diced (Allens)	1/2 cup	45	2.0	10.0	360	(mq)	<1.0	0
white, double diced (Allens)	1/2 cup	45	2.0	10.0	540	(mq)	<1.0	0
white, sliced (A&P)	1/2 cup	45	2.0	11.0	320	(mq)	<1.0	0
white, sliced (Allens)	1/2 cup	45	2.0	10.0	360	(mq)	<1.0	0
white, sliced 'No Salt Added' (Pathmark)	1 cup	100	3.0	20.0	15	(mq)	0.0	0
white, small, sliced (Finast)	1/2 cup	55	1.0	13.0	375	(mq)	0.0	0
white, small, whole (Finast)	1/2 cup	55	1.0	13.0	375	(mq)	0.0	0
white, whole (A&P)	1/2 cup	45	2.0	11.0	320	(mq)	<1.0	0
white, whole 'No Salt Added' (Pathmark)	1 cup	100	3.0	20.0	15	(mq)	0.0	0
whole (Bush's Best)	1/2 cup	40	1.0	8.0	340	na	0.0	na
whole, w/liquid	1 cup	120	4.1	26.0	903	4.8	0.5	0
whole, w/liquid	1/2 cup	60	2.0	13.0	452	>.4 c	0.2	0
whole, w/liquid (Del Monte)	1/2 cup	45	1.0	10.0	355	(mq)	0.0	0
w/liquid	4 oz	45	1.5	9.8	341	>.3 c	0.2	0
POTATO, FINNISH YELLOW, raw (Frieda's)	3.5 oz	100	3.3	22.0	na	(mq)	na	0
POTATO, FREEZE-DRIED								
hash brown, prepared (Mountain House)	1 cup	150	2.0	36.0	(mq)	(mq)	0.0	na
POTATO, FROZEN								
fried	9 oz	419	6.5	63.8	58	>1.3 c	16.5	0
fried, cottage cut, heated in oven	4 oz	247	3.9	38.6	51	>.8 c	9.3	0
fried, partially fried in oil, heated in oven	4 oz	252	3.9	38.4	35	4.8	9.9	0
fried, partially fried in oil, heated in oven	1.75 oz	111	1.7	17.0	15	2.1	4.4	0

Food Name	Serv. Size	Total Cal.	Prot. GMS	Carbs GMS	Sod. MGS	Fiber GMS	Fat GMS	Chol. MGS
hash brown, prepared in vegetable oil	4 oz	247	3.6	31.9	39	2.3 c	13.0	0
hash brown, w/butter sauce, prepared	4 oz	202	2.8	27.4	115	(mq)	10.0	26
puffs, partially fried in oil, prepared	4 oz	252	3.8	34.6	846	>.7 c	12.2	0
whole, peeled	10 oz	221	6.7	49.6	71	>1.1 c	0.5	0
whole, peeled, boiled, drained	4 oz	74	2.2	16.5	23	>.4 c	0.1	0
(A&P)								
fried, crinkle cut	3.5 oz	140	2.0	25.0	25	(mq)	4.0	0
fried, regular	3.5 oz	140	2.0	25.0	25	(mq)	4.0	0
fried, shoestring	3.5 oz	170	2.0	24.0	50	(mq)	6.0	0
fried, steak fries	3.5 oz	140	2.0	24.0	30	(mq)	4.0	0
hash brown	3.5 oz	80	2.0	17.0	20	(mq)	0.0	0
morsels	3.5 oz	140	2.0	23.0	30	(mq)	4.0	0
(Heinz)								
fried, crinkle cut 'Deep Fries'	3 oz	150	2.0	22.0	30	(mq)	6.0	0
fried 'Deep Fries'	3 oz	160	2.0	23.0	20	(mq)	6.0	0
fried, shoestring 'Deep Fries'	3 oz	200	2.0	25.0	20	(mq)	10.0	0
hash brown, w/butter and onions 'Deep Fries'	3 oz	110	1.0	14.0	80	(mq)	7.0	5
(MicroMagic)								
fried	3 oz	290	3.0	40.0	30	(mq)	13.0	na
fried, skinny	3 oz	350	4.0	49.0	40	(mq)	15.0	na
sticks 'Tater Sticks'	4 oz	390	2.0	43.0	620	(mq)	22.0	na
(Ore-Ida)								
fried, cottage cut	3 oz	120	2.0	19.0	25	(mq)	5.0	0
fried 'Country Style Dinner Fries'	3 oz	110	2.0	19.0	30	(mq)	3.0	0
fried, crinkle cut 'Golden Crinkles'	3 oz	120	2.0	19.0	35	(mq)	4.0	0
fried, crinkle cut 'Lites'	3 oz	90	1.0	16.0	35	(mq)	2.0	0
fried, crinkle cut, microwave	3.5 oz	180	2.0	26.0	35	(mq)	8.0	0
fried, crinkle cut 'Pixie Crinkles'	3 oz	140	2.0	21.0	40	(mq)	6.0	0
fried 'Crisp Crowns'	3 oz	160	2.0	20.0	525	(mq)	9.0	0
fried 'Crispers!'	3 oz	230	2.0	25.0	545	(mq)	15.0	0
fried, French, extra crispy 'Nacho Crispers'	3 oz	180	2.0	21.0	280	na	10.0	0
fried, French 'Fast Fries'	3 oz	150	2.0	23.0	230	na	7.0	0
fried 'Golden Fries'	3 oz	120	2.0	19.0	35	(mq)	4.0	0
fried 'Lites'	3 oz	90	2.0	16.0	30	(mq)	2.0	0
fried, shoestring	3 oz	140	2.0	21.0	30	(mq)	6.0	0
fried, shoestring 'Lites'	3 oz	90	1.0	15.0	25	(mq)	4.0	0
fried, wedges 'Home Style Potato Wedges'	3 oz	100	2.0	17.0	45	(mq)	3.0	0
fried, w/onions 'Crispy Crowns'	3 oz	170	1.0	20.0	570	(mq)	9.0	0
hash brown 'Golden Patties'	2.5 oz	140	1.0	15.0	295	(mq)	8.0	0
hash brown, microwave	2 oz	130	1.0	12.0	170	(mq)	8.0	0
hash brown, shredded	3 oz	70	1.0	15.0	40	(mq)	<1.0	0
hash brown 'Southern Style'	3 oz	70	1.0	16.0	35	(mq)	<1.0	0

Food Name	Serv. Size	Total Cal.	Prot. GMS	Carbs GMS	Sod. MGS	Fiber GMS	Fat GMS	Chol. MGS
hash brown, w/cheddar 'Cheddar Browns'	3 oz	90	2.0	13.0	415	(mq)	2.0	10
mashed, natural butter flavor, prepared w/2% milk	1/2 cup	170	4.0	23.0	230	na	5.0	5
mashed, natural butter flavor, unprepared	2.25 oz	100	1.0	14.0	140	na	3.0	5
puffs, bacon flavored 'Tater Tots'	3 oz	140	2.0	19.0	625	(mq)	6.0	0
puffs 'Tater Tots'	3 oz	140	1.0	19.0	550	(mq)	7.0	0
puffs 'Tater Tots' microwave	4 oz	200	2.0	29.0	670	(mq)	9.0	0
puffs, w/onion 'Tater Tots'	3 oz	140	2.0	19.0	715	(mq)	6.0	0
whole, small	3 oz	70	2.0	16.0	45	(mq)	<1.0	0
(Quick 'n Crispy)								
fried, crinkle cut	4 oz	370	3.0	44.0	50	(mq)	19.0	na
fried, shoestring	4 oz	390	3.0	48.0	50	(mq)	20.0	na
fried, thin cuts	4 oz	370	3.0	44.0	50	(mq)	19.0	na
wedges	4 oz	280	3.0	36.0	40	(mq)	13.0	na
(Seabrook)								
diced and hash-shred	4 oz	80	2.0	19.0	41	(mq)	0.0	0
fried	3 oz	120	2.0	20.0	25	(mq)	4.0	na
fried, cottage cut	2.8 oz	110	1.0	17.0	14	(mq)	4.0	na
fried, crinkle cut	3 oz	120	2.0	20.0	24	(mq)	4.0	na
fried, shoestring	3 oz	140	2.0	20.0	45	(mq)	6.0	na
white, whole, boiled	3.2 oz	60	2.0	13.0	5	(mq)	0.0	0
(Southern) white, whole	3.5 oz	69	2.0	15.0	20	(mq)	0.1	0
POTATO CHIPS AND SNACKS								
(Allens)								
barbecue flavor	1 oz	150	2.0	14.0	280	(mq)	9.0	0
hot flavor	1 oz	150	2.0	14.0	200	(mq)	9.0	0
potato sticks, shoestring, canned	1 oz	140	2.0	16.0	190	(mq)	8.0	na
potato sticks, shoestring, canned 'No Salt'	1 oz	140	1.0	16.0	10	(mq)	8.0	na
regular flavor	1 oz	160	2.0	14.0	270	(mq)	10.0	0
(Bachman)								
'Kettle Cooked'	1 oz	140	2.0	16.0	115	(mq)	8.0	0
pasta snack chip 'Pastapazazz'	1 oz	150	2.0	15.0	340	(mq)	9.0	na
'Ridge'	1 oz	160	2.0	14.0	260	(mq)	10.0	0
'Ruffled'	1 oz	160	2.0	14.0	260	(mq)	10.0	0
Saratoga-style 'Kettle Cooked'	1 oz	140	2.0	16.0	115	(mq)	8.0	0
sour cream and onion flavor	1 oz	150	2.0	14.0	200	(mq)	9.0	0
'Unsalted'	1 oz	160	2.0	14.0	5	(mq)	10.0	0
vinegar flavor	1 oz	150	2.0	15.0	610	(mq)	9.0	0
(Barbara's Bakery)								
herb and garlic flavor 'True Blues'	1 oz	140	2.0	15.0	120	na	9.0	0
ripple	1 oz	150	2.0	14.0	250	na	10.0	0
'True Blues'	1 oz	150	2.0	15.0	120	na	10.0	0

Food Name	Serv. Size	Total Cal.	Prot. GMS	Carbs GMS	Sod. MGS	Fiber GMS	Fat GMS	Chol. MGS
(Barrel O'Fun)	1 oz	150	2.0	14.0	160	.4	10.0	0
(Cape Cod)								
dill and sour cream flavor	1 oz	150	2.0	16.0	160	(mq)	8.0	0
dill and sour cream flavor 'No Salt'	1 oz	150	2.0	16.0	15	(mq)	8.0	0
'No Salt Added'	1 oz	150	2.0	16.0	0	(mq)	8.0	0
regular flavor	1 oz	150	2.0	16.0	120	(mq)	8.0	0
'Waves'	1 oz	150	2.0	16.0	120	(mq)	8.0	0
(Cottage Fries) 'No Salt Added'	1 oz	160	2.0	14.0	5	(mq)	11.0	0
(Eagle)								
barbecue flavor 'Extra Crunchy'	1 oz	150	2.0	16.0	220	(mq)	8.0	0
barbecue flavor 'Extra Crunchy Louisiana'	1 oz	150	2.0	16.0	140	(mq)	8.0	0
barbecue flavor 'Thins'	1 oz	150	2.0	15.0	220	(mq)	10.0	0
'Eagle Thins'	1 oz	150	2.0	16.0	220	(mq)	10.0	0
'Extra Crunchy'	1 oz	150	2.0	16.0	180	(mq)	8.0	0
'Idaho Russet'	1 oz	150	2.0	16.0	180	(mq)	8.0	0
'Ridged Thins'	1 oz	150	2.0	15.0	220	(mq)	10.0	0
sour cream and onion flavor 'Ridged'	1 oz	150	2.0	15.0	280	(mq)	10.0	0
(Eden Foods)								
brown rice chips	1 oz	130	2.0	19.0	197	na	5.0	na
sea vegetable chips	1 oz	130	1.0	22.0	200	na	5.0	na
wasabi snack chips	1 oz	130	1.0	22.0	200	(mq)	4.0	0
(Featherweight) 'Low Salt'	1 oz	160	2.0	14.0	4	(mq)	11.0	0
(Flavor Tree) sour cream and onion flavor								
potato sticks	1/4 cup	127	3.0	12.5	360	>.1 c	8.3	na
(Funyuns) rings, onion flavor, approx								
11 rings	1 oz	140	2.0	18.0	275	(mq)	6.0	0
(Great Snackers)								
barbecue flavor	1 serving	60	1.0	8.0	170	(mq)	3.0	0
cheddar cheese flavor	1 serving	60	1.0	8.0	170	(mq)	3.0	0
sour cream and onion flavor	.5 oz	70	1.0	10.0	140	na	3.0	0
toasted onion flavor	1 serving	60	1.0	8.0	120	(mq)	3.0	0
(Hain)								
carrot chip	1 oz	150	2.0	16.0	160	(mq)	9.0	0
carrot chip, barbecue	1 oz	140	2.0	16.0	160	(mq)	8.0	0
carrot chip 'No Salt Added'	1 oz	150	2.0	16.0	30	(mq)	7.0	0
(Health Valley)								
'Country'	1 oz	160	2.0	15.0	60	.9	10.0	0
'Country Dip'	1 oz	160	2.0	15.0	60	.9	10.0	0
'Country Dip No Salt Added'	1 oz	160	2.0	15.0	1	.9	10.0	0
'Country Natural No Salt Added'	1 oz	160	2.0	15.0	1	.9	10.0	0
'Country No Salt Added'	1 oz	160	2.0	15.0	1	.9	10.0	0
'Country Ripple'	1 oz	160	2.0	15.0	60	.9	10.0	0
'Country Ripple No Salt Added'	1 oz	160	2.0	15.0	1	.9	10.0	0

Food Name	Serv. Size	Total Cal.	Prot. GMS	Carbs GMS	Sod. MGS	Fiber GMS	Fat GMS	Chol. MGS
'Natural'	1 oz	160	2.0	15.0	60	.9	10.0	0
(Keebler)								
original flavor, lightly seasoned	1 oz	140	1.0	18.0	190	na	7.0	0
sour cream and onion flavor	1 oz	140	2.0	17.0	260	na	7.0	0
(Kettle Chips)								
jalapeño jack flavor	1 oz	150	2.0	15.0	110	na	9.0	0
lightly salted	1 oz	150	2.0	15.0	80	na	9.0	0
New York cheddar flavor	1 oz	150	2.0	15.0	100	na	9.0	0
no salt	1 oz	150	2.0	15.0	10	na	9.0	0
organically grown, w/sea salt	1 oz	150	2.0	15.0	80	na	9.0	0
salsa w/mesquite flavor	1 oz	150	2.0	15.0	120	na	9.0	0
sea salt and vinegar flavor	1 oz	150	2.0	15.0	120	na	9.0	0
yogurt and green onion flavor	1 oz	150	2.0	15.0	120	na	9.0	0
(King Kold)								
au gratin flavor	1 oz	150	2.0	15.0	220	(mq)	8.0	na
barbecue flavor 'BBQ'	1 oz	140	2.0	16.0	360	(mq)	8.0	na
dill flavor	1 oz	150	2.0	16.0	340	(mq)	8.0	na
onion-garlic flavor	1 oz	150	2.0	15.0	420	(mq)	9.0	na
regular flavor	1 oz	150	2.0	16.0	160	(mq)	9.0	0
'Rip-L'	1 oz	150	2.0	16.0	150	(mq)	9.0	0
sour cream and onion flavor	1 oz	150	2.0	15.0	220	(mq)	10.0	na
(Lay's)								
barbecue flavor, approx 15-20 chips	1 oz	150	1.0	15.0	270	1.1	9.0	0
barbecue flavor 'Kansas City Style' approx 15-20 chips	1 oz	150	2.0	15.0	270	1.1	9.0	0
Cajun flavor 'Crunch Tators Amazin Cajun'	1 oz	150	2.0	17.0	150	1.1	8.0	0
cheddar cheese flavor, approx 15-20 chips	1 oz	150	2.0	14.0	1	1.1	10.0	0
'Flamin' Hot' approx 15-20 chips	1 oz	150	2.0	15.0	190	1.1	9.0	0
jalapeño flavor 'Crunch Tators Hoppin' Jalapeño'	1 oz	140	1.0	18.0	200	1.1	7.0	0
mesquite flavor 'Crunch Tators Mighty Mesquite'	1 oz	150	2.0	17.0	135	1.1	8.0	0
original flavor, approx 15-20 chips	1 oz	150	1.0	15.0	170	1.1	10.0	0
original flavor 'Crunch Tators' approx 16 chips	1 oz	150	2.0	17.0	120	1.1	8.0	0
salt and vinegar flavor, approx 15-20 chips	1 oz	150	1.0	14.0	390	1.1	10.0	0
sour cream and onion flavor, approx 15-20 chips	1 oz	160	2.0	15.0	220	1.1	10.0	1
tangy ranch flavor, approx 15-20 chips	1 oz	160	2.0	15.0	210	1.1	10.0	0
'Unsalted'	1 oz	150	2.0	15.0	10	(mq)	10.0	0
(Louise's)								
mesquite barbecue flavor, fat-free	1 oz	100	2.0	23.0	200	na	<1.0	0
original flavor, fat-free	1 oz	100	2.0	23.0	200	na	<1.0	0

Food Name	Serv. Size	Total Cal.	Prot. GMS	Carbs GMS	Sod. MGS	Fiber GMS	Fat GMS	Chol. MGS
vinegar and salt flavor, fat-free	1 oz	100	2.0	23.0	200	na	<1.0	0
(Mr. Phipps)								
tater crisps, barbecue flavor	.5 oz	60	1.0	10.0	160	na	2.0	0
tater crisps, sour cream and onion flavor ...	.5 oz	60	1.0	10.0	150	na	2.0	0
(Munchos) plain, approx 16 chips	1 oz	160	1.0	15.0	230	na	10.0	0
(Nabisco)								
baked, cheddar cheese flavor, cracker								
chips 'Zings'	.5 oz	70	1.0	9.0	140	na	3.0	2
baked, ranch flavor, cracker chips 'Zings' ..	.5 oz	70	1.0	9.0	140	na	3.0	2
cracker chips, baked 'Zings'	.5 oz	70	1.0	10.0	115	na	3.0	0
(O'Boisies)								
regular flavor	1 oz	150	1.0	16.0	180	(mq)	9.0	0
sour cream and onion flavor	1 oz	150	2.0	15.0	190	(mq)	9.0	0
(Planters)								
potato sticks	1 oz	160	1.0	15.0	170	na	10.0	0
potato sticks, barbecue flavor	1 oz	160	1.0	15.0	220	na	10.0	0
(Poore Brothers)								
barbecue flavor	1 oz	150	2.0	15.0	60	2.0	10.0	0
Cajun flavor	1 oz	140	2.0	16.0	55	2.0	8.0	0
dill pickle flavor	1 oz	140	2.0	16.0	95	2.0	8.0	0
grilled steak and onion flavor	1 oz	140	2.0	15.0	110	2.0	8.0	0
jalapeño flavor	1 oz	140	2.0	16.0	100	2.0	9.0	0
Parmesan and garlic flavor	1 oz	140	2.0	16.0	80	2.0	9.0	0
regular flavor	1 oz	140	2.0	17.0	40	2.0	8.0	0
salt and vinegar flavor	1 oz	140	2.0	16.0	125	1.0	9.0	0
unsalted	1 oz	140	2.0	17.0	5	2.0	8.0	0
(Pringle's)								
barbecue flavor 'Light'	1 oz	150	2.0	17.0	125	(mq)	8.0	na
cheese flavor 'Cheez-ums'	1 oz	170	2.0	12.0	200	(mq)	13.0	na
French onion flavor 'Idaho Rippled'	1 oz	170	2.0	13.0	175	(mq)	12.0	na
'Idaho Rippled'	1 oz	170	2.0	13.0	150	(mq)	12.0	na
'Light'	1 oz	150	2.0	17.0	120	(mq)	8.0	na
ranch flavor 'Light'	1 oz	150	2.0	17.0	135	(mq)	8.0	na
'Regular'	1 oz	170	2.0	12.0	170	(mq)	13.0	na
sour cream and onion flavor	1 oz	170	2.0	13.0	135	(mq)	12.0	na
taco and cheddar flavor 'Idaho Rippled' ...	1 oz	170	2.0	13.0	160	(mq)	12.0	na
(Ray's)								
taro chips, salted	1 oz	139	2.0	20.0	167	na	6.0	0
taro chips, unsalted	1 oz	139	2.0	20.0	15	na	6.0	0
(Ruffles)								
barbecue flavor	1 oz	150	1.0	16.0	320	(mq)	9.0	0
Cajun flavor 'Cajun Spice'	1 oz	150	1.0	15.0	240	(mq)	10.0	0
cheddar and sour cream flavor	1 oz	150	2.0	16.0	260	(mq)	9.0	0

Food Name	Serv. Size	Total Cal.	Prot. GMS	Carbs GMS	Sod. MGS	Fiber GMS	Fat GMS	Chol. MGS
'Choice' 40% less fat, approx 16 chips	1 oz	130	2.0	18.0	130	1.0	6.0	0
'Light Choice' 1/3 less fat	1 oz	130	2.0	19.0	140	na	6.0	0
mesquite barbecue flavor 'Mesquite Grille'	1 oz	160	2.0	14.0	260	(mq)	10.0	0
ranch flavor	1 oz	160	2.0	15.0	240	(mq)	10.0	0
regular flavor	1 oz	150	1.0	15.0	190	(mq)	10.0	0
sour cream and onion flavor	1 oz	150	2.0	15.0	240	(mq)	9.0	0
(Schlotzsky's) barbecue, deli style	1 oz	150	2.0	17.0	115	na	6.0	0
(Snacktime)								
jalapeño flavor 'Krunchers!'	1 oz	150	2.0	16.0	270	(mq)	9.0	0
'Krunchers!'	1 oz	150	2.0	16.0	170	(mq)	9.0	0
mesquite barbecue flavor 'Krunchers!'	1 oz	150	2.0	16.0	200	(mq)	9.0	0
(Spicer's)								
barbecue wheat flavor, for weight control ..	1 oz	100	5.0	12.0	75	9.0	5.0	0
natural flavor, for weight control	1 oz	100	4.0	11.0	65	9.0	4.0	0
sour cream and onion flavor, for weight control	1 oz	100	4.0	12.0	150	6.0	4.0	0
(Sun Chips)								
multi-grain snacks, French onion flavor	1 oz	140	3.0	18.0	120	na	7.0	0
multi-grain snacks, harvest cheddar flavor	1 oz	140	2.0	18.0	125	na	7.0	0
multi-grain snacks, original flavor	1 oz	150	2.0	18.0	100	na	8.0	0
(Tato Skins)								
potato skins, baked	1 oz	150	1.0	17.0	160	(mq)	8.0	0
potato skins, cheese and bacon flavor, ...	1 oz	150	1.0	17.0	180	(mq)	8.0	0
potato skins, sour cream and chives flavor	1 oz	150	1.0	17.0	180	(mq)	8.0	0
(Westbrae)								
no salt	1 oz	150	2.0	16.0	10	na	8.0	0
'Ripple'	1 oz	150	2.0	16.0	100	na	8.0	0
salted	1 oz	160	2.0	15.0	100	na	10.0	0
(Wise)								
barbecue flavor	1 oz	150	2.0	14.0	240	(mq)	10.0	0
barbecue flavor 'Ridgies'	1 oz	150	2.0	14.0	240	(mq)	10.0	0
hot flavor	1 oz	160	2.0	14.0	290	(mq)	11.0	0
'New York Deli'	1 oz	160	2.0	14.0	120	(mq)	11.0	0
onion-garlic flavor	1 oz	150	2.0	14.0	250	(mq)	10.0	0
'Plain'	1 oz	150	2.0	14.0	190	(mq)	10.0	0
'Ridgies'	1 oz	150	2.0	14.0	190	(mq)	10.0	0
'Ridgies Super Crispy'	1 oz	150	2.0	14.0	220	(mq)	10.0	0
rings, onion flavor	1 oz	130	<1.0	21.0	360	(mq)	5.0	0
'Rippled'	1 oz	150	2.0	14.0	190	(mq)	10.0	0
sour cream and onion flavor 'Ridgies'	1 oz	160	2.0	14.0	240	(mq)	11.0	na
(Zapp's)								
Cajun flavor 'Lite Kettle'	1 oz	150	2.0	16.0	94	(mq)	8.0	0
Cajun flavor 'Original Kettle'	1 oz	150	2.0	16.0	94	(mq)	8.0	0

Food Name	Serv. Size	Total Cal.	Prot. GMS	Carbs GMS	Sod. MGS	Fiber GMS	Fat GMS	Chol. MGS
jalapeño flavor 'Original Kettle'	1 oz	150	2.0	16.0	85	(mq)	8.0	na
'Lite Kettle'	1 oz	150	2.0	16.0	45	(mq)	8.0	0
'Lite Kettle No Salt Added'	1 oz	150	2.0	16.0	<1	(mq)	8.0	0
mesquite barbecue flavor 'Lite Kettle'	1 oz	150	2.0	16.0	87	(mq)	8.0	0
mesquite barbecue flavor 'Original Kettle'	1 oz	150	2.0	16.0	87	(mq)	8.0	0
'Original Kettle'	1 oz	150	2.0	16.0	45	(mq)	8.0	0
'Original Kettle No Salt Added'	1 oz	150	2.0	16.0	<1	(mq)	8.0	0
sour cream and onion flavor 'Lite Kettle'	1 oz	150	2.0	16.0	79	(mq)	8.0	na
POTATO DISH, CANNED, au gratin								
(Pantry Express)	1/2 cup	120	3.0	17.0	430	1.5	5.0	5
POTATO DISH, FROZEN								
au gratin 'Family Side Dish'								
(Freezer Queen)	4 oz	100	2.0	19.0	440	(mq)	2.0	na
au gratin 'For One' (Birds Eye)	5.5 oz	240	8.0	24.0	590	1.0	13.0	30
au gratin 'One Serving' (Green Giant)	5.5 oz	200	7.0	20.0	560	(mq)	10.0	20
au gratin, side dish (Stouffer's)	5.75 oz	170	5.0	17.0	670	na	9.0	na
baked, butter 'Twice Baked' (Ore-Ida)	5 oz	200	4.0	27.0	350	na	9.0	0
baked, cheddar cheese 'Twice Baked'								
(Ore-Ida)	5 oz	190	4.0	28.0	420	na	7.0	0
baked, ranch 'Twice Baked' (Ore-Ida)	5 oz	180	5.0	28.0	320	na	6.0	0
baked, sour cream and chives								
'Twice Baked' (Ore-Ida)	5 oz	180	4.0	28.0	360	na	6.0	0
baked, stuffed w/cheddar cheese (Oh Boy!)	6 oz	142	4.0	23.0	612	(mq)	4.0	6
baked, stuffed w/cheese flavored topping								
(Green Giant)	5 oz	200	4.0	33.0	520	(mq)	6.0	na
baked, stuffed w/real bacon (Oh Boy!)	6 oz	116	4.0	18.0	641	(mq)	3.0	5
baked, stuffed w/sour cream and chives								
(Green Giant)	5 oz	230	5.0	31.0	580	(mq)	10.0	na
baked, stuffed w/sour cream and chives								
(Oh Boy!)	6 oz	129	3.0	18.0	418	(mq)	5.0	2
baked, topped w/salsa and cheese								
(Ore-Ida)	5.6 oz	160	5.0	25.0	350	na	4.0	10
cheddared, 'Side Dish' (Budget Gourmet)	5.5 oz	230	7.0	22.0	450	(mq)	13.0	35
cheddared, w/broccoli 'Side Dish'								
(Budget Gourmet)	5 oz	130	6.0	18.0	340	(mq)	4.0	25
fried, 'Country Style Dinner Fries' (Ore-Ida)	3 oz	110	2.0	19.0	30	(mq)	3.0	0
fried, w/onions 'Crispy Crowns' (Ore-Ida)	3 oz	170	1.0	20.0	570	(mq)	9.0	0
garden casserole, low-fat, 'Quick Meals'								
(Healthy Choice)	9.25 oz	180	12.0	23.0	360	na	4.0	20
hash brown, w/butter and onions,								
'Deep Fries' (Heinz)	3 oz	110	1.0	14.0	80	(mq)	7.0	5
hash brown, w/cheddar, 'Cheddar Browns'								
(Ore-Ida)	3 oz	90	2.0	13.0	415	(mq)	2.0	10

Food Name	Serv. Size	Total Cal.	Prot. GMS	Carbs GMS	Sod. MGS	Fiber GMS	Fat GMS	Chol. MGS
nacho, 'Side Dish' (Budget Gourmet)	5 oz	180	10.0	14.0	360	(mq)	10.0	30
new, in sour cream sauce, 'Side Dish'								
(Budget Gourmet)	5 oz	120	3.0	15.0	300	(mq)	6.0	20
'O'Brien' (Ore-Ida)	3 oz	60	1.0	14.0	25	(mq)	<1.0	0
puffs, w/bacon-flavored vegetable protein,								
'Tater Tots' (Ore-Ida)	3 oz	140	2.0	19.0	625	(mq)	6.0	0
puffs, w/onion, 'Tater Tots' (Ore-Ida)	3 oz	140	2.0	19.0	715	(mq)	6.0	0
scalloped, side dish (Stouffer's)	5.75 oz	130	4.0	16.0	610	na	6.0	na
shredded, w/cheese sauce and								
vegetables, 'Singles' (Stokely)	4.5 oz	130	5.0	15.0	480	(mq)	6.0	15
sliced, w/cheddar cheese sauce and								
bacon, 'Singles' (Stokely)	4.5 oz	150	3.0	24.0	460	(mq)	5.0	10
three cheese, 'Side Dish'								
(Budget Gourmet)	5.75 oz	230	8.0	25.0	410	(mq)	11.0	30
wedges, hot and spicy, 'Texas Crispers'								
(Ore-Ida)	3 oz	180	2.0	19.0	250	na	10.0	0
w/broccoli and cheese flavor sauce,								
'One Serving' (Green Giant)	5.5 oz	130	4.0	19.0	720	(mq)	5.0	5
w/broccoli and cheese sauce,								
'Family Side Dish' (Freezer Queen)	5.5 oz	140	3.0	25.0	79	(mq)	3.0	na
POTATO DISH, MICROWAVE								
au gratin, 'Microwave Shelf Pack'								
(Green Giant)	1/2 cup	120	3.0	17.0	430	1.5	5.0	5
scalloped, microwave cup (Lunch Bucket)	7.5 oz	160	4.0	20.0	770	na	7.0	35
scalloped, w/ham, micro cup (Hormel)	7.5 oz	260	8.0	21.0	810	(mq)	16.0	25
POTATO DISH MIX								
and cheese, au gratin 'Potatoes &								
Cheese' (Kraft) prepared	1/2 cup	130	4.0	19.0	570	(mq)	5.0	40
and cheese, broccoli au gratin								
(Kraft) prepared	1/2 cup	150	5.0	20.0	530	(mq)	5.0	40
broccoli au gratin 'Potato Medleys'								
(Betty Crocker) dry	1/5 pkg	110	2.0	22.0	550	(mq)	1.0	na
broccoli au gratin 'Potato Medleys'								
(Betty Crocker) prepared w/margarine								
and 2% milk	1/2 cup	140	3.0	23.0	590	(mq)	4.0	(mq)
cheddar, w/mushrooms 'Potato Medleys'								
(Betty Crocker) dry	1/5 pkg	110	2.0	22.0	490	(mq)	1.0	na
cheddar, w/mushrooms 'Potato Medleys'								
(Betty Crocker) prepared w/margarine								
and whole milk	1/2 cup	140	3.0	23.0	530	(mq)	4.0	(mq)
scalloped, w/broccoli 'Potato Medleys'								
(Betty Crocker) dry	1/5 pkg	100	2.0	19.0	460	(mq)	2.0	na

Food Name	Serv. Size	Total Cal.	Prot. GMS	Carbs GMS	Sod. MGS	Fiber GMS	Fat GMS	Chol. MGS
scalloped, w/broccoli 'Potato Medleys'								
(Betty Crocker) prepared	1/2 cup	140	3.0	21.0	500	(mq)	5.0	(mq)
scalloped, w/green beans and								
mushrooms (Betty Crocker) dry	1/5 pkg	110	2.0	20.0	460	(mq)	2.0	na
scalloped, w/green beans and								
mushrooms (Betty Crocker) prepared	1/2 cup	140	3.0	21.0	500	(mq)	5.0	(mq)
'SpudFlakes' (Martha White) prepared								
w/2% milk	1/3 cup	120	2.0	15.0	345	na	6.0	18
w/cheese, scalloped, and ham (Kraft)								
prepared	1/2 cup	150	5.0	20.0	510	(mq)	5.0	15
w/cheese, scalloped 'Potatoes & Cheese'								
(Kraft) prepared	1/2 cup	140	4.0	20.0	500	(mq)	5.0	25
w/cheese, sour cream and chive (Kraft)								
prepared	1/2 cup	150	5.0	20.0	610	(mq)	5.0	10
w/two cheeses 'Potatoes & Cheese'								
(Kraft) prepared	1/2 cup	130	4.0	19.0	540	(mq)	4.0	10
POTATO ENTRÉE, FROZEN								
baked, chicken divan (Weight Watchers)	11.25 oz	280	17.0	38.0	480	na	7.0	30
baked, homestyle turkey								
(Weight Watchers)	11.25 oz	230	17.0	27.0	510	na	7.0	45
baked, vegetable primavera								
(Weight Watchers)	11.15 oz	320	11.0	49.0	500	na	9.0	5
baked, w/broccoli and cheddar								
(Lean Cuisine)	10 3/8 oz	290	14.0	37.0	590	na	9.0	20
baked, w/broccoli and cheese								
(Weight Watchers)	10.5 oz	270	10.0	43.0	570	na	6.0	5
baked, w/broccoli and ham								
(Weight Watchers)	11.5 oz	240	19.0	30.0	520	na	5.0	15
baked, w/cheese sauce and broccoli								
'Light & Healthy' (Budget Gourmet) ...	10.5 oz	300	13.0	40.0	740	na	10.0	30
baked, w/sour cream (Lean Cuisine) ..	10 3/8 oz	230	9.0	38.0	570	na	5.0	15
POTATO FLOUR								
....	1/2 cup	316	7.2	71.9	31	5.5	0.7	0
.... 1 oz		100	2.3	22.7	10	1.8	0.2	0
POTATO MIX								
AU GRATIN								
(Betty Crocker) prepared w/margarine								
and skim milk	1/2 cup	150	4.0	21.0	600	(mq)	5.0	(mq)
(Fantastic Foods) prepared w/whole milk	1/2 cup	156	6.0	25.0	440	(mq)	4.0	(mq)
(Fantastic Foods) prepared w/whole milk								
and salted butter	1/2 cup	196	6.0	25.0	495	(mq)	8.0	(mq)
(French's) tangy, prepared	1/2 cup	130	4.0	20.0	480	(mq)	5.0	na
(General Mills) dry	1/6 pkg	100	2.0	20.0	520	na	1.0	na

Food Name	Serv. Size	Total Cal.	Prot. GMS	Carbs GMS	Sod. MGS	Fiber GMS	Fat GMS	Chol. MGS
(General Mills) homestyle, w/broccoli, dry	1/6 pkg	90	2.0	18.0	490	na	1.0	na
(General Mills) homestyle, w/broccoli, prepared w/margarine and 2% milk	1/2 cup	140	3.0	19.0	550	na	6.0	na
(General Mills) prepared w/margarine and 2% milk	1/2 cup	150	3.0	21.0	580	na	6.0	na
(Idahoan) prepared	1/2 cup	130	3.0	18.0	475	(mq)	5.0	(mq)
(Pillsbury) 'Specialty' tangy, dry	1/6 pkg	90	2.0	19.0	470	1.0	1.0	0
(Pillsbury) tangy, prepared w/butter and whole milk	1/2 cup	140	3.0	20.0	520	1.0	6.0	15
CASSEROLE *(French's)* cheddar and bacon, prepared	1/2 cup	130	4.0	18.0	390	(mq)	5.0	na
COUNTRY STYLE								
(Fantastic Foods) prepared	1/2 cup	85	3.0	19.0	316	(mq)	0.3	na
(Fantastic Foods) prepared w/salted butter	1/2 cup	118	3.0	19.0	362	(mq)	4.0	(mq)
HASH BROWN								
(Betty Crocker) w/onions, prepared	1/6 pkg	110	2.0	24.0	40	(mq)	1.0	na
(Betty Crocker) w/onions, prepared w/margarine	1/2 cup	160	2.0	24.0	100	(mq)	6.0	na
(General Mills)	1/6 pkg	110	2.0	24.0	25	na	<1.0	na
(General Mills) prepared w/margarine	1/2 cup	160	2.0	24.0	100	na	6.0	na
(Idahoan) herb and butter, dry	1/6 pkg	90	2.0	16.0	425	(mq)	2.0	na
(Idahoan) prepared w/unsalted butter	1/2 cup	140	2.0	18.0	50	(mq)	7.0	na
(Idahoan) 'Quick One-Pan' prepared	1/2 cup	140	2.0	18.0	400	(mq)	7.0	na
JULIENNE								
(General Mills) dry	1/6 pkg	90	2.0	17.0	520	na	1.0	na
(General Mills) prepared w/margarine and 2% milk	1/2 cup	130	3.0	19.0	580	na	5.0	na
MASHED								
(Betty Crocker) bacon and cheddar 'Twice Baked' dry	1/6 pkg	110	3.0	19.0	500	(mq)	2.0	na
(Betty Crocker) bacon and cheddar 'Twice Baked' prepared	1/2 cup	210	6.0	21.0	600	(mq)	11.0	(mq)
(Betty Crocker) butter, herbed 'Twice Baked' dry	1/6 pkg	100	2.0	18.0	440	(mq)	2.0	na
(Betty Crocker) butter, herbed 'Twice Baked' prepared	1/2 cup	220	5.0	20.0	540	(mq)	13.0	(mq)
(Betty Crocker) cheddar, mild, w/onion 'Twice Baked' dry	1/6 pkg	100	2.0	18.0	540	(mq)	2.0	na
(Betty Crocker) cheddar, mild, w/onion 'Twice Baked' prepared	1/2 cup	190	5.0	19.0	640	(mq)	11.0	(mq)

Food Name	Serv. Size	Total Cal.	Prot. GMS	Carbs GMS	Sod. MGS	Fiber GMS	Fat GMS	Chol. MGS
(Betty Crocker) cheddar cheese 'Potato Buds' dry	1/12 pkg	110	2.0	20.0	440	na	2.0	na
(Betty Crocker) cheddar cheese 'Potato Buds' prepared	1/2 cup	180	3.0	21.0	510	na	9.0	na
(Betty Crocker) cheddar cheese 'Potato Buds' reduced fat recipe, dry	1/12 pkg	140	3.0	21.0	480	na	5.0	na
(Betty Crocker) 'Potato Buds' prepared	1/2 cup	130	3.0	17.0	360	(mq)	6.0	(mq)
(Betty Crocker) 'Potato Buds' prepared w/o added salt	1/2 cup	130	3.0	17.0	90	(mq)	6.0	(mq)
(Country Store) prepared	1/3 cup	70	1.0	16.0	10	(mq)	0.0	0
(General Mills) American cheese, homestyle, dry	1/6 pkg	100	2.0	20.0	560	na	1.0	na
(General Mills) American cheese, homestyle, prepared w/margarine and 2% milk	1/2 cup	150	3.0	21.0	620	na	6.0	na
(General Mills) cheddar and bacon, dry	1/6 pkg	100	2.0	20.0	480	na	1.0	na
(General Mills) cheddar and bacon, prepared w/margarine and 2% milk	1/2 cup	150	3.0	21.0	540	na	6.0	na
(General Mills) cheddar cheese, homestyle, dry	1/6 pkg	90	2.0	19.0	470	na	1.0	na
(General Mills) cheddar cheese, homestyle, prepared w/margarine and 2% milk	1/2 cup	150	3.0	21.0	530	na	6.0	na
(Hungry Jack) 'Flakes' prepared	1/2 cup	140	3.0	17.0	380	(mq)	7.0	na
(Idahoan) cheddar, spicy, dry	1/6 pkg	90	2.0	17.0	450	(mq)	1.0	na
(Idahoan) cheddar, spicy, prepared	1/2 cup	140	3.0	21.0	500	(mq)	5.0	(mq)
(Pillsbury) cheddar and bacon 'Specialty' dry	1/6 pkg	90	2.0	18.0	430	1.0	1.0	0
(Pillsbury) cheddar and bacon 'Specialty' prepared w/butter and whole milk	1/2 cup	140	3.0	19.0	480	1.0	6.0	15
SCALLOPED								
(Betty Crocker) cheesy, dry	1/6 pkg	90	2.0	19.0	500	(mq)	1.0	na
(Betty Crocker) cheesy, prepared	1/2 cup	140	3.0	20.0	560	(mq)	5.0	(mq)
(Betty Crocker) dry	1/6 pkg	90	2.0	19.0	520	(mq)	1.0	na
(Betty Crocker) prepared	1/2 cup	140	3.0	20.0	580	(mq)	5.0	(mq)
(Betty Crocker) sour cream and chives, dry	1/6 pkg	100	2.0	19.0	460	(mq)	2.0	na
(Betty Crocker) sour cream and chives, prepared	1/2 cup	140	3.0	21.0	520	(mq)	5.0	(mq)
(Betty Crocker) w/ham, dry	1/5 pkg	100	2.0	20.0	470	(mq)	1.0	(mq)
(Betty Crocker) w/ham, prepared	1/2 cup	160	4.0	22.0	540	(mq)	6.0	(mq)
(French's) creamy Italian, prepared	1/2 cup	120	4.0	19.0	430	(mq)	3.0	na

Food Name	Serv. Size	Total Cal.	Prot. GMS	Carbs GMS	Sod. MGS	Fiber GMS	Fat GMS	Chol. MGS
(French's) crispy top, w/savory onion mix, prepared	1/2 cup	140	3.0	20.0	430	na	5.0	na
(French's) real cheese, prepared	1/2 cup	140	4.0	19.0	380	(mq)	5.0	na
(French's) sour cream and chives, prepared	1/2 cup	150	3.0	19.0	550	(mq)	7.0	na
(General Mills) dry	1/6 pkg	90	2.0	19.0	510	na	1.0	na
(General Mills) prepared w/margarine and 2% milk	1/2 cup	140	3.0	20.0	570	na	5.0	na
(General Mills) smoky cheddar, dry	1/6 pkg	100	2.0	20.0	520	na	1.0	na
(General Mills) smoky cheddar, prepared w/margarine and 2% milk	1/2 cup	140	3.0	21.0	580	na	5.0	na
(General Mills) sour cream and chive	1/6 pkg	100	2.0	19.0	460	na	2.0	na
(General Mills) sour cream and chive, prepared w/margarine and 2% milk	1/2 cup	150	3.0	20.0	520	na	6.0	na
(General Mills) w/ham, dry	1/5 pkg	100	2.0	20.0	550	na	1.0	na
(General Mills) w/ham, prepared w/margarine and 2% milk	1/2 cup	170	4.0	22.0	620	na	7.0	na
(Idahoan) prepared	1/2 cup	140	3.0	20.0	425	(mq)	5.0	(mq)
(Idahoan) prepared w/o added salt, w/unsalted butter	1/2 cup	140	3.0	16.0	55	(mq)	7.0	(mq)
(Idahoan) sour cream and chives, dry	1/6 pkg	90	2.0	15.0	340	(mq)	2.0	na
(Idahoan) sour cream and chives, prepared	1/2 cup	130	2.0	18.0	400	(mq)	5.0	(mq)
(Pillsbury) sour cream and chives 'Specialty,' dry	1/6 pkg	100	2.0	18.0	450	1.0	2.0	0
(Pillsbury) sour cream and chives, 'Specialty,' prepared w/butter and whole milk	1/2 cup	150	3.0	20.0	500	1.0	6.0	15
STUFFED								
(Betty Crocker) sour cream and chives 'Twice Baked,' dry	1/6 pkg	90	2.0	17.0	480	(mq)	2.0	na
(Betty Crocker) sour cream and chives 'Twice Baked' prepared	1/2 cup	200	5.0	19.0	570	(mq)	11.0	(mq)
WESTERN								
(Arrowhead Mills) flakes	2 oz	140	5.0	44.0	24	na	0.0	0
(Barbara's Bakery) dry	4 oz	389	7.0	89.0	63	na	1.0	1
(French's) creamy, prepared	1/2 cup	130	3.0	20.0	520	(mq)	4.0	na
(General Mills) cheesy homestyle, dry	1/6 pkg	100	2.0	19.0	500	na	2.0	na
(General Mills) cheesy homestyle, prepared w/margarine and 2% milk	1/2 cup	150	3.0	20.0	560	na	6.0	na
(General Mills) potato buds, dry	1/8 pkg	70	2.0	16.0	20	na	0.0	na
(General Mills) potato buds, prepared	1/2 cup	130	3.0	17.0	360	na	6.0	na

Food Name	Serv. Size	Total Cal.	Prot. GMS	Carbs GMS	Sod. MGS	Fiber GMS	Fat GMS	Chol. MGS
(General Mills) potato buds, prepared w/o salt	1/2 cup	130	3.0	17.0	90	na	6.0	na
(Hungry Jack) flakes	13.3 oz	70	1.0	16.0	25	1.0	0.0	0
(Hungry Jack) flakes, prepared w/margarine, 2% milk, and water	1/2 cup	130	2.0	17.0	85	1.0	6.0	0
(Hungry Jack) flakes, prepared w/margarine, 2% milk, salt, and water	1/2 cup	130	2.0	17.0	260	1.0	6.0	0
(Idaho) granules	13.3 oz	60	1.0	14.0	30	1.0	0.0	0
(Idaho) granules, prepared	1/2 cup	130	2.0	16.0	320	(mq)	6.0	na
(Idaho) granules, prepared w/margarine, 2% milk, and water	1/2 cup	120	2.0	16.0	85	1.0	5.0	0
(Idaho) granules, prepared w/margarine, 2% milk, salt, and water	1/2 cup	120	2.0	16.0	190	1.0	5.0	0
(Idaho Spuds) flakes	13.3 oz	70	1.0	15.0	40	1.0	0.0	0
(Idaho Spuds) flakes, prepared	1/2 cup	140	3.0	17.0	380	(mq)	7.0	na
(Idaho Spuds) flakes, prepared w/margarine, 2% milk, and water	1/2 cup	130	3.0	17.0	105	1.0	6.0	0
(Idaho Spuds) flakes, prepared w/margarine, 2% milk, salt, and water	1/2 cup	130	3.0	16.0	370	1.0	6.0	0
(Idahoan) dry	1/3 cup	80	2.0	18.0	15	2.0	0.0	0
(Idahoan) 'Complete' dry	1/3 cup	100	2.0	19.0	310	2.0	2.0	0
(Pillsbury) cheesy 'Specialty' dry	1/6 pkg	100	2.0	19.0	490	1.0	2.0	0
(Pillsbury) cheesy 'Specialty,' prepared w/butter and whole milk	1/2 cup	150	3.0	20.0	540	1.0	6.0	15
(Pillsbury) creamy white sauce, 'Specialty,' dry	1/6 pkg	100	2.0	19.0	410	1.0	2.0	0
POTATO PANCAKE								
(Idaho) 3-inch diam each, prepared	3 cakes	90	3.0	16.0	420	(mq)	2.0	na
(Kosher Empire) frozen, triangle, latkes w/onions	2 oz	77	1.0	13.0	108	na	2.4	na
(Pillsbury) 'Specialty'	1/8 pkg	70	2.0	16.0	400	1.0	0.0	0
(Pillsbury) 'Specialty' prepared w/water and egg, 3 inch diam each	3 cakes	90	3.0	16.0	420	1.0	2.0	55
POTATO SALAD, CANNED								
(Joan of Arc) German	1/2 cup	120	2.0	23.0	550	1.6	3.0	na
(Joan of Arc) homestyle	1/2 cup	340	4.0	32.0	1070	3.0	22.0	na
(Read) German	1/2 cup	120	2.0	23.0	550	1.6	3.0	na
(Read) homestyle	1/2 cup	340	4.0	32.0	1070	3.0	22.0	na
POTATO SALAD SEASONING (Tone's)	1 tsp	5	0.2	0.3	1498	.1	0.2	0
POTATO STARCH (Featherweight)	1 cup	620	0.0	154.0	51	na	1.0	0
POTATO STICKS. See POTATO CHIPS AND SNACKS.								
POTTED MEAT SPREAD. See also LUNCHEON MEAT, CANNED; SANDWICH SPREAD.								
beef	1 cup	558	39.4	0.0	2925	0	43.2	175

Food Name	Serv. Size	Total Cal.	Prot. GMS	Carbs GMS	Sod. MGS	Fiber GMS	Fat GMS	Chol. MGS
chicken	1 cup	558	39.4	0.0	2925	0	43.2	175
turkey	1 cup	558	39.4	0.0	2925	0	43.2	175
(Hormel)	1 oz	53	4.0	2.0	280	na	4.0	23
(Hormel)	1 tbsp	30	2.0	0.0	145	0	2.0	(mq)
(Libby's)	1.83 oz	110	7.0	0.0	320	0	9.0	(mq)
POULTRY SEASONING								
dry	1 oz	87	2.7	18.6	8	3.2	2.1	0
dry	1 tbsp	11	0.4	2.4	1	.4	0.3	0
dry	1 tsp	5	0.1	1.0	0	.2	0.1	0
PRESERVES. See also FRUIT SPREAD; JAM; JELLY; MARMALADE.								
APPLE BUTTER								
(Bama)	2 tsp	25	0.0	6.0	5	na	0.0	na
(Knudsen & Sons) organic	2 tbsp	25	0.0	6.0	0	na	0.0	na
(Lucky Leaf)	4 oz	200	0.0	49.0	15	na	1.0	0
(Musselman's)	4 oz	200	0.0	49.0	15	na	1.0	0
(Smucker's) 'Autumn Harvest'	1 tsp	12	0.0	3.0	0	(mq)	0.0	0
(Smucker's) cider	1 tsp	12	0.0	3.0	0	(mq)	0.0	0
(Smucker's) natural	1 tsp	12	0.0	3.0	0	(mq)	0.0	0
(Smucker's) 'Simply Fruit'	1 tsp	16	0.0	4.0	0	(mq)	0.0	0
(Smucker's) spiced	1 tsp	12	0.0	3.0	0	na	0.0	na
(Tap'n Apple)	1 oz	45	<1.0	13.2	<1	.5	<.1	0
(White House)	1 oz	50	0.0	12.0	5	(mq)	0.0	0
APRICOT								
(Knott's Berry Farm)	1 tsp	18	0.0	4.0	0	na	0.0	na
(Polaner)	2 tsp	35	0.0	9.0	5	na	0.0	na
APRICOT-PINEAPPLE								
(Knott's Berry Farm)	1 tsp	18	0.0	4.0	0	na	0.0	na
(Knudsen & Sons)	2 tsp	35	<1.0	8.0	na	na	<1.0	na
BING CHERRY (Knott's Berry Farm)	1 tsp	18	0.0	4.0	0	na	0.0	na
BLACK CHERRY (Knudsen & Sons)	2 tsp	35	<1.0	8.0	na	na	<1.0	na
BLACKBERRY								
(Knott's Berry Farm) seedless	1 tsp	18	0.0	4.0	0	na	0.0	na
(Knudsen & Sons)	2 tsp	35	<1.0	8.0	na	na	<1.0	na
(Knudsen & Sons) organic	2 tsp	25	<1.0	7.0	na	na	<1.0	na
(Polaner) seedless	2 tsp	35	0.0	9.0	5	na	0.0	na
BLUEBERRY								
(Knott's Berry Farm)	1 tsp	18	0.0	4.0	0	na	0.0	na
(Knudsen & Sons)	2 tsp	35	<1.0	8.0	na	na	<1.0	na
(Knudsen & Sons) organic	2 tsp	25	<1.0	7.0	na	na	<1.0	na
(Polaner)	2 tsp	35	0.0	9.0	5	na	0.0	na
BOYSENBERRY								
(Knott's Berry Farm)	1 tsp	18	0.0	4.0	0	na	0.0	na
(Knudsen & Sons)	2 tsp	35	<1.0	8.0	na	na	<1.0	na

Food Name	Serv. Size	Total Cal.	Prot. GMS	Carbs GMS	Sod. MGS	Fiber GMS	Fat GMS	Chol. MGS
CONCORD GRAPE *(Knudsen & Sons)* ...	2 tsp	35	<1.0	8.0	na	na	<1.0	na
KADOTA FIG *(Knott's Berry Farm)*	1 tsp	18	0.0	4.0	0	na	0.0	na
PEACH								
(Bama)	2 tsp	30	0.0	8.0	5	na	0.0	na
(Knudsen & Sons)	2 tsp	35	<1.0	8.0	na	na	<1.0	na
(Polaner)	2 tsp	35	0.0	9.0	5	na	0.0	na
PINEAPPLE *(Polaner)*	2 tsp	35	0.0	9.0	5	na	0.0	na
RED CHERRY *(Knott's Berry Farm)* ...	1 tsp	18	0.0	4.0	0	na	0.0	na
RED RASPBERRY								
(Knott's Berry Farm) seedless	1 tsp	18	0.0	4.0	0	na	0.0	na
(Knudsen & Sons)	2 tsp	35	<1.0	8.0	na	na	<1.0	na
(Knudsen & Sons) organic	2 tsp	25	<1.0	7.0	na	na	<1.0	na
(Polaner)	2 tsp	35	0.0	9.0	5	na	0.0	na
(Polaner) seedless	2 tsp	35	0.0	9.0	5	na	0.0	na
(Smucker's) natural ingredients	1 tsp	18	0.0	4.0	0	na	0.0	na
STRAWBERRY								
(Bama)	2 tsp	30	0.0	8.0	5	na	0.0	na
(Knott's Berry Farm) pure, seedless ..	1 tsp	18	0.0	4.0	0	na	0.0	na
(Knudsen & Sons)	2 tsp	35	<1.0	8.0	na	na	<1.0	na
(Knudsen & Sons) organic	2 tsp	25	<1.0	7.0	na	na	<1.0	na
(Polaner)	2 tsp	35	0.0	9.0	5	na	0.0	na
(Smucker's) natural ingredients	1 tsp	18	0.0	4.0	0	na	0.0	na
PRETZELS								
(A & Eagle)	1 oz	110	3.0	22.0	570	(mq)	2.0	0
(Bachman) 'Nutzels'	1 oz	110	3.0	21.0	470	(mq)	2.0	0
(Bachman) 'Petite'	1 oz	110	3.0	21.0	410	(mq)	2.0	0
(Bachman) 'Petite Sodium Free'	1 oz	110	3.0	21.0	2	(mq)	2.0	0
(Estee) 'Unsalted'	5 pretzels	25	<1.0	5.0	5	<1.0	<1.0	0
(Featherweight) 'Low Salt'	20 pretzels	110	3.0	23.0	30	(mq)	1.0	0
(Mister Salty) 'Juniors'	1 oz	110	2.0	22.0	500	(mq)	2.0	na
(Pepperidge Farm) 'Goldfish'	1 oz	110	3.0	20.0	160	1.0	3.0	0
(Rokeach) 'Baldies Unsalted'	1 oz	110	2.0	20.0	30	(mq)	0.0	0
(Rold Gold) 'Tiny Tim'	1 oz	110	2.0	23.0	610	(mq)	1.0	0
BAVARIAN								
(Barbara's Bakery) 1 oz	2 pretzels	110	4.0	21.0	200	na	<1.0	0
(Barbara's Bakery) no salt added, 1 oz	2 pretzels	110	4.0	21.0	10	na	<1.0	0
(Rold Gold) 1 oz	3 pretzels	120	3.0	22.0	430	na	2.0	0
BEER *(Quinlan)*	1 oz	110	2.6	21.6	446	.1	1.4	0
BRAIDS *(Keebler)* 'Butter Pretzels'	1 oz	110	3.0	21.0	620	(mq)	1.0	0
CHEDDAR *(Combos)*	10 nuggets	143	2.9	19.5	335	>.1 c	5.8	3
CHIPS								
'Mr. Phipps' *(Nabisco)* lightly salted, .5 oz	8 chips	60	1.0	11.0	200	0	1.0	0

Food Name	Serv. Size	Total Cal.	Prot. GMS	Carbs GMS	Sod. MGS	Fiber GMS	Fat GMS	Chol. MGS
'Mr. Phipps' *(Nabisco)* original, .5 oz ... 8 chips		60	1.0	10.0	310	0	1.0	0
'Mr. Phipps' *(Nabisco)* sesame, .5 oz .. 8 chips		60	1.0	10.0	250	na	2.0	0
DUTCH STYLE								
.... 7.5-oz pkg		831	20.9	161.7	3578	>.6 c	9.6	0
.... 1 pretzel		62	1.6	12.1	269	>.1 c	0.7	0
(Estee) 'Unsalted' .... 2 pretzels		110	3.0	23.0	30	na	<1.0	0
(Mister Salty) 1 oz .... 2 pretzels		110	3.0	22.0	440	(mq)	1.0	5
(Rokeach) .... 1 oz		110	3.0	24.0	na	(mq)	0.0	na
(Rokeach) 'Unsalted' .... 1 oz		110	2.0	20.0	30	(mq)	0.0	0
HARD								
(Bachman) .... 1 oz		110	3.0	23.0	290	(mq)	<1.0	0
(Bachman) unsalted .... 1 oz		110	3.0	23.0	50	(mq)	<1.0	0
plain, made w/unenriched flour, salted 10 twists		322	4.2	31.7	5	>1.0 c	20.8	0
plain, made w/unenriched flour, unsalted .... 10 twists		229	5.5	47.5	1029	1.9	2.1	0
plain, salted .... 10 twists		229	5.5	47.5	1029	1.9	2.1	0
plain, unsalted .... 10 twists		229	5.5	47.5	173	1.9	2.1	0
whole wheat .... 2 oz		205	6.3	46.0	115	>1.0 c	1.5	0
HONEYSWEET *(Barbara's Bakery)*								
1 oz.......................... 2 pretzels		110	3.0	21.0	200	na	<1.0	0
KNOTS *(Keebler)* 'Butter Pretzels' .... 1 oz		110	3.0	21.0	530	(mq)	1.0	0
LOGS								
(Bachman) .... 1 oz		110	3.0	21.0	470	(mq)	2.0	0
(Quinlan) ● .... 1 oz		103	2.7	21.5	388	.3	0.8	0
MINIS								
(Barbara's Bakery) 1 oz .... 17 pretzels		110	4.0	21.0	290	na	<1.0	0
(Barbara's Bakery) no salt added, 1 oz .... 17 pretzels		110	4.0	21.0	10	na	<1.0	0
(Mister Salty) 1 oz .... 22 pretzels		110	3.0	21.0	450	na	1.0	0
NINE-GRAIN *(Barbara's Bakery)* 1 oz . 2 pretzels		110	4.0	21.0	200	na	<1.0	0
OAT BRAN *(Quinlan)* .... 1 oz		115	3.5	21.8	156	.3	1.5	0
PARTY								
(Delicious) .... 1 oz		110	3.0	23.0	500	na	1.0	0
(Rokeach) 'Party Cannister' .... 1 oz		110	2.0	23.0	na	(mq)	1.0	0
RICE BRAN, 'No-Salt' *(Quinlan)* .... 1 oz		101	2.6	19.5	52	2.0	2.3	0
RINGS								
(Bachman) .... 1 oz		110	3.0	21.0	410	(mq)	2.0	0
(Mister Salty) .... 1 oz		110	3.0	21.0	510	(mq)	2.0	na
(Mister Salty) butter flavor .... 1 oz		110	3.0	21.0	570	(mq)	2.0	na
RODS								
(Bachman) .... 1 oz		110	3.0	21.0	240	(mq)	2.0	0
(Rold Gold) .... 1 oz		110	3.0	22.0	550	(mq)	2.0	0
(Seyfert's) butter flavor .... 1 oz		110	3.0	21.0	530	(mq)	1.0	na

	Serv.	Total	Prot.	Carbs	Sod.	Fiber	Fat	Chol.
STICKS								
(Delicious)	1 oz	110	3.0	23.0	500	na	1.0	1
(Mister Salty)	1 oz	110	3.0	22.0	620	(mq)	1.0	na
(Mister Salty) butter flavor	1 oz	110	3.0	22.0	620	(mq)	1.0	na
(Mister Salty) fat-free	1 oz	110	3.0	23.0	380	<1.0	<1.0	5
(Mister Salty) very thin, 1 oz	92 sticks	110	3.0	22.0	600	1.0	3.0	0
(Pepperidge Farm) 'Snack Sticks'	8 sticks	120	3.0	23.0	430	1.0	3.0	0
(Quinlan)	1 oz	105	2.7	22.3	538	.3	0.6	0
(Rold Gold)	1 oz	110	2.0	23.0	760	(mq)	1.0	0
THINS								
(Bachman)	1 oz	110	3.0	21.0	410	(mq)	2.0	0
(Bachman) 'Thin'n Light'	1 oz	110	3.0	21.0	410	(mq)	2.0	0
(Quinlan)	1 oz	104	2.8	22.0	765	.1	0.6	0
(Quinlan) tiny	1 oz	109	2.6	21.2	601	.2	1.5	0
(Quinlan) tiny 'No-Salt'	1 oz	115	2.7	22.4	10	.2	1.6	0
(Quinlan) 'Ultra Thins'	1 oz	106	2.7	22.5	618	.1	0.6	0
(Rold Gold) baked, 33% less sodium 'Fat Free'	1 oz	110	3.0	23.0	340	1.0	0.0	0
TREATS (Bachman)	1 oz	110	3.0	21.0	410	(mq)	2.0	0
TWISTS								
(Bachman)	1 oz	110	3.0	21.0	410	(mq)	2.0	0
(Delicious)	1 oz	110	3.0	23.0	500	na	1.0	0
(Mister Salty) .5 oz	5 twists	110	3.0	21.0	580	1.0	2.0	0
(Mister Salty) fat-free, 1 oz	9 twists	110	3.0	23.0	380	<1.0	<1.0	5
(Rold Gold) thin, 1 oz	10 twists	110	2.0	23.0	470	(mq)	1.0	0
(Rold Gold) tiny, 1 oz	15 twists	110	2.0	23.0	420	na	1.0	0
(Ultra Slim Fast)	1 oz	100	2.0	21.0	460	3.0	1.0	0
PRICKLY PEAR								
raw, trimmed	1 oz	12	0.2	2.7	1	>.5 c	0.1	0
raw, trimmed, approx 4.8 oz	1 fruit	42	0.8	9.9	5	3.7	0.5	0
raw, untrimmed	1 lb	140	2.5	32.6	18	>6.2 c	1.7	0
PROSCIUTTO. See LUNCHEON MEAT, HAM.								
PRUNE								
dehydrated	4 oz	384	4.2	101.0	6	>3.3 c	0.8	0
dehydrated, cooked	4 oz	128	1.4	33.7	2	>1.1 c	0.3	0
Canned								
in heavy syrup, w/liquid	1 cup	246	2.0	65.1	7	8.9	0.5	0
in heavy syrup, w/liquid	1/2 cup	123	1.0	32.5	3	4.5	0.2	0
in heavy syrup, w/2 tbsp liquid	5 fruits	90	0.8	23.9	3	3.3	0.2	0
pitted, in heavy syrup, w/liquid	4 oz	119	1.0	31.5	3	4.4	0.2	0
PRUNE, DRIED								
pitted	1 cup	385	4.2	101.0	6	11.6	0.8	0
pitted	4 oz	271	3.0	71.1	5	8.2	0.6	0

Food Name	Serv. Size	Total Cal.	Prot. GMS	Carbs GMS	Sod. MGS	Fiber GMS	Fat GMS	Chol. MGS
pitted, approx 3 oz	10 fruits	201	2.2	52.7	3	6.1	0.4	0
pitted, cooked, stewed, sweetened	4 oz	141	1.2	37.3	2	4.5	0.2	0
pitted, cooked, stewed, unsweetened	4 oz	121	1.3	31.8	2	7.5	0.3	0
(Del Monte)	2 oz	120	1.0	31.0	10	(mq)	0.0	0
(Del Monte) 'Moist Pak'	2 oz	120	1.0	30.0	10	(mq)	0.0	0
(Del Monte) pitted	2 oz	140	1.0	35.0	10	(mq)	0.0	0
(Dole)	2 oz	140	1.0	36.0	10	na	1.0	na
(Mariani) pitted, premium	1/4 cup	140	1.0	36.0	10	4.0	0.0	0
(SunSweet)	2 oz	120	1.0	32.0	10	(mq)	0.0	0
(SunSweet) pitted	2 oz	140	1.0	36.0	10	(mq)	0.0	0
PRUNE JUICE								
	6 oz	136	1.2	33.5	8	1.9	0.1	0
(Del Monte) 'Unsweetened'	6 oz	120	1.0	33.0	10	(mq)	0.0	0
(J. Hungerford) 100% juice	9.03 oz	178	1.5	43.9	10	2.5	0.0	0
(Knudsen & Sons) organic	8 oz	170	1.0	42.0	na	na	0.0	na
(Lucky Leaf)	6 oz	150	0.0	36.0	0	(mq)	0.0	0
(Mott's)	6 oz	130	1.0	32.0	8	(mq)	0.0	0
(Mott's) country style	6 oz	130	1.0	32.0	7	(mq)	0.0	0
(Pathmark) 'All Natural'	6 oz	120	1.0	30.0	10	(mq)	0.0	0
(Pathmark) w/prune pulp 'Homestyle'	6 oz	130	1.0	32.0	10	(mq)	0.0	0
(S&W) 'Unsweetened'	6 oz	120	1.0	31.0	20	(mq)	0.0	0
(SunSweet)	6 oz	130	1.0	33.0	20	(mq)	0.0	0
PRUNE WHIP								
cold	1 cup	203	5.7	48.0	213	>.8 c	0.3	0
hot	1 cup	140	4.0	33.2	148	>.5 c	0.2	0
PUDDING, FROZEN								
butterscotch (Rich's)	3 oz	130	2.0	18.0	130	na	6.0	0
chocolate (Rich's)	3 oz	140	2.0	18.0	135	na	7.0	0
vanilla (Rich's)	3 oz	130	2.0	18.0	160	na	6.0	0
PUDDING, READY-TO-SERVE								
ALMOND (Rice Dream) 'Dream Pudding,'								
non-dairy, low fat	4 oz	150	1.0	31.0	30	na	2.0	0
BANANA								
(Del Monte) 'Pudding Cup'	5 oz	180	3.0	30.0	285	na	5.0	na
(Lucky Leaf)	4 oz	150	2.0	24.0	110	na	5.0	na
(Musselman's)	4 oz	150	2.0	24.0	110	na	5.0	na
(Rice Dream) 'Dream Pudding,' non-dairy,								
fat-free	4 oz	120	1.0	30.0	5	na	0.0	0
(Snack Pack)	4.25 oz	145	2.0	22.0	180	0	6.0	-1
(Snack Pack)	4 oz	158	1.5	25.0	163	0	5.7	0
BUTTERSCOTCH								
(Crowley)	4.5 oz	150	3.0	27.0	210	na	3.0	10
(Del Monte) 'Pudding Cup'	5 oz	180	3.0	31.0	285	na	5.0	na

	Serv.	Total	Prot.	Carbs	Sod.	Fiber	Fat	Chol.
(Featherweight)	1/2 cup	100	0.0	21.0	160	na	1.0	0
(Lucky Leaf)	4 oz	170	2.0	26.0	135	na	7.0	na
(Musselman's)	4 oz	170	2.0	26.0	135	na	7.0	na
(Rice Dream) 'Dream Pudding,' non-dairy, fat-free	4 oz	120	1.0	30.0	5	na	0.0	0
(Snack Pack)	4.25 oz	170	2.0	27.0	210	0	6.0	1
(Snack Pack)	4 oz	153	1.7	23.6	211	0	5.7	1
(Swiss Miss)	4 oz	156	2.5	24.1	182	0	5.6	1
(Ultra Slim Fast) 'Lite 'N Tasty'	4 oz	100	2.0	21.0	230	2.0	<1.0	0
(White House)	3.5 oz	113	1.0	20.0	195	na	3.0	na
BUTTERSCOTCH-CHOCOLATE-VANILLA SWIRL (Jell-O)	4 oz	180	3.0	28.0	140	na	5.0	0
CARAMELLO (Hershey's)	4 oz	180	3.0	28.0	170	na	6.0	0
CAROB (Rice Dream) 'Dream Pudding' non-dairy, fat-free	4 oz	130	1.0	31.0	30	na	0.0	0
CHOCOLATE								
(Crowley)	4.5 oz	190	4.0	29.0	100	na	3.0	10
(Del Monte) 'Pudding Cup'	5 oz	190	4.0	31.0	280	na	6.0	na
(Del Monte) 'Pudding Snack Light'	4.25 oz	100	2.0	19.0	85	na	1.0	0
(Estee)	1/2 cup	70	5.0	12.0	85	na	<1.0	2
(Featherweight)	1/2 cup	100	1.0	21.0	110	na	1.0	0
(Hershey's)	4 oz	180	3.0	29.0	260	na	5.0	0
(Jell-O) 'Free'	4 oz	100	3.0	24.0	200	na	0.0	0
(Jell-O) 'Light Pudding Snacks'	4 oz	100	3.0	21.0	125	na	2.0	5
(Jell-O) 'Pudding Snacks'	5.5 oz	230	4.0	38.0	170	na	8.0	0
(Jell-O) 'Pudding Snacks'	4 oz	170	3.0	28.0	130	na	6.0	0
(Lucky Leaf)	4 oz	180	2.0	27.0	100	na	7.0	na
(Musselman's)	4 oz	180	2.0	27.0	100	na	7.0	na
(Pathmark) 'No Frills'	5 oz	200	2.0	30.0	140	na	8.0	na
(Rice Dream) 'Dream Pudding,' non-dairy, fat-free	4 oz	170	1.0	39.0	30	na	0.0	0
(Snack Pack)	4.25 oz	160	2.0	28.0	125	na	5.0	0
(Snack Pack)	4 oz	161	2.3	24.6	178	0	5.9	0
(Snack Pack) fat-free	4 oz	96	2.0	21.2	212	0	0.4	0
(Snack Pack) 'Light'	4 oz	100	3.0	20.1	120	na	2.0	0
(Swiss Miss)	4 oz	166	3.1	25.8	177	0	5.7	1
(Swiss Miss) fat-free	4 oz	99	1.8	22.3	154	0	0.4	1
(Swiss Miss) 'Light'	4 oz	100	3.0	20.1	120	na	(mq)	0
(Swiss Miss) sundae	4 oz	220	2.0	36.0	140	0	7.0	5
(White House)	3.5 oz	120	2.0	22.0	130	na	4.0	na
CHOCOLATE FUDGE								
(Del Monte) 'Pudding Cup'	5 oz	190	4.0	31.0	260	na	6.0	na
(Jell-O) 'Light Pudding Snacks'	4 oz	100	3.0	22.0	125	na	1.0	5

Food Name	Serv. Size	Total Cal.	Prot. GMS	Carbs GMS	Sod. MGS	Fiber GMS	Fat GMS	Chol. MGS
(Jell-O) 'Pudding Snacks'	4 oz	170	3.0	28.0	130	na	6.0	0
(Lucky Leaf)	4 oz	180	2.0	25.0	105	na	8.0	na
(Musselman's)	4 oz	180	2.0	25.0	105	na	8.0	na
(Snack Pack)	4.25 oz	165	2.0	27.0	125	0	6.0	1
(Snack Pack)	4 oz	158	2.3	23.9	178	0	5.9	0
(Swiss Miss)	4 oz	175	3.3	27.9	207	0	5.6	1
(Swiss Miss) fat-free	4 oz	103	1.8	23.3	151	0	0.3	1
(Swiss Miss) 'Light'	4 oz	100	3.0	20.0	120	0	1.0	0
CHOCOLATE FUDGE-MILK CHOCOLATE								
SWIRL (Jell-O)	4 oz	170	3.0	28.0	135	na	6.0	0
CHOCOLATE-ALMOND (Hershey's)	4 oz	180	3.0	29.0	210	na	6.0	0
CHOCOLATE-CARAMEL SWIRL								
(Jell-O) 'Pudding Snacks'	4 oz	170	3.0	28.0	130	na	6.0	0
(Snack Pack)	4 oz	165	2.5	25.3	178	0	5.9	1
(Snack Pack) 4 pack	4 oz	170	2.0	27.0	180	na	6.0	0
(Swiss Miss)	4 oz	165	2.5	25.3	178	0	5.9	1
CHOCOLATE-MARSHMALLOW								
(Snack Pack)	4.25 oz	165	2.0	26.0	125	0	6.0	1
(Snack Pack)	4 oz	155	1.9	23.4	124	0	5.9	0
CHOCOLATE-MINT SWIRL (Jell-O) 'Free'	4 oz	100	3.0	24.0	220	na	0.0	0
CHOCOLATE-PEANUT BUTTER SWIRL								
(Snack Pack)	4 oz	169	2.4	25.7	173	0	6.3	1
(Snack Pack) 4 pack	4 oz	170	3.0	26.0	180	na	7.0	0
CHOCOLATE-VANILLA SWIRL								
(Hershey's) 'Kisses'	4 oz	180	3.0	29.0	210	na	6.0	0
(Hershey's) 'Kisses Free'	4 oz	100	2.0	22.0	180	na	0.0	0
(Jell-O) combo 'Light Pudding Snacks'	4 oz	100	3.0	21.0	125	na	2.0	5
(Jell-O) 'Free'	4 oz	100	3.0	24.0	220	na	0.0	0
(Jell-O) 'Pudding Snacks'	5.5 oz	240	4.0	39.0	180	na	8.0	0
(Jell-O) 'Pudding Snacks'	4 oz	170	3.0	28.0	135	na	6.0	0
CHOCOLATE-VANILLA-CHOCOLATE SWIRL								
(Swiss Miss)	4 oz	172	2.8	26.6	163	0	6.0	1
COCONUT								
(Rice Dream) 'Dream Pudding,' non-dairy,								
low fat	4 oz	150	1.0	32.0	10	na	2.0	0
LEMON								
(Rice Dream) 'Dream Pudding,' non-dairy,								
fat-free	4 oz	120	1.0	30.0	5	na	0.0	0
(Snack Pack)	4.25 oz	150	<1.0	30.0	75	<1.0	4.0	0
(Snack Pack)	4 oz	138	0.1	28.0	85	0	2.8	0
(White House)	3.5 oz	152	0.0	37.0	65	na	1.0	na
MILK CHOCOLATE								
(Jell-O) 'Pudding Snacks'	4 oz	170	4.0	29.0	135	na	6.0	0

Food Name	Serv. Size	Total Cal.	Prot. GMS	Carbs GMS	Sod. MGS	Fiber GMS	Fat GMS	Chol. MGS
(Snack Pack)	4 oz	166	1.8	26.4	166	0	5.9	1
(Snack Pack) 4 pack	4 oz	160	2.0	26.0	170	na	6.0	0
(Swiss Miss)	4 oz	166	1.8	26.4	166	0	2.9	1
MILK CHOCOLATE-CHOCOLATE								
FUDGE SWIRL (Jell-O)	4 oz	170	3.0	28.0	135	na	6.0	0
RICE								
(Crowley)	4.5 oz	125	4.0	22.0	80	na	2.0	10
(Lucky Leaf)	4 oz	120	3.0	20.0	95	na	3.0	na
(Musselman's)	4 oz	120	3.0	20.0	95	na	3.0	na
(White House)	3.5 oz	111	1.0	20.0	135	na	3.0	na
S'MORES SWIRL								
(Snack Pack)	4 oz	154	1.4	24.7	129	0	5.6	1
(Snack Pack) 4 pack	4 oz	150	2.0	25.0	125	na	6.0	0
TAPIOCA								
(Crowley)	4.5 oz	135	4.0	27.0	70	na	1.0	5
(Del Monte) 'Pudding Cup'	5 oz	180	3.0	30.0	250	na	4.0	na
(Jell-O) 'Pudding Snacks'	4 oz	170	3.0	27.0	140	na	4.0	0
(Lucky Leaf)	4 oz	140	1.0	20.0	95	na	6.0	na
(Musselman's)	4 oz	140	1.0	20.0	95	na	6.0	na
(Snack Pack)	4.25 oz	160	2.0	28.0	200	na	4.0	0
(Snack Pack)	4 oz	151	2.0	22.9	134	0	5.7	1
(Snack Pack) fat-free	4 oz	94	2.1	20.7	185	0	0.4	0
(Snack Pack) 'Light'	4 oz	100	2.0	18.1	105	0	2.0	0
(Swiss Miss)	4 oz	138	2.1	23.6	180	0	3.9	1
(Swiss Miss) fat-free	4 oz	99	2.0	22.0	151	0	0.3	1
(Swiss Miss) 'Light'	4 oz	100	2.0	18.1	105	na	2.0	0
(White House)	3.5 oz	131	1.0	19.0	105	na	6.0	na
VANILLA								
(Crowley)	4.5 oz	140	3.0	26.0	130	na	3.0	10
(Del Monte) 'Pudding Cup'	5 oz	180	3.0	32.0	285	na	5.0	na
(Del Monte) 'Pudding Snack Light'	4.25 oz	100	1.0	19.0	200	na	1.0	0
(Estee)	1/2 cup	70	4.0	12.0	65	na	<1.0	2
(Featherweight)	1/2 cup	100	0.0	20.0	150	na	2.0	0
(Jell-O) 'Free'	4 oz	100	3.0	23.0	250	na	0.0	0
(Jell-O) 'Light Pudding Snacks'	4 oz	100	3.0	20.0	130	na	2.0	5
(Jell-O) 'Pudding Snacks'	5.5 oz	250	4.0	38.0	190	na	9.0	0
(Jell-O) 'Pudding Snacks'	4 oz	180	3.0	28.0	140	na	7.0	0
(Lucky Leaf)	4 oz	170	2.0	25.0	135	na	7.0	na
(Musselman's)	4 oz	170	2.0	25.0	135	na	7.0	na
(Pathmark) 'No Frills'	5 oz	200	2.0	28.0	150	na	8.0	na
(Snack Pack)	4.25 oz	170	1.0	28.0	180	na	6.0	0
(Snack Pack)	4 oz	158	1.5	25.0	141	0	5.7	0
(Snack Pack) fat-free	4 oz	93	1.8	20.8	167	0	0.4	1

Food Name	Serv. Size	Total Cal.	Prot. GMS	Carbs GMS	Sod. MGS	Fiber GMS	Fat GMS	Chol. MGS
(Swiss Miss)	4 oz	156	2.5	24.1	181	0	5.6	1
(Swiss Miss) fat-free	4 oz	98	1.6	22.1	162	0	0.4	1
(Swiss Miss) 'Light'	4 oz	100	2.0	18.1	110	na	2.0	0
(Swiss Miss) sundae	4 oz	175	2.0	26.5	174	0	6.8	1
(Ultra Slim Fast) 'Lite 'N Tasty'	4 oz	100	2.0	21.0	230	2.0	<1.0	0
(White House)	3.5 oz	111	1.0	20.0	135	na	3.0	na
VANILLA-CHOCOLATE SWIRL								
(Jell-O) 'Pudding Snacks'	4 oz	180	3.0	28.0	140	na	6.0	0

PUDDING MIX. See also PUDDING/PIE FILLING MIX.

Food Name	Serv. Size	Total Cal.	Prot. GMS	Carbs GMS	Sod. MGS	Fiber GMS	Fat GMS	Chol. MGS
BANANA								
(Jell-O) 'Instant' prepared	1/2 cup	160	4.0	28.0	410	na	4.0	15
(Jell-O) 'Instant Sugar-free' prepared w/2% milk	1/2 cup	80	4.0	11.0	390	na	2.0	10
BANANA CREAM								
(Jell-O) 'Microwave' prepared	1/2 cup	150	4.0	25.0	220	na	4.0	15
(Royal) 'Instant' prepared	1/2 cup	180	4.0	29.0	390	na	5.0	(mq)
(Royal) prepared	1/2 cup	160	4.0	27.0	210	na	4.0	(mq)
BUTTER ALMOND *(Royal)* toasted 'Instant' prepared	1/2 cup	170	4.0	30.0	350	na	4.0	(mq)
BUTTER PECAN *(Jell-O)* 'Instant' prepared	1/2 cup	170	4.0	28.0	410	na	5.0	15
BUTTERSCOTCH								
(D-Zerta) low calorie, prepared w/skim milk	1/2 cup	70	4.0	12.0	65	na	0.0	0
(Featherweight) 'Instant' prepared	1/2 cup	100	4.0	19.0	190	na	0.0	5
(Featherweight) prepared	1/2 cup	12	0.0	3.0	6	na	0.0	0
(Jell-O) 'Instant' prepared	1/2 cup	160	4.0	28.0	450	na	4.0	15
(Jell-O) 'Instant Sugar-free' prepared w/2% milk	1/2 cup	90	4.0	12.0	390	na	2.0	10
(Jell-O) 'Microwave' prepared	1/2 cup	170	4.0	28.0	180	na	4.0	15
(Jell-O) prepared	1/2 cup	170	4.0	30.0	190	na	4.0	15
(Royal) 'Instant' prepared	1/2 cup	180	4.0	29.0	390	na	5.0	(mq)
(Royal) 'Instant Sugar-free' prepared w/2% milk	1/2 cup	100	4.0	16.0	470	na	2.0	(mq)
(Royal) prepared	1/2 cup	160	4.0	27.0	210	na	4.0	(mq)
CHOCOLATE								
(D-Zerta) low calorie, prepared w/skim milk	1/2 cup	60	5.0	11.0	70	na	0.0	0
(Featherweight) 'Instant' prepared	1/2 cup	110	5.0	22.0	190	na	0.0	5
(Featherweight) prepared	1/2 cup	12	0.0	3.0	0	na	0.0	15
(Jell-O) 'Cook 'n Serve Sugar-free' prepared w/skim milk	1/2 cup	70	5.0	13.0	160	na	3.0	na

Food Name	Serv. Size	Total Cal.	Prot. GMS	Carbs GMS	Sod. MGS	Fiber GMS	Fat GMS	Chol. MGS
(Jell-O) 'Cook 'n Serve Sugar-free' prepared w/2% milk	1/2 cup	90	5.0	13.0	160	na	3.0	10
(Jell-O) 'Instant' prepared	1/2 cup	180	4.0	31.0	480	na	4.0	15
(Jell-O) 'Instant Sugar-free' prepared w/2% milk	1/2 cup	90	4.0	13.0	380	na	3.0	10
(Jell-O) 'Microwave' prepared	1/2 cup	170	5.0	28.0	190	na	5.0	15
(Jell-O) prepared	1/2 cup	160	5.0	28.0	170	na	4.0	15
(Royal) dark and sweet, prepared	1/2 cup	180	5.0	33.0	150	na	4.0	(mq)
(Royal) 'Instant' prepared	1/2 cup	190	4.0	35.0	390	na	4.0	(mq)
(Royal) 'Instant Sugar-free' prepared w/2% milk	1/2 cup	110	5.0	17.0	480	na	3.0	(mq)
(Royal) prepared	1/2 cup	180	5.0	33.0	150	na	4.0	(mq)
(Weight Watchers) 'Instant' prepared w/skim milk	1/2 cup	90	6.0	18.0	420	na	1.0	na
CHOCOLATE FUDGE								
(Jell-O) 'Instant' prepared	1/2 cup	180	5.0	31.0	440	na	5.0	15
(Jell-O) 'Instant Sugar-free' prepared w/2% milk	1/2 cup	100	5.0	14.0	330	na	3.0	10
(Jell-O) prepared	1/2 cup	160	5.0	28.0	170	na	4.0	15
CHOCOLATE-CHOCOLATE CHIP *(Royal)* prepared	1/2 cup	190	4.0	35.0	390	na	4.0	(mq)
CHOCOLATE-MINT *(Royal)* 'Instant' prepared	1/2 cup	190	4.0	35.0	390	na	4.0	(mq)
COCONUT, TOASTED *(Royal)* 'Instant' prepared	1/2 cup	170	4.0	30.0	350	na	4.0	(mq)
COCONUT CREAM *(Jell-O)* 'Instant' prepared	1/2 cup	180	4.0	27.0	320	na	6.0	15
EGG								
(Jell-O) custard 'Americana' prepared	1/2 cup	160	5.0	23.0	200	na	5.0	80
(Royal) custard, prepared	1/2 cup	150	4.0	22.0	115	na	5.0	(mq)
FLAN								
(Jell-O) prepared	1/2 cup	150	4.0	26.0	65	na	4.0	15
(Royal) w/caramel sauce, prepared	1/2 cup	150	4.0	22.0	115	na	5.0	(mq)
FRENCH VANILLA								
(Jell-O) 'Instant' prepared	1/2 cup	160	4.0	28.0	400	na	4.0	15
(Jell-O) prepared	1/2 cup	170	4.0	30.0	190	na	4.0	15
KEY LIME *(Royal)* prepared	1/2 cup	160	1.0	30.0	120	na	3.0	(mq)
LEMON								
(Featherweight) custard, prepared	1/2 cup	40	1.0	8.0	40	na	0.0	0
(French's) prepared	1/2 cup	110	1.0	22.0	110	na	1.0	na
(Jell-O) 'Instant' prepared	1/2 cup	170	4.0	29.0	360	na	4.0	15
(Royal) 'Instant' prepared	1/2 cup	180	1.0	29.0	350	na	5.0	(mq)
(Royal) prepared	1/2 cup	160	1.0	30.0	120	na	3.0	(mq)

Food Name	Serv. Size	Total Cal.	Prot. GMS	Carbs GMS	Sod. MGS	Fiber GMS	Fat GMS	Chol. MGS
MILK CHOCOLATE								
(Jell-O) 'Instant' prepared	1/2 cup	180	5.0	31.0	470	na	5.0	15
(Jell-O) 'Microwave' prepared	1/2 cup	160	4.0	27.0	190	na	5.0	15
(Jell-O) prepared	1/2 cup	160	4.0	28.0	170	na	4.0	15
PISTACHIO								
(Jell-O) 'Instant' prepared	1/2 cup	170	4.0	28.0	410	na	5.0	15
(Jell-O) 'Instant Sugar-free' prepared								
w/2% milk	1/2 cup	90	4.0	12.0	390	na	3.0	10
(Royal) nut 'Instant' prepared	1/2 cup	170	4.0	30.0	350	na	4.0	(mq)
RASPBERRY (Salada) pudding and								
pie glaze, prepared	1/2 cup	130	0.0	32.0	5	na	0.0	0
RICE (Jell-O) 'Americana' prepared	1/2 cup	170	5.0	30.0	160	na	4.0	15
STRAWBERRY (Salada) pudding and								
pie glaze, prepared	1/2 cup	130	0.0	32.0	5	na	0.0	0
VANILLA								
(D-Zerta) low calorie, prepared								
w/skim milk	1/2 cup	70	4.0	12.0	65	na	0.0	0
(Featherweight) custard, prepared	1/2 cup	40	1.0	8.0	40	na	0.0	0
(Featherweight) 'Instant' prepared	1/2 cup	100	4.0	19.0	190	na	0.0	5
(Featherweight) prepared	1/2 cup	12	0.0	3.0	6	na	0.0	0
(Jell-O) 'Cook 'n Serve Sugar-free'								
prepared w/skim milk	1/2 cup	60	4.0	11.0	200	na	2.0	na
(Jell-O) 'Cook 'n Serve Sugar-free'								
prepared w/2% milk	1/2 cup	80	4.0	11.0	200	na	2.0	10
(Jell-O) 'Instant' prepared	1/2 cup	170	4.0	29.0	410	na	4.0	15
(Jell-O) 'Instant Sugar-free' prepared								
w/2% milk	1/2 cup	90	4.0	12.0	390	na	2.0	10
(Jell-O) 'Microwave' prepared	1/2 cup	160	4.0	26.0	180	na	4.0	15
(Jell-O) prepared	1/2 cup	160	4.0	26.0	200	na	4.0	15
(Jell-O) tapioca 'Americana' prepared ..	1/2 cup	160	4.0	27.0	170	na	4.0	15
(Royal) 'Instant' prepared	1/2 cup	180	4.0	29.0	390	na	5.0	(mq)
(Royal) 'Instant Sugar-free' prepared								
w/2% milk	1/2 cup	100	4.0	16.0	470	na	2.0	na
(Royal) prepared	1/2 cup	160	4.0	27.0	210	na	4.0	(mq)
(Royal) tapioca, prepared	1/2 cup	160	4.0	27.0	150	na	4.0	(mq)
PUDDING/PIE FILLING MIX. See also PUDDING MIX.								
BANANA (Jell-O) instant, sugar-free,								
prepared w/2% milk	1/2 cup	80	4.0	11.0	390	na	2.0	10
BANANA CREAM								
(Jell-O) instant, prepared	1/2 cup	160	4.0	28.0	410	na	4.0	15
(Jell-O) microwave, prepared	1/2 cup	150	4.0	25.0	220	na	4.0	15
(Jell-O) prepared, w/o crust	1/6 pie	100	3.0	17.0	160	na	3.0	10
(Royal) dry	1 serving	80	0.0	20.0	110	0	0.0	0

Food Name	Serv. Size	Total Cal.	Prot. GMS	Carbs GMS	Sod. MGS	Fiber GMS	Fat GMS	Chol. MGS
(Royal) instant, dry	1 serving	90	0.0	22.0	390	na	0.0	0
BUTTER PECAN *(Jell-O)* instant,								
prepared	1/2 cup	170	4.0	28.0	410	na	5.0	15
BUTTERSCOTCH								
(D-Zerta) reduced calorie, prepared	1/2 cup	70	4.0	12.0	65	na	0.0	0
(Jell-O) instant, prepared	1/2 cup	160	4.0	28.0	450	na	4.0	15
(Jell-O) instant, sugar-free, prepared								
w/2% milk	1/2 cup	90	4.0	12.0	390	na	2.0	10
(Jell-O) microwave, prepared	1/2 cup	170	4.0	28.0	180	na	4.0	15
(Jell-O) prepared	1/2 cup	170	4.0	30.0	190	na	4.0	15
(Nabisco) 'My•T•Fine' prepared	1/2 cup	90	0.0	22.0	190	na	0.0	na
(Royal) instant, dry	1 serving	90	0.0	22.0	400	na	0.0	0
(Royal) prepared	1/2 cup	90	0.0	23.0	180	0	0.0	0
CHERRY-VANILLA *(Royal)* instant, dry	1 serving	90	0.0	23.0	300	0	0.0	0
CHOCOLATE								
(D-Zerta) reduced calorie, prepared	1/2 cup	60	5.0	11.0	70	na	0.0	0
(Jell-O) instant, prepared	1/2 cup	180	4.0	31.0	480	na	4.0	15
(Jell-O) instant, sugar-free, prepared								
w/2% milk	1/2 cup	90	4.0	13.0	380	na	3.0	10
(Jell-O) microwave, prepared	1/2 cup	170	5.0	28.0	190	na	5.0	15
(Jell-O) prepared	1/2 cup	160	5.0	28.0	170	na	4.0	15
(Jell-O) sugar-free, prepared w/2% milk	1/2 cup	90	5.0	13.0	160	na	3.0	10
(Nabisco) 'My•T•Fine' prepared	1/2 cup	100	1.0	23.0	135	0	0.0	0
(Royal) dark and sweet, instant, dry	1 serving	110	1.0	25.0	460	0	0.0	0
(Royal) dark and sweet, prepared	1/2 cup	90	1.0	22.0	95	1.0	0.0	0
(Royal) instant, dry	1 serving	110	1.0	27.0	450	0	0.0	0
(Royal) instant, sugar-free, prepared	1/2 cup	50	0.0	11.0	420	na	0.0	na
(Royal) prepared	1/2 cup	90	1.0	22.0	90	0	0.0	0
CHOCOLATE FUDGE								
(Jell-O) instant, prepared	1/2 cup	180	5.0	31.0	440	na	5.0	15
(Jell-O) instant, sugar-free, prepared								
w/2% milk	1/2 cup	100	5.0	14.0	330	na	3.0	10
(Jell-O) prepared	1/2 cup	160	5.0	28.0	170	na	4.0	15
(Nabisco) 'My•T•Fine' prepared	1/2 cup	100	1.0	24.0	140	1.0	0.0	na
CHOCOLATE-ALMOND								
(Nabisco) 'My•T•Fine' prepared	1/2 cup	100	1.0	23.0	135	na	1.0	0
(Royal) instant, prepared	1/2 cup	120	0.0	26.0	440	na	1.0	na
CHOCOLATE-CHOCOLATE CHIP *(Royal)*								
instant, dry	1 serving	110	1.0	26.0	390	0	1.0	0
CHOCOLATE-PEANUT BUTTER CHIP								
(Royal) instant, dry	1 serving	110	1.0	26.0	480	0	1.0	0
COCONUT, TOASTED *(Royal)* instant,								
prepared	1/2 cup	100	0.0	20.0	450	na	2.0	na

Food Name	Serv. Size	Total Cal.	Prot. GMS	Carbs GMS	Sod. MGS	Fiber GMS	Fat GMS	Chol. MGS
COCONUT CREAM								
(Jell-O) instant, prepared	1/2 cup	180	4.0	27.0	320	na	6.0	15
(Jell-O) prepared, w/o crust	1/6 pie	110	3.0	16.0	140	na	4.0	10
EGG (Royal) custard, prepared	1/2 cup	60	0.0	16.0	75	na	0.0	na
FLAN								
(Jell-O) prepared	1/2 cup	150	4.0	26.0	65	na	4.0	15
(Royal) caramel custard, prepared	1/2 cup	60	0.0	15.0	55	na	0.0	na
FRENCH VANILLA								
(Jell-O) instant, prepared	1/2 cup	160	4.0	28.0	400	na	4.0	15
(Jell-O) prepared	1/2 cup	170	4.0	30.0	190	na	4.0	15
LEMON								
(Jell-O) instant, prepared	1/2 cup	170	4.0	29.0	360	na	4.0	15
(Nabisco) 'My•T•Fine' dry	1 serving	90	0.0	22.0	170	na	0.0	0
(Royal) instant, dry	1 serving	90	0.0	23.0	320	na	0.0	0
MILK CHOCOLATE								
(Jell-O) instant, prepared	1/2 cup	180	5.0	31.0	470	na	5.0	15
(Jell-O) microwave, prepared	1/2 cup	160	4.0	27.0	190	na	5.0	15
(Jell-O) prepared	1/2 cup	160	4.0	28.0	170	na	4.0	15
PISTACHIO								
(Jell-O) instant, prepared	1/2 cup	170	4.0	28.0	410	na	5.0	15
(Jell-O) instant, sugar-free, prepared w/2% milk	1/2 cup	90	4.0	12.0	390	na	3.0	10
(Royal) instant, dry	1 serving	90	0.0	22.0	360	0	1.0	0
STRAWBERRY (Royal) instant, dry	1 serving	100	0.0	24.0	330	na	0.0	0
TAPIOCA (Nabisco) 'My•T•Fine' dry	1 serving	80	0.0	19.0	160	na	0.0	0
VANILLA								
(D-Zerta) reduced calorie, w/aspartame, prepared	1/2 cup	70	4.0	12.0	65	na	0.0	0
(Jell-O) instant, prepared	1/2 cup	170	4.0	29.0	410	na	4.0	15
(Jell-O) instant, sugar-free, prepared w/2% milk	1/2 cup	90	4.0	12.0	390	na	2.0	10
(Jell-O) microwave, prepared	1/2 cup	160	4.0	26.0	180	na	4.0	15
(Jell-O) prepared	1/2 cup	160	4.0	26.0	200	na	4.0	15
(Jell-O) sugar-free, w/aspartame, prepared w/2% milk	1/2 cup	80	4.0	11.0	200	na	2.0	10
(Nabisco) 'My•T•Fine' prepared	1/2 cup	90	0.0	22.0	120	0	0.0	0
(Royal) instant, dry	1 serving	90	0.0	23.0	325	na	0.0	0
VANILLA-CHOCOLATE CHIP (Royal) instant, dry	1 serving	90	0.0	22.0	350	0	1.0	0
PUERTO RICAN CHERRY. See CHERRY, PUERTO RICAN.								
PUFF PASTRY, FROZEN								
sheet (Pepperidge Farm)	1/4 sheet	260	4.0	22.0	290	(mq)	17.0	na
shell, mini (Pepperidge Farm)	1 shell	50	1.0	4.0	40	(mq)	4.0	na

Food Name	Serv. Size	Total Cal.	Prot. GMS	Carbs GMS	Sod. MGS	Fiber GMS	Fat GMS	Chol. MGS
shell, patty *(Pepperidge Farm)*	1 shell	210	3.0	16.0	180	(mq)	15.0	na
shell, ready to bake	1 shell	259	3.4	21.2	117	na	17.9	0
shell, ready to bake	1 oz	156	2.1	12.8	71	na	10.8	0
PUMELO. See POMELO.								
PUMPKIN								
boiled, drained	4 oz	23	0.8	5.5	1	>.9 c	0.1	0
boiled, drained, mashed	1/2 cup	24	0.9	6.0	1	>1.0 c	0.1	0
raw, 1-inch cubes	1/2 cup	15	0.6	3.8	1	1.0	0.1	0
raw, trimmed	1 oz	7	0.3	1.8	<1	>.3 c	<.1	0
raw, untrimmed	1 lb	83	3.2	20.6	3	>3.5 c	0.3	0
PUMPKIN, CANNED								
	1/2 cup	41	1.3	9.9	6	3.4	0.3	0
w/winter squash	4 oz	39	1.2	9.2	6	>1.8 c	0.3	0
(Del Monte)	1/2 cup	35	1.0	9.0	10	(mq)	0.0	0
(Libby's)	1/2 cup	42	1.4	10.1	6	3.8	0.4	0
(Libby's) solid pack	1/2 cup	42	1.4	10.1	6	3.8	0.4	na
(Stokely)	1/2 cup	40	2.0	10.0	15	(mq)	0.0	0
PUMPKIN FLOWER								
boiled, drained	4 oz	17	1.2	3.7	7	>1.0 c	0.1	0
boiled, drained	1/2 cup	10	0.7	2.2	4	.6	0.1	0
raw	1 cup	5	0.3	1.1	2	>.2 c	0.0	0
raw, trimmed	1 oz	4	0.3	0.9	1	>.2 c	<.1	0
raw, trimmed	1/2 cup	3	0.2	0.5	1	>.1 c	<.1	0
raw, untrimmed	1 lb	23	1.6	5.2	7	>1.0 c	0.1	0
PUMPKIN LEAF								
boiled, drained	4 oz	24	3.1	3.8	9	>1.2 c	0.2	0
boiled, drained	1/2 cup	7	1.0	1.2	3	1.0	0.1	0
raw	1/2 cup	4	0.6	0.5	2	>.2 c	0.1	0
raw, trimmed	1 oz	5	0.9	0.7	3	>.3 c	0.1	0
raw, untrimmed	1 lb	36	5.9	4.3	20	>1.9 c	0.7	0
PUMPKIN PIE SPICE								
dried	1 tbsp	19	0.3	3.9	3	.8	0.7	0
dried	1 tsp	6	0.1	1.2	1	.3	0.2	0
PUMPKIN SEED								
dried	1 lb	1817	82.4	59.8	59	>7.5 c	153.9	0
roasted	1 lb	2021	84.1	243.8	82	>162.8 c	88.0	0
roasted	1 cup	285	11.9	34.4	12	>23.0 c	12.4	0
roasted, approx 85 seeds	1 oz	127	5.3	15.3	5	>10.2 c	5.5	0
w/squash seeds, roasted	1 cup	285	11.9	34.4	12	>23.0 c	12.4	0
w/squash seeds, roasted	1 oz	127	5.3	15.3	5	>10.2 c	5.5	0
PUMPKIN SEED, SHELLED								
dried	1 cup	747	33.9	24.6	24	19.0	63.3	0
dried, approx 142 kernels	1 oz	154	7.0	5.1	5	3.9	13.0	0

Food Name	Serv. Size	Total Cal.	Prot. GMS	Carbs GMS	Sod. MGS	Fiber GMS	Fat GMS	Chol. MGS
roasted	1 cup	1184	74.8	30.5	40	14.7	95.6	0
roasted	1 oz	148	9.4	3.8	5	1.9	12.0	0
w/squash seed kernels, dried	1 cup	747	33.9	24.6	25	19.0	63.3	0
w/squash seed kernels, dried, approx 142 kernels	1 oz	154	7.0	5.1	5	3.9	13.0	0
w/squash seed kernels, roasted	1 cup	1185	74.8	30.5	41	14.7	95.6	0
w/squash seed kernels, roasted	1 oz	149	9.4	3.8	6	1.9	12.0	0
PUNCH. See also FRUIT PUNCH; and individual listings.								
(J. Hungerford)	9.03 oz	133	0.0	33.4	2	0	0.0	0
(Squeezit) 'Mean Green Puncher'	6.75 oz	100	0.0	25.0	5	na	0.0	na
(Squeezit) 'Rockin Red Puncher'	6.75 oz	110	0.0	28.0	5	na	0.0	na
PURPLESAURUS REX DRINK MIX								
(Kool-Aid) sugar-free, w/NutraSweet, prepared	8 oz	4	0.0	0.0	5	na	0.0	0
(Kool-Aid) sugar-sweetened, prepared	8 oz	80	0.0	21.0	5	na	0.0	0
(Kool-Aid) unsweetened, prepared w/sugar	8 oz	100	0.0	25.0	5	na	0.0	0
(Kool-Aid) unsweetened, prepared w/o sugar	8 oz	2	0.0	0.0	5	na	0.0	0
PURSLANE/pussley								
boiled, drained	4 oz	20	1.7	4.0	50	>.9 c	0.2	0
boiled, drained	1/2 cup	10	0.9	2.1	26	>.5 c	0.1	0
raw	1 cup	7	0.6	1.5	19	>.3 c	0.0	0
raw, trimmed	1 oz	5	0.4	1.0	13	>.2 c	<.1	0
raw, trimmed	1/2 cup	4	0.3	0.7	10	>.2 c	<.1	0
raw, untrimmed	1 lb	56	4.5	11.8	156	>2.8 c	0.3	0

Q

Food Name	Serv. Size	Total Cal.	Prot. GMS	Carbs GMS	Sod. MGS	Fiber GMS	Fat GMS	Chol. MGS
QUAIL/bobwhite								
breast meat only, raw	1 oz	35	6.4	0.0	16	0	0.8	(mq)
meat and skin, raw	1 oz	54	5.6	0.0	15	0	3.4	(mq)
raw	1 oz	34	6.0	0.0	29	0	0.9	24
QUAIL GIBLETS, raw	3.5 oz	176	21.8	6.7	70	0	6.2	350
QUICHE								
(Nancy's) Classic French, Monterey jack and swiss, w/bacon	1 quiche	520	21.0	30.0	670	1.0	37.0	210
(Nancy's) French baked, broccoli, cheddar	1 quiche	490	17.0	33.0	750	2.0	33.0	165
QUINCE								
raw, trimmed	1 med	52	0.4	14.1	4	1.8	0.1	0
raw, trimmed	1 oz	16	0.1	4.3	1	>.5 c	<.1	0
raw, untrimmed	1 lb	158	1.1	42.3	11	>4.7 c	0.3	0
QUINOA, WHOLE GRAIN								
dry	1/2 cup	318	11.1	58.6	18	5.0	4.9	0

Food Name	Serv. Size	Total Cal.	Prot. GMS	Carbs GMS	Sod. MGS	Fiber GMS	Fat GMS	Chol. MGS
dry	1 oz	106	3.7	19.5	na	(mq)	1.6	0
dry *(Ancient Harvest)*	1/4 cup	159	5.0	28.0	8	5.7	2.0	0
dry *(Eden Foods)*	2 oz	200	8.0	38.0	30	4.3	4.0	0
dry *(Quinoa)*	1/4 cup	159	5.0	28.0	8	5.7	2.0	0
steam-rolled, flakes *(Ancient Harvest)*	1/3 cup	105	2.6	23.0	5	2.8	1.0	0
steam-rolled, flakes *(Quinoa)*	1/3 cup	105	2.6	23.0	5	2.8	1.0	0
QUINOA FLOUR, WHOLE GRAIN								
non-gluten *(Ancient Harvest)*	1/4 cup	132	4.0	24.0	10	4.7	2.0	0
non-gluten *(Quinoa)*	1/4 cup	132	4.0	24.0	10	4.7	2.0	0
QUINOA PASTA. See PASTA.								
QUINOA SEED *(Arrowhead Mills)*	2 oz	200	9.0	35.0	3	5.3	3.0	0

R

Food Name	Serv. Size	Total Cal.	Prot. GMS	Carbs GMS	Sod. MGS	Fiber GMS	Fat GMS	Chol. MGS
RABBIT								
Domesticated								
raw	1 lb	617	91.0	0.0	186	na	25.2	259
raw	1 oz	38	5.6	0.0	11	na	1.5	16
roasted	3 oz	167	24.7	0.0	40	na	6.8	70
roasted, diced	1 cup	216	31.9	0.0	52	0	8.8	90
stewed	3 oz	175	25.8	0.0	31	na	7.2	73
stewed, diced	1 cup	288	42.5	0.0	52	0	11.8	120
Wild								
raw	1 lb	517	98.8	0.0	227	na	10.5	367
raw	1 oz	32	6.1	0.0	14	na	0.7	23
stewed	3 oz	147	28.1	0.0	38	na	3.0	105
stewed, diced	1 cup	242	46.2	0.0	63	0	4.9	172
RACCOON								
roasted	3 oz	217	24.8	0.0	na	na	12.3	na
roasted, diced	1 cup	357	40.9	0.0	(mq)	0	20.3	(mq)
RADICCHIO								
raw	1 med	2	0.1	0.4	2	na	0.0	0
raw, shredded	1/2 cup	5	0.3	0.9	4	na	0.1	0
RADISH								
fresh *(Dole)*	7 med	20	0.0	3.0	35	(mq)	0.0	na
raw, sliced	1/2 cup	10	0.4	2.1	14	.9	0.3	0
raw, 1 inch long, 3/4 inch diam	10 radishes	8	0.3	1.6	11	.7	0.2	0
raw, trimmed	1 oz	5	0.2	1.0	7	.7	0.2	0
raw, untrimmed	1 lb	68	2.5	14.6	98	>2.2 c	2.2	0
RADISH, BLACK/winter radish								
raw, trimmed	1 lb	77	4.5	16.3	82	(mq)	0.5	0

Food Name	Serv. Size	Total Cal.	Prot. GMS	Carbs GMS	Sod. MGS	Fiber GMS	Fat GMS	Chol. MGS
raw, trimmed	1 oz	5	0.3	1.0	5	(mq)	<.1	0

RADISH, ORIENTAL. See DAIKON.

RADISH, WHITE ICICLE

raw	1 med	2	0.2	0.5	3	>.1 c	0.0	0
raw, sliced	1/2 cup	7	0.6	1.3	8	>.4 c	0.1	0
raw, trimmed	1 oz	4	0.3	0.7	5	>.2 c	<.1	0
raw, untrimmed	1 lb	41	3.2	7.7	47	>2.1 c	0.3	0

RADISH, WINTER. See RADISH, BLACK.

| **RADISH LEAVES,** trimmed .... | 1 oz | 15 | 0.8 | 2.8 | (mq) | >.4 c | 0.1 | 0 |

RADISH SEED

sprouted	1 lb	186	17.3	13.9	28	(mq)	11.5	0
sprouted	1 oz	12	1.1	0.9	2	(mq)	0.7	0
sprouted, raw	1/2 cup	8	0.7	0.7	1	>.4 c	0.5	0

RAG GOURD. See GOURD, DISHCLOTH.

| **RAINBOW PUNCH** (Kool-Aid) 'Koolers' | 8.45 oz | 130 | 0.0 | 36.0 | 10 | na | 0.0 | 0 |

RAINBOW PUNCH MIX

(Kool-Aid) sugar-sweetened	8 oz	80	0.0	21.0	20	na	0.0	0
(Kool-Aid) unsweetened, prepared w/sugar	8 oz	100	0.0	25.0	0	na	0.0	0
(Kool-Aid) unsweetened, prepared w/o sugar	8 oz	2	0.0	0.0	0	na	0.0	0

RAINBOW SMELT. See SMELT, RAINBOW.

RAISIN

Dark

seedless	1 cup packed	495	5.3	130.6	20	8.8	0.8	0
seedless	1 cup	435	4.7	114.7	17	7.7	0.7	0
seedless	1 oz	85	0.9	22.4	3	1.5	0.1	0
seedless (Cinderella) Thompson	1/2 cup	250	3.0	66.0	15	5.8	0.0	0
seedless (Dole)	1/2 cup	260	3.0	63.0	25	(mq)	0.0	0
seedless (Finast)	.5 oz	45	0.0	11.0	5	(mq)	0.0	0
seedless (Sun•Maid)	1/2 cup	290	3.0	69.0	15	(mq)	0.0	0
seedless (Sun•Maid) California sun-dried,								
100% natural	1/2 cup	250	3.0	68.0	10	4.5	0.0	na
w/seeds	1 cup packed	488	4.2	129.5	46	11.2	0.9	0
w/seeds	1 cup	429	3.7	113.8	41	9.9	0.8	0
w/seeds	1 oz	84	0.7	22.2	8	.2	0.2	0
w/seeds (Sun•Maid) Muscat	1/2 cup	270	2.0	67.0	25	na	1.0	na

Golden

seedless	1 lb	1368	15.4	360.7	54	15.9	2.1	0
seedless	1 cup packed	498	5.6	131.2	20	5.8	0.8	0
seedless	1 cup	438	4.9	115.3	17	>2.1 c	0.7	0
seedless	1 oz	86	1.0	22.5	3	>.4 c	0.1	0
seedless (Del Monte) natural	3 oz	250	3.0	68.0	15	(mq)	0.0	0
seedless (Dole)	1/2 cup	260	3.0	63.0	25	(mq)	0.0	0
w/seed (Del Monte)	3 oz	260	3.0	68.0	10	(mq)	0.0	0

Food Name	Serv. Size	Total Cal.	Prot. GMS	Carbs GMS	Sod. MGS	Fiber GMS	Fat GMS	Chol. MGS
w/seed (Dole)	1/2 cup	250	3.0	66.0	25	na	0.0	na
w/seed (Sun•Maid) California	1/2 cup	250	3.0	68.0	10	4.5	0.0	na
RASPBERRY/bramble								
trimmed	1 pint	153	2.8	36.1	0	21.2	1.7	0
trimmed	1 cup	60	1.1	14.2	0	8.4	0.7	0
trimmed	1 oz	14	0.3	3.3	tr	1.3	0.2	0
untrimmed	1 lb	215	4.0	50.4	1	20.5	2.4	0
untrimmed	1 pint	154	2.8	36.1	tr	15.3	1.7	0
Canned								
red, in heavy syrup	4 oz	103	0.9	26.5	3	(mq)	0.1	0
red, in heavy syrup, solid and liquid	1/2 cup	116	1.1	29.9	4	4.2	0.2	0
Frozen								
red, in light syrup (Birds Eye) 'Quick Thaw Pouch'	5 oz	100	1.0	25.0	0	4.0	1.0	0
red, sweetened, unthawed	10 oz	293	2.0	74.3	3	12.5	0.5	0
red, sweetened, unthawed	1 cup	258	1.8	65.4	3	11.0	0.4	0
sweetened	10 oz	291	2.0	74.3	1	12.5	0.5	0
sweetened	1/2 cup	128	0.9	32.7	1	6.3	0.2	0
sweetened	4 oz	117	0.8	29.7	1	5.0	0.2	0
RASPBERRY DRINK, W/CRANBERRY								
(A&P)	6 oz	110	<1.0	27.0	0	(tr)	<1.0	0
(Finast)	6 oz	110	0.0	27.0	10	(tr)	0.0	0
(Pathmark)	6 oz	110	0.0	27.0	10	(tr)	0.0	0
(Pathmark) 'Sodium Free'	6 oz	110	0.0	27.0	0	(tr)	0.0	0
RASPBERRY JUICE								
(Apple & Eve) w/cranberry	6 oz	90	0.0	21.0	10	(mq)	0.0	0
(Dole) blend 'Pure & Light Country Raspberry'	6 oz	87	0.3	24.0	15	(tr)	0.2	0
(Santa Cruz Natural) red, organic	8 oz	120	1.0	28.0	na	na	<1.0	na
(Smucker's) red 'Naturally 100%'	8 oz	120	0.0	30.0	10	(tr)	0.0	0
RASPBERRY JUICE COCKTAIL								
(Welch's) 'Orchard,' bottled	10 oz	160	0.0	40.0	10	0	0.0	0
RASPBERRY JUICE FLOAT								
(Knudsen & Sons)	8 oz	130	2.0	31.0	na	na	0.0	na
RASPBERRY LEMONADE								
(Knudsen & Sons)	8 oz	110	<1.0	28.0	na	na	0.0	na
(Santa Cruz Natural) organic	8 oz	60	<1.0	20.0	na	na	<1.0	na
(Santa Cruz Natural) 'Sparkling' organic	8 oz	85	<1.0	20.0	na	na	<1.0	na
RASPBERRY NECTAR (Knudsen & Sons)	8 oz	120	<1.0	30.0	na	na	0.0	na
RASPBERRY PUNCH MIX								
(Kool-Aid) sugar-sweetened, prepared	8 oz	80	0.0	20.0	25	na	0.0	0
(Kool-Aid) unsweetened, prepared w/sugar	8 oz	100	0.0	25.0	25	na	0.0	0

Food Name	Serv. Size	Total Cal.	Prot. GMS	Carbs GMS	Sod. MGS	Fiber GMS	Fat GMS	Chol. MGS
(Kool-Aid) unsweetened, prepared								
w/o sugar	8 oz	2	0.0	0.0	25	na	0.0	0
RASPBERRY SYRUP *(Knudsen & Sons)* ...	1 oz	75	<1.0	18.0	na	na	<1.0	na
RASPBERRY TOPPING, fat-free *(Smucker's)*								
'Light'	2 tbsp	55	0.0	14.0	0	na	0.0	na
RASPBERRY-PEACH JUICE								
(Knudsen & Sons)	8 oz	115	<1.0	28.0	na	na	0.0	na
RAVIOLI ENTRÉE								
CANNED								
Beef								
(Chef Boyardee) 'Sir Chomps'	7.5 oz	170	7.0	32.0	690	4.0	3.0	15
(Chef Boyardee) w/meat sauce 'Smurfs'	7.5 oz	230	9.0	38.0	1160	na	5.0	11
(Estee)	7.5 oz	230	8.0	25.0	100	(mq)	11.0	10
(Finast) w/sauce	7.5 oz	250	7.0	33.0	1165	(mq)	10.0	(mq)
(Franco-American) w/meat sauce								
'RavioliO's'	7.5 oz	250	10.0	35.0	920	(mq)	8.0	(mq)
(Nalley's)	7.5 oz	180	8.0	30.0	1040	(mq)	3.0	(mq)
(Pathmark) bite size, w/tomato sauce								
'No Frills'	7.5 oz	180	7.0	28.0	890	(mq)	4.0	(mq)
(Pathmark) w/tomato sauce 'No Frills' ...	7.5 oz	180	7.0	28.0	890	(mq)	4.0	(mq)
Cheese								
(Buitoni) w/sauce	7.5 oz	190	7.0	27.0	790	(mq)	6.0	5
(Chef Boyardee) 'Sir Chomps'	7.5 oz	170	6.0	38.0	740	6.0	1.0	5
(Pathmark) w/tomato sauce 'No Frills' ..	7.5 oz	185	7.0	27.0	790	(mq)	6.0	(mq)
Chicken								
(Buitoni) meat, w/sauce	7.5 oz	180	7.0	28.0	890	(mq)	4.0	5
(Chef Boyardee)	7.5 oz	180	7.0	29.0	1100	na	4.0	13
(Chef Boyardee) mini	7.5 oz	220	7.0	29.0	1090	na	8.0	na
FROZEN								
(Celentano)	6.5 oz	380	21.0	50.0	510	(mq)	11.0	(mq)
(Celentano) mini	4 oz	250	13.0	39.0	210	(mq)	5.0	(mq)
Cheese								
(Amy's Kitchen) organic	1 cup	215	12.0	26.0	346	3.0	5.0	7
(Buitoni)	4 oz	360	12.0	31.0	220	(mq)	8.0	65
(Healthy Choice) baked	9 oz	250	14.0	44.0	420	na	2.0	20
(Kid Cuisine) mini	8.75 oz	250	6.0	52.0	730	(mq)	2.0	20
(Lean Cuisine) w/tomato sauce	8.5 oz	240	13.0	30.0	590	na	8.0	55
(Smart Ones) Florentine	8.5 oz	130	8.0	22.0	540	na	1.0	5
(Ultra Slim Fast)	12 oz	330	21.0	60.0	770	na	3.0	40
(Weight Watchers) baked	9 oz	240	18.0	27.0	370	na	6.0	30
MICROWAVE								
(Kid's Kitchen) mini microwave cup	7.5 oz	230	10.0	34.0	870	na	6.0	15

Food Name	Serv. Size	Total Cal.	Prot. GMS	Carbs GMS	Sod. MGS	Fiber GMS	Fat GMS	Chol. MGS
Beef								
(Chef Boyardee)	7.5 oz	190	7.0	31.0	1160	2.0	4.0	11
(Chef Boyardee) 'Main Meals'								
microwave cup	10.5 oz	290	12.0	52.0	na	na	4.0	na
(Hormel) w/tomato sauce micro cup	7.5 oz	247	8.0	28.0	951	(mq)	11.0	21
(Libby's) w/sauce 'Diner' microwave cup	7.75 oz	240	13.0	35.0	890	2.2	5.0	15
Cheese, w/rneat sauce (Chef Boyardee)	7.5 oz	200	6.0	37.0	1010	(mq)	3.0	10
REFRIGERATED								
(Contadina) w/beef 'Fresh'	3 oz	270	13.0	30.0	250	na	11.0	75
(Contadina) w/cheese 'Fresh'	3 oz	270	13.0	30.0	360	na	11.0	75
(DiGiorno) w/Italian herb cheese, cooked	1 cup	280	12.0	35.0	490	na	10.0	35
(DiGiorno) w/Italian sausage, cooked	1 cup	270	13.0	34.0	520	na	9.0	40
RAZZLEBERRY JUICE (Knudsen & Sons)	8 oz	90	<1.0	21.0	na	na	0.0	na
RED BEAN, CANNED								
(A&P)	1/2 cup	120	7.0	23.0	400	(mq)	<1.0	0
(Allens)	1/2 cup	115	7.0	20.0	350	(mq)	<1.0	0
(Bush's Best)	1/2 cup	70	5.0	17.0	350	6.0	0.0	na
(Green Giant)	1/2 cup	90	6.0	19.0	340	5.0	1.0	0
(Joan of Arc)	1/2 cup	90	6.0	19.0	340	5.0	1.0	0
(Van Camp's)	1 cup	194	11.0	38.0	928	(mq)	0.6	0
Small								
(B&M) baked style	8 oz	223	9.0	36.0	725	11.0	5.0	5
(Hunt's)	4.48 oz	89	6.2	18.9	713	5.5	0.5	0
RED CABBAGE. See CABBAGE, RED.								
RED CURRY BASE (A Taste of Thai)	1 tbsp	20	0.0	1.0	430	0	1.5	0
RED PERCH. See OCEAN PERCH, ATLANTIC.								
REDFISH. See OCEAN PERCH, ATLANTIC.								
REDHEAD. See SHEEPSHEAD.								
REFRIED BEANS, CANNED								
	1/2 cup	135	7.8	23.3	534	6.7	1.4	0
	4 oz	121	7.1	21.0	481	6.0	1.2	na
(Del Monte)	1/2 cup	130	6.0	20.0	530	(mq)	2.0	na
(Gebhardt)	4 oz	130	7.0	20.0	490	(mq)	2.0	na
(Little Pancho)	1/2 cup	80	6.0	15.0	330	(mq)	0.0	na
(Old El Paso)	1/4 cup	55	3.0	8.0	200	2.5	<1.0	1
(Rosarita)	4.5 oz	109	6.1	19.8	497	6.2	2.8	1
NO-FAT (Rosarita)	4.5 oz	92	7.3	19.5	481	6.2	0.5	0
ORGANIC								
(Bearitos)	1 oz	30	1.7	4.8	61	.3	0.5	0
(Bearitos) no salt	1 oz	29	1.7	4.7	2	.2	0.5	0
(Bearitos) spicy	1 oz	31	1.6	4.9	56	.5	0.6	0
SPICY								
(Del Monte)	1/2 cup	130	6.0	20.0	480	(mq)	2.0	na

Food Name	Serv. Size	Total Cal.	Prot. GMS	Carbs GMS	Sod. MGS	Fiber GMS	Fat GMS	Chol. MGS
(Old El Paso)	1/4 cup	35	1.0	5.0	280	2.0	1.0	1
(Rosarita)	4.5 oz	109	6.4	19.9	530	6.2	2.6	1
VEGETARIAN								
(Old El Paso) spicy	1/4 cup	70	6.0	15.0	730	5.0	1.0	0
(Rosarita)	4.5 oz	118	7.7	20.9	550	6.0	2.3	0
(Rosarita) spicy	4 oz	120	7.0	19.0	470	(mq)	2.0	0
(Rosarita) w/canola oil	4 oz	100	7.0	18.0	480	6.0	2.0	0
(Rosarita) w/soybean oil	4 oz	100	7.0	18.0	480	6.0	2.0	0
W/BACON (Rosarita)	4.5 oz	116	8.2	18.7	489	8.2	3.1	1
W/CHEESE (Old El Paso)	1/4 cup	36	2.0	4.0	280	2.0	1.0	2
W/GREEN CHILIES								
(Little Pancho)	1/2 cup	80	6.0	15.0	330	(mq)	0.0	na
(Old El Paso)	1/4 cup	49	3.0	8.0	252	2.5	<1.0	na
(Rosarita)	4.5 oz	110	6.1	19.7	495	6.0	2.9	1
W/JALAPEÑO (Gebhardt)	4.5 oz	106	6.8	19.0	380	6.0	3.0	1
W/NACHO CHEESE (Rosarita)	4.5 oz	122	7.9	20.6	482	6.2	3.1	1
W/ONION (Rosarita)	4.5 oz	114	6.4	20.8	508	6.2	2.8	1
W/SAUSAGE (Old El Paso)	1/4 cup	180	6.0	8.0	300	(mq)	8.0	(mq)
REFRIED BEANS, DRIED (Rosarita)	1/3 cup	123	7.2	20.5	469	6.9	4.5	0
REFRIED BEANS ENTRÉE (Chi-Chi's)	7.5 oz	250	9.0	29.0	930	na	11.0	5
REFRIED BEANS MIX								
(Fantastic Foods) instant, prepared w/o added ingredients	1/2 cup	157	10.0	28.0	400	(mq)	2.0	0
(Fantastic Foods) instant, prepared w/2 tbsp salted butter	1/2 cup	207	10.0	28.0	469	(mq)	8.0	na
RELISH. See also specific listings.								
CHOWCHOW								
sour, w/cauliflower, onion, mustard	1 cup	70	3.4	9.8	3211	>1.4 c	3.1	0
sweet, w/cauliflower, onion, mustard	1 cup	284	3.7	66.2	1291	>2.2 c	2.2	0
CRANBERRY-ORANGE								
canned	1/2 cup	246	0.4	63.8	44	>.8 c	0.1	0
canned	4 oz	202	0.3	52.4	36	>.7 c	0.1	0
DILL (Vlasic)	1 oz	2	0.0	1.0	415	(mq)	0.0	0
HAMBURGER								
pickle	1/2 cup	157	0.8	42.1	1337	>1.1 c	0.7	0
pickle	1 tbsp	19	0.1	5.2	164	>.1 c	0.1	0
(Heinz)	1 oz	40	0.0	9.0	255	(mq)	0.0	0
HOT DOG								
pickle	1/2 cup	111	1.8	28.5	1331	>1.1 c	0.6	0
pickle	1 tbsp	14	0.2	3.5	164	>.1 c	0.1	0
(Heinz)	1 oz	35	0.0	8.0	200	(mq)	0.0	0
(Vlasic)	1 oz	40	0.0	8.0	255	(mq)	1.0	0

Food Name	Serv. Size	Total Cal.	Prot. GMS	Carbs GMS	Sod. MGS	Fiber GMS	Fat GMS	Chol. MGS
INDIA								
(Heinz)	1 oz	35	0.0	9.0	215	(mq)	0.0	0
(Vlasic)	1 oz	30	0.0	8.0	205	(mq)	0.0	0
JALAPEÑO (Old El Paso)	2 tbsp	16	1.0	4.0	100	1.0	0.0	0
PICCALILLI								
(Claussen)	1 oz	26	0.3	5.6	170	(mq)	0.3	0
(Heinz)	1 oz	30	0.0	7.0	145	(mq)	0.0	0
(Vlasic) hot	1 oz	35	0.0	8.0	165	(mq)	0.0	0
PICKLE								
sweet	1/2 cup	159	0.5	42.8	989	>1.1 c	0.6	0
sweet	1 tbsp	20	0.1	5.3	122	>.1 c	0.1	0
(Claussen)	1 tbsp	14	0.2	2.9	90	(mq)	0.2	0
SWEET								
	1 tbsp	21	0.1	5.1	107	(mq)	0.1	0
chopped	1 cup	338	1.2	83.3	1744	>2.0 c	1.5	0
chopped	1 tbsp	21	0.1	5.1	107	>.1 c	0.1	0
finely cut	1 cup	338	1.2	83.3	1744	>2.0 c	1.5	0
finely cut	1 tbsp	21	0.1	5.1	107	>.1 c	0.1	0
(Heinz)	1 oz	35	0.0	9.0	205	(mq)	0.0	0
(Vlasic)	1 oz	30	0.0	8.0	220	(mq)	0.0	0
RENNIN, enzyme tablet, unsweetened	1 tablet	1	0.0	0.2	234	0	0.0	0
RHUBARB								
frozen	1/2 cup	14	0.4	3.5	1	(mq)	0.1	0
frozen	4 oz	24	0.6	5.8	2	(mq)	0.1	0
frozen, sweetened, cooked	4 oz	132	0.4	35.4	1	2.3	0.1	0
frozen, sweetened, cooked	1/2 cup	139	0.5	37.4	1	2.4	0.1	0
raw, diced	1/2 cup	13	0.6	2.8	2	1.1	0.1	0
raw, trimmed	1 oz	6	0.3	1.3	1	>.2 c	0.1	0
raw, untrimmed	1 lb	71	3.0	15.4	14	>2.4 c	0.7	0
RICE, ARBORIO, dry (Colavita)	1 oz	100	2.0	22.0	5	(mq)	0.0	0
RICE, BASMATI								
BROWN								
(Arrowhead Mills) long grain, dry	2 oz	200	4.0	44.0	3	3.1	1.0	0
(Fantastic Foods) cooked	1/2 cup	102	3.0	22.0	3	(mq)	0.5	0
(Fantastic Foods) cooked, prepared w/1 tbsp salted butter	1/2 cup	115	3.0	22.0	20	(mq)	2.0	(mq)
WHITE								
(Fantastic Foods) cooked	1/2 cup	103	2.0	23.0	1	(mq)	0.0	0
(Fantastic Foods) cooked, prepared w/1 tbsp salted butter	1/2 cup	116	2.0	23.0	18	(mq)	1.0	(mq)
(Texmati) long grain, cooked	1/2 cup	82	3.0	31.0	0	(mq)	0.0	0
RICE, BROWN								
(Lundberg Family) cooked	1 cup	232	4.9	49.7	0	3.3	1.2	na

Food Name	Serv. Size	Total Cal.	Prot. GMS	Carbs GMS	Sod. MGS	Fiber GMS	Fat GMS	Chol. MGS
(Minute) instant	1/2 cup	120	3.0	25.0	5	na	1.0	0
(Uncle Ben's) precooked, prepared	1/2 cup	90	2.0	21.0	11	1.0	1.0	0
LONG GRAIN								
cooked	1/2 cup	109	2.5	22.5	5	1.8	0.9	0
cooked	4 oz	126	2.9	26.0	6	1.9	1.0	0
cooked *(Carolina)*	1/2 cup	110	2.0	23.0	0	(mq)	0.0	0
cooked *(Mahatma)*	1/2 cup	110	2.0	23.0	10	(mq)	0.0	0
cooked *(River)*	1/2 cup	110	2.0	23.0	na	(mq)	0.0	0
cooked *(S&W)*	3.5 oz	119	3.0	26.0	0	(mq)	0.0	0
cooked *(Uncle Ben's)*	2/3 cup	130	3.0	27.0	0	(mq)	1.0	0
dry	1 oz	105	2.3	21.9	2	1.0	0.8	0
dry	1/2 cup	340	7.3	71.1	6	3.2	2.7	0
dry *(Arrowhead Mills)*	2 oz	200	4.0	44.0	3	3.1	1.0	0
quick-cooked *(S&W)*	3.5 oz	110	2.0	25.0	0	(mq)	0.0	0
MEDIUM GRAIN								
cooked	4 oz	127	2.6	26.7	1	>.3 c	0.9	0
cooked	1/2 cup	110	2.3	23.0	1	>.3 c	0.8	0
dry	1/2 cup	344	7.1	72.4	4	>.9 c	2.5	0
dry	1 oz	103	2.1	21.6	1	>.3 c	0.8	0
dry *(Arrowhead Mills)*	2 oz	200	4.0	44.0	3	3.4	1.0	0
SHORT GRAIN *(Arrowhead Mills)* dry	2 oz	200	4.0	44.0	3	3.4	1.0	0
RICE, GLUTINOUS								
cooked	1/2 cup	116	2.4	25.3	6	1.2	0.2	0
cooked	4 oz	110	2.3	23.9	6	1.1	0.2	0
dry	1/2 cup	120	2.2	26.4	0	2.6	0.2	0
dry	1 oz	105	1.9	23.2	2	.8	0.2	0
RICE, WHITE								
LONG GRAIN								
cooked	1/2 cup	194	13.7	52.3	3	.3	5.6	0
cooked	4 oz	111	2.3	24.1	3	.9	0.2	0
cooked *(Carolina)*	1/2 cup	100	2.0	22.0	10	(mq)	0.0	0
cooked *(Finast)*	1/2 cup	115	2.0	26.0	0	(mq)	0.0	0
cooked *(Mahatma)*	1/2 cup	110	2.0	23.0	na	(mq)	0.0	0
cooked *(River)*	1/2 cup	100	2.0	22.0	10	(mq)	0.0	0
cooked *(S&W)*	3.5 oz	106	2.0	23.0	0	(mq)	0.0	0
cooked *(Uncle Ben's)*	2/3 cup	130	3.0	28.0	0	(mq)	1.0	0
cooked *(Water Maid)*	1/2 cup	100	2.0	22.0	10	(mq)	0.0	0
raw, enriched	1/2 cup	336	6.6	73.6	5	1.2	0.6	0
raw, unenriched	1 oz	103	2.0	22.7	1	.3	0.2	0
In cooking bag								
(Minute)	1/2 cup	90	2.0	20.0	0	(mq)	0.0	0
(Success) enriched, cooked	1/2 cup	100	2.0	21.0	0	(mq)	0.0	0
(Uncle Ben's)	1/2 cup	90	2.0	20.0	10	(mq)	<1.0	0

Food Name	Serv. Size	Total Cal.	Prot. GMS	Carbs GMS	Sod. MGS	Fiber GMS	Fat GMS	Chol. MGS
Parboiled								
cooked	1/2 cup	100	2.0	21.8	3	.4	0.2	0
cooked	4 oz	129	2.6	28.0	3	.6	3.1	0
enriched, cooked	1/2 cup	100	2.0	21.8	3	.4	0.2	0
unenriched, dry	1/2 cup	341	6.3	75.2	5	>.3 c	0.5	0
(Uncle Ben's) 'Converted'	2/3 cup	120	2.0	28.0	0	(mq)	<1.0	0
Precooked or instant								
cooked (Carolina) 'Instant'	1/2 cup	110	2.0	23.0	na	(mq)	0.0	0
cooked (Minute) 'Original'	2/3 cup	120	3.0	27.0	5	na	0.0	0
cooked (Minute) 'Premium'	2/3 cup	120	3.0	27.0	0	(mq)	0.0	0
cooked (Uncle Ben's)	2/3 cup	120	3.0	27.0	10	(mq)	<1.0	0
dry	1/2 cup	182	3.7	40.1	3	>.2 c	0.1	0
dry	1 oz	107	2.2	23.7	2	.5	0.1	0
enriched, cooked	1/2 cup	80	1.7	17.4	2	>.1 c	0.1	0
MEDIUM GRAIN								
cooked	1/2 cup	345	6.3	76.0	5	.3	0.5	0
cooked	4 oz	147	2.7	32.4	tr	.1	0.2	0
dry	1 oz	102	1.9	22.5	<1	.4	0.2	0
enriched, dry	1/2 cup	353	6.5	77.8	1	1.4	0.6	0
unenriched, cooked	1/2 cup	133	2.4	29.2	0	>.1 c	0.2	0
unenriched, dry	1/2 cup	353	6.5	77.8	1	>.3 c	0.6	0
SHORT GRAIN								
cooked	1/2 cup	333	6.1	73.6	1	>.3 c	0.5	0
cooked	4 oz	147	2.7	32.6	tr	>.1 c	0.2	0
dry	1/2 cup	130	2.4	28.6	0	2.8	0.2	0
dry	1 oz	101	1.8	22.4	<1	2.2	0.1	0
unenriched, cooked	1/2 cup	133	2.4	29.3	0	>.1 c	0.2	0
unenriched, dry	1/2 cup	358	6.5	79.2	1	>.3 c	0.5	0
RICE, WILD								
cooked	4 oz	115	4.5	24.2	3	2.1	0.4	0
cooked	1/2 cup	83	3.3	17.5	2	1.5	0.3	0
cooked (Fantastic Foods)	1/2 cup	83	3.0	18.0	0	(mq)	0.0	0
dry	1/2 cup	286	11.8	59.9	6	5.0	0.9	0
dry	1 oz	101	4.2	21.2	2	1.5	0.3	0
RICE BEVERAGE								
almond 'Amazake' (Grainaissance)	8 oz	198	4.0	37.0	20	na	4.0	na
apricot 'Amazake' (Grainaissance)	8 oz	158	3.0	36.0	20	na	0.0	na
carob 'Lite' (Rice Dream)	8 oz	150	1.0	32.0	80	na	3.0	0
chocolate flavored (Rice Dream)	8 oz	190	1.0	44.0	80	na	3.0	0
cocoa-almond 'Amazake' (Grainaissance)	8 oz	198	4.0	36.0	20	na	4.0	na
mocha java 'Amazake' (Grainaissance)	8 oz	178	3.0	37.0	20	na	2.0	na
original flavor 'Amazake' (Grainaissance)	8 oz	148	2.0	34.0	20	na	0.0	na
original flavor 'Horchata' (Don José)	8 oz	70	<1.0	6.0	95	na	4.0	0

Food Name	Serv. Size	Total Cal.	Prot. GMS	Carbs GMS	Sod. MGS	Fiber GMS	Fat GMS	Chol. MGS
sesame 'Amazake' *(Grainaissance)*	8 oz	198	4.0	37.0	20	na	1.0	na
strawberry 'Horchata' *(Don José)*	8 oz	70	<1.0	7.0	95	na	3.5	0
vanilla 'Lite' *(Rice Dream)*	8 oz	120	1.0	28.0	80	na	2.0	0
vanilla pecan 'Amazake' *(Grainaissance)*	8 oz	198	4.0	37.0	20	na	4.0	na
RICE BRAN								
crude	1 oz	90	3.8	14.1	1	6.2	5.9	0
crude	1/3 cup	88	3.7	13.9	1	5.9	5.8	0
RICE BRAN OIL								
	1 cup	1927	0.0	0.0	0	0	218.0	0
	1 oz	251	0.0	0.0	0	0	28.4	0
	1 tbsp	120	0.0	0.0	0	0	13.6	0
(Hain)	1 tbsp	120	0.0	0.0	0	0	14.0	0
RICE CAKE								
(Lundberg Family) sodium-free, all flavors	1 cake	60	1.4	14.0	3	na	0.5	na
(Lundberg Family) very low sodium, all flavors	1 cake	60	1.4	14.0	30	na	0.5	na
APPLE CINNAMON								
(Hain) mini	1/2 cup	60	1.0	12.0	10	0	<1.0	0
(Quaker)	1 cake	40	1.0	9.0	0	na	0.0	0
(Quaker) mini	5 cakes	50	1.0	12.0	0	na	0.0	0
BARBEQUE *(Hain)* mini	.5 oz	70	1.0	10.0	50	0	3.0	0
BROWN RICE								
buckwheat	1 cake	34	0.8	7.2	10	.3	0.3	0
buckwheat, unsalted	1 cake	35	0.7	7.3	2	>.2 c	0.3	0
corn	1 cake	35	0.8	7.3	26	.3	0.3	0
multi-grain	1 cake	35	0.8	7.2	23	.3	0.3	0
multi-grain, unsalted	1 cake	34	0.8	7.2	0	>.1 c	0.3	0
plain	1 cake	35	0.7	7.3	29	.4	0.3	0
rye	1 cake	35	0.7	7.2	10	.4	0.3	0
sesame seed	1 cake	35	0.7	7.3	20	>.2 c	0.3	0
sesame seed, unsalted	1 cake	35	0.8	7.2	0	>.2 c	0.3	0
unsalted	1 cake	34	0.8	7.1	26	0	0.3	0
CARAMEL CORN *(Quaker)* mini	5 cakes	50	1.0	12.0	35	na	0.0	0
CAROB COATED								
(Carafection) 'Mint Rice Crisps'	1 oz	139	2.0	17.0	26	na	7.0	na
(Carafection) 'Rice Crisps'	1 oz	139	2.0	17.0	26	na	7.0	na
CHEESE *(Hain)* mini	5 cakes	60	1.0	10.0	80	0	2.0	0
CINNAMON								
(Chico-San) sugar, mini	5 cakes	50	1.0	12.0	0	na	0.0	0
(Quaker) crunch, fat-free	1 cake	50	1.0	11.0	25	na	0.0	0
CORN *(Quaker)*	1 cake	35	0.7	7.4	53	.2	0.2	na
DILL *(Lundberg Family)* creamy, mini	5 cakes	60	1.0	13.0	57	na	<1.0	2
FIVE-GRAIN *(Hain)*	1 cake	40	<1.0	8.0	10	(mq)	<1.0	0

Food Name	Serv. Size	Total Cal.	Prot. GMS	Carbs GMS	Sod. MGS	Fiber GMS	Fat GMS	Chol. MGS
HONEY NUT								
(Chico-San) unglazed, mini	4 cakes	60	1.0	2.0	35	na	1.0	0
(Hain) mini	.5 oz	60	1.0	11.0	30	0	<1.0	0
MUGWORT (Grainaissance) bake & serve								
'Mochi'	2 oz	140	3.0	29.0	2	na	1.3	na
MULTI-GRAIN								
(Chico-San) very low sodium	1 cake	35	1.0	8.0	30	na	0.0	0
(Pritikin) sodium-free	1 cake	35	1.0	7.0	0	na	0.0	0
(Pritikin) very low sodium	1 cake	35	1.0	7.0	30	na	0.0	0
(Quaker)	.32 oz	34	0.9	6.9	29	.4	0.4	0
NACHO CHEESE								
(Hain) mini	.5 oz	70	1.0	10.0	90	0	2.0	5
(Lundberg Family) mini	5 cakes	57	1.0	13.0	116	na	<1.0	<1
PLAIN								
(Chico-San) original	1 cake	35	1.0	8.0	30	na	0.0	0
(Grainaissance) organic bake & serve								
'Mochi'	2 oz	140	3.0	29.0	2	na	1.3	na
(Hain)	1 cake	40	<1.0	8.0	10	(mq)	<1.0	0
(Hain) mini	.5 oz	60	1.0	12.0	20	0	<1.0	0
(Hain) mini, unsalted	.5 oz	60	1.0	12.0	5	0	<1.0	0
(Hain) unsalted	1 cake	40	<1.0	8.0	5	(mq)	<1.0	0
(Konriko) 'Original Unsalted'	1 cake	30	0.0	7.0	<1	(mq)	0.0	0
(Pritikin) sodium-free	1 cake	35	1.0	7.0	0	na	0.0	0
(Pritikin) very low sodium	1 cake	35	1.0	7.0	35	na	0.0	0
(Quaker)	.32 oz	35	0.8	7.1	36	.3	0.3	0
(Quaker) lightly salted	1 cake	35	1.0	7.0	35	na	0.3	0
(Quaker) unsalted	.32 oz	35	0.8	7.2	0	.3	0.3	0
RAISIN-CINNAMON (Grainaissance) bake								
& serve 'Mochi'	2 oz	143	2.9	30.0	77	na	1.2	na
RANCH								
(Hain) mini	.5 oz	70	1.0	9.0	90	(mq)	3.0	0
(Quaker)	1 cake	35	1.4	6.5	52	.8	0.3	0
SESAME								
(Chico-San) original	1 cake	35	1.0	8.0	0	na	0.0	0
(Hain)	1 cake	40	<1.0	8.0	10	(mq)	<1.0	0
(Hain) unsalted	1 cake	40	<1.0	8.0	5	(mq)	<1.0	0
(Pritikin) sodium-free	1 cake	35	1.0	7.0	0	na	0.0	0
(Pritikin) very low sodium	1 cake	35	1.0	7.0	35	na	0.0	0
(Quaker)	.32 oz	35	0.8	7.1	36	.3	0.3	0
(Westbrae) 'Double Sesame'	.28 oz	30	<1.0	6.0	65	na	<1.0	0
SESAME-GARLIC								
(Grainaissance) bake & serve 'Mochi'	2 oz	143	3.2	28.0	25	na	1.9	na
(Westbrae)	.28 oz	30	<1.0	6.0	55	na	<1.0	0

Food Name	Serv. Size	Total Cal.	Prot. GMS	Carbs GMS	Sod. MGS	Fiber GMS	Fat GMS	Chol. MGS
TERIYAKI								
(Hain) mini	.5 oz	50	1.0	12.0	75	0	<1.0	0
(Westbrae)	.28 oz	30	<1.0	6.0	45	na	<1.0	0
WHEAT *(Quaker)*	1 cake	34	1.4	6.7	52	.8	0.3	0
RICE DISH								
CANNED								
Fried *(LaChoy)*	4.903 oz	236	5.1	53.4	1024	1.9	1.1	0
Spanish								
(Featherweight)	7.5 oz	140	4.0	30.0	32	(mq)	0.0	0
(Heinz)	7.25 oz	150	3.0	26.0	1045	(mq)	5.0	na
(Old El Paso)	1/2 cup	70	1.0	15.0	400	1.0	1.0	0
(Van Camp's)	1 cup	160	3.1	27.0	1270	(mq)	4.0	na
FREEZE-DRIED, w/chicken,								
(Mountain House)	1 cup	400	13.0	41.0	241	(mq)	13.0	(mq)
FROZEN								
Country style *(Birds Eye)* 'International								
Rice Recipes'	3.3 oz	90	2.0	19.0	380	1.0	0.0	0
Florentine *(Green Giant)* 'Rice Originals'	1/2 cup	140	4.0	22.0	400	na	4.0	10
French style *(Birds Eye)* 'International Rice								
Recipes'	3.3 oz	110	3.0	23.0	610	(mq)	0.0	0
Fried								
w/chicken *(Chun King)*	8 oz	260	14.0	41.0	1460	(mq)	4.0	(mq)
w/pork *(Chun King)*	8 oz	270	10.0	44.0	1210	(mq)	6.0	(mq)
Medley *(Green Giant)* 'Rice Originals'	1/2 cup	100	3.0	19.0	310	(mq)	1.0	5
Mexican style, w/chicken *(Lean Cuisine)*								
'Lunch Express'	9 1/8 oz	270	12.0	43.0	580	na	5.0	20
Oriental, w/vegetables *(Budget Gourmet)*								
'Side Dish'	5.75 oz	210	4.0	27.0	310	(mq)	10.0	20
Pilaf								
'Rice Originals' *(Green Giant)*	1/2 cup	110	2.0	21.0	530	(mq)	1.0	2
w/green beans *(Budget Gourmet)*								
'Side Dish'	5.5 oz	240	4.0	35.0	350	(mq)	9.0	10
Spanish style *(Birds Eye)* 'International								
Rice Recipes'	3.3 oz	110	3.0	24.0	540	(mq)	0.0	0
White and wild *(Green Giant)* 'Rice								
Originals'	1/2 cup	130	3.0	24.0	540	(mq)	2.0	0
Wild, w/sherry *(Green Giant)* 'Microwave								
Garden Gourmet'	1 pkg	210	6.0	40.0	580	3.0	4.0	10
W/broccoli								
au gratin *(Birds Eye)* 'For One'	5.75 oz	180	6.0	27.0	430	1.0	6.0	5
in cheese flavored sauce *(Green Giant)*	1/2 cup	120	3.0	18.0	510	>.2 c	4.0	na
in cheese sauce *(Green Giant)*								
'One Serving'	5.5 oz	180	5.0	25.0	550	(mq)	6.0	5

Food Name	Serv. Size	Total Cal.	Prot. GMS	Carbs GMS	Sod. MGS	Fiber GMS	Fat GMS	Chol. MGS
'Rice Originals' (Green Giant)	1/2 cup	120	3.0	18.0	510	na	4.0	5
W/peas and mushrooms in sauce,								
(Green Giant) 'One Serving'	5.5 oz	130	4.0	27.0	410	(mq)	2.0	5
W/spinach in cheese sauce								
(Green Giant) 'Italian Blend'	1/2 cup	140	4.0	22.0	400	(mq)	4.0	10
RICE DISH MIX								
(Arrowhead Mills)	2 oz	200	4.0	43.0	0	na	1.0	na
ALFREDO (Country Inn) prepared	1/2 cup	140	4.0	23.0	570	(mq)	4.0	na
AMANDINE (Hain) '3-Grain Goodness'								
prepared	1/2 cup	130	3.0	17.0	260	(mq)	5.0	0
BEEF BROCCOLI								
(Rice-A-Roni) 'Rice & Sauce'	1/4 pkg	120	3.0	24.0	530	na	0.0	na
(Rice-A-Roni) 'Rice & Sauce' prepared	1/2 cup	140	3.0	24.0	550	na	3.0	na
BEEF FLAVOR								
(Finast) dry mix	1.3 oz	130	4.0	26.0	780	(mq)	1.0	na
(Lipton) 'Rice and Sauce' dry mix	1/2 pkg	120	3.0	26.0	570	(mq)	<1.0	na
(Lipton) 'Rice and Sauce' prepared								
w/1 tbsp butter	1/2 cup	150	3.0	26.0	600	(mq)	3.0	(mq)
(Mahatma) prepared	1/2 cup	100	2.0	20.0	340	(mq)	0.0	0
(Minute) microwave, family size, dry mix	1 pkg	140	4.0	28.0	530	na	0.0	0
(Minute) microwave, family size, prepared								
w/salted butter	1/2 cup	160	4.0	28.0	560	na	3.0	10
(Minute) microwave, single size, dry mix	1 pkg	140	4.0	28.0	530	na	0.0	0
(Minute) microwave, single size, prepared								
w/salted butter	1/2 cup	150	4.0	28.0	550	na	2.0	5
(Rice-A-Roni) dry mix	1.13 oz	110	3.0	24.0	560	(mq)	1.0	na
(Rice-A-Roni) prepared	1/2 cup	140	4.0	24.0	610	(mq)	4.0	na
(Success) prepared	1/2 cup	100	2.0	19.0	370	(mq)	0.0	0
W/mushrooms								
(Rice-A-Roni) dry mix	1.27 oz	120	4.0	26.0	710	(mq)	<1.0	na
(Rice-A-Roni) prepared	1/2 cup	150	4.0	26.0	740	(mq)	3.0	na
W/vermicelli (Make-It-Easy) dry mix	1.3 oz	130	3.0	28.0	(mq)	(mq)	1.0	0
BROWN AND WILD								
(Success) prepared	1/2 cup	120	3.0	23.0	500	(mq)	0.0	0
(Uncle Ben's) prepared	1/2 cup	130	4.0	27.0	500	(mq)	1.0	0
Herb (Arrowhead Mills) 'Quick'	2 oz	140	4.0	28.0	128	4.0	1.0	0
Spanish style (Arrowhead Mills) 'Quick'	2 oz	150	4.0	30.0	145	2.8	1.0	0
Vegetable herb (Arrowhead Mills) 'Quick'	2 oz	150	4.0	30.0	85	4.0	1.0	0
W/mushrooms (Uncle Ben's) prepared	1/2 cup	130	4.0	27.0	500	(mq)	1.0	na
CAJUN								
(Lipton) 'Rice and Sauce' dry mix	1/4 pkg	120	4.0	26.0	600	(mq)	<1.0	0
(Lipton) 'Rice and Sauce' prepared								
w/1 tbsp butter	1/2 cup	150	4.0	26.0	630	(mq)	3.0	(mq)

Food Name	Serv. Size	Total Cal.	Prot. GMS	Carbs GMS	Sod. MGS	Fiber GMS	Fat GMS	Chol. MGS
CHICKEN FLAVOR								
(Finast) dry mix	1.6 oz	160	4.0	31.0	950	(mq)	2.0	na
(Lipton) 'Rice and Sauce' dry mix	1/4 pkg	130	3.0	25.0	440	(mq)	1.0	na
(Lipton) 'Rice and Sauce' prepared								
w/1 tbsp butter	1/2 cup	150	3.0	25.0	470	(mq)	4.0	(mq)
(Mahatma) prepared	1/2 cup	100	2.0	20.0	620	(mq)	0.0	0
(Minute) microwave, family size, dry mix	1 pkg	130	3.0	27.0	640	na	1.0	0
(Minute) microwave, family size prepared								
w/salted butter	1/2 cup	160	3.0	27.0	670	na	4.0	10
(Minute) microwave, single size, dry mix	1 pkg	130	3.0	27.0	640	na	1.0	0
(Minute) microwave, single size, prepared								
w/salted butter	1/2 cup	150	3.0	27.0	660	na	3.0	5
(Rice-A-Roni) dry mix	1.13 oz	110	3.0	24.0	520	(mq)	1.0	na
(Rice-A-Roni) prepared	1/2 cup	150	3.0	24.0	560	(mq)	4.0	na
(Success) prepared	1/2 cup	110	3.0	18.0	420	(mq)	2.0	na
Florentine								
(Rice-A-Roni) 'Savory Classics' dry mix	1.12 oz	108	3.7	21.7	874	1.2	0.8	1
(Rice-A-Roni) 'Savory Classics' prepared	1/2 cup	130	4.0	22.0	910	(mq)	4.0	(mq)
Honey-lemon, w/broccoli *(Suzi Wan)*								
prepared	7.5 oz	370	23.0	45.0	640	(mq)	11.0	na
W/broccoli								
(Rice-A-Roni) dry mix	1.23 oz	120	3.0	25.0	670	(mq)	1.0	na
(Rice-A-Roni) prepared	1/2 cup	150	3.0	25.0	710	(mq)	3.0	na
(Suzi Wan) prepared	1/2 cup	120	4.0	23.0	500	(mq)	1.0	na
W/creamy mushroom *(Country Inn)*								
prepared	1/2 cup	140	3.0	25.0	510	(mq)	3.0	na
W/homestyle vegetables *(Country Inn)*								
prepared	1/2 cup	140	4.0	25.0	490	(mq)	3.0	na
W/mushroom								
(Country Inn) 'Mushroom Royale' prepared	1/2 cup	120	4.0	25.0	560	(mq)	1.0	na
(Rice-A-Roni) dry mix	1.17 oz	130	4.0	26.0	790	(mq)	1.0	na
(Rice-A-Roni) prepared	1/2 cup	180	4.0	26.0	840	(mq)	7.0	na
W/mushroom stock *(Country Inn)* prepared	1/2 cup	130	4.0	25.0	560	(mq)	1.0	na
W/vegetables								
(Rice-A-Roni) dry mix	1.2 oz	120	3.0	25.0	760	(mq)	<1.0	na
(Rice-A-Roni) prepared	1/2 cup	140	3.0	25.0	790	(mq)	3.0	na
(Suzi Wan) prepared	1/2 cup	120	3.0	24.0	550	(mq)	1.0	na
W/vegetables and vermicelli *(Make-It-Easy)*								
dry mix	1.3 oz	130	3.0	28.0	(mq)	(mq)	1.0	na
DRUMSTICK								
(Minute) dry mix	1 pkg	120	3.0	25.0	650	na	0.0	0
(Minute) prepared w/salted butter	1/2 cup	150	3.0	25.0	690	na	4.0	10
FLORENTINE *(Country Inn)* prepared	1/2 cup	140	4.0	24.0	380	(mq)	3.0	na

Food Name	Serv. Size	Total Cal.	Prot. GMS	Carbs GMS	Sod. MGS	Fiber GMS	Fat GMS	Chol. MGS
FRIED								
(Minute) dry mix	1 pkg	120	3.0	25.0	550	na	0.0	0
(Minute) prepared w/oil, w/o salt or butter	1/2 cup	160	3.0	25.0	550	na	5.0	0
(Rice-A-Roni) dry mix	1 oz	110	3.0	21.0	670	(mq)	1.0	na
(Rice-A-Roni) prepared	1/2 cup	110	3.0	21.0	700	(mq)	5.0	na
W/almonds								
(Rice-A-Roni) '1/2 less salt' dry mix	1/5 pkg	120	3.0	26.0	460	na	1.0	0
(Rice-A-Roni) '1/2 less salt' prepared	1/2 cup	130	3.0	26.0	470	na	2.0	0
JASMINE, soft (A Taste of Thai)	1/4 cup	160	3.0	36.0	0	0	0.0	0
HERB								
And butter								
(Lipton) 'Rice and Sauce' prepared w/1 tbsp butter	1/2 cup	150	3.0	24.0	470	(mq)	5.0	(mq)
(Rice-A-Roni) dry mix	1 oz	110	2.0	22.0	760	(mq)	1.0	na
(Rice-A-Roni) prepared	1/2 cup	130	2.0	22.0	790	(mq)	4.0	na
Au gratin								
(Country Inn) prepared	1/2 cup	140	4.0	25.0	450	(mq)	3.0	na
(Success) prepared	1/2 cup	100	2.0	20.0	260	(mq)	0.0	0
Wild rice and herbs (Arrowhead Mills)	1/4 pkg	140	4.0	28.0	220	3.0	1.0	na
LONG GRAIN AND WILD								
(Lipton) 'Rice and Sauce Original' dry mix	1/4 pkg	120	4.0	26.0	530	(mq)	<1.0	na
(Lipton) 'Rice and Sauce Original' prepared w/1 tbsp butter	1/2 cup	150	4.0	26.0	560	(mq)	3.0	(mq)
(Mahatma) prepared	1/2 cup	100	2.0	20.0	480	(mq)	0.0	0
(Minute) dry mix	1 pkg	120	3.0	25.0	530	na	0.0	0
(Minute) prepared w/salted butter	1/2 cup	150	3.0	25.0	570	na	4.0	10
(Minute) prepared w/o salt or butter	2/3 cup	120	3.0	27.0	0	na	0.0	0
(Near East) prepared	1/2 cup	130	3.0	21.0	430	(mq)	4.0	na
(Rice-A-Roni) 'Original' dry mix	1.1 oz	110	3.0	23.0	620	(mq)	0.0	na
(Rice-A-Roni) 'Original' prepared	1/2 cup	130	3.0	23.0	660	(mq)	3.0	na
(Uncle Ben's) 'Fast Cooking' prepared	1/2 cup	100	3.0	21.0	410	(mq)	<1.0	na
(Uncle Ben's) 'Fast Cooking' prepared w/salt and butter	1/2 cup	130	3.0	21.0	450	(mq)	4.0	(mq)
(Uncle Ben's) 'Original' prepared w/salt and butter	1/2 cup	120	3.0	22.0	520	(mq)	2.0	(mq)
(Uncle Ben's) 'Original' prepared w/o salt or butter	1/2 cup	100	3.0	22.0	500	(mq)	<1.0	0
Mexican (Old El Paso) prepared	1/2 cup	140	2.0	28.0	370	(mq)	2.0	0
Pilaf								
(Rice-A-Roni) dry mix	1 oz	100	2.0	23.0	510	(mq)	0.0	na
(Rice-A-Roni) prepared	1/2 cup	130	3.0	23.0	550	(mq)	3.0	na

Food Name	Serv. Size	Total Cal.	Prot. GMS	Carbs GMS	Sod. MGS	Fiber GMS	Fat GMS	Chol. MGS
W/chicken and almonds								
(Rice-A-Roni) dry mix	1.2 oz	120	3.0	23.0	660	(mq)	1.0	na
(Rice-A-Roni) prepared	1/2 cup	140	3.0	24.0	690	(mq)	4.0	na
W/chicken sauce								
(Uncle Ben's) prepared w/salt and butter	1/2 cup	160	4.0	27.0	680	(mq)	5.0	(mq)
(Uncle Ben's) prepared w/o salt or butter	1/2 cup	140	4.0	27.0	650	(mq)	2.0	0
ORIENTAL								
(Hain) '3-Grain Goodness' prepared	1/2 cup	120	4.0	15.0	300	(mq)	5.0	na
(Lipton) dry mix	1/4 pkg	120	4.0	26.0	330	(mq)	<1.0	na
(Lipton) prepared w/1 tbsp butter	1/2 cup	150	4.0	26.0	360	(mq)	3.0	(mq)
PILAF								
(Casbah) dry mix	1 oz	90	2.0	20.0	(mq)	(mq)	0.0	0
(Casbah) prepared	1/2 cup	90	2.0	20.0	(mq)	(mq)	0.0	0
(Lipton) 'Rice and Sauce'	1/4 pkg	120	3.0	25.0	400	(mq)	<1.0	na
(Lipton) 'Rice and Sauce' prepared w/1 tbsp margarine	1/2 cup	140	3.0	25.0	440	(mq)	3.0	na
(Lipton) 'Rice and Sauce' prepared w/2 tbsp butter	1/2 cup	170	3.0	25.0	470	(mq)	6.0	(mq)
(Near East) prepared	1/2 cup	140	3.0	21.0	450	(mq)	5.0	na
(Rice-A-Roni) dry mix	1.2 oz	120	4.0	25.0	570	(mq)	0.0	na
(Rice-A-Roni) prepared	1/2 cup	150	4.0	25.0	550	(mq)	4.0	na
(Success) prepared	1/2 cup	120	2.0	24.0	410	(mq)	0.0	0
Beef flavored *(Near East)* prepared	1/2 cup	140	3.0	21.0	470	(mq)	5.0	na
Brown rice								
(Quick Pilaf) Spanish, prepared w/o salt or butter	1/2 cup	98	2.0	21.0	314	(mq)	0.7	na
(Quick Pilaf) Spanish, prepared w/2 tbsp salted butter	1/2 cup	136	2.0	21.0	369	(mq)	5.0	(mq)
(Quick Pilaf) w/miso, prepared w/o salt or butter	1/2 cup	105	3.0	21.0	240	(mq)	1.0	na
(Quick Pilaf) w/miso, prepared w/2 tbsp salted butter	1/2 cup	145	3.0	21.0	295	(mq)	5.5	(mq)
Chicken flavored *(Near East)* prepared	1/2 cup	140	3.0	21.0	420	(mq)	5.0	na
French								
(Minute) microwave, family size, dry mix	1 pkg	110	2.0	24.0	390	na	0.0	0
(Minute) microwave, family size, prepared w/salted butter	1/2 cup	130	2.0	24.0	420	na	3.0	10
(Minute) microwave, single size, dry mix	1 pkg	110	2.0	24.0	390	na	0.0	0
(Minute) microwave, single size, prepared w/salted butter	1/2 cup	120	2.0	24.0	410	na	2.0	5
Garden								
(Rice-A-Roni) 'Savory Classics' dry mix	1.12 oz	113	3.6	22.9	964	1.1	0.8	1
(Rice-A-Roni) 'Savory Classics' prepared	1/2 cup	140	4.0	23.0	1000	(mq)	4.0	(mq)

Food Name	Serv. Size	Total Cal.	Prot. GMS	Carbs GMS	Sod. MGS	Fiber GMS	Fat GMS	Chol. MGS
Lentil *(Near East)* prepared	1/2 cup	170	6.0	21.0	430	(mq)	7.0	na
Nutted								
(Casbah) dry mix	1 oz	160	4.0	30.0	(mq)	(mq)	2.0	0
(Casbah) prepared	1/2 cup	160	4.0	30.0	(mq)	(mq)	2.0	0
Spanish								
(Casbah) dry mix	1 oz	90	2.0	20.0	(mq)	(mq)	0.0	0
(Casbah) prepared	1/2 cup	90	2.0	20.0	(mq)	(mq)	0.0	0
(Country Inn) w/vegetables, prepared	1/2 cup	120	3.0	25.0	280	(mq)	1.0	na
Wheat *(Near East)* Spanish, prepared	1/2 cup	150	3.0	21.0	380	(mq)	6.0	na
RIB ROAST								
(Minute) dry mix	1 pkg	120	3.0	25.0	680	na	0.0	0
(Minute) prepared w/salted butter	1/2 cup	150	3.0	25.0	720	na	4.0	10
RISOTTO								
(Rice-A-Roni) dry mix	1.5 oz	160	4.0	32.0	1070	(mq)	1.0	na
(Rice-A-Roni) prepared	1/2 cup	200	4.0	32.0	1130	(mq)	6.0	na
Chicken and cheese *(Country Inn)* prepared	1/2 cup	120	3.0	23.0	410	(mq)	2.0	na
SPANISH STYLE								
(Arrowhead Mills) quick, dry mix	1/4 pkg	150	4.0	30.0	255	2.0	1.0	na
(Lipton) 'Rice and Sauce' dry mix	1/4 pkg	120	3.0	26.0	540	(mq)	<1.0	na
(Lipton) 'Rice and Sauce' prepared w/1 tbsp butter	1/2 cup	140	3.0	26.0	570	(mq)	3.0	(mq)
(Mahatma) prepared	1/2 cup	100	2.0	20.0	190	(mq)	0.0	0
(Near East) prepared	1/2 cup	170	3.0	24.0	540	(mq)	7.0	na
(Rice-A-Roni) dry mix	.97 oz	110	3.0	22.0	950	(mq)	1.0	na
(Rice-A-Roni) prepared	1/2 cup	150	4.0	25.0	1090	(mq)	4.0	na
STROGANOFF								
(Rice-A-Roni) dry mix	1.35 oz	150	4.0	27.0	770	(mq)	3.0	na
(Rice-A-Roni) prepared	1/2 cup	200	4.0	27.0	810	(mq)	8.0	na
SWEET AND SOUR								
(Suzi Wan) 'Dinner Recipe' prepared	7.5 oz	220	4.0	48.0	240	(mq)	1.0	na
(Suzi Wan) 'Dinner Recipe' prepared w/o butter	1/2 cup	130	3.0	28.0	460	(mq)	1.0	na
(Suzi Wan) 'Dinner Recipe' prepared w/o butter or salt	7.5 oz	340	24.0	49.0	290	(mq)	5.0	(mq)
TERIYAKI								
(Suzi Wan) 'Dinner Recipe' prepared	7.5 oz	180	5.0	39.0	910	(mq)	1.0	na
(Suzi Wan) 'Dinner Recipe' prepared w/o butter	1/2 cup	120	3.0	25.0	690	(mq)	1.0	na
(Suzi Wan) 'Dinner Recipe' prepared w/o butter or salt	7.5 oz	360	22.0	39.0	970	(mq)	12.0	(mq)
THREE-FLAVOR *(Suzi Wan)* prepared	1/2 cup	120	4.0	24.0	570	(mq)	1.0	na

Food Name	Serv. Size	Total Cal.	Prot. GMS	Carbs GMS	Sod. MGS	Fiber GMS	Fat GMS	Chol. MGS
W/ASPARAGUS								
Au gratin *(Country Inn)* prepared	1/2 cup	130	4.0	22.0	310	(mq)	3.0	na
W/hollandaise sauce								
(Lipton) w/hollandaise sauce 'Rice & Sauce' dry mix	1/4 pkg	120	4.0	25.0	460	(mq)	1.0	na
(Lipton) w/hollandaise sauce 'Rice and Sauce' prepared w/butter	1/2 cup	170	4.0	25.0	530	(mq)	7.0	(mq)
(Lipton) w/hollandaise sauce 'Rice and Sauce' prepared w/margarine	1/2 cup	150	4.0	25.0	500	(mq)	4.0	na
W/BROCCOLI								
Amandine *(Country Inn)* prepared	1/2 cup	130	4.0	23.0	600	(mq)	2.0	na
Au gratin								
(Country Inn) prepared	1/2 cup	130	4.0	22.0	300	(mq)	3.0	na
(Rice-A-Roni) 'Savory Classics' dry mix	1.12 oz	129	3.6	20.9	372	1.1	3.4	4
(Rice-A-Roni) 'Savory Classics' prepared	1/2 cup	180	4.0	21.0	440	(mq)	9.0	(mq)
Stir-fry								
(Suzi Wan) prepared w/salt and butter	7.5 oz	370	22.0	37.0	800	(mq)	15.0	na
(Suzi Wan) prepared w/o salt or butter	7.5 oz	200	5.0	37.0	750	(mq)	3.0	na
W/cheddar cheese								
(Minute) microwave, dry mix	1 pkg	140	4.0	26.0	500	na	2.0	5
(Minute) microwave, prepared w/salted butter	1/2 cup	160	4.0	26.0	530	na	5.0	10
W/CAULIFLOWER, AU GRATIN								
(Country Inn) prepared	1/2 cup	130	4.0	23.0	570	(mq)	3.0	na
(Rice-A-Roni) 'Savory Classics' dry mix	.5 oz	141	4.4	22.7	372	1.1	3.6	5
(Rice-A-Roni) 'Savory Classics' prepared	1/2 cup	170	4.0	23.0	410	(mq)	7.0	(mq)
W/CHEESE								
Cheddar								
(Rice-A-Roni) white, w/herbs, prepared	1 cup	130	7.0	52.0	940	1.0	5.0	10
(Rice-A-Roni) zesty 'Savory Classics' dry mix	1.3 oz	151	4.6	24.7	541	.9	3.8	6
(Rice-A-Roni) zesty 'Savory Classics' prepared	1/2 cup	180	5.0	25.0	580	(mq)	7.0	(mq)
Parmesan								
(Rice-A-Roni) creamy, w/herbs 'Savory Classics' dry mix	1.22 oz	145	4.8	22.0	432	.8	4.2	7
(Rice-A-Roni) creamy, w/herbs 'Savory Classics' prepared	1/2 cup	170	5.0	22.0	470	(mq)	7.0	(mq)
(Ultra Slim Fast) w/chicken flavored sauce, prepared	8 oz	240	5.0	56.0	1080	4.0	1.0	na
W/GREEN BEANS, AMANDINE								
(Country Inn) casserole, prepared	1/2 cup	120	3.0	23.0	370	(mq)	2.0	na
(Rice-A-Roni) 'Savory Classics' dry mix	1.25 oz	152	4.8	22.3	416	1.0	4.8	6

Food Name	Serv. Size	Total Cal.	Prot. GMS	Carbs GMS	Sod. MGS	Fiber GMS	Fat GMS	Chol. MGS
(Rice-A-Roni) 'Savory Classics' prepared	1/2 cup	210	5.0	22.0	490	(mq)	11.0	(mq)
W/MUSHROOMS								
(Country Inn) creamy, w/wild rice,								
prepared	1/2 cup	140	3.0	24.0	310	(mq)	3.0	na
(Lipton) 'Rice and Sauce' dry mix	1/4 pkg	120	3.0	26.0	550	(mq)	<1.0	na
(Lipton) 'Rice and Sauce' prepared								
w/1 tbsp butter	1/2 cup	150	3.0	26.0	580	(mq)	3.0	(mq)
W/ORIENTAL STYLE SAUCE								
(Ultra Slim Fast) prepared	8 oz	240	5.0	58.0	900	4.0	1.0	na
W/VEGETABLES								
And cheddar								
(Lipton) dry mix	1/4 pkg	130	3.0	26.0	420	(mq)	2.0	na
(Lipton) prepared w/1 tbsp margarine	1/2 cup	160	3.0	26.0	450	(mq)	5.0	na
(Lipton) prepared w/2 tbsp butter	1/2 cup	180	3.0	26.0	490	(mq)	7.0	(mq)
Medley (Country Inn) prepared	1/2 cup	140	4.0	28.0	390	(mq)	1.0	na
Spring vegetable and cheese								
(Arrowhead Mills) vegetable herb,								
dry mix	1/4 pkg	150	4.0	30.0	150	3.0	1.0	na
(Rice-A-Roni) 'Savory Classics' dry mix	1.22 oz	141	4.4	22.8	388	1.2	3.5	6
(Rice-A-Roni) 'Savory Classics'								
prepared	1/2 cup	170	4.0	23.0	420	(mq)	7.0	(mq)
YELLOW								
(Mahatma) prepared	1/2 cup	100	2.0	21.0	480	(mq)	0.0	0
(Rice-A-Roni) dry mix	1.16 oz	110	2.0	25.0	730	(mq)	0.0	na
(Rice-A-Roni) prepared	1/2 cup	140	2.0	25.0	780	(mq)	4.0	na
(Success) prepared	1/2 cup	100	2.0	21.0	480	(mq)	0.0	0
RICE FLOUR								
brown	1/2 cup	287	5.7	60.4	6	3.6	2.2	0
brown	1 oz	103	2.0	21.7	2	1.3	0.8	0
brown (Arrowhead Mills)	2 oz	200	4.0	44.0	3	3.1	1.0	0
brown (Featherweight)	1 cup	500	11.0	113.0	7	(mq)	1.0	0
white	1/2 cup	289	4.7	63.3	0	1.9	1.1	0
white	1 oz	104	1.7	22.7	tr	.7	0.4	0
RICE SEASONING (Lawry's) Mexican								
'Seasoning Blends'	1 pkg	94	3.9	17.0	3246	>2.1 c	2.0	na
RICE SYRUP (Lundberg Family) organic								
'Sweet Dreams'	1 tbsp	42	<1.0	10.0	2	na	<1.0	na
RIGATONI. See PASTA.								
RIGATONI ENTRÉE								
(Budget Gourmet) w/broccoli and chicken,								
in cream sauce, frozen	10.8 oz	290	19.0	44.0	710	na	7.0	30
(Chef Boyardee) microwave	7.5 oz	210	8.0	31.0	1080	na	6.0	17
(Chef Boyardee) 'Special Recipe,' canned	7.5 oz	210	9.0	33.0	1040	4.0	6.0	20

Food Name	Serv. Size	Total Cal.	Prot. GMS	Carbs GMS	Sod. MGS	Fiber GMS	Fat GMS	Chol. MGS
(Healthy Choice) w/chicken 'Classics' frozen	12.5 oz	360	31.0	50.0	430	na	4.0	60
(Healthy Choice) w/meat sauce, frozen	9.5 oz	260	16.0	34.0	540	na	6.0	30
(Lean Cuisine) baked w/meat sauce and cheese, frozen	9.75 oz	250	18.0	27.0	430	na	8.0	25
(Stouffer's) w/meat sauce, homestyle, frozen	12 oz	400	21.0	49.0	860	na	13.0	na
ROAST BEEF ENTRÉE								
(Libby's) canned, w/gravy	6 oz	210	27.3	6.5	1030	na	8.0	na
(Top Shelf) frozen, tender	10 oz	240	28.0	19.0	880	na	6.0	60
ROAST BEEF HASH								
(Armour) canned	7.5 oz	350	19.0	20.0	1310	na	21.0	na
(Mary Kitchen) canned	7.5 oz	350	20.0	18.0	1142	(mq)	22.0	(mq)
(Stouffer's) frozen	10 oz	380	30.0	16.0	1340	(mq)	22.0	(mq)
ROAST BEEF LUNCHEON MEAT. See LUNCHEON MEAT.								
ROAST BEEF SPREAD, CANNED								
(Hormel)	.5 oz	31	2.0	0.0	(mq)	0	2.0	(mq)
(Underwood)	2 1/8 oz	140	9.0	<1.0	360	na	11.0	45
(Underwood) 'Light'	2 1/8 oz	90	9.0	2.0	210	na	6.0	30
(Underwood) mesquite-smoked	2 1/8 oz	126	9.0	<1.0	300	na	11.0	45
ROCK-A-DILE RED DRINK								
(Kool-Aid) 'Kool Bursts'	6.75 oz	110	0.0	30.0	10	na	0.0	0
(Kool-Aid) 'Koolers'	8.45 oz	130	0.0	34.0	10	na	0.0	0
ROCK-A-DILE RED DRINK MIX								
(Kool-Aid) sugar-free w/NutraSweet, prepared	8 oz	4	0.0	0.0	0	na	0.0	0
(Kool-Aid) sugar-sweetened, prepared	8 oz	70	0.0	18.0	0	na	0.0	0
(Kool-Aid) unsweetened, prepared w/sugar	8 oz	100	0.0	25.0	0	na	0.0	0
(Kool-Aid) unsweetened, prepared w/o sugar	8 oz	2	0.0	0.0	0	na	0.0	0
ROCKET. See ARUGULA.								
ROCKFISH, PACIFIC, MIXED SPECIES								
baked, broiled, or microwaved	4 oz	137	27.3	0.0	87	0	2.3	50
baked, broiled, or microwaved	3 oz	103	20.4	0.0	65	0	1.7	37
raw	1 lb	427	85.1	0.0	272	0	7.1	156
raw	3 oz	80	15.9	0.0	51	0	1.3	30
raw	1 oz	27	5.3	0.0	17	0	0.4	10
ROE, MIXED SPECIES								
dry-heat cooked	3 oz	173	24.3	1.6	99	0	7.0	407
dry-heat cooked	1 oz	58	8.1	0.5	33	0	2.3	136
raw	1 lb	635	101.2	6.8	(mq)	0	29.1	1696
raw	3 oz	119	19.0	1.3	77	0	5.5	318
raw	1 oz	39	6.3	0.4	25	0	1.8	105
raw	1 tbsp	22	3.6	0.2	(mq)	0	1.0	60

Food Name	Serv. Size	Total Cal.	Prot. GMS	Carbs GMS	Sod. MGS	Fiber GMS	Fat GMS	Chol. MGS
ROLL. See also BREAD; BUN; CROISSANT; ENGLISH MUFFIN.								
BUTTER (Pillsbury) 'Butterflake' refrigerated	1 roll	140	3.0	20.0	530	(mq)	5.0	0
BUTTERMILK (Wonder) brown and serve	1 roll	80	2.0	13.0	140	.6	2.0	na
CRESCENT								
(Pepperidge Farm) 'Deli Classic'	1 roll	110	2.0	13.0	150	tr	6.0	15
(Pillsbury) refrigerated	1 roll	100	2.0	11.0	230	(mq)	6.0	5
CLUB (Pepperidge Farm) 'Deli Classic' brown and serve	1 roll	100	3.0	19.0	190	.5	1.0	0
DINNER								
egg	1-oz roll	87	2.7	14.7	155	1.1	1.8	14
oat bran	1-oz roll	67	2.7	11.4	117	1.2	1.3	0
rye	1-oz roll	81	2.9	15.1	253	na	1.0	0
wheat	1-oz roll	77	2.4	13.0	96	na	1.8	0
whole wheat	1-oz roll	75	2.5	14.5	136	na	1.3	0
(Arnold) 'Dinner Party' 24 per pkg	1 roll	51	1.9	9.4	81	.8	1.2	1
(Awrey's)	1 roll	60	2.0	11.0	115	0	1.0	0
(Awrey's) 'Black Forest'	1 roll	50	2.0	10.0	110	0	1.0	0
(Awrey's) cracked wheat	1 roll	50	2.0	10.0	120	0	1.0	0
(Awrey's) crusty	1 roll	70	2.0	12.0	150	0	1.0	0
(Awrey's) poppy seed	1 roll	59	2.0	11.0	115	0	1.0	0
(Awrey's) sesame seed	1 roll	60	2.0	11.0	115	0	1.0	0
(Home Pride) wheat	1 roll	70	3.0	12.0	140	.6	1.0	0
(Home Pride) white	1 roll	80	2.0	14.0	170	.6	2.0	0
(Pepperidge Farm) country style 'Classic'	1 roll	50	2.0	9.0	90	0	1.0	0
(Pepperidge Farm) 'Old Fashioned'	1 roll	50	2.0	7.0	85	tr	2.0	5
(Pepperidge Farm) 'Party'	1 roll	30	1.0	5.0	50	tr	1.0	0
(Roman Meal)	1 roll	69	2.9	13.0	140	1.2	1.2	0
(Wonder)	1 roll	80	2.0	14.0	140	.6	1.0	na
EGG (Levy's) 'Old Country Deli'	1-oz roll	146	5.3	28.1	431	2.0	2.8	11
FINGER (Pepperidge Farm) w/poppy seeds	1 roll	50	2.0	8.0	80	tr	2.0	5
49ER								
(Colombo Brand) sour	1.2-oz roll	90	4.8	16.4	189	(mq)	0.6	na
(Colombo Brand) sweet	1.2-oz roll	96	4.5	15.4	196	(mq)	1.8	na
FRENCH STYLE								
	1 oz	79	2.4	14.2	173	na	1.2	0
(Du Jour) petite, brown and serve	1 roll	230	9.0	45.0	490	1.8	2.0	0
(Francisco) 'International'	1 roll	108	4.2	21.3	285	1.2	1.5	0
(Pepperidge Farm) 'Deli Classic' brown and serve, 3 per pkg	1/2 roll	120	4.0	24.0	250	.5	1.0	0
(Pepperidge Farm) 'Deli Classic' 9 per pkg	1 roll	100	4.0	20.0	230	.5	1.0	0
GEM STYLE (Wonder) brown and serve	1 roll	80	2.0	13.0	140	.6	2.0	na
HARD	1 oz	83	2.8	14.9	154	na	1.2	0

Food Name	Serv. Size	Total Cal.	Prot. GMS	Carbs GMS	Sod. MGS	Fiber GMS	Fat GMS	Chol. MGS
HEARTH								
(Brownberry) 'Hearth' assorted	1 roll	124	4.4	23.7	247	1.5	2.3	7
(Pepperidge Farm) 'Hearth' brown and serve	1 roll	50	2.0	10.0	100	tr	.1.0	0
HOAGIE								
(Pepperidge Farm) soft 'Deli Classic'	1 roll	210	8.0	34.0	320	1.0	5.0	0
(Wonder)	1 roll	400	13.0	73.0	800	3.0	7.0	na
ITALIAN (Du Jour) crusty, brown and serve	1 roll	80	3.0	16.0	200	.6	1.0	0
KAISER								
	1 oz	83	2.8	14.9	154	na	1.2	0
(Arnold) 'Francisco'	1 roll	184	7.0	35.4	338	2.0	2.9	5
(Brownberry) 'Hearth'	1 roll	152	5.4	29.3	318	1.9	2.8	9
LUIGI (Colombo Brand) 'Twin Pack'	2-oz roll	146	7.6	25.4	334	(mq)	1.6	na
ONION (Levy's) 'Old Country Deli'	1-oz roll	153	6.1	30.8	380	1.8	1.9	11
PAN (Wonder)	1 roll	80	2.0	14.0	140	.6	1.0	na
PARKER HOUSE								
(Bridgford)	1-oz roll	85	2.5	15.8	172	(mq)	1.3	0
(Pepperidge Farm)	1 roll	60	2.0	9.0	80	tr	1.0	5
POTATO (Pepperidge Farm) 'Hearty Classic'	1 roll	90	2.0	14.0	125	tr	3.0	0
SANDWICH								
(Arnold) egg 'Dutch'	1 roll	123	4.5	21.6	203	1.9	3.3	1
(Awrey's) oat bran	1 roll	120	4.0	22.0	250	1.0	2.0	0
(Pepperidge Farm) onion, w/poppy seeds	1 roll	150	5.0	26.0	260	.5	3.0	0
(Pepperidge Farm) potato	1 roll	160	4.0	28.0	260	1.0	4.0	0
(Pepperidge Farm) salad 'Deli Classic'	1 roll	110	4.0	16.0	150	(mq)	4.0	10
(Pepperidge Farm) soft 'Family'	1 roll	100	4.0	18.0	190	.5	2.0	0
(Pepperidge Farm) w/sesame seeds	1 roll	140	5.0	23.0	230	.5	3.0	0
SOURDOUGH (Pepperidge Farm) French style	1 roll	100	4.0	19.0	240	.5	1.0	0
STEAK								
(Colombo Brand) sour	2.6-oz roll	200	10.1	35.1	413	(mq)	2.2	na
(Colombo Brand) sweet	2.6-oz roll	206	10.0	34.2	439	(mq)	3.3	na
TWIST (Pepperidge Farm) golden 'Heat 'n Serve'	1 roll	110	2.0	14.0	150	tr	5.0	5
ROLL, MIX								
(Dromedary) dry mix	1/8 pkg	209	6.0	41.0	363	(mq)	2.0	na
(Dromedary) prepared	2 rolls	239	6.0	41.0	410	(mq)	5.0	na
(Krusteaz) prepared	1 roll	150	3.0	28.0	190	na	3.0	0
(Pillsbury) prepared	2 rolls	270	4.0	25.0	420	(mq)	17.0	na
(Pillsbury) 'Hot Roll Mix' dry mix	1/16 pkg	100	3.0	21.0	200	na	0.0	0
(Pillsbury) 'Hot Roll Mix' prepared	1 roll	120	4.0	21.0	210	na	2.0	15

Food Name	Serv. Size	Total Cal.	Prot. GMS	Carbs GMS	Sod. MGS	Fiber GMS	Fat GMS	Chol. MGS
ROLL, SWEET. See also BUN, SWEET; DANISH PASTRY.								
APPLE								
(Break Cake) 4.5 oz	2 rolls	380	8.0	75.0	460	na	5.0	0
(Break Cake) multi-pak, 1.4 oz	1 roll	120	2.0	24.0	150	na	2.0	0
APPLE CINNAMON, old fashioned								
(Aunt Fanny's) individual	2 oz	180	4.0	34.0	125	1.5	1.0	5
CARAMEL NUT (Aunt Fanny's) individual	2 oz	190	4.0	33.0	125	1.0	6.0	5
CHEESE	1 oz	102	2.0	12.4	101	na	5.2	16
CHERRY								
(Break Cake) 4.5 oz	2 rolls	400	8.0	79.0	390	na	3.0	0
(Break Cake) multi-pak, 1.4 oz	1 roll	130	2.0	25.0	125	na	2.0	0
CINNAMON								
(Aunt Fanny's) duos, individual	1.9 oz	180	4.0	32.0	150	1.0	5.0	5
(Aunt Fanny's) individual	2 oz	190	4.0	34.0	160	1.0	5.0	5
(Aunt Fanny's) rectangular 11-oz size	2 oz	181	3.0	33.0	64	na	4.0	6
(Awrey's) homestyle	1 roll	240	4.0	40.0	200	1.0	7.0	5
(Awrey's) swirl 'Grande'	1 roll	340	4.0	46.0	370	1.0	16.0	10
(Break Cake) 4.5 oz	2 rolls	420	9.0	73.0	430	na	10.0	0
(Break Cake) multi-pak, 1.3 oz	1 roll	120	3.0	22.0	125	na	3.0	0
(Hungry Jack) refrigerated dough w/icing, prepared	2 rolls	290	3.0	37.0	570	(mq)	14.0	na
(Pillsbury) refrigerated dough w/icing, prepared	1 roll	110	1.0	17.0	260	(mq)	5.0	0
CINNAMON NUT (Break Cake) 3 oz	2 rolls	330	5.0	52.0	220	na	11.0	na
CINNAMON RAISIN (Aunt Fanny's) rectangular 11-oz size	2 oz	181	4.0	34.0	83	na	3.0	8
DIXIE FRUIT ROLL (Aunt Fanny's) individual	2 oz	180	3.0	34.0	120	1.0	4.0	5
PECAN								
(Aunt Fanny's) rectangular 11-oz size	2 oz	184	4.0	32.0	79	na	4.0	8
(Break Cake) multi-pak, 1.3 oz	1 roll	120	2.0	22.0	120	na	3.0	0
RAISIN CINNAMON (Break Cake) multi-pak, 1.25 oz	1 roll	120	2.0	21.0	110	na	3.0	0
STRAWBERRY (Aunt Fanny's) rectangular 11-oz size	2 oz	190	4.0	35.0	140	na	4.0	5
ROLL, SWEET, FROZEN								
APPLE (Weight Watchers) sweet 'Microwave'	1/2 pkg	160	3.0	27.0	100	(mq)	4.0	5
CHEESE (Weight Watchers) 'Microwave'	1/2 pkg	180	5.0	32.0	210	(mq)	4.0	5
CINNAMON								
(Pepperidge Farm) 2 per pkg	1 roll	280	4.0	34.0	190	(mq)	14.0	na
(Sara Lee) all butter	2-oz roll	230	3.0	31.0	220	(mq)	11.0	na
(Sara Lee) all butter, w/icing packet	.5-oz pkt	50	0.0	12.0	0	(mq)	0.0	0
(Weight Watchers) glazed	2.1 oz	180	4.0	31.0	170	na	5.0	5
STRAWBERRY (Weight Watchers) 'Microwave'	1/2 pkg	170	3.0	29.0	90	(mq)	5.0	20

Food Name	Serv. Size	Total Cal.	Prot. GMS	Carbs GMS	Sod. MGS	Fiber GMS	Fat GMS	Chol. MGS
ROLL DOUGH, FROZEN								
unraised, enriched, 2 x 2 3/8 inches	1 roll	75	2.1	13.3	135	>.1 c	1.4	1
unraised, unenriched, 2 x 2 3/8 inches	1 roll	75	2.1	13.3	135	>.1 c	1.4	1
ROMAN BEAN. See CRANBERRY BEAN.								
ROOT BEER. See SOFT DRINKS AND MIXERS.								
ROOT BEER FLOAT (Skipper's)	1 serving	302	3.0	33.0	66	na	10.0	10
ROQUETTE. See ARUGULA.								
ROSE APPLE								
raw	100 gm	25	0.6	5.7	0	>1.1 c	0.3	0
trimmed	1 oz	7	0.2	1.6	tr	>.3 c	0.1	0
untrimmed	1 lb	76	1.8	17.3	1	>3.3 c	0.9	0
ROSE COCO BEAN. See CRANBERRY BEAN.								
ROSEFISH. See OCEAN PERCH, ATLANTIC.								
ROSELLE								
raw, trimmed	1 cup	28	0.6	6.4	3	>.7 c	0.4	0
trimmed	1 oz	14	0.3	3.2	2	>.3 c	0.2	0
untrimmed	1 lb	136	2.7	31.3	16	>3.2 c	1.8	0
ROSEMARY								
dried	1 oz	94	1.4	18.2	14	>5.0 c	4.3	0
dried	1 tbsp	11	0.2	2.1	2	>.6 c	0.5	0
dried	1 tsp	4	0.1	0.8	1	>.2 c	0.2	0
dried (Durkee)	1 tsp	5	0.0	0.0	0	0	tr	na
dried (Laurel Leaf)	1 tsp	5	0.0	0.0	0	0	tr	na
dried (Spice Islands)	1 tsp	5	0.1	0.8	1	>.2 c	0.2	0
ROTINI. See PASTA.								
ROTINI ENTRÉE, FROZEN								
(Green Giant) cheddar 'Microwave Garden Gourmet'	1 pkg	230	9.0	32.0	570	4.5	10.0	20
(Mrs. Paul's) seafood 'Light'	9 oz	240	12.0	34.0	570	(mq)	6.0	25
(Weight Watchers) three cheese, w/vegetables	9 oz	270	14.0	34.0	500	na	8.0	5
ROTINI ENTRÉE MIX								
(Velveeta) w/cheese and broccoli, dry mix	1/4 box	210	1.0	24.0	730	na	8.0	25
(Velveeta) w/cheese and broccoli, prepared	1/2 cup	210	10.0	24.0	730	na	8.0	25
RUCULO. See ARUGULA.								
RUGULA. See ARUGULA.								
RUM. See ALCOHOLIC BEVERAGES.								
RUTABAGA								
boiled, drained	4 oz	39	1.2	8.8	20	1.8	0.2	0
boiled, drained, cubed	1/2 cup	33	1.1	7.4	17	1.5	0.2	0
boiled, drained, mashed	1/2 cup	47	1.5	10.5	24	2.2	0.3	0

Food Name	Serv. Size	Total Cal.	Prot. GMS	Carbs GMS	Sod. MGS	Fiber GMS	Fat GMS	Chol. MGS
raw, cubed	1/2 cup	25	0.8	5.7	14	1.8	0.1	0
raw, trimmed	1 oz	10	0.3	2.3	6	>.3 c	0.1	0
raw, untrimmed	1 lb	140	4.6	31.4	77	>4.2 c	0.8	0
RUTABAGA, CANNED *(Allens)* diced	1/2 cup	20	1.0	4.0	260	(mq)	<1.0	0
RYE								
flakes	1/2 cup	281	12.4	58.6	5	>1.3 c	2.1	0
flakes *(Arrowhead Mills)*	2 oz	190	7.0	42.0	1	7.6	1.0	0
whole grain	1 cup	567	25.0	117.9	10	>2.5 c	4.2	0
whole grain	1 oz	95	4.2	19.8	2	>.4 c	0.7	0
whole grain *(Arrowhead Mills)*	2 oz	190	7.0	42.0	1	7.6	1.0	0
RYE CAKE *(Quaker)* 'Grain Cakes'	.32-oz piece	35	1.4	6.5	52	.8	0.3	0
RYE FLOUR								
dark	1/2 cup	207	9.0	44.0	1	14.5	1.7	0
dark	1 oz	92	4.0	19.5	<1	(mq)	0.8	0
light	1/2 cup	187	4.3	40.9	1	7.4	0.7	0
light	1 oz	104	2.4	22.7	<1	4.1	0.4	0
medium	1/2 cup	181	4.8	39.5	2	7.4	0.9	0
medium	1 oz	100	2.7	22.0	1	4.1	0.5	0
(Arrowhead Mills) whole grain	2 oz	190	9.0	39.0	1	7.6	1.0	0
(Krusteaz)	1 cup	351	11.0	73.0	1	3.0	2.0	0
(Pillsbury) 'Bohemian Style' w/wheat flour	1 cup	400	11.0	86.0	0	(mq)	1.0	0
(Pillsbury's Best)	1 cup	400	12.0	83.0	0	(mq)	2.0	0
(Robin Hood) stone ground	1 cup	360	13.0	86.0	10	13.0	2.0	0

RYE WHISKEY. See ALCOHOLIC BEVERAGES.

S

Food Name	Serv. Size	Total Cal.	Prot. GMS	Carbs GMS	Sod. MGS	Fiber GMS	Fat GMS	Chol. MGS
SABLEFISH/skil								
cooked	3 oz	213	14.6	0.0	61	0	16.7	54
raw	1 lb	886	60.8	0.0	254	0	69.4	222
raw	3 oz	166	11.4	0.0	48	0	13.0	42
raw	1 oz	55	3.8	0.0	16	0	4.3	14
raw, approx 6.8 oz	1/2 fillet	376	25.9	0.0	108	0	29.5	95
smoked	4 oz	291	20.0	0.0	836	0	22.8	73
smoked	3 oz	218	15.0	0.0	626	0	17.1	54
SACCHARIN. See SUGAR, ALTERNATIVE.								
SAFFLOWER OIL								
'Hi-Oleic' *(Hain)*	1 tbsp	120	0.0	0.0	0	0	14.0	0
high oleic *(Spectrum Naturals)*	1 tbsp	120	0.0	0.0	0	(tr)	14.0	(tr)
high oleic, unrefined *(Spectrum Naturals)*	1 tbsp	120	0.0	0.0	0	(tr)	14.0	(tr)
linoleic	1/2 cup	964	0.0	0.0	0	0	109.0	0

Food Name	Serv. Size	Total Cal.	Prot. GMS	Carbs GMS	Sod. MGS	Fiber GMS	Fat GMS	Chol. MGS
linoleic	1 tbsp	120	0.0	0.0	0	0	13.6	0
oleic	1/2 cup	964	0.0	0.0	0	0	109.0	0
oleic	1 tbsp	120	0.0	0.0	0	0	13.6	0
organic, unrefined *(Spectrum Naturals)*	1 tbsp	120	0.0	0.0	0	(tr)	14.0	(tr)
over 70% oleic	1 cup	1927	0.0	0.0	0	0	218.0	na
over 70% oleic	1 tbsp	124	0.0	0.0	0	0	14.0	na
SAFFLOWER SEED, dried, kernels	1 oz	147	4.6	9.7	1	>.7 c	10.9	0
SAFFLOWER SEED MEAL,								
partially defatted	1 oz	97	10.1	13.8	1	>2.2 c	0.7	0
SAFFRON								
dried	1 oz	88	3.2	18.5	42	>1.0 c	1.7	0
dried	1 tbsp	7	0.2	1.4	3	.1	0.1	0
dried	1 tsp	2	0.1	0.5	1	tr	0.0	0
SAGE								
ground	1 oz	89	3.0	17.2	3	5.1	3.6	0
ground	1 tbsp	6	0.2	1.2	0	.4	0.3	0
ground	1 tsp	2	0.1	0.4	0	.1	0.1	0
ground *(Durkee)*	1 tsp	3	0.0	0.0	0	0	tr	na
ground *(Laurel Leaf)*	1 tsp	3	0.0	0.0	0	0	tr	na
ground *(Spice Islands)*	1 tsp	4	0.1	0.6	<1	.1	0.1	0
SALAD DRESSING								
BACON *(Kraft)* creamy 'Reduced Calorie'	1 tbsp	30	0.0	2.0	150	na	2.0	0
BACON AND TOMATO								
(Estee)	1 tbsp	8	<1.0	1.0	35	na	<1.0	5
(Kraft)	1 tbsp	70	0.0	1.0	130	na	7.0	0
(Kraft) 'Reduced Calorie'	1 tbsp	30	0.0	2.0	150	na	2.0	0
BLUE CHEESE								
	1 cup	1235	11.8	18.1	2680	na	128.1	42
	1 tbsp	77	0.7	1.1	167	na	8.0	3
(Ayla's Organics) fat free	2 tbsp	30	1.0	4.0	140	0	0.0	0
(Estee)	1 tbsp	8	<1.0	1.0	50	na	<1.0	0
(Featherweight) 'Neu Bleu'	1 tbsp	4	0.0	1.0	110	na	0.0	0
(Hidden Valley Ranch) 'Lowfat'	1 tbsp	10	0.0	3.0	140	na	0.0	0
(Kraft) chunky	1 tbsp	60	1.0	2.0	230	na	6.0	5
(Kraft) chunky 'Reduced Calorie'	1 tbsp	30	0.0	2.0	240	na	2.0	5
(Kraft) 'Free'	1 tbsp	16	0.0	4.0	120	na	0.0	0
(Lawry's) 'Classic'	1 tbsp	186	0.1	1.9	385	>.1 c	2.0	na
(Litehouse) country, dressing and dip, refrigerated	1 tbsp	76	1.0	0.0	84	na	8.0	na
(Litehouse) 'Lite' dressing and dip, refrigerated	1 tbsp	33	1.0	1.0	86	na	3.0	na
(Litehouse) 'Original' dressing and dip, refrigerated	1 tbsp	77	1.0	0.0	82	na	8.0	na

Food Name	Serv. Size	Total Cal.	Prot. GMS	Carbs GMS	Sod. MGS	Fiber GMS	Fat GMS	Chol. MGS
(Roka)	1 tbsp	60	1.0	1.0	170	na	6.0	10
(Roka) 'Reduced Calorie'	1 tbsp	16	1.0	1.0	280	na	1.0	5
(S&W Nutradiet)	1 tbsp	25	0.0	2.0	200	na	2.0	0
(Skipper's) premium	1 pouch	222	1.0	4.0	240	na	23.0	8
(T. Marzetti)	1 tbsp	90	1.0	1.0	180	na	9.0	2
(T. Marzetti) chunky, refrigerated	1 tbsp	78	1.0	1.0	159	na	8.0	14
(T. Marzetti) 'Lite' refrigerated	1 tbsp	45	0.0	0.0	150	na	5.0	5
(Wish-Bone) chunky	1 tbsp	75	0.4	0.7	149	na	7.9	1
(Wish-Bone) chunky 'Lite'	1 tbsp	40	0.3	1.5	197	na	3.7	1
(Wish-Bone) chunky, lite 'Food Service'	.5 oz	40	0.0	1.0	200	na	4.0	0
(Wish-Bone) 'Healthy Sensation!'	.5 oz	20	na	4.0	140	na	na	0
BUTTERMILK								
(Hain) 'Old Fashioned'	1 tbsp	70	(mq)	(mq)	100	na	7.0	0
(Hollywood) 'Old Fashion'	1 tbsp	75	0.0	1.0	40	0	8.0	0
(Kraft) creamy	1 tbsp	80	0.0	1.0	120	0	8.0	5
(Kraft) creamy 'Reduced Calorie'	1 tbsp	30	0.0	1.0	125	na	3.0	5
(Seven Seas) 'Buttermilk Recipe'	1 tbsp	80	0.0	1.0	130	na	8.0	5
(T. Marzetti) and herbs	1 tbsp	95	0.0	0.0	150	na	10.0	3
(T. Marzetti) bacon, refrigerated	1 tbsp	93	0.0	0.0	127	na	10.0	2
(T. Marzetti) blue cheese, refrigerated	1 tbsp	90	1.0	1.0	161	na	10.0	5
CAESAR								
(Estee)	2 tbsp	8	<1.0	<1.0	130	na	<1.0	2
(Hain) creamy	1 tbsp	60	0.0	1.0	220	na	6.0	5
(Hain) creamy 'Low Salt'	1 tbsp	60	0.0	1.0	15	na	6.0	5
(Hollywood)	1 tbsp	70	1.0	2.0	65	0	7.0	0
(Kraft) golden	1 tbsp	70	0.0	1.0	180	na	7.0	0
(Lawry's) 'Classic'	1 tbsp	130	0.8	1.0	337	>.1 c	13.5	na
(Litehouse) dressing and dip, refrigerated	1 tbsp	57	0.0	0.0	84	na	6.0	na
(T. Marzetti)	1 tbsp	80	0.0	1.0	170	na	8.0	2
(T. Marzetti) house	1 tbsp	75	<1.0	<1.0	180	na	8.0	1
(T. Marzetti) refrigerated	1 tbsp	75	0.0	0.0	178	na	8.0	0
(Weight Watchers)	1 tbsp	4	0.0	1.0	200	na	0.0	0
(Wish-Bone)	1 tbsp	77	0.4	0.9	248	na	8.0	1
(Wish-Bone) w/olive oil 'Lite'	.5 oz	30	0.0	1.0	170	na	3.0	0
CALIFORNIA FRENCH								
(Catalina) nonfat 'Free'	1 tbsp	16	0.0	3.0	120	na	0.0	0
(T. Marzetti)	1 tbsp	90	1.0	5.0	100	na	6.0	4
(T. Marzetti) 'Fat-Free'	1 tbsp	16	<1.0	4.0	140	na	0.0	0
(T. Marzetti) 'Light'	1 tbsp	40	0.0	3.0	180	na	3.0	2
CELERY SEED								
(T. Marzetti) and onion	1 tbsp	75	0.0	9.0	90	na	6.0	0
(T. Marzetti) refrigerated	1 tbsp	72	0.0	5.0	101	na	5.0	0

Food Name	Serv. Size	Total Cal.	Prot. GMS	Carbs GMS	Sod. MGS	Fiber GMS	Fat GMS	Chol. MGS
CHEESE								
(Featherweight)	1 tbsp	20	0.0	1.0	70	na	2.0	0
(Hain) vinaigrette	1 tbsp	55	0.0	0.0	130	na	6.0	5
(Hollywood)	1 tbsp	80	0.0	2.0	60	0	8.0	0
CHINESE VINEGAR								
(Lawry's) w/sesame and ginger 'Classic'	1 tbsp	145	0.2	2.4	325	0	15.0	0
CITRUS (Hain) tangy 'Canola'	1 tbsp	50	0.0	1.0	75	na	5.0	0
CREAMY								
(Estee)	1 tbsp	4	0.0	1.0	13	na	0.0	0
(Hain)	1 tbsp	80	0.0	0.0	100	na	8.0	0
(Hain) 'No Salt Added'	1 tbsp	80	0.0	1.0	25	na	8.0	0
(Hollywood)	1 tbsp	90	0.0	2.0	140	0	9.0	0
(Kraft) no oil 'Reduced Calorie'	1 tbsp	4	0.0	1.0	220	na	0.0	0
(Kraft) 'Reduced Calorie'	1 tbsp	25	0.0	1.0	120	na	2.0	0
(Kraft) w/real sour cream	1 tbsp	50	0.0	1.0	120	na	5.0	0
(Kraft) zesty	1 tbsp	50	0.0	1.0	260	na	5.0	0
(Kraft) zesty 'Reduced Calorie'	1 tbsp	20	0.0	1.0	230	na	2.0	0
(Lawry's) w/Parmesan cheese 'Classic'	1 oz	156	0.0	4.5	178	>.1 c	15.1	na
(Life) egg-free 'All Natural'	1 tbsp	39	<1.0	2.0	4	na	4.0	0
(Pathmark)	1 tbsp	70	0.0	1.0	260	na	7.0	0
(Pathmark) zesty	1 tbsp	70	0.0	1.0	370	na	8.0	0
(Pathmark) zesty 'Reduced Calorie'	1 tbsp	6	0.0	1.0	190	na	0.0	0
(Rancher's Choice)	1 tbsp	90	0.0	1.0	140	na	10.0	5
(Rancher's Choice) 'Reduced Calorie'	1 tbsp	30	0.0	1.0	150	na	3.0	5
(S&W Nutradiet)	1 tbsp	10	0.0	1.0	180	na	1.0	na
(S&W Nutradiet) no oil	1 tbsp	2	0.0	0.0	290	na	0.0	0
(Seven Seas)	1 tbsp	70	0.0	1.0	240	na	7.0	0
(Wish-Bone)	1 tbsp	56	0.1	1.5	149	na	5.5	<1
(Wish-Bone) 'Lite'	1 tbsp	26	0.1	2.0	148	na	2.0	<1
(Weight Watchers) 'Single Serve' 1 packet	1 tbsp	9	0.0	2.0	430	na	0.0	0
CUCUMBER								
(Featherweight) creamy	1 tbsp	4	0.0	1.0	80	na	0.0	0
(Hain) dill, creamy	1 tbsp	80	0.0	0.0	210	na	8.0	5
(Kraft) creamy	1 tbsp	70	0.0	1.0	190	na	8.0	0
(Kraft) creamy 'Reduced Calorie'	1 tbsp	25	0.0	1.0	220	na	2.0	0
(Weight Watchers) creamy	1 tbsp	18	(mq)	4.0	85	na	0.0	na
DIJON								
(Estee) creamy	1 tbsp	8	<1.0	<1.0	100	na	<1.0	5
(Featherweight) creamy	1 tbsp	20	0.0	1.0	80	na	2.0	0
(Great Impressions) mustard	1 tbsp	57	0.4	0.3	103	na	6.1	18
(Hain) vinaigrette	1 tbsp	50	0.0	1.0	180	na	5.0	5
(Hollywood) vinaigrette	1 tbsp	60	0.0	2.0	40	0	6.0	0
(Wish-Bone) vinaigrette 'Classic'	1 tbsp	60	0.2	1.0	171	na	6.1	<1

Food Name	Serv. Size	Total Cal.	Prot. GMS	Carbs GMS	Sod. MGS	Fiber GMS	Fat GMS	Chol. MGS
(Wish-Bone) vinaigrette 'Lite Classic'	1 tbsp	30	0.1	1.1	176	na	2.8	0
DILL								
(Ayla's Organics) creamy, fat free	2 tbsp	15	0.0	3.0	140	0.0	0.0	0
(Nasoya) creamy 'Vegi-Dressing'	1 tbsp	40	1.0	1.0	50	na	3.0	0
FRENCH								
(Ayla's Organics) fat free	2 tbsp	10	0.0	3.0	150	0.0	0.0	0
(Catalina)	1 tbsp	60	0.0	4.0	180	na	5.0	0
(Catalina) 'Reduced Calorie'	1 tbsp	18	0.0	3.0	120	na	1.0	0
(Estee)	1 tbsp	4	0.0	1.0	10	na	0.0	0
(Estee) creamy	2 tbsp	10	0.0	2.0	130	na	0.0	0
(Featherweight)	1 tbsp	14	0.0	3.0	15	na	0.0	0
(Great Impressions) w/green pepper, low calorie	1 tbsp	64	0.2	4.1	188	na	5.2	0
(Hain) creamy	1 tbsp	60	0.0	1.0	80	na	6.0	0
(Hain) spicy mustard 'Canola'	1 tbsp	50	1.0	1.0	190	na	5.0	5
(Hollywood) creamy	1 tbsp	70	0.0	2.0	45	0	7.0	0
(Kraft)	1 tbsp	60	0.0	2.0	125	na	6.0	0
(Kraft) 'Miracle'	1 tbsp	70	0.0	3.0	240	na	6.0	0
(Kraft) nonfat 'Free'	1 tbsp	20	0.0	4.0	120	na	0.0	0
(Kraft) 'Reduced Calorie'	1 tbsp	20	0.0	3.0	120	na	1.0	0
(Litehouse) country herb, dressing and marinade, refrigerated	1 tbsp	54	0.0	2.0	196	na	5.0	na
(Pathmark) creamy	1 tbsp	60	0.0	2.0	90	na	5.0	0
(Pathmark) 'Reduced Calorie'	1 tbsp	20	0.0	3.0	160	na	1.0	0
(Pritikin) style, fat-free, sodium-free	1 tbsp	10	0.0	3.0	0	na	0.0	0
(S&W Nutradiet)	1 tbsp	18	0.0	3.0	120	na	0.0	0
(Seven Seas) creamy	1 tbsp	60	0.0	2.0	240	na	6.0	0
(Seven Seas) 'French! Light'	1 tbsp	35	0.0	2.0	210	na	3.0	0
(T. Marzetti) country	1 tbsp	72	0.0	4.0	110	na	6.0	6
(T. Marzetti) 'Frenchette'	1 tbsp	10	0.0	3.0	140	na	0.0	0
(T. Marzetti) honey, refrigerated	1 tbsp	74	0.0	5.0	115	na	6.0	0
(T. Marzetti) honey blue, refrigerated	1 tbsp	70	0.0	5.0	122	na	6.0	1
(T. Marzetti) honey 'Lite' refrigerated	1 tbsp	48	0.0	5.0	118	na	3.0	0
(T. Marzetti) 'Light'	1 tbsp	16	0.0	3.0	160	na	1.0	0
(Ultra Slim Fast) 'Cholesterol Free'	1 tbsp	20	0.0	4.0	105	na	<1.0	0
(Weight Watchers) low-calorie	1 tbsp	10	0.0	2.0	170	na	0.0	0
(Wish-Bone) creamy, garlic	1 tbsp	55	0.1	1.8	158	>.1 c	5.3	0
(Wish-Bone) 'Deluxe'	1 tbsp	60	0.1	2.3	83	na	5.4	0
(Wish-Bone) 'Deluxe Food Service'	1 tbsp	61	0.1	2.4	86	0	5.6	0
(Wish-Bone) garlic	1 tbsp	55	0.1	1.8	158	>.1 c	5.3	0
(Wish-Bone) 'Healthy Sensation!'	.5 oz	20	0.0	4.0	120	na	na	0
(Wish-Bone) 'Lite'	1 tbsp	31	0.0	2.1	70	0	2.5	0
(Wish-Bone) 'Lite Sweet 'n Spicy'	1 tbsp	18	0.0	3.2	110	na	0.5	0

Food Name	Serv. Size	Total Cal.	Prot. GMS	Carbs GMS	Sod. MGS	Fiber GMS	Fat GMS	Chol. MGS
(Wish-Bone) low-calorie 'Lite'	1 tbsp	30	0.1	1.9	67	na	2.5	0
(Wish-Bone) red, low-calorie 'Lite'	1 tbsp	17	0.2	3.2	155	na	0.4	0
(Wish-Bone) style 'Lite'	.5 oz	18	0.0	3.0	140	na	na	0
(Wish-Bone) style, lite 'Food Service'	.5 oz	30	0.0	2.0	75	na	3.0	0
(Wish-Bone) sweet 'n spicy	.5 oz	70	0.0	3.0	160	na	6.0	0
(Wish-Bone) sweet 'n spicy 'Lite'	.5 oz	18	0.0	4.0	130	na	na	0
FRUIT SALAD								
(Great Impressions) orange marmalade	1 tbsp	87	0.2	5.4	48	na	7.1	11
(Knott's Berry Farm)	1 tbsp	50	2.0	3.0	75	na	5.0	na
GARLIC								
(Ayla's Organics) and onion, fat free	2 tbsp	10	0.0	2.0	140	0	0.0	0
(Ayla's Organics) creamy, fat free	2 tbsp	30	1.0	4.0	140	0	0.0	0
(Estee) creamy	1 tbsp	2	0.0	0.0	10	na	0.0	0
(Hain) and sour cream	1 tbsp	70	0.0	0.0	100	na	7.0	0
(Kraft) creamy	1 tbsp	50	0.0	1.0	170	na	5.0	0
(Life) w/tofu 'All Natural' dressing and dip	1 tbsp	70	<1.0	1.4	0	(mq)	7.1	75
(Nasoya) herb 'Vegi-Dressing'	1 tbsp	40	1.0	1.0	50	na	3.0	0
(Pritikin) and herb, fat-free, sodium-free	1 tbsp	6	0.0	2.0	0	na	0.0	0
(T. Marzetti) Italian, refrigerated	1 tbsp	81	0.0	1.0	73	na	9.0	9
(Wish-Bone) creamy	1 tbsp	74	0.1	0.5	158	>.6 c	8.0	0
(Wish-Bone) Sierra	.5 oz	80	0.0	1.0	125	na	8.0	na
GINGER PLUM VINAIGRETTE								
(Simply Delicious) 'Un-Dressing'	1 tbsp	36	0.0	1.0	199	na	4.0	0
HERB								
(Featherweight)	1 tbsp	6	0.0	1.0	5	na	0.0	0
(Featherweight) garden	1 tbsp	25	0.0	2.0	65	na	2.0	0
(Hain) savory 'No Salt Added'	1 tbsp	90	0.0	0.0	25	na	10.0	0
(Marie's) vinaigrette, fat-free 'Lite & Zesty'	1 tbsp	16	0.0	4.0	130	na	0.0	0
(Pritikin) vinaigrette, fat-free, sodium-free	1 tbsp	8	0.0	2.0	0	na	0.0	0
(Seven Seas) and spice 'Viva'	1 tbsp	60	0.0	1.0	170	na	6.0	0
(Seven Seas) and spice 'Viva Herbs & Spices! Light'	1 tbsp	30	0.0	1.0	200	na	3.0	0
(Simply Delicious) garlic vinaigrette 'Un-Dressing'	1 tbsp	43	0.0	1.0	132	na	4.0	0
(Wish-Bone) creamy 'Classics'	1 tbsp	70	0.0	1.2	228	na	7.3	0
HOMESTYLE								
(Dorothy Lynch)	1 tbsp	55	0.1	5.0	85	na	3.8	0
(Dorothy Lynch) 'Reduced Calorie'	1 tbsp	30	0.0	7.0	80	na	<1.0	0
HONEY AND SESAME (Hain)	1 tbsp	60	0.0	2.0	210	na	5.0	0
HONEY MUSTARD								
(Knott's Berry Farm) 'Peggy Jane's'	1 tbsp	60	0.0	2.0	40	na	6.0	na
(Litehouse) dressing and dip, refrigerated	1 tbsp	67	0.0	2.0	55	na	7.0	na

Food Name	Serv. Size	Total Cal.	Prot. GMS	Carbs GMS	Sod. MGS	Fiber GMS	Fat GMS	Chol. MGS
(Simply Delicious) vinaigrette 'Un-Dressing'	1 tbsp	41	0.0	2.0	122	na	4.0	0
(T. Marzetti) Dijon	1 tbsp	67	0.0	3.0	51	na	6.0	7
(T. Marzetti) Dijon, refrigerated	1 tbsp	68	0.0	3.0	103	na	6.0	9
(Wish-Bone) Dijon 'Healthy Sensation!'	1 tbsp	25	0.0	5.0	140	na	0.0	0
ITALIAN								
(Ayla's Organics) fat free	2 tbsp	10	0.0	2.0	140	0	0.0	0
(Estee)	2 tbsp	4	0.0	1.0	130	na	0.0	0
(Featherweight)	1 tbsp	4	0.0	1.0	120	na	0.0	0
(Hain) 'Canola'	1 tbsp	50	0.0	1.0	150	na	5.0	0
(Hain) 'Traditional'	1 tbsp	80	0.0	0.0	330	na	8.0	0
(Hain) 'Traditional No Salt Added'	1 tbsp	60	0.0	1.0	20	na	6.0	0
(Hollywood)	1 tbsp	90	0.0	1.0	300	0	9.0	0
(Kraft) 'Deliciously Light'	1 tbsp	35	0.0	1.0	115	na	3.0	0
(Kraft) house	1 tbsp	60	0.0	1.0	115	na	6.0	0
(Kraft) house 'Reduced Calorie'	1 tbsp	30	0.0	1.0	115	na	2.0	0
(Kraft) nonfat 'Free'	1 tbsp	6	0.0	1.0	210	na	0.0	0
(Kraft) oil-free 'Reduced Calorie'	1 tbsp	4	0.0	1.0	220	na	0.0	0
(Kraft) 'Presto'	1 tbsp	70	0.0	1.0	150	na	7.0	0
(Kraft) zesty	1 tbsp	50	0.0	1.0	260	na	5.0	0
(Kraft) zesty 'Reduced Calorie'	1 tbsp	20	0.0	1.0	230	na	2.0	0
(Marie's) vinaigrette, fat-free 'Lite & Zesty'	1 tbsp	16	0.0	4.0	135	na	0.0	0
(Nasoya) 'Vegi-Dressing'	1 tbsp	40	1.0	1.0	50	na	3.0	0
(Ott's)	1 tbsp	80	<.1	0.2	87	tr	9.1	<1
(Pritikin) fat-free, sodium-free	1 tbsp	8	0.0	2.0	0	na	0.0	0
(Seven Seas) 'Free Viva'	1 tbsp	4	0.0	1.0	220	na	0.0	0
(Seven Seas) 'Viva'	1 tbsp	50	0.0	1.0	240	na	5.0	0
(Seven Seas) 'Viva Italian! Light'	1 tbsp	30	0.0	1.0	230	na	3.0	0
(Skipper's) gourmet	1 pouch	140	0.0	2.0	200	na	15.0	0
(Skipper's) lo-cal	1 pouch	17	0.0	2.0	680	na	1.0	0
(T. Marzetti) 'Fat-Free'	1 tbsp	5	0.0	1.0	270	na	0.0	0
(T. Marzetti) 'Frenchette'	1 tbsp	6	0.0	2.0	280	na	0.0	0
(T. Marzetti) gusto	1 tbsp	58	0.0	0.0	204	na	8.0	0
(T. Marzetti) 'Light'	1 tbsp	35	0.0	1.0	300	na	3.0	0
(T. Marzetti) w/olive oil	1 tbsp	60	0.0	1.0	220	na	7.0	0
(Ultra Slim Fast) 'Cholesterol Free'	1 tbsp	6	0.0	1.0	105	na	<1.0	0
(Wish-Bone)	1 tbsp	46	0.0	1.5	280	na	4.5	0
(Wish-Bone) blended	.5 oz	35	0.0	1.0	210	na	4.0	0
(Wish-Bone) 'Food Service'	.5 oz	45	0.0	2.0	290	na	5.0	0
(Wish-Bone) 'Healthy Sensation!'	1 tbsp	6	0.0	1.0	140	na	0.0	0
(Wish-Bone) 'Lite'	1 tbsp	7	0.2	0.9	212	na	0.3	0
(Wish-Bone) lite 'Food Service'	.5 oz	6	0.0	1.0	250	na	na	0
(Wish-Bone) 'Robusto'	1 tbsp	47	0.1	1.8	288	na	4.5	0

Food Name	Serv. Size	Total Cal.	Prot. GMS	Carbs GMS	Sod. MGS	Fiber GMS	Fat GMS	Chol. MGS
(Weight Watchers) style	1 tbsp	6	0.0	1.0	200	na	0.0	na
(Weight Watchers) style 'Single Serve'								
1 packet	.75 oz	8	0.0	2.0	270	na	0.0	na
ITALIAN, CREAMY								
(Estee)	2 tbsp	14	<1.0	2.0	130	na	<1.0	0
(Kraft)	1 tbsp	60	0.0	1.0	115	na	6.0	0
(Kraft) 'Deliciously Light'	1 tbsp	25	0.0	1.0	120	na	2.0	0
(Kraft) 'Reduced Calorie'	1 tbsp	25	0.0	1.0	120	na	2.0	0
(Kraft) w/real sour cream	1 tbsp	50	0.0	1.0	120	na	5.0	0
(Litehouse) dressing and dip, refrigerated	1 tbsp	60	0.0	0.0	76	na	6.0	na
(Seven Seas) 'Viva Creamy Italian! Light'	1 tbsp	45	0.0	1.0	230	na	4.0	0
(T. Marzetti)	1 tbsp	80	0.0	1.0	100	na	8.0	4
(Weight Watchers)	1 tbsp	12	0.0	3.0	85	na	0.0	na
(Weight Watchers) whipped	1 tbsp	50	0.0	2.0	80	na	5.0	5
(Wish-Bone)	.5 oz	60	0.0	1.0	150	na	6.0	0
(Wish-Bone) 'Food Service'	.5 oz	25	0.0	4.0	140	na	na	0
(Wish-Bone) 'Lite'	.5 oz	25	0.0	4.0	140	na	na	0
LEMON TAHINI VINAIGRETTE								
(Simply Delicious) 'Un-Dressing'	1 tbsp	43	0.0	1.0	170	na	4.0	9
LIME CILANTRO VINAIGRETTE								
(Simply Delicious) 'Un-Dressing'	1 tbsp	41	0.0	1.0	116	na	4.0	0
MAYONNAISE TYPE. See also MAYONNAISE.								
(A&P)	1 tbsp	70	<1.0	2.0	100	na	7.0	0
(Bama)	1 tbsp	50	0.0	3.0	105	0	4.0	na
(Finast)	1 tbsp	70	0.0	2.0	90	0	7.0	na
(Kraft) 'Miracle Whip'	1 tbsp	70	0.0	2.0	85	0	7.0	5
(Kraft) 'Miracle Whip Light'	1 tbsp	40	0.0	3.0	120	0	3.0	0
(Kraft) nonfat 'Miracle Whip Free'	1 tbsp	15	0.0	3.0	105	0	0.0	0
(P&Q)	1 tbsp	50	<1.0	3.0	110	0	5.0	8
(Pathmark) 'No Frills'	1 tbsp	50	0.0	3.0	120	0	5.0	5
(Spin Blend)	1 tbsp	60	0.0	3.0	110	0	5.0	10
(Spin Blend) cholesterol free	1 tbsp	40	0.0	2.0	110	0	4.0	0
(Weight Watchers) whipped	1 tbsp	45	0.0	3.0	100	0	4.0	0
(Weight Watchers) whipped, fat-free	1 tbsp	12	0.0	4.0	125	na	0.0	0
(Weight Watchers) whipped, light	1 tbsp	50	0.0	1.0	100	na	5.0	5
(Weight Watchers) whipped, low-sodium	1 tbsp	50	0.0	1.0	45	na	5.0	5
OIL AND VINEGAR								
W/balsamic vinegar *(Great Impressions)*	1 tbsp	67	<1.0	2.3	367	na	6.5	0
W/Cabernet *(Lawry's)* 'Classics'	1 tbsp	138	0.0	4.9	178	0	13.7	na
W/olive oil								
(Kraft)	1 tbsp	70	0.0	1.0	210	0	8.0	0
(Wish-Bone) Italian 'Classic'	1 tbsp	34	0.0	1.7	190	0	3.0	0
(Wish-Bone) 'Lite Classic'	.5 oz	20	0.0	2.0	170	na	2.0	0

Food Name	Serv. Size	Total Cal.	Prot. GMS	Carbs GMS	Sod. MGS	Fiber GMS	Fat GMS	Chol. MGS
(Wish-Bone) vinaigrette	1 tbsp	28	0.0	1.8	111	0	2.3	0
(Wish-Bone) vinaigrette 'Lite'	1 tbsp	16	0.1	1.9	111	0	0.9	0
W/red wine vinegar								
(Estee)	1 tbsp	2	0.0	0.0	10	0	0.0	0
(Featherweight)	1 tbsp	6	0.0	1.0	100	0	0.0	0
(Great Impressions)	1 tbsp	64	<1.0	2.5	277	na	6.1	0
(Kraft)	1 tbsp	60	0.0	4.0	200	na	4.0	0
(Pathmark)	1 tbsp	70	0.0	2.0	235	na	7.0	0
(Seven Seas) 'Free'	1 tbsp	6	0.0	1.0	190	na	0.0	0
(Seven Seas) 'Viva'	1 tbsp	70	0.0	1.0	290	na	7.0	0
(Seven Seas) 'Viva Red Wine!'	1 tbsp	45	0.0	1.0	190	na	4.0	0
W/white wine vinegar *(Great Impressions)*	1 tbsp	63	<1.0	0.8	242	na	6.6	0
ONION AND CHIVES								
.*(Kraft)* creamy	1 tbsp	70	0.0	1.0	150	na	7.0	0
(Wish-Bone) 'Lite'	1 tbsp	37	0.2	1.6	164	na	3.3	0
ORIENTAL STYLE *(Featherweight)*	1 tbsp	20	0.0	1.0	75	na	2.0	0
PARMESAN *(Hidden Valley Ranch)* Italian 'Lowfat'	1 tbsp	16	0.0	3.0	140	na	1.0	0
PARMESAN PEPPERCORN								
(T. Marzetti)	1 tbsp	81	<1.0	<1.0	129	na	9.0	6
(T. Marzetti) refrigerated	1 tbsp	85	0.0	1.0	154	na	9.0	5
PEPPERCORN								
(Litehouse) dressing and dip, refrigerated	1 tbsp	67	0.0	0.0	66	na	7.0	na
(Simply Delicious) pink, vinaigrette 'Un-Dressing'	1 tbsp	40	0.0	1.0	148	na	4.0	0
(T. Marzetti) cracked, refrigerated	1 tbsp	62	0.0	0.0	135	na	7.0	13
(Weight Watchers) creamy	1 tbsp	8	0.0	2.0	85	na	0.0	na
POPPYSEED								
(Great Impressions)	1 tbsp	131	0.1	8.0	130	na	11.0	0
(Hain) 'Rancher's'	1 tbsp	60	0.0	0.0	105	na	7.0	5
(Knott's Berry Farm) 'Peggy Jane's'	1 tbsp	60	0.0	4.0	90	na	5.0	na
(Litehouse) dressing and dip, refrigerated	1 tbsp	65	0.0	3.0	83	na	6.0	na
(T. Marzetti)	1 tbsp	72	<1.0	5.0	146	na	6.0	8
(T. Marzetti) refrigerated	1 tbsp	65	0.0	5.0	97	na	5.0	5
POTATO SALAD *(T. Marzetti)*	1 tbsp	80	0.0	3.0	170	na	7.0	9
RANCH								
(Hidden Valley Ranch) honey Dijon 'Lowfat'	1 tbsp	20	0.0	3.0	140	na	1.0	0
(Hidden Valley Ranch) original 'Light'	1 tbsp	40	0.0	2.0	140	na	4.0	5
(Kraft) nonfat 'Free'	1 tbsp	16	0.0	3.0	150	na	0.0	0
(Litehouse) country, dressing and dip, refrigerated	1 tbsp	61	0.0	1.0	75	na	7.0	na
(Litehouse) dressing and dip, refrigerated	1 tbsp	59	0.0	1.0	67	na	6.0	na

Food Name	Serv. Size	Total Cal.	Prot. GMS	Carbs GMS	Sod. MGS	Fiber GMS	Fat GMS	Chol. MGS
(Litehouse) jalapeño, dressing and dip, refrigerated	1 tbsp	60	0.0	1.0	80	na	6.0	na
(Litehouse) 'Lite' dressing and dip, refrigerated	1 tbsp	35	1.0	1.0	80	na	3.0	na
(Pritikin) fat-free, sodium-free	1 tbsp	16	0.0	4.0	0	na	0.0	0
(Seven Seas) 'Buttermilk Recipe Ranch! Light'	1 tbsp	50	0.0	1.0	135	na	5.0	0
(Seven Seas) 'Free'	1 tbsp	16	0.0	4.0	120	na	0.0	0
(Seven Seas) 'Viva'	1 tbsp	80	0.0	1.0	135	na	8.0	5
(Seven Seas) 'Viva Ranch! Light'	1 tbsp	50	0.0	2.0	125	na	5.0	5
(Skipper's) house	1 pouch	188	1.0	2.0	302	na	20.0	0
(T. Marzetti)	1 tbsp	90	0.0	0.0	92	na	2.0	3
(T. Marzetti) buttermilk, refrigerated	1 tbsp	93	0.0	1.0	127	na	10.0	2
(T. Marzetti) buttermilk 'Lite' refrigerated	1 tbsp	45	0.0	2.0	135	na	5.0	3
(T. Marzetti) Caesar	1 tbsp	95	<1.0	1.0	150	na	10.0	3
(T. Marzetti) 'Fat-Free'	1 tbsp	12	<1.0	3.0	220	na	0.0	0
(T. Marzetti) garden	1 tbsp	100	0.0	1.0	165	na	10.0	4
(T. Marzetti) honey Dijon	1 tbsp	89	<1.0	1.0	100	na	9.0	14
(T. Marzetti) honey Dijon, refrigerated	1 tbsp	79	<1.0	1.0	101	na	8.0	14
(T. Marzetti) 'Light'	1 tbsp	40	0.0	2.0	166	na	4.0	4
(T. Marzetti) Parmesan, refrigerated	1 tbsp	86	0.0	1.0	120	na	9.0	6
(T. Marzetti) peppercorn	1 tbsp	85	0.0	1.0	13	na	9.0	4
(T. Marzetti) peppercorn 'Fat-Free'	1 tbsp	14	0.0	3.0	173	na	0.0	0
(T. Marzetti) style	1 tbsp	90	1.0	5.0	100	na	6.0	4
(Weight Watchers) creamy	1 tbsp	25	0.0	6.0	100	na	0.0	0
(Weight Watchers) creamy 'Single Serve'	1 pkt	35	0.0	8.0	140	na	0.0	0
(Wish-Bone)	1 tbsp	78	0.1	1.1	156	na	8.3	4
(Wish-Bone) 'Food Service'	.5 oz	80	0.0	1.0	105	na	8.0	5
(Wish-Bone) 'Healthy Sensation!'	1 tbsp	16	0.0	3.0	140	na	0.0	0
(Wish-Bone) 'Lite'	1 tbsp	42	0.2	2.5	148	na	3.5	5
RED WINE VINAIGRETTE								
(Wish-Bone)	1 tbsp	51	0.0	4.2	216	(tr)	3.8	0
(Wish-Bone) 'Lite'	.5 oz	20	0.0	2.0	140	na	2.0	0
ROMANO								
(T. Marzetti) cheese Italian	1 tbsp	80	0.0	0.0	135	na	8.0	2
(T. Marzetti) cheese Italian, refrigerated	1 tbsp	77	<1.0	<1.0	183	na	8.0	3
RUSSIAN								
(Ayla's Organics) fat-free	2 tbsp	10	0.0	3.0	140	0	0.0	0
(Featherweight)	1 tbsp	6	0.0	1.0	125	(mq)	0.0	0
(Kraft)	1 tbsp	60	0.0	4.0	130	(mq)	5.0	0
(Kraft) creamy	1 tbsp	60	0.0	2.0	150	(mq)	5.0	5
(Kraft) 'Reduced Calorie'	1 tbsp	30	0.0	4.0	130	(mq)	1.0	0
(Kraft) w/pure honey, low-calorie	1 tbsp	60	0.0	4.0	130	(mq)	5.0	0

Food Name	Serv. Size	Total Cal.	Prot. GMS	Carbs GMS	Sod. MGS	Fiber GMS	Fat GMS	Chol. MGS
(S&W Nutradiet)	1 tbsp	25	0.0	4.0	120	(mq)	1.0	0
(Weight Watchers) whipped	1 tbsp	50	0.0	2.0	80	na	5.0	5
(Wish-Bone)	1 tbsp	46	0.1	6.0	147	(mq)	2.5	0
(Wish-Bone) 'Food Service'	1 tbsp	47	0.1	6.0	147	(mq)	2.5	0
(Wish-Bone) 'Lite'	1 tbsp	22	0.1	3.9	126	(mq)	0.6	0
SAN FRANCISCO *(Lawry's)* w/Romano cheese 'Classic'	1 oz	136	0.6	2.0	547	>.1 c	14.0	na
SANTA FE *(Wish-Bone)*	.5 oz	70	0.0	1.0	105	na	7.0	5
SESAME SEED								
(Ayla's Organics) toasted, fat-free	2 tbsp	20	0.0	3.0	190	0	0.0	0
(Nasoya) garlic 'Vegi-Dressing'	1 tbsp	40	1.0	1.0	50	(mq)	3.0	0
(Wish-Bone) vinaigrette 'Food Service'	.5 oz	35	0.0	3.0	260	na	2.0	0
SOUR CREAM								
(Crowley) nondairy	1 oz	40	1.0	1.0	5	0	4.0	0
(Friendship) 'Sour Treat'	1 oz	36	1.0	2.0	15	na	3.0	0
SOUR CREAM AND CHIVES								
(Litehouse) vinaigrette, refrigerated	1 tbsp	63	0.0	1.0	72	na	7.0	na
SPINACH SALAD *(T. Marzetti)* refrigerated	1 tbsp	35	0.0	2.0	100	na	3.0	0
SWEET AND SAUCY *(T. Marzetti)*	1 tbsp	65	0.0	4.0	180	na	5.0	0
SWEET AND SOUR								
(T. Marzetti)	1 tbsp	72	0.0	5.0	100	na	6.0	0
(T. Marzetti) 'Fat-Free'	1 tbsp	20	0.0	5.0	130	na	0.0	0
(T. Marzetti) 'Light'	1 tbsp	45	0.0	5.0	105	na	3.0	0
(T. Marzetti) refrigerated	1 tbsp	72	0.0	5.0	99	na	6.0	0
SWISS CHEESE VINAIGRETTE *(Hain)*	1 tbsp	60	0.0	0.0	160	na	7.0	5
THOUSAND ISLAND								
(Estee)	1 tbsp	8	0.0	2.0	30	(mq)	0.0	0
(Featherweight)	1 tbsp	18	0.0	3.0	70	(mq)	0.0	0
(Hain)	1 tbsp	50	0.0	0.0	85	(mq)	5.0	0
(Hollywood)	1 tbsp	60	0.0	3.0	15	0	6.0	5
(Kraft)	1 tbsp	60	0.0	2.0	150	(mq)	5.0	5
(Kraft) and bacon	1 tbsp	60	0.0	2.0	100	(mq)	6.0	0
(Kraft) nonfat 'Free'	1 tbsp	20	0.0	5.0	135	(mq)	0.0	0
(Kraft) 'Reduced Calorie'	1 tbsp	20	0.0	3.0	135	(mq)	1.0	0
(Litehouse) dressing and dip, refrigerated	1 tbsp	65	0.0	1.0	99	na	7.0	na
(S&W Nutradiet)	1 tbsp	25	0.0	2.0	105	(mq)	2.0	na
(Seven Seas) creamy	1 tbsp	50	0.0	2.0	150	(mq)	5.0	5
(Seven Seas) 'Thousand Island! Light'	1 tbsp	30	0.0	3.0	160	(mq)	2.0	5
(Skipper's)	1 pouch	160	0.0	8.0	415	na	14.0	6
(T. Marzetti)	1 tbsp	74	0.0	2.0	120	na	7.0	5
(T. Marzetti) 'Fat-Free'	1 tbsp	17	0.0	4.0	172	na	0.0	0
(T. Marzetti) 'Frenchette'	1 tbsp	20	0.0	3.0	155	na	0.0	4
(T. Marzetti) 'Light'	1 tbsp	35	0.0	3.0	155	na	3.0	4

Food Name	Serv. Size	Total Cal.	Prot. GMS	Carbs GMS	Sod. MGS	Fiber GMS	Fat GMS	Chol. MGS
(T. Marzetti) refrigerated	1 tbsp	82	0.0	6.0	93	na	5.0	0
(Ultra Slim Fast) 'Cholesterol Free'	1 tbsp	18	0.0	4.0	95	na	<1.0	0
(Weight Watchers) whipped	1 tbsp	50	0.0	2.0	80	na	5.0	5
(Wish-Bone)	1 tbsp	63	0.1	3.1	158	(mq)	5.6	7
(Wish-Bone) 'Food Service'	1 tbsp	40	0.2	2.6	107	0	3.2	9
(Wish-Bone) 'Healthy Sensation!'	.5 oz	20	0.0	4.0	135	na	na	0
(Wish-Bone) 'Lite'	1 tbsp	36	.0.2	1.9	99	(mq)	3.0	9
(Wish-Bone) lite 'Food Service'	.5 oz	20	na	4.0	140	na	na	0
TOMATO								
(Featherweight) zesty	1 tbsp	2	0.0	0.0	5	0	0.0	0
(Hain) vinaigrette, garden 'Canola'	1 tbsp	60	0.0	1.0	150	na	6.0	0
(Weight Watchers) vinaigrette	1 tbsp	8	0.0	2.0	150	na	0.0	0
VEGETABLE *(T. Marzetti)* dressing and dip, refrigerated	1 tbsp	88	0.0	1.0	120	na	10.0	2
VINTAGE *(Lawry's)* w/sherry wine 'Classic'	1 tbsp	110	4.3	2.5	415	>.1 c	10.5	0
WHITE WINE								
(Lawry's) w/Chardonnay 'Classic'	1 tbsp	153	0.0	2.7	178	>.1 c	15.7	0
(Marie's) fat-free 'Lite & Zesty'	1 tbsp	20	0.0	5.0	135	na	0.0	0
SALAD DRESSING MIX								
BACON *(Lawry's)* dry mix	1 pkg	65	5.2	9.1	1820	>.5 c	0.8	na
BLUE CHEESE								
(Hain) 'No Oil' prepared	1 tbsp	14	1.0	1.0	180	na	1.0	5
(Hidden Valley Ranch) dry mix	1 pkg	112	4.0	19.0	1931	na	2.0	0
(Weight Watchers) dry mix	1 tbsp	8	0.0	1.0	110	na	0.0	na
BLUE CHEESE AND HERBS								
(Good Seasons) dry mix	1 pkg	4	0.0	1.0	150	na	0.0	0
BUTTERMILK								
(Hain) 'No Oil' prepared	1 tbsp	11	1.0	1.0	150	na	<1.0	0
(Hidden Valley Ranch) original recipe, dry mix, .4 oz	1 pkg	25	3.0	na	2167	na	0.0	0
(Good Seasons) 'Farm Style' dry mix	1 pkg	4	0.0	1.0	95	na	0.0	0
CAESAR								
(Lawry's) dry mix	1 pkg	75	3.4	8.7	1962	>.3 c	3.1	na
(Hain) 'No Oil' prepared	1 tbsp	6	0.0	1.0	200	na	<1.0	0
CHEESE AND GARLIC								
(Good Seasons) dry mix	1 pkg	4	0.0	1.0	170	na	0.0	0
(Hain) 'No Oil' prepared	1 tbsp	6	<1.0	1.0	180	na	<1.0	0
DILL *(Good Seasons)* 'Classic' dry mix	1 tbsp	2	0.0	0.0	150	na	0.0	0
FRENCH								
(Hain) 'No Oil' prepared	1 tbsp	12	0.0	3.0	340	na	0.0	0
(Weight Watchers) style, dry mix	1 tbsp	3	0.0	1.0	150	na	0.0	0
GARLIC AND HERBS *(Good Seasons)* dry mix	1 pkg	4	0.0	1.0	190	na	0.0	0

Food Name	Serv. Size	Total Cal.	Prot. GMS	Carbs GMS	Sod. MGS	Fiber GMS	Fat GMS	Chol. MGS
HERB								
(Good Seasons) 'Classic' dry mix	1 pkg	2	0.0	0.0	150	na	0.0	0
(Hain) 'No Oil' prepared	1 tbsp	2	0.0	1.0	140	na	0.0	0
(Hidden Valley Ranch) creamy, dry mix	1 pkg	76	3.0	16.0	1931	na	0.0	0
HONEY MUSTARD *(Good Seasons)*								
dry mix	1 tbsp	6	0.0	1.0	125	na	0.0	0
ITALIAN								
(Good Seasons) dry mix	1 pkg	2	0.0	1.0	170	na	0.0	0
(Good Seasons) 'Lite' prepared	1 tbsp	25	0.0	1.0	180	na	3.0	0
(Good Seasons) mild	1 tbsp	70	0.0	1.0	190	na	8.0	0
(Good Seasons) 'No Oil' prepared	1 tbsp	6	0.0	2.0	30	na	0.0	0
(Good Seasons) zesty, dry mix	1 pkg	2	0.0	1.0	120	na	0.0	0
(Good Seasons) zesty 'Lite' prepared	1 tbsp	25	0.0	1.0	135	na	3.0	0.
(Hain) 'No Oil' prepared	1 tbsp	2	0.0	1.0	170	na	0.0	0
(Lawry's) dry mix	1 pkg	45	1.6	9.3	2255	>.3 c	0.2	na
(Lawry's) w/cheese, dry mix	1 pkg	74	2.2	11.6	1624	>.2 c	2.1	na
(Weight Watchers) dry mix	1 tbsp	2	0.0	0.0	140	na	0.0	na
ITALIAN, CREAMY *(Weight Watchers)*								
dry mix	1 tbsp	3	0.0	1.0	180	na	0.0	na
ITALIAN CHEESE								
(Good Seasons) dry mix	1 pkg	4	0.0	1.0	130	na	0.0	0
(Good Seasons) 'Lite' prepared	1 tbsp	25	0.0	1.0	135	na	3.0	0
LEMON AND HERBS *(Good Seasons)*								
dry mix	1 pkg	2	0.0	1.0	140	na	0.0	0
PEPPERCORN								
(Hidden Valley Ranch) original recipe, prepared	1 tbsp	58	0.0	1.0	110	na	3.0	4
RANCH								
(Good Seasons) dry mix	1 pkg	4	0.0	1.0	70	na	0.0	0
(Good Seasons) 'Lite' prepared	1 tbsp	30	1.0	2.0	115	na	2.0	5
(Hidden Valley Ranch) 'Original' dry mix	1 pkg	93	3.0	18.0	2211	na	1.0	0
(Hidden Valley Ranch) reduced calorie, dry mix	1 pkg	98	3.0	17.0	2301	na	2.0	0
(Hidden Valley Ranch) w/bacon, dry mix	1.2 oz	118	7.0	1.0	1953	na	2.0	0
RUSSIAN *(Weight Watchers)* dry mix	1 tbsp	4	0.0	1.0	120	na	0.0	na
SPICY PEANUT *(A Taste of Thai)* dry mix	1 tbsp	40	1.0	6.0	360	1.0	1.5	0
THOUSAND ISLAND								
(Hain) 'No Oil' prepared	1 tbsp	12	0.0	3.0	150	na	0.0	<1
(Weight Watchers) dry mix	1 tbsp	4	0.0	1.0	140	na	0.0	na
SALAD MIX. See also PASTA DISH MIX; PASTA SALAD MIX.								
(Saco Foods) 'Easy Caesar' unprepared	.75 oz	98	2.0	7.0	246	na	7.0	4
SALAD SEASONING *(Schilling)*								
'Salad Supreme'	1 tsp	11	0.7	0.5	2807	(mq)	0.1	0

Food Name	Serv. Size	Total Cal.	Prot. GMS	Carbs GMS	Sod. MGS	Fiber GMS	Fat GMS	Chol. MGS
SALAD TOPPING								
(Salad Nibbler) crouton topping,								
buttermilk ranch	1 oz	128	7.0	13.0	241	na	5.0	2.0
(Salad Nibbler) crouton topping,								
seasoned cheddar	1 oz	129	6.0	13.0	224	na	6.0	2.0
(Special Edition) sesame salad nuggets	1 tbsp	35	<1.0	3.0	115	na	2.5	na
(Special Edition) sesame salad nuggets,								
garlic and cheese	1 tbsp	40	<1.0	3.0	130	na	2.5	na
SALAMI. See LUNCHEON MEAT.								
SALISBURY STEAK DINNER. See BEEF DINNER, FROZEN.								
SALISBURY STEAK ENTRÉE. See BEEF ENTRÉE, FROZEN; BEEF ENTRÉE, PACKAGED.								
SALMON, ALTERNATIVE, smoked								
(Mox Lox)	1.5 oz	25	2.0	3.0	380	na	<1.0	5
SALMON, ATLANTIC								
Farmed								
dry-heat cooked	3 oz	175	18.8	0.0	52	0	10.5	54
raw	3 oz	156	16.9	0.0	50	0	9.2	50
Wild								
dry-heat cooked	3 oz	155	21.6	0.0	48	0	6.9	60
raw	3 oz	121	16.9	0.0	37	0	5.4	47
SALMON, CANNED								
CHUM								
(Bumble Bee)	1 cup	306	47.3	0.0	(mq)	0	11.4	(mq)
(Bumble Bee) w/liquid	3.5 oz	160	20.0	0.0	490	na	8.0	60
COHO *(Deming's)* boiled	1/2 cup	140	22.0	0.0	450	0	5.0	(mq)
MIXED *(Libby's)* skinless, boneless	3.25 oz	110	16.0	1.0	420	na	4.0	50
PINK								
Alaska, w/liquid *(Deming's)*	1/2 cup	140	20.0	0.0	450	0	6.0	65
chunk, skinless, boneless, in spring water								
(Chicken of the Sea)	2 oz	60	10.0	0.0	280	na	2.0	na
chunk, skinless, boneless, w/liquid								
(Deming's)	3.25 oz	120	17.0	0.0	420	0	5.0	(mq)
skinless, boneless, w/liquid *(Bumble Bee)*	3.5 oz	120	17.0	0.0	420	na	5.0	25
solids, w/bone and liquid	3 oz	118	16.8	0.0	64	0	5.1	47
w/liquid	4 oz	158	22.4	0.0	628	0	6.9	(mq)
w/liquid *(Bumble Bee)*	1 cup	310	45.1	0.0	851	0	13.0	(mq)
w/liquid *(Bumble Bee)*	3.5 oz	160	20.0	0.0	490	na	8.0	50
w/liquid *(Del Monte)*	1/2 cup	160	22.0	0.0	660	0	7.0	(mq)
w/liquid *(Featherweight)*	2 oz	70	11.0	0.0	45	0	3.0	20
w/liquid *(Libby's)*	7.75 oz	310	45.0	0.0	790	0	13.0	(mq)
SOCKEYE								
(Bumble Bee)	1 cup	376	44.7	0.0	1148	0	20.5	(mq)
(Libby's)	7.75 oz	380	45.0	0.0	760	0	21.0	(mq)

Food Name	Serv. Size	Total Cal.	Prot. GMS	Carbs GMS	Sod. MGS	Fiber GMS	Fat GMS	Chol. MGS
Alaska *(Deming's)*	1/2 cup	170	20.0	0.0	450	0	9.0	65
Alaska, med *(Deming's)*	1/2 cup	150	21.0	0.0	450	0	7.0	65
blueback *(Rubinstein's)*	1/2 cup	170	20.0	0.0	450	0	9.0	(mq)
blueback *(S&W Nutradiet)*	1/2 cup	188	22.0	0.0	45	0	11.0	(mq)
blueback 'Fancy' *(S&W)*	1/2 cup	190	25.0	0.0	590	0	10.0	(mq)
skinless, boneless, w/liquid *(Bumble Bee)*	3.5 oz	130	17.0	0.0	420	na	6.0	30
solids, w/bone, drained	3 oz	130	17.4	0.0	457	0	6.2	37
solids, w/bone, drained, w/o salt	3 oz	130	17.4	0.0	64	0	6.2	37
w/liquid *(Bumble Bee)*	3.5 oz	180	20.0	0.0	490	na	10.0	60
w/liquid *(Del Monte)*	1/2 cup	180	23.0	0.0	660	0	9.0	(mq)
SALMON, CHINOOK/king/lox/smoked								
dry-heat cooked	3 oz	196	21.9	0.0	51	0	11.4	72
raw	1 lb	816	91.0	0.0	213	0	47.4	299
raw	3 oz	153	17.0	0.0	40	0	8.9	56
raw, approx 7 oz	1/2 fillet	356	39.7	0.0	93	0	20.7	131
smoked	3 oz	99	15.5	0.0	666	0	3.7	20
smoked, lox	4 oz	133	20.7	0.0	2268	0	4.9	26
smoked, lox	3 oz	99	15.5	0.0	1700	0	3.7	20
SALMON, CHUM/dog/keta								
dry-heat cooked	3 oz	131	21.9	0.0	54	0	4.1	81
raw	1 lb	544	91.3	0.0	449	0	17.1	336
raw	3 oz	102	17.1	0.0	43	0	3.2	63
raw	1 oz	34	5.7	0.0	14	0	1.1	21
raw, approx 7 oz	1/2 fillet	238	39.9	0.0	99	0	7.5	147
raw, fillet portions *(Peter Pan Seafoods)*	3.5 oz	120	20.1	na	50	na	3.8	74
raw, sides, w/pinbone, *(Peter Pan Seafoods)*	3.5 oz	120	20.1	na	50	na	3.8	74
raw, solids, w/bone, drained, w/o salt	3 oz	120	18.2	0.0	64	0	4.7	33
raw, steaks *(Peter Pan Seafoods)*	3.5 oz	120	20.1	na	50	na	3.8	74
SALMON, COHO/silver								
Farmed								
dry-heat cooked	3 oz	151	20.7	0.0	44	0	7.0	54
raw	3 oz	136	18.1	0.0	40	0	6.5	43
Wild								
dry-heat cooked	3 oz	118	19.9	0.0	49	0	3.7	47
moist-heat cooked	3 oz	156	23.3	0.0	45	0	6.4	48
raw	1 lb	662	98.1	0.0	211	0	27.0	177
raw	3 oz	124	18.4	0.0	39	0	5.0	38
raw	1 oz	41	7.6	0.0	13	0	1.7	11
raw, approx 7 oz	1/2 fillet	289	42.8	0.0	91	0	11.7	89
SALMON, DOG. See SALMON, CHUM.								
SALMON, FROZEN, steak, w/o seasoning								
mix *(SeaPak)*	8-oz pkg	270	46.0	0.0	115	0	9.0	170

Food Name	Serv. Size	Total Cal.	Prot. GMS	Carbs GMS	Sod. MGS	Fiber GMS	Fat GMS	Chol. MGS
SALMON, HUMPBACK. See SALMON, PINK.								
SALMON, KETA. See SALMON, CHUM.								
SALMON, KING. See SALMON, CHINOOK.								
SALMON, PINK/humpback								
dry-heat cooked	3 oz	127	21.7	0.0	73	0	3.8	57
raw	1 lb	527	90.4	0.0	302	0	15.6	236
raw	3 oz	99	17.0	0.0	57	0	2.9	44
raw	1 oz	33	5.7	0.0	19	0	1.0	15
SALMON, RED. See SALMON, SOCKEYE.								
SALMON, REDEYE. See SALMON, SOCKEYE.								
SALMON, SILVER. See SALMON, COHO.								
SALMON, SMOKED. See SALMON, CHINOOK.								
SALMON, SOCKEYE/red/redeye								
dry-heat cooked	4 oz	245	31.0	0.0	75	0	12.4	99
dry-heat cooked	3 oz	184	23.2	0.0	56	0	9.3	74
raw	1 lb	763	96.6	0.0	211	0	38.8	283
raw	3 oz	143	18.1	0.0	40	0	7.3	53
raw	1 oz	48	6.0	0.0	13	0	2.4	18
raw, approx 7 oz	1/2 fillet	333	42.2	0.0	93	0	17.0	123
SALSA. See also SAUCE.								
(Hot Cha Cha) 'Texas'	1 oz	6	0.3	2.5	2	.4	0.0	0
(La Victoria) 'Brava'	1 tbsp	6	<1.0	1.0	100	(mq)	<1.0	0
(La Victoria) 'Casera'	1 tbsp	4	<1.0	1.0	80	(mq)	<1.0	0
(La Victoria) 'Supreme'	2 tbsp	10	0.0	2.0	220	na	0.0	na
(La Victoria) 'Victoria'	1 tbsp	4	<1.0	1.0	80	(mq)	<1.0	0
BURRITO (Del Monte)	1/4 cup	20	0.0	4.0	355	(mq)	0.0	0
EXTRA CHUNKY (Rosarita)								
'de Mexico Style'	2 tbsp	30	1.0	7.0	280	na	<1.0	0
GREEN CHILI								
(Del Monte) mild	1/4 cup	20	0.0	3.0	590	(mq)	0.0	0
(Hain) hot	1/4 cup	22	1.0	4.0	480	(mq)	0.0	0
(La Victoria)	2 tbsp	10	0.0	2.0	150	na	0.0	na
(Nabisco) hot	1 tbsp	6	0.0	2.0	190	na	0.0	0
(Nabisco) medium 'Green Chile Salsa'	1 tbsp	6	0.0	1.0	190	na	0.0	0
(Nabisco) mild 'Green Chile Salsa'	1 tbsp	8	0.0	2.0	190	na	0.0	0
(Old El Paso) 'Thick 'n Chunky'	2 tbsp	3	0.0	1.0	270	(mq)	0.0	0
(Ortega) hot	1 oz	10	0.0	2.0	180	(mq)	0.0	0
(Ortega) medium	1 oz	8	0.0	2.0	180	(mq)	0.0	0
(Ortega) mild	1 oz	8	0.0	2.0	180	(mq)	0.0	0
(Rosarita) mild	1.093 oz	7	0.3	1.5	167	.3	0.1	0
(Territorial House)	.5 oz	4	<1.0	<1.0	80	na	<1.0	na
HOT								
(Chi-Chi's)	1 oz	8	2.0	2.0	153	na	2.0	2

Food Name	Serv. Size	Total Cal.	Prot. GMS	Carbs GMS	Sod. MGS	Fiber GMS	Fat GMS	Chol. MGS
(Enrico's) 'Chunky Style'	2 tbsp	8	1.0	2.0	34	(mq)	0.0	0
(Enrico's) 'Chunky Style No Salt Added'	2 tbsp	8	1.0	2.0	10	(mq)	0.0	0
(Old El Paso) 'Thick 'n Chunky'	2 tbsp	6	<1.0	1.0	170	(mq)	<1.0	0
(Pablo's) 'Deli Style'	1 oz	10	1.0	2.0	250	na	0.0	0
(Rosarita) chunky	3 tbsp	25	1.0	6.0	300	<1.0	<1.0	0
JALAPEÑO								
(La Victoria) green	1 tbsp	4	<1.0	1.0	105	(mq)	<1.0	0
(La Victoria) red	1 tbsp	6	<1.0	1.0	95	(mq)	<1.0	0
MEDIUM								
(Chi-Chi's)	1 oz	7	2.0	2.0	135	na	2.0	2
(Litehouse) 'Zesty'	1 tbsp	4	0.0	1.0	110	na	0.0	na
(Old El Paso) 'Thick 'n Chunky'	2 tbsp	6	<1.0	1.0	170	(mq)	<1.0	0
(Ortega) thick and chunky	1 tbsp	4	0.0	1.0	150	na	0.0	0
(Pace) 'Thick & Chunky'	2 tbsp	4	<1.0	<1.0	101	na	<1.0	na
(Rosarita) chunky	3 tbsp	25	1.0	6.0	350	<1.0	<1.0	0
(Rosarita) 'Traditional'	1.093 oz	7	0.3	1.6	234	.5	0.1	0
MILD								
(Chi-Chi's)	1 oz	7	2.0	2.0	116	na	2.0	2
(Enrico's) 'Chunky Style'	2 tbsp	8	1.0	2.0	34	(mq)	0.0	0
(Enrico's) 'Chunky Style No Salt Added'	2 tbsp	8	1.0	2.0	10	(mq)	0.0	0
(Hain)	1/2 cup	20	1.0	4.0	410	(mq)	0.0	0
(Hunt's) 'Homestyle'	1.093 oz	27	0.5	6.2	236	.6	0.2	0
(Old El Paso) 'Thick 'n Chunky'	2 tbsp	6	<1.0	1.0	170	(mq)	<1.0	0
(Pablo's) 'Deli Style'	1 oz	10	1.0	2.0	250	na	0.0	0
(Pace) and dip, mild 'Chunky'	2 tbsp	4	<1.0	<1.0	101	na	<1.0	na
(Pace) 'Thick & Chunky'	2 tbsp	4	<1.0	<1.0	101	na	<1.0	na
(Rosarita) 'Casa Mamita'	1.129 oz	7	0.4	1.2	170	.4	0.1	0
(Rosarita) chunky	3 tbsp	25	1.0	6.0	340	<1.0	<1.0	0
(Rosarita) roasted	1.093 oz	10	0.5	1.7	233	.6	0.3	0
(Rosarita) 'Traditional'	1.093 oz	7	0.6	1.4	247	.5	0.1	0
OMELETTE *(La Victoria)*	1 tbsp	6	<1.0	1.0	95	(mq)	<1.0	0
PICANTE								
(Del Monte) hot	1/2 cup	20	0.0	4.0	385	(mq)	0.0	0
(Del Monte) hot and chunky	1/4 cup	15	0.0	3.0	405	(mq)	0.0	0
(La Victoria) medium	2 tbsp	5	0.0	1.0	180	na	0.0	na
(La Victoria) mild	2 tbsp	10	1.0	2.0	230	na	0.0	na
(LàCasita) mild, chunky	2 oz	16	<1.0	4.0	226	na	0.0	0
(Old El Paso) hot	2 tbsp	10	<1.0	2.0	160	na	<1.0	0
(Old El Paso) medium	2 tbsp	10	<1.0	2.0	160	na	<1.0	0
(Old El Paso) mild	2 tbsp	10	<1.0	2.0	160	na	<1.0	0
(Ortega)	1 oz	10	0.0	2.0	300	(mq)	0.0	0
(Rosarita)	1.093 oz	7	0.4	1.3	247	.2	0.1	0

Food Name	Serv. Size	Total Cal.	Prot. GMS	Carbs GMS	Sod. MGS	Fiber GMS	Fat GMS	Chol. MGS
RANCHERA								
(La Victoria)	1 tbsp	6	<1.0	1.0	85	(mq)	<1.0	0
(Ortega)	1 oz	12	0.0	3.0	250	(mq)	0.0	0
ROJA (Del Monte) mild	1/4 cup	20	0.0	4.0	510	(mq)	0.0	0
TACO								
(Nabisco) 'Hot Thick and Smooth'	1 tbsp	8	0.0	2.0	105	0	0.0	0
(Nabisco) 'Medium Thick and Smooth'	1 tbsp	8	0.0	2.0	105	0	0.0	0
(Nabisco) 'Mild Thick and Smooth'	1 tbsp	8	0.0	2.0	115	0	0.0	0
(Ortega) hot	1 oz	10	0.0	2.0	300	(mq)	0.0	0
(Ortega) mild	1 oz	10	0.0	2.0	290	(mq)	0.0	0
(Rosarita) medium, chunky	3 tbsp	25	1.0	6.0	310	<1.0	<1.0	0
(Rosarita) mild	2 oz	27	1.0	6.1	304	.1	0.1	<1
(Rosarita) mild, chunky	3 tbsp	25	1.0	6.0	300	<1.0	<1.0	0
TOMATILLO								
(Rosarita) green 'de Mexico Style'	2 tbsp	20	1.0	4.0	190	na	<1.0	0
(Rosarita) medium	1.093 oz	8	0.1	1.8	188	.5	0.2	0
TRADITIONAL (Rosarita) 'de Mexico Style'	2 tbsp	12	1.0	3.0	350	na	0.0	0
VERDE (Old El Paso) 'Thick 'n Chunky'	2 tbsp	10	<1.0	2.0	135	(mq)	<1.0	0
VERY LOW SODIUM (Pritikin)	1/4 cup	25	1.0	5.0	15	na	0.0	0
SALSIFY/oyster plant /vegetable oyster								
boiled, drained	4 oz	77	3.1	17.4	18	3.5	0.2	0
boiled, drained, sliced	1/2 cup	46	1.9	10.5	11	2.1	0.1	0
raw, sliced	1/2 cup	55	2.2	12.5	13	2.2	0.1	0
raw, trimmed	1 oz	23	0.9	5.3	6	>.5 c	0.1	0
raw, untrimmed	1 lb	325	13.0	73.4	79	>7.1 c	0.8	0
SALSIFY, BLACK/scorzonera								
raw	1 lb	372	15.0	84.4	91	(mq)	0.1	0
raw	1 oz	23	0.9	5.3	6	(mq)	tr	0
SALT								
iodized (Morton)	1 tsp	0	0.0	0.0	2300	0	0.0	0
kosher (Morton)	1 tsp	0	0.0	0.0	1880	0	0.0	0
mixture 'Lite Salt' (Morton)	1 tsp	<1	0.0	tr	1100	0	0.0	0
non-iodized (Morton)	1 tsp	0	0.0	0.0	2300	0	0.0	0
plain	1 cup	0	0.0	0.0	112398	0	0.0	0
plain	1 tbsp	0	0.0	0.0	6976	0	0.0	0
plain	1 tsp	0	0.0	0.0	2325	0	0.0	0
sea (Hain)	1 tsp	0	0.0	0.0	2255	0	0.0	0
SALT, ALTERNATIVE								
Plain								
(Estee) 'Salt-It'	1/8 tsp	0	0.0	0.0	0	0	0.0	0
(Featherweight)	1/4 tsp	0	0.0	0.0	0	0	0.0	0
(Lawry's) 'Salt-Free'	1 tsp	10	0.3	1.8	2	>.4 c	0.2	0
(Morton)	1 tsp	<1	0.0	0.1	<1	na	0.0	0

Food Name	Serv. Size	Total Cal.	Prot. GMS	Carbs GMS	Sod. MGS	Fiber GMS	Fat GMS	Chol. MGS
Seasoned								
(Estee) 'Seasoned Salt-It'	1/8 tsp	0	0.0	0.0	0	na	0.0	0
(Featherweight)	1/4 tsp	0	0.0	0.0	0	0	0.0	0
(Health Valley) all-purpose 'Instead of Salt'	1 tsp	11	0.5	1.5	3	0	0.5	0
(Lawry's) 'Salt-Free'	1 tsp	3	0.1	0.6	7	>.1 c	<.1	0
(Morton)	1 tsp	2	<.1	0.5	<1	na	<.1	0
SALT PORK, cured (Hormel)	2 oz	320	4.0	0.0	1800	0	33.0	40
SALT SEASONING								
(Lawry's)	1 tsp	4	0.1	0.6	1367	>.1 c	0.1	0
(Lawry's) 'Hot 'n Spicy'	1 tsp	3	0.1	1.5	79	>.1 c	0.1	0
(Lawry's) 'Lite'	1 tsp	8	0.3	1.7	357	>.1 c	<.1	0
(Morton)	1 tsp	4	<1.0	<1.0	1300	na	<.1	0
(Morton) 'Nature's Seasons'	1 tsp	3	<.1	<1.0	1400	na	<.1	0
(Schilling)	1 tsp	4	0.2	0.6	980	na	na	0
(Schilling) 'Salt 'n Spice'	1 tsp	3	0.2	0.6	939	na	na	0
SANDWICH								
BEEF								
(Hot Pockets) frozen, pocket, and cheddar	5 oz	370	17.0	36.0	1390	(mq)	17.0	60
(Lean Pockets) frozen, pocket, and								
broccoli	1 pkg	250	11.0	30.0	760	(mq)	8.0	(mq)
(Manwich) extra thick and chunky,								
prepared	1 sandwich	330	17.0	36.0	870	3.0	13.0	50
(Manwich) Mexican, prepared	1 sandwich	310	17.0	30.0	690	2.0	13.0	50
(Manwich) original, prepared	1 sandwich	320	17.0	31.0	590	2.0	13.0	50
(Manwich) 'Sloppy Joe' prepared ..	1 sandwich	310	17.0	31.0	620	1.0	13.0	50
(Tyson) frozen, barbecue, microwave	1 sandwich	200	15.0	29.0	600	na	2.7	30
CANADIAN BACON								
(Quick Meal) muffin, w/egg and cheese ..	4.5 oz	250	16.0	29.0	680	na	8.0	115
CHEESEBURGER								
(Kid Cuisine) frozen	6.25 oz	400	12.0	47.0	550	(mq)	19.0	40
(Kid Cuisine) frozen, double 'Mega Meal'	9.1 oz	480	20.0	55.0	1040	na	20.0	na
(MicroMagic) frozen	4.75 oz	450	17.0	29.0	790	(mq)	25.0	80
CHICKEN								
(Banquet) patties, breast meat 'Microwave'	4 oz	310	16.0	31.0	664	(mq)	14.0	(mq)
(BestFresh) breast, teriyaki,								
charbroiled	1 sandwich	490	34.0	45.0	1030	6.0	20.0	60
(BestFresh) w/cucumber yogurt								
dressing	1 sandwich	390	24.0	38.0	960	1.0	15.0	70
(Hot Pockets) frozen, pocket, and cheddar	5 oz	310	16.0	38.0	720	(mq)	11.0	(mq)
(Kid Cuisine)	8.2 oz	470	16.0	61.0	830	na	17.0	40
(Lean Pockets) frozen, pocket, Oriental ..	1 pkg	250	14.0	35.0	840	(mq)	6.0	(mq)
(Lean Pockets) frozen, pocket, Parmesan	1 pkg	270	19.0	35.0	750	(mq)	6.0	(mq)

Food Name	Serv. Size	Total Cal.	Prot. GMS	Carbs GMS	Sod. MGS	Fiber GMS	Fat GMS	Chol. MGS
(Lean Pockets) frozen, pocket, white meat only 'Fajita'	1 sandwich	250	13.0	36.0	810	na	6.0	30
(Lean Pockets) frozen, pocket, white meat only, glazed 'Supreme'	1 sandwich	240	10.0	35.0	630	na	7.0	30
(MicroMagic) frozen	4.5 oz	390	13.0	42.0	650	(mq)	16.0	35
(Quick Meal)	4.3 oz	320	16.0	40.0	640	na	11.0	65
(Quick Meal) biscuit	4.2 oz	310	13.0	36.0	900	na	13.0	50
(Quick Meal) grilled	4.7 oz	300	21.0	35.0	620	na	9.0	60
(Tyson) boneless, grilled	3.5 oz	200	15.0	25.0	470	na	5.0	32
(Tyson) breast, boneless, grilled .	3.5 oz	150	17.0	2.0	400	na	8.0	44
(Tyson) frozen, barbecue 'Microwave'	4 oz	230	16.0	27.0	510	(mq)	6.0	(mq)
(Tyson) frozen, breast 'Microwave'	3.5 oz	275	14.0	27.0	(mq)	(mq)	12.0	(mq)
(Tyson) frozen, mini 'Microwave'	3.5 oz	230	12.0	39.0	(mq)	(mq)	5.0	(mq)
(Ultimate 200) grilled	4 oz	200	18.0	22.0	420	na	5.0	20
EGG								
(Jimmy Dean) frozen, w/egg and cheese	1 biscuit	300	11.0	28.0	890	2.0	16.0	95
(Jimmy Dean) frozen, w/ham and cheese	1 biscuit	240	13.0	26.0	720	1.0	10.0	100
(Jimmy Dean) w/sausage and cheese	1 biscuit	390	14.0	28.0	1040	2.0	27.0	115
(Swanson) frozen, w/beefsteak and cheese 'Great Starts'	4.9 oz	360	17.0	27.0	730	(mq)	20.0	(mq)
(Swanson) frozen, w/Canadian bacon and cheese 'Great Starts'	5.2 oz	420	16.0	37.0	1845	(mq)	22.0	(mq)
(Swanson) frozen, w/Canadian bacon and cheese 'Great Starts'	4.1 oz	290	15.0	25.0	770	(mq)	15.0	(mq)
(Swanson) frozen, w/sausage and cheese 'Great Starts'	5.5 oz	460	18.0	35.0	1310	(mq)	28.0	(mq)
ENGLISH MUFFIN *(Weight Watchers)*	4 oz	240	14.0	29.0	540	na	8.0	15
FISH FILLET *(Quick Meal)*	5.2 oz	430	16.0	56.0	910	na	16.0	68
HAM AND CHEESE								
(Hot Pockets) frozen, pocket	5 oz	360	19.0	36.0	1320	(mq)	16.0	90
(Owens) refrigerated 'Border Breakfasts' ..	2 oz	150	7.0	14.0	600	(mq)	6.0	(mq)
(Swanson) refrigerated, bagel 'Great Starts'	3 oz	240	12.0	28.0	600	(mq)	8.0	(mq)
(Ultimate 200) frozen, pocket	4 oz	200	14.0	24.0	490	na	6.0	5
(Weight Watchers) bagel	3 oz	210	13.0	28.0	460	na	6.0	15
HAMBURGER *(MicroMagic)* frozen	4 oz	350	13.0	26.0	500	(mq)	18.0	55
HOT DOG								
(Kid Cuisine)	6.7 oz	450	13.0	27.0	880	na	19.0	40
(Kid Cuisine) 'Mega Meal'	8.25 oz	500	16.0	52.0	1260	na	25.0	na
OMELET								
(Weight Watchers) 'Classic'	3.84 oz	210	14.0	22.0	410	na	7.0	30
(Weight Watchers) 'Garden'	3.60 oz	210	9.0	28.0	480	na	6.0	15

Food Name	Serv. Size	Total Cal.	Prot. GMS	Carbs GMS	Sod. MGS	Fiber GMS	Fat GMS	Chol. MGS
PIZZA								
(Amy's Kitchen) frozen, pocket, cheese								
calzone, organic	4.5 oz	313	15.0	41.0	272	4.0	9.0	24
(Hot Pockets) frozen, pocket, pepperoni	5 oz	380	17.0	40.0	1240	(mq)	17.0	45
(Hot Pockets) frozen, pocket, sausage	5 oz	360	15.0	40.0	590	(mq)	16.0	65
(Lean Pockets) frozen, pocket 'Deluxe'	1 pkg	280	14.0	34.0	500	(mq)	9.0	na
(Lean Pockets) frozen, pocket, sausage								
and pepperoni 'Deluxe'	1 sandwich	300	13.0	37.0	670	na	11.0	35
(Ultimate 200) pocket 'Deluxe'	4 oz	200	15.0	25.0	400	na	5.0	5
PORK *(Quick Meal)* barbecue	4.3 oz	350	16.0	40.0	550	na	14.0	65
RIB *(Swanson)* hot, smothered	10.25 oz	340	13.0	50.0	690	na	10.0	25
SAUSAGE								
(Jimmy Dean) refrigerated,								
microwave	1 sandwich	160	5.0	10.0	360	na	11.0	na
(Owens) refrigerated, biscuit								
'Border Breakfasts'	2 oz	210	6.0	14.0	400	(mq)	14.0	(mq)
(Owens) refrigerated, biscuit, smoked								
'Border Breakfasts'	2 oz	200	4.0	15.0	786	(mq)	6.0	(mq)
(Owens) refrigerated, biscuit, w/egg								
and cheese 'Border Breakfasts'	2.5 oz	250	8.0	15.0	500	(mq)	15.0	(mq)
(Quick Meal) biscuit	3.7 oz	350	10.0	29.0	870	na	22.0	40
(Quick Meal) biscuit, w/cheese	4.3 oz	420	13.0	31.0	1060	na	27.0	60
(Quick Meal) biscuit, w/egg	4.5 oz	350	11.0	30.0	780	na	21.0	110
(Quick Meal) muffin, w/egg and cheese	5.1 oz	76	3.0	5.0	143	na	4.0	26
(Swanson) frozen, biscuit, w/egg								
'Great Starts'	4.7 oz	410	14.0	36.0	1180	(mq)	22.0	(mq)
(Weight Watchers) frozen, biscuit								
'Microwave'	3 oz	220	11.0	19.0	560	na	11.0	70
SUBMARINE *(BestFresh)* 'Deluxe'	1 sandwich	790	39.0	59.0	2070	8.0	44.0	105
TURKEY								
(BestFresh) smoked	1 sandwich	580	39.0	49.0	1770	7.0	26.0	80
(Healthy Deli) w/corned beef 'Doubledecker'	1 oz	30	5.1	0.6	195	0	0.7	12
(Healthy Deli) w/ham 'Doubledecker'	1 oz	30	4.8	0.8	185	0	0.9	11
(Hot Pockets) pocket, frozen, w/ham and								
cheese	5 oz	320	17.0	37.0	780	(mq)	11.0	(mq)
(Lean Pockets) pocket, frozen, w/broccoli								
and cheese	1 sandwich	260	13.0	32.0	680	na	9.0	30
VEGETABLE								
(Ken & Robert's) pocket, barbecue								
style 'Truly Amazing'	5 oz	320	11.0	50.0	560	1.5	10.0	0
(Ken & Robert's) pocket, broccoli								
cheddar 'Truly Amazing'	5 oz	275	11.0	37.0	540	.1	9.0	0

Food Name	Serv. Size	Total Cal.	Prot. GMS	Carbs GMS	Sod. MGS	Fiber GMS	Fat GMS	Chol. MGS
(Ken & Robert's) pocket, Greek style								
'Truly Amazing'	5 oz	270	11.0	35.0	500	tr	10.0	0
(Ken & Robert's) pocket, Indian style								
'Truly Amazing'	5 oz	300	9.6	41.0	500	.9	12.0	0
(Ken & Robert's) pocket, Oriental style								
'Truly Amazing'	5 oz	295	9.6	40.8	572	.9	12.0	0
(Ken & Robert's) pocket, pizza style								
'Truly Amazing'	5 oz	315	12.0	42.0	620	1.2	12.0	0
(Ken & Robert's) pocket, Tex Mex style								
'Truly Amazing'	5 oz	310	11.0	43.0	595	.3	11.0	0
SANDWICH SEASONING MIX, dry								
(Manwich)	.25 oz	20	<1.0	5.0	350	<1.0	<1.0	0
SANDWICH SPREAD. See also LUNCHEON MEAT, CANNED; POTTED MEAT SPREAD.								
'Chub' *(Oscar Mayer)*	1 oz	67	2.0	4.3	273	0	4.7	10
pork and beef	1 oz	67	2.2	3.4	287	0	4.9	11
pork and beef	1 tbsp	35	1.1	1.8	152	0	2.6	6
SAPODILLA								
approx 7.5 oz	1 med	141	0.8	33.9	20	9.0	1.9	0
pulp	1 cup	200	1.1	48.1	29	12.7	2.7	0
trimmed	1 oz	24	0.1	5.7	3	1.5	0.3	0
untrimmed	1 lb	300	1.6	72.5	44	19.2	4.0	0
SAPOTE/marmalade plum								
trimmed	1 oz	38	0.6	9.6	3	>.5 c	0.2	0
trimmed, approx 11.2 oz	1 med	301	4.8	76.0	23	5.8	1.4	0
untrimmed	1 lb	431	6.8	108.7	31	>6.1 c	1.9	0
SARDINE								
ATLANTIC								
in soybean oil, drained	3.75-oz can	191	22.6	0.0	465	0	10.5	131
in soybean oil, drained	2 oz	118	14.8	0.0	286	0	6.5	81
in soybean oil, drained, approx .8 oz	2 med	50	5.9	0.0	121	0	2.8	34
BRISLING, w/liquid *(Underwood)*	3.75-oz can	260	19.0	1.0	450	0	20.0	(mq)
MAINE								
in mustard sauce, drained *(Beach Cliff)*	3 oz	227	13.0	4.0	350	na	18.0	na
in soybean oil, drained *(Beach Cliff)*	3 oz	240	16.0	0.0	20	na	20.0	na
in tomato sauce, drained *(Beach Cliff)*	3 oz	210	15.0	0.0	350	na	17.0	na
in water, drained *(Beach Cliff)*	3 oz	230	17.0	1.0	350	na	18.0	na
MIXED								
'Kippered Snacks' *(Brunswick)*	3.5 oz	185	16.0	1.0	610	0	14.0	(mq)
in mustard sauce *(Underwood)*	3.75 oz	220	16.0	2.0	650	na	16.0	(mq)
in oil *(Featherweight)*	1 7/8 oz	130	19.0	1.0	65	0	10.0	45
in soya oil, drained *(Underwood)*	3.75 oz	230	16.0	1.0	400	na	18.0	na
in Tabasco sauce, drained *(Underwood)*	3 oz	220	16.0	1.0	400	na	16.0	(mq)
in tomato sauce *(Del Monte)*	1/2 cup	360	19.0	45.0	540	(mq)	12.0	(mq)

Food Name	Serv. Size	Total Cal.	Prot. GMS	Carbs GMS	Sod. MGS	Fiber GMS	Fat GMS	Chol. MGS
in tomato sauce *(Underwood)*	3.75 oz	220	16.0	2.0	500	na	16.0	(mq)
in water *(Featherweight)*	1 7/8 oz	95	9.0	1.0	65	0	7.0	20
NORWAY								
in mild sardine oil, drained *(Empress)*	3.75-oz can	260	19.0	1.0	(mq)	0	20.0	(mq)
in mild sardine oil, w/liquid *(Empress)*	3.75-oz can	460	19.0	1.0	(mq)	0	42.0	(mq)
NORWEGIAN BRISLING *(S&W)*	1.5 oz	130	10.0	0.0	220	0	10.0	(mq)
PACIFIC								
in tomato sauce, drained	13 oz	659	60.5	0.0	1532	.3	44.3	226
in tomato sauce, drained	2 oz	101	9.3	1.0	235	2.2	6.8	35
in tomato sauce, drained, approx 1.3 oz	1 med	68	6.2	0.0	157	.2	4.6	23

SAUCE. See also APPLESAUCE; BARBECUE SAUCE; CRANBERRY SAUCE; SALSA; TOMATO SAUCE.

ALFREDO SAUCE

Food Name	Serv. Size	Total Cal.	Prot. GMS	Carbs GMS	Sod. MGS	Fiber GMS	Fat GMS	Chol. MGS
(Betty Crocker) 'Recipe Sauces'	4 oz	190	1.0	8.0	650	na	17.0	20
(Contadina)	4 oz	350	6.0	6.0	500	na	34.0	100
(Contadina) 'Fresh' refrigerated	6 oz	540	9.0	10.0	620	na	53.0	85
(Contadina) 'Light' refrigerated	3.33 oz	150	7.0	7.0	460	na	10.0	40
(DiGiorno) reduced fat 'Lighter Varieties'	1/4 cup	180	5.0	15.0	580	na	11.0	35
(DiGiorno) refrigerated	2 oz	200	4.0	2.0	490	na	20.0	55
(Progresso) 'Authentic Pasta Sauces'	1/2 cup	340	13.0	6.0	1080	na	30.0	95

APPLE-APRICOT SAUCE

Food Name	Serv. Size	Total Cal.	Prot. GMS	Carbs GMS	Sod. MGS	Fiber GMS	Fat GMS	Chol. MGS
(Lucky Leaf/Musselman's) 'Fruit n' Sauce'	4 oz	90	0.0	22.0	20	(mq)	0.0	0

APPLE-CHERRY SAUCE

(Lucky Leaf/Musselman's) 'Fruit n' Sauce'	4 oz	100	0.0	24.0	20	(mq)	0.0	0

APPLE-CRANBERRY SAUCE

(Lucky Leaf/Musselman's) 'Fruit n' Sauce'	4 oz	80	0.0	19.0	15	(tr)	0.0	0

APPLE-PEACH SAUCE

(Lucky Leaf/Musselman's) 'Fruit n' Sauce'	4 oz	90	0.0	22.0	20	(mq)	0.0	0

APPLE-PINEAPPLE SAUCE

(Lucky Leaf/Musselman's) 'Fruit n' Sauce'	4 oz	110	0.0	26.0	20	(mq)	0.0	0

APPLE-STRAWBERRY SAUCE

(Lucky Leaf/Musselman's) 'Fruit n' Sauce'	4 oz	100	0.0	24.0	20	(mq)	0.0	0

BASIL-HERB SAUCE *(Golden Dipt)*

'Nature Bay'	2 grams	8	0.0	1.0	36	na	0.0	0

BEARNAISE SAUCE *(Great Impressions)*

	2 tbsp	192	0.5	0.2	148	na	21.0	48

BEEF SAUCE

(Ragu) barbecue 'Beef Tonight'	4 oz	70	2.0	15.0	580	na	<1.0	0
(Ragu) skillet lasagna 'Beef Tonight'	4 oz	60	3.0	9.0	630	na	1.0	5
(Ragu) Stroganoff 'Beef Tonight'	4 oz	130	1.0	6.0	770	na	12.0	10

BOLOGNESE SAUCE

(Contadina)	5 oz	130	8.0	0.0	500	na	7.0	25
(Contadina) 'Fresh' refrigerated	7.5 oz	230	22.0	12.0	600	(mq)	11.0	50
(Progresso) 'Authentic Pasta Sauces'	1/2 cup	150	10.0	12.0	520	2.6	8.0	20

Food Name	Serv. Size	Total Cal.	Prot. GMS	Carbs GMS	Sod. MGS	Fiber GMS	Fat GMS	Chol. MGS
BROWN GRAVY SAUCE *(LaChoy)*	3.139 oz	284	2.2	68.5	400	0	0.1	0
BROWNING SAUCE *(Gravymaster)*	1 tsp	12	0.5	2.4	<1	tr	tr	0
CACCIATORE SAUCE *(Recipe Sauces)* ..	3.9 oz	40	1.0	9.0	570	na	<1.0	0
CARBONARA SAUCE *(DiGiorno)*								
refrigerated	2 oz	200	4.0	3.0	380	na	19.0	40
CHARDONNAY SAUCE *(Golden Dipt)*								
'Nature Bay'	1 oz	60	0.0	1.0	160	na	6.0	0
CHEDDAR CHEESE SAUCE								
(J. Hungerford) 'Stadium'	2.011 oz	80	1.0	6.0	500	0	5.0	4
(Lucky Leaf/Musselman's)	4 oz	220	3.0	12.0	1000	0	18.0	(mq)
(Lucky Leaf/Musselman's) aged	4 oz	240	5.0	11.0	920	0	20.0	(mq)
(Lucky Leaf/Musselman's) aged, mild	4 oz	200	5.0	9.0	790	0	18.0	(mq)
(Lucky Leaf/Musselman's) aged, sharp ...	4 oz	230	9.0	6.0	850	0	17.0	(mq)
CHEESE SAUCE								
(Snow's) Welsh rarebit	1/2 cup	170	9.0	10.0	460	na	11.0	na
(White House) aged	3.5 oz	213	4.0	10.0	810	0	18.0	(mq)
CHICKEN SAUCE								
(Ragu) cacciatore 'Chicken Tonight'	4 oz	70	1.0	12.0	490	na	2.0	0
(Ragu) country French 'Chicken Tonight' ..	4 oz	140	1.0	6.0	730	na	12.0	5
(Ragu) creamy, primavera 'Chicken Tonight'	4 oz	90	1.0	9.0	650	na	6.0	5
(Ragu) creamy, w/mushrooms								
'Chicken Tonight'	4 oz	110	1.0	5.0	650	na	10.0	5
(Ragu) herbed, w/wine 'Chicken Tonight' ..	4 oz	100	2.0	13.0	610	na	4.0	5
(Ragu) honey mustard, light								
'Chicken Tonight'	4 oz	50	1.0	12.0	420	na	<1.0	0
(Ragu) sweet and sour 'Chicken Tonight' ..	4 oz	80	0.0	19.0	280	na	0.0	0
(Ragu) sweet and spicy, light								
'Chicken Tonight'	4 oz	50	2.0	10.0	390	na	<1.0	0
CHILI SAUCE								
(Chef Boyardee) hot dog, w/beef	1 oz	30	1.0	4.0	140	(mq)	1.0	na
(Del Monte) tomato	1/4 cup	70	1.0	17.0	835	(mq)	0.0	0
(El Molino) green, mild	2 tbsp	10	0.0	2.0	210	(mq)	0.0	0
(Featherweight)	1 tbsp	8	0.0	2.0	10	(mq)	0.0	0
(Gebhardt) hot dog	2 tbsp	20	1.0	2.0	150	(mq)	1.0	na
(Heinz)	1 oz	30	0.0	7.0	430	0	0.0	0
(Hunt's)	1.199 oz	35	0.3	8.0	393	.7	0.1	0
(Las Palmas) red	1/2 cup	25	1.0	3.0	670	0	1.0	0
(Manwich) 'Chili Fixin's'	5.3 oz	110	6.0	20.0	900	5.0	<1.0	0
(S&W) 'Chili Makin's'	1/2 cup	100	5.0	20.0	782	(mq)	1.0	0
(Wolf Brand) hot dog	1.25 oz	44	1.5	4.4	199	>.4 c	2.3	na
CHOCOLATE SAUCE								
(Chocolate Mountain)	2 tbsp	120	1.0	20.0	80	na	4.0	4

Food Name	Serv. Size	Total Cal.	Prot. GMS	Carbs GMS	Sod. MGS	Fiber GMS	Fat GMS	Chol. MGS
CLAM SAUCE								
Red								
(Buitoni)	5 oz	190	8.0	28.0	560	(mq)	6.0	20
(Contadina) 'Fresh' refrigerated	7.5 oz	120	7.0	15.0	800	(mq)	4.0	35
(Ferrara)	4 oz	70	5.0	8.0	320	(mq)	2.0	10
(Progresso)	1/2 cup	70	5.0	7.0	560	(mq)	3.0	(mq)
White								
(Contadina) 'Fresh' refrigerated	6 oz	290	8.0	13.0	800	(mq)	23.0	94
(Ferrara)	4 oz	80	5.0	4.0	570	(mq)	5.0	10
(Progresso)	1/2 cup	110	9.0	1.0	280	(mq)	8.0	(mq)
COCKTAIL SAUCE								
(Del Monte)	1/4 cup	70	1.0	17.0	765	na	0.0	0
(Estee)	1 tbsp	10	<1.0	2.0	35	na	<1.0	0
(Golden Dipt) extra hot	1 tbsp	20	0.0	5.0	210	na	0.0	0
(Golden Dipt) regular	1 tbsp	20	0.0	5.0	210	na	0.0	0
(Great Impressions)	1 tbsp	21	0.2	4.7	182	na	0.1	0
(Great Impressions) 'Brandy Glow'	1 tbsp	68	0.2	1.6	106	na	6.7	10
(Great Impressions) 'Low Salt'	1 tbsp	21	0.2	4.8	6	na	0.1	0
(Sauceworks)	1 tbsp	14	0.0	3.0	170	na	0.0	0
(Skipper's)	1 tbsp	20	0.0	5.0	216	na	0.0	0
(Stokely)	1 tbsp	18	0.0	5.0	90	na	0.0	0
CRANBERRY-ORANGE SAUCE								
(Ocean Spray) crushed, for chicken 'Cran•Fruit'	2 oz	90	0.0	23.0	10	na	0.0	na
CRANBERRY-RASPBERRY SAUCE								
(Ocean Spray) crushed, for chicken 'Cran•Fruit'	2 oz	90	0.0	23.0	10	na	0.0	na
CREOLE SAUCE								
(Enrico's) Cajun 'Light'	4 oz	76	2.0	9.0	284	na	2.8	0
(Golden Dipt) cooking sauce	1 oz	20	0.0	2.0	190	na	1.0	0
DIABLO SAUCE (Escoffier)	1 tbsp	20	0.0	4.0	160	na	0.0	0
DIJONAISSE SAUCE (Golden Dipt) cooking sauce	1 oz	52	0.0	2.0	130	na	4.0	0
ENCHILADA SAUCE								
(Gebhardt)	3 tbsp	25	<1.0	3.0	170	<1.0	1.0	<1
(La Victoria)	1 cup	80	1.0	10.0	1520	(tr)	5.0	0
(Rosarita)	3 oz	20	0.0	4.0	430	(tr)	0.0	0
Green (Old El Paso)	2 tbsp	11	<1.0	3.0	200	0	0.0	0
Hot								
(Del Monte)	1/2 cup	45	1.0	11.0	1090	(tr)	0.0	0
(El Molino)	2 tbsp	16	0.0	2.0	100	(tr)	1.0	0
(Las Palmas)	1/2 cup	25	1.0	3.0	670	0	1.0	0
(Old El Paso)	1/4 cup	30	<1.0	4.0	250	(tr)	1.0	0

Food Name	Serv. Size	Total Cal.	Prot. GMS	Carbs GMS	Sod. MGS	Fiber GMS	Fat GMS	Chol. MGS
(Ortega)	1 oz	12	0.0	3.0	280	(tr)	0.0	0
Mild								
(Del Monte)	1/2 cup	45	1.0	11.0	1150	(tr)	0.0	0
(Old El Paso)	1/4 cup	25	<1.0	4.0	250	(tr)	1.0	0
(Ortega)	1 oz	12	0.0	3.0	280	(tr)	0.0	0
(Rosarita)	2.5 oz	25	<1.0	3.0	230	<1.0	1.0	0
FAJITA SAUCE (Tio Sancho) 'Skillet Sauce'	1 oz	14	0.5	1.8	590	>.1 c	0.5	0
FORESTIERA SAUCE (Contadina) 'Fresh' refrigerated	7.5 oz	270	6.0	15.0	830	na	9.0	15
FOUR CHEESE SAUCE								
(Contadina)	4 oz	300	8.0	7.0	400	na	27.0	80
(Contadina) 'Fresh' refrigerated	6 oz	470	12.0	8.0	500	0	45.0	147
(DiGiorno) refrigerated	2 oz	170	4.0	3.0	340	na	16.0	45
FRENCH WHITE SAUCE (Golden Dipt) cooking sauce	1 oz	55	0.0	3.0	210	na	4.0	0
GARLIC-CHILI PEPPER SAUCE								
(A Taste of Thai)	1 tbsp	10	0.0	2.0	220	0	0.0	0
GARLIC-HERB SAUCE (Golden Dipt) 'Nature Bay'	2 grams	8	0.0	1.0	87	na	0.0	0
GUAVA SAUCE, cooked	1/2 cup	43	0.4	11.3	5	4.3	0.2	0
HERB AND GARLIC SAUCE (Lawry's) w/lemon juice	1/4 cup	36	3.6	3.8	3688	<.1	0.4	na
HOLLANDAISE SAUCE								
(Great Impressions)	2 tbsp	192	0.5	0.3	107	(mq)	21.0	48
HONEY SOY SAUCE								
(Golden Dipt) cooking sauce	1 oz	90	0.0	5.0	250	na	8.0	0
(Golden Dipt) 'Nature Bay'	1 oz	90	0.0	5.0	250	na	8.0	0
HORSERADISH SAUCE								
(Great Impressions)	1 tbsp	74	0.0	1.4	199	(mq)	7.6	1
(Heinz)	1 tbsp	74	0.2	2.0	113	(mq)	7.4	na
(Life) strong 'All Natural'	1/2 tbsp	7	<1.0	<1.0	2	(mq)	<1.0	0
(Sauceworks)	1 tbsp	50	0.0	2.0	105	(mq)	5.0	5
HOT DOG SAUCE (Just Rite)	2 oz	60	2.0	6.0	220	<1.0	3.0	7
HOT PEPPER SAUCE								
(Gebhardt) 'Louisiana Style'	1/2 tsp	0	0.0	(tr)	45	(tr)	0.0	0
(Tabasco)	1/4 tsp	<1	tr	<1.0	9	(tr)	tr	0
HOT SAUCE (Gebhardt)	1/2 tsp	<1	<1.0	<1.0	55	<1.0	<1.0	0
JALAPEÑO CHEESE SAUCE								
(Pablo's) 'Deli Style'	1 oz	59	2.0	4.0	470	na	4.0	5
(White House)	3.5 oz	193	3.0	10.0	890	(tr)	16.0	(mq)
LEMON BUTTER-DILL SAUCE								
(Golden Dipt) cooking sauce	1 oz	110	0.0	5.0	180	na	10.0	0

Food Name	Serv. Size	Total Cal.	Prot. GMS	Carbs GMS	Sod. MGS	Fiber GMS	Fat GMS	Chol. MGS
LEMON-DILL SAUCE *(Golden Dipt)*								
'Nature Bay'	1 oz	110	0.0	3.0	150	na	11.0	0
LOBSTER SAUCE *(Progresso)* rock	1/2 cup	120	4.0	11.0	430	2.0	8.0	10
MARINARA SAUCE								
(Angela Mia)	4.409 oz	47	1.9	9.0	503	3.1	1.5	0
(Buitoni)	1/2 cup	70	1.0	11.0	570	(mq)	3.0	0
(DiGiorno) refrigerated	5 oz	110	3.0	12.0	680	na	6.0	5
(Millina's Finest) organic, fat-free	4 oz	48	2.0	9.0	210	na	0.5	na
(Millina's Finest) Zinfandel, organic, fat-free	4 oz	44	2.0	9.0	215	na	0.5	na
(Pathmark) 'All Natural'	1/2 cup	80	2.0	12.0	710	(mq)	2.0	0
(Pathmark) 'No Frills'	1/2 cup	80	2.0	12.0	620	(mq)	3.0	0
(Prego)	4 oz	100	1.0	10.0	620	(mq)	6.0	0
(Progresso)	1/2 cup	90	4.0	9.0	520	(mq)	5.0	1
(Progresso) 'Authentic Pasta Sauces'	1/2 cup	110	4.0	10.0	250	2.4	6.0	4
(Rokeach)	3 oz	60	1.0	9.0	257	(mq)	2.0	0
(Westbrae)	4 oz	40	2.0	7.0	370	na	<1.0	0
(Westbrae) w/mushrooms	4 oz	50	2.0	7.0	380	na	29.0	0
MESQUITE SAUCE *(Lawry's)* w/lime juice	1/4 cup	24	3.0	3.0	4142	>.1 c	0.4	0
MUSHROOM SAUCE *(Quincy's)*	3 oz	27	1.0	5.0	366	na	<1.0	na
NACHO CHEESE SAUCE								
(J. Hungerford)	2.011 oz	120	2.0	7.0	440	0	9.0	5
(J. Hungerford) 'Stadium'	2.011 oz	80	1.0	6.0	410	0	5.0	4
(Kaukauna)	1 oz	80	3.0	4.0	330	0	6.0	8
(Lucky Leaf)	4 oz	220	4.0	11.0	1010	0	18.0	(mq)
(Musselman's)	4 oz	220	4.0	11.0	1010	0	18.0	(mq)
(Pablo's) 'Deli Style'	1 oz	59	2.0	4.0	470	na	4.0	5
(White House)	3.5 oz	193	3.0	10.0	890	0	16.0	(mq)
NEWBURG SAUCE *(Snow's)* w/sherry	1/3 cup	120	3.0	10.0	520	na	8.0	na
ORANGE SAUCE *(LaChoy)* Mandarin	1 tbsp	24	<.1	6.1	38	.1	tr	0
ORANGE-DIJON SAUCE *(Golden Dipt)*								
'Nature Bay'	1 oz	110	0.0	6.0	200	na	9.0	0
OREGANO-HERB SAUCE *(Golden Dipt)*								
'Nature Bay'	2 grams	6	0.0	1.0	88	na	0.0	0
PARMIGIANA SAUCE *(Betty Crocker)*								
'Recipe Sauces'	3.9 oz	50	2.0	9.0	430	na	1.0	0
PASTA SAUCE/spaghetti sauce								
(Angela Mia)	4.409 oz	49	1.5	10.6	607	2.5	0.5	0
(Campbell's) 'Homestyle'	4 oz	40	2.0	10.0	360	2.0	0.0	0
(Enrico's) 'All Natural'	4 oz	60	2.0	9.0	345	(mq)	1.0	0
(Hunt's) 'Homestyle'	4 oz	60	2.0	10.0	530	2.0	2.0	0
(Hunt's) 'Olde Country'	4 oz	60	2.0	8.0	560	na	2.0	0
(Progresso)	1/2 cup	110	3.0	13.0	660	(mq)	5.0	2
(Ragu) 'Old World Style'	4 oz	80	2.0	9.0	740	na	4.0	0

Food Name	Serv. Size	Total Cal.	Prot. GMS	Carbs GMS	Sod. MGS	Fiber GMS	Fat GMS	Chol. MGS
(Ragu) 'Slow Cooked Homestyle'	4 oz	110	2.0	15.0	510	na	5.0	0
(Ragu) 'Thick & Hearty'	4 oz	100	2.0	15.0	460	(mq)	3.0	0
Garden								
(Prego) combination	4 oz	80	2.0	14.0	420	(mq)	2.0	na
(Pritikin) chunky	1/2 cup	50	2.0	11.0	30	na	0.0	0
(Ragu) harvest 'Todays Recipe'	4 oz	50	2.0	8.0	370	na	1.0	0
Garlic and herb								
(Healthy Choice)	4 oz	40	2.0	9.0	350	na	<1.0	0
(Hunt's) 'Classic'	4.409 oz	58	1.9	9.5	598	1.8	2.1	0
(Hunt's) 'Light'	4.409 oz	39	2.2	7.3	379	2.6	0.8	0
(Hunt's) 'Olde Country'	4.409 oz	63	2.3	8.9	522	3.3	2.7	0
Garlic and onion								
(Campbell's) extra	4 oz	50	2.0	12.0	320	2.0	<1.0	0
(Del Monte)	1/2 cup	70	1.0	10.0	430	na	2.0	na
(Healthy Choice) chunky	4 oz	40	2.0	10.0	350	na	0.0	0
(Prego)	4 oz	110	1.0	16.0	510	(mq)	4.0	na
Italian								
(Campbell's)	4 oz	50	2.0	12.0	360	2.0	0.0	0
(Healthy Choice) vegetable, chunky	4 oz	40	1.0	9.0	350	na	0.0	0
(Hunt's) vegetable 'Olde Country'	4.409 oz	64	2.5	9.0	616	2.8	2.6	0
(Pastorelli) 'Italian Chef'	4 oz	81	3.0	11.0	430	>1.1 c	3.0	na
(Ragu) 'Fresh Italian'	4 oz	90	2.0	13.0	490	(mq)	3.0	0
(Ragu) garden combination 'Chunky Gardenstyle'	4 oz	110	2.0	15.0	500	na	5.0	0
Meat								
(Chef Boyardee) w/ground beef 'Jars'	4 oz	90	2.0	14.0	605	(mq)	3.0	(mq)
(Hunt's)	4.444 oz	65	1.9	10.9	604	1.9	2.3	3
(Hunt's) 'Homestyle'	4.409 oz	56	2.2	6.9	596	1.6	2.6	2
(Hunt's) 'Light'	4.409 oz	45	2.1	7.9	437	2.9	1.2	2
(Hunt's) 'Olde Country'	4.409 oz	56	2.5	7.2	474	2.7	2.6	0
(Ragu) 'Homestyle'	4 oz	110	2.0	15.0	510	na	5.0	2
Meat flavor								
(Chef Boyardee)	3.75 oz	80	2.0	11.0	650	(mq)	3.0	na
(Chef Boyardee) 'Original'	3.75 oz	120	3.0	13.0	650	(mq)	6.0	na
(Contadina) 'Original Recipe'	1/2 cup	100	2.7	17.2	430	na	3.2	2
(Del Monte)	1/2 cup	70	2.0	9.0	440	na	2.0	na
(Hunt's)	4 oz	70	2.0	12.0	570	(mq)	2.0	na
(P&Q)	1/2 cup	70	1.0	11.0	510	(mq)	2.0	na
(Pathmark) 'All Natural'	1/2 cup	80	2.0	11.0	790	(mq)	3.0	na
(Pathmark) 'No Frills'	1/2 cup	90	2.0	11.0	620	(mq)	5.0	na
(Prego)	4 oz	140	2.0	20.0	660	(mq)	6.0	na
(Progresso)	1/2 cup	110	4.0	13.0	660	(mq)	5.0	5
(Weight Watchers)	1/3 cup	50	2.0	9.0	440	(mq)	1.0	na

Food Name	Serv. Size	Total Cal.	Prot. GMS	Carbs GMS	Sod. MGS	Fiber GMS	Fat GMS	Chol. MGS
Meatless								
(Chef Boyardee) 'Jars'	4 oz	60	1.0	11.0	790	(mq)	1.0	na
(P&Q)	1/2 cup	70	1.0	14.0	540	(mq)	1.0	na
(Pathmark) 'All Natural'	1/2 cup	70	2.0	11.0	710	(mq)	2.0	na
(Pathmark) 'No Frills'	1/2 cup	80	1.0	11.0	583	(mq)	3.0	na
Mushroom								
(Campbell's)	4 oz	50	2.0	11.0	330	2.0	<1.0	0
(Campbell's) 'Healthy Request'	4 oz	50	2.0	11.0	330	2.0	<1.0	0
(Contadina) 'Original Recipe'	1/2 cup	90	2.1	17.5	430	na	2.3	0
(Del Monte)	1/2 cup	70	1.0	11.0	440	na	2.0	na
(Healthy Choice) chunky	4 oz	45	2.0	10.0	350	na	0.0	0
(Hunt's)	4.444 oz	65	1.9	10.9	604	1.9	2.3	0
(Hunt's) 'Homestyle'	4.409 oz	56	2.2	6.9	586	1.6	2.6	0
(Hunt's) 'Light'	4.409 oz	39	2.2	7.3	379	2.6	0.8	0
(Hunt's) 'Olde Country'	4.409 oz	53	2.1	7.0	542	2.7	2.7	0
(Prego) w/extra spice 'Extra Chunky'	4 oz	100	2.0	17.0	450	(mq)	3.0	na
(Ragu) chunky 'Todays Recipe'	4 oz	50	2.0	8.0	370	na	1.0	0
(Ragu) 'Homestyle'	4 oz	110	2.0	15.0	530	na	2.0	0
(Ragu) super 'Chunky Gardenstyle'	4 oz	110	2.0	15.0	500	na	5.0	0
(Ragu) 'Thick & Hearty'	4 oz	100	2.0	15.0	460	—	3.0	0
Mushroom and green pepper								
(Enrico's) 'All Natural'	4 oz	60	2.0	9.0	345	(mq)	1.0	0
(Enrico's) 'All Natural No Salt Added'	4 oz	60	2.0	9.0	30	(mq)	1.0	0
(Prego) 'Extra Chunky'	4 oz	100	2.0	14.0	410	(mq)	4.0	na
(Ragu) 'Chunky Gardenstyle'	4 oz	110	2.0	15.0	500	na	5.0	0
Mushroom and onion								
(Prego) 'Extra Chunky'	4 oz	100	2.0	13.0	490	(mq)	4.0	na
(Ragu) 'Chunky Gardenstyle'	4 oz	110	2.0	15.0	560	na	5.0	0
Mushroom and tomato								
(DiGiorno) w/plum tomatoes, refrigerated	5 oz	100	3.0	20.0	240	na	1.0	0
(Millina's Finest) organic, fat-free	4 oz	45	2.0	9.0	198	na	0.5	na
(Prego) 'Extra Chunky'	4 oz	110	1.0	14.0	500	(mq)	5.0	na
Mushroom flavor								
(Chef Boyardee)	3.75 oz	60	1.0	11.0	790	(mq)	1.0	na
(Chef Boyardee) 'Jars'	4 oz	70	1.0	11.0	655	(mq)	2.0	na
(Chef Boyardee) 'Original'	3.75 oz	80	1.0	13.0	680	(mq)	3.0	na
(Enrico's)	4 oz	60	2.0	9.0	(mq)	(mq)	1.0	0
(Enrico's) w/fresh mushrooms	4 oz	60	2.0	9.0	336	(mq)	1.0	0
(Featherweight)	4 oz	60	2.0	11.0	310	(mq)	1.0	0
(Hunt's)	4 oz	70	2.0	12.0	560	(mq)	2.0	0
(P&Q)	1/2 cup	70	1.0	14.0	580	(mq)	1.0	na
(Pathmark) 'All Natural'	1/2 cup	70	2.0	11.0	730	(mq)	2.0	na
(Prego)	4 oz	130	2.0	20.0	630	(mq)	5.0	na

Food Name	Serv. Size	Total Cal.	Prot. GMS	Carbs GMS	Sod. MGS	Fiber GMS	Fat GMS	Chol. MGS
(Progresso)	1/2 cup	110	3.0	13.0	630	(mq)	5.0	5
(Weight Watchers)	1/3 cup	40	1.0	9.0	430	(mq)	0.0	0
No salt added								
(Eden Foods) organic	4 oz	80	3.0	14.0	0	na	2.0	na
(Enrico's) 'All Natural No Salt Added'	4 oz	60	2.0	9.0	30	(mq)	1.0	0
(Prego) 'No Salt Added'	4 oz	110	2.0	11.0	25	(mq)	6.0	na
Original *(Pritikin)*	1/2 cup	60	2.0	14.0	35	na	1.0	0
Parmesan, 'Classic' *(Hunt's)*	4.409 oz	50	1.8	7.8	634	1.8	2.1	0
Primavera								
(Progresso) creamy 'Authentic Pasta Sauces'	1/2 cup	190	5.0	8.0	410	1.0	17.0	54
(Westbrae)	4 oz	60	2.0	7.0	490	na	3.0	0
(Westbrae) no salt	4 oz	40	2.0	7.0	105	na	0.0	0
Sausage and green pepper *(Prego)* 'Extra Chunky'	4 oz	160	3.0	19.0	500	(mq)	8.0	(mq)
Sicilian *(Progresso)* 'Authentic Pasta Sauces'	1/2 cup	30	<1.0	2.0	660	<1.0	2.5	0
Sweet pepper and onion *(Millina's Finest)* organic, fat-free	4 oz	41	2.0	7.0	305	na	0.5	na
Three cheese *(Prego)*	4 oz	100	3.0	17.0	410	na	2.0	(mq)
Tomato and basil								
(Hunt's) 'Classic'	4.409 oz	48	1.8	7.5	613	3.9	2.1	0
(Millina's Finest) organic, fat-free	4 oz	46	2.0	9.0	232	na	0.5	na
Tomato and herb								
(Ragu) 'Homestyle'	4 oz	110	2.0	15.0	510	na	5.0	0
(Ragu) 'Ragu Fine Italian'	4 oz	90	2.0	13.0	490	na	3.0	0
(Ragu) 'Today's Recipe'	4 oz	50	2.0	8.0	370	na	1.0	0
Tomato chunks *(Hunt's)* 'Chunky Style'	4 oz	50	1.0	12.0	470	na	<1.0	0
Tomato-based								
(Prego) and basil	4 oz	100	2.0	18.0	370	(mq)	2.0	na
(Prego) and onion 'Extra Chunky'	4 oz	110	2.0	14.0	490	(mq)	5.0	na
Tomatoes, garlic, and onion *(Ragu)* 'Chunky Gardenstyle'	4 oz	110	2.0	15.0	500	na	5.0	0
Traditional								
(Contadina) 'Original Recipe'	1/2 cup	90	2.0	17.0	440	na	2.3	0
(Del Monte)	1/2 cup	70	1.0	11.0	430	na	2.0	na
(Healthy Choice)	4 oz	40	2.0	9.0	380	na	<1.0	0
(Hunt's) 'Homestyle'	4.409 oz	56	2.2	3.9	596	1.6	2.6	0
(Hunt's) 'Light'	4.409 oz	39	2.2	7.3	421	2.6	0.8	0
(Hunt's) 'Olde Country'	4.409 oz	53	2.1	7.0	542	2.7	2.7	0
(Hunt's) 'Traditional'	4 oz	70	2.0	12.0	530	(mq)	2.0	0
Zinfandel wine *(Sutter Home)*	1/2 cup	100	2.0	11.0	520	na	5.0	0

Food Name	Serv. Size	Total Cal.	Prot. GMS	Carbs GMS	Sod. MGS	Fiber GMS	Fat GMS	Chol. MGS
PEPPER STEAK SAUCE *(Betty Crocker)*								
'Recipe Sauces'	3.8 oz	50	1.0	8.0	270	na	2.0	0
PEPPER-DILL SAUCE *(Golden Dipt)*								
'Nature Bay'	2 grams	8	0.0	1.0	96	na	0.0	0
PESTO SAUCE								
(Contadina) refrigerated 'Fresh'	2.33 oz	350	6.0	6.0	420	(mq)	34.0	10
(DiGiorno) refrigerated	2.3 oz	340	8.0	5.0	430	na	32.0	20
PICANTE SAUCE								
(Estee)	2 tbsp	8	<1.0	2.0	60	(mq)	0.0	0
(Gebhardt)	1 tbsp	4	0.0	1.0	120	(mq)	0.0	0
(Wise)	2 tbsp	12	0.0	3.0	130	(mq)	0.0	0
All varieties								
(Old El Paso)	2 tbsp	8	<1.0	2.0	310	(mq)	<1.0	0
(Old El Paso) 'Chunky'	2 tbsp	7	0.0	2.0	270	(mq)	0.0	0
Extra mild *(Pace)* 'Thick & Chunky'	2 tsp	3	0.3	0.5	111	na	0.1	na
Hot								
(Chi-Chi's)	1 oz	10	2.0	2.0	268	na	2.0	2
(Guiltless Gourmet)	1 oz	8	0.0	1.0	133	<1.0	0.0	0
(Pace) 'Thick & Chunky'	2 tsp	3	0.3	0.5	111	na	0.1	na
(Rosarita) chunky	3 tbsp	18	<1.0	4.0	515	<1.0	<1.0	0
(Rosarita) zesty jalapeño	1.093 oz	8	0.4	1.7	246	.7	0.2	0
Medium								
(Chi-Chi's)	1 oz	8	2.0	2.0	192	na	2.0	2
(Guiltless Gourmet)	1 oz	8	0.0	1.0	133	<1.0	0.0	0
(Pace) 'Thick & Chunky'	2 tsp	3	0.3	0.5	111	na	0.1	na
(Rosarita) chunky	3 tbsp	16	<1.0	4.0	650	<1.0	(mq)	0
(Rosarita) zesty jalapeño	1.093 oz	9	0.4	1.7	254	.6	0.2	0
Mild								
(Azteca)	1 tbsp	4	0.0	1.0	85	(mq)	0.0	0
(Chi-Chi's)	1 oz	9	2.0	2.0	198	na	2.0	2
(Guiltless Gourmet)	1 oz	8	0.0	1.0	133	<1.0	0.0	0
(Hunt's) 'Homestyle'	1.093 oz	11	0.5	2.1	256	.5	0.2	0
(Pace) 'Thick & Chunky'	2 tsp	3	0.3	0.5	111	na	0.1	na
(Rosarita)	3.5 oz	45	2.0	9.0	1015	(mq)	<1.0	0
(Rosarita) chunky	3 tbsp	25	1.0	5.0	630	<1.0	<1.0	0
(Rosarita) zesty jalapeño	1.093 oz	8	0.5	1.7	239	.5	0.1	0
PIZZA SAUCE								
(Angela Mia)	2.222 oz	27	1.4	5.2	190	1.8	0.6	0
(Angela Mia) super heavy								
'Premium Choice'	2.258 oz	28	2.5	5.8	36	2.9	0.5	0
(Chef Boyardee) w/cheese	2.63 oz	70	1.0	7.0	385	(mq)	4.0	(mq)
(Chef Boyardee) w/cheese 'Jars'	3.88 oz	90	1.0	10.0	565	(mq)	6.0	(mq)
(Contadina) original 'Quick & Easy'	1/4 cup	30	1.0	5.0	330	(mq)	1.0	na

Food Name	Serv. Size	Total Cal.	Prot. GMS	Carbs GMS	Sod. MGS	Fiber GMS	Fat GMS	Chol. MGS
(Contadina) 'Pizza Squeeze'	1/4 cup	30	1.0	5.0	330	(mq)	1.0	na
(Contadina) w/Italian cheese	1/4 cup	30	1.0	5.0	380	(mq)	1.0	(mq)
(Contadina) w/pepperoni	1/4 cup	40	1.0	5.0	360	(mq)	2.0	(mq)
(Eden Foods) and pasta sauce, organic	4 oz	80	3.0	10.0	320	na	3.0	na
(Enrico's) 'Homemade Style All Natural'	4 oz	60	2.0	9.0	(mq)	(mq)	1.0	0
(Enrico's) 'Homemade Style All Natural No Salt'	4 oz	60	2.0	9.0	30	(mq)	1.0	0
(Hunt's)	2.363 oz	32	1.8	4.9	416	1.5	1.1	0
(Hunt's)	2.222 oz	21	1.3	3.8	251	1.6	0.5	0
(Pastorelli) 'Italian Chef'	4 oz	90	3.0	12.0	430	(mq)	3.0	na
(Pizza Quick)	3 tbsp	35	1.0	3.0	330	(mq)	2.0	0
(Pizza Quick) traditional	1.7 oz	35	1.0	3.0	330	na	2.0	0
PLUM SAUCE (LaChoy) tangy	1 oz	45	0.1	10.8	17	(mq)	0.1	0
RIB SAUCE (Dip 'n Joy) 'Saucy Rib'	1 oz	60	0.0	14.0	250	na	0.0	0
RIGOLLETO SAUCE (DiGiorno) refrigerated	5 oz	110	2.0	9.0	660	na	8.0	0
ROBERT SAUCE (Escoffier) 'Sauce Robert'	1 tbsp	20	0.0	5.0	70	tr	0.0	0
SANDWICH SAUCE								
(Hormel) 'Not-so-Sloppy Sloppy Joe'	2.24 oz	70	1.0	16.0	730	na	1.0	5
(Libby's) 'Sloppy Joe'	2.5 oz	45	1.0	10.0	na	na	<1.0	440
(Manwich)	2.5 oz	40	1.0	10.0	390	na	<1.0	na
(Manwich) bold	2.222 oz	62	0.5	13.1	802	.8	1.1	0
(Manwich) extra thick and chunky	2.5 oz	60	1.0	15.0	640	na	<1.0	na
(Manwich) Mexican	2.258 oz	26	1.2	5.0	552	.8	0.2	0
(Manwich) Mexican 'Sloppy Joe'	2.5 oz	35	1.0	9.0	460	na	<1.0	0
(Manwich) thick and chunky	2.293 oz	44	1.4	8.6	737	.8	0.5	0
SEAFOOD COCKTAIL SAUCE (Heinz)	1/4 cup	60	1.0	13.0	680	na	0.0	0
SEAFOOD SAUCE								
(Great Impressions) Creole	1 tbsp	21	0.2	4.7	182	na	0.1	0
(Great Impressions) dipping	1 tbsp	17	0.6	2.2	129	na	0.7	0
(Great Impressions) dipping, Polynesian	1 tbsp	38	<1.0	9.5	127	na	<1.0	0
SEASONING SAUCE (A Taste of Thai)	1 tbsp	15	2.0	1.0	1760	0	0.0	0
SHOYU. See SOY SAUCE.								
SHRIMP SAUCE (Tone's) 'Craboil'	1 tsp	10	0.3	1.2	1	.3	0.6	1
SOY SAUCE								
shoyu	1 tbsp	9	0.9	1.5	3314	0	tr	0
shoyu, low-sodium	1 tbsp	9	0.9	1.5	600	0	tr	0
tamari	1 tbsp	11	1.9	1.0	1005	0	<.1	0
(Eden Foods) shoyu, organic	1/2 tsp	2	0.0	0.0	140	na	0.0	na
(Eden Foods) shoyu, organic, reduced sodium	1/2 tsp	2	0.0	0.0	80	na	0.0	na
(Kikkoman)	1 tbsp	10	na	0.9	892	0	tr	0
(Kikkoman) 'Lite'	1 tbsp	11	na	1.3	600	0	tr	0

Food Name	Serv. Size	Total Cal.	Prot. GMS	Carbs GMS	Sod. MGS	Fiber GMS	Fat GMS	Chol. MGS
(LaChoy)	1 tsp	<1	0.2	0.3	429	0	0.0	0
(LaChoy) 'Lite'	1 tsp	<1	0.2	0.3	220	0	0.0	0
(Westbrae) mild	1/2 tsp	2	1.0	1.0	85	na	0.0	0
(Westbrae) organic	1/2 tsp	2	1.0	1.0	105	na	0.0	0
(Westbrae) tamari	1/2 tsp	2	1.0	1.0	170	na	0.0	0
(Westbrae) wheat-free	1/2 tsp	3	1.0	1.0	140	na	0.0	0
SPAGHETTI SAUCE. See PASTA SAUCE.								
STEAK SAUCE								
(A.1.)	1 tbsp	18	0.0	4.0	160	na	0.0	0
(A.1.) bold	1 tbsp	18	0.0	4.0	160	na	0.0	0
(Heinz) '57'	1 tbsp	16	0.0	4.0	190	0	0.0	0
(Heinz) hickory smoke '57'	1 tbsp	16	0.0	4.0	180	0	0.0	0
(Heinz) traditional	1 tbsp	12	0.2	2.6	200	na	0.0	0
(Hunt's)	1 tbsp	10	0.3	2.3	256	.3	0.1	0
(Lea & Perrins)	1 oz	40	<1.0	10.0	220	na	<1.0	na
STIR-FRY SAUCE								
(Kikkoman)	1 tsp	6	0.3	2.3	120	tr	tr	0
(LaChoy) Mandarin	4.48 oz	71	2.3	15.6	851	1.3	0.2	0
(LaChoy) sweet and sour	4.797 oz	146	2.2	34.8	821	1.5	0.1	0
(LaChoy) Szechwan	4.55 oz	73	2.8	16.0	612	2.1	0.2	0
(Lawry's)	1/4 cup	120	1.9	19.6	1128	>.2 c	3.8	na
STROGANOFF SAUCE *(Betty Crocker)*								
'Recipe Sauces'	4 oz	60	1.0	6.0	540	na	4.0	10
SWEET AND SOUR SAUCE								
(A Taste of Thai) tangy, hot	2 tbsp	30	0.0	8.0	95	0	0.0	0
(Betty Crocker) 'Recipe Sauces'	4.1 oz	130	<1.0	32.0	360	na	0.0	0
(Contadina)	1/2 cup	150	<1.0	32.0	430	.1	3.0	0
(Great Impressions) Hawaiian	2 tbsp	102	0.0	25.5	<1	na	0.0	0
(Great Impressions) hot	2 tbsp	102	0.0	25.5	<1	na	0.0	0
(Great Impressions) regular	2 tbsp	102	0.0	25.5	<1	na	0.0	0
(Hickory Farms) Hawaiian	2 tbsp	102	0.0	25.5	2	na	0.0	0
(Hickory Farms) regular	2 tbsp	102	0.0	25.5	<1	na	0.0	0
(Kikkoman)	1 tbsp	18	na	4.0	63	na	0.0	0
(LaChoy)	1 tbsp	30	na	7.0	320	na	na	0
(LaChoy) duck sauce	1 tbsp	26	<.1	6.9	59	0	tr	0
(Lawry's)	1/4 cup	549	3.4	11.7	4056	>.4 c	7.5	na
(Sauceworks)	1 tbsp	25	0.0	5.0	50	na	0.0	0
SZECHUAN SAUCE *(LaChoy)* hot and spicy	1 oz	48	0.1	12.0	141	0	0.2	0
TACO SAUCE								
(Estee)	2 tbsp	14	<1.0	3.0	25	(mq)	0.0	0
(Hain) and dip	4 tbsp	25	1.0	5.0	350	na	1.0	5
(Lawry's) 'Sauce'n Seasoner'	1/4 cup	40	0.7	7.6	636	0	0.6	0
(Old El Paso)	2 tbsp	15	1.0	3.0	300	1.0	0.0	0

Food Name	Serv. Size	Total Cal.	Prot. GMS	Carbs GMS	Sod. MGS	Fiber GMS	Fat GMS	Chol. MGS
(Rosarita)	.1764 oz	2	0.1	0.4	40	.1	0.0	0
Chunky (Lawry's)	1/4 cup	22	0.9	4.0	549	>.4 c	0.4	0
Green (La Victoria)	1 tbsp	0	0.0	1.0	90	na	0.0	na
Hot								
(Chi-Chi's)	1 oz	18	2.0	4.0	254	na	2.0	1
(Del Monte)	1/4 cup	15	0.0	4.0	440	(mq)	0.0	0
(Old El Paso)	2 tbsp	10	<1.0	2.0	130	(mq)	<1.0	na
(Ortega)	1 oz	12	0.0	3.0	210	(mq)	0.0	0
Medium								
(Heinz)	1 tbsp	6	0.0	1.0	(mq)	(mq)	0.0	0
(Old El Paso)	2 tbsp	10	<1.0	2.0	130	(mq)	<1.0	0
Mild								
(Del Monte)	1/2 cup	15	0.0	4.0	480	(mq)	0.0	0
(Enrico's) 'No Salt Added'	2 tbsp	14	1.0	3.0	25	(mq)	0.0	0
(Heinz)	1 tbsp	6	0.0	1.0	(mq)	(mq)	0.0	0
(Old El Paso)	2 tbsp	10	<1.0	2.0	130	(mq)	<1.0	na
(Ortega)	1 oz	12	0.0	3.0	220	(mq)	0.0	0
Red								
(El Molino) mild	2 tbsp	10	0.0	2.0	170	(mq)	0.0	0
(La Victoria)	1 tbsp	5	0.0	1.0	80	na	0.0	na
Thick, chunky (Chi-Chi's)	1 oz	12	2.0	3.0	140	na	2.0	2
Western style (Ortega)	1 oz	8	0.0	2.0	180	(mq)	0.0	0
TAMARI SAUCE. See SOY SAUCE.								
TARTAR SAUCE								
(Best Foods)	1 tbsp	70	0.0	0.0	220	na	8.0	5
(Best Foods) reduced fat	1 tbsp	30	0.0	3.0	210	na	2.0	0
(Golden Dipt)	1 tbsp	70	0.0	2.0	100	na	7.0	10
(Golden Dipt) 'Lite'	1 tbsp	50	0.0	4.0	40	na	4.0	5
(Great Impressions)	1 tbsp	86	0.2	1.2	76	na	9.0	10
(Heinz)	2 tbsp	140	0.0	4.0	240	na	14.0	5
(Hellmann's)	1 tbsp	70	0.0	0.0	220	na	8.0	5
(Kraft) nonfat 'Free'	1 tbsp	10	0.0	3.0	120	na	0.0	0
(Life) egg-free 'All Natural'	1 tbsp	38	<1.0	<1.0	2	na	4.0	0
(Sauceworks)	1 tbsp	50	0.0	2.0	85	na	5.0	5
(Sauceworks) natural lemon and herb flavor	1 tbsp	70	0.0	0.0	85	na	8.0	5
(Skipper's)	1 tbsp	65	0.0	0.0	102	na	7.0	4
(Weight Watchers)	1 tbsp	35	0.0	3.0	80	na	3.0	5
TERIYAKI SAUCE								
(Betty Crocker) 'Recipe Sauces'	3.9 oz	60	2.0	13.0	860	na	<1.0	0
(Golden Dipt) ginger marinade	1 oz	120	1.0	12.0	920	na	7.0	0
(Kikkoman)	1 tbsp	15	na	2.7	630	na	tr	tr
(Kikkoman) 'Baste & Glaze'	1 tbsp	27	na	6.0	420	na	tr	0

Food Name	Serv. Size	Total Cal.	Prot. GMS	Carbs GMS	Sod. MGS	Fiber GMS	Fat GMS	Chol. MGS
(LaChoy)	1/2 tsp	5	<1.0	1.0	290	<1.0	<1.0	0
(LaChoy) basting sauce	1/2 tsp	2	<1.0	<1.0	110	<1.0	<1.0	0
(LaChoy) 'Lite'	1/2 tsp	5	<1.0	1.0	85	<1.0	<1.0	0
(LaChoy) 'Sauce and Marinade'	1 oz	30	1.0	5.0	1640	na	0.0	na
(LaChoy) stir-fry sauce	4.621 oz	105	2.3	24.3	1152	1.6	0.1	0
(LaChoy) thick and rich	1 oz	41	0.7	9.4	509	<.1.0	0.1	<1
(Lawry's) barbecue marinade	1/8 cup	82	4.1	13.7	6115	>.1 c	1.1	na
(Lawry's) w/pineapple juice	1/4 cup	72	6.4	11.0	7100	>.1 c	0.4	na
VEGETABLE SAUCE								
(Contadina) refrigerated, garden 'Light'	.5 oz	50	2.0	10.0	620	na	0.0	0
WORCESTERSHIRE SAUCE								
(French's) regular	1 tbsp	10	0.0	2.0	160	na	0.0	0
(French's) smoky	1 tbsp	10	0.0	2.0	160	na	0.0	0
(Heinz)	1 tsp	0	0.0	0.0	55	na	0.0	0
(Lea & Perrins)	1 tsp	5	<1.0	1.0	55	na	<1.0	0
(Lea & Perrins) white wine	1 tsp	4	<1.0	1.0	40	na	<1.0	0
(Life) 'All Natural'	1/2 tbsp	5	<1.0	1.0	2	na	<1.0	0
SAUCE MIX								
ALFREDO SAUCE								
(French's) 'Pasta Toss' dry mix	2 tsp	25	1.0	2.0	310	na	2.0	na
(Lawry's) 'Pasta Alfredo' dry mix	1 pkg	226	8.0	19.2	3222	>.6 c	13.3	na
BEARNAISE SAUCE dry mix	.9-oz pkg	90	3.5	14.8	841	>.1 c	2.2	tr
BEEF SAUTÉ SAUCE *(Lipton)* golden, dry mix	1/6 pkg	120	3.0	24.0	520	na	2.0	na
CHEESE SAUCE								
(French's) prepared	1/4 cup	80	3.0	7.0	430	na	4.0	(mq)
(McCormick/Schilling) dry mix	1/4 pkg	35	2.0	3.5	477	na	1.5	na
(McCormick/Schilling) nacho, dry mix	1/4 pkg	42	3.0	4.5	409	na	1.5	na
CHICKEN SAUCE								
(Lawry's) southwest 'Seasoning Blends' dry mix	1 pkg	71	1.1	16.0	3947	na	0.3	na
(McCormick/Schilling) cacciatore 'Sauce Blends' dry mix	1 pkg	132	3.6	28.0	1092	(mq)	4.8	na
(McCormick/Schilling) Creole 'Sauce Blends' dry mix	1 pkg	140	2.0	24.0	1084	(mq)	4.8	na
(McCormick/Schilling) curry 'Sauce Blends' dry mix	1 pkg	152	2.4	24.0	1288	(mq)	5.6	na
(McCormick/Schilling) Dijon 'Sauce Blends' dry mix	1 pkg	156	3.2	20.0	1414	(mq)	6.8	na
(McCormick/Schilling) mesquite marinade 'Sauce Blends' dry mix	1 pkg	132	1.6	24.0	2068	(mq)	3.0	na
(McCormick/Schilling) teriyaki 'Sauce Blends' dry mix	1 pkg	172	6.8	28.0	1380	(mq)	3.6	na

Food Name	Serv. Size	Total Cal.	Prot. GMS	Carbs GMS	Sod. MGS	Fiber GMS	Fat GMS	Chol. MGS
CURRY SAUCE, prepared . . . . 1/2 cup	135	5.3	12.9	638	>.2 c	7.4	18
HOLLANDAISE SAUCE							
(McCormick/Schilling) dry mix . . . . . . 1/4 pkg	51	1.0	3.5	170	(mq)	3.8	na
LEMON BUTTER SAUCE							
(Weight Watchers) dry mix . . . . 1 tbsp	6	1.0	1.0	90	na	0.0	na
MUSHROOM SAUCE dry mix . . . . 1-oz pkg	99	4.1	15.5	1766	>.3 c	2.7	0
PASTA SAUCE							
(Estee) prepared w/margarine and							
skim milk . . . . 4 oz	60	2.0	9.0	30	(mq)	1.0	0
(Featherweight) prepared w/margarine							
and skim milk . . . . 4 oz	60	2.0	11.0	310	(mq)	1.0	0
(French's) cheese and garlic 'Pasta Toss'							
dry mix . . . . 2 tsp	25	1.0	2.0	320	(mq)	2.0	na
(French's) Italian 'Pasta Toss' dry mix . . . . 2 tsp	25	1.0	2.0	340	(mq)	2.0	na
(French's) Italian style, prepared . . . . . . 5/8 cup	100	2.0	15.0	790	(mq)	4.0	na
(French's) Romanoff 'Pasta Toss' dry mix . 2 tsp	30	1.0	1.0	310	(mq)	2.0	na
(French's) w/mushrooms, prepared . . . . 5/8 cup	100	2.0	13.0	1050	(mq)	4.0	na
(Lawry's) 'Rich & Thick' dry mix . . . . 1 pkg	147	3.5	28.1	2172	>.5 c	2.2	na
(Lawry's) w/imported mushrooms, dry mix 1 pkg	143	5.2	26.0	2015	>2.1 c	1.5	na
(McCormick/Schilling) dry mix . . . . 1/4 pkg	32	1.0	6.0	615	(mq)	0.3	na
(Prego) prepared w/margarine and							
skim milk . . . . 4 oz	130	2.0	20.0	630	(mq)	5.0	na
(Ragu) prepared w/margarine and							
skim milk . . . . 4 oz	80	2.0	9.0	740	(mq)	4.0	0
PEANUT SAUCE (A Taste of Thai) dry mix 2 tbsp	25	1.0	4.0	115	(mq)	0.5	0
PESTO SAUCE (French's) 'Pasta Toss'							
dry mix . . . . 2 tsp	20	1.0	1.0	280	(mq)	1.0	na
SANDWICH SAUCE (Manwich) dry mix .2469 oz	22	0.2	5.3	351	.3	0.1	0
SEAFOOD SAUCE (Progresso) prepared 1/2 cup	110	5.0	12.0	445	2.3	6.0	11
SOUR CREAM SAUCE							
(McCormick/Schilling) dry mix . . . . 1/4 pkg	44	1.3	4.0	272	na	2.8	na
STROGANOFF SAUCE							
(Lawry's) dry mix . . . . 1 pkg	123	4.5	25.5	2814	>.8 c	0.3	na
(Natural Touch) prepared . . . . 4 oz	90	4.0	10.0	na	na	3.0	na
SWEET AND SOUR SAUCE, dry mix . . 2-oz pkg	220	0.6	54.5	584	na	0.1	na
TACO SAUCE (Tio Sancho) 'Dinner Kit'							
dry mix . . . . 2-oz pkg	62	1.6	13.4	750	>.5 c	0.2	na
TERIYAKI SAUCE dry mix . . . . 1.6-oz pkg	130	4.1	27.6	4784	na	0.9	na
WHITE SAUCE prepared . . . . 1/2 cup	121	5.1	10.7	398	>.1 c	6.7	17
SAUERKRAUT, CANNED							
(A&P) . . . . 1/2 cup	20	1.0	5.0	800	(mq)	<1.0	na
(Allens) w/liquid, shredded . . . . 1/2 cup	21	1.0	5.0	880	(mq)	<1.0	na
(Bush's Best) 'Bavarian Kraut' . . . . 1/2 cup	60	1.0	15.0	400	3.0	0.0	na

Food Name	Serv. Size	Total Cal.	Prot. GMS	Carbs GMS	Sod. MGS	Fiber GMS	Fat GMS	Chol. MGS
(Bush's Best) 'Kraut' deli style	1/2 cup	20	1.0	5.0	680	na	0.0	na
(Bush's Best) 'Kraut' shredded	1/2 cup	20	1.0	5.0	680	na	0.0	na
(Claussen)	1/2 cup	17	0.6	3.2	517	(mq)	0.2	0
(Del Monte)	1/2 cup	25	1.0	6.0	775	(mq)	0.0	0
(Eden Foods) organic	1/2 cup	25	2.0	4.0	580	2.8	<1.0	na
(Finast)	1/2 cup	30	1.0	6.0	800	(mq)	0.0	0
(Pathmark)	1/2 cup	20	0.0	4.0	880	(mq)	0.0	0
(Snow Floss)	1/2 cup	28	1.0	4.0	780	1.0	0.0	0
(Stokely) 'Bavarian'	1/2 cup	30	1.0	7.0	780	(mq)	0.0	0
(Stokely) w/liquid, shredded and chopped	1/2 cup	20	1.0	4.0	810	(mq)	0.0	0
(Vlasic) 'Old Fashioned'	1 oz	4	0.0	1.0	280	(mq)	0.0	0
SAUERKRAUT JUICE								
canned	1 cup	24	1.7	5.6	1905	0	0.0	0
canned or bottled (Biotta)	6 oz	21	1.1	4.0	1482	(mq)	0.1	0
canned or bottled (S&W)	5 oz	14	1.0	3.0	1120	(mq)	0.0	0
SAUSAGE. See also individual listings.								
(Hickory Farms) 'Safari'	1 oz	98	5.0	1.0	343	0	9.0	14
(Hillshire Farm) 'Country Recipe'	2 oz	180	7.0	2.0	490	0	16.0	(mq)
(Hormel)	3 oz	290	12.0	1.0	(mq)	0	27.0	(mq)
(JM) .5-oz patties, cooked	1 patty	70	2.0	1.0	170	0	6.0	(mq)
(JM) raw	1 oz	130	3.0	1.0	180	0	14.0	(mq)
(Jones Dairy Farm)	1 patty	155	5.5	tr	281	0	14.4	36
(Jones Dairy Farm) 'Golden Brown'	1 patty	155	4.6	tr	250	0	14.7	29
(Jones Dairy Farm) 'Golden Brown' mild	1 link	100	2.6	tr	150	0	9.8	18
(Jones Dairy Farm) 'Golden Brown' spicy	1 link	100	2.8	tr	159	0	9.5	18
Brown and serve								
(Eckrich) 'Lean Supreme Heat 'n Serve'	2 links	120	7.0	1.0	440	0	10.0	(mq)
(Hormel)	2 links	140	6.0	0.0	430	0	13.0	(mq)
(Hormel) uncooked	2 links	180	7.0	0.0	411	0	17.0	(mq)
(Jones Dairy Farm) 'Light'	1 link	60	3.5	1.0	150	0	4.1	16
(Swift) 'Country Recipe'	1 link	130	4.0	1.0	240	0	12.0	(mq)
(Swift) 'Country Recipe'	1 patty	130	4.0	1.0	240	0	12.0	(mq)
(Swift) microwave	1 link	120	4.0	1.0	270	0	12.0	(mq)
(Swift) 'Premium Original'	1 link	130	3.0	1.0	260	0	12.0	(mq)
(Swift) 'Premium Original'	1 patty	120	4.0	1.0	270	0	12.0	(mq)
(Swift) smoked flavor	1 link	120	4.0	1.0	280	0	11.0	(mq)
Roll								
(Eckrich) minced	1-oz slice	80	4.0	1.0	300	0	7.0	(mq)
(Jones Dairy Farm) 'Cello Roll'	1 slice	105	3.7	tr	200	0	9.6	24
BEEF								
(Eckrich)	1 oz	100	3.0	<1.0	270	0	9.0	(mq)
(Eckrich) 'Lean Supreme'	1 oz	80	4.0	1.0	230	0	7.0	(mq)

Food Name	Serv. Size	Total Cal.	Prot. GMS	Carbs GMS	Sod. MGS	Fiber GMS	Fat GMS	Chol. MGS
(Eckrich) 'Smok-Y-Links'	2 links	160	6.0	2.0	350	0	14.0	(mq)
(Hillshire Farm) 'Bun Size'	2 oz	180	8.0	2.0	570	0	16.0	(mq)
(Hillshire Farm) 'Flavorseal'	2 oz	180	7.0	2.0	490	0	16.0	(mq)
(Jones Dairy Farm) 'Golden Brown'	1 link	75	3.8	tr	159	0	6.1	18
(Oscar Mayer) 'Smokies' 1.5-oz links	1 link	124	5.4	0.7	429	0	11.0	27
(Swift) 'Premium Brown 'N Serve'	1 link	120	4.0	1.0	250	0	12.0	(mq)
BEEF AND CHEDDAR *(Hillshire Farms)*								
'Flavorseal'	2 oz	190	8.0	1.0	500	0	15.0	(mq)
CHEESE								
(Hormel) 'Smokie Cheezers'	2 links	168	9.0	1.0	623	0	15.0	(mq)
(Oscar Mayer) 'Smokies'	1.5 oz	126	5.7	0.7	452	0	11.2	28
Hot								
(Eckrich) 'Smok-Y-Links'	2 links	150	6.0	1.0	360	0	14.0	(mq)
(Hillshire Farm) 'Flavorseal'	2 oz	180	7.0	2.0	510	0	16.0	(mq)
Maple-flavored *(Eckrich)* 'Smok-Y-Links'	2 links	160	6.0	2.0	390	0	14.0	(mq)
W/ham *(Eckrich)* 'Smok-Y-Links'	2 links	160	6.0	2.0	500	0	15.0	(mq)
HOT								
(JM) .5-oz patties, cooked	1 patty	70	2.0	1.0	170	0	6.0	(mq)
(JM) patties, raw	1 oz	130	3.0	1.0	180	0	14.0	(mq)
(OHSE) 'Hot Links'	1 oz	80	4.0	4.0	310	0	3.0	(mq)
ITALIAN STYLE								
cooked	3 oz	268	16.6	1.3	765	0	21.3	65
cooked	2.4 oz	216	13.4	1.0	618	0	17.2	52
pork, cooked	1 oz	92	5.7	0.4	261	0	7.3	22
pork, raw	1 oz	98	4.0	0.2	207	0	8.9	22
raw	4 oz	391	16.1	0.7	826	0	35.4	86
raw	3.2 oz	315	13.0	0.6	665	0	28.5	69
Hot *(Hillshire Farm)* 'Links'	2 oz	180	7.0	1.0	(mq)	0	17.0	(mq)
Mild *(Hillshire Farm)* 'Links'	2 oz	190	7.0	1.0	(mq)	0	17.0	(mq)
Smoked *(Hillshire Farm)* 'Flavorseal'	2 oz	200	7.0	1.0	500	0	18.0	(mq)
MAPLE-FLAVORED *(Swift)* brown and serve	1 link	120	3.0	1.0	260	0	12.0	(mq)
NEW ENGLAND STYLE								
(Eckrich)	1 oz	35	5.0	1.0	370	(tr)	1.0	(mq)
(Light & Lean)	2 slices	90	10.0	0.0	(mq)	0	6.0	(mq)
(Oscar Mayer) .8-oz slices	1 slice	29	3.9	0.4	291	(tr)	1.3	14
PICKLED								
(Penrose) beer, .5-oz links	1 link	40	2.0	1.0	220	0	3.0	(mq)
(Penrose) firecracker, 1.5-oz links	1 link	120	6.0	1.0	620	0	10.0	(mq)
(Penrose) firecracker, .5-oz links	1 link	40	2.0	1.0	220	0	3.0	(mq)
(Penrose) firecracker, giant, 2.1-oz links	1 link	170	9.0	1.0	870	0	14.0	(mq)
(Penrose) hot, .5-oz links	1 link	40	2.0	1.0	220	0	3.0	(mq)
(Penrose) Polish, .5-oz links	1 link	40	2.0	1.0	220	0	3.0	(mq)
(Penrose) red hot, .5-oz links	1 link	40	2.0	1.0	220	0	3.0	(mq)

Food Name	Serv. Size	Total Cal.	Prot. GMS	Carbs GMS	Sod. MGS	Fiber GMS	Fat GMS	Chol. MGS
POLISH STYLE								
....	1 oz	92	4.0	0.5	248	0	8.1	20
10-inch sausage	1 link	740	32.0	3.7	1989	0	65.2	159
PORK								
4-inch links, cooked	1 link	48	2.5	0.1	168	0	4.1	11
4-inch links, raw	1 link	117	3.3	0.3	187	0	11.3	19
fresh, cooked	1 oz	105	5.6	0.3	367	0	8.8	24
fresh, raw	2 oz	238	6.7	0.6	380	0	23.0	39
patties, 1/4 inch x 3 7/8 inch diam, cooked	1 patty	100	5.3	0.3	349	0	8.4	22
patties, 1/4 inch x 3 7/8 inch diam, raw	1 patty	238	6.7	0.6	380	0	23.0	39
(Hormel) 'Little Sizzlers'	2 links	103	6.0	0.0	172	0	9.0	(mq)
(Hormel) 'Little Sizzlers'	1 oz	130	3.0	2.0	192	na	13.0	19
(Hormel) 'Midget Links'	2 links	143	7.0	0.0	327	0	13.0	(mq)
(Jimmy Dean) cooked	1 oz	120	4.0	<1.0	240	na	11.0	na
(Jimmy Dean) links	2 links	180	7.0	<1.0	380	na	17.0	na
(Jimmy Dean) 'Light'	1.2 oz	80	7.0	<1.0	230	na	7.0	25
(Jimmy Dean) patties	1 patty	140	5.0	<1.0	300	na	13.0	na
(JM) 'Tasty Link' cooked	1.4 oz	190	6.0	1.0	290	0	18.0	(mq)
(JM) 'Tasty Link' raw	1.8 oz	260	6.0	1.0	380	0	26.0	(mq)
(Jones Dairy Farm)	1 link	140	2.9	tr	176	0	13.7	24
(Jones Dairy Farm) 'Golden Brown Light'	1 link	55	3.3	0.5	132	0	4.2	16
(Jones Dairy Farm) 'Light'	1 link	70	4.2	1.0	232	0	5.0	21
(Oscar Mayer) 'Little Friers' cooked	8.9 oz	989	40.7	2.8	2641	0	90.3	210
(Oscar Mayer) 'Little Friers' cooked	1 link	82	3.4	0.2	219	0	7.5	17
(Tyson) country, whole hog	3.5 oz	320	13.0	1.0	905	na	29.0	49
PORK AND BACON (JM) 'Tasty Link' raw	1.8 oz	220	6.0	1.0	340	0	21.0	(mq)
PORK AND BEEF								
fresh, cooked	1 oz	112	3.9	0.8	228	0	10.3	(mq)
fresh, 1/4 inch x 3 7/8-inch diam patties, cooked	1 patty	107	3.7	0.7	217	0	9.8	19
fresh, 2 inch x 3/4-inch diam links, cooked	1 link	51	1.8	0.4	105	0	4.7	9
smoked, 4 inch x 1 1/8-inch diam links ...	1 link	228	9.1	1.0	643	0	20.6	48
smoked, 2 inch x 3/4-inch diam links	1 link	54	2.1	0.2	151	0	4.8	11
smoked, w/flour and nonfat dry milk added, 4 inch x 1 1/8-inch diam links	1 link	182	9.5	2.7	741	0	14.6	59
smoked, w/flour and nonfat dry milk added, 2 inch x 3/4-inch diam links	1 link	43	2.2	0.6	174	0	3.4	14
smoked, w/nonfat dry milk added, 4 inch x 1 1/8-inch diam links	1 link	213	9.0	1.3	798	0	18.8	44
smoked, w/nonfat dry milk added, 2 inch x 3/4-inch diam links	1 link	50	2.1	0.3	188	0	4.4	10
SAGE (Jimmy Dean) cooked	1 oz	120	4.0	<1.0	240	na	11.0	na

Food Name	Serv. Size	Total Cal.	Prot. GMS	Carbs GMS	Sod. MGS	Fiber GMS	Fat GMS	Chol. MGS
SMOKED								
(Eckrich) 'Lean Supreme'	1 oz	70	4.0	1.0	230	0	6.0	(mq)
(Eckrich) 'Skinless'	1 link	180	7.0	2.0	420	0	16.0	(mq)
(Hillshire Farm) 'Bun Size'	2 oz	180	8.0	2.0	570	0	16.0	(mq)
(Hillshire Farm) 'Flavorseal'	2 oz	190	7.0	1.0	500	0	17.0	(mq)
(Hillshire Farm) 'Links'	2 oz	190	8.0	1.0	520	0	18.0	(mq)
(Hillshire Farm) 'Lite'	2 oz	160	8.0	2.0	(mq)	0	13.0	(mq)
(Hormel) 'Smokies'	2 links	160	9.0	2.0	597	0	14.0	(mq)
(OHSE)	1 oz	80	4.0	1.0	320	0	7.0	(mq)
(Oscar Mayer) 'Big & Juicy Smokie Links'								
2.7-oz links	1 link	227	9.3	1.2	757	0	20.5	48
(Oscar Mayer) 'Little Smokies' .3-oz links	1 link	27	1.2	0.1	92	0	2.5	6
(Oscar Mayer) 'Smokie Links' 1.5-oz links	1 link	126	5.4	0.6	426	0	11.3	28
(Pilgrim's Pride)	3 oz	144	13.1	2.5	890	0	9.1	64
SWEDISH STYLE (Hickory Farms)	1 oz	100	5.0		380	0	9.0	20
TURKEY								
(Butterball)	1 oz	50	4.0	<1.0	250	0	4.0	(mq)
(Jimmy Dean) 'Light'	1.2 oz	80	6.0	<1.0	230	na	7.0	25
(Louis Rich) cooked	1 link	46	5.4	0.1	234	0	2.7	18
(Louis Rich) 85% fat-free, cooked	24 gm	45	6.0	<1.0	235	na	3.0	20
(Norbest) 'Tasti-Lean' chub or links	1 oz	53	4.6	0.3	179	0	2.8	(mq)
Breakfast type								
(Hudson's) ground	1 oz	65	4.3	0.0	180	0	5.3	(mq)
(Louis Rich) 85% fat-free	1 oz	55	6.0	<1.0	230	na	3.0	25
(Louis Rich) ground, cooked	1 oz	56	5.9	0.2	215	0	3.5	22
(Mr. Turkey)	1 oz	58	4.6	0.4	181	0	4.3	16
Smoked								
(Louis Rich)	1 oz	43	4.5	0.7	249	0	2.4	19
(Louis Rich) 90% fat-free	1 oz	40	5.0	<1.0	250	na	2.0	20
(Louis Rich) w/cheese	1 oz	47	4.7	0.7	269	0	2.8	18
(Louis Rich) w/cheddar, 90% fat-free	1 oz	45	5.0	<1.0	270	na	3.0	20
(Mr. Turkey)	1 oz	47	4.5	0.5	230	0	3.4	19
TURKEY AND PORK (Jimmy Dean) 'Light'	1.2 oz	80	6.0	<1.0	230	na	7.0	25
W/BACON (Swift) brown and serve	1 link	120	4.0	1.0	270	0	11.0	(mq)
W/HAM (Swift) brown and serve	1 link	130	3.0	1.0	260	0	13.0	(mq)
SAUSAGE, ALTERNATIVE								
(Heartline) 'Italian Sausage Style'	2 oz	176	19.0	9.0	680	na	7.0	0
(Heartline) 'Pepperoni Style' lite	.5 oz	22	5.0	1.0	135	3.0	0.0	0
Canned (Worthington) 'Saucettes'	2 links	140	10.0	5.0	350	(mq)	9.0	0
Frozen								
(Morningstar Farms) links,								
'Breakfast Links'	3 links	190	12.0	3.0	500	(mq)	14.0	0

Food Name	Serv. Size	Total Cal.	Prot. GMS	Carbs GMS	Sod. MGS	Fiber GMS	Fat GMS	Chol. MGS
(Morningstar Farms) patties, 'Breakfast Patties'	2 patties	190	15.0	7.0	710	(mq)	12.0	0
(Worthington) links, 'Prosage'	3 links	190	13.0	4.0	570	(mq)	14.0	0
(Worthington) patties, 'Prosage'	2 patties	210	18.0	4.0	780	(mq)	14.0	0
(Worthington) roll, 'Prosage' 3/8-inch slice	2 slices	180	13.0	4.0	570	(mq)	12.0	0
SAUSAGE, CANNED								
(Hormel) hot	1 patty	150	7.0	0.0	549	0	13.0	(mq)
(Hormel) mild	1 patty	150	7.0	0.0	541	0	13.0	(mq)
SAUSAGE SEASONING, pork *(Tone's)*	1 tsp	12	0.4	2.7	1	.7	0.3	0
SAUSAGE STICK								
(Hickory Farms) 'Sportsman Stick'	1 oz	138	9.0	4.0	1075	0	10.0	40
BEEF								
(Pemmican) Pepperoni	1.1 oz	170	8.0	2.0	500	0	14.0	(mq)
(Pemmican) Tabasco	1.1 oz	120	5.0	2.0	410	0	10.0	(mq)
(Pemmican) Teriyaki	1.1 oz	150	8.0	5.0	410	0	11.0	(mq)
SMOKED								
(Slim Jim) 'Big Slim'	.52 oz	80	3.0	1.0	220	0	7.0	(mq)
(Slim Jim) 'Giant Slim'	1.1 oz	180	7.0	2.0	470	0	16.0	(mq)
(Slim Jim) 'Jumbo Jim'	1 oz	150	8.0	2.0	430	0	12.0	(mq)
(Slim Jim) 'Super Slim'	.7 oz	110	4.0	1.0	300	0	10.0	(mq)
Mild *(Slim Jim)* 'Handi-Paks'	.31 oz	50	2.0	1.0	130	0	4.0	(mq)
Nacho *(Slim Jim)* 'Super Slim'	.31 oz	40	2.0	1.0	160	0	3.0	(mq)
Pepperoni *(Slim Jim)* 'Handi-Paks'	.31 oz	50	2.0	1.0	130	0	4.0	(mq)
Spicy								
(Slim Jim) 'Handi-Paks'	.31 oz	50	2.0	1.0	130	0	4.0	(mq)
(Pemmican)	.8 oz	110	5.0	1.0	410	0	10.0	(mq)
Tabasco *(Slim Jim)* 'Handi-Paks'	.31 oz	50	2.0	1.0	130	0	4.0	(mq)
SUMMER SAUSAGE								
Beef *(Hickory Farms)*	1 oz	100	5.0	1.0	345	0	8.0	20
Smoked *(Slim Jim)*	.5 oz	80	3.0	1.0	200	0	7.0	(mq)
Teriyaki *(Pemmican)*	.8 oz	110	5.0	1.0	410	0	10.0	(mq)
SAUSAGE TACO refrigerated *(Owens)* 'Border Breakfasts'	2.17 oz	190	7.0	11.0	345	(mq)	12.0	65
SAVORY								
ground	1 oz	77	1.9	19.5	7	>4.3 c	1.7	0
ground	1 tbsp	12	0.3	3.0	1	>.7 c	0.3	0
ground	1 tsp	4	0.1	1.0	0	>.2 c	0.1	0
ground *(Durkee)*	1 tsp	5	0.0	0.0	0	0	tr	na
ground *(Laurel Leaf)*	1 tsp	5	0.0	0.0	0	0	tr	na
ground *(Spice Islands)*	1 tsp	5	0.1	1.0	<1	>.2 c	0.1	0

SAVOY CABBAGE. See CABBAGE, SAVOY.

SCALLION. See ONION, GREEN.

Food Name	Serv. Size	Total Cal.	Prot. GMS	Carbs GMS	Sod. MGS	Fiber GMS	Fat GMS	Chol. MGS
SCALLOP, ALTERNATIVE								
canned *(Worthington)*								
'Vegetable Skallops'	1/2 cup	90	15.0	4.0	430	(mq)	2.0	0
canned *(Worthington)* 'Vegetable Skallops'								
no salt	1/2 cup	80	13.0	4.0	80	(mq)	1.0	0
mixed species, made from surimi	3 oz	84	10.9	9.0	676	0	0.4	19
SCALLOP, MIXED SPECIES								
breaded, fried	4 oz	244	20.5	11.5	526	>.2 c	12.4	69
fried, frozen *(Mrs. Paul's)*	3 oz	200	9.0	22.0	410	(mq)	8.0	(mq)
raw	1 lb	400	76.1	10.7	730	0	3.4	152
raw	3 oz	75	14.3	2.0	137	0	0.7	28
raw	1 oz	25	4.8	0.7	46	0	0.2	9
SCALLOP SQUASH. See SQUASH, SCALLOP.								
SCORZONERA. See SALSIFY, BLACK.								
SCRAPPLE								
	1 oz	60	2.5	4.1	268	0	3.8	12
(Jones Dairy Farm)	1 slice	65	2.7	4.2	165	0	3.7	24
SCOTCH. See ALCOHOLIC BEVERAGES.								
SCHAV. See SOUP.								
SCREWDRIVER. See ALCOHOLIC BEVERAGES.								
SCROD ENTRÉE, FROZEN								
baked 'Microwave Entrees' *(Gorton's)*	1 pkg	320	22.0	17.0	420	(mq)	18.0	80
SCUP/sea bream								
dry-heat cooked	3 oz	115	20.6	0.0	46	0	3.0	57
raw	1 lb	477	85.6	0.0	191	0	12.4	(mq)
raw	3 oz	89	16.0	0.0	36	0	2.3	44
raw	1 oz	30	5.4	0.0	12	0	0.8	(mq)
SEA BASS. See BASS, SEA, MIXED SPECIES.								
SEA BREAM. See SCUP.								
SEA DEVIL. See MONKFISH.								
SEA PERCH. See OCEAN PERCH, ATLANTIC.								
SEA TROUT. See TROUT, SEA, MIXED SPECIES.								
SEAFOOD ENTRÉE, CANNED. See individual listings.								
SEAFOOD ENTRÉE, FROZEN. See also individual listings.								
(Armour) w/natural herbs 'Classics Lite'	10 oz	190	13.0	29.0	1020	(mq)	2.0	35
(Budget Gourmet) Newburg	10 oz	350	17.0	43.0	660	(mq)	12.0	70
(Budget Gourmet) scallop and shrimp								
'Mariner'	11.5 oz	320	16.0	43.0	690	na	9.0	70
(Cajun Cookin') gumbo	17 oz	330	16.0	51.0	1330	(mq)	7.0	(mq)
(Gorton's) clam 'Crunchy Clam Strips'								
microwave, 5.8-oz pkg	2.9 oz	270	8.0	20.0	350	na	17.0	20
(Pillsbury) casserole 'Microwave Classic'	1 pkg	420	15.0	37.0	950	(mq)	24.0	(mq)

Food Name	Serv. Size	Total Cal.	Prot. GMS	Carbs GMS	Sod. MGS	Fiber GMS	Fat GMS	Chol. MGS
(Swanson) Creole, w/rice 'Homestyle Recipe'	9 oz	240	7.0	40.0	810	(mq)	6.0	(mq)
SEAFOOD FRYING MIX								
(Golden Dipt)	2/3 oz	60	1.0	14.0	600	(mq)	0.0	0
(Golden Dipt) fish fry	2/3 oz	60	2.0	14.0	430	(mq)	0.0	0
(Golden Dipt) fish fry, Cajun style	2/3 oz	60	2.0	14.0	470	(mq)	0.0	0
SEAFOOD SALAD. See also individual listings.								
(Longacre) w/crabmeat 'Saladfest'	1 oz	45	1.0	3.0	130	na	3.0	5
SEAFOOD SEASONING MIX								
(Featherweight)	1/4 pkg	18	1.0	8.0	10	(mq)	0.0	0
(Golden Dipt) all-purpose	1/4 tsp	2	0.0	0.0	85	na	0.0	0
(Golden Dipt) blackened redfish	1/4 tsp	2	0.0	0.0	140	na	0.0	0
(Golden Dipt) fish, broiled	1/4 tsp	2	0.0	0.0	125	na	0.0	0
(Golden Dipt) lemon pepper	1/4 tsp	8	1.0	1.0	115	na	0.0	0
(Golden Dipt) shrimp and crab, Cajun style	1/4 tsp	2	0.0	0.0	200	na	0.0	0
(Schilling) Chesapeake Bay	1/2 tsp	2	0.1	0.2	202	na	0.1	0
SEASONING AND COATING MIX. See also individual listings.								
(Golden Dipt) breading	1 oz	90	3.0	20.0	630	(mq)	0.0	0
(Shake 'N Bake) country mild recipe	1/4 pkt	80	1.0	10.0	500	na	4.0	0
(Shake 'N Bake) Italian herb recipe	1/4 pkt	80	2.0	14.0	610	na	1.0	0
For chicken								
(Oven Fry) 'Extra Crispy'	1/4 pkt	120	3.0	21.0	840	na	2.0	0
(Oven Fry) 'Home Style Flour Recipe'	1/4 pkt	90	1.0	15.0	980	na	2.0	0
(Shake 'N Bake) hot and spicy	1/4 pkt	80	2.0	15.0	380	na	2.0	0
(Shake 'N Bake) 'Original Barbecue Recipe'	1/4 pkt	90	1.0	18.0	840	na	2.0	0
(Shake 'N Bake) 'Original Recipe'	1/4 pkt	80	2.0	14.0	450	na	2.0	0
For fish *(Shake 'N Bake)* 'Original Recipe'	1/4 pkt	70	1.0	14.0	410	na	1.0	0
For pork								
(Oven Fry) 'Extra Crispy'	1/8 pkt	60	2.0	10.0	350	na	1.0	0
(Shake 'N Bake) hot and spicy	1/8 pkt	45	1.0	8.0	220	na	1.0	0
(Shake 'N Bake) 'Original Barbecue Recipe'	1/8 pkt	35	0.0	8.0	260	na	0.0	0
(Shake 'N Bake) 'Original Recipe'	1/8 pkt	40	1.0	8.0	310	na	1.0	0
SEAWEED								
Dried								
agar	1 oz	87	1.8	22.9	29	2.2	0.1	0
nori	1 lb	158	26.4	23.2	217	>1.2 c	1.3	0
nori	1 oz	10	1.6	1.4	14	>.1 c	0.1	0
spirulina	1 oz	82	16.3	6.8	297	>1.0 c	2.2	0
Raw								
agar	1 lb	116	2.5	30.6	40	2.2	0.1	0
agar	1 oz	7	0.2	1.9	3	.1	tr	0

Food Name	Serv. Size	Total Cal.	Prot. GMS	Carbs GMS	Sod. MGS	Fiber GMS	Fat GMS	Chol. MGS
Irish moss	1 lb	222	6.9	55.8	303	(mq)	0.7	0
Irish moss	1 oz	14	0.4	3.5	19	(mq)	<.1	0
kelp	1 lb	195	7.6	43.4	1056	6.0	2.5	0
kelp	100 gm	43	1.7	9.6	233	1.3	0.6	0
kelp	1 oz	12	0.5	2.7	66	.4	0.2	0
laver	1 lb	158	26.4	23.2	217	1.2	1.3	0
laver	100 gm	35	5.8	5.1	48	.3	0.3	0
laver	1 oz	10	1.6	1.4	14	.1	0.1	0
spirulina	1 lb	120	26.9	11.0	444	1.5	1.8	0
spirulina	1 oz	8	1.7	0.7	28	.1	0.1	0
wakame	1 lb	206	13.7	41.5	3957	2.5	2.9	0
wakame	1 oz	13	0.9	2.6	247	.2	0.2	0

SELTZER. See SOFT DRINKS AND MIXERS.

SEMOLINA

Food Name	Serv. Size	Total Cal.	Prot. GMS	Carbs GMS	Sod. MGS	Fiber GMS	Fat GMS	Chol. MGS
enriched	1/2 cup	311	5.7	68.6	6	3.3	0.5	0
unenriched	1/2 cup	109	2.3	23.7	1	.3	0.2	0
whole grain	1 cup	602	21.2	121.6	2	6.5	1.8	0
whole grain	1 oz	102	3.6	20.6	<1	1.1	0.3	0

SESAME BUTTER. See also TAHINI MIX.

Food Name	Serv. Size	Total Cal.	Prot. GMS	Carbs GMS	Sod. MGS	Fiber GMS	Fat GMS	Chol. MGS
gourmet *(Roaster Fresh)*	1 oz	168	5.0	6.0	3	na	15.0	na
made from raw and stone ground kernels	1 oz	162	5.1	7.4	21	2.6	13.6	0
made from raw and stone ground kernels	1 tbsp	86	2.7	3.9	11	1.4	7.2	0
made from roasted kernels	1 oz	169	4.8	6.0	33	2.6	15.3	0
made from roasted kernels	1 tbsp	89	2.5	3.2	17	1.4	8.1	0
made from unroasted kernels	1 oz	172	5.1	5.1	0	2.6	16.0	0
made from unroasted kernels	1 tbsp	85	2.5	2.5	0	1.3	7.9	0
organic *(Arrowhead Mills)*	1 oz	170	6.0	4.0	<1	2.6	17.0	0
organic, Mid-Eastern *(Westbrae)*	2 tbsp	220	9.0	3.0	na	na	20.0	0
organic 'Natural' *(Westbrae)*	2 tbsp	220	6.0	6.0	35	na	19.0	0
paste	1 oz	169	5.1	7.2	3	1.5	14.4	0
paste	1 tbsp	95	2.9	4.1	2	.9	8.1	0

SESAME FLOUR

Food Name	Serv. Size	Total Cal.	Prot. GMS	Carbs GMS	Sod. MGS	Fiber GMS	Fat GMS	Chol. MGS
high-fat	1 oz	149	8.7	7.6	12	>1.8 c	10.5	0
low-fat	1 oz	95	14.2	10.1	11	>1.4 c	0.5	0
partially defatted	1 oz	108	11.5	10.0	12	>1.7 c	3.4	0

SESAME MEAL, partially defatted | 1 oz | 161 | 4.8 | 7.4 | 11 | >1.1 c | 13.6 | 0

SESAME OIL

Food Name	Serv. Size	Total Cal.	Prot. GMS	Carbs GMS	Sod. MGS	Fiber GMS	Fat GMS	Chol. MGS
	1/2 cup	964	0.0	0.0	0	0	109.0	0
	1 oz	251	0.0	0.0	0	0	28.4	0
	1 tbsp	120	0.0	0.0	0	0	13.6	0
(Eden Foods) hot pepper	1 tbsp	120	0.0	0.0	0	na	14.0	na
(Eden Foods) toasted	1 tbsp	120	0.0	0.0	0	na	14.0	na
(Eden Foods) unrefined	1 tbsp	120	0.0	0.0	0	na	14.0	na

Food Name	Serv. Size	Total Cal.	Prot. GMS	Carbs GMS	Sod. MGS	Fiber GMS	Fat GMS	Chol. MGS
(Hain)	1 tbsp	120	0.0	0.0	0	0	14.0	0
(Spectrum Naturals)	1 tbsp	120	0.0	0.0	0	(tr)	14.0	(tr)
(Spectrum Naturals) unrefined	1 tbsp	120	0.0	0.0	0	(tr)	14.0	(tr)
SESAME SEASONING								
(Schilling) all-purpose 'Parsley Patch'	1 tsp	15	0.6	1.0	2	na	1.0	0
SESAME SEED/sim sim								
Decorticated								
dried	1 tbsp	47	2.1	0.8	3	.2	4.4	0
dried	1 tsp	16	.7	.3	1	.1	1.5	0
Kernels								
dried	1 cup	882	39.6	14.1	59	>4.4 c	82.2	0
dried	1 oz	167	7.5	2.7	11	>.8 c	15.5	0
dried	1 tbsp	47	2.1	0.8	3	.2	4.4	0
dried	1 tsp	16	0.7	0.3	1	.1	1.5	0
dried *(Arrowhead Mills)*	1 oz	160	6.0	4.0	3	3.7	14.0	0
dried, toasted	1 oz	161	4.8	7.4	11	4.8	13.6	0
Whole								
dried	1 lb	2598	80.4	106.4	51	53.5	225.3	0
dried	1 cup	825	25.5	33.8	16	17.0	71.5	0
dried	1 oz	162	5.0	6.6	3	3.3	14.1	0
dried	1 tbsp	52	1.6	2.1	1	1.1	4.5	0
dried *(Arrowhead Mills)*	1 oz	160	5.0	6.0	4	3.1	14.0	0
dried *(Durkee)*	1 tsp	13	0.0	0.0	0	0	<0.1	na
dried *(Laurel Leaf)*	1 tsp	13	0.0	0.0	0	0	<0.1	na
roasted	1 oz	160	4.8	7.3	3	4.0	13.6	0
SESAME STICKS								
(Barbara's Bakery)	1 oz	130	3.0	20.0	255	na	4.0	na
(Flavor Tree)	1/4 cup	133	3.1	10.6	358	>.1 c	9.1	0
(Flavor Tree) 'No Salt'	1/4 cup	131	3.2	13.4	7	>.1 c	8.1	0
SESBANIA FLOWER. See KATURAY.								
SHAD, AMERICAN								
dry-heat cooked	3 oz	214	18.5	0.0	55	0	15.0	82
raw	1 lb	891	76.8	0.0	233	0	62.5	(mq)
raw	3 oz	167	14.4	0.0	43	0	11.7	64
raw	1 oz	56	4.8	0.0	14	0	3.9	(mq)
SHAKE 'N BAKE. See SEASONING AND COATING MIX.								
SHALLOT								
freeze-dried	1 oz	99	3.5	22.9	17	>1.3 c	0.1	0
freeze-dried	1/4 cup	13	0.4	2.9	2	>.2 c	0.0	0
freeze-dried	1 tbsp	3	0.1	0.7	1	tr	0.0	0
raw	100 gm	72	2.5	16.8	12	>.7 c	0.1	0
raw	1 tbsp	7	0.3	1.7	1	>.1 c	0.0	0
raw, trimmed	1 oz	20	0.7	4.8	3	>.2 c	<.1	0

Food Name	Serv. Size	Total Cal.	Prot. GMS	Carbs GMS	Sod. MGS	Fiber GMS	Fat GMS	Chol. MGS
raw, untrimmed	1 lb	287	10.0	67.1	48	>2.8 c	0.4	0
SHARK								
Mako, boneless steak, raw								
(Peter Pan Seafoods)	3.5 oz	87	19.1	na	79	na	1.2	51
Mixed species								
batter-dipped, fried	3 oz	194	15.8	5.4	104	na	11.7	50
raw	1 lb	591	95.2	0.0	360	0	20.5	232
raw	3 oz	110	17.8	0.0	67	0	3.8	43
raw	1 oz	37	5.9	0.0	22	0	1.3	14
SHEANUT OIL								
	1/2 cup	964	0.0	0.0	0	0	109.0	0
	1 oz	251	0.0	0.0	0	0	28.4	0
	1 tbsp	120	0.0	0.0	0	0	13.6	0
SHEEPSHEAD/California sheepshead/fathead/redhead								
baked	6.6-oz fillet	234	48.4	0.0	136	0	3.0	(mq)
baked	4 oz	143	29.5	0.0	83	0	1.8	(mq)
baked	3 oz	107	22.1	0.0	62	0	1.4	54
broiled	6.6-oz fillet	234	48.4	0.0	136	0	3.0	(mq)
broiled	4 oz	143	29.5	0.0	83	0	1.8	(mq)
microwaved	6.6-oz fillet	234	48.4	0.0	136	0	3.0	(mq)
microwaved	4 oz	143	29.5	0.0	83	0	1.8	(mq)
raw	1 lb	490	91.7	0.0	324	0	10.9	(mq)
raw	3 oz	92	17.2	0.0	60	0	2.0	43
raw	1 oz	31	5.7	0.0	20	0	0.7	(mq)
roasted	4 oz	143	29.5	0.0	83	0	1.8	(mq)
SHELLIE BEAN, CANNED								
w/liquid	1/2 cup	37	2.2	7.6	407	4.2	0.2	0
w/liquid	4 oz	34	2.0	7.0	379	3.9	0.2	0
(Stokely)	1/2 cup	35	2.0	7.0	470	(mq)	0.0	0
SHERBET. See also FRUIT BAR, FROZEN; ICE BARS AND DESSERTS; SORBET.								
all flavors (Sealtest)	1/2 cup	130	1.0	28.0	30	na	1.0	5
orange	1/2 cup	132	1.1	29.2	44	>.3 c	1.9	5
orange	1 oz	40	0.3	8.6	13	tr	0.6	2
orange (Borden)	1/2 cup	110	1.0	25.0	40	na	1.0	(mq)
orange (Darigold)	1/2 cup	120	1.0	26.0	25	na	1.0	(mq)
vanilla-orange 'Cubic Scoops' (Sealtest)	4 oz	130	2.0	22.0	40	(tr)	4.0	15
vanilla-red raspberry 'Cubic Scoops' (Sealtest)	4 oz	130	2.0	22.0	40	(tr)	4.0	15
SHERBET BAR								
all flavors 'Fat-Free' (Fudgsicle)	1 bar	70	2.0	14.0	45	na	0.0	0
all flavors 'Sugar-Free' (Fudgsicle)	1 bar	35	2.0	6.0	50	na	1.0	5
chocolate (Fudgsicle)	1 bar	70	2.0	12.0	70	na	1.0	na

Food Name	Serv. Size	Total Cal.	Prot. GMS	Carbs GMS	Sod. MGS	Fiber GMS	Fat GMS	Chol. MGS
chocolate, w/nuts 'Sugar-Free Fudge								
Nut Dip' *(Fudgsicle)* .... 1 bar		130	2.0	12.0	40	(mq)	8.0	5
orange .... 2.75-oz bar		91	0.7	20.1	30	>.2 c	1.3	3
w/cream, all flavors 'Sugar-Free'								
(Creamsicle) .... 1 bar		25	1.0	5.0	20	na	1.0	na
SHORT RIBS ENTRÉE, FROZEN								
(Armour) boneless 'Classics' .... 9.75 oz		380	24.0	34.0	790	(mq)	16.0	90
(Stouffer's) in gravy .... 9 oz		350	30.0	12.0	900	na	20.0	(mq)
(Tyson) 'Gourmet Selection' .... 11 oz		470	25.0	38.0	950	(mq)	24.0	(mq)
SHORTENING								
COMMERCIAL								
hydrogenated soybean oil and								
cottonseed oil .... 1 cup		1812	0.0	0.0	0	0	205.0	0
hydrogenated soybean oil and								
cottonseed oil .... 1 tbsp		113	0.0	0.0	0	0	12.8	0
lard and vegetable oil .... 1 cup		1845	0.0	0.0	0	0	205.0	115
lard and vegetable oil .... 1 tbsp		115	0.0	0.0	0	0	12.8	7
(Wesson) 'Crystal' .... 1 tbsp		122	0.0	0.0	0	0	13.5	0
(Wesson) 'Lo-Melt' .... 1 tbsp		122	0.0	0.0	0	0	13.5	0
(Wesson) 'Super' .... 1 tbsp		122	0.0	0.0	0	0	13.5	0
(Wesson) 'Wesgold' .... 1 tbsp		122	0.0	0.0	0	0	13.5	0
(Wesson) 'Wespour' .... 1 tbsp		122	0.0	0.0	0	0	13.5	0
For baking								
hydrogenated soybean, palm, and								
cottonseed oils .... 1 cup		1812	0.0	0.0	0	0	205.0	0
hydrogenated soybean, palm, and								
cottonseed oils .... 1 tbsp		113	0.0	0.0	0	0	12.8	0
For bread								
hydrogenated soybean oil and								
cottonseed oil .... 1 cup		1812	0.0	0.0	0	0	205.0	0
hydrogenated soybean oil and								
cottonseed oil .... 1 tbsp		113	0.0	0.0	0	0	12.8	0
For cakes and frostings								
hydrogenated soybean and								
cottonseed oils .... 1 cup		1812	0.0	0.0	0	0	205.0	0
hydrogenated soybean and								
cottonseed oils .... 1 tbsp		113	0.0	0.0	0	0	12.8	0
hydrogenated soybean oil .... 1 cup		1812	0.0	0.0	0	0	205.0	0
hydrogenated soybean oil .... 1 tbsp		113	0.0	0.0	0	0	12.8	0
For confectionery								
fractionated palm oil .... 1 cup		1927	0.0	0.0	0	0	218.0	0
fractionated palm oil .... 1 tbsp		120	0.0	0.0	0	0	13.6	0

Food Name	Serv. Size	Total Cal.	Prot. GMS	Carbs GMS	Sod. MGS	Fiber GMS	Fat GMS	Chol. MGS
hydrogenated coconut and/or palm								
kernel oil	1 cup	1812	0.0	0.0	0	0	205.0	0
hydrogenated coconut and/or palm								
kernel oil	1 tbsp	113	0.0	0.0	0	0	12.8	0
Heavy duty, for frying								
beef tallow and cottonseed oil	1 cup	1845	0.0	0.0	0	0	205.0	205
beef tallow and cottonseed oil	1 tbsp	115	0.0	0.0	0	0	12.8	13
hydrogenated palm oil	1 cup	1812	0.0	0.0	0	0	205.0	0
hydrogenated palm oil	1 tbsp	113	0.0	0.0	0	0	12.8	0
hydrogenated soybean and								
cottonseed oils	1 cup	1812	0.0	0.0	0	0	205.0	0
hydrogenated soybean and								
cottonseed oils	1 tbsp	113	0.0	0.0	0	0	12.8	0
hydrogenated soybean oil, 30% linoleic	1 cup	1812	0.0	0.0	0	0	205.0	0
hydrogenated soybean oil, 30% linoleic	1 tbsp	113	0.0	0.0	0	0	12.8	0
hydrogenated soybean oil, under								
1% linoleic	1 cup	1812	0.0	0.0	0	0	205.0	0
hydrogenated soybean oil, under								
1% linoleic	1 tbsp	113	0.0	0.0	0	0	12.8	0
Multi-purpose								
hydrogenated soybean and palm oils	1 cup	1812	0.0	0.0	0	0	205.0	0
hydrogenated soybean and palm oils	1 tbsp	113	0.0	0.0	0	0	12.8	0
HOUSEHOLD								
hydrogenated soybean and								
cottonseed oils	1 cup	1812	0.0	0.0	0	0	205.0	0
hydrogenated soybean and								
cottonseed oils	1 tbsp	113	0.0	0.0	0	0	12.8	0
hydrogenated soybean oil and palm oil	1 cup	1812	0.0	0.0	0	0	205.0	0
hydrogenated soybean oil and palm oil	1 tbsp	113	0.0	0.0	0	0	12.8	0
lard and vegetable oil	1 cup	1845	0.0	0.0	0	0	205.0	115
lard and vegetable oil	1 tbsp	115	0.0	0.0	0	0	12.8	7
(Crisco) vegetable	1 tbsp	110	0.0	0.0	0	0	12.0	0
(Crisco) vegetable, butter flavor	1 tbsp	110	0.0	0.0	0	0	12.0	0
(Finast) vegetable	1 tbsp	110	0.0	0.0	0	0	13.0	0
(Finast) vegetable, butter flavor	1 tbsp	110	0.0	0.0	0	0	12.0	0
(Wesson)	1 tbsp	100	0.0	0.0	0	0	12.0	0
SHOYU. See SAUCE, SOY.								
SHRIMP, ALTERNATIVE								
made from surimi	1 lb	458	56.2	41.4	3198	0	6.7	163
made from surimi	1 oz	29	3.5	2.6	200	0	0.4	10
made from surimi	3 oz	86	10.5	7.8	599	0	1.3	31
SHRIMP, MIXED SPECIES								
boiled	4 oz	112	23.7	(mq)	254	0	1.2	221

Food Name	Serv. Size	Total Cal.	Prot. GMS	Carbs GMS	Sod. MGS	Fiber GMS	Fat GMS	Chol. MGS
boiled, .8-oz size	4 shrimp	22	4.6	(mq)	49	0	0.2	43
breaded, fried	3 oz	206	18.2	9.8	292	>.1 c	10.4	150
breaded, fried	1.1 oz	73	6.4	3.4	103	<.1	3.7	53
breaded, fried, .8-oz size	4 shrimp	73	6.4	3.4	103	0	3.7	53
fried	4 oz	274	24.3	13.0	390	>.2 c	13.9	201
moist-heat cooked	3 oz	84	17.8	0.0	190	0	0.9	166
moist-heat cooked, .8-oz size	4 shrimp	22	4.6	0.0	49	0	0.2	43
poached	4 oz	112	23.7	(mq)	254	0	1.2	221
poached, .8-oz size	4 shrimp	22	4.6	(mq)	49	0	0.2	43
raw	1 lb	481	92.1	4.1	673	0	7.8	692
raw	3 oz	90	17.3	0.8	126	0	1.5	129
raw, .8-oz size	4 shrimp	30	5.7	0.3	41	0	0.5	43
steamed	4 oz	112	23.7	(mq)	254	0	1.2	221
steamed, .8-oz size	4 shrimp	22	4.6	(mq)	49	0	0.2	43
Canned								
drained	1 cup	154	29.5	1.3	216		2.5	221
drained	3 oz	102	19.6	0.9	144	0	1.7	147
drained	4 oz	136	26.2	1.2	192	0	2.2	196
drained (Louisiana Brand)	2 oz	58	12.0	0.0	(mq)	0	1.0	(mq)
large, drained (ShopRite)	2 oz	50	10.0	0.0	720	0	1.0	(mq)
SHRIMP CHOW MEIN, canned								
(LaChoy)	3/4 cup	35	4.0	4.0	940	2.0	1.0	50
(LaChoy) 'Bi-Pack'	8.536 oz	60	3.9	10.2	935	2.9	1.0	30
(LaChoy) 'Bi-Pack'	3/4 cup	50	3.0	7.0	860	2.0	1.0	19
SHRIMP COCKTAIL								
(Booth) w/garlic butter sauce and vegetable rice	10 oz	400	13.0	40.0	750	(mq)	25.0	(mq)
(Budget Gourmet) w/fettuccine	9.5 oz	375	10.0	38.0	660	(mq)	20.0	145
(LaChoy) w/lobster sauce 'Fresh & Lite'	10 oz	240	12.0	36.4	946	2.8	6.2	118
(Mrs. Paul's) w/clams and linguini 'Light'	10 oz	240	12.0	36.0	750	(mq)	5.0	40
(Sau-Sea)	4 oz	113	7.0	19.0	1020	na	1.0	102
(SeaPak) 'Super Valu' heat and serve	4 oz	210	12.0	30.0	730	(mq)	4.0	80
SHRIMP ENTRÉE, FROZEN								
BAY, BABY (Armour) 'Classics Lite'	9.75 oz	220	12.0	31.0	890	(mq)	6.0	105
BATTERED								
(SeaPak) 'Shrimp 'n Batter'	4 oz	260	11.0	20.0	470	(mq)	15.0	20
(SeaPak) w/crabmeat stuffing	4 oz	260	8.0	27.0	780	(mq)	13.0	(mq)
BREADED								
(Gorton's) original seasoning	2.7 oz	200	9.0	15.0	450	na	12.0	50
(Gorton's) popcorn style	2.7 oz	220	8.0	16.0	450	na	14.0	50
(Gorton's) scampi seasoning	2.7 oz	210	9.0	16.0	440	na	12.0	50
(Mrs. Paul's) fried	3 oz	200	9.0	16.0	430	(mq)	11.0	(mq)

Food Name	Serv. Size	Total Cal.	Prot. GMS	Carbs GMS	Sod. MGS	Fiber GMS	Fat GMS	Chol. MGS
BUTTERFLY								
(Gorton's) 'Specialty'	4 oz	160	19.0	16.0	540	na	<1.0	(mq)
(SeaPak) breaded 'Mikado'	4 oz	160	12.0	26.0	170	(mq)	1.0	110
BUTTERFLY/ROUND (SeaPak) breaded	4 oz	150	14.0	20.0	(mq)	(mq)	1.0	(mq)
CAJUN STYLE (Mrs. Paul's) 'Light'	9 oz	230	9.0	37.0	740	(mq)	5.0	60
CREOLE								
(Armour) 'Classics Lite'	11.25 oz	260	6.0	53.0	900	(mq)	2.0	45
(Cajun Cookin')	12 oz	390	17.0	55.0	1130	(mq)	11.0	(mq)
(Healthy Choice)	11.25 oz	230	8.0	45.0	430	na	2.0	60
CRISP (Gorton's) 'Specialty'	4 oz	280	9.0	26.0	740	(mq)	15.0	(mq)
CRUNCHY								
(Gorton's) 'Crunchy Shrimp' microwave	2 oz	160	7.0	12.0	380	na	9.0	40
(Gorton's) whole 'Microwave Specialty'	5 oz	380	14.0	35.0	870	(mq)	20.0	65
ETOUFFEE (Cajun Cookin')	17 oz	360	19.0	52.0	1170	(mq)	9.0	(mq)
FETTUCCINE ALFREDO (Booth)	10 oz	260	19.0	28.0	620	(mq)	8.0	(mq)
JAMBALAYA (Cajun Cookin')	12 oz	450	20.0	43.0	800	(mq)	20.0	(mq)
MARINARA								
(Healthy Choice)	10.5 oz	260	10.0	51.0	320	na	1.0	60
(Smart Ones) w/linguini	8 oz	150	8.0	26.0	390	na	<1.0	60
NEW ORLEANS, w/wild rice (Booth)	10 oz	230	13.0	35.0	950	(mq)	5.0	(mq)
ORIENTAL, w/pineapple rice (Booth)	10 oz	190	11.0	30.0	950	(mq)	3.0	(mq)
PRIMAVERA								
(Booth) w/fettucini	10 oz	200	16.0	28.0	760	(mq)	3.0	(mq)
(Mrs. Paul's) 'Light'	9.5 oz	180	11.0	28.0	840	(mq)	3.0	125
(Right Course)	9 5/8 oz	240	12.0	32.0	590	(mq)	7.0	50
SCAMPI (Gorton's) 'Microwave Entrées'	1 pkg	390	10.0	21.0	470	(mq)	30.0	(mq)
STIR-FRY (Shanghai)	10.3 oz	170	18.0	19.0	1200	na	2.0	55
SHRIMP ENTRÉE, PACKAGED								
(Ultra Slim Fast) creole	12 oz	240	12.0	45.0	730	na	4.0	80
(Ultra Slim Fast) marinara	12 oz	290	17.0	53.0	880	na	3.0	70
SHRIMP PASTE, canned	1 tsp	13	1.5	0.1	10	0	0.7	12
SHRIMP SALAD								
(Longacre) 'Saladfest'	1 oz	45	2.0	2.0	150	na	3.0	25
(Longacre) 'Saladfest' w/seafood	1 oz	42	2.0	2.0	160	na	3.0	15
SICAMA. See JICAMA.								
SILVER HAKE. See WHITING, MIXED SPECIES.								
SIM SIM. See SESAME SEED.								
SISYMBRIUM SEED								
whole, dried	1 cup	235	9.0	43.1	68	>22.0 c	3.4	0
whole, dried	1 oz	90	3.5	16.5	26	>8.4 c	1.3	0
SKIL. See SABLEFISH.								
SKUNK CABBAGE. See CABBAGE, SKUNK.								
SLIMEHEAD. See ORANGE ROUGHY.								

Food Name	Serv. Size	Total Cal.	Prot. GMS	Carbs GMS	Sod. MGS	Fiber GMS	Fat GMS	Chol. MGS
SLOPPY JOE SEASONING MIX								
(French's)	1/8 pkg	16	0.0	4.0	390	(mq)	0.0	0
(Lawry's) 'Seasoning Blends'	1 pkg	126	2.8	27.7	3442	>.8 c	0.4	0
(Schilling)	1/4 pkg	26	0.5	6.0	750	(mq)	0.5	0
SMELT, RAINBOW								
broiled	4 oz	141	25.6	0.0	87	0	3.5	102
dry-heat cooked	4 oz	141	25.6	0.0	87	0	3.5	102
dry-heat cooked	3 oz	105	19.2	0.0	65	0	2.6	77
microwaved	4 oz	141	25.6	0.0	87	0	3.5	102
raw	1 lb	440	80.0	0.0	272	0	11.0	318
raw	3 oz	82	15.0	0.0	51	0	2.1	59
raw	1 oz	27	5.0	0.0	17	0	0.7	20
SNACK. See CORN CHIPS AND SNACKS; SNACK BAR; SNACK MIX.								
SNACK BAR. See also DIET BAR.								
(Barbara's Bakery)								
apple, real fruit, .5 oz	1 bar	50	0.0	11.0	0	na	0.0	0
apricot, real fruit, .5 oz	1 bar	50	0.0	11.0	0	na	0.0	0
cherry, real fruit, .5 oz	1 bar	50	0.0	11.0	0	na	0.0	0
grape, real fruit, .5 oz	1 bar	50	0.0	11.0	0	na	0.0	0
raspberry, real fruit, .5 oz	1 bar	50	0.0	11.0	1	na	0.0	0
(Bear Valley)								
carob-cocoa, food bar 'Pemmican'	3.75 oz	440	16.0	68.0	80	7.0	12.0	0
coconut almond, food bar 'Meal Pack'	3.75 oz	400	13.0	56.0	80	6.0	12.0	0
fruit 'n nut, food bar 'Pemmican'	3.75 oz	420	17.0	59.0	90	9.0	13.0	0
sesame lemon, food bar 'Meal Pack'	3.75 oz	410	17.0	57.0	85	4.0	13.0	0
(Carnation)								
chocolate chip, breakfast bar	1 bar	200	6.0	20.0	180	1.4	11.0	<1
chocolate crunch, breakfast bar	1 bar	190	6.0	20.0	150	1.2	10.0	<1
peanut butter chocolate chip, breakfast bar	1 bar	200	6.0	20.0	170	1.4	11.0	<1
peanut butter crunch, breakfast bar	1 bar	190	6.0	20.0	180	1.0	10.0	<1
(Earth Grains)								
banana apple walnut 'Bagel Power Bar'	1 bar	270	12.0	45.0	280	na	6.0	0
citrus almond w/mixed fruit 'Bagel Power Bar'	1 bar	260	12.0	45.0	280	na	4.0	0
fruit and nut 'Bagel Power Bar'	1 bar	240	9.0	48.0	280	na	3.0	0
(Glenny's)								
apple-cinnamon	1.25 oz	120	1.0	28.0	15	na	<1.0	na
caramel	1.25 oz	120	1.0	29.0	65	na	<1.0	na
chocolate	1.25 oz	120	1.0	28.0	20	na	<1.0	na
raspberry	1.25 oz	120	1.0	29.0	15	na	<1.0	na
(Health Valley)								
apple, fat-free	1 bar	140	3.0	33.0	10	3.7	0.0	0
'Apple Bakes'	1 bar	100	2.0	16.0	27	2.8	3.0	0

Food Name	Serv. Size	Total Cal.	Prot. GMS	Carbs GMS	Sod. MGS	Fiber GMS	Fat GMS	Chol. MGS
apricot, fat-free	1 bar	140	3.0	33.0	10	3.7	0.0	0
date, fat-free	1 bar	140	3.0	33.0	10	3.7	0.0	0
'Date Bakes'	1 bar	100	3.0	16.0	25	2.8	3.0	0
'Fruit & Fitness'	1 bar	200	4.0	39.0	234	4.8	3.0	0
'Oat Bran, Fig & Nut Bakes'	1 bar	110	2.0	19.0	18	3.1	3.0	0
oat bran, raisin, and cinnamon	1 bar	140	3.0	32.0	12	6.3	2.0	0
'Oat Bran Apricot Bakes'	1 bar	100	2.0	19.0	18	2.9	2.0	0
'Oat Bran Jumbo Fruit and Nut Bars'	1 bar	150	4.0	29.0	11	8.4	4.0	0
'Oat Bran Jumbo Fruit Bars'	1 bar	170	4.0	28.0	9	6.7	5.0	0
raisin, fat-free	1 bar	140	3.0	33.0	10	3.7	0.0	0
'Raisin Bakes'	1 bar	100	2.0	16.0	19	2.8	3.0	0
rice bran, almond, and date	1 bar	190	4.0	29.0	6	5.6	6.0	0
(Kudos)								
peaches and cream 'Pan Squares'	1 square	150	2.0	22.0	105	2.0	6.0	na
peanut butter and chocolate chip 'Pan Squares'	1 square	170	3.0	20.0	105	2.0	9.0	na
strawberry and cream cheese 'Pan Squares'	1 square	150	2.0	22.0	105	2.0	6.0	na
(Tiger's Milk) peanut butter and honey, carob coated	1 bar	160	6.0	23.0	90	na	5.0	na
(Weider)								
'Sportsfood Enerquench Bar'	1 bar	200	6.0	44.0	80	na	1.0	na
'Sportsfood Protein Bar'	1 bar	160	10.0	21.0	140	na	4.0	na

SNACK BAR MIX, PREPARED

Food Name	Serv. Size	Total Cal.	Prot. GMS	Carbs GMS	Sod. MGS	Fiber GMS	Fat GMS	Chol. MGS
(Betty Crocker)								
caramel oatmeal 'Supreme Dessert'	1 bar	110	1.0	15.0	65	na	5.0	0
chocolate and toffee 'Supreme Dessert'	1 bar	110	1.0	17.0	55	na	4.0	10
chocolate peanut butter 'Supreme Dessert'	1 bar	110	1.0	14.0	100	na	5.0	10
date 'Classic'	1 bar	60	1.0	9.0	35	(mq)	2.0	0
lemon-Sunkist 'Supreme Dessert' prepared w/4 eggs	1 bar	110	1.0	17.0	65	na	4.0	30
M&M cookie bars 'Supreme Dessert'	1 bar	110	1.0	16.0	80	na	5.0	10
raspberry 'Supreme Dessert'	1 bar	100	1.0	16.0	95	na	4.0	0

SNACK MIX

Food Name	Serv. Size	Total Cal.	Prot. GMS	Carbs GMS	Sod. MGS	Fiber GMS	Fat GMS	Chol. MGS
(Doo Dads) original recipe, 1 oz	1/2 cup	129	2.9	18.2	360	1.9	5.2	0
(Flavor Tree)								
'Party Mix'	1/4 cup	163	3.4	12.3	407	>.1 c	11.0	0
'Party Mix No Salt'	1 1/2 cup	163	3.9	13.2	8	>.1 c	10.8	0
(Pepperidge Farm)								
cheese, super cheddar 'Goldfish Party Mix'	1 oz	140	4.0	15.0	330	na	7.0	15
'Classic'	1 oz	140	4.0	14.0	360	1.0	8.0	0
lightly smoked	1 oz	150	4.0	13.0	350	1.0	8.0	0

Food Name	Serv. Size	Total Cal.	Prot. GMS	Carbs GMS	Sod. MGS	Fiber GMS	Fat GMS	Chol. MGS
nutty deluxe, cashews and almonds								
'Goldfish'	1/2 cup	180	5.0	20.0	330	2.0	9.0	25
original, honey roasted peanuts 'Goldfish'	1/2 cup	170	5.0	21.0	360	2.0	8.0	5
spicy	1 oz	140	4.0	14.0	340	1.0	8.0	5
(Ralston)								
barbecue 'Chex' 2/3 cup	1 oz	130	3.0	18.0	380	na	5.0	0
'Chex Traditional' 2/3 cup	1 oz	120	3.1	18.5	288	>.5 c	4.9	0
cool sour cream and onion 'Chex' 2/3 cup	1 oz	130	3.0	19.0	300	(mq)	5.0	na
golden cheddar 'Chex' 2/3 cup	1 oz	130	3.0	19.0	300	(mq)	5.0	na
nacho cheese 'Chex' 2/3 cup	1 oz	130	3.0	19.0	430	(mq)	5.0	na
(Ritz) traditional, baked	1 oz	130	2.0	18.0	310	na	6.0	0
SNAPPER, RED, MIXED SPECIES								
broiled	4 oz	145	3.0	0.0	65	0	2.0	53
dry-heat cooked	4 oz	145	3.0	0.0	65	0	2.0	53
dry-heat cooked	3 oz	109	22.4	0.0	48	0	1.5	40
microwaved	4 oz	145	3.0	0.0	65	0	2.0	53
raw	1 lb	452	93.0	0.0	291	0	6.1	168
raw	3 oz	85	17.4	0.0	54	0	1.1	31
raw	1 oz	28	5.8	0.0	18	0	0.4	10

SNOW PEAS. See PEAS, SNOW.

SOBA NOODLE. See NOODLE, JAPANESE.

SODA. See SOFT DRINKS AND MIXERS.

SODA, CLUB. See SOFT DRINKS AND MIXERS.

SOFT DRINKS AND MIXERS. See also WATER, SPARKLING, FLAVORED.

Food Name	Serv. Size	Total Cal.	Prot. GMS	Carbs GMS	Sod. MGS	Fiber GMS	Fat GMS	Chol. MGS
(A&W)								
cream soda	1 oz	14	0.1	3.6	2	0	tr	0
cream soda, 'Diet'	1 oz	<1	0.1	0.0	4	0	<.1	0
root beer	1 oz	15	<.1	3.5	5	0	<.1	0
root beer, 'Diet'	1 oz	<1	0.1	0.0	4	0	tr	0
(Canada Dry)								
collins mixer	8 oz	80	0.0	20.0	17	0	0.0	0
ginger ale	8 oz	90	0.0	21.0	7	0	0.0	0
ginger ale, 'Golden'	8 oz	100	0.0	24.0	24	0	0.0	0
grape, 'Concord'	8 oz	130	0.0	32.0	21	0	0.0	0
half and half	8 oz	110	0.0	26.0	17	0	0.0	0
tonic	8 oz	90	0.0	22.0	7	0	0.0	0
whiskey sour mixer	8 oz	90	0.0	22.0	17	0	0.0	0
(Coca Cola)								
cherry cola	6 oz	76	0.0	20.0	4	0	0.0	0
cherry cola, 'Diet'	6 oz	<1	0.0	0.2	4	0	0.0	0
cola, caffeine-free	6 oz	77	0.0	20.0	4	0	0.0	0
cola, 'Classic'	6 oz	72	0.0	19.0	7	0	0.0	0
cola, diet, caffeine-free	6 oz	<1	0.0	0.2	4	0	0.0	0

Food Name	Serv. Size	Total Cal.	Prot. GMS	Carbs GMS	Sod. MGS	Fiber GMS	Fat GMS	Chol. MGS
cola, diet, w/caffeine	6 oz	<1	0.0	0.2	4	0	0.0	0
cola, w/caffeine	6 oz	77	0.0	20.0	4	0	0.0	0
(Dr. Diablo) cola	12 oz	140	0.0	38.0	14	0	0.0	0
(Dr. Pepper)								
cola	12 oz	150	0.0	38.4	18	0	0.0	0
cola, caffeine-free	12 oz	150	0.0	38.4	18	0	0.0	0
diet	12 oz	3	0.0	0.2	18	0	0.0	0
diet, caffeine-free	12 oz	3	0.0	0.2	18	0	0.0	0
(Fanta)								
ginger ale	6 oz	63	0.0	16.0	14	0	0.0	0
grape	6 oz	86	0.0	22.0	7	0	0.0	0
orange	6 oz	88	0.0	23.0	7	0	0.0	0
root beer	6 oz	78	0.0	20.0	10	0	0.0	0
(Fresca) citrus	6 oz	2	0.0	0.2	tr	0	0.0	0
(Health Valley)								
ginger ale	12 oz	153	1.0	35.0	30	0	1.0	0
root beer, 'Old Fashioned'	12 oz	120	1.0	26.0	12	0	1.0	0
root beer, sarsaparilla	12 oz	153	1.0	35.0	27	0	1.0	0
wild berry	12 oz	142	1.0	33.0	27	0	1.0	0
(Hires)								
cream soda, caffeine-free	6 oz	90	<1.0	24.0	40	0	<1.0	na
cream soda, 'Diet' caffeine-free	6 oz	2	<1.0	<1.0	45	0	<1.0	na
root beer, caffeine-free	6 oz	90	<1.0	23.0	55	0	<1.0	na
root beer, 'Diet' caffeine-free, w/NutraSweet	6 oz	2	<1.0	<1.0	70	0	<1.0	na
(Jolt) cola	6 oz	85	0.0	20.7	10	0	0.0	0
(Mello Yello)								
citrus	6 oz	87	0.0	22.0	14	0	0.0	0
citrus, diet	6 oz	3	0.0	0.2	<1	0	0.0	0
(Mountain Dew)								
citrus	12 oz	179	0.0	44.4	31	0	0.0	0
citrus, diet	12 oz	4	0.0	0.7	<1	0	0.0	0
(Mr. Pibb) cola	6 oz	71	0.0	19.0	10	0	0.0	0
(Mug)								
root beer	12 oz	168	0.0	42.0	39	0	0.0	0
root beer, 'Diet'	12 oz	4	0.0	1.2	39	0	0.0	0
(Natural 90 Diet) all flavors	6 oz	2	0.0	<1.0	10	0	0.0	0
(Pathmark) cola, 'No Frills Sugar-free'	8 oz	0	0.0	tr	(mq)	0	0.0	0
(Pepsi)								
cherry cola, 'Diet Wild Cherry'	12 oz	1	0.0	na	2	0	0.0	0
cherry cola, 'Wild Cherry'	12 oz	163	0.0	43.2	2	0	0.0	0
cola, caffeine-free	12 oz	160	0.0	39.6	2	0	0.0	0
cola, clear 'Diet Crystal' w/NutraSweet	6 oz	0	0.0	0.0	35	0	0.0	na
cola, diet, caffeine-free	12 oz	<1	0.0	0.2	2	0	0.0	0

Food Name	Serv. Size	Total Cal.	Prot. GMS	Carbs GMS	Sod. MGS	Fiber GMS	Fat GMS	Chol. MGS
cola, diet, w/caffeine	12 oz	<1	0.0	0.2	2	0	0.0	0
cola, 'Light'	12 oz	<1	0.0	0.1	2	0	0.0	0
cola, w/caffeine	12 oz	160	0.0	39.6	2	0	0.0	0
(Santa Cruz Naturals) ginger ale, organic								
'Sparkling'	8 oz	155	<1.0	36.0	na	0	<1.0	na
(Schweppes)								
blackberry, 'Royal'	6 oz	35	0.0	8.0	5	0	0.0	0
citrus, tropical 'Royal'	6 oz	35	0.0	8.0	5	0	0.0	0
club soda	6 oz	0	0.0	0.0	25	0	0.0	0
collins mixer	6 oz	75	0.0	18.0	51	0	0.0	0
ginger ale	6 oz	65	0.0	16.0	10	0	0.0	0
ginger ale, raspberry	6 oz	65	0.0	16.0	10	0	0.0	0
ginger ale, raspberry 'Diet'	6 oz	2	0.0	<1.0	55	0	0.0	0
ginger ale, 'Sugar-free'	6 oz	2	0.0	<1.0	39	0	0.0	0
ginger beer	6 oz	70	0.0	17.0	30	0	0.0	0
grape	6 oz	95	0.0	23.0	15	0	0.0	0
grapefruit	6 oz	80	0.0	20.0	28	0	0.0	0
kiwi-passion fruit, 'Royal'	6 oz	35	0.0	8.0	5	0	0.0	0
lemon, bitter	6 oz	82	0.0	20.0	13	0	0.0	0
lemon, sour	6 oz	79	0.0	19.0	12	0	0.0	0
lemon-lime	6 oz	72	0.0	18.0	30	0	0.0	0
orange, sparkling	6 oz	88	0.0	22.0	17	0	0.0	0
peaches and cream, 'Royal'	6 oz	35	0.0	8.0	5	0	0.0	0
root beer	6 oz	76	0.0	19.0	17	0	0.0	0
seltzer, all flavors	6 oz	0	0.0	0.0	5	0	0.0	0
seltzer, 'Low Sodium'	6 oz	0	0.0	0.0	7	0	0.0	0
seltzer, 'Sodium-free'	6 oz	0	0.0	0.0	5	0	0.0	0
strawberry-banana, 'Royal'	6 oz	35	0.0	8.0	5	0	0.0	0
tonic	6 oz	64	0.0	16.0	8	0	0.0	0
tonic, 'Diet'	6 oz	2	0.0	<1.0	45	0	0.0	0
vanilla bean, 'Royal'	6 oz	35	0.0	8.0	5	0	0.0	0
Vichy water	6 oz	0	0.0	0.0	76	0	0.0	0
wild cherry, 'Royal'	6 oz	35	0.0	8.0	5	0	0.0	0
wild raspberry, 'Royal'	6 oz	35	0.0	8.0	5	0	0.0	0
(7•Up)								
cherry citrus	12 oz	148	0.0	38.7	32	0	0.0	0
cherry citrus, diet	12 oz	4	0.0	tr	32	0	0.0	0
lemon-lime	12 oz	144	0.0	36.2	32	0	0.0	0
lemon-lime, diet	12 oz	4	0.0	0.0	32	0	0.0	0
(Shasta)								
apple, 'Yoshi Apple'	8 oz	130	0.0	31.0	30	0	0.0	na
berry, 'Luigi Berry'	8 oz	130	0.0	32.0	30	0	0.0	na
black cherry	12 oz	162	0.0	44.0	29	0	0.0	0

Food Name	Serv. Size	Total Cal.	Prot. GMS	Carbs GMS	Sod. MGS	Fiber GMS	Fat GMS	Chol. MGS
cherry, 'Princess Toadstool Cherry'	8 oz	130	0.0	31.0	30	0	0.0	na
cherry cola	12 oz	140	0.0	38.0	22	0	0.0	0
citrus mist	12 oz	170	0.0	46.0	19	0	0.0	0
club soda	12 oz	0	0.0	0.0	46	0	0.0	0
cola	12 oz	147	0.0	40.0	3	0	0.0	0
cola, 'Free'	12 oz	151	0.0	41.0	2	0	0.0	0
collins mixer	12 oz	118	0.0	32.0	23	0	0.0	0
cream soda, 'Creme'	12 oz	154	0.0	42.0	23	0	0.0	0
ginger ale	12 oz	120	0.0	33.0	23	0	0.0	0
grape	12 oz	177	0.0	48.0	34	0	0.0	0
lemon-lime	12 oz	146	0.0	39.0	19	0	0.0	0
orange	12 oz	177	0.0	48.0	28	0	0.0	0
red berry	12 oz	158	0.0	43.0	20	0	0.0	0
root beer	12 oz	154	0.0	42.0	31	0	0.0	0
strawberry	12 oz	147	0.0	40.0	36	0	0.0	0
tonic	12 oz	121	0.0	33.0	17	0	0.0	0
(Slice)								
lemon-lime	12 oz	150	0.0	38.4	69	0	0.0	0
lemon-lime, 'Diet'	12 oz	16	0.0	2.4	69	0	0.0	0
orange, 'Diet'	12 oz	12	0.0	2.3	2	0	0.0	0
orange, Mandarin	12 oz	193	0.0	50.4	<1	0	0.0	0
(Snapple)								
'Amazin' Grape'	8 oz	120	0.0	28.0	5	0	0.0	0
'Cherry Lime Rickey'	8 oz	110	0.0	27.0	0	0	0.0	0
'Creme D'Vanilla'	8 oz	130	0.0	33.0	0	0	0.0	0
'French Cherry'	8 oz	120	0.0	29.0	0	0	0.0	0
'Kiwi Peach'	8 oz	120	0.0	29.0	0	0	0.0	0
'Kiwi Strawberry'	8 oz	130	0.0	33.0	5	0	0.0	0
'Mango Madness'	8 oz	130	0.0	33.0	5	0	0.0	0
'Passion Supreme'	8 oz	120	0.0	29.0	0	0	0.0	0
'Peach Melba'	8 oz	120	0.0	31.0	0	0	0.0	0
'Raspberry'	8 oz	120	0.0	31.0	0	0	0.0	0
'Tru Root Beer'	8 oz	110	0.0	29.0	0	0	0.0	0
(Spree)								
cherry-lime	12 oz	158	0.0	43.0	2	0	0.0	0
cola	12 oz	147	0.0	40.0	1	0	0.0	0
ginger ale	12 oz	120	0.0	33.0	1	0	0.0	0
grapefruit	12 oz	154	0.0	42.0	1	0	0.0	0
lemon-lime	12 oz	154	0.0	42.0	1	0	0.0	0
lemon-tangerine	12 oz	165	0.0	45.0	1	0	0.0	0
lime, Mandarin	12 oz	154	0.0	42.0	1	0	0.0	0
root beer	12 oz	154	0.0	42.0	2	0	0.0	0
tropical blend	12 oz	146	0.0	41.0	2	0	0.0	0

Food Name	Serv. Size	Total Cal.	Prot. GMS	Carbs GMS	Sod. MGS	Fiber GMS	Fat GMS	Chol. MGS
(Sprite)								
lemon-lime	6 oz	71	0.0	18.0	23	0	0.0	0
lemon-lime, diet	6 oz	2	0.0	0.0	tr	0	0.0	0
(Squirt)								
citrus	1 oz	13	tr	3.2	2	0	tr	na
citrus, 'Diet'	1 oz	<1	tr	0.1	1	0	tr	na
citrus berry, 'Ruby Red'	8 oz	120	0.0	30.0	25	0	0.0	na
(Tab)								
cola, caffeine-free	6 oz	<1	0.0	0.2	4	0	0.0	0
cola, w/caffeine	6 oz	<1	0.0	0.2	4	0	0.0	0
(Vernor's)								
ginger	3.5 oz	40	0.1	10.0	4	0	0.1	na
ginger, 'Diet'	3.5 oz	<1	0.1	0.1	7	0	0.1	na
(Wink) grapefruit	8 oz	120	0.0	30.0	19	0	0.0	0
(Yoo-Hoo) chocolate	9 oz	140	3.0	27.0	130	0	1.0	(tr)
SOLE								
dry-heat cooked	3 oz	99	20.5	0.0	89	0	1.3	58
raw	3 oz	77	16.0	0.0	69	0	1.0	41
SOLE, FROZEN								
Dinner *(Healthy Choice)* au gratin	11 oz	270	16.0	40.0	470	na	5.0	55
Entrée								
(Gorton's) in lemon butter 'Microwave Entrees'	1 pkg	380	25.0	17.0	560	(mq)	24.0	120
(Gorton's) seafood stuffed 'Select' approx 5 oz	1 fillet	160	16.0	18.0	730	na	3.0	50
(Healthy Choice) w/lemon butter sauce	8.25 oz	230	16.0	33.0	430	na	4.0	45
Fillet								
(Booth) Atlantic	4 oz	90	19.0	0.0	180	0	1.0	(mq)
(Gorton's) 'Fishmarket Fresh'	5 oz	110	24.0	1.0	140	0	1.0	(mq)
(Mrs. Paul's) breaded 'Light'	1 fillet	240	16.0	20.0	450	(mq)	10.0	50
(SeaPak)	4 oz	90	20.0	0.0	135	0	1.0	(mq)
(Van de Kamp's) breaded 'Light'	1 fillet	250	17.0	18.0	480	(mq)	12.0	45
(Van de Kamp's) 'Natural'	4 oz	100	22.0	0.0	105	0	2.0	35
SOMEN NOODLE. See NOODLE, JAPANESE.								
SORBET. See also FRUIT BARS, FROZEN; ICE BARS AND DESSERTS; SHERBET.								
(Baskin-Robbins)								
fruit whip	1 scoop	80	0.0	24.0	20	na	0.0	0
red raspberry	1 scoop	140	0.0	34.0	25	na	0.0	(mq)
(Cascadian Farms)								
blackberry	1 oz	25	0.6	21.2	na	na	0.1	na
raspberry	1 oz	28	0.7	20.9	na	na	0.2	na
strawberry	1 oz	26	0.6	22.0	na	na	0.1	na
(Dole)								
Mandarin orange	4 oz	110	0.5	28.0	9	fiber	0.1	na
peach	4 oz	120	0.6	28.0	11	na	0.6	0

Food Name	Serv. Size	Total Cal.	Prot. GMS	Carbs GMS	Sod. MGS	Fiber GMS	Fat GMS	Chol. MGS
pineapple	4 oz	120	0.5	28.0	11	na	0.1	0
raspberry	4 oz	110	0.4	28.0	12	na	<.1	0
strawberry	4 oz	110	0.5	28.0	1	na	0.1	0
(Frusen Glädjé) raspberry	1/2 cup	140	0.0	36.0	10	na	0.0	0
(Häagen Dazs)								
blueberry, and vanilla ice cream	1/2 cup	190	3.0	25.0	35	na	8.0	(mq)
Key lime, and vanilla ice cream	1/2 cup	200	2.0	29.0	30	na	7.0	(mq)
lemon 'Ice Cream Shop'	4 oz	140	1.0	34.0	5	na	0.0	na
orange, and vanilla ice cream	1/2 cup	190	3.0	27.0	35	na	8.0	(mq)
orange 'Ice Cream Shop'	4 oz	113	1.0	30.0	7	na	0.0	na
raspberry, and vanilla ice cream	1/2 cup	180	2.0	23.0	35	na	8.0	(mq)
raspberry 'Ice Cream Shop'	4 oz	93	0.0	22.0	7	na	0.0	na
SORGHUM								
broomcorn, whole grain	100 gm	327	9.9	72.9	1	>3.2 c	2.9	0
whole grain	1 cup	650	21.7	143.3	na	>4.6 c	6.3	0
whole grain	1 oz	96	3.2	21.2	na	>.7 c	0.9	0
SORGHUM SYRUP								
	1/2 cup	424	0.0	112.2	na	0	0.0	0
	1 tbsp	53	0.0	4.0	na	0	0.0	0
SORREL								
boiled, drained	4 oz	23	2.1	3.3	3	>.8 c	0.7	0
raw, trimmed	1 oz	6	0.6	0.9	1	>.2 c	0.2	0
raw, trimmed, chopped	1/2 cup	15	1.3	2.1	3	1.9	0.5	0
raw, untrimmed	1 lb	70	6.4	10.2	13	>2.5 c	2.2	0
SOUP, CANNED, CONDENSED								
(NOTE: Unless otherwise specified, PREPARED = prepared as directed w/water.)								
ASPARAGUS, CREAM OF								
prepared	1 cup	87	2.3	10.7	981	.7	4.1	5
prepared w/whole milk	8 oz	161	6.3	16.4	1042	.7	8.2	22
unprepared	10.75 oz	210	5.6	26.0	2385	1.2	9.9	12
(Campbell's) prepared	8 oz	80	2.0	10.0	820	(mq)	4.0	5
BEAN								
(Campbell's) 'Homestyle' prepared	8 oz	130	6.0	25.0	700	(mq)	1.0	na
W/bacon								
(Campbell's) 'Healthy Request'	4 oz	140	6.0	22.0	470	6.0	4.0	5
(Campbell's) 'Healthy Request' prepared	8 oz	140	6.0	21.0	470	(mq)	4.0	5
(Campbell's) prepared	8 oz	140	6.0	21.0	840	(mq)	4.0	5
W/frankfurters								
prepared	1 cup	188	10.0	22.0	1093	>1.5 c	7.0	13
unprepared	11.25 oz	455	24.2	53.4	2653	>3.6 c	16.9	30
W/pork								
prepared	1 cup	172	7.9	22.8	951	8.6	5.9	3
unprepared	11.5 oz	418	19.2	55.3	2309	20.9	14.4	6

Food Name	Serv. Size	Total Cal.	Prot. GMS	Carbs GMS	Sod. MGS	Fiber GMS	Fat GMS	Chol. MGS
BEEF								
(Campbell's) prepared	8 oz	80	5.0	10.0	830	(mq)	2.0	10
W/bouillon (Campbell's) prepared	8 oz	16	3.0	1.0	820	na	0.0	0
W/broth (Campbell's) prepared	8 oz	16	3.0	1.0	820	na	0.0	0
W/vegetables (Campbell's) 'Healthy Request'	4 oz	70	5.0	9.0	490	na	2.0	5
BEEF MUSHROOM								
prepared	1 cup	73	5.8	6.3	942	>.5 c	3.0	7
unprepared	10.75 oz	186	14.0	15.9	2358	>.9 c	7.3	15
BEEF NOODLE								
prepared	1 cup	83	4.8	9.0	952	0	3.1	5
unprepared	10.75 oz	204	11.7	21.8	2315	1.8	7.5	12
(Campbell's) prepared	8 oz	70	4.0	7.0	830	(mq)	3.0	15
(Campbell's) 'Homestyle' prepared	8 oz	80	5.0	7.0	810	(mq)	4.0	20
W/ground beef (Campbell's) prepared	8 oz	90	4.0	10.0	820	(mq)	4.0	25
BLACK BEAN								
prepared	1 cup	116	5.6	19.8	1198	4.5	1.5	0
unprepared	11 oz	282	13.7	48.1	2910	21.2	3.7	0
BROCCOLI, CREAM OF								
(Campbell's) prepared	8 oz	80	1.0	8.0	790	(mq)	5.0	na
(Campbell's) prepared w/whole milk	8 oz	140	5.0	14.0	850	(mq)	7.0	(mq)
CELERY, CREAM OF								
prepared	1 cup	90	1.7	8.8	949	.7	5.6	15
prepared w/whole milk	1 cup	164	5.7	14.5	1009	.7	9.7	32
unprepared	10.75 oz	220	4.0	21.4	2309	1.8	13.6	34
(Campbell's) prepared	8 oz	100	2.0	8.0	820	(mq)	7.0	5
CHEESE								
prepared	1 cup	156	5.4	10.5	958	0	10.5	30
prepared w/whole milk	1 cup	231	9.5	16.2	1019	0	14.6	48
unprepared	11 oz	378	13.2	25.6	2331	2.5	25.4	72
Cheddar (Campbell's) prepared	8 oz	110	4.0	10.0	810	na	6.0	10
Nacho								
(Campbell's) prepared	8 oz	110	4.0	8.0	740	na	8.0	na
(Campbell's) prepared w/whole milk	8 oz	180	8.0	13.0	800	na	12.0	(mq)
CHICKEN								
W/barley (Campbell's) prepared	8 oz	70	3.0	10.0	850	(mq)	2.0	(mq)
W/dumplings								
prepared	1 cup	96	5.6	6.1	860	.7	5.5	34
unprepared	10.5 oz	235	13.6	14.7	2095	1.8	13.4	80
(Campbell's) 'Chicken 'n Dumplings' prepared	8 oz	80	4.0	9.0	960	(mq)	3.0	25
W/rice								
prepared	1 cup	60	3.5	7.2	815	0	1.9	7
unprepared	10.5 oz	146	8.6	17.4	1982	1.5	4.7	15
(Campbell's) prepared	8 oz	60	2.0	7.0	790	(mq)	3.0	10

Food Name	Serv. Size	Total Cal.	Prot. GMS	Carbs GMS	Sod. MGS	Fiber GMS	Fat GMS	Chol. MGS
(Campbell's) 'Healthy Request'	4 oz	60	2.0	7.0	480	na	2.0	10
(Campbell's) 'Healthy Request' prepared	8 oz	60	2.0	7.0	480	(mq)	3.0	10
CHICKEN, CREAM OF								
prepared	1 cup	117	3.4	9.3	986	.2	7.4	10
unprepared	10.75 oz	284	8.3	22.5	2397	.6	17.9	24
(Campbell's) prepared	8 oz	110	2.0	9.0	810	na	7.0	10
(Campbell's) 'Healthy Request'	4 oz	70	2.0	11.0	490	na	2.0	10
(Campbell's) 'Healthy Request' prepared	8 oz	70	2.0	11.0	490	na	2.0	10
W/broccoli								
(Campbell's)	4 oz	110	3.0	9.0	710	na	7.0	10
(Campbell's) prepared	8 oz	110	3.0	9.0	710	na	7.0	10
CHICKEN BROTH								
prepared	1 cup	39	4.9	0.9	776	0	1.4	0
unprepared	10.75 oz	95	13.5	2.3	1909	0	3.2	3
(Campbell's) prepared	8 oz	30	1.0	2.0	710	na	2.0	0
CHICKEN GUMBO								
prepared	1 cup	56	2.6	8.4	954	2.0	1.4	5
unprepared	10.75 oz	137	6.4	20.3	2321	4.7	3.5	9
CHICKEN MUSHROOM								
prepared	1 cup	132	4.4	9.3	942	>.2 c	9.1	10
unprepared	10.75 oz	332	10.7	23.2	2358	.6	22.3	24
Creamy *(Campbell's)* prepared	8 oz	120	3.0	8.0	920	(mq)	8.0	15
CHICKEN NOODLE								
prepared	1 cup	75	4.1	9.4	1106	.7	2.5	7
unprepared	10.5 oz	182	9.6	22.7	2256	1.8	5.5	15
(Campbell's) prepared	8 oz	60	3.0	8.0	900	(mq)	2.0	15
(Campbell's) 'Healthy Request'	4 oz	60	3.0	8.0	460	na	2.0	15
(Campbell's) 'Healthy Request' prepared	8 oz	60	3.0	8.0	440	(mq)	2.0	15
(Campbell's) 'Homestyle' prepared	8 oz	70	3.0	8.0	880	(mq)	3.0	15
Broth and noodles *(Campbell's)* prepared	8 oz	45	1.0	8.0	860	(mq)	1.0	10
Creamy								
(Campbell's)	4 oz	120	4.0	10.0	800	na	7.0	na
(Campbell's) prepared	8 oz	120	4.0	10.0	800	na	7.0	10
(Campbell's) prepared w/2% milk	8 oz	180	8.0	16.0	850	na	9.0	na
Curly noodle *(Campbell's)* prepared	8 oz	80	3.0	11.0	800	(mq)	3.0	15
Double noodle in broth								
(Campbell's)	4 oz	90	4.0	13.0	700	na	2.0	na
(Campbell's) prepared	8 oz	90	4.0	13.0	700	na	2.0	na
Ring noodle *(Campbell's)* 'Noodle-O's'								
prepared	8 oz	70	3.0	9.0	820	(mq)	2.0	20
CHICKEN VEGETABLE								
prepared	1 cup	75	3.6	8.6	945	1.0	2.8	10
unprepared	10.5 oz	182	8.8	20.9	2298	>.3 c	6.9	21

Food Name	Serv. Size	Total Cal.	Prot. GMS	Carbs GMS	Sod. MGS	Fiber GMS	Fat GMS	Chol. MGS
(Campbell's) prepared	8 oz	70	3.0	8.0	850	(mq)	3.0	10
CHILI BEEF								
prepared	1 cup	170	6.7	21.5	1035	9.5	6.6	13
unprepared	11.25 oz	412	16.2	52.1	2514	>3.5 c	16.0	32
(Campbell's) prepared	8 oz	140	5.0	20.0	840	(mq)	5.0	10
CLAM CHOWDER								
Manhattan style								
prepared	1 cup	78	2.2	12.2	578	1.5	2.2	2
unprepared	10.75 oz	186	5.3	29.7	1394	3.7	5.4	6
(Campbell's) prepared	8 oz	70	2.0	10.0	820	(mq)	2.0	0
(Campbell's) 'Seashore Soups'	4 oz	70	2.0	10.0	820	na	2.0	5
(Doxsee) prepared	7.5 oz	70	3.0	11.0	780	(mq)	2.0	(mq)
(Snow's)	3.75 oz	70	3.0	9.0	630	na	2.0	na
(Snow's) prepared	7.5 oz	70	3.0	11.0	780	(mq)	2.0	(mq)
New England style								
prepared	8 oz	95	4.8	12.4	915	1.5	2.9	5
prepared w/whole milk	8 oz	164	9.5	16.6	992	1.5	6.6	22
(Campbell's) prepared	8 oz	80	3.0	12.0	870	(mq)	3.0	5
(Campbell's) prepared w/whole milk	8 oz	150	7.0	17.0	930	(mq)	7.0	(mq)
(Campbell's) 'Seashore Soups'	4 oz	80	3.0	12.0	870	na	3.0	5
(Gorton's) prepared w/whole milk	1/4 can	140	7.0	17.0	740	(mq)	5.0	15
(Snow's)	3.75 oz	70	5.0	8.0	620	na	2.0	na
(Snow's) prepared w/whole milk	7.5 oz	140	8.0	13.0	670	(mq)	6.0	(mq)
CONSOMMÉ								
Beef	10.5 oz	72	13.0	4.3	1550	0	0.0	0
Beef, w/gelatin								
prepared	1 cup	29	5.4	1.8	637	na	0.0	0
unprepared	10.5 oz	71	13.0	4.3	1550	na	0.0	0
(Campbell's) prepared	8 oz	25	4.0	2.0	750	na	0.0	0
CORN, CREAM OF, GOLDEN								
(Campbell's)	4 oz	110	2.0	18.0	700	na	3.0	5
(Campbell's) prepared	8 oz	110	2.0	18.0	700	na	3.0	5
(Campbell's) prepared w/2% milk	8 oz	160	6.0	23.0	760	na	5.0	10
CORN CHOWDER, NEW ENGLAND								
(Snow's)	3.75 oz	80	2.0	13.0	590	na	2.0	na
(Snow's) prepared w/whole milk	7.5 oz	150	5.0	18.0	640	na	6.0	na
FISH CHOWDER, NEW ENGLAND								
(Snow's)	3.75 oz	60	5.0	6.0	560	na	2.0	na
(Snow's) prepared w/whole milk	7.5 oz	130	9.0	11.0	620	(mq)	6.0	(mq)
GREEN PEA								
prepared	1 cup	165	8.6	26.5	988	2.8	2.9	0
prepared w/whole milk	1 cup	239	12.6	32.2	1046	2.8	7.0	18
unprepared	11.25 oz	399	20.9	64.4	2399	7.0	7.1	0

Food Name	Serv. Size	Total Cal.	Prot. GMS	Carbs GMS	Sod. MGS	Fiber GMS	Fat GMS	Chol. MGS
(Campbell's) prepared	8 oz	160	8.0	25.0	820	(mq)	3.0	5
MINESTRONE								
prepared	1 cup	82	4.3	11.2	911	1.0	2.5	2
unprepared	10.5 oz	203	10.4	27.3	2217	2.4	6.1	3
(Campbell's) prepared	8 oz	80	3.0	13.0	900	(mq)	2.0	0
MUSHROOM								
Beefy *(Campbell's)* prepared	8 oz	60	4.0	5.0	960	(mq)	3.0	10
Golden *(Campbell's)* prepared	8 oz	70	2.0	9.0	870	(mq)	3.0	5
W/beef stock								
prepared	1 cup	85	3.2	9.3	969	.7	4.0	7
unprepared	10.75 oz	207	7.7	22.6	2358	.3	9.8	18
MUSHROOM, CREAM OF								
prepared	1 cup	129	2.3	9.3	1032	.5	9.0	2
prepared w/whole milk	1 cup	203	6.1	15.0	1076	.5	13.6	20
unprepared	10.75 oz	314	4.9	22.6	2470	.9	23.1	3
(Campbell's) prepared	8 oz	100	2.0	8.0	820	(mq)	7.0	0
(Campbell's) 'Healthy Request'	4 oz	60	1.0	9.0	480	na	2.0	5
(Campbell's) 'Healthy Request' prepared	8 oz	60	1.0	9.0	480	(mq)	2.0	5
MUSHROOM BARLEY								
prepared	1 cup	73	1.9	11.7	891	.7	2.3	0
unprepared	10.75 oz	186	4.6	29.3	2227	1.8	5.5	0
(Rokeach) prepared	1 cup	85	3.4	17.3	904	(mq)	0.2	na
ONION								
prepared	1 cup	58	3.8	8.2	1053	1.0	1.7	0
unprepared	10.5 oz	137	9.1	19.9	2563	2.1	4.2	0
unprepared	8 oz	113	7.5	16.4	2116	1.7	3.5	0
French *(Campbell's)* prepared	8 oz	60	2.0	9.0	900	(mq)	2.0	5
ONION, CREAM OF								
prepared	1 cup	107	2.8	12.7	927	>.5 c	5.3	15
prepared w/whole milk	1 cup	186	6.8	18.4	1004	.7	9.4	32
unprepared	10.75 oz	268	6.7	31.7	2318	1.2	12.8	37
(Campbell's) prepared	8 oz	100	2.0	12.0	830	(mq)	5.0	15
(Campbell's) prepared w/half water, half milk	8 oz	140	4.0	15.0	860	(mq)	7.0	(mq)
OYSTER STEW								
prepared	1 cup	58	2.1	4.1	981	0	3.8	14
prepared w/whole milk	1 cup	135	6.2	9.8	1041	0	7.9	32
unprepared	10.5 oz	143	5.1	9.9	2384	0	9.3	33
(Campbell's) prepared	8 oz	70	2.0	5.0	840	(mq)	5.0	25
(Campbell's) prepared w/whole milk	8 oz	140	6.0	10.0	890	(mq)	9.0	(mq)
PASTA								
Alphabet *(Campbell's)* prepared	8 oz	80	3.0	10.0	800	(mq)	3.0	10
Chicken and stars *(Campbell's)* prepared	8 oz	60	3.0	7.0	870	(mq)	2.0	10

Food Name	Serv. Size	Total Cal.	Prot. GMS	Carbs GMS	Sod. MGS	Fiber GMS	Fat GMS	Chol. MGS
Teddy bears in chicken broth								
(Campbell's)	4 oz	60	2.0	11.0	770	na	1.0	5
(Campbell's) prepared	8 oz	60	2.0	11.0	770	na	1.0	5
PEPPER POT								
prepared	1 cup	104	6.4	9.4	971	.5	4.6	10
unprepared	10.5 oz	250	15.5	22.8	2360	>1.2 c	11.3	24
(Campbell's) prepared	8 oz	90	5.0	9.0	970	(mq)	4.0	40
POTATO, CREAM OF								
prepared	1 cup	73	1.8	11.5	1000	.5	2.4	5
prepared w/whole milk	1 cup	149	5.8	17.2	1061	.5	6.4	22
unprepared	10.75 oz	180	4.2	27.9	2431	1.2	5.7	15
(Campbell's) prepared	8 oz	80	1.0	12.0	870	(mq)	3.0	5
(Campbell's) prepared w/tofu, 1 tbsp oil	8 oz	120	3.0	15.0	900	(mq)	4.0	(mq)
SCOTCH BROTH								
prepared	1 cup	80	5.0	9.5	1012	1.2	2.6	5
unprepared	10.5 oz	197	12.1	23.0	2461	>.9 c	6.4	12
(Campbell's) prepared	8 oz	80	4.0	9.0	870	na	3.0	10
SEAFOOD CHOWDER, NEW ENGLAND								
(Snow's)	3.75 oz	60	4.0	6.0	640	na	2.0	na
(Snow's) prepared w/whole milk	7.5 oz	140	8.0	14.0	670	na	6.0	(mq)
SHRIMP, CREAM OF								
prepared	1 cup	90	2.8	8.2	976	.2	5.2	17
prepared w/whole milk	1 cup	164	6.8	13.9	1037	.3	9.3	35
unprepared	10.75 oz	220	6.8	19.9	2373	.6	12.6	40
(Campbell's) prepared	8 oz	90	2.0	8.0	810	na	6.0	20
(Campbell's) prepared w/whole milk	8 oz	160	5.0	13.0	860	na	10.0	(mq)
(Campbell's) 'Seashore Soups'	4 oz	90	2.0	8.0	810	na	6.0	20
(Campbell's) 'Seashore Soups' prepared w/2% milk	4 oz	140	5.0	13.0	810	na	10.0	20
SPLIT PEA								
W/egg barley (Rokeach) prepared	1 cup	132	8.2	23.6	757	(mq)	0.5	na
W/ham								
prepared	1 cup	190	10.3	28.0	1007	>.7 c	4.4	8
unprepared	11.5 oz	460	25.0	67.8	2445	>1.6 c	10.7	20
W/ham and bacon (Campbell's) prepared	8 oz	160	9.0	24.0	780	(mq)	4.0	5
STOCKPOT								
prepared	1 cup	99	4.9	11.5	1047	>.5 c	3.9	5
unprepared	11 oz	243	11.8	27.9	2546	>1.3 c	9.5	9
TOMATO								
prepared	1 cup	85	2.0	16.6	871	.5	1.9	0
prepared w/whole milk	1 cup	161	6.1	22.3	932	.5	6.0	17
unprepared	10.75 oz	207	5.0	40.3	2120	1.2	4.7	0
(Campbell's) prepared	8 oz	90	1.0	17.0	680	(mq)	2.0	0

Food Name	Serv. Size	Total Cal.	Prot. GMS	Carbs GMS	Sod. MGS	Fiber GMS	Fat GMS	Chol. MGS
(Campbell's) prepared w/whole milk	8 oz	150	5.0	22.0	740	(mq)	4.0	(mq)
(Campbell's) 'Healthy Request'	4 oz	90	1.0	17.0	430	na	2.0	0
(Campbell's) 'Healthy Request' prepared	8 oz	90	1.0	17.0	430	(mq)	2.0	0
(Campbell's) 'Healthy Request' prepared w/half 2% milk, half water	8 oz	140	5.0	22.0	490	na	3.0	5
(Campbell's) 'Healthy Request' prepared w/skim milk	4 oz	130	5.0	22.0	490	na	2.0	5
(Campbell's) 'Healthy Request' prepared w/whole milk	8 oz	150	5.0	22.0	490	(mq)	4.0	10
Italian, w/basil and oregano								
(Campbell's)	4 oz	90	1.0	21.0	740	na	0.0	0
(Campbell's) prepared	8 oz	90	1.0	21.0	740	na	0.0	0
Zesty (Campbell's) prepared	8 oz	100	1.0	20.0	760	(mq)	2.0	na
TOMATO, CREAM OF								
(Campbell's) 'Homestyle' prepared	8 oz	110	1.0	20.0	810	(mq)	3.0	5
(Campbell's) 'Homestyle' prepared w/whole milk	8 oz	180	5.0	25.0	860	(mq)	7.0	(mq)
TOMATO BEEF W/NOODLES								
prepared	1 cup	139	4.5	21.1	917	1.5	4.3	5
unprepared	10.75 oz	342	10.8	51.5	2230	>.3 c	10.4	9
TOMATO BISQUE								
prepared w/milk	1 cup	198	6.3	29.4	1109	>.8 c	6.6	23
unprepared	11 oz	300	5.5	57.6	2546	2.5	6.1	12
(Campbell's) prepared	8 oz	120	2.0	22.0	820	(mq)	3.0	5
TOMATO RICE								
prepared	1 cup	119	2.1	21.9	815	1.5	2.7	2
unprepared	11 oz	290	5.1	53.3	1981	4.1	6.6	3
(Campbell's) 'Old Fashioned' prepared	8 oz	110	1.0	22.0	730	(mq)	2.0	0
TURKEY NOODLE								
prepared	1 cup	68	3.9	8.6	815	.7	2.0	5
unprepared	10.75 oz	168	9.5	21.0	1983	1.8	4.8	12
(Campbell's) prepared	8 oz	70	3.0	9.0	880	(mq)	2.0	15
TURKEY VEGETABLE								
prepared	1 cup	72	3.1	8.6	906	.5	3.0	2
unprepared	10.5 oz	179	7.5	21.0	2202	1.5	7.4	3
(Campbell's) prepared	8 oz	70	2.0	8.0	710	(mq)	3.0	10
VEGETABLE								
(Campbell's) prepared	8 oz	90	3.0	14.0	830	(mq)	2.0	0
(Campbell's) 'Homestyle' prepared	8 oz	60	2.0	9.0	880	(mq)	2.0	0
(Campbell's) 'Old Fashioned' prepared	8 oz	60	2.0	9.0	880	(mq)	2.0	0
Hearty, w/pasta								
(Campbell's)	4 oz	70	3.0	15.0	800	na	<1.0	0
(Campbell's) prepared	8 oz	70	3.0	15.0	800	na	<1.0	0

Food Name	Serv. Size	Total Cal.	Prot. GMS	Carbs GMS	Sod. MGS	Fiber GMS	Fat GMS	Chol. MGS
Vegetarian								
prepared	1 cup	72	2.1	12.0	822	.5	1.9	0
unprepared	10.5 oz	176	5.1	29.1	2003	1.5	4.7	0
(Campbell's) prepared	8 oz	80	2.0	13.0	790	(mq)	2.0	0
W/beef broth								
prepared	1 cup	82	3.0	13.1	810	.5	1.9	2
unprepared	10.5 oz	197	7.2	31.9	1970	3.7	4.7	3
W/beef stock								
(Campbell's) 'Healthy Request'	4 oz	90	3.0	14.0	500	na	2.0	5
(Campbell's) 'Healthy Request' prepared	8 oz	90	3.0	14.0	500	(mq)	2.0	5
VEGETABLE BEEF								
prepared	1 cup	78	5.6	10.2	956	.5	1.9	5
unprepared	10.75 oz	192	13.6	24.7	2327	4.9	4.6	12
(Campbell's) prepared	8 oz	70	4.0	10.0	780	(mq)	2.0	10
(Campbell's) 'Healthy Request' prepared	8 oz	70	4.0	10.0	470	(mq)	2.0	10
WON TON *(Campbell's)* prepared	8 oz	40	2.0	5.0	850	(mq)	1.0	10
SOUP, CANNED, READY-TO-SERVE								
BEAN								
(Grandma Brown's)	1 cup	190	9.0	30.9	700	9.8	3.4	<1
W/ham								
(Campbell's) 'Chunky Old Fashioned'	11 oz	290	14.0	38.0	1110	(mq)	9.0	na
(Campbell's) 'Chunky Old Fashioned'	9 5/8 oz	250	12.0	33.0	960	(mq)	8.0	na
(Campbell's) 'Home Cookin'	9.5 oz	180	12.0	25.0	890	(mq)	4.0	(mq)
(Campbell's) 'Home Cookin'	10.75 oz	210	14.0	29.0	1000	(mq)	4.0	(mq)
(Healthy Choice)	7.5 oz	220	12.0	35.0	480	na	4.0	5
(Hormel) 'Hearty Soup'	7.5 oz	190	9.0	29.0	640	na	4.0	23
BEEF								
(Progresso)	10.5 oz	180	15.0	17.0	840	(mq)	6.0	35
(Progresso)	9.5 oz	160	13.0	15.0	760	(mq)	5.0	35
Bouillon	8 oz	17	2.7	0.1	782	0	0.5	0
Broth *(College Inn)*	7 oz	16	3.0	1.0	960	na	0.0	0
Chunky								
(Campbell's) 'Chunky'	10.75 oz	200	15.0	24.0	1100	(mq)	5.0	(mq)
(Campbell's) 'Chunky'	9.5 oz	170	13.0	21.0	970	(mq)	4.0	(mq)
Fat-free *(Health Valley)*	6.9 oz	10	1.0	2.0	290	0	0.0	0
Fat-free, no salt added *(Health Valley)*	6.9 oz	10	1.0	2.0	5	0	0.0	0
Hearty								
(Healthy Choice) 'Hearty Beef'	7.5 oz	120	9.0	17.0	580	na	2.0	20
(Progresso)	9.5 oz	160	15.0	15.0	820	(mq)	4.0	35
Stroganoff style *(Campbell's)* 'Chunky'	10.75 oz	320	15.0	28.0	1230	(mq)	16.0	(mq)
W/barley								
(Progresso)	10.5 oz	150	13.0	16.0	870	3.0	5.0	30
(Progresso)	9.5 oz	140	12.0	16.0	780	3.0	4.0	30

Food Name	Serv. Size	Total Cal.	Prot. GMS	Carbs GMS	Sod. MGS	Fiber GMS	Fat GMS	Chol. MGS
W/broth								
(College Inn)	1 cup	18	2.0	1.0	1280	0	0.0	(mq)
(Health Valley)	7.5 oz	17	1.0	2.0	420	0	1.0	1
(Health Valley) 'No Salt Added'	7.5 oz	17	1.0	2.0	0	0	1.0	1
(Progresso) seasoned	4 oz	10	2.0	<1.0	380	0	<1.0	0
(Swanson)	7.25 oz	18	2.0	0.0	750	0	1.0	(mq)
W/minestrone								
(Progresso)	10.5 oz	180	15.0	18.0	1000	(mq)	6.0	35
(Progresso)	9.5 oz	170	13.0	16.0	910	(mq)	5.0	30
W/noodles (Progresso)	9.5 oz	170	15.0	18.0	1030	(mq)	4.0	40
W/tomato juice	1 oz	11	0.2	2.6	40	0	0.0	0
W/vegetables								
(Lipton) 'Hearty Ones'	11 oz	229	10.4	40.0	921	(mq)	3.0	29
(Progresso)	10.5 oz	170	17.0	18.0	880	(mq)	3.0	40
(Progresso)	9.5 oz	150	15.0	16.0	790	(mq)	3.0	35
W/vegetables and pasta								
(Campbell's) 'Home Cookin'	10.75 oz	140	12.0	18.0	1060	(mq)	2.0	(mq)
(Campbell's) 'Home Cookin'	9.5 oz	120	10.0	16.0	940	(mq)	2.0	(mq)
BERRY								
Blueberry (Great Impressions)	6 oz	95	0.4	22.5	92	(mq)	0.3	0
Three berry (Great Impressions)	6 oz	107	0.5	25.8	90	(mq)	0.2	0
BLACK BEAN								
(Health Valley)	7.5 oz	160	7.0	24.0	285	17.0	3.0	0
(Health Valley) 'No Salt Added'	7.5 oz	160	7.0	24.0	20	17.0	3.0	0
(Health Valley) w/vegetables, fat-free	7.5 oz	70	9.0	9.0	290	17.0	0.0	0
BORSCHT								
(Gold's)	8 oz	100	4.0	21.0	1280	(mq)	0.0	0
(Rokeach)	1 cup	96	0.8	23.0	985	>.3 c	0.3	0
(Rokeach) 'Unsalted'	1 cup	103	0.8	23.0	50	>.5 c	0.3	0
Low-calorie								
(Gold's)	8 oz	20	1.0	5.0	1160	(mq)	<1.0	0
(Manischewitz)	1 cup	20	1.0	4.0	725	(mq)	0.0	0
(Rokeach) 'Diet'	1 cup	29	0.8	5.8	897	>.8 c	0.2	0
W/beets (Manischewitz)	1 cup	80	1.0	20.0	660	(mq)	0.0	0
BROCCOLI, CREAM OF (Andersen's)	7.5 oz	170	5.0	20.0	670	na	8.0	na
CHERRY (Great Impressions)	6 oz	123	0.6	29.6	88	(mq)	0.2	0
CHICKEN								
(Progresso) 'Homestyle'	9.5 oz	110	11.0	12.0	740	na	3.0	20
Broth								
(Campbell's) 'Healthy Request'	8 oz	16	3.0	1.0	470	na	0.0	0
(Campbell's) 'Low Sodium'	10.5 oz	30	3.0	2.0	85	0	1.0	(mq)
(College Inn)	1 cup	35	1.0	0.0	1320	0	3.0	(mq)
(College Inn)	7 oz	35	1.0	0.0	990	0	3.0	5

Food Name	Serv. Size	Total Cal.	Prot. GMS	Carbs GMS	Sod. MGS	Fiber GMS	Fat GMS	Chol. MGS
(College Inn) lower salt	7 oz	20	1.0	0.0	550	0	2.0	5
(Hain)	8.75 oz	70	2.0	0.0	870	0	6.0	5
(Health Valley) fat-free	6.9 oz	20	4.0	1.0	290	0	0.0	0
(Hain) 'No Salt Added'	8.75 oz	60	3.0	0.0	75	0	5.0	5
(Health Valley)	7.5 oz	35	4.0	1.0	410	0	2.0	2
(Health Valley) 'No Salt Added'	7.5 oz	35	4.0	1.0	0	0	2.0	2
(Pritikin) defatted	1 cup	18	3.0	1.0	160	0	1.0	0
(Progresso)	4 oz	8	2.0	0.0	360	0	0.0	5
(Swanson)	7.25 oz	30	2.0	2.0	900	0	2.0	(mq)
(Swanson) 'Natural Goodness'	7.25 oz	20	2.0	1.0	580	0	1.0	(mq)
Chunky								
(Campbell's) 'Chunky Old Fashioned'	10.75 oz	180	12.0	21.0	1220	na	5.0	(mq)
(Campbell's) 'Chunky Old Fashioned'	9.5 oz	150	10.0	18.0	1070	na	4.0	(mq)
(Healthy Choice) 'Hearty Chicken'	7.5 oz	150	9.0	17.0	530	na	5.0	35
Hearty								
(Progresso)	10.5 oz	130	14.0	9.0	960	na	4.0	30
(Progresso)	9.5 oz	130	13.0	11.0	900	na	4.0	25
Nuggets, w/vegetables and noodles								
(Campbell's) 'Chunky'	10.75 oz	190	11.0	24.0	1060	(mq)	6.0	(mq)
(Campbell's) 'Chunky'	9.5 oz	170	9.0	21.0	940	(mq)	6.0	(mq)
W/meatballs *(Progresso)* 'Chickarina'	9.5 oz	130	8.0	13.0	820	(mq)	5.0	20
W/noodles								
(Campbell's) 'Home Cookin'	10.75 oz	140	13.0	12.0	1150	(mq)	4.0	(mq)
(Campbell's) 'Home Cookin'	9.5 oz	110	11.0	10.0	1020	(mq)	3.0	(mq)
(Campbell's) 'Low Sodium'	10.75 oz	170	13.0	17.0	90	(mq)	5.0	(mq)
W/ribbon pasta *(Pritikin)*	1 cup	80	6.0	13.0	180	1.0	1.0	5
W/rice								
(Campbell's) 'Chunky'	9.5 oz	140	10.0	16.0	1060	(mq)	4.0	30
(Healthy Choice)	7.5 oz	140	5.0	18.0	510	na	4.0	15
(Hormel) 'Hearty Soup'	7.5 oz	110	5.0	17.0	890	na	2.0	6
W/wild rice *(Progresso)*	9.5 oz	120	6.0	17.0	850	na	3.0	20
CHICKEN, CREAM OF *(Progresso)*	9.5 oz	190	10.0	12.0	970	(mq)	11.0	35
CHICKEN BARLEY *(Progresso)*	9.25 oz	100	10.0	12.0	740	3.5	2.0	20
CHICKEN GUMBO, w/sausage								
(Campbell's) 'Home Cookin'	10.75 oz	140	11.0	15.0	1090	(mq)	4.0	(mq)
(Campbell's) 'Home Cookin'	9.5 oz	120	9.0	13.0	960	(mq)	3.0	(mq)
CHICKEN MINESTRONE								
(Campbell's) 'Home Cookin'	10.75 oz	180	15.0	17.0	950	(mq)	6.0	(mq)
(Campbell's) 'Home Cookin'	9.5 oz	160	13.0	15.0	840	(mq)	5.0	(mq)
(Progresso)	10.5 oz	140	12.0	14.0	1060	(mq)	4.0	20
(Progresso)	9.5 oz	130	12.0	12.0	870	(mq)	3.0	20
CHICKEN MUSHROOM, CREAMY								
(Campbell's) 'Chunky'	10.5 oz	270	12.0	13.0	1280	(mq)	19.0	(mq)

Food Name	Serv. Size	Total Cal.	Prot. GMS	Carbs GMS	Sod. MGS	Fiber GMS	Fat GMS	Chol. MGS
(Campbell's) 'Chunky'	9 3/8 oz	240	10.0	12.0	1140	(mq)	17.0	(mq)
CHICKEN NOODLE								
(Hain)	9.5 oz	120	9.0	11.0	980	(mq)	4.0	20
(Hain) 'No Salt Added'	9.5 oz	120	9.0	12.0	90	(mq)	4.0	25
(Healthy Choice) 'Old Fashioned								
Chicken Noodle'	7.5 oz	90	5.0	9.0	520	na	3.0	20
(Hormel) 'Hearty Soup'	7.5 oz	110	7.0	14.0	690	na	3.0	18
(Lipton) 'Hearty Ones Homestyle'	11 oz	227	10.1	37.4	989	(mq)	4.0	37
(Progresso)	10.5 oz	120	12.0	8.0	970	(mq)	4.0	40
(Progresso)	9.5 oz	120	11.0	10.0	920	(mq)	4.0	40
(Progresso) 'Healthy Classics'	8 oz	80	7.0	10.0	460	na	2.0	15
(Weight Watchers)	10.5 oz	80	6.0	9.0	1230	(mq)	2.0	(mq)
Chunky								
(Campbell's) 'Chunky'	10.75 oz	200	14.0	20.0	1140	(mq)	7.0	(mq)
(Campbell's) 'Chunky'	9.5 oz	180	12.0	18.0	1000	(mq)	7.0	(mq)
Hearty *(Campbell's)* 'Healthy Request'	8 oz	80	9.0	7.0	470	na	2.0	25
CHICKEN RICE								
(Campbell's) 'Home Cookin'	10.75 oz	150	14.0	10.0	1090	(mq)	6.0	(mq)
(Campbell's) 'Home Cookin'	9.5 oz	130	12.0	9.0	960	(mq)	5.0	(mq)
(Progresso)	10.5 oz	120	9.0	12.0	990	(mq)	4.0	25
(Progresso)	9.5 oz	130	9.0	16.0	750	(mq)	3.0	25
Chunky	8 oz	127	12.3	13.0	888	1.0	3.2	12
Hearty *(Campbell's)* 'Healthy Request'	8 oz	110	5.0	15.0	480	na	3.0	10
W/vegetables *(Progresso)* 'Healthy Classics'	8 oz	80	7.0	11.0	440	na	2.0	10
CHICKEN VEGETABLE								
(Hain)	9.5 oz	120	8.0	14.0	930	(mq)	4.0	15
(Hain) 'No Salt Added'	9.5 oz	130	8.0	14.0	100	(mq)	4.0	20
(Campbell's) 'Chunky'	9.5 oz	170	10.0	19.0	1080	(mq)	6.0	25
(Campbell's) 'Chunky Low Sodium'	10.75 oz	240	15.0	21.0	95	(mq)	11.0	10
(Campbell's) 'Home Cookin'	10.75 oz	180	11.0	25.0	970	na	4.0	na
(Pritikin)	1 cup	70	5.0	12.0	150	2.0	1.0	5
(Progresso)	9.5 oz	140	9.0	17.0	800	(mq)	4.0	25
Chunky								
(Health Valley)	7.5 oz	125	7.0	20.0	425	4.0	2.0	11
(Health Valley) 'No Salt Added'	7.5 oz	125	7.0	20.0	60	4.0	2.0	11
Hearty *(Campbell's)* 'Healthy Request'	8 oz	120	7.0	16.0	420	na	3.0	10
CHILI BEEF								
(Campbell's) 'Chunky'	11 oz	290	21.0	37.0	1120	(mq)	7.0	(mq)
(Campbell's) 'Chunky'	9.75 oz	260	18.0	33.0	990	(mq)	6.0	(mq)
(Healthy Choice) thick and hearty	7.5 oz	150	11.0	22.0	560	na	1.0	15
CLAM CHOWDER								
Manhattan style								
(Campbell's) 'Chunky'	10.75 oz	160	7.0	24.0	1110	(mq)	4.0	(mq)

Food Name	Serv. Size	Total Cal.	Prot. GMS	Carbs GMS	Sod. MGS	Fiber GMS	Fat GMS	Chol. MGS
(Campbell's) 'Chunky'	9.5 oz	150	7.0	21.0	980	(mq)	4.0	(mq)
(Health Valley)	7.5 oz	110	6.0	15.0	510	13.4	2.0	15
(Health Valley) 'No Salt Added'	7.5 oz	110	6.0	15.0	60	13.4	2.0	15
(Progresso)	9.5 oz	120	13.0	13.0	800	(mq)	2.0	10
New England style								
(Campbell's) 'Chunky'	10.75 oz	290	9.0	26.0	1200	(mq)	17.0	(mq)
(Campbell's) 'Chunky'	9.5 oz	260	8.0	23.0	1060	(mq)	15.0	(mq)
(Campbell's) 'Healthy Request'	8 oz	100	4.0	14.0	490	na	3.0	10
(Campbell's) 'Home Cookin'	10.75 oz	260	8.0	15.0	1240	na	18.0	na
(Gorton's) 'New England Style'	7.5 oz	140	7.0	17.0	720	na	5.0	20
(Hain)	9.25 oz	180	8.0	26.0	780	(mq)	4.0	25
(Hormel) 'Hearty Soup'	7.5 oz	130	5.0	16.0	790	na	5.0	30
(Progresso)	10.5 oz	220	7.0	21.0	1050	(mq)	12.0	20
(Progresso)	9.25 oz	220	8.0	20.0	950	(mq)	12.0	(mq)
(Weight Watchers)	7.5 oz	90	5.0	16.0	450	na	0.0	5
CORN AND VEGETABLE, fat-free								
(Health Valley)	7.5 oz	70	4.0	13.0	290	3.0	0.0	0
CORN CHOWDER								
(Campbell's) 'Chunky'	10.75 oz	340	14.0	23.0	1200	(mq)	21.0	(mq)
(Campbell's) 'Chunky'	9.5 oz	300	12.0	21.0	1060	(mq)	19.0	(mq)
(Progresso)	9.25 oz	200	5.0	22.0	840	(mq)	10.0	10
CRAB	8 oz	76	5.5	10.3	1235	.7	1.5	10
CREOLE								
(Campbell's) 'Chunky'	10.75 oz	240	11.0	31.0	910	na	8.0	na
(Campbell's) 'Chunky'	9.5 oz	220	10.0	28.0	800	na	7.0	na
ESCAROLE, in chicken broth *(Progresso)*	9.25 oz	30	2.0	2.0	1100	(mq)	1.0	5
GAZPACHO	8 oz	56	8.7	0.8	1183	3.7	2.2	0
HAM AND BEAN								
(Campbell's) w/butterbeans 'Chunky'	10.75 oz	280	12.0	34.0	1180	(mq)	10.0	(mq)
(Progresso)	9.5 oz	140	11.0	28.0	950	8.0	2.0	10
LEMON *(Great Impressions)*	6 oz	90	0.2	22.1	109	(mq)	<1.0	0
LENTIL								
(Health Valley)	7.5 oz	170	9.0	28.0	435	17.0	2.0	0
(Health Valley) 'No Salt Added'	7.5 oz	170	9.0	28.0	25	17.0	2.0	0
(Progresso)	10.5 oz	140	10.0	24.0	1000	6.5	4.0	0
(Progresso)	9.5 oz	140	10.0	25.0	840	6.5	4.0	0
(Progresso) 'Healthy Classics'	8 oz	120	7.0	19.0	420	na	1.0	0
Hearty								
(Campbell's) 'Home Cookin'	10.75 oz	170	11.0	28.0	930	(mq)	2.0	na
(Campbell's) 'Home Cookin'	9.5 oz	140	9.0	24.0	820	(mq)	1.0	na
Vegetarian								
(Hain)	9.5 oz	160	9.0	25.0	690	(mq)	3.0	5
(Hain) 'No Salt Added'	9.5 oz	160	9.0	24.0	65	(mq)	3.0	5

Food Name	Serv. Size	Total Cal.	Prot. GMS	Carbs GMS	Sod. MGS	Fiber GMS	Fat GMS	Chol. MGS
W/carrots, fat-free *(Health Valley)*	7.5 oz	70	8.0	10.0	290	15.0	0.0	0
W/ham	8 oz	139	9.3	20.2	1319	>1.4 c	2.8	7
W/sausage *(Progresso)*	9.5 oz	170	8.0	21.0	840	5.0	8.0	20
MACARONI AND BEAN								
(Progresso)	10.5 oz	150	9.0	27.0	1020	8.0	4.0	0
(Progresso)	9.5 oz	140	8.0	25.0	920	(mq)	5.0	0
MENUDO *(Old El Paso)*	1/2 can	476	15.0	14.0	770	2.0	52.0	176
MINESTRONE								
(Campbell's) 'Chunky'	9.5 oz	160	6.0	24.0	870	(mq)	4.0	0
(Campbell's) 'Healthy Request'	8 oz	90	4.0	13.0	420	na	2.0	2
(Campbell's) 'Home Cookin'	10.75 oz	140	4.0	22.0	1220	(mq)	3.0	na
(Campbell's) 'Home Cookin'	9.5 oz	120	4.0	20.0	1080	(mq)	3.0	na
(Hain)	9.5 oz	170	8.0	27.0	1060	(mq)	2.0	0
(Hain) 'No Salt Added'	9.5 oz	160	7.0	28.0	35	(mq)	4.0	0
(Health Valley)	7.5 oz	130	6.0	19.0	637	12.5	3.0	0
(Health Valley) 'No Salt Added'	7.5 oz	130	6.0	19.0	80	12.5	3.0	0
(Health Valley) 'Real Italian Fat-Free'	7.5 oz	80	8.0	12.0	290	4.0	0.0	0
(Healthy Choice)	7.5 oz	160	6.0	30.0	520	na	2.0	0
(Hormel) 'Hearty Soup'	7.5 oz	100	5.0	17.0	460	na	1.0	5
(Lipton) 'Hearty Ones'	11 oz	189	8.0	36.1	821	(mq)	3.2	6
(Progresso)	10.5 oz	120	7.0	25.0	930	7.0	3.0	0
(Progresso)	9.5 oz	130	7.0	22.0	1010	6.0	4.0	0
(Progresso) chunky, hearty	9.25 oz	110	7.0	16.0	740	(mq)	2.0	5
(Progresso) chunky, zesty	9.5 oz	150	7.0	19.0	1130	4.0	8.0	10
(Progresso) 'Healthy Classics'	8 oz	120	4.0	19.0	490	na	2.0	0
MUSHROOM, CREAM OF								
(Campbell's) 'Low Sodium'	10.5 oz	210	3.0	18.0	55	(mq)	14.0	(mq)
(Hain)	9.25 oz	110	4.0	16.0	740	(mq)	4.0	15
(Progresso)	9.25 oz	160	4.0	14.0	1120	(mq)	10.0	15
(Weight Watchers)	10.5 oz	90	3.0	14.0	1250	(mq)	2.0	na
MUSHROOM BARLEY								
(Hain)	9.5 oz	100	4.0	17.0	600	(mq)	2.0	10
(Health Valley)	7.5 oz	100	5.0	16.0	394	8.5	2.0	0
(Health Valley) 'No Salt Added'	7.5 oz	100	5.0	16.0	20	8.5	2.0	0
PEPPER STEAK								
(Campbell's) 'Chunky'	9.5 oz	160	12.0	21.0	920	(mq)	3.0	(mq)
(Campbell's) 'Chunky'	10.75 oz	180	14.0	24.0	1050	(mq)	3.0	(mq)
POTATO, CREAM OF *(Andersen's)*	7.5 oz	200	4.0	25.0	630	na	10.0	na
POTATO LEEK								
(Health Valley)	7.5 oz	130	4.0	23.0	360	7.4	2.0	0
(Health Valley) 'No Salt Added'	7.5 oz	130	4.0	23.0	20	7.4	2.0	0
SCHAV *(Gold's)*	8 oz	25	2.0	4.0	1380	na	0.0	15

Food Name	Serv. Size	Total Cal.	Prot. GMS	Carbs GMS	Sod. MGS	Fiber GMS	Fat GMS	Chol. MGS
SIRLOIN BURGER								
(Campbell's) 'Chunky'	10.75 oz	220	12.0	23.0	1240	na	9.0	(mq)
(Campbell's) 'Chunky'	9.5 oz	200	11.0	20.0	1090	na	8.0	(mq)
SPLIT PEA								
(Andersen's)	7.5 oz	130	9.0	24.0	770	na	0.0	na
(Campbell's) 'Low Sodium'	10.75 oz	230	12.0	37.0	30	(mq)	4.0	(mq)
(Grandma Brown's)	1 cup	208	11.7	31.0	522	5.8	4.1	<1
(Hain)	9.5 oz	170	11.0	28.0	970	(mq)	1.0	0
(Hain) 'No Salt Added'	9.5 oz	170	11.0	29.0	40	(mq)	1.0	0
(Progresso)	9.5 oz	160	11.0	27.0	1050	4.5	3.0	5
Green								
(Health Valley)	7.5 oz	190	11.0	34.0	276	14.7	0.3	0
(Health Valley) 'No Salt Added'	7.5 oz	190	11.0	34.0	25	14.7	0.3	0
(Hain) vegetarian	9.5 oz	170	11.0	28.0	970	(mq)	1.0	0
(Hain) vegetarian 'No Salt Added'	9.5 oz	170	13.0	27.0	70	(mq)	1.0	0
(Progresso)	10.5 oz	201	12.0	31.0	920	(mq)	3.0	na
W/ham								
(Campbell's) 'Chunky'	10.5 oz	230	12.0	33.0	1080	(mq)	6.0	(mq)
(Campbell's) 'Chunky'	9.5 oz	210	11.0	30.0	950	(mq)	5.0	(mq)
(Campbell's) 'Home Cookin'	10.75 oz	230	16.0	38.0	1310	(mq)	1.0	(mq)
(Campbell's) 'Home Cookin'	9.5 oz	200	14.0	34.0	1150	(mq)	1.0	(mq)
(Healthy Choice)	7.5 oz	170	10.0	25.0	460	na	3.0	10
(Progresso)	10.5 oz	160	11.0	24.0	980	6.0	5.0	15
(Progresso)	9.5 oz	150	11.0	23.0	880	5.0	5.0	15
STEAK AND POTATO								
(Campbell's) 'Chunky'	10.75 oz	200	14.0	24.0	1140	(mq)	5.0	(mq)
(Campbell's) 'Chunky'	9.5 oz	170	12.0	21.0	1000	(mq)	4.0	(mq)
TOMATO								
(Health Valley)	7.5 oz	100	2.0	17.0	450	1.2	3.0	0
(Health Valley) 'No Salt Added'	7.5 oz	100	2.0	17.0	40	1.2	3.0	0
(Healthy Choice) 'Tomato Garden'	7.5 oz	130	4.0	22.0	510	na	3.0	5
(Progresso)	9.5 oz	120	4.0	20.0	1100	(mq)	3.0	0
Beef, w/rotini *(Progresso)*	9.5 oz	170	12.0	18.0	930	(mq)	6.0	30
Garden								
(Campbell's) 'Home Cookin'	10.75 oz	150	2.0	29.0	930	(mq)	3.0	na
(Campbell's) 'Home Cookin'	9.5 oz	130	2.0	25.0	820	(mq)	2.0	na
W/tomato pieces *(Campbell's)* 'Low Sodium'	10.5 oz	190	4.0	30.0	45	(mq)	6.0	(mq)
W/tortellini *(Progresso)*	9.25 oz	130	5.0	16.0	1040	(mq)	5.0	10
TOMATO VEGETABLE, fat-free								
(Health Valley)	7.5 oz	50	5.0	8.0	290	3.0	0.0	0
TORTELLINI								
(Progresso)	9.5 oz	90	5.0	11.0	930	(mq)	3.0	10

Food Name	Serv. Size	Total Cal.	Prot. GMS	Carbs GMS	Sod. MGS	Fiber GMS	Fat GMS	Chol. MGS
(Progresso) Creamy	9.25 oz	240	5.0	17.0	910	(mq)	16.0	35
TURKEY	8 oz	135	10.2	14.1	923	>.9 c	4.4	9
TURKEY RICE								
(Hain)	9.5 oz	100	8.0	10.0	970	(mq)	3.0	20
(Hain) 'No Salt Added'	9.5 oz	120	7.0	13.0	85	(mq)	4.0	15
TURKEY VEGETABLE								
(Campbell's) 'Chunky'	9 3/8 oz	150	9.0	16.0	1060	(mq)	6.0	(mq)
(Weight Watchers)	10.5 oz	70	4.0	10.0	1020	(mq)	2.0	(mq)
VEGETABLE								
(Campbell's) 'Chunky'	10.75 oz	160	4.0	28.0	1100	(mq)	4.0	0
(Campbell's) 'Chunky'	9.5 oz	150	4.0	25.0	970	(mq)	4.0	0
(Health Valley)	7.5 oz	110	4.0	20.0	296	4.0	1.0	0
(Health Valley) 'No Salt Added'	7.5 oz	110	4.0	20.0	40	4.0	1.0	0
(Healthy Choice) 'Country Vegetable'	7.5 oz	120	3.0	23.0	540	na	1.0	0
(Progresso)	9.5 oz	80	4.0	15.0	1190	3.5	2.0	5
(Progresso) 'Healthy Classics'	8 oz	80	4.0	13.0	450	na	1.0	5
Country								
(Campbell's) 'Home Cookin'	10.75 oz	120	4.0	20.0	1070	(mq)	2.0	na
(Campbell's) 'Home Cookin'	9.5 oz	100	3.0	18.0	940	(mq)	2.0	na
(Hormel) 'Hearty Soup'	7.5 oz	90	4.0	14.0	730	na	2.0	2
Five bean, chunky								
(Health Valley)	7.5 oz	110	4.0	21.0	448	10.6	2.0	0
(Health Valley) 'No Salt Added'	7.5 oz	110	4.0	21.0	56	10.6	2.0	0
Fourteen garden vegetables, fat-free								
(Health Valley)	7.5 oz	50	4.0	9.0	260	3.0	0.0	0
Hearty *(Campbell's)* 'Healthy Request'	8 oz	90	3.0	17.0	480	na	1.0	0
Italian, w/pasta								
(Hain)	9.5 oz	160	4.0	25.0	910	(mq)	5.0	20
(Hain) 'Low Sodium'	9.5 oz	140	4.0	22.0	90	(mq)	6.0	20
Mediterranean *(Campbell's)* 'Chunky'	9.5 oz	170	4.0	24.0	1010	(mq)	6.0	na
Vegetarian								
chunky *(Weight Watchers)*	10.5 oz	100	3.0	18.0	1250	(mq)	2.0	0
(Hain)	9.5 oz	140	4.0	22.0	920	(mq)	4.0	0
(Hain) 'No Salt Added'	9.5 oz	150	5.0	23.0	45	(mq)	5.0	0
W/barley, fat-free *(Health Valley)*	7.5 oz	60	4.0	11.0	270	4.0	0.0	0
W/beef stock *(Weight Watchers)*	10.5 oz	90	4.0	13.0	1370	(mq)	2.0	(mq)
VEGETABLE BEEF								
(Campbell's) 'Chunky Low Sodium'	10.75 oz	180	14.0	19.0	90	(mq)	5.0	(mq)
(Campbell's) 'Chunky Old Fashioned'	10.75 oz	190	13.0	20.0	1100	(mq)	6.0	25
(Campbell's) 'Chunky Old Fashioned'	9.5 oz	160	12.0	17.0	970	(mq)	5.0	25
(Campbell's) hearty	8 oz	120	8.0	17.0	460	na	2.0	15
(Campbell's) 'Home Cookin'	10.75 oz	140	13.0	17.0	1160	(mq)	3.0	(mq)
(Campbell's) 'Home Cookin'	9.5 oz	120	11.0	15.0	1020	(mq)	2.0	(mq)

Food Name	Serv. Size	Total Cal.	Prot. GMS	Carbs GMS	Sod. MGS	Fiber GMS	Fat GMS	Chol. MGS
(Hormel) 'Hearty Soup'	7.5 oz	90	6.0	15.0	730	na	1.0	5
(Healthy Choice) 'Vegetable Beef'	7.5 oz	130	8.0	21.0	530	na	1.0	15
VEGETABLE BROTH								
(Hain)	9.5 oz	45	1.0	10.0	1180	na	0.0	0
(Hain) 'Low Sodium'	9.5 oz	40	1.0	8.0	85	na	<1.0	0
SOUP, FROZEN								
ASPARAGUS, CREAM OF								
(Kettle Ready)	6 oz	62	0.8	5.1	406	(mq)	4.3	na
(Myers)	9.75 oz	152	11.0	10.0	992	(mq)	8.0	na
BARLEY BEAN *(Tabatchnick)*	7.5 oz	130	6.0	22.0	217	(mq)	2.0	0
BEAN								
Northern bean *(Tabatchnick)*	7.5 oz	164	8.0	29.0	240	(mq)	2.0	0
Savory, w/ham *(Kettle Ready)*	6 oz	113	6.8	20.2	459	(mq)	3.6	(mq)
W/beef and vegetables, hearty								
(Kettle Ready)	6 oz	85	4.2	10.7	448	(mq)	3.0	(mq)
BLACK BEAN, w/ham *(Kettle Ready)*	6 oz	154	8.1	23.0	613	(mq)	6.2	(mq)
BROCCOLI, CREAM OF								
(Kettle Ready)	6 oz	94	0.9	6.4	417	(mq)	7.2	na
(Myers)	9.75 oz	174	8.0	11.0	905	(mq)	11.0	na
(Tabatchnick)	7.5 oz	90	4.0	10.0	285	(mq)	4.0	4
CABBAGE *(Tabatchnick)*	7.5 oz	110	2.0	21.0	185	(mq)	2.0	0
CAULIFLOWER, CREAM OF *(Kettle Ready)*	6 oz	93	2.3	5.5	445	(mq)	7.0	na
CHEDDAR CHEESE, CREAM OF								
(Kettle Ready)	6 oz	158	4.1	7.3	616	>.1 c	12.5	na
(Kettle Ready) w/broccoli	6 oz	137	4.0	4.7	533	na	11.3	na
CHEESE, w/broccoli *(Myers)*	9.75 oz	325	12.0	19.0	1257	(mq)	23.0	na
CHICKEN *(Tabatchnick)*	7.5 oz	65	2.0	10.0	255	na	2.0	0
CHICKEN, CREAM OF *(Kettle Ready)*	6 oz	98	5.7	5.0	668	na	6.2	(mq)
CHICKEN GUMBO *(Kettle Ready)*	6 oz	94	3.5	12.1	473	(mq)	3.5	(mq)
CHICKEN NOODLE								
(Kettle Ready)	6 oz	94	5.0	12.0	569	(mq)	3.0	(mq)
(Myers)	9.75 oz	87	8.0	5.0	1046	(mq)	5.0	(mq)
CHILI								
(Kettle Ready)	6 oz	161	11.7	14.0	454	(mq)	6.5	na
(Kettle Ready) jalapeño	6 oz	173	11.0	14.7	531	(mq)	8.0	na
CLAM CHOWDER								
Boston *(Kettle Ready)*	6 oz	131	3.5	13.0	417	(mq)	7.3	(mq)
Manhattan style *(Kettle Ready)*	6 oz	69	3.6	8.0	549	(mq)	2.6	(mq)
New England style								
(Kettle Ready)	6 oz	116	3.0	11.4	373	(mq)	6.5	(mq)
(Myers)	9.75 oz	152	7.0	21.0	910	(mq)	5.0	(mq)
(Stouffer's)	8 oz	180	8.0	16.0	790	(mq)	9.0	(mq)
(Tabatchnick)	7.5 oz	98	6.0	14.0	255	(mq)	2.0	0

Food Name	Serv. Size	Total Cal.	Prot. GMS	Carbs GMS	Sod. MGS	Fiber GMS	Fat GMS	Chol. MGS
CORN CHOWDER w/broccoli *(Kettle Ready)*	6 oz	102	1.4	13.0	323	(mq)	5.0	na
LENTIL *(Tabatchnick)*	7.5 oz	170	11.0	27.0	240	(mq)	2.0	0
MINESTRONE								
(Kettle Ready) hearty	6 oz	104	3.3	15.2	577	(mq)	4.4	na
(Tabatchnick)	7.5 oz	137	8.0	24.0	265	(mq)	2.0	0
MUSHROOM, CREAM OF								
(Kettle Ready)	6 oz	85	0.6	6.2	371	(mq)	6.4	na
(Tabatchnick)	6 oz	75	3.0	11.0	325	(mq)	2.0	3
MUSHROOM BARLEY								
(Tabatchnick)	7.5 oz	92	2.0	16.0	234	(mq)	2.0	0
(Tabatchnick) 'No Salt'	7.5 oz	97	4.0	18.0	77	(mq)	1.0	0
ONION, French *(Kettle Ready)*	6 oz	42	0.7	5.0	562	(mq)	2.2	na
PEA								
(Tabatchnick)	7.5 oz	175	10.0	31.0	290	(mq)	1.0	0
(Tabatchnick) 'No Salt'	7.5 oz	175	10.0	31.0	79	(mq)	1.0	0
SEAFOOD BISQUE *(Myers)*	9.75 oz	163	9.0	13.0	1393	na	8.0	(mq)
SPINACH, CREAM OF								
(Myers)	9.75 oz	174	9.0	10.0	905	(mq)	11.0	na
(Stouffer's)	8 oz	210	7.0	12.0	1020	(mq)	15.0	na
(Tabatchnick)	7.5 oz	85	5.0	12.0	200	(mq)	2.0	4
SPLIT PEA W/HAM *(Kettle Ready)*	6 oz	155	11.1	25.3	483	(mq)	4.4	(mq)
TOMATO RICE *(Tabatchnick)*	6 oz	73	2.0	14.0	300	(mq)	1.0	0
TOMATO TORTELLINI *(Kettle Ready)*	6 oz	122	3.5	15.0	447	(mq)	5.4	na
VEGETABLE								
(Kettle Ready) garden	6 oz	85	2.6	12.3	296	(mq)	3.0	na
(Tabatchnick)	7.5 oz	97	4.0	18.0	190	(mq)	1.0	0
(Tabatchnick) 'No Salt'	7.5 oz	92	2.0	16.0	77	(mq)	2.0	0
VEGETABLE BEEF *(Myers)*	9.75 oz	120	9.0	8.0	1030	(mq)	6.0	(mq)
ZUCCHINI *(Tabatchnick)*	6 oz	80	3.0	12.0	285	(mq)	2.0	3
SOUP, MICROWAVE								
BEAN								
W/bacon and ham *(Campbell's)*	7.5 oz	230	8.0	38.0	830	(mq)	5.0	(mq)
W/ham, chowder *(Hormel)* 'Micro-Cup Hearty Soups'	1 pkg	191	10.0	31.0	664	(mq)	3.0	30
BEEF, w/vegetable *(Hormel)* 'Micro-Cup Hearty Soups'	1 pkg	71	5.0	12.0	811	(mq)	1.0	9
CHICKEN								
W/rice *(Campbell's)* 'Microwave'	7.5 oz	100	3.0	14.0	820	(mq)	4.0	(mq)
W/vegetables and rice *(Hormel)* 'Micro-Cup Hearty Soups'	1 pkg	114	5.0	16.0	1025	(mq)	3.0	7
CHICKEN NOODLE								
(Campbell's) 'Microwave'	7.5 oz	100	5.0	11.0	870	(mq)	4.0	(mq)
(Hormel) 'Micro-Cup Hearty Soups'	1 pkg	108	7.0	14.0	686	(mq)	3.0	22

Food Name	Serv. Size	Total Cal.	Prot. GMS	Carbs GMS	Sod. MGS	Fiber GMS	Fat GMS	Chol. MGS
(Lunch Bucket) microwave cup	7.25 oz	90	4.0	13.0	810	na	2.0	25
(Weight Watchers) microwave cup	7.5 oz	90	8.0	13.0	450	na	1.0	15
CHILI BEEF (Campbell's) 'Microwave'	7.5 oz	190	7.0	32.0	870	(mq)	4.0	(mq)
CLAM CHOWDER, New England (Hormel)								
'Micro-Cup Hearty Soups'	1 pkg	118	5.0	15.0	882	(mq)	5.0	30
MINESTRONE (Hormel) 'Micro-Cup								
Hearty Soups'	1 pkg	104	7.0	15.0	903	(mq)	2.0	10
NOODLE								
Beef flavor (Campbell's) 'Cup Microwave'	1.35 oz	130	6.0	23.0	1270	(mq)	2.0	(mq)
Chicken flavor (Campbell's)								
'Cup Microwave'	1.35 oz	140	7.0	22.0	1340	(mq)	3.0	na
Pork flavor, w/vegetables (Campbell's)								
'Hearty Microwave'	1.7 oz	180	7.0	32.0	1320	(mq)	2.0	na
W/chicken broth (Campbell's)								
'Cup Microwave'	1.35 oz	130	6.0	23.0	1360	(mq)	2.0	na
VEGETABLE, country								
(Hormel) 'Micro-Cup Hearty Soups'	1 pkg	89	5.0	13.0	865	(mq)	2.0	1
(Lunch Bucket) microwave cup	7.25 oz	70	1.0	15.0	740	na	1.0	0
VEGETABLE BEEF								
(Campbell's) 'Microwave'	7.5 oz	100	5.0	16.0	830	(mq)	2.0	(mq)
(Weight Watchers) microwave cup	7.5 oz	90	8.0	13.0	450	na	1.0	10
SOUP MIX								
(NOTE: Unless otherwise specified, PREPARED = prepared as directed w/water.)								
ASPARAGUS, prepared	8 oz	52	2.0	7.9	707	.3	1.5	0
ASPARAGUS, CREAM OF, prepared	8 oz	58	2.2	8.9	800	na	1.7	0
BEAN W/BACON, prepared	1 cup	106	5.5	16.4	927	9.0	2.2	3
BEEF								
Beef flavor, w/noodles								
(Campbell's) 'Ramen Noodle' prepared	6 oz	160	5.0	32.0	890	(mq)	1.0	na
(Estee) prepared	6 oz	20	1.0	3.0	140	(mq)	<1.0	<1
(Lipton) 'Cup-A-Soup' prepared	6 oz	44	1.7	7.6	746	na	0.7	na
(Lipton) 'Hearty' prepared	6 oz	107	3.5	20.2	698	>.2 c	1.4	na
Beef flavor, w/noodles and vegetables								
(Campbell's) prepared	6 oz	220	7.0	44.0	1600	(mq)	2.0	na
Broth								
cubed	1 cube	6	0.6	0.6	864	0	0.1	0
cubed, prepared	6 oz	5	0.6	0.6	869	0	0.1	0
powder, prepared	8 oz	20	1.3	1.9	1362	0	0.7	0
Hearty (Soup Starter) 'Homestyle'	.945 oz	90	2.0	20.0	740	na	<1.0	0
Vegetable (Soup Starter) 'Homestyle'	.91 oz	90	3.0	18.0	790	na	<1.0	0
W/noodles (Ultra Slim Fast) 1 envelope,								
prepared	6 oz	45	5.0	7.0	700	2.0	<1.0	5
BEEF NOODLE, prepared	8 oz	40	2.2	6.0	1042	.8	0.8	3

Food Name	Serv. Size	Total Cal.	Prot. GMS	Carbs GMS	Sod. MGS	Fiber GMS	Fat GMS	Chol. MGS
BLACK BEAN								
(Fantastic Foods) 'Jumpin' black beans, prepared	10 oz	170	12.0	40.0	490	13.0	1.0	0
BROCCOLI								
Creamy								
(Lipton) 'Cup-A-Soup' prepared	6 oz	62	1.1	9.1	610	>.3 c	2.4	na
(Lipton) 'Cup-A-Soup Food Service' prepared	6 oz	62	1.7	8.9	658	(mq)	2.3	na
(Ultra Slim Fast) 1 envelope, prepared	6 oz	75	5.0	14.0	800	2.0	<1.0	0
Golden *(Lipton)* 'Cup-A-Soup Lite' prepared	6 oz	42	1.3	16.3	427	(mq)	1.2	1
W/cheese *(Lipton)* 'Cup-A-Soup' prepared	6 oz	70	1.7	9.8	595	(mq)	3.4	na
BOUILLON								
Beef flavor								
cubed	1 cube	6	0.6	0.6	864	(tr)	0.1	tr
cubed *(Steero)*	1 cube	6	<1.0	1.0	930	(tr)	<1.0	na
cubed *(Wyler's)*	1 cube	6	<1.0	1.0	930	(tr)	<1.0	na
instant *(Featherweight)*	1 tsp	18	0.0	2.0	10	(tr)	1.0	5
instant *(Lite-Line)* 'Low Sodium'	1 tsp	12	<1.0	2.0	5	(tr)	<1.0	na
instant *(Steero)*	1 tsp	6	<1.0	1.0	930	(tr)	<1.0	na
instant *(Weight Watchers)* 'Broth Mix'	1 pkt	8	1.0	1.0	930	(tr)	0.0	0
instant *(Wyler's)*	1 tsp	6	<1.0	1.0	930	(tr)	<1.0	na
powder	1 pkt	14	1.0	1.4	1019	0	0.5	1
powder, prepared	8 oz	19	1.3	1.9	1359	0	0.7	1
Brown								
(G. Washington's) 'Seasoning & Broth'	.14 oz	6	0.0	1.0	1015	(tr)	0.0	0
(G. Washington's) 'Seasoning & Broth' kosher	.14 oz	6	0.0	1.0	1110	(tr)	0.0	0
Chicken flavor								
cubed	1 cube	9	0.7	1.1	1152	(tr)	0.2	1
cubed *(Steero)*	1 cube	8	<1.0	1.0	990	(tr)	<1.0	na
cubed *(Wyler's)*	1 cube	8	<1.0	1.0	900	(tr)	<1.0	na
instant *(Featherweight)*	1 tsp	18	0.0	2.0	5	(tr)	1.0	5
instant *(Lite-Line)* 'Low Sodium'	1 tsp	12	<1.0	2.0	5	(tr)	<1.0	na
instant *(Steero)*	1 tsp	8	<1.0	1.0	990	(tr)	<1.0	na
instant *(Weight Watchers)* 'Broth Mix'	1 pkt	8	1.0	1.0	990	(tr)	0.0	0
instant *(Wyler's)*	1 tsp	8	<1.0	1.0	900	(tr)	<1.0	na
Golden								
(G. Washington's) 'Seasoning & Broth'	.13 oz	6	0.0	1.0	935	(tr)	0.0	0
(G. Washington's) 'Seasoning & Broth' kosher	.13 oz	6	0.0	1.0	1015	(tr)	0.0	0
Onion flavor								
(G. Washington's) 'Seasoning and Broth'	.18 oz	12	1.0	2.0	695	(tr)	0.0	0
(Wyler's) instant	1 tsp	10	<1.0	1.0	670	(tr)	<1.0	0

Food Name	Serv. Size	Total Cal.	Prot. GMS	Carbs GMS	Sod. MGS	Fiber GMS	Fat GMS	Chol. MGS
Vegetable flavor								
(G. Washington's) 'Seasoning & Broth'	.18 oz	12	1.0	2.0	715	(tr)	0.0	0
(Wyler's) instant	1 tsp	6	<1.0	1.0	910	(tr)	<1.0	0
CAULIFLOWER, prepared	8 oz	69	2.9	10.7	843	>.2 c	1.7	0
CELERY, prepared	8 oz	63	2.6	9.8	838	>.2 c	1.6	0
CHEESE								
(Fantastic Noodles) creamy cheddar								
w/noodles, prepared	7 oz	178	7.0	21.0	578	(mq)	8.0	na
(Hain) cheese and broccoli, prepared	6 oz	310	7.0	19.0	980	(mq)	22.0	na
(Hain) 'Savory Soup & Sauce Mix' prepared	6 oz	250	6.0	20.0	890	na	16.0	na
CHICKEN								
prepared	8 oz	107	1.8	13.3	1185	.3	5.3	3
(Soup Starter) 'Homestyle'	.735 oz	70	2.0	15.0	770	na	<1.0	10
Broth								
cubed	1 cube	10	0.7	1.1	1152	0	0.2	1
cubed, prepared	6 oz	9	0.7	1.1	593	0	0.2	0
(Lipton) 'Cup-A-Soup' prepared	6 oz	20	0.4	3.3	605	na	0.6	1
Creamy, w/vegetables (Lipton) prepared	6 oz	93	1.7	14.4	708	(mq)	3.1	na
Creamy, w/white meat (Campbell's) prepared	6 oz	90	3.0	12.0	1020	na	4.0	(mq)
Florentine (Lipton) 'Lite'	6 oz	42	10.0	7.6	481	na	0.5	6
Hearty								
(Lipton) 'Country Style'	6 oz	69	3.8	11.1	688	na	1.1	na
(Lipton) 'Supreme' prepared	6 oz	107	2.0	11.4	848	na	5.9	na
Lemon (Lipton) 'Cup-A-Soup Lite' prepared	6 oz	48	2.0	9.1	419	na	0.4	4
W/corn (Lipton) 'Country' prepared	6 oz	133	3.3	17.5	704	>.2 c	5.5	na
W/noodles (Ultra Slim Fast) 1 envelope,								
prepared	6 oz	45	5.0	6.0	970	2.0	<1.0	5
CHICKEN, CREAM OF								
(Lipton) 'Cup-A-Soup' prepared	6 oz	84	1.4	9.7	757	na	4.4	na
(Lipton) 'Food Service' prepared	6 oz	84	1.7	9.4	840	na	4.4	na
CHICKEN LEEK								
creamy (Ultra Slim Fast) 1 envelope,								
prepared	6 oz	50	5.0	7.0	1070	2.0	<1.0	2
CHICKEN NOODLE								
prepared	1 cup	53	3.0	7.4	1284	.8	1.2	3
(Campbell's) 'Lowfat Block' prepared	1 cup	160	5.0	32.0	940	(mq)	1.0	na
(Campbell's) 'Quality Recipe' prepared	1 cup	100	5.0	16.0	710	(mq)	2.0	na
(Campbell's) 'Ramen Noodle' prepared	1 cup	190	5.0	26.0	970	(mq)	8.0	na
(Estee) 'Instant' prepared	6 oz	25	1.0	4.0	135	(mq)	<1.0	<1
(Lipton) 'Cup-A-Soup' prepared	6 oz	48	3.0	6.6	635	(mq)	1.1	na
(Lipton) 'Supreme' prepared	6 oz	107	1.7	11.8	757	(mq)	5.9	na
(Mrs. Grass) 'Chickeny Rich'	1/4 pkg	70	2.0	10.0	900	(mq)	2.0	na
Creamy, hearty (Lipton) prepared	7 oz	179	5.1	21.4	639	(mq)	8.2	na

Food Name	Serv. Size	Total Cal.	Prot. GMS	Carbs GMS	Sod. MGS	Fiber GMS	Fat GMS	Chol. MGS
Hearty								
(Lipton) prepared	1 cup	83	4.4	13.3	753	(mq)	1.3	na
(Lipton) prepared	7 oz	118	4.8	21.2	655	(mq)	1.5	na
W/meat								
(Campbell's) white meat	6 oz	90	6.0	12.0	770	(mq)	2.0	(mq)
(Lipton) 'Cup' prepared	6 oz	46	2.6	6.6	660	(mq)	1.0	(mq)
(Lipton) 'Value Pack' prepared	6 oz	46	2.6	6.6	660	(mq)	1.0	(mq)
(Lipton) white meat, diced, prepared	1 cup	81	4.3	12.1	795	(mq)	1.8	(mq)
W/rice (Lipton) prepared	6 oz	47	2.2	7.7	667	(mq)	0.8	na
W/vegetables								
(Campbell's) prepared	1 cup	270	6.0	38.0	1470	(mq)	10.0	na
(Campbell's) lowfat, prepared	1 cup	220	7.0	44.0	1500	(mq)	2.0	na
(Lipton) 'Cup' prepared	6 oz	47	2.5	7.8	566	>.2 c	0.6	8
(Lipton) hearty, prepared	1 cup	75	3.0	12.3	687	(mq)	1.6	na
CHICKEN RICE, prepared	8 oz	61	2.5	9.3	981	0	1.4	3
CHICKEN VEGETABLE, prepared	8 oz	50	2.7	7.8	807	>.3 c	0.8	3
CHILI PEPPER (A Taste of Thai) hot and sour,								
prepared	1 cup	40	0.0	5.0	1330	0	2.0	0
CLAM CHOWDER								
Manhattan style (Golden Dipt)	1/4 pkg	80	2.0	13.0	700	(mq)	2.0	3
New England style (Golden Dipt)	1/4 pkg	70	2.0	12.0	680	(mq)	2.0	2
CONSOMMÉ, w/gelatin, prepared	1 cup	17	2.2	2.1	3299	0	0.0	0
GINGER (A Taste of Thai) tangy coconut,								
prepared	1 cup	250	3.0	3.0	1050	0	1.5	0
GREEN PEA								
(Lipton) 'Cup-A-Soup' prepared	6 oz	113	4.2	14.4	553	>.2 c	4.2	na
(Lipton) 'Cup-A-Soup Food Service'								
prepared	6 oz	115	3.5	15.1	635	>.7 c	4.5	na
HERB (Lipton) savory, w/garlic								
'Recipe Secrets' prepared	8 oz	35	<1.0	7.0	490	na	<1.0	na
LEEK								
Creamy (Ultra Slim Fast) 1 envelope								
prepared	6 oz	80	5.0	15.0	780	2.0	<1.0	0
LENTIL (Hain) 'Savory Soup Mix' prepared	6 oz	130	4.0	20.0	810	(mq)	2.0	na
LOBSTER BISQUE (Golden Dipt)								
prepared	1/4 pkg	30	1.0	5.0	560	na	1.0	2
MINESTRONE								
(Hain) 'Savory Soup Mix' prepared	6 oz	110	4.0	20.0	870	(mq)	1.0	na
(Manischewitz) prepared	6 oz	50	3.0	9.0	160	(mq)	<1.0	na
MUSHROOM								
(Estee) 'Instant' prepared	6 oz	40	1.0	3.0	115	(mq)	2.0	10
(Hain) 'Savory Soup & Recipe Mix'								
prepared	6 oz	210	4.0	11.0	710	(mq)	15.0	na

Food Name	Serv. Size	Total Cal.	Prot. GMS	Carbs GMS	Sod. MGS	Fiber GMS	Fat GMS	Chol. MGS
(Hain) 'Savory Soup & Recipe Mix No Salt Added' prepared	6 oz	250	5.0	15.0	180	(mq)	20.0	na
Beef flavor *(Lipton)* prepared	1 cup	38	1.7	6.7	763	(mq)	0.5	na
MUSHROOM, CREAM OF *(Lipton)*								
'Cup-A-Soup' prepared	6 oz	71	1.3	9.1	756	(mq)	3.2	na
NOODLE								
(Campbell's) 'Quality Soup & Recipe' prepared	1 cup	110	5.0	19.0	700	(mq)	2.0	na
(Lipton) 'Cup-A-Soup Ring Noodle' prepared	6 oz	47	2.7	7.6	650	(mq)	0.7	na
(Lipton) 'Giggle Noodle' prepared	1 cup	77	2.9	11.4	784	(mq)	2.1	na
(Lipton) 'Ring-O-Noodle' prepared	1 cup	71	2.7	10.4	784	(mq)	2.0	na
Beef flavor								
(Cup O'Noodles) prepared	1 cup	290	8.0	33.0	1490	(mq)	14.0	na
(Oodles of Noodles) prepared	1 cup	390	9.0	49.0	1810	(mq)	18.0	na
(Top Ramen) prepared	1 cup	390	9.0	49.0	1810	(mq)	18.0	na
Beefy, w/vegetables *(Lipton)* prepared	1 cup	85	2.5	16.7	810	(mq)	0.9	na
Chicken flavor								
(Cup O'Noodles) prepared	1 cup	300	9.0	32.0	1790	(mq)	16.0	na
(Cup O'Noodles) 'Hearty' prepared	1 cup	300	8.0	35.0	1210	(mq)	14.0	na
(Oodles of Noodles) prepared	1 cup	400	10.0	48.0	1910	(mq)	18.0	na
(Top Ramen) prepared	1 cup	400	10.0	48.0	1910	(mq)	18.0	na
Hearty *(Campbell's)* 'Quality Soup & Recipe' prepared	1 cup	90	4.0	15.0	840	(mq)	1.0	na
Hearty, w/vegetables *(Lipton)* prepared	1 cup	75	3.0	12.3	687	(mq)	1.6	na
Oriental								
(Campbell's) 'Ramen Noodle' prepared	1 cup	190	5.0	26.0	930	(mq)	8.0	na
(Campbell's) 'Ramen Noodle Lowfat Block' prepared	1 cup	150	5.0	31.0	940	(mq)	1.0	na
(Oodles of Noodles) prepared	1 cup	390	10.0	49.0	1660	(mq)	18.0	na
(Top Ramen) prepared	1 cup	390	10.0	49.0	1660	(mq)	18.0	na
Oriental, w/vegetables								
(Campbell's) 'Cup-A-Ramen' prepared	1 cup	270	6.0	38.0	1210	(mq)	10.0	na
(Campbell's) 'Cup-A-Ramen Lowfat' prepared	1 cup	220	7.0	44.0	1400	(mq)	2.0	na
Pork flavor								
(Campbell's) 'Ramen Noodle' prepared	1 cup	200	5.0	26.0	860	(mq)	8.0	na
(Campbell's) 'Ramen Noodle Lowfat Block' prepared	1 cup	150	4.0	31.0	1140	(mq)	1.0	na
(Oodles of Noodles) prepared	1 cup	390	10.0	51.0	2060	(mq)	20.0	na
(Top Ramen) prepared	1 cup	390	10.0	51.0	2060	(mq)	20.0	na
Pork flavor, w/old-fashioned vegetables								
(Cup O'Noodles) 'Hearty' prepared	6 oz	290	6.0	34.0	1250	(mq)	15.0	na

Food Name	Serv. Size	Total Cal.	Prot. GMS	Carbs GMS	Sod. MGS	Fiber GMS	Fat GMS	Chol. MGS
Pork flavor, w/seafood (Cup O'Noodles)								
'Hearty' prepared .... 1 cup		300	7.0	34.0	1170	(mq)	15.0	na
Pork flavor, w/shrimp (Cup O'Noodles)								
prepared .... 1 cup		300	10.0	32.0	1480	(mq)	14.0	na
W/chicken broth								
(Campbell's) 'Cup 2 Minute Soup' prepared	6 oz	90	4.0	15.0	910	(mq)	2.0	na
(Campbell's) 'Double Noodle'	1.78 oz	200	8.0	36.0	770	na	2.0	na
(Campbell's) 'Double Noodle' prepared ...	8 oz	200	8.0	36.0	770	na	2.0	na
ONION								
(Campbell's) 'Quality Soup & Recipe'								
prepared .... 1 cup		30	1.0	7.0	700	(mq)	0.0	0
(Estee) prepared	6 oz	25	1.0	4.0	140	(mq)	<1.0	0
(Hain) 'Savory Soup, Dip & Recipe Mix'								
prepared	6 oz	50	2.0	6.0	900	(mq)	2.0	na
(Hain) 'Savory Soup, Dip & Recipe Mix'								
no salt, prepared	6 oz	50	1.0	9.0	470	(mq)	1.0	na
(Lipton) prepared .... 1 cup		20	0.7	4.3	632	(mq)	0.2	na
(Lipton) 'Cup-A-Soup' prepared	6 oz	27	0.9	4.7	665	>.1 c	0.5	na
(Mrs. Grass) 'Soup & Dip Mix' prepared	1/4 pkg	35	1.0	6.0	1070	(mq)	<1.0	0
Beefy (Lipton) prepared .... 1 cup		29	0.8	4.2	803	(mq)	1.0	na
Creamy								
(Lipton) 'Cup-A-Soup' prepared	6 oz	70	1.2	9.5	678	>.2 c	3.2	na
(Ultra Slim Fast) 1 envelope, prepared ...	6 oz	45	5.0	7.0	1180	2.0	<1.0	0
Golden, w/chicken broth (Lipton) prepared	1 cup	62	1.1	11.0	716	(mq)	1.5	na
Mushroom (Lipton) prepared	1 cup	41	1.4	6.8	684	(mq)	0.9	na
ORIENTAL (Lipton) 'Cup-A-Soup Lite'								
prepared	6 oz	45	1.5	5.8	457	na	1.7	3
OXTAIL prepared	8 oz	71	2.8	9.0	1210	.5	2.6	3
POTATO LEEK (Hain) 'Savory Soup Mix'								
prepared	6 oz	260	4.0	20.0	690	(mq)	18.0	na
SEAFOOD CHOWDER (Golden Dipt) ...	1/4 pkg	70	2.0	12.0	730	na	2.0	2
SHRIMP								
Bisque (Golden Dipt) dry mix	1/4 pkg	30	1.0	5.0	570	na	1.0	2
W/vegetables								
(Campbell's) 'Cup-A-Ramen' prepared ...	1 cup	280	6.0	40.0	1190	(mq)	10.0	na
(Campbell's) 'Lowfat' prepared	1 cup	230	7.0	45.0	1290	(mq)	2.0	na
SPLIT PEA								
Green								
(Hain) 'Savory Soup Mix' prepared	6 oz	310	4.0	16.0	940	(mq)	10.0	na
(Manischewitz) prepared	6 oz	45	3.0	9.0	320	(mq)	<1.0	0
Fat-free, thick and creamy (Fantastic Foods)								
'Splittin Pea'	10 oz	145	13.0	31.0	490	3.0	1.0	0
W/carrots (Health Valley)	7.5 oz	80	9.0	17.0	290	12.5	0.0	0

Food Name	Serv. Size	Total Cal.	Prot. GMS	Carbs GMS	Sod. MGS	Fiber GMS	Fat GMS	Chol. MGS
TOMATO								
(Estee) 'Instant' prepared	6 oz	40	1.0	5.0	95	(mq)	<1.0	0
(Hain) 'Savory Soup & Recipe Mix' prepared	6 oz	220	3.0	19.0	770	(mq)	14.0	na
(Lipton) 'Cup-A-Soup' prepared	6 oz	103	2.5	21.2	524	(mq)	0.9	na
(Lipton) 'Cup-A-Soup Food Service' prepared	6 oz	100	2.8	20.1	563	(mq)	0.9	na
Creamy *(Ultra Slim Fast)* 1 envelope, prepared	6 oz	60	5.0	10.0	990	2.0	<1.0	0
Creamy, w/herb *(Lipton)* 'Cup-A-Soup Lite' prepared	6 oz	66	1.6	14.1	305	(mq)	0.3	2
Minestrone *(Cous•cous)*	10 oz	200	9.0	41.0	590	na	0.0	na
TOMATO VEGETABLE								
prepared	8 oz	56	2.0	10.2	1146	.5	0.9	0
W/noodles *(Fantastic Noodles)* prepared	7 oz	158	5.0	20.0	434	(mq)	8.0	na
VEGETABLE								
(Campbell's) 'Quality Soup & Recipe' prepared	1 cup	40	1.0	8.0	710	(mq)	0.0	0
(Hain) 'Savory Soup Mix' prepared	6 oz	80	2.0	13.0	730	(mq)	1.0	na
(Hain) 'Savory Soup Mix No Salt Added' prepared	6 oz	80	2.0	13.0	330	(mq)	1.0	na
(Lipton) prepared	1 cup	39	1.6	6.9	640	>.4 c	0.5	na
(Manischewitz) prepared	6 oz	50	3.0	9.0	65	(mq)	<1.0	0
Country *(Lipton)* prepared	1 cup	80	2.6	15.7	803	(mq)	0.7	na
Curry, w/noodles *(Fantastic Noodles)* prepared	7 oz	150	5.0	18.0	472	(mq)	7.0	na
Garden *(Lipton)* 'Lots-A-Noodles Cup-A-Soup' prepared	7 oz	123	4.3	23.1	720	(mq)	1.5	na
Harvest								
(Lipton) 'Country Style' prepared	6 oz	95	2.0	18.9	569	>.5 c	1.2	na
(Lipton) 'Cup-A-Soup Country Style' prepared	6 oz	91	1.7	18.8	459	>.5 c	1.2	na
Hearty *(Ultra Slim Fast)* 1 envelope, prepared	6 oz	45	5.0	5.0	850	2.0	<1.0	0
Miso, w/noodles *(Fantastic Noodles)* prepared	7 oz	152	5.0	19.0	434	(mq)	7.0	na
Noodle, w/meatballs *(Lipton)* 'Country Style' prepared	6 oz	95	4.9	15.4	764	>.5 c	1.6	na
Parmesan *(Cous•cous)*	10 oz	200	9.0	35.0	550	na	3.0	na
Spring *(Lipton)* 'Cup-A-Soup' prepared	6 oz	33	1.1	5.9	746	>.3 c	0.8	6
VEGETABLE BEEF, prepared	8 oz	53	2.9	8.0	1002	.5	1.1	0
VIRGINIA PEA								
(Lipton) prepared	6 oz	113	4.7	14.6	664	>.4 c	4.1	<1

Food Name	Serv. Size	Total Cal.	Prot. GMS	Carbs GMS	Sod. MGS	Fiber GMS	Fat GMS	Chol. MGS
(Lipton) 'Country Style' prepared	6 oz	148	5.3	17.3	828	>.8 c	6.4	na
SOUR CREAM								
	1 cup	493	7.3	9.8	123	0	48.2	102
	1 oz	61	0.9	1.2	15	0	5.9	13
	1 tbsp	26	0.4	0.5	6	0	2.5	5
(Bison)	1 oz	50	1.0	1.0	15	0	5.0	20
(Breakstone's)	1 tbsp	30	0.0	1.0	5	0	3.0	10
(Crowley)	1 oz	50	1.0	1.0	15	0	5.0	20
(Darigold)	1 tbsp	23	0.9	1.1	5	0	2.8	5
(Friendship)	2 tbsp	55	1.0	1.0	15	0	5.0	42
(Knudsen) 'Hampshire'	1 oz	60	1.0	1.0	10	0	6.0	20
(Sealtest)	1 tbsp	30	0.0	1.0	5	0	3.0	10
French onion *(Crowley)*	1 oz	50	1.0	1.0	130	0	5.0	20
Pasteurized, 100% natural *(Alta•Dena)*	1 oz	60	1.0	1.0	15	0	6.0	na
W/acidophilus, cultured *(Alta•Dena)* 'Kefir'	1 oz	70	1.0	1.0	40	0	6.0	na
W/chives *(Land O'Lakes)* 'Light'	2 tbsp	40	2.0	4.0	150	na	2.0	5
HALF AND HALF								
(Breakstone's) 'Light Choice'	1 tbsp	25	1.0	1.0	10	0	2.0	5
(Sealtest) 'Light'	1 tbsp	25	1.0	1.0	10	0	2.0	5
Cultured	1 tbsp	20	0.4	0.6	6	0	1.8	6
LIGHT/LOW-FAT								
(Crowley)	1 oz	30	1.0	2.0	25	0	2.0	5
(Friendship) 'Lite Delite'	2 tbsp	35	1.0	2.0	25	0	2.0	8
(Knudsen)	1 oz	40	1.0	2.0	20	0	3.0	10
(Land O'Lakes) 'Light'	2 tbsp	40	2.0	4.0	35	na	2.0	5
(Naturally Yours) 'Real•Dairy' no fat	2 tbsp	15	3.0	1.0	15	na	0.0	0
(Weight Watchers)	2 tbsp	35	2.0	2.0	40	0	2.0	(mq)
SOUR CREAM, ALTERNATIVE/NONDAIRY								
	1 cup	479	5.5	15.3	235	0	44.9	0
	1 oz	59	0.7	1.9	29	0	5.5	0
(Crowley) dressing	1 oz	40	1.0	1.0	5	0	4.0	0
(Pet)	1 tbsp	25	<1.0	<1.0	25	0	2.0	<1
Cultured								
	1 cup	479	5.5	15.2	235	0	44.9	40
	1 oz	58	0.7	1.9	29	0	5.5	0
(Light n' Lively) nonfat	1 tbsp	10	1.0	1.0	30	na	0.0	10
SOURSOP. See GUANABANA.								
SOY BEVERAGE								
(Edensoy) 'Extra' original	8.45 oz	140	10.0	14.0	110	na	4.0	na
(Edensoy) original	8.45 oz	140	10.0	14.0	120	na	4.0	0
(Health Valley) fat-free 'Soy Moo'	1 cup	110	7.0	19.0	25	0	0.0	0
(Soyamel) powdered mix, prepared	8 oz	130	7.0	10.0	210	na	7.0	0
(WestSoy) 'Lite' plain	8 oz	100	4.0	16.0	100	na	2.0	0

Food Name	Serv. Size	Total Cal.	Prot. GMS	Carbs GMS	Sod. MGS	Fiber GMS	Fat GMS	Chol. MGS
(WestSoy) 'Natural' original	8 oz	150	7.0	18.0	115	na	5.0	0
(WestSoy) 'Natural' unsweetened	8 oz	100	7.0	5.0	40	na	5.0	0
(WestSoy) 'Plus' plain	8 oz	150	6.0	18.0	140	na	5.0	0
ALMOND FLAVOR								
(WestSoy) 'Lite'	6 oz	160	5.0	26.0	140	na	4.0	0
(WestSoy) 'Natural'	6 oz	250	7.0	31.0	140	(mq)	11.0	0
BANANA FLAVOR *(WestSoy)* 'Lite'								
creamy banana	6 oz	160	5.0	26.0	140	na	3.0	0
CAROB FLAVOR								
(Ah Soy)	6 oz	160	4.0	30.0	120	(mq)	3.0	0
(Edensoy)	8.45 oz	160	6.0	30.0	125	na	5.0	0
(WestSoy) 'Plus'	8 oz	160	6.0	21.0	80	na	5.0	0
Malted								
(WestSoy) 'Lite'	6 oz	160	5.0	27.0	140	na	3.0	0
(WestSoy) 'Natural'	6 oz	270	7.0	37.0	120	(mq)	11.0	0
CHOCOLATE FLAVOR *(Ah Soy)*	6 oz	160	5.0	29.0	120	(mq)	3.0	0
COCOA FLAVOR								
(WestSoy) 'Lite'	8 oz	140	3.0	27.0	95	na	2.0	10
(WestSoy) 'Lite' w/mint	6 oz	160	5.0	26.0	140	na	3.0	0
COFFEE FLAVOR *(WestSoy)* 'Natural'								
java malted	6 oz	270	7.0	37.0	140	(mq)	11.0	0
VANILLA FLAVOR								
(Ah Soy)	6 oz	160	5.0	23.0	140	(mq)	5.0	0
(Edensoy) 'Extra'	8.45 oz	150	8.0	25.0	95	3.0	3.0	na
(Edensoy) 'Natural Vanilla'	8.45 oz	150	8.0	25.0	140	na	3.0	0
(WestSoy) 'Lite'	8 oz	110	3.0	20.0	80	na	2.0	0
(WestSoy) 'Lite' vanilla royale	6 oz	160	5.0	26.0	140	na	3.0	0
(WestSoy) 'Plus'	8 oz	150	6.0	20.0	120	na	5.0	0
All natural *(WestSoy)*	8 oz	120	4.0	22.0	140	na	2.5	0
Malted *(WestSoy)* 'Natural'	6 oz	250	7.0	31.0	140	(mq)	11.0	0
SOY FLOUR								
defatted	1 oz	93	13.3	10.9	6	>1.2 c	0.3	0
defatted, stirred	1/2 cup	165	23.5	19.2	10	8.8	0.6	0
full-fat	1 oz	124	9.8	10.0	4	>1.3 c	5.9	0
full-fat *(Arrowhead Mills)*	2 oz	250	20.0	18.0	1	8.1	11.0	0
full-fat, roasted	1 oz	125	9.9	9.5	3	>.6 c	6.2	0
full-fat, roasted, stirred	1/2 cup	185	14.6	14.1	5	>.9 c	9.2	0
full-fat, stirred	1/2 cup	183	14.5	14.8	5	4.0	8.7	0
low-fat	1 oz	92	13.2	10.8	5	>1.2 c	1.9	0
low-fat, stirred	1/2 cup	143	20.5	16.7	8	4.5	3.0	0
SOY MEAL								
defatted, raw	1/2 cup	207	27.4	24.5	2	>3.5 c	1.5	0
defatted, raw	1 oz	96	12.7	11.4	1	3.3	0.7	0

Food Name	Serv. Size	Total Cal.	Prot. GMS	Carbs GMS	Sod. MGS	Fiber GMS	Fat GMS	Chol. MGS
SOY MILK. See SOY BEVERAGE.								
SOY PROTEIN CONCENTRATE								
acid wash extracted	1 oz	93	16.3	8.7	252	>1.1 c	0.1	0
acid/water wash extracted	1 oz	94	16.5	8.8	255	>1.1 c	0.1	0
alcohol extracted	1 oz	93	16.3	8.7	1	>1.1 c	0.1	0
SOY PROTEIN ISOLATE								
	1 oz	95	22.6	2.1	281	1.6	1.0	0
potassium type	1 oz	91	22.6	2.9	14	>.1 c	0.2	0
w/potassium	1 oz	96	22.9	0.2	14	>.1 c	1.0	0
w/sodium	1 oz	96	22.9	0.2	281	>.1 c	1.0	0
SOYBEAN								
Dried								
boiled	4 oz	196	18.9	11.2	1	>2.3 c	10.2	0
boiled	1/2 cup	149	14.3	8.5	1	5.2	7.7	0
dry-roasted	1/2 cup	387	34.0	28.1	2	7.0	18.6	0
dry-roasted	1 oz	128	11.2	9.3	1	>1.5 c	6.1	0
raw	1/2 cup	387	33.9	28.1	2	11.6	18.5	0
raw	1 oz	118	10.3	8.6	1	3.5	5.7	0
raw *(Arrowhead Mills)*	2 oz	230	19.0	19.0	2	13.2	10.0	0
roasted	1/2 cup	405	30.3	28.9	140	>4.0 c	21.8	0
roasted	1 oz	134	10.0	9.5	46	>1.3 c	7.2	0
Green								
boiled, drained	4 oz	160	14.0	12.5	na	>2.1 c	7.3	0
boiled, drained	1/2 cup	127	11.1	9.9	13	3.8	5.8	0
raw	1/2 cup	188	16.6	14.1	19	5.4	8.7	0
raw, in pods	1 lb	353	31.1	26.6	na	>4.0 c	16.4	0
raw, shelled	1 oz	42	3.7	3.1	na	>.6 c	1.9	0
Kernels, roasted/toasted								
whole	1 cup	489	40.0	33.0	4	3.9	25.9	0
whole	1 oz	129	10.5	8.7	1	1.0	6.8	0
Mature								
boiled	1/2 cup	149	14.3	8.5	1	5.2	7.7	0
dry-roasted	1/2 cup	387	34.0	28.1	2	7.0	18.6	0
raw	1/2 cup	387	33.9	28.1	2	8.7	18.5	0
roasted	1/2 cup	405	30.3	28.9	140	>4.0 c	21.8	0
Mature, sprouted								
boiled, drained	1 cup	48	6.6	4.6	5	>1.0 c	1.8	0
raw	1 lb	580	59.4	50.7	62	>10.4 c	30.4	0
raw	1/2 cup	43	4.6	3.3	5	>.8 c	2.3	0
steamed	1/2 cup	38	4.0	3.1	5	.4	2.1	0
stir-fried	3.5 oz	125	13.1	9.4	14	>2.5 c	7.1	0
SOYBEAN, FERMENTED. See also MISO.								
natto	1/2 cup	187	15.6	12.6	6	>1.4 c	9.7	0

Food Name	Serv. Size	Total Cal.	Prot. GMS	Carbs GMS	Sod. MGS	Fiber GMS	Fat GMS	Chol. MGS
natto	1 oz	60	5.0	4.1	2	0	3.1	0
SOYBEAN CURD CAKE. See TOFU.								
SOYBEAN FLAKES (Arrowhead Mills)	2 oz	250	20.0	18.0	2	8.1	11.0	0
SOYBEAN LECITHIN OIL								
	1/2 cup	964	0.0	0.0	0	0	109.0	0
	1 oz	251	0.0	0.0	0	0	28.4	0
	1 tbsp	120	0.0	0.0	0	0	13.6	0
SOYBEAN OIL								
	1 cup	1927	0.0	0.0	0	0	218.0	0
hydrogenated	1 cup	1927	0.0	0.0	0	0	218.0	0
hydrogenated	1 oz	251	0.0	0.0	0	0	28.4	0
hydrogenated	1 tbsp	120	0.0	0.0	0	0	13.6	0
(Hain)	1 tbsp	120	0.0	0.0	0	0	14.0	0
(IGA)	1 tbsp	120	0.0	0.0	0	0	14.0	0
SOYBEAN-COTTONSEED OIL								
hydrogenated	1/2 cup	964	0.0	0.0	0	0	109.0	0
hydrogenated	1 oz	251	0.0	0.0	0	0	28.4	0
hydrogenated	1 tbsp	120	0.0	0.0	0	0	13.6	0
SPAGHETTI. See PASTA.								
SPAGHETTI ENTRÉE, CANNED								
W/beef (Chef Boyardee) 'Beef-O-Getti'	7.5 oz	220	7.0	27.0	1240	(mq)	9.0	(mq)
W/beef, in tomato sauce (Chef Boyardee)	7.5 oz	240	7.0	30.0	1120	(mq)	9.0	(mq)
W/frankfurters (Van Camp's) 'Spaghettee Weenee'	1 cup	243	9.4	34.7	1128	>.5 c	7.4	(mq)
W/frankfurters, in tomato sauce (Franco-American) 'SpaghettiOs'	7.5 oz	220	8.0	26.0	1000	(mq)	9.0	(mq)
W/meatballs								
(Estee)	7.5 oz	240	9.0	19.0	130	(mq)	14.0	30
(Featherweight)	7.5 oz	160	12.0	23.0	400	(mq)	3.0	20
(Nalley's)	7.5 oz	190	10.0	29.0	950	(mq)	4.0	(mq)
W/meatballs, in sauce (Buitoni)	7.5 oz	190	9.0	21.0	940	(mq)	8.0	20
W/meatballs, in tomato sauce								
(Chef Boyardee)	7.5 oz	230	8.0	30.0	970	(mq)	9.0	(mq)
(Franco-American)	7 3/8 oz	220	10.0	28.0	870	(mq)	8.0	(mq)
(Franco-American) 'SpaghettiOs'	7 3/8 oz	220	9.0	25.0	950	(mq)	9.0	(mq)
(Pathmark) 'No Frills'	7.5 oz	200	9.0	22.0	860	(mq)	8.0	(mq)
W/tomato and cheese sauce								
(Franco-American) 'SpaghettiOs'	7.5 oz	170	5.0	33.0	860	(mq)	2.0	na
W/tomato sauce, rings (Finast)	7.5 oz	150	4.0	31.0	480	(mq)	1.0	na
SPAGHETTI ENTRÉE, FREEZE-DRIED								
(Mountain House) w/meat and sauce, prepared	1 cup	260	12.0	41.0	(mq)	(mq)	5.0	(mq)

Food Name	Serv. Size	Total Cal.	Prot. GMS	Carbs GMS	Sod. MGS	Fiber GMS	Fat GMS	Chol. MGS
SPAGHETTI ENTRÉE, FROZEN								
Parmesan, w/Italian-style green beans								
(Stouffer's)	10.25 oz	240	10.0	30.0	810	na	9.0	na
W/beef (Dining Lite)	9 oz	220	12.0	25.0	440	(mq)	8.0	20
W/beef sauce and mushrooms (Le Menu)								
'LightStyle'	9 oz	280	12.0	45.0	450	(mq)	6.0	15
W/Italian-style meatballs (Swanson)								
'Homestyle Recipe'	13 oz	490	23.0	60.0	940	(mq)	18.0	(mq)
W/meat sauce								
(Banquet) 'Casserole'	8 oz	270	14.0	35.0	1250	(mq)	8.0	(mq)
(Freezer Queen) 'Single Serve'	10 oz	350	14.0	47.0	610	(mq)	12.0	(mq)
(Kid Cuisine)	9.25 oz	310	9.0	43.0	690	(mq)	12.0	35
(Lean Cuisine)	11.5 oz	290	15.0	45.0	500	na	6.0	20
(Stouffer's)	12 7/8 oz	320	16.0	38.0	560	na	12.0	na
(Weight Watchers)	10 oz	240	16.0	28.0	490	na	7.0	5
W/meatballs								
(Banquet)	10 oz	290	11.0	44.0	580	(mq)	10.0	30
(Morton)	10 oz	200	6.0	39.0	1090	(mq)	3.0	10
(Stouffer's) 19.5-oz pkg	1/2 pkg	290	14.0	37.0	790	na	9.0	na
(Stouffer's) 12 5/8-oz pkg	1 pkg	440	22.0	53.0	960	na	16.0	na
(Swanson)	12.5 oz	390	14.0	46.0	1100	(mq)	17.0	(mq)
W/meatballs and sauce (Lean Cuisine)	9.5 oz	290	20.0	36.0	550	na	7.0	30
SPAGHETTI ENTRÉE, MICROWAVE								
(Lunch Bucket) 'Spaghetti 'n Meatsauce'								
microwave cup	7.5 oz	240	9.0	39.0	870	na	5.0	30
Rings (Kid's Kitchen) microwave cup	7.5 oz	180	8.0	35.0	930	na	1.0	10
Rings and franks in tomato sauce								
(Kid's Kitchen) microwave cup	7.5 oz	290	12.0	33.0	960	na	12.0	30
W/meatballs								
(Chef Boyardee) 'Microwave'	7.5 oz	230	7.0	29.0	1060	(mq)	10.0	20
(Hormel) micro cup	7.5 oz	210	10.0	27.0	930	na	7.0	20
(Kid's Kitchen) microwave cup	7.5 oz	220	11.0	26.0	880	na	8.0	20
W/meatballs, in sauce (Libby's) 'Diner'	7.75 oz	190	10.0	31.0	870	2.2	3.0	15
SPAGHETTI ENTRÉE, PACKAGED								
Spaghettini (Top Shelf)	1 serving	240	13.0	35.0	1020	(mq)	5.0	5
W/beef and mushroom sauce								
(Ultra Slim Fast)	12 oz	370	20.0	49.0	990	na	10.0	25
W/meat sauce (Top Shelf)	10 oz	260	14.0	37.0	980	na	6.0	20
SPAGHETTI ENTRÉE MIX								
(Kraft) 'Mild American Dinner' prepared	1 cup	300	10.0	50.0	630	(mq)	7.0	0
(Kraft) 'Tangy Italian Style Dinner' prepared	1 cup	310	11.0	49.0	670	(mq)	8.0	5
Low-fat, w/whole wheat noodles								
(Fantastic Foods) 'All-O-Round'	10 oz	211	10.0	45.0	275	na	2.0	4

Food Name	Serv. Size	Total Cal.	Prot. GMS	Carbs GMS	Sod. MGS	Fiber GMS	Fat GMS	Chol. MGS
W/condensed meat sauce								
(Chef Boyardee) 'Dinner' prepared ...	3.25 oz	250	12.0	37.0	595	(mq)	6.0	(mq)
W/meat sauce								
(Chef Boyardee) 'Dinner' prepared	7.9 oz	240	12.0	42.0	1155	(mq)	3.0	(mq)
(Kraft) 'Dinner' prepared	1 cup	360	12.0	47.0	880	(mq)	14.0	15
W/mushroom sauce (Chef Boyardee)								
'Dinner' prepared	7.9 oz	210	11.0	41.0	1085	(mq)	1.0	na
SPAGHETTI SEASONING (Tone's)	1 tsp	11	0.2	2.5	469	.1	<.1	tr
SPAGHETTI SQUASH. See SQUASH, SPAGHETTI.								
SPAM. See LUNCHEON MEAT, CANNED.								
SPARE RIB SEASONING MIX,								
'Bag 'n Season' (Schilling)	1 pkg	185	0.3	42.0	3690	na	1.5	2
SPINACH								
boiled, drained	4 oz	26	3.4	4.3	79	2.5	0.3	0
boiled, drained	1/2 cup	21	2.7	3.4	63	2.0	0.2	0
raw	10-oz pkg	62	8.1	9.9	224	7.4	1.0	0
raw (Dole)	3 oz	9	3.0	0.1	107	8.0	0.3	na
raw, chopped	1/2 cup	6	0.8	1.0	22	.7	0.1	0
raw, chopped	1 oz	6	0.8	1.0	22	.7	0.1	0
raw, untrimmed	1 lb	73	9.3	11.4	257	8.5	1.1	0
SPINACH, CANNED								
drained solids	1/2 cup	25	3.0	3.6	29	>.9 c	0.5	0
drained solids, no salt added	4 oz	26	3.2	3.9	31	3.2	0.6	0
w/liquid	4 oz	22	2.4	3.3	362	1.0	0.4	0
w/liquid, low-sodium	4 oz	22	2.4	3.3	85	1.0	0.4	0
(Allens)	1/2 cup	28	2.0	3.0	35	(mq)	<1.0	0
(Allens) chopped	1/2 cup	28	2.0	3.0	330	(mq)	<1.0	0
(Allens) sliced	1/2 cup	28	2.0	3.0	330	(mq)	<1.0	0
(Allens) whole	1/2 cup	28	2.0	3.0	330	(mq)	<1.0	0
(Bush's Best) chopped	1/2 cup	25	2.0	4.0	330	na	0.0	na
(Del Monte) chopped, w/liquid	1/2 cup	25	2.0	4.0	355	(mq)	0.0	0
(Del Monte) whole, w/liquid	1/2 cup	25	2.0	4.0	355	(mq)	0.0	0
(Del Monte) whole, w/liquid,								
'No Salt Added'	1/2 cup	25	2.0	4.0	35	(mq)	0.0	0
(Featherweight)	1/2 cup	35	2.0	4.0	30	(mq)	1.0	0
(Finast)	1/2 cup	25	3.0	4.0	360	(mq)	0.0	0
(Finast) 'No Salt Added'	1/2 cup	25	3.0	4.0	110	(mq)	0.0	0
(Freshlike) cut	1/2 cup	20	2.0	4.0	340	na	0.0	na
(Freshlike) cut, water-packed, w/o salt ..	1/2 cup	20	2.0	4.0	20	na	0.0	na
(Freshlike) cut, water packed, w/o								
sugar or salt	1/2 cup	20	2.0	4.0	20	na	0.0	na
(Pathmark) 'No Frills'	1 cup	45	5.0	8.0	700	(mq)	1.0	0
(Pathmark) 'No Salt Added'	1/2 cup	30	2.0	4.0	35	(mq)	1.0	0

Food Name	Serv. Size	Total Cal.	Prot. GMS	Carbs GMS	Sod. MGS	Fiber GMS	Fat GMS	Chol. MGS
(Pathmark) whole	1/2 cup	30	2.0	4.0	370	(mq)	1.0	0
(S&W) 'Premium Northwest'	1/2 cup	25	2.0	3.0	395	(mq)	0.0	0
(Stokely)	1/2 cup	30	2.0	3.0	420	(mq)	0.0	0
(Veg•All) cut	1/2 cup	20	2.0	4.0	340	na	0.0	na
SPINACH, FROZEN								
Chopped								
boiled, drained	10-oz pkg	62	6.9	11.7	189	>2.4 c	0.5	0
boiled, drained	1/2 cup	27	3.0	5.1	82	>1.0 c	0.2	0
unprepared	10-oz pkg	68	8.3	11.4	210	8.5	0.9	0
unprepared	1 cup	37	4.6	6.2	115	4.7	0.5	0
(A&P)	3.3 oz	20	3.0	4.0	90	(mq)	<1.0	0
(Birds Eye)	3.3 oz	20	3.0	3.0	90	3.0	0.0	0
(Finast)	3.3 oz	20	3.0	3.0	70	(mq)	0.0	0
(Frosty Acres)	3.3 oz	20	3.0	3.0	70	>1.0 c	0.0	0
(Seabrook)	3.3 oz	20	3.0	3.0	70	>1.0 c	0.0	0
(Southern)	3.5 oz	25	3.0	3.5	100	(mq)	0.3	0
Creamed								
(Birds Eye) 'Combination Vegetables'	3 oz	60	2.0	5.0	310	1.0	4.0	0
(Green Giant)	1/2 cup	70	3.0	10.0	480	(mq)	3.0	2
(Stouffer's)	4.5 oz	170	4.0	7.0	380	(mq)	14.0	na
Leaf								
boiled, drained	10-oz pkg	62	6.9	11.7	189	6.6	0.5	0
boiled, drained	4 oz	32	3.6	6.1	98	2.4	0.2	0
unprepared	10-oz pkg	68	8.3	11.4	210	8.5	0.9	0
unprepared	1 cup	37	4.6	6.2	115	4.7	0.5	0
(A&P)	3.3 oz	25	3.0	4.0	100	(mq)	<1.0	0
(Birds Eye) 'Portion Pack'	3.2 oz	20	3.0	3.0	70	2.0	0.0	0
(Birds Eye) whole leaf	3.3 oz	20	3.0	4.0	90	3.0	0.0	0
(Finast)	3.3 oz	20	3.0	4.0	75	(mq)	0.0	0
(Freshlike) cut	3.3 oz	20	3.0	4.0	75	na	0.0	na
(Frosty Acres)	3.3 oz	20	3.0	4.0	75	>1.0 c	0.0	0
(Green Giant) cut, in butter sauce	1/2 cup	40	3.0	6.0	380	3.5	2.0	5
(Green Giant) 'Harvest Fresh'	1/2 cup	25	4.0	5.0	170	3.0	0.0	0
(Green Giant) 'Plain Polybag'	1/2 cup	25	3.0	6.0	100	5.0	0.0	0
(Seabrook) cut	3.3 oz	20	3.0	4.0	77	>1.0 c	0.0	0
(Southern) whole	3.5 oz	25	2.9	3.6	100	(mq)	0.3	0
(Veg•All) cut	3.3 oz	20	3.0	4.0	75	na	0.0	na
SPINACH, NEW ZEALAND								
boiled, drained	4 oz	14	1.5	2.5	121	>.7 c	0.2	0
boiled, drained, chopped	1/2 cup	11	1.2	2.0	96	>.6 c	0.2	0
raw, chopped	1/2 cup	4	0.4	0.7	36	>.2 c	0.1	0
raw, untrimmed	1 lb	47	4.9	8.2	425	>2.3 c	0.7	0

Food Name	Serv. Size	Total Cal.	Prot. GMS	Carbs GMS	Sod. MGS	Fiber GMS	Fat GMS	Chol. MGS
SPINACH ENTRÉE, FROZEN								
au gratin *(Budget Gourmet)*	6 oz	120	5.0	14.0	410	(mq)	5.0	40
creamed *(Stouffer's)*	4.5 oz	190	4.0	8.0	400	na	16.0	na
soufflé *(Stouffer's)*	6 oz	220	9.0	11.0	820	na	15.0	na
SPINACH SALAD, 'Sassy Spinach Kit'								
(Saco)	1/2 cup	157	2.0	14.0	437	1.0	11.0	3
SPIRULINA								
dried	100 gm	290	57.5	23.9	1048	3.6	7.7	0
dried	1 oz	82	16.3	6.8	297	>1.0 c	2.2	0
raw	100 gm	26	5.9	2.4	98	>.3 c	0.4	0
SPLIT PEAS								
boiled	4 oz	134	9.5	23.9	2	2.6	0.4	0
boiled *(A&P)*	1 cup	220	16.0	40.0	15	(mq)	<1.0	0
boiled, mature seeds	1/2 cup	116	8.2	20.7	2	8.1	0.4	0
raw	1 oz	97	7.0	17.1	4	1.6	0.3	0
raw, green *(Arrowhead Mills)*	2 oz	200	14.0	35.0	14	7.5	1.0	0
raw, mature seeds	1/2 cup	334	24.1	59.2	15	25.0	1.1	0
SPONGE GOURD. See GOURD, DISHCLOTH.								
SPORTS DRINK								
CHOCOLATE								
(Weider) 'Dynamic Muscle Builder'	11 oz	220	18.0	36.0	260	na	<1.0	na
(Weider) 'Dynamic Weight Gainer'	11 oz	280	18.0	48.0	320	na	2.0	na
(Weider) high-energy 'Protein Blast'	11.5 oz	270	22.0	44.0	240	na	<1.0	na
(Weider) 'Sports Line Power Shake'								
Dutch chocolate	11 oz	220	15.0	37.0	150	na	<1.0	na
FRUIT PUNCH *(Pro-formance)*	8 oz	99	0.0	26.0	0	na	0.0	na
GRAPE								
(Opti-Carb 140)	16 oz	140	0.0	35.0	9	na	0.0	na
(Pro-formance)	8 oz	99	0.0	26.0	0	na	0.0	na
LEMON								
(Knudsen & Sons) 'Isotonic Sports								
Beverage'	8 oz	60	0.0	21.0	35	na	0.0	na
(Pro-formance)	8 oz	99	0.0	26.0	0	na	0.0	na
LEMONADE								
(Power Burst) advanced performance								
beverage	8 oz	50	0.0	14.0	25	na	0.0	na
LEMON-LIME *(Shasta)* caffeine-free,								
'Body Works'	8 oz	60	0.0	15.0	95	na	0.0	na
ORANGE								
(All Sport) caffeine-free	8 oz	70	0.0	19.0	55	na	0.0	na
(Gatorade)	8 oz	50	0.0	14.0	110	na	0.0	na
(Opti-Carb 140)	16 oz	140	0.0	35.0	9	na	0.0	na
(PowerAde)	8 oz	70	0.0	19.0	70	na	0.0	na

Food Name	Serv. Size	Total Cal.	Prot. GMS	Carbs GMS	Sod. MGS	Fiber GMS	Fat GMS	Chol. MGS
(Pro-formance)	8 oz	99	0.0	26.0	0	na	0.0	na
(Shasta) caffeine-free, 'Body Works'	8 oz	60	0.0	15.0	95	na	0.0	na
(10-K)	8 oz	60	0.0	15.0	55	na	0.0	na
SPORTS DRINK MIX								
(Tiger's Milk)								
'Breakfast Booster' dry	2 level tbsp	70	2.0	14.0	20	na	<1.0	na
'Energy Booster' dry	3 heap tbsp	120	0.0	28.0	10	na	<1.0	na
'Protein Booster' Dutch chocolate, dry	3 heap tbsp	90	8.0	12.0	140	na	<1.0	na
'Protein Booster' vanilla-orange creme, dry	3 heap tbsp	90	8.0	12.0	140	na	<1.0	na
(Weider)								
'Big' chocolate malt, sugar-free, dry	4 scoops	320	18.0	58.0	370	na	2.0	na
'Carbo Energizer' orange, dry	4 scoops	230	0.0	58.0	40	na	0.0	na
'Crash Weight Gain No. 7' vanilla, dry	4 heap tbsp	300	6.0	61.0	84	na	3.0	0
'Dynamic Body Shaper' Dutch chocolate, dry	2 scoops	110	13.0	12.0	170	na	<1.0	na
'Dynamic Muscle Builder' dry	3 heap tbsp	100	18.0	6.0	116	na	0.0	na
'Dynamic Muscle Builder' natural chocolate, dry	2 scoops	120	18.0	9.0	170	na	1.0	na
'Dynamic Muscle Builder' natural vanilla, dry	2 scoops	120	18.0	9.0	180	na	<1.0	na
'Dynamic Weight Gainer' Dutch chocolate, dry	4 scoops	320	18.0	61.0	400	na	<1.0	na
'Dynamic Weight Gainer' peanut butter, dry	4 scoops	330	18.0	61.0	390	na	2.0	na
'90 Plus' vanilla, sugar-free, dry	2 scoops	100	25.0	1.0	150	na	0.0	na
'N2itro-Fire' protein blend, dry	2 tbsp	110	8.0	17.0	100	na	1.0	na
'Victory Explosive Workout' citrus, dry	4 tbsp	190	0.0	48.0	50	na	0.0	na
SPOT								
dry-heat cooked	3 oz	134	20.2	0.0	31	0	5.3	65
raw	1 lb	559	84.0	0.0	130	0	22.2	(mq)
raw	1 oz	35	5.2	0.0	8	0	1.4	(mq)
SPREAD, VEGETARIAN								
	1 cup	953	2.3	54.9	(mq)	(mq)	83.2	187
	1 oz	110	0.3	6.4	(mq)	(mq)	9.6	22
	1 tbsp	60	0.1	3.4	(mq)	(mq)	5.2	12
(Best Foods)	1 tbsp	50	0.0	2.0	170	(mq)	5.0	5
(Hellmann's)	1 tbsp	50	0.0	2.0	170	(mq)	5.0	5
(Kraft)	1 tbsp	50	0.0	3.0	95	(mq)	5.0	5

SPREADS. See CHEESE SPREAD; SPREAD, VEGETARIAN; and individual listings.
SPRING ONION. See ONION, GREEN.

Food Name	Serv. Size	Total Cal.	Prot. GMS	Carbs GMS	Sod. MGS	Fiber GMS	Fat GMS	Chol. MGS
SPRINKLES								
milk chocolate *(Snack Pack)*	3.88 oz	178	2.0	28.4	156	.3	6.3	1
vanilla chocolate *(Snack Pack)*	3.88 oz	166	1.5	26.3	132	.1	6.1	0
SQUAB/pigeon								
Raw								
breast meat only	1 oz	38	6.2	0:0	(mq)	0	1.3	26
giblets	100 gm	154	19.8	1.2	70	0	7.2	350
light meat w/o skin	1 lb	202	32.9	0.0	83	0	6.8	136
meat and skin	1 oz	83	5.2	0.0	(mq)	0	6.7	(mq)
meat and skin, approx 7 oz	1 squab	584	36.8	0.0	(mq)	0	47.4	(mq)
meat only	1 oz	40	5.0	0.0	(mq)	0	2.1	(mq)
SQUASH SEED. See PUMPKIN SEED.								
SQUASH, ACORN/table queen squash								
boiled, mashed	1/2 cup	41	0.8	10.7	4	>1.4 c	0.1	0
boiled, mashed	4 oz	39	0.8	10.0	3	>1.3 c	0.1	0
raw *(Frieda's)*	1 lb	249	8.6	63.5	45	(mq)	0.5	0
raw *(Frieda's)*	1 oz	16	0.5	4.0	3	(mq)	<.1	0
raw, approx 4-inch diam	1 squash	172	3.5	44.9	13	>6.0 c	0.4	0
raw, cubes	1/2 cup	28	0.6	7.3	3	>1.0 c	0.1	0
raw, trimmed	1 oz	11	0.2	3.0	1	>.4 c	<.1	0
raw, untrimmed	1 lb	138	2.8	35.9	11	>4.8 c	0.3	0
SQUASH, BANANA								
baked *(Frieda's)*	1 lb	286	8.2	69.9	45	(mq)	1.8	0
baked *(Frieda's)*	1 oz	18	0.5	4.4	3	(mq)	0.1	0
SQUASH, BUTTERNUT								
baked	4 oz	45	1.0	11.9	5	>1.4 c	0.1	0
baked, cubes	1/2 cup	41	0.9	10.7	4	>1.3 c	0.1	0
boiled, mashed	1/2 cup	47	1.5	12.1	2	>1.0 c	0.1	0
raw, cubes	1/2 cup	32	0.7	8.2	3	>1.0 c	0.1	0
raw, trimmed	1 oz	13	0.3	3.3	1	>.4 c	<.1	0
raw, untrimmed	1 lb	172	3.8	44.6	15	>5.3 c	0.4	0
SQUASH, CORN AND BUTTERNUT								
(Earth's Best)	4.5 oz	90	2.0	15.0	0	na	2.0	na
SQUASH, CROOKNECK								
boiled, drained	4 oz	23	1.0	4.9	1	1.2	0.4	0
boiled, drained, slices	1/2 cup	18	0.8	3.9	1	>.5 c	0.3	0
canned, drained, no salt added	4 oz	15	0.7	3.4	6	1.1	0.1	0
canned, yellow, cut *(Allens)*	1/2 cup	16	1.0	3.0	230	(mq)	<1.0	0
frozen, boiled, drained	4 oz	28	1.5	6.3	7	1.4	0.2	0
frozen, cooked *(Kohl's)*	4 oz	45	1.0	11.0	0	(mq)	<1.0	0
frozen, yellow *(Seabrook)*	3.3 oz	18	1.0	4.0	1	>1.0 c	0.0	0
frozen, yellow *(Southern)*	3.5 oz	21	1.5	4.1	20	(mq)	0.1	0
raw, ends trimmed	1 oz	5	0.3	1.1	1	.3	0.1	0

Food Name	Serv. Size	Total Cal.	Prot. GMS	Carbs GMS	Sod. MGS	Fiber GMS	Fat GMS	Chol. MGS
raw, slices	1/2 cup	12	0.6	2.6	1	>.4 c	0.2	0
raw, untrimmed	1 lb	84	4.2	18.2	7	4.9	1.1	0
SQUASH, HUBBARD								
baked	4 oz	57	2.8	12.3	9	>2.0 c	0.7	0
baked, cubes	1/2 cup	51	2.5	11.0	8	>1.8 c	0.6	0
boiled, mashed	1/2 cup	35	1.8	7.6	6	3.4	0.4	0
boiled, mashed	4 oz	34	1.7	7.3	6	3.4	0.4	0
raw, cubes	1/2 cup	23	1.2	5.1	4	>.8 c	0.3	0
raw, trimmed	1 oz	11	0.6	2.5	2	>.4 c	0.1	0
raw, untrimmed	1 lb	116	5.8	25.3	20	>4.1 c	1.5	0
SQUASH, MARROW/vegetable marrow squash								
raw, trimmed	1 oz	4	0.2	1.0	na	>.1 c	<.1	0
SQUASH, SCALLOP/cymling/pattypan squash								
boiled, drained	4 oz	18	1.2	3.7	1	>.5 c	0.2	0
boiled, drained, mashed	1/2 cup	19	1.2	4.0	1	>.6 c	0.2	0
boiled, drained, slices	1/2 cup	14	0.9	3.0	1	>.4 c	0.2	0
raw, slices	1/2 cup	12	0.8	2.5	1	>.4 c	0.1	0
raw, trimmed	1 oz	5	0.3	1.1	<1	>.2 c	0.1	0
raw, untrimmed	1 lb	81	5.3	17.1	5	>2.5 c	0.9	0
SQUASH, SPAGHETTI								
baked or boiled, drained	4 oz	33	0.7	7.3	20	>1.6 c	0.3	0
baked or boiled, drained	1/2 cup	23	0.5	5.0	14	1.1	0.2	0
raw, cubes	1/2 cup	16	0.3	3.5	9	>.7 c	0.3	0
raw, trimmed	1 oz	9	0.2	2.0	5	>.4 c	0.2	0
raw, untrimmed	1 lb	106	2.1	22.3	55	>4.5 c	1.8	0
SQUASH, STRAIGHTNECK, raw, slices	1/2 cup	12	0.6	2.6	1	>.4 c	0.2	0
SQUASH, SUMMER, all varieties								
boiled, drained	4 oz	23	1.0	4.9	1	1.6	0.4	0
boiled, drained, slices	1/2 cup	18	0.8	3.9	1	1.3	0.3	0
raw, slices	1/2 cup	13	0.8	2.8	1	.8	0.1	0
raw, trimmed	1 oz	6	0.3	1.2	1	.3	0.1	0
raw, untrimmed	1 lb	87	5.1	18.7	8	5.2	0.9	0
SQUASH, WINTER, all varieties								
baked	4 oz	44	1.0	9.9	1	3.2	0.7	0
baked, cubes	1/2 cup	40	0.9	8.9	1	2.9	0.6	0
frozen, cooked (Birds Eye)	4 oz	45	1.0	11.0	0	2.0	0.0	0
frozen, cooked (Seabrook)	4 oz	45	1.0	11.0	2	2.0	0.0	0
raw, cubes	1/2 cup	21	0.8	5.1	2	1.0	0.1	0
raw, trimmed	1 oz	11	0.4	2.5	1	5.0	0.1	0
raw, untrimmed	1 lb	119	4.7	28.4	12	5.8	0.7	0
SQUID, MIXED SPECIES/calamari								
fried	3 oz	149	15.2	6.6	260	>.1 c	6.4	221
raw	1 lb	416	70.7	14.0	199	0	6.3	105º

Food Name	Serv. Size	Total Cal.	Prot. GMS	Carbs GMS	Sod. MGS	Fiber GMS	Fat GMS	Chol. MGS
raw	3 oz	78	13.2	2.6	37	0	1.2	198
raw	1 oz	26	4.4	0.9	12	0	0.4	66
SQUIRREL								
raw	1 oz	34	5.9	0.0	29	0	0.9	23
roasted	4 oz	154	27.4	0.0	107	0	4.1	108
roasted, diced	1 cup	190	33.8	0.0	132	0	5.1	133
STAR APPLE. See CAIMIT.								
STAR FRUIT/carambola								
cubed	1 cup	45	0.7	10.7	3	3.7	0.5	0
trimmed	1 oz	9	0.2	2.2	1	.3	0.1	0
untrimmed	1 lb	142	2.3	33.7	7	5.0	1.5	0
STEAK SEASONING 'Spice Blends'								
(Schilling)	1/4 tsp	1	0.1	0.1	273	na	(tr)	0
STIR-FRY ENTRÉE KIT								
(Tyson)	9 oz	230	22.0	15.0	480	na	9.0	80
(Tyson) 'Yoshida Oriental Sauce'	1.6 oz	100	2.0	22.0	1260	na	1.0	0
STIR-FRY SEASONING (Gilroy)	1 tsp	6	0.2	1.0	5	na	0.0	na
STRAIGHTNECK SQUASH. See SQUASH, STRAIGHTNECK.								
STRAWBERRY								
trimmed	1 pint	96	2.0	22.5	3	8.3	1.2	0
trimmed	1 cup	45	0.9	10.5	1	3.9	0.6	0
trimmed	1 oz	9	0.2	2.0	<1	.7	0.1	0
untrimmed	1 lb	130	2.6	30.0	5	11.1	1.6	0
Canned, in heavy syrup	4 oz	104	0.6	26.7	5	(mq)	0.3	0
Freeze-dried (Mountain House) prepared	1/4 cup	45	1.0	12.0	<1	(mq)	0.0	0
Frozen								
in light syrup, halves 'Quick Thaw Pouch'								
(Birds Eye)	5 oz	90	1.0	22.0	5	1.0	0.0	0
in light syrup, whole (Birds Eye)	4 oz	80	1.0	20.0	0	2.0	0.0	0
sweetened, sliced	10-oz pkg	273	1.5	73.6	9	5.4	0.4	0
sweetened, sliced	1 cup	245	1.4	66.1	8	4.8	0.3	0
sweetened, sliced	4 oz	109	0.6	29.4	3	2.2	0.1	0
sweetened, sliced (Finast)	3.3 oz	125	1.0	30.0	5	(mq)	0.0	0
sweetened, whole	10-oz pkg	222	1.5	59.6	3	5.4	0.4	0
sweetened, whole	1 cup	199	1.3	53.5	3	4.8	0.4	0
sweetened, whole	4 oz	88	0.6	23.8	1	2.1	0.2	0
unsweetened	20-oz pkg	198	2.4	51.8	11	11.9	0.6	0
unsweetened	1 cup	52	0.6	13.6	3	3.1	0.2	0
unsweetened	4 oz	40	0.5	10.4	2	4.8	0.1	0
STRAWBERRY-BANANA NECTAR (Kern's)	6 oz	110	0.0	28.0	0	na	0.0	na
STRAWBERRY COLADA. See ALCOHOLIC BEVERAGES.								
STRAWBERRY DAIQUIRI. See ALCOHOLIC BEVERAGES.								

Food Name	Serv. Size	Total Cal.	Prot. GMS	Carbs GMS	Sod. MGS	Fiber GMS	Fat GMS	Chol. MGS
STRAWBERRY DRINK								
(Snapple) 'Strawberry Passion Awareness'								
real fruit	8 oz	120	0.0	31.0	25	na	0.0	na
STRAWBERRY FLAVOR DRINK								
(Ensure) liquid nutrition	8 oz	250	8.8	34.3	200	na	8.8	5
(Ensure) liquid nutrition 'Plus'	8 oz	355	13.0	47.3	250	na	12.6	5
(Frostee)	8 oz	180	2.0	27.0	150	(tr)	7.0	na
(Sego) 'Lite'	10 oz	150	11.0	17.0	390	(tr)	4.0	5
(Sego) 'Very Strawberry'	10 oz	225	11.0	34.0	360	(tr)	5.0	5
(Squeezit) 'Silly Billy Strawberry'	6.75 oz	90	0.0	23.0	5	na	0.0	na
(Tang)	8.45 oz	120	0.0	32.0	10	na	0.0	0
(10-K)	8 oz	60	0.0	15.0	55	na	0.0	na
STRAWBERRY FLAVOR DRINK MIX, PREPARED								
(Kool-Aid) presweetened	8 oz	80	0.0	20.0	0	(tr)	0.0	0
(Nestlé) 'Quik' 2 1/2 heap tsp w/whole milk	8 oz	220	8.0	32.0	120	(tr)	8.0	(mq)
(Nestlé) 'Quik' 2 1/2 heap tsp w/2% milk	8 oz	200	8.0	32.0	120	(tr)	5.0	(mq)
(Nestlé) 'Quik' 2 1/2 heap tsp w/skim milk	8 oz	160	8.0	32.0	125	(tr)	0.0	na
(Turbo Nutrition) weight gain protein powder,								
2 oz w/whole milk	8 oz	360	36.0	33.0	420	na	9.0	na
(Wylers) 'Crystals'	8 oz	85	0.0	20.7	43	(tr)	0.3	0
STRAWBERRY GUAVA JUICE								
(Knudsen & Sons)	8 oz	105	<1.0	26.0	na	na	0.0	na
STRAWBERRY GUAVA NECTAR								
(Santa Cruz Natural) organic	8 oz	90	<1.0	24.0	na	na	<1.0	na
STRAWBERRY JUICE DRINK								
(Knudsen & Sons) float	8 oz	130	2.0	32.0	na	na	0.0	na
(Tang) 'Fruit Box'	8.45 oz	120	0.0	32.0	10	(tr)	0.0	0
(Wyler's) 'Fruit Slush'	4 oz	157	0.0	39.3	10	(tr)	0.0	0
STRAWBERRY LEMONADE								
(Kern's)	6 oz	110	0.0	28.0	0	na	0.0	na
(Knudsen & Sons)	8 oz	90	<1.0	21.0	na	na	0.0	na
(Santa Cruz Natural) organic	8 oz	60	<1.0	20.0	na	na	<1.0	na
(Snapple)	8 oz	110	0.0	26.0	5	na	0.0	0
STRAWBERRY NECTAR								
(Knudsen & Sons)	8 oz	105	<1.0	29.0	na	na	0.0	na
(Libby's)	6 oz	110	0.0	27.0	0	(mq)	0.0	0
STRAWBERRY PUNCH DRINK								
(Arizona) 'Cowboy Cocktail'	8 oz	120	0.0	30.0	20	na	0.0	na
STRAWBERRY PUNCH MIX								
(Kool-Aid) sugar-sweetened, prepared	8 oz	80	0.0	20.0	0	na	0.0	0
(Kool-Aid) unsweetened, prepared w/sugar	8 oz	100	0.0	25.0	25	na	0.0	0
(Kool-Aid) unsweetened, prepared								
w/o sugar	8 oz	2	0.0	0.0	25	na	0.0	0

Food Name	Serv. Size	Total Cal.	Prot. GMS	Carbs GMS	Sod. MGS	Fiber GMS	Fat GMS	Chol. MGS
STRAWBERRY SYRUP								
(Knott's Berry Farm)	1 oz	120	0.0	30.0	0	na	0.0	na
(Knudsen & Sons)	1 oz	75	<1.0	18.0	na	na	<1.0	na
(S&W) w/saccharin	1 tsp	4	0.0	1.0	25	na	0.0	0
STRAWBERRY TOPPING								
(Kraft)	1 tbsp	50	0.0	14.0	5	na	0.0	0
(Smucker's)	2 tbsp	120	0.0	30.0	0	na	0.0	0
(Smucker's) fat-free 'Light'	2 tbsp	55	0.0	14.0	0	na	0.0	na
STRING BEAN. See GREEN BEAN.								
STROGANOFF DINNER. See BEEF ENTRÉE.								
STRUDEL. See individual listings.								
STUFFED PEPPER								
(Celentano) sweet red, frozen	13 oz	350	28.0	28.0	810	(mq)	20.0	(mq)
(Stouffer's) green, w/beef in tomato								
sauce, frozen	7.75 oz	200	9.0	22.0	650	na	8.0	na
(Stouffer's) single serving	10 oz	220	10.0	28.0	1010	na	8.0	na
STUFFING								
(Betty Crocker)								
chicken, dry	1/6 pkg	110	4.0	21.0	530	na	1.0	na
traditional herb, dry	1/6 pkg	110	4.0	22.0	550	na	1.0	na
traditional herb, prepared w/salted butter	1/2 cup	190	4.0	22.0	640	(mq)	9.0	na
(Brownberry)								
corn, dry	1 oz	103	3.7	20.6	350	1.5	1.6	0
herb, dry	1 oz	100	3.6	20.7	297	1.6	1.3	0
(Croutettes) dry	.7 oz	70	3.0	14.0	260	0	0.0	0
(General Mills)								
chicken, dry	1/6 pkg	110	4.0	21.0	530	na	1.0	na
chicken, prepared w/margarine	1/2 cup	180	4.0	21.0	620	na	9.0	na
traditional herb, dry	1/6 pkg	110	4.0	22.0	550	na	<1.0	na
traditional herb, prepared w/margarine	1/2 cup	180	4.0	22.0	640	na	8.0	na
(Golden Dipt)								
Cajun style, dry	1/4 cup	40	1.0	9.0	590	na	0.0	0
cheddar and French, dry	1/2 cup	80	4.0	9.0	580	na	3.0	14
garden herb, dry	1/4 cup	40	1.0	9.0	330	na	0.0	0
(Golden Grain)								
chicken, dry	1 oz	106	3.9	20.0	637	1.2	1.2	<1
cornbread, dry	1 oz	105	3.3	20.9	774	1.2	1.0	<1
herb and butter, dry	1 oz	104	3.7	19.7	713	1.4	1.1	<1
w/wild rice, dry	1 oz	108	3.6	20.9	611	1.3	1.1	<1
(Pepperidge Farm)								
apple and raisin 'Distinctive Stuffing' dry	1 oz	110	3.0	21.0	410	(mq)	1.0	na
classic chicken 'Distinctive Stuffing' dry	1 oz	110	4.0	20.0	410	(mq)	1.0	na
cornbread, dry	1 oz	110	3.0	22.0	320	(mq)	1.0	na

Food Name	Serv. Size	Total Cal.	Prot. GMS	Carbs GMS	Sod. MGS	Fiber GMS	Fat GMS	Chol. MGS
country style, dry	1 oz	100	4.0	21.0	400	(mq)	1.0	na
cube, dry	1 oz	110	3.0	22.0	400	(mq)	1.0	na
herb, country garden 'Distinctive Stuffing' dry	1 oz	120	4.0	18.0	300	(mq)	4.0	na
herb, dry	1 oz	110	3.0	22.0	380	(mq)	1.0	na
vegetable, harvest, w/almonds 'Distinctive' dry	1 oz	110	4.0	19.0	250	(mq)	3.0	na
wild rice and mushroom 'Distinctive Stuffing' dry	1 oz	130	4.0	17.0	310	(mq)	5.0	na
(Stove Top)								
Americana San Francisco, prepared w/salted butter	1/2 cup	170	4.0	20.0	650	(mq)	9.0	20
beef, prepared w/salted butter	1/2 cup	180	4.0	21.0	590	(mq)	9.0	20
chicken flavor, prepared w/salted butter	1/2 cup	180	4.0	20.0	570	(mq)	9.0	20
cornbread 'Flexible Serving' prepared w/salted butter	1/2 cup	170	4.0	20.0	580	(mq)	9.0	15
cornbread, prepared w/salted butter . . .	1/2 cup	170	3.0	21.0	570	(mq)	9.0	20
cornbread, prepared w/salted margarine	1/2 cup	180	4.0	22.0	590	na	9.0	0
homestyle herb 'Flexible Serving' prepared w/salted butter	1/2 cup	170	4.0	20.0	520	(mq)	9.0	15
long grain and wild rice, prepared w/salted butter	1/2 cup	180	4.0	22.0	560	(mq)	9.0	20
mushroom and onion, prepared w/salted butter	1/2 cup	180	4.0	20.0	490	(mq)	9.0	20
pork 'Flexible Serving' prepared w/salted butter	1/2 cup	170	4.0	20.0	630	(mq)	9.0	15
pork, prepared w/salted butter	1/2 cup	170	4.0	20.0	570	(mq)	9.0	20
savory herbs, prepared w/salted butter	1/2 cup	170	4.0	20.0	590	(mq)	9.0	20
turkey, prepared w/salted butter	1/2 cup	170	4.0	20.0	640	(mq)	9.0	20
turkey, prepared w/salted margarine . . .	1/2 cup	180	4.0	20.0	630	na	9.0	0
STUFFING, FROZEN								
chicken 'Stuffing Originals' *(Green Giant)*	1/2 cup	170	4.0	21.0	670	(mq)	7.0	na
cornbread 'Stuffing Originals' *(Green Giant)*	1/2 cup	170	3.0	25.0	660	(mq)	6.0	na
mushroom 'Stuffing Originals' *(Green Giant)*	1/2 cup	150	4.0	19.0	780	(mq)	7.0	na
wild rice 'Stuffing Originals' *(Green Giant)*	1/2 cup	160	3.0	21.0	540	(mq)	7.0	na
STUFFING MIX, MICROWAVE								
broccoli and cheese, prepared w/salted butter *(Stove Top)*	1/2 cup	170	4.0	20.0	580	(mq)	8.0	15
cornbread, homestyle, prepared w/salted butter *(Stove Top)*	1/2 cup	160	3.0	20.0	450	(mq)	7.0	10

Food Name	Serv. Size	Total Cal.	Prot. GMS	Carbs GMS	Sod. MGS	Fiber GMS	Fat GMS	Chol. MGS
mushroom and onion, prepared								
w/salted butter *(Stove Top)*	1/2 cup	170	4.0	21.0	510	(mq)	7.0	10
STURGEON, MIXED SPECIES								
baked	4 oz	153	23.5	0.0	(mq)	0	5.9	(mq)
broiled	4 oz	153	23.5	0.0	(mq)	0	5.9	(mq)
dry-heat cooked	3 oz	115	17.6	0.0	59	0	4.4	65
microwaved	4 oz	153	23.5	0.0	(mq)	0	5.9	(mq)
raw	1 lb	478	73.2	0.0	(mq)	0	18.3	(mq)
raw	3 oz	89	13.7	0.0	46	0	3.4	51
raw	1 oz	30	4.6	0.0	(mq)	0	1.1	(mq)
smoked	4 oz	196	35.4	0.0	(mq)	0	5.0	(mq)
SUCCOTASH								
boiled, drained	4 oz	130	5.7	27.6	19	>1.5 c	0.9	0
boiled, drained	1/2 cup	110	4.9	23.4	16	>1.3 c	0.8	0
raw	1 lb	451	22.8	88.9	19	11.8	4.6	0
raw	1 oz	28	1.4	5.6	1	.7	0.3	0
Canned								
(S&W) 'Country Style'	1/2 cup	80	4.0	16.0	250	(mq)	1.0	0
(Stokely)	1/2 cup	90	3.0	20.0	300	(mq)	0.0	0
Frozen								
boiled, drained	4 oz	105	4.9	22.6	51	>1.2 c	1.0	0
boiled, drained	1/2 cup	79	3.7	17.0	38	>.9 c	0.8	0
unprepared	1/2 cup	73	3.4	15.6	35	4.9	0.7	0
(Frosty Acres)	3.3 oz	100	4.0	19.0	47	>1.0 c	0.0	0
(Seabrook)	3.3 oz	100	4.0	19.0	47	>1.0 c	0.0	0
SUCKER								
dry-heat cooked	3 oz	101	18.3	0.0	43	0	2.5	45
raw	1 lb	419	76.0	0.0	181	0	10.5	187
SUGAR, ALTERNATIVE								
(Equal) aspartame	1 pkg	4	0.0	<1.0	0	0	0.0	0
(Featherweight) saccharin	1 tablet	0	0.0	0.0	8	0	0.0	0
(Featherweight) saccharin, liquid	3 drops	0	0.0	0.0	0	0	0.0	0
(Nutra Taste) saccharin	1 pkt	4	0.0	1.0	0	na	0.0	na
(NutraSweet) aspartame 'Spoonful'	1 tsp	2	0.0	<1.0	0	na	0.0	na
(S&W Nutradiet) saccharin, liquid	1/8 tsp	0	0.0	0.0	0	0	0.0	0
(Sprinkle Sweet)	1 tsp	2	0.0	0.5	19	0	0.0	0
(Sugar Twin) saccharin	1 pkt	4	0.0	<1.0	0	na	0.0	na
(Sugar Twin) saccharin 'Plus'	1 pkt	3	0.0	<1.0	0	na	0.0	na
(Sweet 'n Low)	1 pkt	4	0.0	1.0	0	0	0.0	0
(Sweet One)	1 pkt	4	0.0	1.0	0	na	0.0	na
(Sweet Plus)	1 pkt	4	0.0	1.0	0	na	0.0	na
(Sweet•10)	1/8 tsp	0	0.0	0.0	2	0	0.0	0
(Weight Watchers) 'Sweet'ner'	1 pkt	4	0.0	1.0	30	0	0.0	0

Food Name	Serv. Size	Total Cal.	Prot. GMS	Carbs GMS	Sod. MGS	Fiber GMS	Fat GMS	Chol. MGS
SUGAR, BEET OR CANE. See also SUGAR, ALTERNATIVE; SUGAR, DEXTROSE; SUGAR, MAP**▶** SUGAR, TURBINADO; SUGAR CANE BATON.								
BROWN								
dark, 'Old Fashioned' (Domino)	1 tsp	16	0.0	4.0	0	na	0.0	na
golden, fresh from Hawaii (C&H)	1 tsp	16	0.0	4.0	0	na	0.0	na
light, 'Brownulated' (Domino)	1 tsp	12	0.0	3.0	0	na	0.0	na
light, golden, packed (Domino)	1 tsp	16	0.0	4.0	0	na	0.0	na
packed	1 cup	827	0.0	214.1	86	0	0.0	0
packed	1 oz	106	0.0	27.3	1	0	0.0	0
unpacked	1 cup	545	0.0	141.1	57	0	0.0	0
CONFECTIONER'S/powdered								
sifted	1 cup	385	0.0	99.5	1	0	0.0	0
sifted	1 oz	109	0.0	28.2	<1	0	0.0	0
sifted, 10-X (Domino)	1/2 cup	240	0.0	60.0	0	na	0.0	na
unsifted	1 cup	462	0.0	119.4	1	0	0.0	0
unsifted	1 tbsp	31	0.0	8.0	tr	0	0.0	0
GRANULATED								
	1 cup	774	0.0	199.8	2	0	0.0	0
	1 oz	109	0.0	28.2	<1	0	0.0	0
	1 tsp	15	0.0	4.0	0	0	0.0	0
cubes 'Dots' (Domino)	1 cube	8	0.0	2.0	0	na	0.0	na
cubes, 1/2 inch	2 cubes	19	0.0	5.0	tr	0	0.0	0
juice, organic (Sucanat)	1 tsp	12	0.0	3.0	0	na	0.0	0
lumps, 1 1/8 x 3/4 x 5/16 inches	1 lump	19	0.0	5.0	tr	0	0.0	0
packet, approx .2 oz	1 pkt	23	0.0	6.0	tr	0	0.0	0
'Packets' (Domino)	1 pkt	16	0.0	4.0	0	na	0.0	na
SUPERFINE, instant dissolving (Domino)	1 tsp	16	0.0	4.0	0	na	0.0	na
SUGAR, DEXTROSE								
anhydrous	100 gm	366	0.0	99.5	0	0	0.0	0
anhydrous	1 oz	104	0.0	28.2	tr	0	0.0	0
crystallized	100 gm	335	0.0	91.0	0	0	0.0	0
crystallized	1 oz	95	0.0	25.8	tr	0	0.0	0
SUGAR, MAPLE								
	100 gm	354	0.1	90.9	11	0	0.2	0
	1-oz piece	100	0.0	25.8	3	0	0.1	0
SUGAR, TURBINADO (Hain)	1 tbsp	50	0.0	12.0	0	0	0.0	0
SUGAR APPLE/sweetsop								
raw, approx 2 7/8-inch diam	1 med	146	3.2	36.6	14	6.8	0.5	0
raw, pulp	1 cup	235	5.2	59.1	23	11.0	0.7	0
trimmed	1/2 cup	118	2.6	29.6	12	3.4	0.4	0
trimmed	1 oz	27	0.6	6.7	3	.8	0.1	0
untrimmed	1 lb	236	5.1	59.0	24	12.8	0.7	0
SUGAR CANE BATON (Frieda's)	1 oz	21	<.1	49.9	na	(tr)	0.1	0

Food Name	Serv. Size	Total Cal.	Prot. GMS	Carbs GMS	Sod. MGS	Fiber GMS	Fat GMS	Chol. MGS
SUGAR CANE JUICE .... 1 oz		21	0.1	5.1	na	tr	tr	0
SUMMER SAUSAGE								
(Eckrich) .... 1-oz slice		80	4.0	1.0	320	0	7.0	(mq)
(Hillshire Farm) .... 2 oz		180	9.0	1.0	670	0	16.0	(mq)
(Hormel) 'Perma-Fresh' .... 2 slices		140	10.0	0.0	706	0	11.0	(mq)
(Hormel) 'Tangy Chub' .... 1 oz		90	5.0	0.0	317	0	7.0	(mq)
(Hormel) 'Thuringer' .... 1 oz		90	4.0	0.0	332	0	9.0	(mq)
BEEF								
(Hillshire Farm) .... 2 oz		190	9.0	1.0	(mq)	0	17.0	(mq)
(Hormel) 'Beefy' .... 1 oz		100	5.0	0.0	313	0	9.0	(mq)
(Lean & Lite) .... 1 oz		43	6.1	1.0	(mq)	0	2.3	18
(Light & Lean) .... 2 slices		100	6.0	0.0	(mq)	0	8.0	(mq)
(OHSE) .... 1 oz		75	5.0	2.0	340	0	5.0	(mq)
(Oscar Mayer) .... .8-oz slice		69	3.5	0.2	331	0	6.1	19
TURKEY (Louis Rich) .... 1-oz slice		55	4.7	0.4	326	0	3.9	21
W/CHEESE (Hillshire Farm) .... 2 oz		200	9.0	1.0	(mq)	0	18.0	(mq)
SUNCHOKE. See ARTICHOKE, JERUSALEM.								
SUN-DRIED TOMATOES, in oil and herbs								
(Bella Sun Luci) .... 2/3 oz		60	2.0	6.0	20	2.0	3.0	0
SUNFISH/calico bass/crappie/pumpkinseed								
dry-heat cooked .... 3 oz		97	21.1	0.0	88	0	0.8	73
raw .... 1 lb		404	88.0	0.0	368	0	3.2	304
raw .... 3 oz		76	16.5	0.0	68	0	0.6	57
raw .... 1 oz		25	5.5	0.0	23	0	0.2	19
SUNFLOWER BUTTER								
.... 1 oz		165	5.6	7.8	1	1.4	13.6	0
.... 1 tbsp		93	3.2	4.4	1	.8	7.6	0
gourmet (Roaster Fresh) .... 1 oz		160	6.0	5.0	1	na	13.6	na
roasted (Maranatha Natural) .... 2 tbsp		170	4.0	8.0	5	na	14.0	0
SUNFLOWER OIL								
hydrogenated .... 1/2 cup		964	0.0	0.0	0	0	109.0	0
hydrogenated .... 1 oz		251	0.0	0.0	0	0	28.4	0
linoleic .... 1/2 cup		964	0.0	0.0	0	0	109.0	0
linoleic .... 1 oz		251	0.0	0.0	0	0	28.4	0
(Hain) .... 1 tbsp		120	0.0	0.0	0	0	14.0	0
(IGA) .... 1 tbsp		120	0.0	0.0	0	0	14.0	0
(Kroger) .... 1 tbsp		122	0.0	0.0	0	0	13.6	0
(Pathmark) .... 1 tbsp		130	0.0	0.0	0	0	14.0	0
(Spectrum Naturals) .... 1 tbsp		120	0.0	0.0	0	(tr)	14.0	(tr)
(Wesson) .... 1 tbsp		122	0.0	0.0	0	0	13.6	0
SUNFLOWER SEED KERNELS								
Dried								
.... 1 cup		821	32.8	27.0	4	15.1	71.4	0

Food Name	Serv. Size	Total Cal.	Prot. GMS	Carbs GMS	Sod. MGS	Fiber GMS	Fat GMS	Chol. MGS
. . . .	1 oz	162	6.5	5.3	1	3.0	14.1	0
in shell	1 lb	1397	55.8	46.0	8	na	121.4	0
(Arrowhead Mills)	1 oz	160	7.0	6.0	3	4.4	13.0	0
(Frito-Lay's)	1 oz	160	7.0	6.0	265	na	14.0	0
Dry-roasted								
. . . .	1 cup	745	24.8	30.8	4	11.5	63.7	0
. . . .	1 oz	165	5.5	6.8	1	2.5	14.1	0
salted	1 cup	745	24.8	30.8	998	8.7	63.7	0
salted	1 oz	165	5.5	6.8	221	1.9	14.1	0
(Fisher)	1 oz	170	6.0	6.0	200	na	15.0	0
(Fisher) in shell	1 oz	170	6.0	6.0	110	na	15.0	0
(Fisher) in shell, salted	1 oz	170	6.0	6.0	110	na	14.0	0
(Flavor House)	1 oz	180	8.0	4.0	200	(mq)	15.0	0
(Pathmark)	1 oz	180	5.0	7.0	150	(mq)	14.0	0
(Planters)	1 oz	160	6.0	6.0	170	na	14.0	0
Oil-roasted								
. . . .	1 cup	830	28.8	19.9	4	9.2	77.6	0
. . . .	1 oz	175	6.1	4.2	1	1.9	16.3	0
salted	1 cup	830	28.8	19.9	814	9.2	77.6	0
salted	1 oz	175	6.1	4.2	171	1.9	16.3	0
(Fisher)	1 oz	170	6.0	4.0	170	na	16.0	0
(Planters)	1 oz	170	6.0	5.0	135	na	15.0	0
Toasted								
. . . .	1 cup	829	23.1	27.6	4	>2.4 c	76.1	0
. . . .	1 oz	176	4.9	5.9	1	>.5 c	16.1	0
salted	1 cup	829	23.1	27.6	821	>2.4 c	76.1	0
salted	1 oz	176	4.9	5.9	174	>.5 c	16.1	0
(Fisher)	1 oz	170	6.0	6.0	0	na	14.0	0
SUNFLOWER SEED FLOUR								
partially defatted	1 cup	261	38.5	28.7	2	4.2	1.3	0
partially defatted	1 oz	92	13.6	10.2	1	1.5	0.5	0
partially defatted	1 tbsp	16	2.4	1.8	0	.3	0.1	0
SUNSHINE JUICE, organic								
(Santa Cruz Natural)	8 oz	100	1.0	23.0	na	na	1.0	na
SURIMI								
. . . .	3 oz	84	12.9	5.8	122	0	0.8	25
leg style 'Classic Seablends' 10% crab								
(Peter Pan Seafoods)	3.5 oz	85	9.8	na	890	na	0.4	31
leg style 'Standard Seablends'								
(Peter Pan Seafoods)	3.5 oz	88	9.0	na	845	na	0.4	34
salad style 'Classic Seablends Combo'								
10% crab *(Peter Pan Seafoods)*	3.5 oz	85	9.8	na	890	na	0.4	31

Food Name	Serv. Size	Total Cal.	Prot. GMS	Carbs GMS	Sod. MGS	Fiber GMS	Fat GMS	Chol. MGS
salad style 'Standard Seablends Combo'								
(Peter Pan Seafoods)	3.5 oz	88	9.0	na	845	na	0.4	34
SURINAM CHERRY. See PITANGA.								
SWAMP CABBAGE. See CABBAGE, SKUNK.								
SWEDISH MEATBALL DINNER/ENTRÉE								
frozen dinner, 'Classics' (Armour)	11.25 oz	330	19.0	23.0	1140	na	18.0	80
frozen entrée, w/parsley noodles, gravy								
'Lean Cuisine' (Stouffer's)	9.25 oz	420	24.0	32.0	740	na	21.0	na
frozen entrée, w/pasta, gravy								
'Lean Cuisine' (Stouffer's)	9 1/8 oz	290	23.0	31.0	550	na	8.0	55
SWEDISH TURNIP								
boiled, drained	4 oz	39	1.2	8.8	20	>1.2 c	0.2	0
boiled, drained, cubed	1/2 cup	29	0.9	6.6	15	>.9 c	0.2	0
boiled, drained, mashed	1/2 cup	41	1.3	9.3	22	>1.3 c	0.2	0
raw, cubed	1/2 cup	25	0.8	5.7	14	>.8 c	0.1	0
raw, trimmed	1 oz	10	0.3	2.3	6	>.3 c	0.1	0
raw, untrimmed	1 lb	140	4.6	31.4	77	>4.2 c	0.8	0
SWEET AND SOUR DINNER (LaChoy) ..	4.48 oz	89	1.1	21.7	838	2.0	0.2	0
SWEET POTATO. See also YAM.								
baked in skin, pulp only	4 oz	117	2.0	27.5	11	3.4	0.1	0
baked in skin, pulp only, 5 inches long,								
2 inches diam	1 potato	118	2.0	27.7	12	3.4	0.1	0
baked in skin, pulp only, mashed	1/2 cup	103	1.7	24.3	10	3.0	0.1	0
boiled, w/o skin	4 oz	119	1.9	27.5	15	>1.0 c	0.3	0
boiled, w/o skin, mashed	1/2 cup	172	2.7	39.8	21	>1.4 c	0.5	0
dehydrated flakes, dry	1 cup	455	5.0	108.0	217	>3.8 c	0.7	0
dehydrated flakes, prepared w/water	1 lb	431	4.5	102.6	204	>3.6 c	0.5	0
dehydrated flakes, prepared w/water	1 cup	242	2.5	57.6	115	>2.0 c	0.3	0
raw, cubes	1 cup	140	2.2	32.3	17	4.0	0.4	0
raw, 5 inches long, 2 inches diam	1 potato	136	2.2	31.6	17	3.9	0.4	0
raw, trimmed	1 oz	30	0.5	6.9	4	.9	0.1	0
raw, untrimmed	1 lb	343	5.4	79.3	44	9.8	1.0	0
SWEET POTATO, CANNED								
Candied								
(Joan of Arc)	1/2 cup	240	1.0	60.0	15	(mq)	0.0	0
(Princella)	1/2 cup	240	1.0	60.0	15	(mq)	0.0	0
(Royal Prince)	1/2 cup	240	1.0	60.0	15	(mq)	0.0	0
(S&W)	1/2 cup	180	1.0	44.0	355	(mq)	0.0	0
In extra heavy syrup (S&W) 'Southern' ...	1/2 cup	139	1.0	31.0	27	(mq)	1.0	0
In heavy syrup								
(Joan of Arc)	1/2 cup	130	1.0	34.0	35	(mq)	0.0	0
(Princella)	1/2 cup	130	1.0	34.0	35	(mq)	0.0	0
(Royal Prince)	1/2 cup	130	1.0	34.0	35	(mq)	0.0	0

Food Name	Serv. Size	Total Cal.	Prot. GMS	Carbs GMS	Sod. MGS	Fiber GMS	Fat GMS	Chol. MGS
In light syrup								
(Finast)	1/2 cup	110	2.0	25.0	45	(mq)	<1.0	0
(Joan of Arc)	1/2 cup	110	1.0	28.0	25	(mq)	0.0	0
(Princella)	1/2 cup	110	1.0	28.0	25	(mq)	0.0	0
(Royal Prince)	1/2 cup	110	1.0	28.0	25	(mq)	0.0	0
In pineapple-orange sauce								
(Joan of Arc)	1/2 cup	210	1.0	54.0	35	(mq)	0.0	0
(Princella)	1/2 cup	210	1.0	54.0	35	(mq)	0.0	0
(Royal Prince)	1/2 cup	210	1.0	54.0	35	(mq)	0.0	0
In syrup								
(Allens) cut	1/2 cup	90	2.0	20.0	20	(mq)	<1.0	0
(Allens) whole	1/2 cup	90	2.0	20.0	40	(mq)	<1.0	0
(Joan of Arc)	1/2 cup	90	1.0	24.0	45	(mq)	0.0	0
(Kohl's) cut	1/2 cup	110	1.0	31.0	30	(mq)	<1.0	0
(Pathmark) 'No Frills'	1/2 cup	105	1.0	25.0	33	(mq)	0.0	0
(Pathmark) 'Southern'	1 cup	230	2.0	55.0	100	(mq)	0.0	0
(Princella)	1/2 cup	90	1.0	24.0	45	(mq)	0.0	0
(Royal Prince)	1/2 cup	90	1.0	24.0	45	(mq)	0.0	0
(Taylor's Brand) whole and cut	1 cup	240	3.0	58.0	56	(mq)	0.0	0
In water (Allens) cut	1/2 cup	70	1.0	16.0	20	(mq)	<1.0	0
SWEET POTATO, FROZEN								
unprepared, cubes	1/2 cup	84	1.5	19.5	5	>.7 c	0.2	0
(Mrs. Paul's) candied	4 oz	170	1.0	42.0	40	(mq)	0.0	0
(Mrs. Paul's) candied, w/apples								
'Sweets 'n Apples'	4 oz	160	1.0	38.0	60	(mq)	0.0	0
SWEET POTATO LEAF								
raw, approx 12 1/4 inches long	1 leaf	6	0.6	1.0	1	>.2 c	0.1	0
raw, chopped	1 cup	12	1.4	2.2	3	>.4 c	0.1	0
raw, trimmed	1 oz	10	1.1	1.8	3	>.3 c	0.1	0
raw, untrimmed	1 lb	149	17.1	27.2	38	>5.1 c	1.3	0
steamed	4 oz	39	2.6	8.3	15	2.1	0.3	0
steamed	1/2 cup	11	0.7	2.3	4	.6	0.1	0

SWEETBREAD. See BEEF, PANCREAS; BEEF, THYMUS; LAMB, PANCREAS; VEAL, PANCREA
VEAL, THYMUS.

SWEETENERS. See SUGAR, ALTERNATIVE; SUGAR, BEET OR CANE; SUGAR, MAPLE;
SUGAR, TURBINADO.

SWEETSOP. See SUGAR APPLE.

SWISS CHARD/chard

boiled, drained	4 oz	23	2.1	4.7	203	>1.1 c	0.1	0
boiled, drained, chopped	1/2 cup	18	1.6	3.6	158	1.9	0.1	0
raw, chopped	1/2 cup	3	0.3	0.7	38	.3	0.0	0
raw, trimmed	1 oz	5	0.5	1.1	60	>.2 c	0.1	0
raw, untrimmed	1 lb	81	7.5	15.6	888	>3.3 c	0.8	0

Food Name	Serv. Size	Total Cal.	Prot. GMS	Carbs GMS	Sod. MGS	Fiber GMS	Fat GMS	Chol. MGS
SWISS STEAK DINNER								
frozen *(Budget Gourmet)*	11.2 oz	450	23.0	40.0	1110	(mq)	22.0	70
frozen *(Swanson)*	10 oz	350	26.0	37.0	700	(mq)	11.0	(mq)
SWISS STEAK SEASONING MIX								
'Bag 'n Season' *(Schilling)*	1 pkg	81	1.9	17.0	2651	na	0.4	1
SWORDFISH								
baked	4 oz	176	28.8	0.0	130	0	5.8	57
broiled	4 oz	176	28.8	0.0	130	0	5.8	57
dry-heat cooked	3 oz	132	21.6	0.0	98	0	4.4	43
frozen, steaks, w/o seasoning mix								
(SeaPak)	6-oz pkg	210	34.0	0.0	155	0	7.0	70
microwaved	4 oz	176	28.8	0.0	130	0	5.8	57
raw	1 lb	548	89.8	0.0	408	0	18.2	178
raw	3 oz	103	16.8	0.0	77	0	3.4	33
raw	1 oz	34	5.6	0.0	26	0	1.1	11
raw *(Peter Pan Seafoods)*	3.5 oz	118	19.1	na	102	na	4.0	39

T

Food Name	Serv. Size	Total Cal.	Prot. GMS	Carbs GMS	Sod. MGS	Fiber GMS	Fat GMS	Chol. MGS
TABBOULEH MIX								
(Casbah) dry	1 oz	126	4.0	28.0	(mq)	(mq)	1.0	0
(Fantastic Foods) prepared w/oil and								
tomatoes	1/2 cup	161	2.0	17.0	250	(mq)	10.0	0
(Fantastic Foods) prepared w/o oil	1/2 cup	85	3.0	17.0	265	na	0.5	na
(Near East) prepared	1/2 cup	170	3.0	20.0	290	(mq)	9.0	0
TABLE QUEEN SQUASH. See SQUASH, ACORN.								
TACO DIP. See DIP, TACO.								
TACO KIT								
(Natural Touch) vegetarian	2 tbsp	90	10.0	6.0	(mq)	(mq)	2.0	0
(Old El Paso) prepared	1 taco	67	2.0	8.0	423	(mq)	3.0	na
(Tio Sancho) 'Dinner Kit' prepared	1 taco	64	1.1	8.1	1	>.5 c	3.1	na
TACO SEASONING MIX								
(Hain)	1/10 pkg	10	1.0	2.0	200	(mq)	0.0	0
(Lawry's) 'Seasoning Blends'	1 pkg	118	3.4	23.6	1441	>1.0 c	1.1	0
(Old El Paso)	1 pkg	100	1.0	21.0	3570	(mq)	1.0	na
(Old El Paso)	1/12 pkg	8	<1.0	2.0	298	(mq)	<1.0	0
(Schilling)	1/4 pkg	31	1.0	6.0	675	(mq)	0.5	0
(Tio Sancho)	1.51 oz	132	2.9	26.0	2623	>2.0 c	1.7	0
(Tio Sancho) 'Dinner Kit' taco seasoning	1.25 oz	104	2.1	20.9	2500	>1.7 c	1.4	na
TACO SHELL								
(Azteca) corn	1 shell	60	1.0	7.0	65	(mq)	3.0	0

Food Name	Serv. Size	Total Cal.	Prot. GMS	Carbs GMS	Sod. MGS	Fiber GMS	Fat GMS	Chol. MGS
(Azteca) flour	1 shell	200	3.0	18.0	130	(mq)	12.0	na
(Chi-Chi's)	1 shell	140	2.0	17.0	5	na	7.0	0
(Gebhardt)	1 shell	50	1.0	7.0	<1	<1.0	2.0	0
(Lawry's)	1 shell	50	0.8	8.0	123	>.2 c	2.1	0
(Lawry's) 'Super'	1 shell	86	1.4	13.0	210	>.4 c	3.6	0
(Old El Paso)	1 shell	50	0.0	6.0	50	.5	3.0	0
(Old El Paso) 'Mini'	3 shells	70	1.0	7.0	60	.5	4.0	0
(Old El Paso) 'Super Size'	1 shell	100	1.0	11.0	95	1.5	6.0	0
(Ortega)	1 shell	50	0.0	8.0	5	(mq)	2.0	0
(Rosarita)	1 shell	50	1.0	7.0	<1	<1.0	2.0	0
(Tio Sancho)	1 shell	64	1.1	8.1	1	>.5 c	3.1	0
(Tio Sancho) 'Super'	1 shell	94	1.6	11.3	2	>.7 c	4.7	0
TAFFY. See CANDY.								
TAHINI MIX								
(Arrowhead Mills) organic	1 oz	170	6.0	4.0	<1	2.6	17.0	0
(Casbah) dry	1 oz	25	2.0	2.0	(mq)	(mq)	5.0	0
(Erewhon) 'Sesame Tahini'	2 tbsp	200	6.0	3.0	65	na	18.0	na
(Maranatha Natural) 'Sesame Tahini'	2 tbsp	210	8.0	3.0	20	na	19.0	0
(Westbrae) raw, organic	2 tbsp	210	8.0	1.0	0	na	19.0	na
(Westbrae) toasted, organic	2 tbsp	220	8.0	3.0	0	na	19.0	na
TAMALE								
(Derby) beef	2 tamales	160	8.0	15.0	570	1.0	7.0	24
(Gebhardt)	2 tamales	290	5.0	19.0	730	2.0	22.0	54
(Gebhardt) jumbo	2 tamales	400	7.0	26.0	1025	3.0	30.0	75
Canned								
(Derby) beef	6.561 oz	253	7.3	20.8	1034	4.0	17.4	23
(Gebhardt)	5.75 oz	269	4.6	18.6	770	2.6	20.7	28
(Gebhardt) beef	4 oz	230	4.0	15.0	620	(mq)	17.0	(mq)
(Gebhardt) jumbo	6.949 oz	332	5.6	24.0	930	3.2	25.2	34
(Hormel)	7.5 oz	280	6.0	19.0	990	na	20.0	35
(Hormel) beef	2 tamales	140	4.0	8.0	550	(mq)	10.0	(mq)
(Hormel) hot 'n spicy	7.5 oz	280	6.0	19.0	990	na	20.0	35
(Libby's) beef, w/sauce	7.5 oz	408	8.9	26.4	1200	na	30.2	43
(Old El Paso)	2 tamales	190	5.0	16.0	380	(mq)	12.0	20
(Van Camp's) w/sauce	1 cup	293	8.3	28.6	1132	>2.2 c	16.2	(mq)
(Wolf Brand)	7.75 oz	328	8.3	24.9	1181	>1.5 c	24.5	(mq)
Frozen								
(Amy's Kitchen) 'Mexican' organic	8 oz	170	6.0	36.0	190	5.0	3.0	0
(Hormel) beef	1 tamale	140	6.0	13.0	555	(mq)	7.0	(mq)
(Patio) dinner	13 oz	470	12.0	58.0	1850	(mq)	21.0	35
TAMALITO (Dennison's) in chili gravy, canned	7.5 oz	310	6.0	37.0	1395	(mq)	16.0	(mq)

Food Name	Serv. Size	Total Cal.	Prot. GMS	Carbs GMS	Sod. MGS	Fiber GMS	Fat GMS	Chol. MGS
TAMARIND/Indian date								
pulp	1 cup	287	3.4	75.0	34	>6.1 c	0.7	0
'Tamarindos' (Frieda's)	3.5 oz	239	2.8	62.5	51	(mq)	0.6	0
trimmed	1 oz	68	0.8	17.7	8	>1.4 c	0.2	0
untrimmed	1 lb	369	4.3	96.4	43	>7.9 c	0.9	0
TANGELO JUICE, fresh	100 gm	41	0.5	9.7	1	0	0.1	0
TANGERINE								
peeled, seeded	1 oz	12	0.2	3.2	<1	>.1 c	0.1	0
sections, w/o membrane	1/2 cup	43	0.6	10.9	2	>.3 c	0.2	0
untrimmed	1 lb	144	2.1	36.6	4	>1.1 c	0.6	0
TANGERINE, CANNED								
in heavy syrup (S&W)	1/2 cup	76	0.0	20.0	10	(mq)	0.0	0
in juice	4 oz	42	0.7	10.9	6	.9	<.1	0
in light syrup	4 oz	69	0.5	18.4	7	.9	0.1	0
in light syrup (A&P)	1/2 cup	80	<1.0	20.0	0	(mq)	<1.0	0
in light syrup (Dole)	1/2 cup	76	0.6	20.0	0	(mq)	0.1	0
in light syrup (Empress)	5.5 oz	100	0.0	25.0	10	(mq)	0.0	0
in light syrup (Finast)	5.5 oz	100	0.0	25.0	na	(mq)	0.0	0
'Natural Style' (S&W)	1/2 cup	60	0.0	15.0	10	(mq)	0.0	0
sections, in water (Featherweight)	1/2 cup	35	0.0	8.0	10	(mq)	0.0	0
unsweetened (S&W Nutradiet)	1/2 cup	28	0.0	7.0	10	(mq)	0.0	0
TANGERINE JUICE								
canned, sweetened	1 cup	125	1.3	29.9	2	.5	0.5	0
canned, sweetened	1 oz	16	0.2	3.7	0	.1	0.1	0
chilled 'Pure & Light Mandarin Tangerine' (Dole)	6 oz	97	0.6	25.0	20	(mq)	0.1	0
fresh	1 cup	106	1.2	25.0	2	.5	0.5	0
fresh	1 oz	13	0.2	3.1	0	.1	0.1	0
frozen concentrate, sweetened, diluted w/3 vol water	1 cup	111	1.0	26.7	2	na	0.3	0
frozen concentrate, sweetened, diluted w/3 vol water	1 oz	14	0.1	3.3	0	na	0.0	0
frozen concentrate, sweetened, undiluted	6 oz	345	3.2	83.1	6	1.3	0.8	0
frozen or chilled (Minute Maid)	6 oz	90	1.0	23.0	0	na	0.0	na
TANGERINE ORANGE DRINK								
'Thirst Quencher Light' (Gatorade)	8 oz	25	0.0	7.0	80	na	0.0	na
TAPIOCA, PEARL								
dry	1 cup	518	0.3	134.8	2	1.6	0.0	0
dry	1 oz	97	<.1	25.1	tr	.3	tr	0
TARO								
cooked	4 oz	161	0.6	39.2	11	>1.0 c	0.1	0
cooked, slices	1/2 cup	94	0.3	22.8	10	3.4	0.1	0
raw, slices	1/2 cup	56	0.8	13.8	6	2.1	0.1	0

Food Name	Serv. Size	Total Cal.	Prot. GMS	Carbs GMS	Sod. MGS	Fiber GMS	Fat GMS	Chol. MGS
raw, trimmed	1 oz	30	0.4	7.5	3	>.2 c	0.1	0
raw, untrimmed	1 lb	419	5.9	103.2	43	>3.1 c	0.8	0
TARO, TAHITIAN								
cooked	4 oz	50	4.7	7.8	61	>2.6 c	0.8	0
cooked, slices	1/2 cup	30	2.8	4.7	37	>1.5 c	0.5	0
raw, slices	1/2 cup	25	1.7	4.3	31	>1.1 c	0.6	0
raw, trimmed	1 lb	181	12.7	31.3	227	>7.9 c	4.4	0
raw, trimmed	1 oz	11	0.8	2.0	14	>.5 c	0.3	0
TARO LEAF								
raw	1 cup	12	1.4	1.9	1	1.0	0.2	0
raw, 11 x 6 1/2 inches	1 leaf	4	0.5	0.7	0	.4	0.1	0
raw, trimmed	1 oz	12	1.4	1.9	1	>.6 c	0.2	0
raw, untrimmed	1 lb	115	13.5	18.3	8	>5.5 c	2.0	0
steamed	4 oz	27	3.1	4.6	2	>.6 c	0.5	0
steamed	1/2 cup	18	2.0	3.0	1	>.4 c	0.3	0
TARO SHOOTS								
cooked	4 oz	16	0.8	3.6	2	>.6 c	0.1	0
cooked, slices	1/2 cup	10	0.5	2.2	1	>.4 c	0.1	0
raw, 15 x 5 inches	1 shoot	9	0.8	1.9	1	>.5 c	0.1	0
raw, slices	1/2 cup	5	0.4	1.0	0	>.3 c	0.0	0
raw, trimmed	1 oz	3	0.3	0.7	<1	>.2 c	<.1	0
raw, untrimmed	1 lb	45	3.7	9.3	4	>2.3 c	0.4	0
TARPON, ATLANTIC								
raw	1 lb	422	94.8	0.0	(mq)	0	1.8	(mq)
raw	1 oz	26	5.0	0.0	(mq)	0	0.1	(mq)
TARRAGON								
ground	1 oz	84	6.5	14.2	18	2.1	2.1	0
ground	1 tbsp	14	1.1	2.4	3	.4	0.4	0
ground	1 tsp	5	0.4	0.8	1	.1	0.1	0
ground *(Durkee)*	1 tsp	10	0.0	0.0	0	0	<0.1	na
ground *(Laurel Leaf)*	1 tsp	10	0.0	0.0	0	0	<0.1	na
ground *(Spice Islands)*	1 tsp	5	0.3	0.7	1	.1	0.1	0
TEA								
Brewed								
prepared w/distilled water	6 oz	2	0.0	0.5	0	0	0.0	0
prepared w/tap water	6 oz	2	0.0	0.5	5	0	0.0	0
(Celestial Seasonings) caffeine-free	8 oz	4	tr	0.8	5	tr	tr	0
(Nestea)	6 oz	0	0.0	0.0	0	0	0.0	0
Instant								
decaffeinated *(Lipton)*	6 oz	0	0.0	0.0	0	0	0.0	0
lemon flavor *(Lipton)*	6 oz	3	0.1	0.6	1	0	0.0	0
regular *(Lipton)*	6 oz	0	0.0	0.0	0	0	0.0	0

Food Name	Serv. Size	Total Cal.	Prot. GMS	Carbs GMS	Sod. MGS	Fiber GMS	Fat GMS	Chol. MGS
TEA, FLAVORED								
(Bigelow)								
'Chinese Fortune'	5.25 oz	1	<.1	0.1	<1	0	tr	0
'Cinnamon Stick'	5.25 oz	1	<.1	0.1	<1	0	tr	0
'Constant Comment'	5.25 oz	1	<.1	0.1	<1	0	tr	0
'Darjeeling'	5.25 oz	1	<.1	0.1	<1	0	tr	0
'Earl Grey'	5.25 oz	1	<.1	0.1	1	0	tr	0
'English Teatime'	5.25 oz	1	<.1	0.1	tr	0	tr	0
'Lemon Lift'	5.25 oz	1	<.1	0.2	<1	0	tr	0
'Plantation Mint'	5.25 oz	1	<.1	0.1	1	0	tr	0
'Raspberry Royale'	5.25 oz	1	<.1	0.1	<1	0	tr	0
(Celestial Seasonings)								
'Amaretto Nights'	8 oz	3	tr	0.6	1	tr	tr	0
apple spice 'Fruit & Tea'	8 oz	3	<.1	0.2	1	tr	tr	0
'Bavarian Chocolate Orange'	8 oz	7	tr	1.6	5	tr	tr	0
'Cinnamon Vienna'	8 oz	2	tr	0.4	2	tr	tr	0
'Classic English Breakfast'	8 oz	3	tr	0.4	<1	tr	tr	0
'Darjeeling Gardens'	8 oz	3	tr	0.5	<1	tr	tr	0
'Extraordinary Earl Grey'	8 oz	3	tr	0.5	<1	tr	tr	0
'Irish Cream Mist'	8 oz	3	tr	0.6	1	tr	tr	0
lemon 'Fruit & Tea'	8 oz	3	tr	0.5	<1	tr	tr	0
mint, Swiss	8 oz	3	tr	0.4	<1	tr	tr	0
'Morning Thunder'	8 oz	3	tr	0.4	<1	tr	tr	0
orange spice 'Fruit & Tea'	8 oz	3	tr	0.4	<1	tr	tr	0
raspberry 'Fruit & Tea'	8 oz	2	tr	0.5	<1	tr	tr	0
(Nestea)								
apple spice	16 oz	180	2.0	44.0	50	na	0.0	0
apple spice	6 oz	66	1.0	16.5	18	na	0.0	0
lemon, natural	16 oz	180	2.0	44.0	50	na	0.0	0
lemon, natural	6 oz	66	1.0	16.5	18	na	0.0	0
lemon, natural, diet	16 oz	180	2.0	44.0	50	na	0.0	0
lemon, natural, diet	6 oz	66	1.0	16.5	18	na	0.0	0
peach	16 oz	180	2.0	44.0	50	na	0.0	0
peach	6 oz	66	1.0	16.5	18	na	0.0	0
raspberry	16 oz	180	2.0	44.0	50	na	0.0	0
raspberry	6 oz	66	1.0	16.5	18	na	0.0	0
tropical	16 oz	180	2.0	44.0	50	na	0.0	0
tropical	6 oz	66	1.0	16.5	18	na	0.0	0
(Tetley)								
'Apple Freeze'	8 oz	79	tr	20.0	<1	na	0.0	na
'Classic'	8 oz	69	tr	17.0	<1	na	0.0	na
'Classic Lemon'	8 oz	108	0.1	27.0	<1	na	0.0	na
'Diet Lemon Frost'	8 oz	10	0.1	2.3	<1	na	0.0	na

Food Name	Serv. Size	Total Cal.	Prot. GMS	Carbs GMS	Sod. MGS	Fiber GMS	Fat GMS	Chol. MGS
'Diet Raspberry Blizzard'	8 oz	10	0.1	2.4	<1	na	0.0	na
'Lemon Frost'	8 oz	89	tr	22.0	<1	na	0.0	na
'Orange Glazier'	8 oz	79	tr	20.0	<1	na	0.0	na
'Peach Chiller'	8 oz	79	tr	20.0	<1	na	0.0	na
'Raspberry Blizzard'	8 oz	95	tr	24.0	<1	na	0.0	na
(Wyler's) 'Fruit Tea Punch'	12 oz	118	0.0	29.6	1	0	0.0	0
TEA, HERBAL								
(Bigelow)								
almond orange	5 oz	<1	<.1	<.1	<1	0	tr	0
'Apple Orchard'	5.25 oz	5	<.1	1.2	1	0	tr	0
apple spice	5 oz	<1	tr	<.1	1	0	tr	0
chamomile	5 oz	<1	<.1	tr	2	0	tr	0
chamomile mint	5 oz	<1	tr	tr	1	0	tr	0
cinnamon orange	5 oz	<1	<.1	0.1	<1	0	tr	0
cranberry apple	5 oz	1	0.1	0.3	1	0	tr	0
'Fruit & Almond'	5.25 oz	1	<.1	<.1	<1	0	tr	0
grains, roasted, w/carob	5 oz	3	<.1	0.6	1	0	tr	0
hibiscus and rose hips	5 oz	1	<.1	0.2	1	0	tr	0
'I Love Lemon'	5.25 oz	1	<.1	<.1	<1	0	tr	0
'Lemon & C'	5 oz	<1	tr	<.1	<1	0	tr	0
'Mint Blend'	5 oz	<1	<.1	0.2	3	0	tr	0
'Mint Medley'	5.25 oz	1	<.1	0.2	<1	0	tr	0
'Orange & C'	5 oz	<1	tr	<.1	<1	0	tr	0
'Orange & Spice'	5.25 oz	1	<.1	<.1	1	0	tr	0
peppermint	5 oz	<1	<.1	<.1	2	0	<.1	0
red raspberry	5 oz	1	0.1	0.2	<1	0	tr	0
spearmint	5 oz	<1	<.1	<.1	1	0	tr	0
'Specially Strawberry'	5 oz	1	0.1	0.2	<1	0	tr	0
'Sweet Dreams'	5.25 oz	1	<.1	0.1	1	0	tr	0
'Take-A-Break'	5.25 oz	1	<.1	0.6	1	0	tr	0
(Celestial Seasonings)								
'Almond Sunset'	8 oz	3	tr	1.1	2	tr	tr	0
chamomile	8 oz	2	tr	0.5	5	tr	tr	0
'Cinnamon Apple Spice'	8 oz	3	tr	0.4	1	tr	tr	0
'Cinnamon Rose'	8 oz	2	tr	1.1	1	tr	tr	0
'Country Peach Spice'	8 oz	3	tr	0.7	3	tr	tr	0
'Cranberry Cove'	8 oz	3	tr	0.7	1	tr	tr	0
'Emperor's Choice'	8 oz	4	<.1	0.9	2	<.1	<.1	0
'Ginseng Plus'	8 oz	3	tr	<.5	4	tr	tr	0
'Grandma's Tummy Mint'	8 oz	2	tr	<.3	7	tr	tr	0
'Lemon Mist'	8 oz	2	tr	<.5	3	tr	tr	0
'Lemon Zinger'	8 oz	4	<.1	0.7	1	tr	tr	0
'Mandarin Orange Spice'	8 oz	5	tr	1.1	2	tr	tr	0

Food Name	Serv. Size	Total Cal.	Prot. GMS	Carbs GMS	Sod. MGS	Fiber GMS	Fat GMS	Chol. MGS
'Mellow Mint'	8 oz	2	tr	0.4	4	tr	tr	0
'Mint Magic'	8 oz	1	tr	0.4	3	tr	tr	0
'Mo's 24'	8 oz	2	<.1	0.2	4	tr	tr	0
'Orange Zinger'	8 oz	5	tr	1.2	1	tr	tr	0
peppermint	8 oz	2	tr	1.1	8	tr	tr	0
'Raspberry Patch'	8 oz	4	tr	1.1	1	tr	tr	0
'Red Zinger'	8 oz	4	tr	1.1	2	<.1	tr	0
'Roastaroma'	8 oz	11	<.1	2.0	4	<.1	<.1	0
'Sleepytime'	8 oz	5	tr	1.1	2	<.1	tr	0
spearmint	8 oz	5	<.1	0.2	6	<.1	<.1	0
'Strawberry Fields'	8 oz	4	tr	0.8	1	tr	tr	0
'Sunburst C'	8 oz	3	tr	1.1	6	<.1	tr	0
'Wild Forest Blackberry'	8 oz	2	tr	1.8	1	tr	tr	0
(Lipton)								
'Almond Pleasure'	8 oz	4	0.0	1.0	0	0	0.0	0
chamomile	8 oz	4	0.0	1.0	0	0	0.0	0
cinnamon apple	8 oz	2	0.0	<1.0	0	0	0.0	0
'Citrus Sunset'	8 oz	4	0.0	1.0	0	0	0.0	0
'Gentle/Tangy Orange'	8 oz	4	0.0	1.0	0	0	0.0	0
'Lemon Soother'	8 oz	4	0.0	1.0	0	0	0.0	0
'Toasty Spice'	8 oz	6	0.0	1.0	0	0	0.0	0
TEA, ICED								
BOTTLE, BOX, OR CAN								
(Arizona)								
'Diet'	8 oz	4	0.0	0.0	15	na	0.0	na
'Diet' with lemon	8 oz	4	0.0	0.0	15	na	0.0	na
raspberry flavor, sun-brewed style	8 oz	95	0.0	25.0	20	na	0.0	na
(Lipton) w/lemon, aseptic box	8.45 oz	96	1.6	24.0	20	0	0.3	0
(Nestea)								
	8 oz	90	0.0	22.0	35	na	0.0	na
diet	8 oz	4	0.0	1.0	35	na	0.0	na
(Shasta)	12 oz	124	0.0	34.0	28	0	0.0	0
(Snapple)								
cranberry	8 oz	110	0.0	27.0	10	na	0.0	0
'Diet'	8 oz	0	0.0	1.0	10	na	0.0	0
lemon	8 oz	110	0.0	27.0	10	na	0.0	0
mango	8 oz	110	0.0	27.0	5	na	0.0	0
mint	8 oz	120	0.0	29.0	10	na	0.0	0
old fashioned	8 oz	80	0.0	20.0	10	na	0.0	0
orange	8 oz	110	0.0	27.0	10	na	0.0	0
peach	8 oz	110	0.0	27.0	10	na	0.0	0
peach 'Diet'	8 oz	0	0.0	1.0	10	na	0.0	0
raspberry	8 oz	120	0.0	29.0	10	na	0.0	0

Food Name	Serv. Size	Total Cal.	Prot. GMS	Carbs GMS	Sod. MGS	Fiber GMS	Fat GMS	Chol. MGS
raspberry 'Diet'	8 oz	0	0.0	1.0	10	na	0.0	0
strawberry	8 oz	100	0.0	26.0	10	na	0.0	0
w/lemon, 'Diet'	8 oz	4	<1.0	<1.0	15	na	<1.0	na
(Tetley)								
brewed	8 oz	74	0.0	19.0	20	na	0.0	na
brewed, w/lemon	8 oz	74	0.0	19.0	20	na	0.0	na
sweetened	8 oz	74	0.0	19.0	20	na	0.0	na
(Veryfine)								
peach kiwi flavored, brewed, 'Chillers'	8 oz	80	0.0	18.0	5	0	0.0	0
w/lemon	8 oz	80	<1.0	16.0	10	0	0.0	0
PREPARED FROM MIX								
(Crystal Light)								
w/NutraSweet	8 oz	4	0.0	0.0	0	na	0.0	0
w/Nutrasweet, decaffeinated	8 oz	4	0.0	0.0	0	0	0.0	0
(Lipton)								
lemon flavor	6 oz	55	0.0	14.3	1	0	0.0	0
lemon flavor, decaffeinated	6 oz	55	0.0	14.2	<1	0	0.0	0
lemon flavor, w/NutraSweet	8 oz	5	0.1	1.2	2	0	0.0	0
'Sugar-free'	8 oz	1	0.0	0.3	6	0	0.0	0
'Sugar-free' decaffeinated	8 oz	1	0.0	0.3	5	0	0.0	0
(Nestea)								
'Ice Teasers' all flavors	8 oz	6	0.0	1.0	0	0	0.0	0
lemon flavor	8 oz	6	0.0	1.0	0	0	0.0	0
lemon flavor, sugar-free	8 oz	4	0.0	1.0	0	0	0.0	0
lemon flavor, sugar-free, decaffeinated	2 tsp	6	0.0	1.0	0	0	0.0	0
'100%'	8 oz	2	0.0	0.0	0	na	0.0	na
'100%' decaffeinated	8 oz	0	0.0	0.0	0	0	0.0	0
sugar-free	8 oz	6	0.0	1.0	5	na	0.0	na
w/sugar and lemon	8 oz	70	0.0	19.0	0	na	0.0	na
(Pathmark)								
lemon flavor, low-calorie	8 oz	4	0.0	1.0	0	0	0.0	0
lemon flavor, low-calorie, decaffeinated	8 oz	4	0.0	1.0	0	0	0.0	0
lemon flavor, sugar-sweetened, decaffeinated	2 tbsp	80	0.0	20.0	0	0	0.0	0
TEA FLAVORED DRINK *(10-K)*	8 oz	60	0.0	15.0	55	na	0.0	na
TEASEED OIL								
	1 cup	1927	0.0	0.0	0	0	218.0	0
	1 oz	251	0.0	0.0	0	0	28.4	0
	1 tbsp	120	0.0	0.0	0	0	13.6	0
TEFF FLOUR, whole-grain								
(Arrowhead Mills)	2 oz	200	7.0	41.0	6	7.7	1.0	0
TEFF SEED *(Arrowhead Mills)*	1/2 cup	165	15.7	14.1	5	>2.5 c	6.4	0
TEMPEH	1 oz	56	5.4	4.8	2	>.8 c	2.2	0

Food Name	Serv. Size	Total Cal.	Prot. GMS	Carbs GMS	Sod. MGS	Fiber GMS	Fat GMS	Chol. MGS
TENDERGREEN. See MUSTARD SPINACH.								
TEQUILA. See ALCOHOLIC BEVERAGES.								
TEQUILA SUNRISE. See ALCOHOLIC BEVERAGES.								
TERIYAKI MARINADE								
(Lawry's)	2 tbsp	72	6.4	11.0	7100	.2	0.4	0
(Lawry's) barbecue	1/4 cup	164	8.0	27.4	12330	.1	2.3	na
TERRAPIN, diamond back, raw	100 gm	111	18.6	0.0	50	0	3.5	50
THURINGER CERVELAT								
(Hillshire Farm)	2 oz	180	9.0	1.0	650	0	15.0	(mq)
(Hormel) 'Old Smokehouse'	1 oz	90	4.0	1.0	328	0	8.0	(mq)
(Hormel) 'Old Smokehouse Chub'	1 oz	100	5.0	0.0	332	0	9.0	(mq)
(Hormel) 'Old Smokehouse Sliced'	1 oz	100	5.0	0.0	321	0	9.0	(mq)
(Hormel) 'Viking Club Cervelat'	1 oz	90	5.0	0.0	325	0	8.0	(mq)
(JM) beef	1-oz slice	80	5.0	1.0	340	0	7.0	(mq)
(JM) 'Cervelat'	1-oz slice	70	4.0	1.0	260	0	6.0	(mq)
THYME								
ground	1 oz	78	2.6	18.1	16	5.3	2.1	0
ground	1 tbsp	12	0.4	2.8	2	.8	0.3	0
ground	1 tsp	4	0.1	0.9	1	.3	0.1	0
ground (Durkee)	1 tsp	5	0.0	0.0	0	0	tr	na
ground (Laurel Leaf)	1 tsp	5	0.0	0.0	0	0	tr	na
ground (Spice Islands)	1 tsp	5	0.1	1.0	1	.4	0.1	0
TILEFISH								
broiled	4 oz	167	27.8	0.0	67	0	5.3	(mq)
dry-heat cooked	4 oz	167	27.8	0.0	67	0	5.3	(mq)
dry-heat cooked	3 oz	125	20.8	0.0	50	0	4.0	54
microwaved	4 oz	167	27.8	0.0	67	0	5.3	(mq)
raw	1 lb	433	79.4	0.0	239	0	10.5	(mq)
raw	3 oz	82	14.9	0.0	45	0	2.0	43
raw	1 oz	27	5.0	0.0	15	0	0.7	(mq)
TOASTED SESAME OIL. See SESAME OIL.								
TOASTER BISCUIT. See BISCUIT, TOASTER.								
TOASTER MUFFIN/PASTRY. See MUFFIN/PASTRY, TOASTER.								
TOFFEE. See CANDY.								
TOFU/soybean curd cake								
raw	1 oz	22	2.3	0.5	2	.3	1.4	0
raw	1/2 cup	94	10.0	2.3	9	1.5	5.9	0
Flavored								
Chinese five-spice (Nasoya)	5 oz	150	15.0	2.0	15	(mq)	8.0	0
French, country herb (Nasoya)	5 oz	150	15.0	2.0	15	(mq)	8.0	0
pasteurized (Frieda's)	4.2 oz	86	9.6	2.9	8	(mq)	(mq)	0
Freeze-dried/koyadofu	1 oz	136	13.6	4.1	2	>.1 c	8.6	0
Fried	1 oz	77	4.9	3.0	5	>.1 c	5.7	0

Food Name	Serv. Size	Total Cal.	Prot. GMS	Carbs GMS	Sod. MGS	Fiber GMS	Fat GMS	Chol. MGS
Grilled/yakidofu	1 oz	25	2.2	0.3	5	(mq)	1.7	0
Okara	1 oz	22	0.9	3.6	3	>1.2 c	0.5	0
Salted and fermented/fuyu	1 oz	33	2.3	1.5	814	>.1 c	2.3	0
Silken *(Mori-Nu)*	1/2 pkg	90	10.0	4.0	50	na	4.0	0
TOFU PATTY, FROZEN								
garden *(Natural Touch)*	.2.5-oz patty	90	10.0	3.0	260	(mq)	4.0	0
okara *(Natural Touch)*	.2.25-oz patty	160	11.0	7.0	420	(mq)	10.0	0
TOFU SPREAD								
green chili 'Tofu Topper' canned								
(Natural Touch)	2 tbsp	50	2.0	2.0	(mq)	(mq)	4.0	0
herb and spice 'Tofu Topper' canned								
(Natural Touch)	2 tbsp	50	2.0	2.0	(mq)	(mq)	4.0	0
Mexican 'Tofu Topper' canned								
(Natural Touch)	2 tbsp	60	2.0	2.0	(mq)	(mq)	5.0	0
TOM COLLINS. See ALCOHOLIC BEVERAGES.								
TOMATILLO/ground husk tomato								
fresh *(Frieda's)*	3.5 oz	25	1.4	4.2	na	(mq)	0.5	0
raw	1 med	11	0.3	2.0	0	na	0.4	0
raw, chopped	1/2 cup	.21	0.6	3.8	1	na	0.7	0
TOMATO. See also TOMATO, SUN-DRIED.								
Green								
raw, 2 3/5-inch diam	1 tomato	30	1.5	6.3	16	1.8	0.3	0
trimmed	1 oz	7	0.3	1.4	4	>.1 c	0.1	0
untrimmed	1 lb	99	5.0	21.1	55	>2.1 c	0.8	0
Red								
boiled	1/2 cup	32	1.3	7.0	13	1.2	0.5	0
boiled	4 oz	31	1.2	6.6	12	1.1	0.5	0
raw, chopped	1/2 cup	19	0.8	4.2	8	1.2	0.3	0
raw, 2 3/5 inch diam, 4.75 oz	1 tomato	26	1.0	5.7	11	1.6	0.4	0
raw, trimmed	1 oz	6	0.2	1.3	3	.4	0.1	0
raw, untrimmed	1 lb	88	3.5	19.2	36	5.4	1.4	0
stewed	1 cup	80	2.0	13.2	460	1.7	2.7	0
stewed	4 oz	90	2.2	14.8	516	1.9	3.0	0
TOMATO, CANNED								
(A&P)								
sliced	1/2 cup	35	1.0	8.0	350	(mq)	<1.0	0
whole	1/2 cup	25	1.0	6.0	220	(mq)	<1.0	0
(Angela Mia)								
chopped, 'Premium Choice'	4 oz	24	1.7	4.1	254	1.2	0.4	0
crushed	4 oz	25	2.5	5.1	463	2.0	0.2	0
crushed, chunky	4 oz	26	2.0	5.1	378	2.0	0.3	0
crushed, 'Premium Choice'	2.222 oz	29	1.7	5.6	25	.9	0.4	0

Food Name	Serv. Size	Total Cal.	Prot. GMS	Carbs GMS	Sod. MGS	Fiber GMS	Fat GMS	Chol. MGS
(Contadina)								
crushed, in purée	1/2 cup	30	1.0	6.0	350	(mq)	<1.0	0
Italian style	1/2 cup	35	1.0	8.0	250	(mq)	<1.0	0
Italian style, pear	1/2 cup	25	1.0	5.0	220	(mq)	<1.0	0
'Recipe Ready'	1/2 cup	25	1.0	5.0	570	na	0.2	0
stewed	1/2 cup	35	1.0	8.0	350	(mq)	<1.0	0
stewed, Mexican style	1/2 cup	35	1.0	8.0	230	na	0.3	0
whole, peeled	1/2 cup	25	1.0	5.0	260	(mq)	<1.0	0
w/jalapeños	1/2 cup	35	1.0	8.0	250	(mq)	<1.0	0
(Del Monte)								
stewed	1/2 cup	35	1.0	8.0	355	(mq)	0.0	0
stewed, 'No Salt Added'	1/2 cup	35	1.0	8.0	45	(mq)	0.0	0
wedges, w/liquid	1/2 cup	30	1.0	8.0	355	(mq)	0.0	0
whole, peeled, w/liquid	1/2 cup	25	1.0	5.0	220	(mq)	0.0	0
(Eden Foods) crushed, organic,								
no salt added	4 oz	35	2.0	6.0	0	na	0.0	0
(Featherweight)	1/2 cup	20	1.0	4.0	<1	(mq)	0.0	0
(Finast)								
sliced	1/2 cup	35	1.0	9.0	355	(mq)	0.0	0
whole, peeled	1/2 cup	25	1.0	6.0	195	(mq)	0.0	0
(Hunt's)								
choice cut	4 oz	19	1.1	4.0	278	.5	0.0	0
crushed	4 oz	31	0.9	7.2	317	1.1	0.4	0
crushed, 'Angela Mia'	4 oz	35	1.0	7.0	260	<1.0	<1.0	0
crushed, Italian flavored	4 oz	40	2.0	9.0	460	<1.0	<1.0	0
diced, in juice	4 oz	19	1.1	4.0	477	.5	0.1	0
diced, in juice, 'No Salt Added'	4 oz	20	1.1	4.1	8	.5	0.1	0
diced, in purée	4 oz	23	1.3	4.7	304	.6	0.2	0
diced, w/green chilies	.3527 oz	2	0.1	0.2	33	.1	0.1	0
pear shaped	4.868 oz	21	1.5	4.1	285	1.2	0.1	0
pear shaped	4.832 oz	21	1.5	4.1	373	.6	0.1	0
pear shaped	4.656 oz	20	1.4	3.9	360	.6	0.1	0
pear shaped, Italian flavored	4 oz	20	1.0	5.0	320	<1.0	<1.0	0
peeled, choice cut	4 oz	20	1.0	5.0	460	1.0	<1.0	0
stewed	4 oz	33	1.2	6.7	357	.8	0.1	0
stewed, 'Food Service'	4 oz	29	1.2	6.7	262	.8	0.1	0
stewed, Italian flavored	4 oz	35	1.0	8.0	400	<1.0	<1.0	0
stewed, 'No Salt Added'	1/2 cup	35	1.0	8.0	20	(mq)	0.0	0
whole	4 oz	20	1.0	5.0	415	(mq)	0.0	0
whole, Italian flavored	4 oz	25	1.0	6.0	420	<1.0	<1.0	0
whole, 'No Salt Added'	4 oz	20	1.0	5.0	20	(mq)	0.0	0
whole, peeled	5.608 oz	24	1.7	4.7	433	.7	0.3	0
whole, peeled	5.22 oz	22	1.6	4.4	333	.6	0.1	0

Food Name	Serv. Size	Total Cal.	Prot. GMS	Carbs GMS	Sod. MGS	Fiber GMS	Fat GMS	Chol. MGS
whole, peeled	5.009 oz	22	1.5	4.2	387	.6	0.1	0
whole, peeled	4.832 oz	21	1.5	4.1	373	.6	0.1	0
whole, peeled, 'No Salt Added'	4.832 oz	21	1.5	4.1	9	.6	0.1	0
(Old El Paso) w/green chilies	1/4 cup	14	0.0	3.0	480	(mq)	0.0	0
(Ortega) w/jalapeños	1 oz	8	0.0	1.0	120	(mq)	0.0	0
(Pathmark)								
crushed	1/2 cup	40	1.0	9.0	210	(mq)	0.0	0
crushed, 'No Frills'	1 cup	90	3.0	20.0	510	(mq)	0.0	0
'No Frills'	1 cup	50	2.0	11.0	440	(mq)	0.0	0
sliced	1/2 cup	35	1.0	9.0	360	(mq)	0.0	0
whole, peeled, 'No Salt Added'	1/2 cup	25	1.0	6.0	20	(mq)	0.0	0
whole, peeled, w/tomato juice	1/2 cup	25	1.0	6.0	220	(mq)	0.0	0
(S&W)								
aspic, supreme	1/2 cup	60	1.0	16.0	860	(mq)	0.0	0
cut, peeled 'Ready-Cut'	1/2 cup	25	1.0	6.0	220	(mq)	0.0	0
diced, in rich purée	1/2 cup	35	1.0	8.0	290	(mq)	0.0	0
Italian, sliced	1/2 cup	35	1.0	9.0	355	(mq)	0.0	0
Mexican style	1/2 cup	40	1.0	8.0	360	(mq)	0.0	0
sliced	1/2 cup	35	1.0	9.0	355	(mq)	0.0	0
stewed, '50% Salt Reduced'	1/2 cup	35	1.0	9.0	180	(mq)	0.0	0
whole, peeled	1/2 cup	25	1.0	6.0	220	(mq)	0.0	0
whole, peeled, Italian-style pear, w/basil	1/2 cup	25	1.0	5.0	200	(mq)	0.0	0
(S&W Nutradiet) whole	1/2 cup	25	1.0	5.0	20	(mq)	0.0	0
(Stokely)								
stewed	1/2 cup	35	1.0	8.0	220	(mq)	0.0	0
whole	1/2 cup	25	1.0	5.0	190	(mq)	0.0	0
TOMATO, PICKLED, kosher (Claussen)	1 oz	5	0.2	1.0	330	(mq)	0.0	0
TOMATO-BEEF COCKTAIL (Beefamato)	6 oz	80	1.0	19.0	240	(mq)	0.0	na
TOMATO-CHILE COCKTAIL (Snap-E-Tom)	6 oz	40	2.0	7.0	980	(mq)	0.0	0
TOMATO-CLAM COCKTAIL (Clamato)	6 oz	96	1.0	23.0	815	(mq)	0.0	na
TOMATO JUICE								
(A&P)	6 oz	30	1.0	7.0	550	(mq)	0.0	0
(Biotta)	6 oz	28	1.3	5.8	277	(mq)	0.1	0
(Campbell's)	6 oz	40	1.0	8.0	540	(mq)	0.0	0
(Featherweight)	6 oz	35	1.0	8.0	10	(mq)	0.0	0
(Hunt's)	9.03 oz	33	2.1	6.5	608	.8	0.2	0
(Hunt's)	7.16 oz	28	1.8	5.5	513	.7	0.2	0
(Hunt's)	6 oz	30	1.0	7.0	640	(mq)	0.0	0
(Hunt's)	5.467 oz	22	1.4	4.2	399	.5	0.1	0
(Hunt's) 'No Salt Added'	6 oz	45	2.0	11.0	30	(mq)	0.0	0
(Knudsen & Sons) organic	8 oz	50	<1.0	10.0	na	na	0.0	na
(Libby's)	6 oz	35	2.0	7.0	500	na	0.0	na
(Pathmark)	6 oz	30	1.0	6.0	510	(mq)	0.0	0

Food Name	Serv. Size	Total Cal.	Prot. GMS	Carbs GMS	Sod. MGS	Fiber GMS	Fat GMS	Chol. MGS
(Pathmark) frozen, diluted	6 oz	35	1.0	8.0	450	(mq)	0.0	0
(S&W) 'California'	6 oz	35	1.0	8.0	600	(mq)	0.0	0
(S&W Nutradiet)	6 oz	35	1.0	8.0	20	(mq)	0.0	0
(Stokely)	4 oz	20	1.0	4.0	330	(mq)	0.0	0
(Welch's)	6 oz	35	1.0	7.0	550	0	0.0	0
TOMATO PASTE								
(Contadina)	2 oz	50	2.0	11.0	40	na	<1.0	na
(Contadina) Italian style	2 oz	65	2.0	12.0	520	na	1.0	na
(Hunt's)	1.164 oz	24	1.4	4.9	81	.7	0.2	0
(Hunt's) 'Food Service'	1.164 oz	24	1.4	4.9	101	.7	0.2	0
(Hunt's) Italian style	1.164 oz	25	1.5	4.7	255	.8	0.4	0
(Hunt's) 'No Salt Added'	1.164 oz	24	1.4	4.9	11	.7	0.2	0
(Hunt's) w/garlic	2 oz	50	2.0	11.0	440	2.0	<1.0	0
(Hunt's) w/garlic	1.164 oz	26	1.6	5.1	247	.8	0.3	0
TOMATO POWDER								
ground	1 oz	86	3.7	21.2	38	>1.9 c	0.1	0
ground	100 gm	302	12.9	74.7	134	>6.7 c	0.4	0
TOMATO PURÉE								
(Angela Mia)	2.187 oz	16	0.9	2.9	21	.4	0.3	0
(Contadina)	1/2 cup	40	2.0	8.0	35	na	<1.0	na
(Contadina) w/crushed tomatoes	1/2 cup	30	1.0	6.0	350	na	<1.0	na
(Hunt's)	2.187 oz	23	1.6	4.3	98	.7	0.3	0
(Hunt's) 'Food Service'	2.222 oz	26	1.5	5.0	22	.8	0.4	0
TOMATO SAUCE								
CANNED								
(A&P)	1/2 cup	45	2.0	9.0	600	(mq)	<1.0	0
(Contadina)	1/2 cup	30	1.0	7.0	580	(mq)	<1.0	0
(Del Monte)	1 cup	70	3.0	16.0	1330	(mq)	1.0	0
(Finast)	1/2 cup	45	2.0	9.0	650	(mq)	0.0	0
(Health Valley)	1 cup	70	2.4	13.0	460	.3	0.5	0
(Hunt's)	4 oz	30	1.0	7.0	730	(mq)	0.0	0
(Hunt's)	2.187 oz	16	1.0	2.6	360	.1	0.2	0
(Pathmark)	1/2 cup	40	2.0	9.0	620	(mq)	0.0	0
(S&W)	1/2 cup	40	2.0	9.0	620	(mq)	0.0	0
(Stokely)	1/2 cup	30	1.0	7.0	810	(mq)	0.0	0
Casera *(Hunt's)*	2.187 oz	22	0.7	5.2	293	.8	0.1	0
Chunky								
(Hunt's) chili	2.222 oz	21	1.0	4.1	320	1.4	0.4	0
(Hunt's) 'Food Service'	2.187 oz	15	1.1	2.8	360	.5	0.2	0
(Hunt's) Italian	2.222 oz	29	1.0	4.5	293	1.4	1.1	0
(Hunt's) Mexican	2.222 oz	19	0.7	3.8	369	1.2	0.4	0
(Hunt's) tomato	2.187 oz	13	0.7	2.9	405	1.1	0.1	0
Garden vegetable *(Contadina)*	5 oz	80	2.0	9.0	580	na	3.0	0

Food Name	Serv. Size	Total Cal.	Prot. GMS	Carbs GMS	Sod. MGS	Fiber GMS	Fat GMS	Chol. MGS
Herb flavored *(Hunt's)*	4 oz	70	2.0	12.0	470	2.0	2.0	<1
Hot, Maya *(Hunt's)*	1.058 oz	6	0.3	1.1	174	.2	0.2	0
Italian style								
(Contadina)	1/2 cup	30	1.0	7.0	670	(mq)	<1.0	0
(Contadina) sausage	5 oz	110	5.0	8.0	570	na	6.0	15
(Hunt's)	4 oz	60	2.0	11.0	520	(mq)	2.0	na
(Hunt's)	2.222 oz	26	1.1	5.2	251	1.4	0.5	0
(Rokeach)	3 oz	60	1.0	8.0	243	(mq)	2.0	0
Low sodium *(Rokeach)*	3 oz	50	1.0	8.0	124	(mq)	2.0	0
Marinara								
(Buitoni)	1/2 cup	70	1.0	11.0	570	(mq)	3.0	0
(Contadina)	4 oz	80	2.0	8.0	460	na	4.0	0
(Pathmark) 'No Frills'	1/2 cup	80	1.0	12.0	620	(mq)	3.0	0
(Rokeach)	3 oz	60	1.0	9.0	257	(mq)	2.0	0
'Meatloaf Fixin's' *(Hunt's)*	2 oz	20	<1.0	5.0	580	<1.0	<1.0	0
No salt added								
(Del Monte)	1 cup	70	3.0	16.0	50	(mq)	1.0	0
(Finast)	8 oz	90	4.0	18.0	10	(mq)	0.0	0
(Health Valley)	1 cup	70	2.4	13.0	43	.3	0.5	0
(Hunt's)	4 oz	35	1.0	8.0	25	(mq)	0.0	0
(Hunt's)	2.187 oz	16	1.0	2.6	11	.1	0.2	0
(Pathmark)	1/2 cup	45	2.0	9.0	25	(mq)	0.0	0
Pesto *(Contadina)*	2.33 oz	350	7.0	5.0	440	na	34.0	10
Plum *(Contadina)*	5 oz	80	2.0	8.0	420	na	4.0	5
'Special'								
(Hunt's)	4 oz	35	1.0	8.0	320	(mq)	0.0	0
(Hunt's)	2.187 oz	21	0.8	3.8	144	.6	0.6	0
'Thick and Zesty' *(Contadina)*	1/2 cup	40	2.0	8.0	650	(mq)	<1.0	0
W/bits *(Hunt's)*	4 oz	30	1.0	7.0	620	2.0	<1.0	0
W/garlic								
(Hunt's)	4 oz	70	2.0	10.0	480	2.0	2.0	0
(Hunt's)	2.258 oz	29	1.0	4.9	269	1.8	1.0	0
W/green chilies *(Old El Paso)*	1/4 cup	14	<1.0	3.0	480	(mq)	<1.0	0
W/herbs *(Hunt's)*	2.187 oz	33	1.3	4.9	255	.8	1.3	0
W/jalapeños *(Old El Paso)*	1/4 cup	11	1.0	2.0	150	(mq)	1.0	0
W/mushrooms *(Hunt's)*	4 oz	25	1.0	6.0	710	2.0	<1.0	0
W/onions								
(Del Monte)	1 cup	100	3.0	23.0	1150	(mq)	1.0	0
(Hunt's)	4 oz	40	1.0	9.0	650	2.0	<1.0	0
REFRIGERATED								
(Contadina) 'Light'	.5 oz	50	2.0	9.0	570	na	0.0	0
(Contadina) marinara 'Fresh'	7.5 oz	100	4.0	12.0	700	(mq)	4.0	0
(Contadina) plum w/basil 'Fresh'	7.5 oz	100	3.0	14.0	700	(mq)	4.0	5

Food Name	Serv. Size	Total Cal.	Prot. GMS	Carbs GMS	Sod. MGS	Fiber GMS	Fat GMS	Chol. MGS
TOMATOES, SUN-DRIED. See SUN-DRIED TOMATOES.								
TOMATOSEED OIL								
.... 1/2 cup		964	0.0	0.0	0	0	109.0	0
.... 1 oz		251	0.0	0.0	0	0	28.4	0
.... 1 tbsp		120	0.0	0.0	0	0	13.6	0
TONIC. See SOFT DRINKS AND MIXERS.								
TORSK. See CUSK.								
TORTELLINI DISH/ENTRÉE, FROZEN								
(Birds Eye) in tomato sauce 'For One' ... 5.5 oz		210	11.0	31.0	500	0	5.0	30
(Budget Gourmet) 'Side Dish' .... 5.5 oz		180	7.0	25.0	400	(mq)	9.0	15
(Green Giant) marinara 'One Serving' ... 5.5 oz		260	8.0	37.0	660	(mq)	9.0	25
(Green Giant) Provençal 'Microwave Garden Gourmet' .... 1 pkg		260	10.0	44.0	840	3.0	6.0	15
(Le Menu) and meat sauce 'LightStyle' ... 8 oz		250	11.0	34.0	480	(mq)	8.0	15
(Stouffer's) in Alfredo sauce .... 8 7/8 oz		580	26.0	35.0	830	na	37.0	na
(Stouffer's) w/tomato sauce .... 9.25 oz		360	18.0	39.0	720	na	15.0	na
(Top Shelf) in marinara sauce .... 10 oz		211	10.0	37.0	663	(mq)	3.0	35
(Top Shelf) w/shrimp and seafood ...... 10 oz		278	16.0	36.0	1341	(mq)	8.0	89
(Weight Watchers) .... 9 oz		310	14.0	50.0	570	na	6.0	15
TORTELLINI PASTA, NONDAIRY								
regular (Tofutti) frozen .... 2 oz		210	12.0	32.0	158	(mq)	4.0	0
spinach (Tofutti) frozen .... 2 oz		210	12.0	32.0	158	(mq)	4.0	0
TORTELLINI PASTA, REFRIGERATED								
CHEESE (DiGiorno) approx 1 cup cooked 1/3 pkg		270	13.0	41.0	240	na	6.0	35
CHICKEN AND HERB (DiGiorno) approx 1 cup cooked .... 1/3 pkg		240	14.0	37.0	230	na	5.0	40
EGG								
w/cheese, 'Fresh' (Contadina) .... 4.5 oz		380	21.0	60.0	570	(mq)	6.0	70
w/cheese, 'Fresh' (Contadina) .... 3 oz		260	13.0	39.0	310	na	6.0	40
w/chicken and prosciutto, 'Fresh' (Contadina) .... 4.5 oz		370	24.0	53.0	560	(mq)	7.0	75
w/meat, 'Fresh' (Contadina) .... 4.5 oz		380	22.0	60.0	580	(mq)	6.0	75
MOZZARELLA GARLIC (DiGiorno) approx 1 cup cooked .... 1/3 pkg		260	13.0	35.0	270	na	8.0	40
SAUSAGE, Italian, 'Fresh' (Contadina) .... 3 oz		260	11.0	37.0	290	na	7.0	65
SPINACH								
w/cheese, 'Fresh' (Contadina) .... 4.5 oz		380	21.0	60.0	590	(mq)	6.0	70
w/cheese, 'Fresh' (Contadina) .... 3 oz		260	13.0	38.0	360	na	6.0	45
w/chicken and prosciutto, 'Fresh' (Contadina) .... 4.5 oz		340	24.0	53.0	580	(mq)	7.0	75
w/meat, 'Fresh' (Contadina) .... 4.5 oz		380	22.0	60.0	610	(mq)	6.0	75
W/CHICKEN AND PROSCIUTTO								
(Contadina) .... 3 oz		250	15.0	34.0	370	na	6.0	50

Food Name	Serv. Size	Total Cal.	Prot. GMS	Carbs GMS	Sod. MGS	Fiber GMS	Fat GMS	Chol. MGS
W/MEAT								
(Contadina) 'Fresh'	3 oz	260	13.0	39.0	380	na	6.0	45
(DiGiorno) approx 1 cup cooked	1/3 pkg	280	12.0	38.0	360	na	9.0	40
TORTILLA, CORN								
(Azteca)	1 tortilla	45	1.0	9.0	10	0	0.0	0
(Old El Paso)	1 tortilla	60	1.0	10.0	170	na	1.0	0
TORTILLA, FLOUR								
(Azteca) 9-inch diam	1 tortilla	130	3.0	23.0	180	0	3.0	0
(Azteca) 7-inch diam	1 tortilla	80	2.0	14.0	110	0	2.0	0
(Mission) 'Light'	1 tortilla	70	2.0	16.0	280	4.0	1.0	0
(Old El Paso)	1 tortilla	150	4.0	27.0	360	na	3.0	0
Burrito style								
(Garcia's)	1 tortilla	220	5.0	37.0	220	2.0	5.0	0
(Mission) 'Premium'	1 tortilla	230	6.0	40.0	395	na	6.0	0
(Tyson)	1 tortilla	173	5.0	29.0	40	na	4.0	0
(Tyson) large, heat-pressed	1 tortilla	182	5.0	33.0	90	na	4.0	0
(Tyson) small, hand-stretched	1 tortilla	106	3.0	19.0	50	na	2.0	0
Fajita style								
(Fry's) extra soft	1 tortilla	100	2.0	17.0	160	na	2.0	0
(Garcia's)	1 tortilla	100	2.0	17.0	220	<1.0	2.5	0
(Tyson)	1 tortilla	84	3.0	18.0	20	na	2.0	0
Taco size								
(Mission) soft	1 tortilla	150	4.0	25.0	255	na	4.0	0
(Tyson) soft	1 tortilla	121	4.0	20.0	30	na	3.0	0
TORTILLA CHIPS. See also CORN CHIPS AND SNACKS.								
(Bachman)								
nacho	1 oz	140	2.0	18.0	210	(mq)	6.0	0
'No Salt'	1 oz	140	2.0	19.0	0	(mq)	6.0	0
(Barbara's Bakery)								
yellow corn, organic	1 oz	140	2.0	18.0	120	na	7.0	0
yellow corn, organic, no salt added	1 oz	140	2.0	18.0	15	na	7.0	0
(Bearitos)								
blue corn 'Organic'	1 oz	146	2.9	17.4	29	.6	7.0	0
blue corn 'Organic No Salt'	1 oz	137	2.6	17.1	3	1.0	6.5	0
yellow corn 'Organic'	1 oz	143	2.1	18.1	58	1.1	6.4	0
yellow corn 'Organic No Salt'	1 oz	148	2.2	17.2	2	1.4	7.2	0
(Bravos)								
nacho cheese flavored, jalapeño	1 oz	150	2.0	19.0	170	(mq)	7.0	0
nacho cheese flavored, round, crispy	1 oz	150	2.0	18.0	180	(mq)	8.0	0
nacho cheese flavored, strips	1 oz	140	2.0	18.0	220	(mq)	7.0	0
(Buenitos)								
'Tortilla Chips'	1 oz	150	2.0	18.0	80	3.6	8.0	0
'Tortilla Chips, No Salt Added'	1 oz	150	2.0	18.0	1	3.6	8.0	0

Food Name	Serv. Size	Total Cal.	Prot. GMS	Carbs GMS	Sod. MGS	Fiber GMS	Fat GMS	Chol. MGS
(Doritos)								
'Cool Ranch'	1 oz	140	2.0	18.0	170	1.5	7.0	0
'Cool Ranch Light'	1 oz	120	2.0	21.0	240	(mq)	4.0	0
'Jumpin' Jack'	1 oz	140	2.0	18.0	220	1.5	7.0	0
nacho cheese	1 oz	140	2.0	18.0	240	(mq)	7.0	0
nacho cheese 'Light'	1 oz	120	2.0	21.0	290	(mq)	4.0	0
salsa and cheese 'Thins'	1 oz	150	2.0	17.0	180	na	8.0	0
'Salsa Rio'	1 oz	140	2.0	18.0	190	1.5	7.0	0
taco	1 oz	140	2.0	18.0	250	1.5	7.0	0
toasted corn	1 oz	140	2.0	19.0	80	1.5	7.0	0
white corn, lightly salted 'Thins'	1 oz	140	2.0	19.0	135	na	7.0	0
(Eagle) ranch	1 oz	140	2.0	17.0	190	(mq)	8.0	1
(Featherweight)								
'Low Salt'	1 oz	150	2.0	18.0	10	(mq)	8.0	0
nacho	1 oz	150	2.0	18.0	45	(mq)	8.0	0
(Guiltless Gourmet)								
white corn, baked, salted	1 oz	110	3.0	22.0	160	2.0	1.5	0
yellow corn, baked, salted	1 oz	110	3.0	22.0	140	3.0	1.5	0
yellow corn, baked, unsalted	1 oz	110	3.0	22.0	25	3.0	1.5	0
(Hain)								
sesame	1 oz	140	2.0	19.0	190	(mq)	7.0	0
sesame, cheese	1 oz	160	2.0	20.0	270	(mq)	8.0	5
sesame, 'No Salt Added'	1 oz	140	2.0	19.0	0	(mq)	7.0	5
taco	1 oz	160	2.0	15.0	320	(mq)	11.0	5
(Keebler)								
cinnamon crispaña, flour 'Chacho's'	1 oz	140	2.0	19.0	70	na	7.0	0
original, restaurant style 'Chacho's'	1 oz	140	3.0	18.0	180	na	7.0	5
(Kettle Ties)								
blue corn, lightly salted	1 oz	140	3.0	18.0	80	2.0	6.0	0
blue corn, no salt	1 oz	140	3.0	18.0	2	2.0	6.0	0
yellow corn, lightly salted	1 oz	140	2.0	19.0	80	2.0	7.0	0
yellow corn, no salt	1 oz	140	2.0	19.0	3	2.0	7.0	0
(La Famous)								
'No Salt Added'	1 oz	140	2.0	18.0	5	(mq)	7.0	0
plain	1 oz	140	2.0	18.0	180	(mq)	7.0	0
(Laura Scudder's)								
lightly salted 'Restaurant Style'	1 oz	140	2.0	18.0	90	(mq)	7.0	0
nacho, jalapeño 'Strips'	1 oz	150	2.0	19.0	170	(mq)	7.0	0
nacho, 'Triangles'	1 oz	140	2.0	18.0	220	(mq)	7.0	0
picante 'Restaurant Style Strips'	1 oz	150	2.0	19.0	190	(mq)	7.0	0
(Old El Paso)								
crispy	1 oz	150	2.0	17.0	105	.5	8.0	0
white, round 'NaChips' low sodium	1 oz	160	2.0	17.0	5	na	9.0	0

Food Name	Serv. Size	Total Cal.	Prot. GMS	Carbs GMS	Sod. MGS	Fiber GMS	Fat GMS	Chol. MGS
(Planters)								
nacho cheese	1 oz	150	2.0	18.0	160	na	8.0	0
traditional	1 oz	150	2.0	18.0	150	na	8.0	0
(Slimchips) fat-free	.4 oz	44	<1.0	10.0	60	<.5	<.5	0
(Tio Sancho)								
'Microwave Snacks'	.4 oz	567	8.5	74.4	590	>4.0 c	26.1	na
nacho	.5 oz	70	4.1	0.7	282	>.1 c	5.7	na
(Tostitos)								
nacho, sharp	1 oz	150	2.0	17.0	200	(mq)	8.0	0
white corn, baked 'Cool Ranch'	1 oz	130	2.0	21.0	170	na	3.0	0
white corn, baked, no salt	1 oz	110	2.0	24.0	0	na	1.0	0
white corn, baked 'Original'	1 oz	110	2.0	24.0	140	na	1.0	0
(Wise) nacho cheese flavored, crispy, round	1 oz	150	2.0	18.0	180	na	8.0	na
TORULA YEAST. See YEAST, TORULA.								
TOSTACO SHELL *(Old El Paso)*	1 shell	100	1.0	11.0	10	1.0	5.0	0
TOSTADA SHELL								
(Lawry's)	1 shell	73	1.2	9.5	147	>.4 c	3.5	0
(Old El Paso)	1 shell	55	<1.0	6.0	65	.5	3.0	0
(Ortega)	1 shell	50	0.0	8.0	5	(mq)	2.0	0
(Pancho Villa)	1 shell	55	<1.0	6.0	65	na	3.0	0
(Rosarita)	1 shell	60	1.0	8.0	<1	<1.0	3.0	0
(Tio Sancho)	1 shell	67	1.2	8.4	1	>.5 c	3.2	0
TOWEL GOURD. See GOURD, DISHCLOTH.								
TRAIL MIX								
(Harmony) 'Delux Super'	1/4 cup	150	3.0	23.0	35	3.0	7.0	0
(Harmony) nut and berry mix	1/4 cup	160	5.0	21.0	0	3.0	8.0	0
TREE FERN								
cooked	4 oz	45	0.3	12.5	6	.7	0.1	0
cooked, chopped	1/2 cup	28	0.2	7.8	4	2.6	0.1	0
TRITICALE								
whole grain	1/2 cup	323	12.5	69.2	5	>2.5 c	2.0	0
whole grain	1 oz	95	3.7	20.4	1	5.1	0.6	0
TRITICALE FLOUR								
whole grain	1/2 cup	220	8.6	47.5	1	9.5	1.2	0
whole grain	1 oz	96	3.7	20.7	<1	4.1	0.5	0
TROPICAL CITRUS DRINK								
chilled *(Five Alive)*	6 oz	90	0.0	21.0	20	na	0.0	na
frozen, prepared *(Five Alive)*	6 oz	90	0.0	21.0	0	na	0.0	na
TROPICAL FRUIT DRINK								
bottled 'Thirst Quencher' *(Gatorade)*	8 oz	50	0.0	14.0	110	na	0.0	na
mix 'Thirst Quencher' prepared *(Gatorade)*	8 oz	60	0.0	15.0	110	na	0.0	na
TROPICAL FRUIT JUICE								
bottled *(Juicy Juice)*	6 oz	110	1.0	26.0	10	na	0.0	na

Food Name	Serv. Size	Total Cal.	Prot. GMS	Carbs GMS	Sod. MGS	Fiber GMS	Fat GMS	Chol. MGS
boxed (Juicy Juice) .... 8.45 oz		150	1.0	36.0	10	na	0.0	na
TROPICAL LIME COOLER								
(Knudsen & Sons) .... 8 oz		130	<1.0	32.0	na	na	0.0	na
TROPICAL NECTAR, can or bottle (Kern's) 6 oz		110	0.0	27.0	5	na	0.0	na
TROPICAL ORANGE DRINK, 'Fruit Box'								
(Tang) .... 8.45 oz		150	0.0	37.0	10	na	0.0	0
TROPICAL PASSION JUICE								
(Knudsen & Sons) .... 8 oz		80	<1.0	20.0	na	na	0.0	na
TROPICAL PUNCH								
Can, bottle, or box								
(Knudsen & Sons) .... 8 oz		105	<1.0	33.0	na	na	0.0	na
(Kool-Aid) 'Koolers' .... 8.45 oz		130	0.0	35.0	10	na	0.0	0
(Minute Maid) .... 6 oz		90	0.0	22.0	20	na	0.0	na
(Santa Cruz Natural) organic .... 8 oz		110	<1.0	26.0	na	na	<1.0	na
Mix								
(Kool-Aid) sugar-free, w/NutraSweet,								
prepared .... 8 oz		4	0.0	0.0	10	na	0.0	0
(Kool-Aid) sugar-sweetened, prepared .... 8 oz		80	0.0	21.0	0	na	0.0	0
(Kool-Aid) unsweetened, prepared w/sugar 8 oz		100	0.0	25.0	0	na	0.0	0
(Kool-Aid) unsweetened, prepared w/o								
sugar .... 8 oz		2	0.0	0.0	0	na	0.0	0
TROPICAL SALAD (Sun Fresh) chilled,								
packed in light syrup .... 3.5 oz		88	1.2	18.7	39	2.3	0.9	1
TROUT, MIXED SPECIES								
dry-heat cooked .... 3 oz		161	22.6	0.0	57	0	7.2	63
raw .... 1 lb		673	94.2	0.0	236	0	30.0	264
raw .... 3 oz		126	17.6	0.0	44	0	5.6	49
raw .... 1 oz		42	5.9	0.0	15	0	1.9	16
raw, approx 2.8 oz .... 1 fillet		117	16.4	0.0	41	0	5.2	46
TROUT, RAINBOW								
farmed, dry-heat cooked .... 3 oz		144	20.6	0.0	36	0	6.1	58
farmed, raw .... 3 oz		117	17.7	0.0	30	0	4.6	50
wild, dry-heat cooked .... 3 oz		127	19.5	0.0	48	0	4.9	59
wild, raw .... 3 oz		101	17.4	0.0	26	0	2.9	50
wild, raw, approx 2.8 oz .... 1 fillet		189	32.6	0.0	49	0	5.5	94
TROUT, SEA, MIXED SPECIES								
raw .... 1 lb		472	76.0	0.0	263	0	16.4	376
raw .... 3 oz		88	14.2	0.0	49	0	3.1	71
raw .... 1 oz		29	4.7	0.0	16	0	1.0	24
TUMERIC. See TURMERIC.								
TUNA, ALBACORE. See TUNA, CANNED; TUNA, FROZEN.								
TUNA, ALTERNATIVE, frozen 'Tuno'								
(Worthington) .... 2 oz		100	5.0	3.0	310	(mq)	7.0	0

Food Name	Serv. Size	Total Cal.	Prot. GMS	Carbs GMS	Sod. MGS	Fiber GMS	Fat GMS	Chol. MGS
TUNA, BLUEFIN								
dry-heat cooked	4 oz	209	33.9	0.0	57	0	7.1	56
dry-heat cooked	3 oz	156	25.4	0.0	43	0	5.3	42
raw	1 lb	652	105.8	0.0	177	0	22.2	173
raw	3 oz	122	19.8	0.0	33	0	4.2	32
raw	1 oz	41	6.6	0.0	11	0	1.4	11
TUNA, CANNED								
LIGHT								
In canola oil, chunk (Chicken of the Sea)	2 oz	160	12.0	<1.0	250	na	12.0	na
In oil								
drained	3 oz	168	24.8	0.0	301	0	7.0	15
drained, approx 6 oz	1 can	339	49.8	0.0	605	0	14.0	31
w/o salt, drained	3 oz	168	24.8	0.0	43	0	7.0	15
w/o salt, drained, approx 6 oz	1 can	339	49.8	0.0	86	0	14.0	31
In pure vegetable oil, chunk, w/liquid								
(Chicken of the Sea)	2 oz	160	12.0	<1.0	250	na	12.0	na
In soybean oil								
chunk, drained	1 oz	56	8.3	0.0	100	0	2.3	5
chunk, drained (A&P)	2 oz	150	13.0	<1.0	310	0	13.0	(mq)
chunk, drained (Bumble Bee)	2 oz	110	12.0	0.0	310	0	12.0	30
chunk, drained (Finast)	2 oz	150	13.0	<1.0	310	0	13.0	(mq)
chunk, drained (Star-Kist)	2 oz	150	13.0	<1.0	310	0	13.0	25
chunk 'Fancy' drained (S&W)	2 oz	140	13.0	0.0	450	0	10.0	(mq)
solid, drained (Progresso)	1/3 cup	150	13.0	<1.0	400	0	13.0	(mq)
solid, drained (Star-Kist)	2 oz	150	13.0	<1.0	310	0	13.0	25
w/o salt, drained	1 oz	56	8.3	0.0	14	0	2.3	5
In spring water, chunk, w/liquid								
(Chicken of the Sea)	2 oz	60	12.0	<1.0	250	na	1.0	na
In water								
chunk, drained (Bumble Bee)	2 oz	50	12.0	0.0	310	0	1.0	30
chunk, drained (Finast)	2 oz	60	13.0	<1.0	310	0	<1.0	(mq)
chunk, drained (Pathmark)	2 oz	70	15.0	0.0	310	0	2.0	(mq)
chunk, drained (Star-Kist)	2 oz	60	13.0	<1.0	310	0	<1.0	25
chunk, diet, drained (Star-Kist)	2 oz	65	14.0	<1.0	35	0	<1.0	25
chunk 'Fancy' drained (S&W)	2 oz	60	13.0	0.0	500	0	1.0	(mq)
chunk 'No Salt Added' drained								
(Weight Watchers)	2 oz	60	14.0	<1.0	210	0	<1.0	25
chunk '60% Less Salt' drained (Star-Kist)	2 oz	65	14.0	<1.0	120	0	1.0	25
drained	3 oz	111	25.1	0.0	303	0	0.4	15
drained	1 oz	37	8.4	0.0	101	0	0.1	(mq)
drained, approx 6.3 oz	1 can	216	48.8	0.0	587	0	0.8	30
drained (A&P)	2 oz	60	13.0	<1.0	310	0	<1.0	(mq)
drained (Empress)	2 oz	60	12.0	0.0	310	0	1.0	(mq)

Food Name	Serv. Size	Total Cal.	Prot. GMS	Carbs GMS	Sod. MGS	Fiber GMS	Fat GMS	Chol. MGS
solid, drained *(Star-Kist)*	2 oz	60	14.0	<1.0	310	0	<1.0	25
solid 'Prime Catch' drained *(Star-Kist)*	2 oz	60	14.0	<1.0	310	0	<1.0	25
w/o salt, drained	3 oz	111	25.1	0.0	43	0	0.4	15
w/o salt, drained	1 oz	37	8.4	0.0	14	0	0.1	(mq)
w/o salt, drained, approx 6.3 oz	1 can	216	48.8	0.0	83	0	0.8	30
WHITE								
In oil								
drained	3 oz	158	22.5	0.0	337	0	6.9	26
drained, approx 6.3 oz	1 can	331	47.2	0.0	705	0	14.4	55
w/o salt, drained	3 oz	158	22.5	0.0	43	0	6.9	26
w/o salt, drained, approx 6.3 oz	1 can	331	47.2	0.0	89	0	14.4	55
In soybean oil								
chunk, drained	1 oz	53	7.5	0.0	112	0	2.3	9
chunk, drained *(A&P)*	2 oz	150	13.0	<1.0	310	0	10.0	(mq)
chunk, drained *(Bumble Bee)*	2 oz	110	12.0	0.0	310	0	12.0	330
chunk, drained *(Star-Kist)*	2 oz	140	14.0	<1.0	310	0	10.0	25
solid, albacore, drained *(Bumble Bee)*	2 oz	100	14.0	0.0	310	0	8.0	30
solid, albacore, drained *(Finast)*	2 oz	145	14.0	<1.0	320	0	10.0	(mq)
solid, albacore, drained *(S&W)*	2 oz	160	13.0	0.0	450	0	12.0	(mq)
solid, albacore, drained *(Star-Kist)*	2 oz	140	14.0	<1.0	310	0	10.0	25
w/o salt, drained	1 oz	53	7.5	0.0	14	0	2.3	0
In spring water, solid, fancy albacore								
(Chicken of the Sea)	2 oz	60	14.0	<1.0	250	na	1.0	na
In water								
chunk, diet, drained *(Star-Kist)*	2 oz	70	15.0	<1.0	30	0	1.0	25
chunk, drained *(A&P)*	2 oz	100	12.0	<1.0	310	0	5.0	(mq)
chunk, drained *(Bumble Bee)*	2 oz	60	12.0	0.0	310	0	2.0	30
chunk '60% Less Salt' drained *(Star-Kist)*	2 oz	70	15.0	<1.0	120	0	<1.0	25
drained	3 oz	116	22.7	0.0	333	0	2.1	36
drained, approx 6.1 oz	1 can	234	45.9	0.0	674	0	4.2	72
solid, albacore, drained *(A&P)*	2 oz	70	15.0	<1.0	310	0	<1.0	(mq)
solid, albacore, drained *(Bumble Bee)*	2 oz	60	14.0	0.0	310	0	2.0	30
solid, albacore, drained *(Finast)*	2 oz	70	15.0	<1.0	310	0	1.0	(mq)
solid, albacore, drained *(Pathmark)*	2 oz	70	15.0	0.0	310	0	2.0	(mq)
solid, albacore, drained *(Star-Kist)*	2 oz	70	15.0	<1.0	310	0	1.0	25
solid, albacore, drained *(Weight Watchers)*	2 oz	70	15.0	<1.0	210	0	1.0	25
w/o salt, drained	3 oz	116	22.7	0.0	43	0	2.1	36
w/o salt, drained	1 oz	39	7.6	0.0	14	0	0.7	12
w/o salt, drained, approx 6.1 oz	1 can	234	45.9	0.0	86	0	4.2	72
TUNA, FROZEN								
(Peter Pan Seafoods) albacore, white,								
steaks, skinless, boneless, raw	3.5 oz	102	18.8	na	51	na	4.9	54

Food Name	Serv. Size	Total Cal.	Prot. GMS	Carbs GMS	Sod. MGS	Fiber GMS	Fat GMS	Chol. MGS
(Peter Pan Seafoods) yellowfin, steaks,								
skinless, boneless, raw	3.5 oz	131	23.4	na	61	na	4.1	45
(SeaPak) steak, w/o seasoning mix	6-oz pkg	180	40.0	0.0	65	0	2.0	75
TUNA, SKIPJACK/aku/arctic bonito/katsuo/oceanic bonito. See also BONITO.								
dry-heat cooked	3 oz	112	24.0	0.0	40	0	1.1	51
raw	1 lb	468	99.8	0.0	167	0	4.6	213
raw	3 oz	88	18.7	0.0	31	0	0.9	40
raw	1 oz	29	6.2	0.0	10	0	0.3	13
raw, approx 7 oz	1/2 fillet	204	43.6	0.0	73	0	2.0	93
TUNA, YELLOWFIN/ahi								
dry-heat cooked	3 oz	118	25.5	0.0	40	0	1.0	na
raw	1 lb	492	106.0	0.0	168	0	4.3	203
raw	3 oz	92	19.9	0.0	31	0	0.8	38
raw	1 oz	31	6.6	0.0	10	0	0.3	13
TUNA ENTRÉE, FROZEN								
noodle casserole *(Stouffer's)*	10 oz	280	17.0	33.0	1090	na	15.0	na
noodle casserole *(Weight Watchers)*	9 oz	230	15.0	27.0	550	na	7.0	20
pie *(Banquet)*	7 oz	540	17.0	44.0	810	(mq)	33.0	30
TUNA ENTRÉE, MIX								
au gratin, dry mix *(Tuna Helper)*	1/5 pkg	180	6.0	27.0	800	(mq)	5.0	na
buttery rice, dry mix *(Tuna Helper)*	1/5 pkg	160	4.0	32.0	830	(mq)	2.0	na
cheesy noodle, dry mix *(Tuna Helper)*	1/5 pkg	160	5.0	27.0	810	(mq)	4.0	na
creamy broccoli, dry mix *(Tuna Helper)*	1/5 pkg	200	6.0	35.0	800	na	4.0	na
fettuccine Alfredo, dry mix *(Tuna Helper)*	1/5 pkg	160	6.0	28.0	760	(mq)	3.0	na
mushroom, creamy, dry mix								
(Tuna Helper)	1/5 pkg	140	5.0	28.0	580	(mq)	1.0	na
noodle, creamy, dry mix *(Tuna Helper)*	1/5 pkg	210	5.0	29.0	790	(mq)	8.0	na
pot pie, dry mix *(Tuna Helper)*	1/6 pkg	290	4.0	31.0	730	(mq)	17.0	na
salad, dry mix *(Tuna Helper)*	1/5 pkg	140	5.0	28.0	580	(mq)	1.0	na
tetrazzini, dry mix *(Tuna Helper)*	1/5 pkg	160	6.0	26.0	620	(mq)	3.0	na
TUNA LUNCH KIT								
'Charlie's Lunch Kit' w/1 mayo packet								
(Star-Kist)	4.6 oz	290	24.0	16.0	780	na	15.0	na
'Charlie's Lunch Kit' w/2 mayo packets								
(Star-Kist)	5 oz	370	24.0	16.0	845	na	15.0	na
TUNA MIX								
classic Italian 'Tuna Mix-ins' dry mix								
(Bumble Bee)	1 oz	25	0.0	5.0	5	na	0.0	0
garden and herb 'Tuna Mix-ins' dry mix								
(Bumble Bee)	1 oz	25	0.0	5.0	5	na	0.0	0
lemon herb 'Tuna Mix-ins' dry mix								
(Bumble Bee)	1 oz	25	0.0	6.0	5	na	0.0	0

Food Name	Serv. Size	Total Cal.	Prot. GMS	Carbs GMS	Sod. MGS	Fiber GMS	Fat GMS	Chol. MGS
zesty tomato 'Tuna Mix-ins' dry mix								
(Bumble Bee) ...... 1 oz		25	0.0	5.0	5	na	0.0	0
TUNA SALAD								
(Longacre) ...... 1 oz		58	2.0	3.0	130	na	4.0	10
(Longacre) 'Saladfest' ...... 1 oz		52	3.0	2.0	180	na	4.0	10
TUNA SALAD SPREAD (Libby's)								
'Spreadables' ...... 1.9 oz		80	5.0	5.0	220	1.9	5.0	na
TUNKA. See GOURD, WHITE.								
TURBOT, DOMESTIC								
raw ...... 1 lb		845	65.2	0.0	363	0	62.8	209
raw ...... 1 oz		53	4.1	0.0	23	0	3.9	13
raw, approx 7.2 oz ...... 1/2 fillet		380	29.3	0.0	163	0	28.2	94
TURBOT, EUROPEAN								
dry-heat cooked ...... 3 oz		104	17.5	0.0	163	0	3.2	53
raw ...... 1 lb		432	72.8	0.0	678	0	13.4	(mq)
raw ...... 3 oz		81	13.6	0.0	127	0	2.5	41
raw ...... 1 oz		27	4.6	0.0	43	0	0.8	(mq)
raw, approx 7.2 oz ...... 1/2 fillet		194	32.7	0.0	306	0	6.0	98
TURKEY, ALL CLASSES								
BACK MEAT W/SKIN								
raw ...... 1 lb		896	81.6	0.0	304	0	59.2	336
raw ...... 1 oz		56	5.1	0.0	19	0	3.7	21
roasted ...... 4 oz		276	30.2	0.0	83	0	16.3	103
BREAST MEAT W/SKIN								
raw ...... 1 lb		720	99.2	0.0	272	0	32.0	288
raw ...... 1 oz		45	6.2	0.0	17	0	2.0	18
roasted ...... 4 oz		214	32.6	0.0	71	0	8.4	84
DARK MEAT ONLY								
raw ...... 1 lb		560	91.2	0.0	352	0	19.2	320
raw ...... 1 oz		35	5.7	0.0	22	0	1.2	20
roasted ...... 1 cup		262	40.0	0.0	111	0	10.1	119
roasted ...... 4 oz		212	32.4	0.0	90	0	8.2	96
DARK MEAT W/SKIN								
raw ...... 1 lb		720	86.4	0.0	320	0	40.0	320
raw ...... 1 oz		45	5.4	0.0	20	0	2.5	20
roasted ...... 4 oz		251	31.2	0.0	86	0	13.1	101
LEG MEAT W/SKIN								
raw ...... 1 lb		656	88.0	0.0	336	0	30.4	320
raw ...... 1 oz		41	5.5	0.0	21	0	1.9	20
roasted ...... 4 oz		236	31.6	0.0	87	0	11.1	96
LIGHT MEAT ONLY								
raw ...... 1 lb		528	107.2	0.0	288	0	6.4	272
raw ...... 1 oz		33	6.7	0.0	18	0	0.4	17

Food Name	Serv. Size	Total Cal.	Prot. GMS	Carbs GMS	Sod. MGS	Fiber GMS	Fat GMS	Chol. MGS
roasted	4 oz	178	33.9	0.0	73	0	3.7	78
roasted, diced	1 cup	220	41.9	0.0	90	0	4.5	97
LIGHT MEAT W/SKIN								
raw	1 lb	72.0	97.6	0.0	272	0	33.6	288
raw	1 oz	45	6.1	0.0	17	0	2.1	18
roasted	4 oz	223	32.4	0.0	71	0	9.4	86
NECK MEAT ONLY								
raw	1 lb	608	91.2	0.0	416	0	24.0	352
raw	1 oz	38	5.7	0.0	26	0	1.5	22
simmered	4 oz	204	30.4	0.0	64	0	8.2	138
SKIN ONLY								
raw	1 lb	1760	57.6	0.0	160	0	168.0	576
raw	1 oz	110	3.6	0.0	10	0	10.5	26
roasted	1 oz	125	5.6	0.0	15	0	11.2	32
WING MEAT W/SKIN								
raw	1 lb	896	91.2	0.0	256	0	56.0	320
raw	1 oz	56	5.7	0.0	16	0	3.5	20
roasted	4 oz	260	31.0	0.0	69	0	14.1	92
TURKEY, ALTERNATIVE								
(Worthington) roll, smoked, frozen	4 slices	180	13.0	5.0	820	(mq)	12.0	0
(Worthington) sliced, smoked, frozen	4 slices	180	13.0	5.0	820	(mq)	12.0	0
(Worthington) 'Turkee Slices' canned	2 slices	130	9.0	3.0	430	(mq)	9.0	0
(Worthington) '209' canned, drained	2 slices	120	8.0	3.0	(mq)	(mq)	8.0	0
TURKEY, BONELESS. See also LUNCHEON MEAT.								
BREAST								
(Butterball) 'Slice 'n Serve'	1 oz	35	5.0	<1.0	230	0	1.0	(mq)
(Longacre) 'Gourmet'	1 oz	35	5.0	1.0	300	0	1.0	15
(Longacre) 'Gourmet Low Salt'	1 oz	30	6.0	1.0	150	0	<1.0	10
(Longacre) 'Premium'	1 oz	30	4.0	1.0	250	0	1.0	10
(Longacre) 'Salt Watchers'	1 oz	32	7.0	0.0	10	0	<1.0	15
(Mr. Turkey)	1 oz	31	5.8	0.3	233	0	0.7	10
Barbecue seasoned *(Butterball)* Slice 'n Serve	1 oz	40	5.0	1.0	210	0	2.0	(mq)
Browned								
(Longacre) glazed 'Gourmet'	1 oz	35	5.0	1.0	240	0	1.0	15
(Longacre) glazed 'Premium'	1 oz	30	4.0	1.0	300	0	1.0	10
(Longacre) roasted 'Gourmet'	1 oz	35	5.0	1.0	260	0	1.0	15
(Longacre) roasted 'Premium'	1 oz	30	4.0	1.0	300	0	1.0	10
Golden								
(Boar's Head)	1 oz	35	6.0	<1.0	200	0	1.0	20
(Boar's Head) skinless	1 oz	30	6.0	<1.0	(mq)	0	<1.0	10
Hickory smoked *(Butterball)* 'Slice 'n Serve'	1 oz	35	5.0	1.0	250	0	1.0	(mq)
Honey roasted *(Louis Rich)*	1 oz	32	4.9	1.2	315	0	0.8	11

Food Name	Serv. Size	Total Cal.	Prot. GMS	Carbs GMS	Sod. MGS	Fiber GMS	Fat GMS	Chol. MGS
Lean, lite								
(Longacre) 'Deli'	1 oz	35	6.0	0.0	160	0	1.0	15
(Longacre) skinless 'Deli'	1 oz	35	6.0	0.0	160	0	<1.0	15
(Longacre) smoked 'Deli'	1 oz	35	6.0	0.0	160	0	1.0	15
Skinless								
(Longacre) 'Catering'	1 oz	35	6.0	<1.0	280	0	<1.0	15
(Longacre) 'Gourmet'	1 oz	30	5.0	1.0	260	0	<1.0	15
(Longacre) 'Premium'	1 oz	30	4.0	1.0	250	0	<1.0	10
(Norbest) 'Blue Label'	1 oz	26	5.1	0.4	252	0	0.4	(mq)
(Norbest) 'Norfresh'	1 oz	27	5.2	0.5	269	0	0.3	(mq)
(Norbest) 'Norfresh Blue Label'	1 oz	24	4.4	0.7	253	0	0.3	(mq)
(Norbest) 'Norfresh Yellow Label'	1 oz	24	4.4	0.4	284	0	0.5	(mq)
(Norbest) 'Orange Label'	1 oz	26	5.1	0.5	239	0	0.2	(mq)
(Norbest) salt-free 'Blue Label'	1 oz	33	7.7	<.1	13	0	0.3	(mq)
(Norbest) 'Tan Label'	1 oz	24	4.3	0.5	354	0	0.5	(mq)
(Norbest) 'Yellow Label'	1 oz	26	4.3	0.8	272	0	0.5	(mq)
Smoked								
(Healthy Deli) 'Gourmet'	1 oz	31	5.8	0.4	170	0	0.5	11
(Hormel) 'Perma-Fresh'	2 slices	60	10.0	0.0	540	0	2.0	(mq)
(Longacre)	1 oz	35	6.0	0.0	240	0	1.0	15
(Norbest) 'Gold Label'	1 oz	29	6.4	0.1	270	0	<.6	(mq)
(OHSE)	1 oz	30	5.0	1.0	340	0	1.0	(mq)
W/skin								
(Norbest) 'Blue Label'	1 oz	28	5.1	0.2	239	0	0.7	(mq)
(Norbest) 'Norfresh Orange Label'	1 oz	26	5.3	0.1	256	0	0.3	(mq)
(Norbest) 'Norfresh Yellow Label'	1 oz	25	4.8	0.1	244	0	0.5	(mq)
(Norbest) 'Orange Label'	1 oz	28	5.7	0.1	232	0	0.3	(mq)
(Norbest) prebrowned 'Orange Label'	1 oz	29	5.1	0.2	259	0	0.8	(mq)
(Norbest) salt-free 'Blue Label'	1 oz	35	7.5	0.2	13	0	0.5	(mq)
(Norbest) smoked 'Orange Label'	1 oz	30	5.3	0.9	284	0	0.5	(mq)
(Norbest) 'Yellow Label'	1 oz	26	5.1	0.1	271	0	0.4	(mq)
BREAST AND LIGHT MEAT								
(Longacre) browned and roasted	1 oz	40	5.0	1.0	240	0	2.0	15
(Longacre) 'Deli Chef'	1 oz	35	5.0	1.0	240	0	1.0	15
(Longacre) skinless 'Deli Chef'	1 oz	40	4.0	1.0	240	0	2.0	15
BREAST AND THIGH (Norbest) 'Blue Label'	1 oz	31	5.8	0.2	238	0	0.9	(mq)
DARK MEAT (Norbest) ham flavor, hickory smoked	1 oz	39	4.6	0.1	335	0	2.2	(mq)
OVEN COOKED (OHSE)	1 oz	30	5.0	1.0	190	0	1.0	(mq)
ROLL								
(Norbest) white meat 'Orange Label'	1 oz	29	4.1	0.5	299	0	0.9	(mq)
(Norbest) white and dark meat 'Orange Label'	1 oz	36	4.0	0.3	314	0	2.0	(mq)

Food Name	Serv. Size	Total Cal.	Prot. GMS	Carbs GMS	Sod. MGS	Fiber GMS	Fat GMS	Chol. MGS
SMOKED *(Louis Rich)*	1 oz	32	5.4	0.4	284	0	1.0	14
W/PORK *(Healthy Favorites)*								
'Breakfast Strips'	11 grams	18	1.8	0.4	145	0	1.0	9
TURKEY, CANNED								
(Hormel) chunk	6.75 oz	230	37.0	0.0	1278	0	10.0	(mq)
(Hormel) chunk	2.5 oz	80	13.0	1.0	420	0	3.0	45
(Swanson) white	2.5 oz	80	17.0	1.0	260	0	1.0	(mq)
(Tyson) 'Wholesale Club Item'	3.5 oz	120	23.0	0.0	360	na	3.0	na
TURKEY, FROZEN/REFRIGERATED								
BREAST								
Cooked								
(Land O'Lakes)	3 oz	100	20.0	0.0	55	0	1.0	50
(Longacre) 'Cook-N-Bag'	1 oz	38	8.0	<1.0	85	0	<1.0	15
(Louis Rich)	1 oz	47	8.1	0.1	21	0	1.5	21
(Louis Rich) barbecue	1 oz	33	5.3	0.9	315	0	1.0	12
(Louis Rich) hen, w/o wings	1 oz	50	7.9	0.1	19	0	2.0	19
(Louis Rich) hickory smoked	1 oz	33	5.4	0.8	346	0	1.0	13
(Louis Rich) honey roasted	1 oz	33	5.3	1.1	318	0	0.8	12
(Louis Rich) oven roasted	1 oz	31	5.3	0.4	296	0	0.9	13
(Louis Rich) roast	1 oz	42	8.3	0.2	20	0	0.8	19
(Louis Rich) slices	1 oz	39	8.4	0.1	24	0	0.5	17
(Louis Rich) smoked	1 oz	33	5.7	0.2	268	0	1.0	11
(Louis Rich) steaks	1 oz	39	8.4	0.1	24	0	0.5	17
(Louis Rich) tenderloins	1 oz	39	8.5	0.2	24	0	0.5	18
(Mr. Turkey) barbecue, quarter 'Chub'	1 oz	34	5.4	1.0	251	0	1.0	11
(Mr. Turkey) oven roasted, quarter 'Chub'	1 oz	34	5.8	0.4	266	0	1.0	12
(Mr. Turkey) smoked, quarter 'Chub'	1 oz	35	6.1	0.3	263	0	1.0	10
(Tyson) skinless, boneless 'Wholesale Club Item'	3.5 oz	160	30.0	0.0	65	na	3.0	70
w/skin, roasted, broth pre-basted	4 oz	143	25.1	0.0	450	0	3.9	48
Raw								
(Longacre) 'Cook-N-Bag'	1 oz	27	6.0	<1.0	120	0	<1.0	10
(Longacre) 'Ready-to-Cook'	1 oz	39	8.0	0.0	150	0	<1.0	(mq)
(Norbest) steaks, cubed	4 oz	135	27.8	<.1	81	0	2.0	(mq)
(Norbest) strips and tips 'Tasti-Lean'	4 oz	135	27.8	<.1	81	0	2.0	(mq)
(Norbest) tenderloin 'Tasti-Lean Tenders'	4 oz	135	27.8	<.1	81	0	2.0	(mq)
(Norbest) w/gravy	4 oz	115	20.7	1.1	492	0	2.4	(mq)
CUTLET *(Norbest)* raw 'Tasti-Lean'	4 oz	135	27.8	<.1	81	0	2.0	(mq)
DARK MEAT *(Butterball)* w/o skin, roasted, approx 3.5 oz	2 slices	195	25.0	na	90	0	10.0	130
DRUMSTICK								
(Land O'Lakes)	3 oz	120	17.0	0.0	85	0	5.0	(mq)
(Louis Rich) cooked	1 oz	56	7.9	0.1	22	0	2.6	27

Food Name	Serv. Size	Total Cal.	Prot. GMS	Carbs GMS	Sod. MGS	Fiber GMS	Fat GMS	Chol. MGS
(Louis Rich) cooked 'Fresh Turkey Cuts'	1 oz	55	8.0	<1.0	25	na	3.0	30
HINDQUARTER ROAST *(Land O'Lakes)*	3 oz	140	17.0	0.0	80	0	8.0	(mq)
LIGHT AND DARK MEAT								
roasted, then seasoned	4 oz	176	24.2	3.5	771	na	6.6	(mq)
seasoned raw, then roasted	1 lb	544	79.8	29.0	3075	na	10.0	(mq)
seasoned raw, then roasted	1 oz	34	5.0	1.8	192	na	0.6	(mq)
(Butterball) w/skin, roasted, approx 3.5 oz	2 slices	195	27.0	na	115	0	10.0	100
LIGHT MEAT *(Butterball)* w/o skin, roasted, approx 3.5 oz	2 slices	160	30.0	na	130	0	4.0	80
THIGH								
w/skin, roasted, pre-basted w/broth	4 oz	178	21.3	0.0	496	0	9.7	70
(Land O'Lakes)	3 oz	150	17.0	0.0	75	0	10.0	(mq)
(Louis Rich) cooked	1 oz	64	7.5	0.1	20	0	3.7	27
(Louis Rich) cooked 'Fresh Turkey Cuts'	1 oz	65	7.0	<1.0	20	na	4.0	30
WHOLE								
(Louis Rich) w/o giblets, cooked	1 oz	52	7.7	0.1	23	0	2.3	22
(Louis Rich) w/o giblets, cooked 'Fresh Whole Turkey'	1 oz	50	8.0	<1.0	25	na	2.0	25
(Norbest) boneless, cooked	1 oz	42	6.2	0.3	105	0	1.5	(mq)
(Norbest) boneless, smoked, cooked	1 oz	42	6.4	0.3	218	0	1.6	(mq)
WING								
(Land O'Lakes)	3 oz	120	18.0	0.0	65	0	5.0	(mq)
(Louis Rich) cooked	1 oz	54	7.2	0.1	20	0	2.7	31
(Louis Rich) cooked 'Drumettes'	1 oz	51	7.8	0.1	20	0	2.2	29
(Louis Rich) cooked 'Fresh Turkey Cuts'	1 oz	55	7.0	<1.0	20	na	3.0	30
(Louis Rich) drumettes, cooked 'Fresh Turkey Cuts'	1 oz	50	8.0	<1.0	20	na	2.0	30
(Louis Rich) portions, cooked	1 oz	54	6.9	0.1	17	0	2.9	29
(Louis Rich) portions, cooked 'Fresh Turkey Cuts'	1 oz	55	7.0	<1.0	20	na	3.0	30
W/GRAVY *(Norbest)* raw	4 oz	115	20.3	1.1	600	0	2.7	(mq)
YOUNG								
(Land O'Lakes)	3 oz	130	17.0	<1.0	55	0	7.0	65
(Land O'Lakes) butter-basted	3 oz	140	17.0	<1.0	135	0	8.0	85
(Land O'Lakes) self-basting, w/broth	3 oz	120	18.0	<1.0	145	0	5.0	77
TURKEY, FRYER-ROASTER								
BACK MEAT ONLY								
raw	1 lb	544	94.4	0.0	288	0	16.0	336
raw	1 oz	34	5.9	0.0	18	0	1.0	21
roasted	4 oz	193	31.8	0.0	83	0	6.4	108
BACK MEAT W/SKIN								
raw	1 lb	688	89.6	0.0	272	0	336.0	384

Food Name	Serv. Size	Total Cal.	Prot. GMS	Carbs GMS	Sod. MGS	Fiber GMS	Fat GMS	Chol. MGS
raw	1 oz	43	5.6	0.0	17	0	2.1	24
roasted	4 oz	231	29.7	0.0	79	0	11.6	122
BREAST MEAT ONLY								
raw	1 lb	496	112.0	0.0	224	0	3.2	288
raw	1 oz	31	7.0	0.0	14	0	0.2	18
roasted	4 oz	153	34.1	0.0	59	0	0.8	94
BREAST MEAT W/SKIN								
raw	1 lb	560	107.2	0.0	224	0	12.8	320
raw	1 oz	35	6.7	0.0	14	0	0.8	20
roasted	4 oz	174	33.0	0.0	60	0	3.6	102
DARK MEAT ONLY								
raw	1 lb	496	92.8	0.0	320	0	12.8	368
raw	1 oz	31	5.8	0.0	20	0	0.8	23
roasted	4 oz	184	32.7	0.0	90	0	4.9	127
roasted, diced	1 cup	227	40.4	0.0	111	0	6.0	157
DARK MEAT W/SKIN								
raw	1 lb	592	91.2	0.0	304	0	22.4	400
raw	1 oz	37	5.7	0.0	19	0	1.4	25
roasted	4 oz	206	31.4	0.0	86	0	8.0	133
LEG MEAT ONLY								
raw	1 lb	496	92.8	0.0	320	0	11.2	384
raw	1 oz	31	5.8	0.0	20	0	0.7	24
roasted	4 oz	180	33.1	0.0	92	0	4.3	135
LEG MEAT W/SKIN								
raw	1 lb	528	91.2	0.0	320	0	16.0	400
raw	1 oz	33	5.7	0.0	20	0	1.0	25
roasted	4 oz	193	32.3	0.0	91	0	6.1	79
LIGHT MEAT ONLY								
raw	1 lb	496	110.4	0.0	240	0	1.6	304
raw	1 oz	31	6.9	0.0	15	0	0.1	19
roasted	4 oz	159	34.2	0.0	64	0	1.3	98
roasted, diced	1 cup	196	42.3	0.0	78	0	1.6	120
LIGHT MEAT W/SKIN								
raw	1 lb	608	104.0	0.0	224	0	17.6	352
raw	1 oz	38	6.5	0.0	14	0	1.1	22
roasted	4 oz	186	32.6	0.0	65	0	5.2	108
SKIN ONLY								
raw	1 lb	1280	75.2	0.0	160	0	107.2	624
raw	1 oz	80	4.7	0.0	10	0	6.7	39
WING MEAT ONLY								
raw	1 lb	480	102.4	0.0	288	0	4.8	368
raw	1 oz	30	6.4	0.0	18	0	0.3	23
roasted	4 oz	185	35.0	0.0	88	0	3.9	116

Food Name	Serv. Size	Total Cal.	Prot. GMS	Carbs GMS	Sod. MGS	Fiber GMS	Fat GMS	Chol. MGS
WING MEAT W/SKIN								
raw	1 lb	720	94.4	0.0	256	0	35.2	448
raw	1 oz	45	5.9	0.0	16	0	2.2	28
roasted	4 oz	235	31.4	0.0	83	0	11.2	130
TURKEY, GROUND								
Cooked								
	4 oz	260	27.7	0.0	94	0	15.6	78
approx 2.9 oz	1 patty	193	22.4	0.0	88	0	10.8	84
yield from 1 lb raw	11.6 oz	754	80.4	0.0	273	0	45.5	227
(Hudson's)	1 oz	55	5.0	0.0	35	0	3.7	(mq)
(Longacre)	1 oz	60	5.0	0.0	20	0	4.0	30
(Louis Rich) 85% fat-free	1 oz	60	7.0	<1.0	30	na	3.0	30
(Louis Rich) 90% fat-free	1 oz	50	7.0	<1.0	30	na	3.0	25
(Louis Rich) 90% fat-free, natural flavorings	1 oz	50	7.0	<1.0	35	na	2.0	25
(Mr. Turkey)	1 oz	54	4.5	0.0	27	0	4.0	20
Raw								
	1 lb	676	79.2	0.0	426	0	37.5	358
	1 oz	40	4.9	0.0	27	0	2.1	21
(Norbest)	1 oz	45	5.2	0.1	34	0	2.6	(mq)
(Louis Rich) w/natural flavoring	1 oz	50	7.5	0.0	33	0	2.2	24
TURKEY, YOUNG HEN								
BACK MEAT W/SKIN								
raw	1 lb	992	80.0	0.0	272	0	72.0	304
raw	1 oz	62	5.0	0.0	17	0	4.5	19
roasted	4 oz	288	29.9	0.0	78	0	17.7	96
BREAST MEAT W/SKIN								
raw	1 lb	752	97.6	0.0	256	0	38.4	288
raw	1 oz	47	6.1	0.0	16	0	2.4	18
roasted	4 oz	220	32.7	0.0	66	0	8.9	82
DARK MEAT ONLY								
raw	1 lb	592	91.2	0.0	336	0	22.4	288
raw	1 oz	37	5.7	0.0	21	0	1.4	18
roasted	4 oz	218	32.2	0.0	85	0	8.8	91
roasted, diced	1 cup	269	39.8	0.0	105	0	10.9	112
DARK MEAT W/SKIN								
raw	1 lb	784	84.8	0.0	304	0	46.4	288
raw	1 oz	49	5.3	0.0	19	0	2.9	18
roasted	4 oz	263	31.0	0.0	82	0	14.5	95
LEG MEAT W/SKIN								
raw	1 lb	688	88.0	0.0	320	0	33.6	288
raw	1 oz	43	5.5	0.0	20	0	2.1	18
roasted	4 oz	242	31.4	0.0	83	0	11.9	93

Food Name	Serv. Size	Total Cal.	Prot. GMS	Carbs GMS	Sod. MGS	Fiber GMS	Fat GMS	Chol. MGS
LIGHT MEAT ONLY								
raw	1 lb	528	107.2	0.0	272	0	8.0	256
raw	1 oz	33	6.7	0.0	17	0	0.5	16
roasted	4 oz	183	33.9	0.0	68	0	4.2	77
roasted, diced	1 cup	225	41.8	0.0	84	0	5.2	95
LIGHT MEAT W/SKIN								
raw	1 lb	752	97.6	0.0	256	0	36.8	288
raw	1 oz	47	6.1	0.0	16	0	2.3	18
roasted	4 oz	235	32.5	0.0	66	0	10.7	84
SKIN ONLY								
roasted	1 oz	137	5.4	0.0	12	0	12.6	30
WING MEAT W/SKIN								
raw	1 lb	960	91.2	0.0	224	0	62.4	288
raw	1 oz	60	5.7	0.0	14	0	3.9	18
roasted	4 oz	270	31.0	0.0	64	0	15.3	87
TURKEY, YOUNG TOM								
BACK MEAT W/SKIN								
raw	1 lb	81.6	83.2	0.0	320	0	51.2	352
raw	1 oz	51	5.2	0.0	20	0	3.2	22
roasted	4 oz	270	30.4	0.0	87	0	15.5	107
BREAST MEAT W/SKIN								
raw	1 lb	688	99.2	0.0	288	0	28.8	112
raw	1 oz	43	6.2	0.0	18	0	1.8	7
roasted	4 oz	214	32.4	0.0	76	0	8.4	85
DARK MEAT ONLY								
raw	1 lb	560	91.2	0.0	368	0	19.2	336
raw	1 oz	35	5.7	0.0	23	0	1.2	21
roasted	4 oz	210	32.5	0.0	93	0	7.9	100
roasted, diced	1 cup	259	40.1	0.0	115	0	9.8	123
DARK MEAT W/SKIN								
raw	1 lb	688	86.4	0.0	336	0	35.2	352
raw	1 oz	43	5.4	0.0	21	0	2.2	22
roasted	4 oz	245	31.3	0.0	91	0	12.3	103
LEG MEAT W/SKIN								
raw	1 lb	640	88.0	0.0	352	0	28.8	352
raw	1 oz	40	5.5	0.0	22	0	1.8	22
roasted	4 oz	234	31.7	0.0	91	0	10.9	102
LIGHT MEAT ONLY								
raw	1 lb	512	105.6	0.0	304	0	6.4	288
raw	1 oz	32	6.6	0.0	19	0	0.4	18
roasted	4 oz	175	33.9	0.0	77	0	3.3	78
roasted, diced	1 cup	216	41.8	0.0	95	0	4.1	97

Food Name	Serv. Size	Total Cal.	Prot. GMS	Carbs GMS	Sod. MGS	Fiber GMS	Fat GMS	Chol. MGS
LIGHT MEAT W/SKIN								
raw	1 lb	704	97.6	0.0	288	0	32.0	304
raw	1 oz	44	6.1	0.0	18	0	2.0	19
roasted	4 oz	217	32.3	0.0	76	0	8.7	85
SKIN ONLY								
raw	1 lb	1664	60.8	0.0	176	0	157.0	432
raw	1 oz	104	3.8	0.0	11	0	9.8	27
roasted	1 oz	120	5.7	0.0	17	0	10.6	33
WING MEAT W/SKIN								
raw	1 lb	848	92.8	0.0	272	0	51.2	320
raw	1 oz	53	5.8	0.0	17	0	3.2	20
roasted	4 oz	251	31.1	0.0	75	0	13.0	92
TURKEY BREAST								
BARBECUED *(Louis Rich)* skinless	1 oz	30	6.0	<1.0	280	na	<1.0	10
HONEY ROASTED								
(Louis Rich) 95% fat-free	1-oz slice	35	5.0	1.0	315	na	1.0	10
(Louis Rich) skinless	1 oz	30	6.0	<1.0	295	na	<1.0	10
OVEN ROASTED								
(Louis Rich) 'Carving Board'	22 grams	21	4.5	0.1	272	0	0.3	9
(Louis Rich) 'Fresh Turkey Cuts'	1 oz	45	8.0	<1.0	20	na	2.0	20
(Louis Rich) 96% fat-free 'Deli-Thin'	1 slice	10	2.0	<1.0	130	na	<1.0	5
(Louis Rich) 97% fat-free	1-oz slice	30	5.0	1.0	315	na	<1.0	10
(Louis Rich) 97% fat-free 'Deli-Thin'	1 slice	10	2.0	<1.0	125	na	<1.0	5
(Louis Rich) roast 'Fresh Turkey Cuts'	1 oz	40	8.0	<1.0	20	na	<1.0	20
(Louis Rich) skinless	1 oz	25	6.0	<1.0	275	na	<1.0	10
(Louis Rich) slices 'Fresh Turkey Cuts'	1 oz	40	8.0	<1.0	25	na	<1.0	15
(Louis Rich) steaks 'Fresh Turkey Cuts'	1 oz	40	8.0	<1.0	25	na	<1.0	20
(Louis Rich) tenderloins 'Fresh Turkey Cuts'	1 oz	40	8.0	<1.0	25	na	<1.0	20
SMOKED								
(Louis Rich) 'Carving Board'	10 grams	9	2.0	0.1	124	0	0.1	4
(Louis Rich) 96% fat-free	1 oz	35	6.0	<1.0	270	na	1.0	10
(Louis Rich) 97% fat-free 'Deli-Thin'	1 slice	10	2.0	<1.0	110	na	<1.0	5
(Louis Rich) 98% fat-free	1-oz slice	20	4.0	<1.0	210	na	<1.0	10
(Louis Rich) skinless	1 oz	30	6.0	<1.0	330	na	<1.0	10
TURKEY DINNER, FROZEN								
(Banquet)	10.5 oz	390	18.0	35.0	1110	(mq)	20.0	40
(Banquet) 'Extra Helping'	19 oz	750	29.0	68.0	1980	(mq)	42.0	65
(Morton)	10 oz	230	15.0	28.0	1300	(mq)	6.0	45
(Swanson)	11.5 oz	350	21.0	42.0	1090	(mq)	11.0	(mq)
(Swanson) 'Hungry Man'	17 oz	550	36.0	61.0	1810	(mq)	18.0	(mq)
BREAST								
(Budget Gourmet) Dijon	11.2 oz	340	20.0	37.0	860	(mq)	12.0	65
(Budget Gourmet) sliced	11.1 oz	290	16.0	36.0	1200	(mq)	9.0	45

Food Name	Serv. Size	Total Cal.	Prot. GMS	Carbs GMS	Sod. MGS	Fiber GMS	Fat GMS	Chol. MGS
(Healthy Choice) medallions, w/vegetables 'Classics'	12.5 oz	350	29.0	45.0	480	na	6.0	60
(Le Menu) sliced, w/mushroom gravy	10.5 oz	300	22.0	38.0	1020	(mq)	7.0	(mq)
(Swanson) w/pasta	11.25 oz	310	22.0	36.0	670	na	9.0	35
DIVAN *(Le Menu)* 'LightStyle'	10 oz	260	25.0	23.0	420	(mq)	7.0	60
SLICED								
(Freezer Queen)	10 oz	280	16.0	36.0	1210	(mq)	8.0	(mq)
(Le Menu) 'LightStyle'	10 oz	210	21.0	21.0	540	(mq)	5.0	30
TETRAZZINI *(Healthy Choice)*	12.6 oz	340	23.0	49.0	490	na	6.0	40
W/DRESSING AND GRAVY								
(Armour) 'Classics'	11.5 oz	320	19.0	34.0	1280	(mq)	12.0	50
(Banquet) w/dressing and gravy 'Healthy Balance'	11.25 oz	270	16.0	41.0	750	na	5.0	40
TURKEY ENTRÉE								
(Dinty Moore) w/dressing and gravy 'American Classics'	10 oz	290	28.0	33.0	910	na	5.0	40
(Hormel) and vegetables 'Health Selections' microwave cup	7.25 oz	220	15.0	35.0	420	na	2.0	20
(Libby's) w/dressing and gravy 'Diner' microwave cup	7 oz	170	11.0	15.0	830	1.2	7.0	35
(Mountain House) tetrazzini, freeze-dried, prepared	1 cup	200	13.0	20.0	(mq)	(mq)	8.0	(mq)
(Turkey by George) hickory barbecue	5 oz	190	28.0	8.0	840	na	5.0	65
(Turkey by George) Italian Parmesan	5 oz	170	28.0	3.0	860	na	5.0	70
(Turkey by George) lemon pepper	5 oz	160	28.0	4.0	830	na	4.0	60
(Turkey by George) mustard tarragon	5 oz	180	29.0	3.0	830	na	6.0	80
(Ultra Slim Fast) glazed, w/dressing	10.5 oz	340	28.0	49.0	570	na	5.0	50
(Ultra Slim Fast) medallions, in herb sauce	12 oz	280	23.0	33.0	950	na	6.0	40
TURKEY ENTRÉE, FROZEN								
À LA KING *(Budget Gourmet)* w/rice	10 oz	390	20.0	36.0	740	(mq)	18.0	75
BREAST								
(Healthy Choice) sliced, w/dressing and gravy 'Classics'	10 oz	270	27.0	30.0	530	na	4.0	50
(Lean Cuisine) sliced, w/dressing	7 7/8 oz	200	16.0	23.0	590	na	5.0	25
(Lean Cuisine) sliced, w/mushroom sauce and rice	8 oz	230	17.0	24.0	540	na	7.0	35
(Stouffer's) roast, w/stuffing and gravy	7 7/8 oz	270	19.0	27.0	920	na	9.0	na
(Tyson) 'Gourmet Selections'	11.5 oz	380	19.0	51.0	1350	(mq)	11.0	(mq)
(Weight Watchers) stuffed	8.5 oz	270	18.0	31.0	520	na	8.0	60
CASSEROLE *(Pillsbury)* 'Microwave Classic'	1 pkg	430	20.0	31.0	880	(mq)	25.0	(mq)
CROQUETTES *(Freezer Queen)* breaded, w/gravy	7 oz	250	13.0	19.0	940	(mq)	13.0	(mq)

Food Name	Serv. Size	Total Cal.	Prot. GMS	Carbs GMS	Sod. MGS	Fiber GMS	Fat GMS	Chol. MGS
DIJON *(Lean Cuisine)* .... 9.5 oz		210	20.0	20.0	590	na	6.0	45
GLAZED *(Le Menu)* 'LightStyle' .... 8.25 oz		260	18.0	34.0	720	(mq)	6.0	35
HOMESTYLE *(Lean Cuisine)* w/vegetables								
and pasta .... 9 3/8 oz		230	21.0	25.0	550	na	5.0	50
MEDALLIONS *(Smart Ones)* roasted,								
w/mushroom sauce .... 8.5 oz		200	13.0	35.0	440	na	1.0	25
PIE								
(Banquet) .... 7 oz		510	16.0	39.0	860	(mq)	31.0	40
(Banquet) 'Supreme Microwave' .... 7 oz		430	15.0	30.0	740	(mq)	27.0	35
(Mrs. Paterson's) w/broccoli 'Aussie Pie' 5.5 oz		460	16.0	42.0	790	na	26.0	95
(Stouffer's) .... 10 oz		410	16.0	3.0	750	na	24.0	na
(Swanson) 'Hungry Man' .... 16 oz		650	24.0	57.0	1470	(mq)	36.0	(mq)
(Swanson) 'Pot Pie' .... 7 oz		380	11.0	36.0	720	(mq)	21.0	(mq)
(Tyson) .... 9 oz		370	13.0	39.0	981	na	18.0	34
ROASTED *(Healthy Choice)* and mushrooms								
in gravy .... 8.5 oz		200	18.0	26.0	380	na	3.0	40
SLICED								
(Banquet) w/gravy 'Cookin' Bags' .... 5 oz		100	7.0	5.0	(mq)	na	6.0	(mq)
(Banquet) w/gravy 'Family Entrees' ...... 8 oz		150	12.0	8.0	(mq)	na	8.0	(mq)
(Freezer Queen) w/dressing and gravy								
'Single Serve' .... 9 oz		230	17.0	32.0	1130	(mq)	5.0	(mq)
(Freezer Queen) w/gravy 'Cook-In-Pouch' 5 oz		70	7.0	6.0	880	na	2.0	(mq)
(Freezer Queen) w/gravy 'Family Suppers' 7 oz		110	9.0	8.0	1160	na	5.0	(mq)
(Right Course) in mild curry sauce,								
w/rice pilaf .... 8.75 oz		320	23.0	40.0	570	(mq)	8.0	50
TETRAZZINI *(Stouffer's)* .... 10 oz		400	22.0	26.0	960	na	23.0	na
W/DRESSING								
(Freezer Queen) w/dressing and gravy								
'Deluxe Family' .... 7 oz		160	12.0	18.0	1130	(mq)	5.0	(mq)
(Tyson) 'Looney Tunes Elmer Fudd' ... 6.55 oz		260	10.0	40.0	510	na	7.0	18
W/DRESSING AND POTATOES								
(Swanson) 'Homestyle Recipe' .... 9 oz		290	18.0	30.0	1010	(mq)	11.0	(mq)
W/GRAVY *(Tyson)* 'Gourmet Selections' .. 9.5 oz		320	19.0	34.0	900	na	12.0	35
W/VEGETABLES *(Healthy Choice)*								
low fat 'Homestyle' .... 9.5 oz		230	24.0	28.0	470	na	3.0	35
WHITE MEAT *(Le Menu)* w/stuffing and								
gravy .... 8 oz		200	19.0	19.0	610	(mq)	5.0	25
TURKEY FAT								
.... 1 cup		1846	0.0	0.0	0	0	204.6	209
.... 1 oz		255	0.0	0.0	0	0	28.3	29
.... 1 tbsp		115	0.0	0.0	0	0	12.8	13
TURKEY GIBLETS								
raw .... 1 oz		37	5.5	0.6	25	0	1.2	80

Food Name	Serv. Size	Total Cal.	Prot. GMS	Carbs GMS	Sod. MGS	Fiber GMS	Fat GMS	Chol. MGS
raw: 1 gizzard, 1 heart, and 1 liver,								
approx 8.6 oz . . . . 1 pkt	315	47.2	5.1	212	0	10.2	688
simmered . . . . 4 oz	189	30.1	2.4	67	0	5.8	474
simmered, chopped or diced . . . . 1 cup	243	38.5	3.0	85	0	7.4	606
simmered, w/giblet fat . . . . 1 cup	242	38.5	3.0	86	0	7.4	606
TURKEY GIZZARD								
raw . . . . 1 oz	33	5.4	0.2	23	0	1.0	45
raw, approx 4 oz . . . . 1 gizzard	132	21.6	0.7	90	0	4.2	179
simmered . . . . 1 cup	236	42.7	0.9	78	0	5.6	336
simmered . . . . 4 oz	185	33.4	0.7	61	0	4.4	263
TURKEY HAM SALAD								
(Longacre) . . . . 1 oz	53	2.0	3.0	190	na	4.0	10
(Longacre) 'Saladfest' . . . . 1 oz	58	2.0	2.0	270	na	4.0	10
TURKEY HEART								
raw . . . . 1 oz	41	5.2	0.2	25	0	2.0	33
raw, approx 1 oz . . . . 1 heart	41	5.2	0.2	25	0	2.0	33
simmered . . . . 1 cup	257	38.8	3.0	80	0	8.9	328
simmered . . . . 4 oz	201	30.3	2.3	62	0	6.9	256
TURKEY LIVER								
raw . . . . 1 oz	39	5.7	1.2	27	0	1.1	132
raw, approx 3.6 oz . . . . 1 liver	140	20.4	4.2	98	0	4.1	475
simmered . . . . 1 cup	237	33.6	4.8	90	0	8.3	876
simmered . . . . 4 oz	192	27.2	3.9	73	0	6.7	710
TURKEY NUGGET								
(Louis Rich) 80% fat-free, breaded,								
cooked . . . . 3/4 oz	60	3.0	3.0	155	na	4.0	10
TURKEY SALAD								
(Longacre) . . . . 1 oz	70	3.0	3.0	200	na	5.0	10
(Longacre) 'Saladfest' . . . . 1 oz	68	3.0	2.0	180	na	5.0	15
TURKEY SEASONING MIX								
(Schilling) roast 'Bag'n Season' . . . . 1 pkg	146	6.0	20.0	1935	na	5.0	na
TURKEY SPREAD								
(Libby's) 'Spreadables' . . . . 1.9 oz	100	5.0	6.0	260	1.9	6.0	15
(Underwood) chunky 'Light' . . . . 2 1/8 oz	75	11.0	2.0	330	na	2.0	25
TURKEY STICK								
(Louis Rich) cooked, breaded,								
80% fat-free . . . . .95 oz	80	4.0	5.0	195	na	5.0	10
(Louis Rich) cooked, prepared . . . . 1 oz	81	4.1	4.8	197	(mq)	5.0	12
(The Turkey Store) breast meat, cheese								
'Gobble Stix' . . . . 1 stick	30	6.0	0.5	na	na	0.8	10
(The Turkey Store) breast meat, smoked								
'Gobble Stix' . . . . 1 stick	25	5.0	0.1	na	na	0.2	10

Food Name	Serv. Size	Total Cal.	Prot. GMS	Carbs GMS	Sod. MGS	Fiber GMS	Fat GMS	Chol. MGS
TURMERIC								
ground	1 oz	100	2.2	18.4	11	>1.9 c	2.8	0
ground	1 tbsp	24	0.5	4.4	3	1.4	0.7	0
ground	1 tsp	8	0.2	1.4	1	.5	0.2	0
ground (Durkee)	1 tsp	9	0.0	0.0	0	0	tr	na
ground (Laurel Leaf)	1 tsp	9	0.0	0.0	0	0	tr	na
ground (Spice Islands)	1 tsp	7	0.2	1.3	<1	>.1 c	0.2	0
TURNIP								
boiled, drained	4 oz	20	0.8	5.6	57	2.3	0.1	0
boiled, drained, cubed	1/2 cup	14	0.6	3.8	39	1.6	0.1	0
boiled, drained, mashed	1/2 cup	21	0.8	5.6	58	2.3	0.1	0
raw, cubed	1/2 cup	18	0.6	4.1	44	1.2	.0.1	0
raw, trimmed	1 oz	8	0.3	1.8	19	.5	<.1	0
raw, untrimmed	1 lb	100	3.3	22.9	248	6.6	0.4	0
Canned								
(Allens) diced	1/2 cup	16	2.0	2.0	25	(mq)	<1.0	0
(Stokely)	1/2 cup	20	2.0	3.0	350	(mq)	0.0	0
Frozen								
boiled, drained	4 oz	26	1.7	4.9	41	>.8 c	0.3	0
mashed	3 1/3 oz	15	1.0	2.8	23	1.7	0.2	0
(Southern) diced	3.5 oz	17	1.0	2.9	50	(mq)	0.2	0
TURNIP GREENS								
boiled, drained	4 oz	23	1.3	4.9	33	3.5	0.3	0
boiled, drained, chopped	1/2 cup	14	0.8	3.1	21	2.2	0.2	0
raw, chopped	1/2 cup	8	0.4	1.6	11	.7	0.1	0
raw, untrimmed	1 lb	85	4.8	18.2	126	7.6	1.0	0
TURNIP GREENS, CANNED								
Chopped								
(Allens)	1/2 cup	21	2.0	3.0	15	(mq)	<1.0	0
(Bush's Best)	1/2 cup	20	2.0	3.0	310	na	0.0	na
W/diced turnips								
(Allens) chopped	1/2 cup	19	2.0	1.0	15	(mq)	<1.0	0
(Bush's Best)	1/2 cup	25	1.0	4.0	370	2.0	0.0	na
(Stokely)	1/2 cup	20	2.0	0.0	340	(mq)	0.0	0
W/liquid	1/2 cup	16	1.6	2.8	324	1.5	0.4	0
TURNIP GREENS, FROZEN								
boiled, drained	10 oz	66	7.4	11.0	33	>2.3 c	0.9	0
boiled, drained	4 oz	34	3.8	5.6	17	>1.2 c	0.5	0
boiled, drained	1/2 cup	25	2.8	4.1	12	>.8 c	0.3	0
chopped	10 oz	62	7.0	10.4	34	6.8	0.9	0
chopped	1/2 cup	18	2.0	3.0	10	2.0	0.3	0
chopped (Frosty Acres)	3.3 oz	20	2.0	4.0	10	>1.0 c	0.0	0
chopped (Seabrook)	3.3 oz	20	2.0	4.0	11	>1.0 c	0.0	0

Food Name	Serv. Size	Total Cal.	Prot. GMS	Carbs GMS	Sod. MGS	Fiber GMS	Fat GMS	Chol. MGS
chopped *(Southern)*	3.5 oz	25	2.5	3.6	70	(mq)	0.3	0
w/turnips	10 oz	60	7.0	9.7	51	6.8	0.5	0
w/turnips *(Seabrook)*	3.3 oz	20	3.0	3.0	na	(mq)	0.0	0
w/turnips, boiled, drained	4 oz	19	2.4	3.3	17	>.6 c	0.2	0

TURNIP-ROOTED PARSLEY. See PARSLEY ROOT.

TURNOVER. See also PASTRY.

Food Name	Serv. Size	Total Cal.	Prot. GMS	Carbs GMS	Sod. MGS	Fiber GMS	Fat GMS	Chol. MGS
apple, frozen *(Pepperidge Farm)*	1 turnover	300	3.0	34.0	210	(mq)	17.0	na
apple, refrigerated *(Pillsbury)*	1 turnover	170	2.0	23.0	320	(mq)	8.0	0
blueberry, frozen *(Pepperidge Farm)*	1 turnover	310	3.0	32.0	230	(mq)	19.0	na
cherry, frozen *(Pepperidge Farm)*	1 turnover	310	3.0	32.0	280	(mq)	19.0	na
cherry, refrigerated *(Pillsbury)*	1 turnover	170	2.0	23.0	320	(mq)	8.0	0
peach, frozen *(Pepperidge Farm)*	1 turnover	310	3.0	34.0	260	(mq)	18.0	na
raspberry, frozen *(Pepperidge Farm)*	1 turnover	310	4.0	36.0	260	(mq)	17.0	na

TURTLE, GREEN

Food Name	Serv. Size	Total Cal.	Prot. GMS	Carbs GMS	Sod. MGS	Fiber GMS	Fat GMS	Chol. MGS
canned	100 gm	106	23.4	0.0	68	0	0.7	50
raw	100 gm	89	19.8	0.0	68	0	0.5	50

TUSK. See CUSK.

U

Food Name	Serv. Size	Total Cal.	Prot. GMS	Carbs GMS	Sod. MGS	Fiber GMS	Fat GMS	Chol. MGS

UDON NOODLE. See NOODLE, JAPANESE.
ULTRA SLIM FAST. See DIET DRINK.
UMEBOSHI PLUM. See PLUM, JAPANESE.

V

Food Name	Serv. Size	Total Cal.	Prot. GMS	Carbs GMS	Sod. MGS	Fiber GMS	Fat GMS	Chol. MGS
VANILLA BAKING CHIPS *(Hershey's)*	1/4 cup	240	3.0	25.0	65	na	14.0	na
VANILLA EXTRACT, pure *(Virginia Dare)*	1 tsp	10	0.0	0.3	0	0	0.0	0

VANILLA FLAVOR DRINK, CANNED

Food Name	Serv. Size	Total Cal.	Prot. GMS	Carbs GMS	Sod. MGS	Fiber GMS	Fat GMS	Chol. MGS
(Ensure) liquid nutrition	8 oz	250	8.8	34.3	200	na	8.8	5
(Ensure) liquid nutrition 'Plus'	8 oz	355	13.0	47.3	250	na	12.6	5
(Ensure) liquid nutrition, w/fiber	8 oz	260	9.4	38.3	200	na	8.8	5
(Sego) 'Lite'	10 oz	150	11.0	17.0	390	na	4.0	5
(Sego) 'Lite French Vanilla'	10 oz	150	11.0	17.0	390	na	4.0	5
(Sego) 'Very Vanilla'	10 oz	225	11.0	34.0	360	na	5.0	5
(Sustacal) liquid food, nutritionally complete	8 oz	240	14.5	33.0	220	na	5.5	na

Food Name	Serv. Size	Total Cal.	Prot. GMS	Carbs GMS	Sod. MGS	Fiber GMS	Fat GMS	Chol. MGS
VEAL								

(NOTE: TRIMMED = Lean; separable fat removed. UNTRIMMED = Separable fat not removed.)

BRAINS

Food Name	Serv. Size	Total Cal.	Prot. GMS	Carbs GMS	Sod. MGS	Fiber GMS	Fat GMS	Chol. MGS
braised	3 oz	116	9.8	0.0	133	0	8.2	2635
pan-fried	3 oz	181	12.3	0.0	150	0	14.2	1802
raw	1 oz	33	2.9	0.0	36	na	2.3	445
GROUND								
broiled	1 cup	200	28.3	0.0	96	0	8.8	119
broiled	3 oz	146	20.7	0.0	71	na	6.4	88
raw	1 cup	325	43.7	0.0	185	0	15.3	185
raw	1 oz	40	5.4	0.0	23	na	1.9	23
HEART								
braised	3 oz	158	24.7	0.1	49	0	5.7	150
raw	1 oz	31	4.8	0.0	22	0	1.1	29
simmered	4 oz	368	57.7	0.3	116	0	13.4	349
KIDNEYS								
braised	3 oz	139	22.4	0.0	94	na	4.8	672
raw	1 oz	28	4.4	0.2	50	na	0.9	102
LEG								
Trimmed								
braised	3 oz	173	31.2	0.0	57	0	4.3	115
pan-fried	3 oz	156	28.2	0.0	65	0	3.9	91
raw	1 oz	30	6.0	0.0	18	0	0.5	22
roasted	3 oz	127	23.9	0.0	58	0	2.9	88
Untrimmed								
braised	3 oz	179	30.7	0.0	57	0	5.4	114
pan-fried	3 oz	179	27.0	0.0	65	0	7.1	89
raw	1 oz	33	5.9	0.0	18	0	0.9	22
roasted	3 oz	136	23.5	0.0	58	0	4.0	88
LEG AND SHOULDER								
raw, trimmed	1 oz	31	5.7	0.0	23	0	0.7	24
trimmed, braised	3 oz	160	29.7	0.0	79	0	3.7	123
LIVER								
braised	3 oz	140	18.4	2.3	45	na	5.9	477
pan-fried	3 oz	208	25.3	3.3	112	na	9.7	281
raw	4 oz	152	20.3	5.2	70	na	5.0	350
raw	1 oz	38	5.0	1.3	17	na	1.2	87
LOIN								
Trimmed								
braised	3 oz	192	28.5	0.0	71	0	7.8	106
raw	1 oz	32	5.7	0.0	25	0	0.9	22
roasted	3 oz	149	22.4	0.0	82	0	5.9	90
stewed	4 oz	256	38.1	0.0	95	0	10.4	142

Food Name	Serv. Size	Total Cal.	Prot. GMS	Carbs GMS	Sod. MGS	Fiber GMS	Fat GMS	Chol. MGS
Untrimmed
braised	3 oz	241	25.7	0.0	68	0	14.6	100
raw	1 oz	46	5.3	0.0	24	0	2.6	22
roasted	3 oz	184	21.1	0.0	79	0	10.5	88
stewed	4 oz	322	34.2	0.0	91	0	19.5	134
LUNGS
braised	3 oz	88	15.9	0.0	48	0	2.2	224
raw	1 oz	25	4.6	0.0	30	0	0.6	64
PANCREAS
braised	3 oz	218	24.7	0.0	58	0	12.4	na
raw	1 oz	51	4.2	0.0	19	0	3.7	48
RIB
Trimmed
braised	3 oz	185	29.3	0.0	84	0	6.6	122
raw	1 lb	544	90.6	0.0	431	0	17.6	376
raw	1 oz	34	5.6	0.0	27	0	1.1	23
roasted	3 oz	150	21.9	0.0	82	0	6.3	98
stewed	4 oz	247	39.1	0.0	112	0	8.9	163
Untrimmed
braised	3 oz	213	27.6	0.0	81	0	10.6	118
raw	1 lb	735	85.6	0.0	404	0	40.9	372
raw	1 oz	45	5.3	0.0	25	0	2.5	23
roasted	3 oz	194	20.4	0.0	78	0	11.9	94
stewed	4 oz	285	36.8	0.0	108	0	14.2	158
SHOULDER, ARM
Trimmed
braised	3 oz	171	30.4	0.0	77	0	4.5	132
braised, approx 5.6 oz	1 steak	321	57.1	0.0	143	0	8.5	248
raw	1 oz	29	5.6	0.0	24	0	0.6	23
roasted	3 oz	139	22.2	0.0	77	0	4.9	93
roasted, approx 9.6 oz	1 steak	447	71.2	0.0	248	0	15.8	298
Untrimmed
braised	3 oz	201	28.6	0.0	74	0	8.7	126
braised, approx 6.1 oz	1 steak	409	58.2	0.0	151	0	17.7	257
raw	1 oz	37	5.4	0.0	23	0	1.5	23
roasted	3 oz	156	21.6	0.0	77	0	7.0	92
SHOULDER, BLADE
Trimmed
braised	3 oz	168	27.8	0.0	86	0	5.5	134
diced, braised	1 cup	277	45.7	0.0	141	0	9.1	221
diced, roasted	1 cup	239	35.9	0.0	143	0	9.6	167
diced, stewed	1 cup	277	45.7	0.0	141	0	9.1	221
raw	1 lb	513	89.1	0.0	440	0	14.8	408

Food Name	Serv. Size	Total Cal.	Prot. GMS	Carbs GMS	Sod. MGS	Fiber GMS	Fat GMS	Chol. MGS
raw	1 oz	32	5.5	0.0	27	0	0.9	25
roasted	3 oz	145	21.8	0.0	87	0	5.8	101
stewed	4 oz	224	37.0	0.0	115	0	7.3	179
Untrimmed								
braised	3 oz	191	26.6	0.0	83	0	8.6	130
diced, braised	1 cup	315	43.8	0.0	137	0	14.1	214
diced, roasted	1 cup	260	35.2	0.0	140	0	12.1	164
diced, stewed	1 cup	315	43.8	0.0	137	0	14.1	214
raw	1 lb	585	87.2	0.0	431	0	23.6	408
raw	1 oz	36	5.4	0.0	27	0	1.5	25
roasted	3 oz	158	21.4	0.0	85	0	7.4	99
stewed	4 oz	255	35.4	0.0	111	0	11.4	174
SHOULDER, WHOLE								
Trimmed								
braised	3 oz	169	28.6	0.0	82	0	5.2	110
diced, braised	1 cup	279	47.2	0.0	136	0	8.5	182
diced, roasted	1 cup	238	36.1	0.0	136	0	9.3	160
diced, stewed	1 cup	279	47.2	0.0	136	0	8.5	182
raw	1 lb	508	89.8	0.0	417	0	13.6	390
raw	1 oz	31	5.5	0.0	26	0	0.8	24
roasted	3 oz	144	21.9	0.0	82	0	5.6	97
stewed	4 oz	226	38.2	0.0	110	0	6.9	147
Untrimmed								
braised	3 oz	194	27.2	0.0	81	0	8.6	107
diced, braised	1 cup	319	44.9	0.0	133	0	14.2	176
diced, roasted	1 cup	258	35.4	0.0	134	0	11.8	158
diced, stewed	1 cup	319	44.9	0.0	133	0	14.2	176
raw	1 lb	590	87.4	0.0	413	0	24.0	395
raw	1 oz	36	5.4	0.0	25	0	1.5	24
roasted	3 oz	156	21.5	0.0	82	0	7.2	96
stewed	4 oz	259	36.4	0.0	108	0	11.5	143
SIRLOIN								
Trimmed								
braised	3 oz	173	28.9	0.0	69	0	5.5	96
diced, braised	1 cup	286	47.5	0.0	113	0	9.1	158
diced, roasted	1 cup	235	36.8	0.0	119	0	8.7	146
diced, stewed	1 cup	286	47.5	0.0	113	0	9.1	158
raw	1 lb	499	91.6	0.0	363	0	11.7	358
raw	1 oz	31	5.7	0.0	22	0	0.7	22
roasted	3 oz	143	22.4	0.0	72	0	5.3	88
stewed	4 oz	231	38.5	0.0	92	0	7.4	128
Untrimmed								
braised	3 oz	214	26.6	0.0	67	0	11.2	92

Food Name	Serv. Size	Total Cal.	Prot. GMS	Carbs GMS	Sod. MGS	Fiber GMS	Fat GMS	Chol. MGS
diced, braised	1 cup	353	43.8	0.0	111	0	18.4	151
diced, roasted	1 cup	283	35.2	0.0	116	0	14.6	143
diced, stewed	1 cup	353	43.8	0.0	111	0	18.4	151
raw	1 lb	689	86.5	0.0	345	0	35.4	354
raw	1 oz	43	5.3	0.0	21	0	2.2	22
roasted	3 oz	172	21.4	0.0	71	0	8.9	87
stewed	4 oz	286	35.4	0.0	90	0	14.9	122
SPLEEN								
braised	3 oz	110	20.5	0.0	49	0	2.5	380
raw	1 oz	27	5.1	0.0	27	0	0.6	95
THYMUS								
braised	3 oz	148	26.8	0.0	56	0	3.7	399
raw	1 oz	28	5.0	0.0	23	0	0.7	75
TONGUE								
braised	3 oz	172	22.0	0.0	54	0	8.6	202
raw	1 oz	37	4.8	0.5	23	0	1.5	17
TOP ROUND								
Trimmed								
braised	4 oz	230	41.6	0.0	76	0	5.8	159
diced, braised	1 cup	284	51.4	0.0	94	0	7.1	189
diced, roasted	1 cup	210	39.3	0.0	95	0	4.7	144
diced, stewed	1 cup	284	51.4	0.0	94	0	7.1	189
pan-fried in vegetable oil	4 oz	208	37.6	0.0	87	0	5.2	121
roasted	4 oz	170	31.8	0.0	77	0	3.8	177
stewed	4 oz	230	41.6	0.0	76	0	5.8	159
Untrimmed								
diced, roasted	1 cup	224	38.8	0.0	95	0	6.5	144
diced, stewed	1 cup	295	50.6	0.0	94	0	8.9	188
pan-fried in vegetable oil	4 oz	239	36.0	0.0	86	0	9.5	119
roasted	4 oz	181	31.4	0.0	77	0	5.3	117
stewed	4 oz	239	41.0	0.0	76	0	7.2	152
VEAL ENTRÉE, FROZEN								
MARSALA (Le Menu) 'LightStyle'	10 oz	230	22.0	28.0	700	(mq)	3.0	75
PARMIGIANA								
(Armour) 'Classics'	11.25 oz	400	18.0	34.0	1320	(mq)	22.0	55
(Le Menu)	11.5 oz	390	24.0	36.0	840	(mq)	17.0	(mq)
(Morton)	10 oz	260	10.0	35.0	1510	(mq)	8.0	35
(Swanson)	12.25 oz	430	20.0	42.0	1010	(mq)	20.0	(mq)
(Swanson) 'Homestyle Recipe'	10 oz	330	19.0	33.0	960	(mq)	13.0	(mq)
(Swanson) 'Hungry Man'	18.25 oz	590	32.0	57.0	1840	(mq)	26.0	(mq)
(Ultimate 200)	8.2 oz	150	22.0	5.0	550	na	4.0	50
Breaded								
(Banquet) 'Cookin' Bags'	4 oz	230	10.0	20.0	(mq)	(mq)	11.0	(mq)

Food Name	Serv. Size	Total Cal.	Prot. GMS	Carbs GMS	Sod. MGS	Fiber GMS	Fat GMS	Chol. MGS
(Banquet) 'Family Entrées'	8 oz	370	18.0	33.0	(mq)	(mq)	18.0	(mq)
(Freezer Queen)	5 oz	220	11.0	17.0	560	(mq)	12.0	(mq)
(Freezer Queen) 'Cook-In-Pouch'	5 oz	220	11.0	17.0	560	(mq)	12.0	(mq)
(Freezer Queen) 'Deluxe Family Suppers'	7 oz	300	17.0	22.0	820	(mq)	15.0	(mq)
Platter *(Freezer Queen)*	10 oz	400	22.0	32.0	870	(mq)	20.0	(mq)
W/pasta Alfredo *(Stouffer's)* homestyle	9.25 oz	350	28.0	26.0	1060	na	15.0	na
STEAK								
(Hormel)	4 oz	130	22.0	2.0	(mq)	na	4.0	(mq)
(Hormel) breaded	4 oz	240	17.0	13.0	(mq)	(mq)	13.0	(mq)
VEGETABLE. See individual listings.								
VEGETABLE DISH, CANNED. See also individual listings.								
Corn, beans, and carrots, w/pasta, in tomato sauce *(Green Giant)*	1/2 cup	80	2.0	17.0	330	3.0	2.0	0
Green beans, potatoes, and mushrooms, in sauce *(Green Giant)*	1/2 cup	50	1.0	9.0	430	2.0	2.0	0
Snap beans, potatoes, and mushrooms, in sauce *(Green Giant)*	1/2 cup	50	1.0	9.0	430	2.0	2.0	0
String beans, potatoes, and mushrooms, in sauce *(Green Giant)*	1/2 cup	50	1.0	9.0	430	2.0	2.0	0
VEGETABLE DISH, FROZEN. See also individual listings.								
Broccoli, cauliflower, carrots								
(Birds Eye) 'Butter Sauce'	3.3 oz	45	2.0	6.0	290	2.0	2.0	5
(Birds Eye) 'Cheese Sauce'	4.5 oz	110	5.0	11.0	410	2.0	5.0	5
(Birds Eye) 'Farm Fresh'	4 oz	35	2.0	7.0	40	3.0	0.0	0
(Green Giant) 'Butter Sauce'	1/2 cup	30	2.0	4.0	240	3.0	1.0	5
(Green Giant) in cheese sauce	1/2 cup	60	3.0	9.0	490	2.0	2.0	2
(Green Giant) 'One Serving'	1 pkg	30	3.0	7.0	40	3.0	0.0	0
(Stokely) 'Singles' w/baby carrots	3 oz	25	2.0	5.0	25	(mq)	1.0	0
(Stokely) w/baby carrots, in cheese sauce	4 oz	70	4.0	8.0	180	(mq)	3.0	15
Broccoli, cauliflower, peppers, w/red peppers 'Farm Fresh' *(Birds Eye)*	4 oz	30	3.0	5.0	25	3.0	0.0	0
Broccoli, corn, peppers, w/red peppers 'Farm Fresh' *(Birds Eye)*	4 oz	60	3.0	14.0	15	3.0	1.0	0
Broccoli, green beans, onions, peppers, w/pearl onions and red peppers *(Birds Eye)*	4 oz	35	2.0	7.0	15	3.0	0.0	0
Broccoli, peppers, bamboo shoots, mushrooms, w/red peppers *(Birds Eye)*	4 oz	30	3.0	5.0	20	3.0	0.0	0
Broccoli and carrots, w/rotini, in cheese sauce *(Green Giant)*	1 pkg	100	5.0	17.0	440	3.0	2.0	5
Brussels sprouts, cauliflower, carrots *(Birds Eye)*	4 oz	40	3.0	8.0	30	4.0	0.0	0
Cauliflower, broccoli, carrots, in cheese sauce *(Freezer Queen)*	5 oz	60	2.0	10.0	360	(mq)	1.0	na

Food Name	Serv. Size	Total Cal.	Prot. GMS	Carbs GMS	Sod. MGS	Fiber GMS	Fat GMS	Chol. MGS
Cauliflower, carrots, snow peas, w/baby carrots and snow pea pods *(Birds Eye)*	4 oz	40	2.0	8.0	35	3.0	0.0	0
Cauliflower, zucchini, carrots, peppers, w/red peppers *(Birds Eye)*	4 oz	30	2.0	6.0	25	2.0	0.0	0
Peas, carrots, water chestnuts, w/sugar snap peas and baby carrots *(Birds Eye)*	3.2 oz	50	2.0	11.0	20	4.0	0.0	0
Zucchini, carrots, onions, mushrooms, w/pearl onions *(Birds Eye)*	4 oz	30	1.0	7.0	15	1.0	0.0	0
VEGETABLE ENTRÉE								
Chinese style, w/chicken, frozen								
(Budget Gourmet)	10 oz	280	11.0	47.0	590	na	7.0	10
Country style, w/beef tips *(Ultra Slim Fast)*	12 oz	230	21.0	26.0	960	na	5.0	45
Italian style, w/chicken, frozen								
(Budget Gourmet)	10.25 oz	310	14.0	50.0	690	na	8.0	30
Pot pie, frozen								
(Amy's Kitchen) organic	8 oz	347	9.0	45.0	260	3.0	16.0	na
(Morton) w/beef	7 oz	430	11.0	27.0	740	(mq)	31.0	30
(Morton) w/chicken	7 oz	420	14.0	27.0	740	(mq)	28.0	35
(Morton) w/turkey	7 oz	420	14.0	27.0	740	(mq)	28.0	40
Stir-fry, frozen *(Shanghai)*	5.1 oz	75	6.0	11.0	510	na	1.0	0
VEGETABLE FLAKES *(French's)*								
dehydrated	1 tbsp	12	0.0	3.0	20	(mq)	0.0	0
VEGETABLE JUICE								
cocktail, canned	6 oz	35	1.1	8.3	664	1.5	0.2	0
cocktail, canned	1/2 cup	23	0.8	5.5	442	1.0	0.1	0
(Biotta) 'Breuss Juice'	6 oz	67	1.9	13.2	147	(mq)	0.1	0
(Biotta) 'Cocktail'	6 oz	50	1.7	10.1	497	(mq)	0.1	0
(Knudsen & Sons) 'Very Veggie'	8 oz	40	<1.0	8.0	na	na	0.0	na
(Knudsen & Sons) 'Very Veggie' low sodium	8 oz	40	2.0	8.0	32	na	0.0	na
(Knudsen & Sons) 'Very Veggie' organic	8 oz	40	2.0	8.0	na	na	0.0	na
(Knudsen & Sons) 'Very Veggie' spicy	8 oz	40	2.0	8.0	560	na	0.0	na
(Smucker's) hearty	8 oz	58	0.6	13.0	714	(mq)	<.1	0
(Smucker's) hot and spicy	8 oz	58	0.6	13.0	650	(mq)	<.1	0
(V•8)	6 oz	35	1.0	8.0	560	(mq)	0.0	0
(V•8) 'Light'n Tangy'	6 oz	40	1.0	8.0	240	na	0.0	0
(V•8) 'No Salt Added'	6 oz	35	1.0	8.0	45	(mq)	0.0	0
(V•8) 'Picante' mild	6 oz	35	1.0	8.0	520	na	0.0	0
(V•8) spicy hot	6 oz	35	1.0	8.0	650	(mq)	0.0	0
(Veryfine) '100%'	6 oz	32	1.6	6.0	600	(mq)	0.0	0
VEGETABLE MARROW SQUASH. See SQUASH, MARROW.								
VEGETABLE OIL. See also individual listings.								
(Crisco)	1 tbsp	120	0.0	0.0	0	0	14.0	0
(Finast)	1 tbsp	120	0.0	0.0	0	0	14.0	0

Food Name	Serv. Size	Total Cal.	Prot. GMS	Carbs GMS	Sod. MGS	Fiber GMS	Fat GMS	Chol. MGS
(Hain) 'All Blend'	1 tbsp	120	0.0	0.0	0	0	14.0	0
(Hain) w/garlic 'Garlic & Oil'	1 tbsp	120	0.0	0.0	0	0	14.0	0
(Kroger)	1 tbsp	122	0.0	0.0	0	0	13.6	0
(Pathmark)	1 tbsp	120	0.0	0.0	0	0	14.0	0
(Pathmark) 'No Frills'	1 tbsp	130	0.0	0.0	0	0	14.0	0
(Puritan)	1 tbsp	120	0.0	0.0	0	0	14.0	0
(Wesson)	1 tbsp	120	0.0	0.0	0	0	14.0	0

VEGETABLE OIL SPRAY. See COOKING SPRAY.

VEGETABLE OIL SPREAD. See MARGARINE SPREAD.

VEGETABLE OYSTER. See SALSIFY.

VEGETABLE SPONGE. See GOURD, DISHCLOTH.

VEGETABLE STICKS, breaded, frozen

Food Name	Serv. Size	Total Cal.	Prot. GMS	Carbs GMS	Sod. MGS	Fiber GMS	Fat GMS	Chol. MGS
(Farm Rich)	4 oz	240	4.0	34.0	980	(mq)	10.0	na

VEGETABLES, MIXED, CANNED

Food Name	Serv. Size	Total Cal.	Prot. GMS	Carbs GMS	Sod. MGS	Fiber GMS	Fat GMS	Chol. MGS
drained	4 oz	53	2.9	10.5	169	2.7	0.3	0
drained	1/2 cup	39	2.1	7.6	122	>1.1 c	0.2	0
w/liquid	4 oz	41	1.6	8.1	254	>1.3 c	0.3	0
w/liquid	1/2 cup	40	2.0	7.0	355	(mq)	0.0	0
(A&P) 'Eastern'	1/2 cup	45	2.0	8.0	330	(mq)	<1.0	0
(A&P) 'No Salt Added'	1/2 cup	40	1.0	9.0	20	(mq)	<1.0	0
(A&P) 'Western'	1/2 cup	40	1.0	9.0	380	(mq)	<1.0	0
(Bush's Best) 'Mixed Greens'	1/2 cup	20	2.0	3.0	300	na	0.0	na
(Featherweight)	1/2 cup	40	2.0	8.0	25	(mq)	0.0	0
(Finast)	1/2 cup	40	1.0	8.0	390	(mq)	0.0	0
(Finast) 'No Salt Added'	1/2 cup	40	2.0	8.0	25	(mq)	0.0	0
(Freshlike) water packed, w/o salt	1/2 cup	35	2.0	8.0	25	na	0.0	na
(Freshlike) water packed, w/o sugar or salt	1/2 cup	35	2.0	8.0	25	na	0.0	na
(Green Giant) 'Garden Medley'	1/2 cup	35	1.0	9.0	350	1.0	0.0	0
(Green Giant) 'Pantry Express'	1/2 cup	35	1.0	8.0	300	1.0	<1.0	0
(LaChoy) 'Chinese'	1/2 cup	12	1.0	2.0	30	1.1	0.1	0
(LaChoy) 'Chop Suey'	1/2 cup	9	0.7	2.0	330	1.0	0.1	0
(LaChoy) 'Fancy Mix'	1/2 cup	12	1.0	2.0	30	1.0	<1.0	0
(P&Q) 'Chunky Eastern'	1/2 cup	40	2.0	8.0	330	(mq)	<1.0	0
(P&Q) 'Chunky Western'	1/2 cup	40	1.0	9.0	380	(mq)	<1.0	0
(Pathmark)	1/2 cup	35	2.0	8.0	320	(mq)	0.0	0
(Pathmark) 'No Salt Added'	1/2 cup	35	2.0	7.0	25	(mq)	0.0	0
(S&W) 'Old Fashioned Harvest'	1/2 cup	35	1.0	6.0	380	(mq)	0.0	0
(Stokely)	1/2 cup	40	2.0	8.0	300	(mq)	0.0	0
(Stokely) 'No Salt or Sugar Added'	1/2 cup	40	2.0	8.0	25	(mq)	0.0	0
(Veg•All) 'Homestyle Large Cut'	1/2 cup	35	2.0	9.0	380	na	0.0	na
(Veg•All) 'Lite'	1/2 cup	35	2.0	8.0	25	na	0.0	na
(Veg•All) 'Original'	1/2 cup	35	2.0	8.0	320	na	0.0	na

Food Name	Serv. Size	Total Cal.	Prot. GMS	Carbs GMS	Sod. MGS	Fiber GMS	Fat GMS	Chol. MGS
VEGETABLES, MIXED, FROZEN								
boiled, drained	10-oz pkg	162	7.9	36.0	96	10.5	0.4	0
boiled, drained	4 oz	67	3.2	14.8	40	4.3	0.2	0
boiled, drained	1/2 cup	54	2.6	11.9	32	3.5	0.1	0
(A&P)	3.3 oz	65	3.0	13.0	55	(mq)	<1.0	0
(Birds Eye)	3.3 oz	60	3.0	13.0	40	2.0	0.0	0
(Birds Eye) 'Portion Pack'	3 oz	50	2.0	12.0	35	2.0	0.0	0
(Freshlike)	3.3 oz	70	3.0	13.0	45	na	0.0	na
(Frosty Acres)	3.3 oz	65	3.0	13.0	50	>1.0 c	0.0	0
(Green Giant)	1/2 cup	40	2.0	9.0	40	2.0	0.0	0
(Green Giant) 'Harvest Fresh'	1/2 cup	40	2.0	9.0	125	2.0	0.0	0
(Green Giant) 'Plain Polybag'	1/2 cup	40	2.0	9.0	40	2.0	0.0	0
(Health Valley)	1/2 cup	68	3.0	14.0	39	1.9	0.0	0
(Seabrook)	3.3 oz	65	3.0	13.0	50	>1.0 c	0.0	0
(Southern)	3.5 oz	69	3.2	13.9	60	(mq)	0.0	0
(Stokely) 'Singles'	3 oz	60	2.0	12.0	40	(mq)	1.0	0
(Veg•All)	3.3 oz	70	3.0	13.0	45	na	0.0	na
CALIFORNIA STYLE								
(A&P) 'California Blend'	3.3 oz	25	2.0	5.0	25	(mq)	<1.0	0
(Freshlike) 'California Blend'	3.3 oz	30	2.0	6.0	20	na	0.0	na
(Green Giant) 'American Mixtures'	1/2 cup	25	2.0	6.0	40	2.0	0.0	0
(Veg•All) 'California Blend'	3.3 oz	30	2.0	6.0	20	na	0.0	na
CHINESE STYLE								
(Birds Eye) chow mein, w/Oriental sauce 'Custom Cuisine'	4.6 oz	80	3.0	14.0	570	1.0	2.0	0
(Birds Eye) chow mein, w/seasoned sauce	3.3 oz	90	2.0	12.0	370	1.0	4.0	0
(Birds Eye) 'Stir-Fry'	3.3 oz	35	2.0	8.0	540	2.0	0.0	0
CHUCKWAGON STYLE								
(Freshlike) 'Chuckwagon Blend'	3.3 oz	70	2.0	16.0	5	na	1.0	na
(Veg•All) 'Chuckwagon Blend'	3.3 oz	70	2.0	16.0	5	na	1.0	na
COUNTRY STYLE								
(Birds Eye) 'International Rice Recipes'	3.3 oz	90	2.0	19.0	380	1.0	0.0	0
(Freshlike) 'Country Blend'	3.3 oz	50	2.0	12.0	15	na	0.0	na
(Green Giant) 'American Mixtures Heartland'	1/2 cup	25	1.0	6.0	35	2.0	0.0	0
(Veg•All) 'Country Blend'	3.3 oz	50	2.0	12.0	15	na	0.0	na
DUTCH STYLE (Frosty Acres)	3.2 oz	30	2.0	5.0	30	(mq)	0.0	0
FOR BEEF								
(Birds Eye) Oriental style, w/sauce	4.6 oz	90	6.0	11.0	350	2.0	4.0	0
(Birds Eye) w/cream mushroom 'Custom Cuisine'	4.6 oz	60	3.0	9.0	450	2.0	2.0	5

Food Name	Serv. Size	Total Cal.	Prot. GMS	Carbs GMS	Sod. MGS	Fiber GMS	Fat GMS	Chol. MGS
FOR CHICKEN								
(Birds Eye) w/tomato basil sauce	4.6 oz	110	5.0	17.0	360	1.0	3.0	0
(Birds Eye) w/wild rice, in white wine sauce	4.6 oz	100	3.0	19.0	510	1.0	0.0	0
FOR CHICKEN OR FISH (Birds Eye)								
w/Dijon mustard sauce	4.6 oz	70	4.0	9.0	310	1.0	3.0	5
FOR CHICKEN OR SHRIMP (Birds Eye)								
w/delicate herb sauce	4.6 oz	90	3.0	8.0	460	2.0	5.0	0
FOR SOUP								
(Freshlike)	3.3 oz	50	2.0	11.0	40	na	0.0	na
(Veg•All)	3.3 oz	50	2.0	11.0	40	na	0.0	na
FOR STEW								
(A&P)	4 oz	60	1.0	13.0	30	(mq)	<1.0	0
(Freshlike) 5-ways	3.3 oz	50	1.0	12.0	40	na	0.0	na
(Freshlike) 4-ways	3.3 oz	50	1.0	11.0	40	na	0.0	na
(Frosty Acres)	3 oz	42	3.0	10.0	21	(mq)	0.0	0
(Kohl's)	3.3 oz	50	1.0	10.0	30	(mq)	<1.0	0
(Ore-Ida)	3 oz	60	1.0	12.0	40	(mq)	<1.0	0
(Veg•All) 5-ways	3.3 oz	50	1.0	12.0	40	na	0.0	na
(Veg•All) 4-ways	3.3 oz	50	1.0	11.0	40	na	0.0	na
FRENCH STYLE (Birds Eye)								
'International Recipes'	3.3 oz	110	3.0	23.0	610	na	0.0	0
IN BUTTER SAUCE								
(Finast)	3.3 oz	70	4.0	15.0	340	(mq)	4.0	na
(Green Giant)	1/2 cup	60	2.0	11.0	300	2.0	2.0	5
ITALIAN STYLE								
(A&P) blend	3.3 oz	40	2.0	8.0	35	(mq)	<1.0	0
(Birds Eye) 'International Recipes'	3.3 oz	100	2.0	11.0	490	2.0	5.0	0
(Freshlike) 'Italian Blend'	3.3 oz	30	2.0	7.0	20	na	0.0	na
(Freshlike) 'Italian Blend' food service	3.3 oz	25	1.0	5.0	20	na	0.0	na
(Veg•All) 'Italian Blend'	3.3 oz	30	2.0	7.0	20	na	0.0	na
(Veg•All) 'Italian Blend' food service	3.3 oz	25	1.0	5.0	20	na	0.0	na
JAPANESE STYLE								
(Birds Eye) 'International Recipes'	3.3 oz	90	2.0	10.0	420	2.0	5.0	0
(Birds Eye) 'Stir-Fry'	3.3 oz	30	2.0	7.0	510	2.0	0.0	0
LE SUEUR STYLE (Green Giant)								
'Valley Combinations'	1/2 cup	70	4.0	12.0	400	2.0	2.0	0
MANHATTAN STYLE (Green Giant)								
'American Mixtures'	1/2 cup	25	2.0	5.0	15	2.0	0.0	0
MIDWESTERN STYLE								
(Freshlike) 'Midwestern Blend'	3.3 oz	40	2.0	8.0	30	na	0.0	na
(Veg•All) 'Midwestern Blend'	3.3 oz	40	2.0	8.0	30	na	0.0	na

Food Name	Serv. Size	Total Cal.	Prot. GMS	Carbs GMS	Sod. MGS	Fiber GMS	Fat GMS	Chol. MGS
NEW ENGLAND STYLE								
(Birds Eye) 'International Recipes'	3.3 oz	130	3.0	14.0	430	2.0	7.0	0
(Green Giant) 'American Mixtures'	1/2 cup	70	3.0	14.0	75	4.0	1.0	0
ORIENTAL STYLE								
(A&P) blend	3.3 oz	25	2.0	5.0	15	(mq)	<1.0	0
(Birds Eye) 'International Recipes'	3.3 oz	70	2.0	8.0	300	1.0	4.0	0
(Freshlike) 'Oriental Blend'	3.3 oz	25	3.0	5.0	10	na	0.0	na
(Frosty Acres)	3.2 oz	25	2.0	5.0	15	(mq)	0.0	0
(Veg•All) 'Oriental Blend'	3.3 oz	25	3.0	5.0	10	na	0.0	na
SAN FRANCISCO STYLE								
(Birds Eye) 'International Recipes'	3.3 oz	100	2.0	11.0	400	1.0	5.0	0
(Green Giant) 'American Mixtures'	1/2 cup	25	1.0	7.0	35	2.0	0.0	0
SANTA FE STYLE (Green Giant)								
'American Mixtures'	1/2 cup	70	2.0	16.0	0	2.0	1.0	0
SCANDINAVIAN STYLE								
(Freshlike) 'Scandinavian Blend'	3.3 oz	45	2.0	9.0	30	na	0.0	na
(Veg•All) 'Scandinavian Blend'	3.3 oz	45	2.0	9.0	30	na	0.0	na
SEATTLE STYLE (Green Giant)								
'American Mixtures'	1/2 cup	25	2.0	7.0	35	2.0	0.0	0
SPANISH STYLE (Birds Eye)								
'International Recipes'	3.3 oz	110	3.0	24.0	540	na	0.0	0
WESTERN STYLE (Green Giant)								
'American Mixtures'	1/2 cup	60	2.0	12.0	25	2.0	2.0	0
WINTER VEGETABLES								
(A&P) blend	3.3 oz	24	2.0	6.0	190	(mq)	<1.0	0
(Freshlike) 'Winter Blend'	3.3 oz	25	3.0	5.0	25	na	0.0	na
(Veg•All) 'Winter Blend'	3.3 oz	25	3.0	5.0	25	na	0.0	na
W/PASTA								
(Birds Eye) cheese tortellini, in tomato sauce 'For One'	5.5 oz	210	11.0	31.0	500	0	5.0	30
(Birds Eye) in Stroganoff sauce 'Custom Cuisine'	4.6 oz	120	5.0	15.0	700	0	5.0	30
(Birds Eye) in white cheese sauce 'Custom Cuisine'	4.6 oz	150	7.0	19.0	440	1.0	6.0	15
(Birds Eye) primavera style, w/seasoned sauce	3.3 oz	120	5.0	14.0	340	2.0	5.0	5
(Stokely) rotini, in cheddar cheese sauce 'Singles'	4 oz	100	4.0	15.0	380	(mq)	3.0	10
(Stokely) shells, in Italian style sauce 'Singles'	4 oz	170	3.0	5.0	270	(mq)	15.0	5
W/TERIYAKI SAUCE (Stokely) 'Singles'	4 oz	100	3.0	24.0	580	(mq)	0.0	0
W/WHITE AND WILD RICE, pilaf (Stokely) 'Singles'	4 oz	80	3.0	17.0	290	(mq)	0.0	5

Food Name	Serv. Size	Total Cal.	Prot. GMS	Carbs GMS	Sod. MGS	Fiber GMS	Fat GMS	Chol. MGS
VEGETABLES, MIXED, MICROWAVE								
(Green Giant) 'Microwave Shelf-Pack'	1/2 cup	35	1.0	8.0	300	1.0	<1.0	0
(Pantry Express) 'Microwave Shelf-Pack'	1/2 cup	35	1.0	8.0	300	1.0	<1.0	0
VEGETARIAN ENTRÉE. See also individual listings.								
(Amy's Kitchen) Salisbury steak, organic, frozen 'Country Dinner'	11 oz	482	12.0	48.0	760	4.0	19.0	32
(Ken & Robert's) patty, frozen 'Truly Amazing'	2.5-oz patty	110	5.0	19.0	390	na	2.0	0
(LaChoy) chow mein, w/o meat, canned	3/4 cup	35	2.0	6.0	820	2.2	0.4	0
(Natural Touch) patty, frozen 'Dinner Entree'	3 oz	230	20.0	6.0	300	(mq)	14.0	0
(Tofutti) tortellini, meatless, frozen	2 oz	220	12.0	38.0	110	(mq)	2.0	0
(Worthington) roast, frozen 'Dinner Roast'	2 oz	120	7.0	5.0	440	(mq)	8.0	0
VEGETARIAN ENTRÉE MIX. See also individual listings.								
(Tofu Classics) stroganoff, creamy, prepared w/tofu	1/2 cup	94	7.0	11.0	264	(mq)	3.0	0
(Tofu Classics) stroganoff, creamy, prepared w/tofu and salted butter	1/2 cup	127	7.0	11.0	310	(mq)	7.0	(mq)
VEGETARIAN FOODS. See BACON, ALTERNATIVE; BEEF, ALTERNATIVE; BEEF JERKY, ALTERNATIVE; BURGER, ALTERNATIVE; BURGER MIX, VEGETARIAN; CHICKEN, ALTERNATIVE; CRAB, ALTERNATIVE; FISH FILLET, ALTERNATIVE; HAM, ALTERNATIVE; LUNCHEON MEAT, ALTERNATIVE; MEAT, ALTERNATIVE; MEAT LOAF MIX, ALTERNATIVE; SAUSAGE, ALTERNATIVE; SCALLOP, ALTERNATIVE; SPREAD, VEGETARIAN; TUNA, ALTERNATIVE; TURKEY, ALTERNATIVE VEGETARIAN ENTRÉE; and individual listings.								
VENISON. See DEER; MOOSE.								
VIENNA SAUSAGE, CANNED								
beef and pork	1 oz	79	2.9	0.6	270	0	7.1	15
2 inches long, 7/8 inch diam	1 sausage	45	1.6	0.3	152	0	4.0	8
(Armour) chicken, in beef stock 'Premium' lite	2 oz	150	6.0	1.0	400	na	13.0	na
(Armour) hot and spicy	2.5 oz	190	6.0	3.0	860	na	17.0	na
(Armour) in barbecue sauce	2.5 oz	190	6.0	4.0	760	na	17.0	na
(Armour) in beef stock	2 oz	180	5.0	1.0	530	na	17.0	na
(Armour) in beef stock, lite	2 oz	150	6.0	1.0	400	na	13.0	na
(Armour) smoked	2 oz	180	5.0	1.0	530	na	17.0	na
(Hormel)	1 oz	69	3.0	2.0	225	na	7.0	15
(Hormel) chicken	1 oz	56	3.0	1.0	220	na	5.0	27
(Hormel) w/o broth	4 links	200	7.0	1.0	479	0	18.0	(mq)
(Libby's) chicken, in beef broth	2 oz	130	7.0	3.0	560	na	10.0	na
(Libby's) in barbecue sauce	2.5 oz	180	8.0	2.0	420	0	15.0	(mq)
(Libby's) in beef broth	2 oz	160	6.0	1.0	330	0	15.0	(mq)
VINE SPINACH/basella								
raw	1 lb	86	8.2	15.4	(mq)	>3.2 c	1.4	0
raw	3.5 oz	19	1.8	3.4	24	>.7 c	0.3	0

Food Name	Serv. Size	Total Cal.	Prot. GMS	Carbs GMS	Sod. MGS	Fiber GMS	Fat GMS	Chol. MGS
VINEGAR								
APPLE CIDER								
. . . .	1 cup	34	0.0	14.2	2	0	0.0	0
. . . .	1 tbsp	2	0.0	0.9	0	0	0.0	0
(Great Impressions)	1 tbsp	7	0.0	0.9	<1	0	0.0	0
(Hain)	1 tbsp	2	0.0	4.0	1	0	0.0	0
(Heinz)	.51 oz	2	0.0	0.0	1	0	0.0	0
(Heinz) gourmet 'Decanter'	.51 oz	4	0.0	0.0	0	na	0.0	na
(Indian Summer)	1 cup	40	<1.0	14.0	5	0	<1.0	0
(Lucky Leaf)	1 oz	4	0.0	2.0	0	0	0.0	0
(Musselman's)	1 oz	4	0.0	2.0	0	0	0.0	0
(Spectrum Naturals) filtered	1 tbsp	7	0.0	2.0	55	(tr)	0.0	0
(Spectrum Naturals) unfiltered	1 tbsp	7	0.0	2.0	55	(tr)	0.0	0
(White House)	1 oz	4	0.0	2.0	5	0	0.0	0
BROWN RICE								
(Spectrum Naturals) organic	1 tbsp	0	0.0	0.0	0	(tr)	0.0	0
(Spectrum Naturals) organic, seasoned . .	1 tbsp	10	0.0	2.0	240	(tr)	0.0	0
WHITE								
. . . .	1 cup	29	0.0	12.0	2	0	0.0	0
. . . .	1 tbsp	2	0.0	0.8	0	0	0.0	0
(Heinz)	1 tbsp	2	0.0	0.0	1	0	0.0	0
(Indian Summer)	1 cup	30	<1.0	12.0	5	0	<1.0	0
(Lucky Leaf)	1 oz	4	0.0	2.0	0	0	0.0	0
(Musselman's)	1 oz	4	0.0	2.0	0	0	0.0	0
(Spectrum Naturals) organic	1 tbsp	0	0.0	0.0	0	(tr)	0.0	0
WINE								
(Great Impressions) basil	1 tbsp	7	0.0	0.6	<1	0	0.0	0
(Great Impressions) paprika, hot	1 tbsp	6	0.0	0.6	<1	0	0.0	0
(Great Impressions) raspberry	1 tbsp	7	0.0	1.0	<1	0	0.0	0
(Heinz) gourmet 'Decanter'	.51 oz	4	0.0	0.0	0	na	0.0	na
(Heinz) tarragon, gourmet 'Decanter'	.51 oz	2	0.0	0.0	0	na	0.0	na
(Lucky Leaf) red	1 oz	0	0.0	0.0	0	0	0.0	0
(Musselman's) red	1 oz	0	0.0	0.0	0	0	0.0	0
(Regina) all varieties	1 oz	4	0.0	0.0	0	0	0.0	0
(Spectrum Naturals) garlic, organic	1 tbsp	0	0.0	0.0	0	(tr)	0.0	0
(Spectrum Naturals) Italian herb, organic	1 tbsp	0	0.0	0.0	0	(tr)	0.0	0
(Spectrum Naturals) raspberry, organic . .	1 tbsp	10	2.0	0.0	0	(tr)	0.0	0
(Spectrum Naturals) red, organic	1 tbsp	0	0.0	0.0	0	(tr)	0.0	0
(Spectrum Naturals) white, organic	1 tbsp	0	0.0	0.0	0	(tr)	0.0	0
VITA JUICE *(Knudsen & Sons)*	8 oz	90	1.0	21.0	na	na	0.0	na
VODKA. See ALCOHOLIC BEVERAGES.								

W

Food Name	Serv. Size	Total Cal.	Prot. GMS	Carbs GMS	Sod. MGS	Fiber GMS	Fat GMS	Chol. MGS
WAFFLE, FROZEN								
(Aunt Jemima) 'Original' 2.5 oz	1 waffle	173	4.3	27.8	591	1.5	5.6	6
(Downyflake)	2 waffles	120	3.0	20.0	420	(mq)	3.0	0
(Downyflake) 'Crisp & Healthy'	1 waffle	80	2.0	16.0	180	1.0	1.0	0
(Downyflake) 'Hot-N-Buttery'	2 waffles	180	4.0	27.0	620	(mq)	6.0	na
(Downyflake) 'Jumbo'	2 waffles	170	4.0	30.0	570	(mq)	4.0	0
(Eggo) 'Homestyle'	1 waffle	120	3.0	16.0	250	(mq)	5.0	10
(Eggo) 'Nutri-Grain'	1 waffle	130	3.0	18.0	250	2.0	5.0	0
(Roman Meal)	2 waffles	280	5.0	33.0	680	3.0	14.0	4
APPLE (Eggo) 'Fruit Top'	3.1 oz	190	3.0	32.0	250	na	6.0	0
APPLE CINNAMON								
(Aunt Jemima) 2.5 oz	1 waffle	176	4.5	28.8	616	2.0	5.6	6
(Downyflake) 'Crisp & Healthy'	1 waffle	80	2.0	16.0	180	1.0	1.0	0
(Eggo)	1 waffle	130	3.0	18.0	250	(mq)	5.0	na
(Van's)	1 waffle	75	2.8	8.4	68	3.3	2.0	0
BLUEBERRY								
(Aunt Jemima) 2.5 oz	1 waffle	175	4.2	29.2	684	1.3	5.2	5
(Downyflake)	2 waffles	180	4.0	32.0	570	(mq)	4.0	0
(Eggo)	1 waffle	130	3.0	18.0	250	(mq)	5.0	na
(Eggo) 'Fruit Top'	3.1 oz	190	3.0	32.0	250	na	6.0	0
(Krusteaz) 1.2 oz	1 waffle	110	3.0	19.0	210	2.0	3.0	3
BUTTERMILK								
(Aunt Jemima) 2.5 oz	1 waffle	179	4.4	28.7	615	1.3	5.8	7
(Downyflake)	2 waffles	190	5.0	32.0	750	(mq)	5.0	0
(Downyflake) 'Jumbo'	2 waffles	170	4.0	30.0	630	na	4.0	na
(Eggo)	1 waffle	120	3.0	16.0	250	(mq)	5.0	10
(Krusteaz) 1.2 oz	1 waffle	100	3.0	16.0	190	2.0	2.0	4
GOLDEN (Krusteaz) 1.2 oz	1 waffle	100	2.0	16.0	190	2.0	2.0	3
HONEY ALMOND (Van's)	1 waffle	75	2.8	8.4	68	3.3	2.0	0
MULTIGRAIN								
(Downyflake)	2 waffles	250	6.0	28.0	500	3.5	4.0	0
(Van's)	1 waffle	75	2.8	8.4	68	3.3	2.0	0
OAT BRAN								
(Aunt Jemima)	2.5 oz	154	5.9	29.4	676	3.0	2.8	na
(Downyflake)	2 waffles	260	6.0	30.0	650	3.0	13.0	0
(Eggo) 'Common Sense'	1 waffle	110	3.0	16.0	220	2.0	4.0	0
(Eggo) w/fruit and nut 'Common Sense'	1 waffle	120	3.0	17.0	220	2.0	5.0	0
(Van's) 'Belgian'	1 waffle	89	3.3	11.0	124	na	2.0	0
ORIGINAL (Van's) 'Belgian'	1 waffle	86	2.6	14.0	54	na	2.0	0
PEACH (Eggo) 'Fruit Top'	3.1 oz	190	3.0	30.0	240	na	6.0	0
RAISIN BRAN (Eggo) 'Nutri-Grain'	1 waffle	130	3.0	18.0	250	2.0	5.0	0

Food Name	Serv. Size	Total Cal.	Prot. GMS	Carbs GMS	Sod. MGS	Fiber GMS	Fat GMS	Chol. MGS
RICE BRAN *(Downyflake)*	2 waffles	210	5.0	25.0	230	3.5	11.0	0
SEVEN GRAIN *(Van's)* 'Belgian'	1 waffle	88	3.3	9.9	81	na	2.0	0
STRAWBERRY								
(Eggo)	1 waffle	130	3.0	18.0	250	(mq)	5.0	na
(Eggo) 'Fruit Top'	1 waffle	190	3.0	31.0	230	na	6.0	0
WHOLE-GRAIN WHEAT *(Aunt Jemima)*	1 waffle	154	5.9	29.4	676	3.0	2.8	na
WAFFLE BREAKFAST, FROZEN								
(Swanson) Belgian, w/sausage								
'Great Starts'	2.85 oz	280	7.0	21.0	420	(mq)	19.0	(mq)
(Swanson) Belgian, w/strawberries								
and sausage	3.5 oz	210	3.0	31.0	240	(mq)	8.0	(mq)
(Swanson) w/bacon 'Great Starts'	2.2 oz	230	7.0	19.0	710	(mq)	14.0	(mq)
WAFFLE MIX. See PANCAKE/WAFFLE MIX.								
WALNUT, BLACK								
Dried								
....	1 oz	172	6.9	3.4	0	1.4	16.1	0
chopped	1 cup	759	30.4	15.1	1	6.3	70.7	0
finely ground	1 cup	486	19.5	9.7	1	4.0	45.3	0
in shell	1 lb	661	26.5	13.2	2	5.4	61.6	0
Raw *(Planters)*	1 oz	180	7.0	3.0	0	na	17.0	0
Shelled *(Fisher)*	1 oz	170	7.0	3.0	0	na	16.0	0
WALNUT, ENGLISH								
Dried								
....	1 lb	1310	29.2	37.4	21	9.8	126.3	0
halves	1 cup	642	14.3	18.3	10	4.8	61.9	0
halves, approx 14	1 oz	182	4.1	5.2	3	1.4	17.6	0
in shell	1 lb	1310	29.2	37.4	21	9.8	126.3	0
pieces or chips	1 cup	770	17.2	22.0	12	5.8	74.2	0
(Diamond)	1 oz	192	5.0	4.0	na	(mq)	19.0	0
(Fisher) chopped	1 oz	180	4.0	5.0	0	na	18.0	0
(Fisher) ground	1 oz	180	4.0	5.0	0	na	18.0	0
(Planters) halves	1 oz	190	4.0	3.0	0	(mq)	20.0	0
(Planters) pieces	1 oz	190	4.0	3.0	0	(mq)	20.0	0
(Planters) whole	1 oz	190	4.0	3.0	0	(mq)	20.0	0
Raw *(Fisher)*	1 oz	180	4.0	5.0	0	na	18.0	0
WALNUT, PERSIAN								
Dried, in shell	1 lb	1310	29.2	37.4	21	9.8	126.3	0
Dried, shelled								
halves	1 cup	642	14.3	18.3	10	4.8	61.9	0
halves, approx 14	1 oz	182	4.1	5.2	3	1.4	17.6	0
pieces or chips	1 cup	770	17.2	22.0	12	5.8	74.2	0
(Diamond)	1 oz	192	5.0	4.0	na	(mq)	19.0	0
(Planters) halves	1 oz	190	4.0	3.0	0	(mq)	20.0	0

Food Name	Serv. Size	Total Cal.	Prot. GMS	Carbs GMS	Sod. MGS	Fiber GMS	Fat GMS	Chol. MGS
(Planters) pieces	1 oz	190	4.0	3.0	0	(mq)	20.0	0
(Planters) whole	1 oz	190	4.0	3.0	0	(mq)	20.0	0
WALNUT OIL								
....	1 cup	1927	0.0	0.0	0	0	218.0	0
....	1 tbsp	120	0.0	0.0	0	0	13.6	0
(Hain)	1 tbsp	120	0.0	0.0	0	0	14.0	0
(Spectrum Naturals)	1 tbsp	120	0.0	0.0	0	(tr)	14.0	(tr)
WATER, BOTTLED								
(Perrier)	1 cup	0	0.0	0.0	2	0	0.0	0
(Perrier)	6.5-oz bottle	0	0.0	0.0	2	0	0.0	0
(Poland Spring)	1 cup	0	0.0	0.0	2	0	0.0	0
distilled *(Arrowhead)*	1 liter	0	0.0	0.0	0	0	0.0	0
drinking *(Arrowhead)*	1 liter	0	0.0	0.0	16	0	0.0	0
fluoridated *(Arrowhead)*	1 liter	0	0.0	0.0	16	0	0.0	0
mineral *(Perrier)*	1 liter	0	0.0	0.0	19	0	0.0	0
sparkling, natural, unflavored								
(Clearly Canadian)	6 oz	0	0.0	0.0	3	na	0.0	na
spring *(Arrowhead)*	1 liter	0	0.0	0.0	9	0	0.0	0
spring, Arizona Tule *(Arrowhead)*	1 liter	0	0.0	0.0	7	0	0.0	0
Vichy *(Schweppes)*	6 oz	0	0.0	0.0	76	0	0.0	0
WATER, SPARKLING, FLAVORED. See also SOFT DRINKS AND MIXERS.								
BLACK CHERRY								
'Refresher' *(Quest)*	10 oz	2	0.0	0.0	40	na	0.0	na
'Refresher' *(Quest)*	8 oz	2	0.0	0.0	35	na	0.0	na
BLACKBERRY, 'Mountain Blackberry'								
(Clearly Canadian)	6 oz	70	0.0	16.0	10	na	0.0	na
CHERRY, 'Wild Cherry' *(Clearly Canadian)* ..	6 oz	70	0.0	16.0	10	na	0.0	na
CHERRY-BLACKBERRY, w/juice *(Cascadia)*	6 oz	2	0.0	0.0	0	na	0.0	na
CRANBERRY, 'Coastal Cranberry'								
(Clearly Canadian)	6 oz	70	0.0	16.0	10	na	0.0	na
GRAPEFRUIT, w/juice *(Cascadia)*	6 oz	2	0.0	0.0	0	na	0.0	na
GUAVA-BERRY, w/juice *(Cascadia)*	6 oz	2	0.0	0.0	0	na	0.0	na
LEMONAID, w/juice *(Cascadia)*	6 oz	2	0.0	0.0	0	na	0.0	na
LEMON-LIME *(H2OH!)*	6 oz	0	0.0	0.0	0	na	0.0	na
LOGANBERRY, 'Western Loganberry'								
(Clearly Canadian)	6 oz	70	0.0	16.0	10	na	0.0	na
NATURAL BERRY *(H2OH!)*	6 oz	0	0.0	0.0	0	na	0.0	na
PEACH, 'Orchard Peach' *(Clearly Canadian)*	6 oz	70	0.0	16.0	10	na	0.0	na
PEACH-CITRUS								
'Refresher' *(Quest)*	10 oz	2	0.0	0.0	40	na	0.0	na
'Refresher' *(Quest)*	8 oz	2	0.0	0.0	35	na	0.0	na
RASPBERRY								
'Country Raspberry' *(Clearly Canadian)* ...	6 oz	70	0.0	16.0	10	na	0.0	na

Food Name	Serv. Size	Total Cal.	Prot. GMS	Carbs GMS	Sod. MGS	Fiber GMS	Fat GMS	Chol. MGS
'Refresher' *(Quest)*	10 oz	2	0.0	0.0	40	na	0.0	na
'Refresher' *(Quest)*	8 oz	2	0.0	0.0	35	na	0.0	na
RED RASPBERRY								
'Refresher' *(Quest)*	10 oz	2	0.0	0.0	40	na	0.0	na
'Refresher' *(Quest)*	8 oz	2	0.0	0.0	35	na	0.0	na
STRAWBERRY-KIWI								
'Refresher' *(Quest)*	10 oz	2	0.0	0.0	40	na	0.0	na
'Refresher' *(Quest)*	8 oz	2	0.0	0.0	35	na	0.0	na
TANGERINE-LIME								
'Refresher' *(Quest)*	10 oz	2	0.0	0.0	40	na	0.0	na
'Refresher' *(Quest)*	8 oz	2	0.0	0.0	35	na	0.0	na
WATER CHESTNUT, CHINESE/matai								
approx 1.7 oz	4 fruits	38	0.5	8.6	5	1.1	0.0	0
slices	1/2 cup	66	0.9	14.8	9	1.9	0.1	0
trimmed	1 oz	30	0.4	6.8	4	>.2 c	<.1	0
untrimmed	1 lb	369	4.9	83.6	50	>2.8 c	0.4	0
Canned								
sliced, w/liquid	1/2 cup	35	0.6	8.7	6	1.8	0.0	0
w/liquid	4 oz	57	1.0	14.1	9	>.7 c	0.1	0
w/liquid	4 fruits	14	0.3	3.5	2	.7	0.0	0
(LaChoy)	1.28 oz	18	0.3	4.5	3	(mq)	<.1	0
(LaChoy) chopped	.6349 oz	9	0.2	2.2	2	.9	0.1	0
(LaChoy) sliced	1/4 cup	18	<1.0	4.0	3	<1.0	<1.0	0
(LaChoy) sliced	.776 oz	11	0.2	2.7	3	1.1	0.1	0
(LaChoy) whole	4 fruits	14	<1.0	4.0	2	<1.0	<1.0	0
(LaChoy) whole	.6702 oz	10	0.2	2.3	2	.9	0.1	0
WATER CONVOLVULUS. See CABBAGE, SKUNK.								
WATERCRESS								
chopped	1/2 cup	2	0.4	0.2	7	.4	0.0	0
fresh	1 sprig	0	0.1	0.0	1	.1	0.0	0
trimmed	1 oz	3	0.7	0.4	12	.7	<.1	0
untrimmed	1 lb	46	9.6	5.4	170	9.6	0.4	0
WATERMELON								
diced	1 cup	51	1.0	11.5	3	.6	0.7	0
diced	1/2 cup	25	0.5	5.7	2	.3	0.3	0
sliced, 1/16 of 10-inch-diam fruit	1 slice	154	3.0	34.6	10	1.9	2.1	0
trimmed	1 oz	9	0.2	2.0	1	.1	0.1	0
untrimmed	1 lb	74	1.5	16.9	5	.9	1.0	0
WATERMELON SEED, DRIED								
in hard coat	1 lb	935	47.5	25.7	166	>5.1 c	79.5	0
kernels	1 cup	602	30.6	16.5	107	>3.3 c	51.2	0
kernels	1 oz	158	8.1	4.3	28	>.9 c	13.4	0

Food Name	Serv. Size	Total Cal.	Prot. GMS	Carbs GMS	Sod. MGS	Fiber GMS	Fat GMS	Chol. MGS
WAX BEAN, CANNED								
(Allens)	1/2 cup	15	1.0	3.0	260	(mq)	<1.0	0
(Del Monte) golden, cut	1/2 cup	20	0.0	4.0	355	(mq)	0.0	0
(Del Monte) golden, French style	1/2 cup	20	0.0	4.0	355	(mq)	0.0	0
(Stokely)	1/2 cup	20	1.0	4.0	360	(mq)	0.0	0
(Stokely) 'No Salt or Sugar'	1/2 cup	20	1.0	4.0	5	(mq)	0.0	0
WAX BEAN, FROZEN								
(Frosty Acres)	3 oz	25	2.0	5.0	1	>1.0 c	0.0	0
(Seabrook) cut	3 oz	25	2.0	5.0	1	>1.0 c	0.0	0
WELSH ONION. See ONION, WELSH.								
WELSH RAREBIT								
(Snow's) canned	1/2 cup	170	9.0	10.0	460	na	11.0	(mq)
(Stouffer's) frozen	5 oz	270	13.0	9.0	460	na	20.0	na
WESTERN DINNER, FROZEN								
(Banquet)	11 oz	630	28.0	40.0	720	(mq)	41.0	90
(Morton)	10 oz	290	14.0	29.0	1450	(mq)	14.0	35
(Swanson)	11.5 oz	430	22.0	43.0	1060	(mq)	19.0	(mq)
WHEAT, SPROUTED								
	1/3 cup	71	2.7	15.3	6	.4	0.5	0
	1 oz	56	2.1	12.1	5	(mq)	0.4	0
WHEAT, WHOLE GRAIN								
DURUM								
	1 cup	650	26.3	136.6	3	(mq)	4.7	0
	1/2 cup	325	13.1	68.3	2	>2.2 c	2.4	0
	1 oz	96	3.9	20.2	<1	(mq)	0.7	0
HARD RED								
spring	1 cup	631	29.6	130.6	4	24.2	3.7	0
spring	1/2 cup	316	14.8	65.3	2	12.1	1.8	0
spring	1 oz	93	4.4	19.3	<1	>.6 c	0.5	0
spring or winter (Arrowhead Mills)	2 oz	190	8.0	41.0	1	8.3	1.0	0
winter	1 cup	628	24.2	136.7	4	24.2	3.0	0
winter	1/2 cup	314	12.1	68.3	2	12.1	1.5	0
winter	1 oz	93	3.6	20.2	<1	>.6 c	0.4	0
HARD WHITE								
	1 cup	656	21.7	145.7	na	(mq)	3.3	0
	1/2 cup	328	10.9	72.9	2	>2.2 c	1.6	0
	1 oz	97	3.2	21.5	na	(mq)	0.5	0
SOFT RED								
for pastry (Arrowhead Mills)	2 oz	190	8.0	41.0	1	8.3	1.0	0
winter	1 cup	556	17.4	124.7	4	>2.9 c	2.6	0
winter	1/2 cup	278	8.7	62.4	2	>1.4 c	1.3	0
winter	1 oz	94	2.9	21.0	<1	>.5 c	0.4	0

Food Name	Serv. Size	Total Cal.	Prot. GMS	Carbs GMS	Sod. MGS	Fiber GMS	Fat GMS	Chol. MGS
SOFT WHITE								
....	1 cup	571	18.0	126.6	na	(mq)	3.3	0
....	1/2 cup	286	9.0	63.3	2	>1.4 c	1.7	0
....	1 oz	96	3.0	21.4	na	(mq)	0.6	0
WHEAT BRAN								
crude	1/2 cup	65	4.7	19.4	1	12.8	1.3	0
crude	1 oz	61	4.4	18.3	<1	12.0	1.2	0
crude	2 tbsp	15	1.1	4.5	0	3.0	0.3	0
crude (Arrowhead Mills)	2 oz	50	10.0	30.0	3	24.4	2.0	0
toasted (Kretschmer)	1 oz	57	5.7	14.8	2	11.4	2.3	0
unprocessed (Quaker)	2 tbsp	8	1.0	3.8	0	3.3	0.2	0
WHEAT CAKE								
(Quaker) 'Grain Cakes'	1 cake	34	1.4	6.7	52	.8	0.3	0
(Quaker) lightly salted	1 cake	35	1.0	7.0	50	na	0.0	0
WHEAT FLAKES (Arrowhead Mills)	2 oz	210	8.0	42.0	1	6.7	1.0	0
WHEAT FLOUR								
RYE								
(Pillsbury's Best) medium-colored	1 cup	400	12.0	83.0	0	9	2.0	0
(Pillsbury's Best) w/wheat 'Bohemian Style'	1 cup	400	11.0	86.0	0	na	1.0	0
WHITE								
(Drifted Snow)	1 cup	400	11.0	87.0	0	(mq)	1.0	0
(Softasilk)	1/4 cup	100	2.0	23.0	0	(mq)	0.0	0
(Wondra)	1 cup	400	11.0	87.0	0	(mq)	1.0	0
All-purpose								
enriched	1/2 cup	226	6.4	47.3	1	1.7	0.6	0
enriched	1 oz	103	2.9	21.6	<1	.8	0.3	0
enriched, calcium-fortified	1/2 cup	226	6.4	47.3	1	>.2 c	0.6	0
(Ballard)	1 cup	400	11.0	87.0	0	(mq)	1.0	0
(Ceresota)	4 oz	390	12.5	82.5	0	(mq)	1.0	0
(Gold Medal)	1 cup	400	11.0	87.0	0	(mq)	1.0	0
(Heckers)	4 oz	390	12.5	82.5	0	(mq)	1.0	0
(Pillsbury's Best)	1 cup	400	11.0	87.0	0	(mq)	1.0	0
(Red Band)	1 cup	390	10.0	85.0	0	(mq)	1.0	0
(Robin Hood)	1 cup	400	13.0	85.0	0	(mq)	1.0	0
(White Deer)	1 cup	400	11.0	87.0	0	(mq)	1.0	0
All-purpose, unbleached								
enriched	1/2 cup	226	6.4	47.3	1	>.2 c	0.6	0
(Arrowhead Mills)	2 oz	200	7.0	53.0	1	(mq)	1.0	0
(Gold Medal)	1 cup	400	11.0	87.0	0	(mq)	1.0	0
(Pillsbury's Best)	1 cup	400	12.0	86.0	0	(mq)	1.0	0
(Robin Hood)	1 cup	400	13.0	85.0	0	(mq)	1.0	0
Bread								
enriched	1/2 cup	249	8.3	50.0	1	1.7	1.1	0

Food Name	Serv. Size	Total Cal.	Prot. GMS	Carbs GMS	Sod. MGS	Fiber GMS	Fat GMS	Chol. MGS
enriched	1 oz	102	3.4	20.6	<1	(mq)	0.5	0
(Gold Medal) 'Better for Bread'	1 cup	400	14.0	83.0	0	(mq)	1.0	0
(Pillsbury's Best)	1 cup	400	14.0	83.0	0	(mq)	2.0	0
Cake								
enriched	1/2 cup	195	4.4	42.1	1	.9	0.5	0
enriched	1 oz	103	2.3	22.1	<1	(mq)	0.2	0
Self-rising								
enriched	1/2 cup	219	6.1	46.0	787	2.0	0.6	0
enriched	1 oz	100	2.8	21.0	360	<.1	0.3	0
(Aunt Jemima) enriched	1 oz	109	3.0	23.6	368	>.1 c	0.3	0
(Ballard)	1 cup	380	9.0	84.0	1290	(mq)	1.0	0
(Gold Medal)	1 cup	380	10.0	83.0	1520	(mq)	1.0	0
(Pillsbury's Best)	1 cup	380	9.0	84.0	1290	2	1.0	0
(Pillsbury's Best) unbleached	1 cup	380	9.0	84.0	1290	2	1.0	0
(Red Band)	1 cup	380	9.0	83.0	1520	(mq)	1.0	0
(Robin Hood)	1 cup	380	10.0	83.0	1520	(mq)	1.0	0
Shake and blend (Pillsbury's Best)	2 tbsp	50	1.0	11.0	0	na	0.0	0
Tortilla mix								
enriched	1/3 cup	150	3.6	24.8	250	>.1 c	3.9	0
enriched	1 oz	115	2.7	19.0	192	<.1	3.0	0
WHOLE GRAIN								
	1/2 cup	203	8.2	43.5	3	7.3	1.1	0
	1 oz	96	3.9	20.6	1	3.6	0.5	0
(Arrowhead Mills) pastry	2 oz	180	6.0	41.0	1	6.8	1.0	0
(Arrowhead Mills) stone ground	2 oz	200	8.0	40.0	1	6.7	1.0	0
(Ceresota)	4 oz	400	15.0	80.0	0	(mq)	2.0	0
(Gold Medal)	1 cup	350	16.0	78.0	0	10.0	2.0	0
(Gold Medal) blend	1 cup	380	14.0	84.0	0	8.0	2.0	0
(Heckers)	4 oz	400	15.0	80.0	0	(mq)	2.0	0
(Krusteaz)	1 cup	450	17.0	90.0	5	15.0	2.0	0
(Pillsbury's Best)	1 cup	400	15.0	80.0	10	(mq)	2.0	0
WHEAT GERM								
crude	1/4 cup	104	6.7	15.0	3	3.8	2.8	0
crude	1 oz	102	6.6	14.7	3	4.3	2.8	0
toasted	1 cup	431	32.9	56.1	4	14.6	12.1	0
toasted	1 oz	108	8.3	14.1	1	3.7	3.0	0
(Arrowhead Mills) raw	2 oz	210	15.0	26.0	1	6.5	6.0	0
(Kretschmer)	1 oz	103	9.3	12.3	2	3.3	3.4	0
(Kretschmer) honey crunch	1 oz	105	7.6	15.2	2	3.0	2.8	0
WHEAT GERM OIL								
	1 cup	1927	0.0	0.0	0	0	218.0	0
	1 tbsp	120	0.0	0.0	0	0	13.6	0
(Spectrum Naturals) unrefined	1 tbsp	120	0.0	0.0	0	(tr)	14.0	(tr)

Food Name	Serv. Size	Total Cal.	Prot. GMS	Carbs GMS	Sod. MGS	Fiber GMS	Fat GMS	Chol. MGS
WHEAT GLUTEN (Arrowhead Mills)								
'Vita 1' toasted	1 oz	100	15.0	9.0	1	.9	1.0	0
WHEAT NUTS								
macadamia flavor, w/o salt	1 oz	176	3.2	7.9	13	1.5	16.0	0
other flavors, w/o salt	1 oz	184	3.7	5.9	26	1.5	17.7	0
unflavored, w/salt added	1 oz	177	3.9	6.7	143	1.5	16.4	0
WHEAT PILAF MIX, dry mix (Casbah)	1 oz	100	3.0	20.0	(mq)	(mq)	0.0	0
WHELK								
moist-heat cooked	3 oz	234	40.5	13.2	350	0	0.7	110
raw	1 lb	623	108.1	35.2	934	0	1.8	294
raw	3 oz	116	20.3	6.6	175	0	0.3	55
raw	1 oz	39	6.8	2.2	54	0	0.1	18
WHEY								
Acid								
dry	1 cup	193	6.7	41.9	552	0	0.3	2
dry	1 oz	96	3.3	20.8	274	0	0.2	(tr)
dry	1 tbsp	10	0.3	2.1	28	0	0.0	0
fluid	1 quart	235	7.5	50.4	473	0	0.9	5
fluid	1 cup	59	1.9	12.6	118	0	0.2	1
fluid	1 oz	7	0.2	1.5	14	0	<.1	(tr)
Sweet								
dry	1 cup	512	18.8	108.0	1565	0	1.5	9
dry	1 oz	100	3.7	21.1	306	0	0.3	2
dry	1 tbsp	26	1.0	5.6	81	0	0.1	0
fluid	1 quart	263	8.4	50.6	526	0	3.5	20
fluid	1 cup	66	2.1	12.6	132	0	0.9	5
fluid	1 oz	8	0.2	1.5	15	0	0.1	<1
WHIPPED TOPPING. See CREAM TOPPING.								
WHISKEY. See ALCOHOLIC BEVERAGES.								
WHISKEY SOUR. See ALCOHOLIC BEVERAGES.								
WHITE BEAN								
boiled	4 oz	158	11.0	28.5	7	>2.8 c	0.4	0
boiled	1/2 cup	125	8.8	22.6	5	5.7	0.3	0
raw	1/2 cup	336	23.6	60.9	16	15.4	0.9	0
raw	1 oz	94	6.6	17.1	5	>1.7 c	0.2	0
small, boiled	4 oz	161	10.2	29.3	2	5.0	0.7	0
small, boiled	1/2 cup	128	8.1	23.2	2	>2.2 c	0.6	0
small, raw	1/2 cup	363	22.8	67.2	13	>2.9 c	1.3	0
small, raw	1 oz	95	6.0	17.6	3	2.9	0.3	0
WHITE BEAN, CANNED								
	1/2 cup	153	9.5	28.7	7	6.3	0.4	0
w/liquid	4 oz	133	8.2	24.9	515	>.8 c	0.3	0
WHITE-FLOWERED GOURD. See GOURD, BOTTLE.								

Food Name	Serv. Size	Total Cal.	Prot. GMS	Carbs GMS	Sod. MGS	Fiber GMS	Fat GMS	Chol. MGS
WHITE GOURD. See GOURD, WHITE.								
WHITEFISH								
dry-heat cooked	3 oz	146	20.8	0.0	55	0	6.4	65
dry-heat cooked, approx 7 oz	1 fillet	265	37.7	0.0	100	0	11.6	119
raw	1 lb	610	86.6	0.0	232	0	26.6	272
raw	3 oz	114	16.2	0.0	43	0	5.0	51
raw	1 oz	38	5.4	0.0	14	0	1.7	17
raw, approx 7 oz	1 fillet	265	37.8	0.0	101	0	11.6	119
smoked	4 oz	122	26.5	0.0	1156	0	1.1	37
smoked	3 oz	92	19.9	0.0	866	0	0.8	28
smoked	1 oz	30	6.6	0.0	285	0	0.3	9
WHITING, MIXED SPECIES/silver hake								
dry-heat cooked	4 oz	130	26.6	0.0	150	0	1.9	95
dry-heat cooked	3 oz	98	20.0	0.0	112	0	1.4	7
raw	1 lb	408	83.1	0.0	326	0	6.0	303
raw	3 oz	77	15.6	0.0	61	0	1.1	57
raw	1 oz	26	5.2	0.0	20	0	0.4	19
WHITING, MIXED SPECIES, FROZEN								
(Booth)	4 oz	100	19.0	0.0	90	0	1.0	(mq)
(Booth) 'Individually Wrapped'	4 oz	80	19.0	0.0	85	0	1.0	(mq)
WILD BERRY DRINK								
(Hi-C)	6 oz	92	0.1	22.5	17	(tr)	0.1	0
(Hi-C) aseptic box or chilled	6 oz	90	0.0	22.0	20	na	0.0	na
(Hi-C) boxed	8.45 oz	129	0.1	31.7	24	(tr)	0.1	0
(Hi-C) chilled	6 oz	90	0.0	22.0	20	na	0.0	na
(Tropicana) 'Juice Sparkler'	8 oz	110	(tr)	27.0	15	(tr)	0.0	0
WINE. See ALCOHOLIC BEVERAGES.								
WINE, COOKING. See also ALCOHOLIC BEVERAGES.								
Burgundy (Regina)	1/4 cup	2	<1.0	<1.0	365	0	<1.0	0
Marsala (Holland House)	1 oz	9	0.0	2.3	186	0	0.0	0
red (Holland House)	1 oz	6	0.0	1.5	186	0	0.0	0
Sauternes (Regina)	1/4 cup	2	<1.0	<1.0	365	0	<1.0	0
sherry (Holland House)	1 oz	5	0.0	1.2	186	0	0.0	0
sherry (Regina)	1/4 cup	20	<1.0	5.0	70	0	<1.0	0
vermouth (Holland House)	1 oz	2	0.0	<1.0	186	0	0.0	0
white (Holland House)	1 oz	2	0.0	<1.0	186	0	0.0	0
WINGED BEAN/goa bean								
boiled, drained	4 oz	43	6.0	3.6	5	>1.6 c	0.7	0
immature seeds, boiled, drained	1/2 cup	12	1.6	1.0	1	>.4 c	0.2	0
immature seeds, raw, approx .6 oz	1 pod	8	1.1	0.7	1	>.4 c	0.1	0
immature seeds, slices, raw	1 cup	22	3.1	1.9	2	>1.1 c	0.4	0
mature seeds, boiled, drained	1/2 cup	126	9.1	12.8	11	>2.1 c	5.0	0
mature seeds, raw	1/2 cup	372	27.0	38.0	35	>6.2 c	14.9	0

Food Name	Serv. Size	Total Cal.	Prot. GMS	Carbs GMS	Sod. MGS	Fiber GMS	Fat GMS	Chol. MGS
trimmed, raw	1 oz	14	2.0	1.2	1	>.7 c	0.2	0
untrimmed, raw	1 lb	218	30.9	19.2	17	>11.4 c	3.9	0
WINGED BEAN, DRIED								
boiled	4 oz	167	12.0	16.9	15	>2.8 c	6.6	0
boiled	1/2 cup	126	9.1	12.8	11	>2.1 c	5.0	0
raw	1/2 cup	372	27.0	38.0	35	14.1	14.9	0
raw	1 oz	116	8.4	11.8	11	4.4	4.6	0
WINGED BEAN LEAVES								
trimmed	1 lb	336	26.5	64.0	na	>11.3 c	5.0	0
trimmed	1 oz	21	1.7	4.0	na	>.7 c	0.3	0
WOLF FISH/ocean catfish								
dry-heat cooked	3 oz	105	19.1	0.0	93	0	2.6	50
frozen *(Booth)*	4 oz	115	20.0	0.0	85	0	20.0	(mq)
raw	1 lb	437	79.4	0.0	386	0	10.8	209
raw	3 oz	82	14.9	0.0	72	0	2.0	39
raw	1 oz	27	5.0	0.0	24	0	0.7	13
raw, approx 5.4 oz	1/2 fillet	147	26.8	0.0	130	0	3.7	70
WON TON SKIN								
	1 oz	83	2.8	16.4	162	na	0.4	3
	1 wrapper	23	0.8	4.6	46	na	0.1	1
(Nasoya)	1 wrapper	23	1.0	4.5	19	(mq)	0.0	0
WON TON SOUP. See SOUP.								

Y

Food Name	Serv. Size	Total Cal.	Prot. GMS	Carbs GMS	Sod. MGS	Fiber GMS	Fat GMS	Chol. MGS
YAM								
boiled and drained, or baked	4 oz	132	1.7	31.2	9	(mq)	0.2	0
boiled and drained, or baked, cubed	1/2 cup	79	1.0	18.8	5	2.7	0.1	0
raw, cubed	1/2 cup	89	1.1	20.9	7	3.1	0.1	0
raw, trimmed	1 oz	33	0.4	7.9	3	(mq)	<.1	0
raw, untrimmed	1 lb	460	6.0	108.8	37	(mq)	0.7	0
Mountain/Hawaiian								
raw, approx 8.25 inches long	1 yam	281	5.6	68.5	55	>1.9 c	0.4	0
raw, cubed	1/2 cup	46	0.9	11.1	9	>.3 c	0.1	0
raw, trimmed	1 oz	19	0.4	4.6	4	>.1 c	<.1	tr
raw, untrimmed	1 lb	253	5.0	61.4	49	>1.7 c	0.4	0
steamed	4 oz	93	2.0	22.7	14	>.6 c	0.1	0
steamed, cubed	1/2 cup	59	1.2	14.4	9	>.4 c	0.1	0
YAM, CANNED *(Bush's Best)*	1/2 cup	120	1.0	28.0	20	na	0.0	na
YAM BEAN TUBER. See JICAMA.								

Food Name	Serv. Size	Total Cal.	Prot. GMS	Carbs GMS	Sod. MGS	Fiber GMS	Fat GMS	Chol. MGS
YARDLONG BEAN/asparagus bean								
boiled, drained	4 oz	53	2.9	10.4	5	>1.7 c	0.1	0
boiled, drained, approx 13.25 inches long	1 pod	7	0.4	1.3	1	>.2 c	0.0	0
boiled, drained, sliced	1 cup	49	2.6	9.6	4	1.6	0.1	0
boiled, drained, sliced	1/2 cup	25	1.3	4.8	2	>.8 c	0.1	0
mature, boiled	1/2 cup	101	7.1	18.1	4	>1.4 c	0.4	0
mature, raw	1/2 cup	291	20.4	52.0	14	>4.0 c	1.1	0
raw, approx 13.25 inches long	1 pod	6	0.3	1.0	0	>.1 c	0.1	0
raw, sliced	1 cup	43	2.5	7.6	4	>.6 c	0.4	0
raw, sliced	1/2 cup	22	1.3	3.8	2	(mq)	0.2	0
raw, trimmed	1 oz	13	0.8	2.4	1	(mq)	0.1	0
raw, untrimmed	1 lb	203	12.1	36.0	17	(mq)	1.7	0
Dried								
boiled	4 oz	134	9.4	23.9	6	>1.8 c	0.5	0
boiled	1/2 cup	102	7.1	18.1	4	>1.4 c	0.4	0
raw	1/2 cup	292	20.4	52.0	14	>4.0 c	1.1	0
raw	1 oz	98	6.9	17.6	5	>1.4 c	0.4	0
YEAST, BAKER'S								
active dry	1 oz	79	10.3	10.9	15	0	0.5	0
active dry	1 tbsp	35	4.6	4.6	6	3.3	0.6	0
active dry	.25-oz pkg	21	2.7	2.7	4	1.9	0.3	0
compressed	100 gm	105	8.4	18.1	30	9.3	1.9	0
compressed	.6-oz cake	18	1.4	3.1	5	1.6	0.3	0
compressed, fortified	1 oz	24	3.4	3.1	4	>.2 c	0.1	0
compressed, not fortified	1 oz	24	3.4	3.1	4	>.2 c	0.1	0
YEAST, BREWER'S								
debittered	1 oz	79	10.9	10.8	34	>.5 c	0.3	0
debittered	1 tbsp	23	3.1	3.1	10	>.1 c	0.1	0
(Fleischmann's) 'Active Dry/RapidRise'	1/4 oz	20	3.0	3.0	10	(mq)	0.0	0
(Red Star) 'Active Dry'	1/4 oz	15	2.0	2.0	5	(mq)	0.0	0
YEAST, TORULA	1 oz	78	10.8	10.4	4	>.9 c	0.3	0
YELLOW BEAN								
mature, boiled	1/2 cup	127	8.1	22.2	4	>1.0 c	1.0	0
mature, raw	1/2 cup	338	21.6	59.5	12	>2.7 c	2.5	0
Dried								
boiled	4 oz	163	10.4	28.7	6	>1.3 c	1.2	0
boiled	1/2 cup	126	8.1	22.2	4	>1.0 c	1.0	0
raw	1/2 cup	338	21.6	59.5	12	>2.7 c	2.6	0
raw	1 oz	98	6.2	17.2	3	>.8 c	0.7	0
YELLOW MOMBIN. See JOBO.								
YELLOWEYE BEAN (B&M) canned, baked style	8 oz	326	15.0	50.0	770	15.0	7.0	4
YELLOW-EYED PEAS. See BLACK-EYED PEAS.								

Food Name	Serv. Size	Total Cal.	Prot. GMS	Carbs GMS	Sod. MGS	Fiber GMS	Fat GMS	Chol. MGS
YELLOWTAIL, MIXED SPECIES								
dry-heat cooked	3 oz	159	25.2	0.0	43	0	5.7	60
raw	1 lb	662	105.0	0.0	177	0	23.8	(mq)
raw	3 oz	124	19.7	0.0	33	0	4.4	47
raw	1 oz	41	6.6	0.0	11	0	1.5	(mq)
YOGURT								
(Colombo) 'Fruit on the Bottom' all flavors	8 oz	230	7.0	36.0	140	(mq)	6.0	(mq)
(Colombo) 'Nonfat Fruit on the Bottom' all flavors	8 oz	190	8.0	38.0	140	(mq)	<1.0	5
(Colombo) 'Nonfat Lite Minipack' all flavors	4.4 oz	100	5.0	20.0	70	(mq)	0.0	(mq)
(Crowley) 'Sundae Style' all flavors	8 oz	250	9.0	47.0	170	(mq)	2.0	10
(Crowley) 'Swiss Style' all flavors	8 oz	240	8.0	48.0	150	(mq)	2.0	10
(Dannon) 'Extra Smooth' all flavors	4.4 oz	130	5.0	24.0	80	(mq)	2.0	10
(Dannon) 'Hearty Nuts & Raisins' all flavors except vanilla	8 oz	260	11.0	48.0	120	(mq)	3.0	10
(Knudsen) 'Lowfat' all flavors except strawberry	8 oz	240	11.0	43.0	135	(mq)	4.0	15
(Light n' Lively) 'Free' all flavors except strawberry	4.4 oz	50	4.0	8.0	60	(mq)	0.0	0
(Ripple) '70' fat-free, all flavors	6 oz	70	5.0	13.0	85	(mq)	0.0	5
(Yoplait) 'Fat-free' all flavors	6 oz	150	7.0	31.0	95	(mq)	0.0	5
(Yoplait) 'Light' all flavors	6 oz	90	7.0	14.0	100	(mq)	0.0	5
(Yoplait) 'Light' all flavors	4 oz	60	5.0	9.0	65	(mq)	0.0	5
APPLE CRISP *(New Country)* 'Lowfat'	6 oz	150	5.0	30.0	85	(mq)	2.0	(mq)
BANANA								
(Dannon) 'Sprinkl'ins' lowfat	4.1 oz	140	5.0	24.0	80	na	2.0	5
(Yoplait) 'Custard Style'	6 oz	180	7.0	30.0	105	na	3.0	na
BANANA BERRY								
(Light n' Lively) lowfat, 1% milkfat, cultured	4.4 oz	130	5.0	24.0	75	na	1.0	10
BERRIES *(Yoplait)* 'Breakfast' w/wheat, raisins, and walnuts	6 oz	200	8.0	39.0	125	na	2.0	na
BLACK CHERRY								
(Alta•Dena) 'Blended European Style'	8 oz	190	8.0	38.0	140	na	<1.0	na
(Alta•Dena) 'Naja' fruit-on-the-bottom	8 oz	240	12.0	40.0	150	na	4.0	na
(Breyers) 'Lowfat'	8 oz	260	9.0	49.0	120	(mq)	3.0	10
(Knudsen) 'Cal 70'	6 oz	70	5.0	12.0	75	(mq)	0.0	5
(Light n' Lively)	8 oz	230	9.0	44.0	125	(mq)	2.0	15
(Light n' Lively) '100'	8 oz	100	8.0	17.0	100	(mq)	0.0	0
(Mountain High) 'Honey Light' natural	8 oz	190	9.0	35.0	140	na	1.0	5
(TCBY) 'Light'	8 oz	100	8.0	17.0	180	na	0.0	na

Food Name	Serv. Size	Total Cal.	Prot. GMS	Carbs GMS	Sod. MGS	Fiber GMS	Fat GMS	Chol. MGS
BLUEBERRY								
(Alta•Dena) 'Maya' fruit-on-the-bottom	8 oz	280	11.0	39.0	170	na	9.0	na
(Breyers) 'Lowfat'	8 oz	250	9.0	48.0	120	(mq)	2.0	10
(Dannon) 'Blended' fat-free	6 oz	160	7.0	33.0	105	na	0.0	5
(Dannon) 'Light' nonfat	8 oz	100	9.0	19.0	135	na	0.0	<5
(Knudsen) 'Cal 70'	6 oz	70	6.0	11.0	80	(mq)	0.0	5
(Light n' Lively)	8 oz	240	8.0	46.0	130	(mq)	2.0	10
(Light n' Lively)	4.4 oz	130	5.0	26.0	79	(mq)	1.0	5
(Light n' Lively) 'Free' nonfat	4.4 oz	50	4.0	8.0	60	na	0.0	0
(Light n' Lively) '100'	8 oz	90	8.0	15.0	110	(mq)	0.0	0
(Mountain High) 'Honey Light' natural	8 oz	190	9.0	35.0	140	na	<1.0	5
(Mountain High) w/other natural flavors	8 oz	220	10.0	31.0	140	(mq)	6.0	(mq)
(New Country) 'Supreme'	6 oz	150	5.0	31.0	90	(mq)	2.0	(mq)
(TCBY)	8 oz	220	9.0	42.0	150	na	2.0	na
(TCBY) 'Light' nonfat, w/aspartame	8 oz	100	8.0	17.0	210	na	0.0	na
(Weight Watchers) 'Ultimate 90'	8 oz	90	10.0	13.0	120	na	0.0	5
(Yogi) 'Sundae' cheesecake, w/gelatin	5.6 oz	50	6.0	14.0	75	na	<1.0	4
(Yoplait) 'Fruit-on-the-Bottom'	6 oz	170	7.0	35.0	105	na	0.0	5
(Yoplait) 'Light' fat-free	6 oz	90	5.0	16.0	70	na	0.0	5
(Yoplait) 'Original' 99% fat-free	6 oz	180	8.0	32.0	130	na	2.0	na
(Yoplait) 'Parfait Style' blueberry and vanilla	6 oz	200	8.0	34.0	120	na	3.0	na
BOYSENBERRY (Yoplait) 'Original'								
99% fat-free	6 oz	180	8.0	32.0	130	na	2.0	na
CAPPUCCINO (Dannon) 'Light' nonfat	8 oz	100	9.0	16.0	135	na	0.0	<5
CHERRIES JUBILEE (Weight Watchers)								
'Ultimate 90'	8 oz	90	10.0	13.0	120	na	0.0	5
CHERRY								
(Dannon) 'Sprinkl'ins' lowfat	4.1 oz	140	5.0	24.0	80	na	2.0	5
(Light n' Lively)	4.4 oz	140	5.0	27.0	70	(mq)	1.0	5
(New Country) 'Supreme'	6 oz	150	5.0	32.0	90	(mq)	2.0	(mq)
(Yoplait) 'Breakfast Yogurt' w/almonds	6 oz	200	8.0	38.0	90	2.0	3.0	10
(Yoplait) 'Custard Style'	6 oz	180	7.0	30.0	95	(mq)	4.0	20
(Yoplait) 'Light' fat-free	6 oz	90	5.0	16.0	70	na	0.0	5
(Yoplait) 'Original' 99% fat-free	6 oz	180	8.0	32.0	130	na	2.0	na
(Yoplait) 'Parfait Style' cherry and vanilla	6 oz	200	8.0	34.0	120	na	3.0	na
CHERRY-VANILLA								
(Dannon) 'Light' nonfat	8 oz	100	9.0	18.0	135	na	0.0	<5
(Dannon) 'Sprinkl'ins' lowfat	4.1 oz	140	5.0	24.0	95	na	2.0	5
(Lite-Line) 'Swiss Style 1%'	8 oz	240	10.0	45.0	150	(mq)	2.0	(mq)
(TCBY)	8 oz	220	9.0	42.0	150	na	2.0	na
(Yogi) w/gelatin 'Sundae'	5.6 oz	50	6.0	14.0	75	na	<1.0	4
(Yoplait) fat-free 'Light Custard Style'	6 oz	90	6.0	17.0	85	na	0.0	5

Food Name	Serv. Size	Total Cal.	Prot. GMS	Carbs GMS	Sod. MGS	Fiber GMS	Fat GMS	Chol. MGS
COFFEE								
(Bison) 'Lowfat'	8 oz	210	11.0	33.0	160	0	4.0	10
(Dannon) 'Fresh Flavors'	8 oz	200	10.0	34.0	140	0	3.0	10
(Friendship) 'Lowfat'	8 oz	210	11.0	35.0	170	0	3.0	14
CRANBERRY-RASPBERRY								
(Weight Watchers) 'Ultimate 90'	8 oz	90	10.0	13.0	120	na	0.0	5
FRUIT CRUNCH (New Country) 'Lowfat'	6 oz	150	5.0	30.0	90	(mq)	2.0	(mq)
GRAPE								
(Dannon) lowfat 'Sprinkl'ins'	4.1 oz	140	5.0	24.0	110	na	2.0	5
(Light n' Lively)	4.4 oz	130	6.0	24.0	70	(mq)	1.0	10
HAWAIIAN SALAD (New Country) 'Lowfat'	6 oz	150	5.0	31.0	90	(mq)	2.0	(mq)
LEMON								
(Alta·Dena) 'Naja' fruit-on-the-bottom	8 oz	240	12.0	40.0	150	na	4.0	na
(Bison) 'Lowfat'	8 oz	210	11.0	33.0	160	na	4.0	10
(Dannon) 'Fresh Flavors'	8 oz	200	10.0	34.0	140	na	3.0	10
(Knudsen) 'Cal 70'	6 oz	70	6.0	12.0	125	na	0.0	0
(Light n' Lively) '100'	8 oz	100	9.0	16.0	150	na	0.0	5
(Mountain High) 'Natural'	8 oz	220	10.0	31.0	140	na	6.0	na
(New Country) 'Supreme'	6 oz	150	5.0	31.0	90	na	2.0	(mq)
(Weight Watchers) 'Ultimate 90'	1 cup	90	10.0	13.0	120	na	0.0	5
(Yoplait) 'Original' 99% fat-free	6 oz	180	8.0	32.0	130	na	2.0	na
LEMON CHIFFON								
(Dannon) 'Blended' fat-free	6 oz	150	8.0	30.0	110	na	0.0	5
(Dannon) 'Light' non-fat	8 oz	100	9.0	15.0	135	na	0.0	<5
(Yogi) 'Sundae' w/gelatin	5.6 oz	50	6.0	14.0	75	na	<1.0	4
MIXED BERRIES								
(Alta·Dena) 'Blended European Style'	8 oz	190	8.0	39.0	140	na	<1.0	na
(Breyers) 'Lowfat'	8 oz	250	9.0	48.0	120	(mq)	2.0	10
(New Country) 'Lowfat'	6 oz	150	5.0	31.0	85	(mq)	2.0	(mq)
(Yoplait) 'Custard Style'	6 oz	180	7.0	30.0	95	(mq)	4.0	20
(Yoplait) 'Original' 99% fat-free	6 oz	180	8.0	32.0	130	na	2.0	na
ORANGE								
(Dannon) 'Fruit-on-the-Bottom'	8 oz	230	9.0	44.0	130	na	3.0	10
(New Country) 'Supreme'	6 oz	150	5.0	31.0	90	na	2.0	(mq)
ORANGE-PINEAPPLE (Yogi) 'Sundae' w/gelatin	5.6 oz	50	6.0	14.0	75	na	<1.0	4
PEACH								
(Alta·Dena) 'Naja' fruit-on-the-bottom	8 oz	240	12.0	40.0	150	na	4.0	na
(Alta·Dena) nonfat, fruit-on-the-bottom	8 oz	190	12.0	36.0	128	na	<1.0	na
(Breyers) 'Lowfat'	8 oz	250	9.0	48.0	120	(mq)	2.0	10
(Carnation) 'Smooth'n Creamy' fruit on the bottom	8 oz	250	8.0	47.0	130	na	3.0	na
(Dannon) 'Fruit-on-the-Bottom'	8 oz	230	9.0	44.0	140	na	3.0	10

Food Name	Serv. Size	Total Cal.	Prot. GMS	Carbs GMS	Sod. MGS	Fiber GMS	Fat GMS	Chol. MGS
(Dannon) 'Light' nonfat	8 oz	100	9.0	17.0	135	na	0.0	5
(Knudsen) 'Cal 70'	6 oz	70	6.0	11.0	95	(mq)	0.0	0
(Light n' Lively)	8 oz	240	9.0	46.0	120	(mq)	2.0	15
(Light n' Lively)	4.4 oz	130	5.0	26.0	65	(mq)	1.0	10
(Light n' Lively) '100'	8 oz	100	9.0	16.0	115	(mq)	0.0	5
(Lite-Line) 'Swiss Style 1%'	8 oz	230	10.0	42.0	150	(mq)	2.0	(mq)
(Mountain High) 'Natural'	8 oz	220	10.0	31.0	140	na	6.0	na
(New Country) 'Lowfat' 'n cream	6 oz	150	5.0	31.0	90	(mq)	2.0	(mq)
(TCBY)	8 oz	220	9.0	36.0	150	na	2.0	na
(Weight Watchers) 'Ultimate 90'	8 oz	90	10.0	13.0	120	na	0.0	5
(Yogi) 'Sundae' peachy peach, w/gelatin	5.6 oz	50	6.0	14.0	75	na	<1.0	4
(Yoplait) 'Crunch 'N Yogurt' nonfat, w/granola	7 oz	220	8.0	43.0	125	na	2.0	5
(Yoplait) 'Fruit-on-the-Bottom'	6 oz	170	7.0	35.0	105	na	0.0	5
(Yoplait) 'Light' fat-free	6 oz	90	5.0	17.0	70	na	0.0	5
(Yoplait) 'Light Custard Style' fat-free	6 oz	90	6.0	17.0	85	na	0.0	5
(Yoplait) 'Original' 99% fat-free	6 oz	180	8.0	32.0	130	na	2.0	na
(Yoplait) 'Parfait Style' peach and vanilla	6 oz	200	8.0	34.0	120	na	3.0	na
PIÑA COLADA								
(Yoplait)	6 oz	190	8.0	32.0	110	(mq)	3.0	10
(Yoplait) 'Original' 99% fat-free	6 oz	180	8.0	32.0	130	na	2.0	na
PINEAPPLE								
(Breyers) 'Lowfat'	8 oz	250	9.0	50.0	120	(mq)	2.0	10
(Knudsen) 'Cal 70'	6 oz	70	6.0	12.0	125	(mq)	0.0	0
(Light n' Lively)	8 oz	230	9.0	47.0	120	(mq)	2.0	10
(Light n' Lively)	4.4 oz	130	5.0	26.0	65	(mq)	1.0	5
(Yoplait) 'Original' 99% fat-free	6 oz	180	8.0	32.0	130	na	2.0	na
PLAIN								
(Alta•Dena) nonfat	8 oz	100	13.0	13.0	160	na	<1.0	na
(Bison) 'Lowfat'	8 oz	150	12.0	17.0	180	0	4.0	10
(Bison) 'Nonfat'	8 oz	120	12.0	16.0	170	0	0.0	0
(Breyers) 'Lowfat'	8 oz	140	12.0	16.0	170	0	3.0	20
(Colombo)	8 oz	160	9.0	13.0	160	0	8.0	(mq)
(Colombo) 'Nonfat Lite'	8 oz	110	11.0	17.0	160	0	<1.0	5
(Crowley)	8 oz	160	10.0	14.0	150	0	8.0	30
(Crowley) 'Lowfat'	8 oz	140	12.0	17.0	180	0	2.0	10
(Crowley) 'Nonfat'	8 oz	120	13.0	17.0	180	0	<1.0	<1
(Dannon) 'Lowfat'	8 oz	140	10.0	16.0	160	0	4.0	15
(Dannon) 'Nonfat'	8 oz	110	11.0	16.0	160	0	0.0	5
(Friendship) 'Lowfat 1.5%'	8 oz	150	12.0	17.0	190	0	3.0	14
(Knudsen)	8 oz	200	12.0	16.0	170	0	9.0	35
(Knudsen) 'Lowfat'	8 oz	160	12.0	17.0	180	0	5.0	25
(Lite-Line) 'Swiss Style 1.5%'	8 oz	140	12.0	18.0	150	0	2.0	(mq)

Food Name	Serv. Size	Total Cal.	Prot. GMS	Carbs GMS	Sod. MGS	Fiber GMS	Fat GMS	Chol. MGS
(Meadow Gold) lowfat, 2% milkfat	8 oz	160	12.0	16.0	160	0	5.0	(mq)
(Mountain High)	8 oz	200	12.0	16.0	140	0	9.0	(mq)
(Weight Watchers) 'Nonfat'	8 oz	90	10.0	13.0	135	0	<1.0	5
(Yoplait)	6 oz	130	10.0	15.0	140	0	3.0	15
(Yoplait) fat-free	8 oz	120	13.0	17.0	170	na	0.0	10
(Yoplait) 'Nonfat'	8 oz	120	13.0	18.0	160	0	0.0	5
(Yoplait) 'Original' 98% fat-free	6 oz	120	10.0	15.0	150	na	2.0	15
RAINBOW PUNCH *(Yoplait)* 'Trix'	6 oz	190	9.0	31.0	120	na	3.0	na
RASPBERRY								
(Alta•Dena) 'Blended European Style'	8 oz	180	8.0	37.0	140	na	<1.0	na
(Dannon) 'Blended' fat-free	6 oz	150	8.0	30.0	110	na	0.0	5
(Dannon) 'Fruit-on-the-Bottom'	8 oz	240	9.0	45.0	140	na	3.0	10
(Dannon) 'Light' nonfat	8 oz	100	9.0	18.0	135	na	0.0	5
(Meadow Gold) 'Sundae Style' lowfat, natural	8 oz	250	10.0	42.0	160	na	4.0	na
(Mountain High) 'Honey Light' natural	8 oz	190	9.0	35.0	140	na	<1.0	5
(TCBY)	8 oz	220	9.0	42.0	150	na	2.0	na
(Weight Watchers) 'Ultimate 90'	8 oz	90	10.0	13.0	120	na	0.0	5
(Yoplait) fat-free 'Light'	6 oz	90	5.0	16.0	70	na	0.0	5
(Yoplait) 'Fruit-on-the-Bottom'	6 oz	170	7.0	35.0	105	na	0.0	5
(Yoplait) 'Original' 99% fat-free	6 oz	180	8.0	32.0	130	na	2.0	na
RED RASPBERRY								
(Alta•Dena) 'Naja' fruit-on-the-bottom	8 oz	240	12.0	40.0	150	na	4.0	na
(Breyers) 'Lowfat'	8 oz	250	9.0	48.0	120	(mq)	2.0	10
(Carnation) 'Smooth'n Creamy' fruit on the bottom	8 oz	250	8.0	47.0	130	na	3.0	na
(Knudsen) 'Cal 70'	6 oz	70	6.0	11.0	80	(mq)	0.0	5
(Light n' Lively)	8 oz	230	9.0	43.0	130	(mq)	2.0	10
(Light n' Lively)	4.4 oz	130	5.0	24.0	70	(mq)	1.0	5
(Light n' Lively) 'Free' nonfat	4.4 oz	50	4.0	8.0	60	(mq)	0.0	0
(Light n' Lively) '100'	8 oz	90	8.0	15.0	105	(mq)	0.0	0
(Meadow Gold) lowfat, 1.5% milkfat	8 oz	250	10.0	42.0	160	(mq)	4.0	(mq)
(New Country) 'Supreme'	6 oz	150	5.0	31.0	90	(mq)	2.0	(mq)
STRAWBERRY								
(Alta•Dena) 'Blended European Style'	8 oz	180	8.0	37.0	140	na	<1.0	na
(Alta•Dena) 'Maya' fruit-on-the-bottom	8 oz	280	11.0	39.0	170	na	9.0	na
(Alta•Dena) 'Naja' fruit-on-the-bottom	8 oz	240	12.0	40.0	150	na	4.0	na
(Breyers) 'Lowfat'	8 oz	250	9.0	48.0	120	(mq)	2.0	10
(Carnation) 'Smooth'n Creamy' fruit on the bottom	8 oz	230	8.0	44.0	115	na	3.0	na
(Colombo)	8 oz	210	8.0	29.0	140	(mq)	7.0	(mq)
(Crowley) 'Nonfat'	8 oz	190	12.0	35.0	190	(mq)	<1.0	<1
(Dannon) 'Blended' fat-free	6 oz	150	8.0	30.0	110	na	0.0	5

Food Name	Serv. Size	Total Cal.	Prot. GMS	Carbs GMS	Sod. MGS	Fiber GMS	Fat GMS	Chol. MGS
(Dannon) 'Fruit-on-the-Bottom'	8 oz	230	9.0	45.0	140	na	3.0	10
(Dannon) 'Light' nonfat	8 oz	100	9.0	17.0	135	na	0.0	5
(Dannon) 'Sprinkl'ins' lowfat	4.1 oz	140	5.0	24.0	95	na	2.0	5
(Knudsen) 'Cal 70'	6 oz	70	6.0	11.0	85	(mq)	0.0	0
(Knudsen) 'Lowfat'	8 oz	250	10.0	45.0	135	(mq)	4.0	15
(Light n' Lively)	8 oz	240	9.0	45.0	130	(mq)	2.0	15
(Light n' Lively)	4.4 oz	130	5.0	25.0	70	(mq)	1.0	10
(Light n' Lively) 'Free'	4.4 oz	50	4.0	8.0	60	(mq)	0.0	0
(Light n' Lively) '100'	8 oz	90	8.0	15.0	105	(mq)	0.0	5
(Lite-Line) 'Lowfat 1%'	8 oz	240	10.0	46.0	150	(mq)	2.0	(mq)
(Mountain High) 'Honey Light' natural	8 oz	190	9.0	35.0	140	na	<1.0	5
(New Country) 'Supreme'	6 oz	150	5.0	30.0	90	(mq)	2.0	(mq)
(TCBY)	8 oz	220	9.0	43.0	150	na	2.0	na
(Weight Watchers) 'Ultimate 90'	8 oz	90	10.0	13.0	120	na	0.0	5
(Yoplait) 'Custard Style'	6 oz	180	7.0	30.0	105	na	3.0	na
(Yoplait) 'Fruit-on-the-Bottom'	6 oz	170	7.0	35.0	105	na	0.0	5
(Yoplait) 'Light' fat-free	6 oz	90	5.0	16.0	70	na	0.0	5
(Yoplait) 'Light Custard Style' fat-free	6 oz	90	6.0	17.0	85	na	0.0	5
(Yoplait) 'Original' 99% fat-free	6 oz	180	8.0	32.0	130	na	2.0	na
(Yoplait) 'Parfait Style' strawberry and vanilla	6 oz	200	8.0	34.0	120	na	3.0	na
STRAWBERRY CHEESECAKE (Yogi) 'Sundae' w/gelatin	5.6 oz	50	6.0	14.0	75	na	<1.0	4
STRAWBERRY FRUIT BASKET (Knudsen) 'Cal 70'	6 oz	70	6.0	11.0	75	(mq)	0.0	5
STRAWBERRY FRUIT CUP								
(Dannon) 'Light' nonfat	8 oz	100	9.0	17.0	135	na	0.0	5
(Light n' Lively)	8 oz	240	9.0	47.0	120	(mq)	2.0	15
(Light n' Lively)	4.4 oz	130	5.0	26.0	65	(mq)	1.0	10
(Light n' Lively) 'Free' nonfat	4.4 oz	50	4.0	8.0	55	(mq)	0.0	0
(Light n' Lively) '100'	8 oz	90	8.0	15.0	100	(mq)	0.0	0
(New Country) 'Lowfat'	6 oz	150	5.0	30.0	85	(mq)	2.0	(mq)
STRAWBERRY-ALMOND (Yoplait) 'Breakfast Yogurt'	6 oz	200	8.0	38.0	90	2.0	3.0	10
STRAWBERRY-BANANA								
(Alta•Dena) nonfat, fruit-on-the-bottom	8 oz	180	12.0	35.0	128	na	<1.0	na
(Breyers) 'Lowfat'	8 oz	250	9.0	50.0	120	(mq)	2.0	10
(Carnation) 'Smooth'n Creamy' fruit on the bottom	8 oz	240	9.0	42.0	125	na	4.0	na
(Dannon) 'Fruit-on-the-Bottom'	8 oz	230	9.0	44.0	140	na	3.0	10
(Dannon) 'Light' nonfat	8 oz	100	9.0	17.0	135	na	0.0	<5
(Dannon) lowfat 'Sprinkl'ins'	4.1 oz	140	5.0	24.0	95	na	2.0	5
(Knudsen) 'Cal 70'	6 oz	70	6.0	12.0	80	(mq)	0.0	0

Food Name	Serv. Size	Total Cal.	Prot. GMS	Carbs GMS	Sod. MGS	Fiber GMS	Fat GMS	Chol. MGS
· (Light n' Lively)	8 oz	260	9.0	52.0	120	(mq)	2.0	10
(Light n' Lively)	4.4 oz	140	5.0	29.0	65	(mq)	1.0	5
(Light n' Lively) 'Free' nonfat	4.4 oz	50	4.0	8.0	60	na	0.0	0
(Mountain High) 'Honey Light' natural	8 oz	190	9.0	35.0	140	na	<1.0	5
(New Country)	6 oz	150	5.0	31.0	85	(mq)	2.0	(mq)
(TCBY)	8 oz	220	9.0	43.0	150	na	2.0	na
(Weight Watchers) 'Ultimate 90'	8 oz	90	10.0	13.0	120	na	0.0	5
(Yoplait) 'Breakfast' w/wheat and walnuts	6 oz	200	8.0	40.0	110	na	2.0	na
(Yoplait) 'Fruit-on-the-Bottom'	6 oz	170	7.0	35.0	105	na	0.0	5
(Yoplait) 'Light' fat-free	6 oz	90	5.0	16.0	70	na	0.0	5
(Yoplait) 'Original' 99% fat-free	6 oz	180	8.0	32.0	130	na	2.0	na
(Yoplait) 'Trix' bash	6 oz	190	9.0	31.0	120	na	3.0	na
STRAWBERRY-RHUBARB (Yoplait)	6 oz	190	8.0	32.0	110	(mq)	3.0	10
TRIPLE CHERRY (Yoplait) 'Trix'	6 oz	190	9.0	31.0	120	na	3.0	na
TROPICAL FRUIT								
(Dannon) 'Light' nonfat	8 oz	100	5.0	18.0	135	na	0.0	<5
(Ripple) '70'	6 oz	70	5.0	13.0	85	(mq)	0.0	5
(Weight Watchers) 'Ultimate 90'	8 oz	90	10.0	13.0	120	na	0.0	5
(Yoplait) 'Breakfast' w/wheat, raisins, and nuts	6 oz	200	8.0	41.0	110	na	3.0	na
VANILLA								
(Bison) 'Lowfat'	8 oz	210	11.0	33.0	160	0	4.0	10
(Breyers) 'Lowfat' vanilla bean	8 oz	230	11.0	41.0	150	0	3.0	20
(Colombo) French	8 oz	215	8.0	30.0	140	0	7.0	(mq)
(Colombo) 'Nonfat Lite'	8 oz	160	10.0	30.0	140	0	<1.0	5
(Crowley) 'Lowfat'	8 oz	200	12.0	33.0	170	0	2.0	10
(Dannon) 'Blended' French, fat-free	6 oz	150	7.0	31.0	100	na	0.0	5
(Dannon) 'Fresh Flavors'	8 oz	200	10.0	34.0	140	0	3.0	10
(Dannon) 'Fresh Flavors'	4.4 oz	110	5.0	20.0	90	0	2.0	5
(Dannon) 'Hearty Nuts & Raisins' w/wheat	8 oz	270	9.0	48.0	120	(mq)	5.0	10
(Dannon) 'Light' nonfat	8 oz	100	9.0	16.0	135	na	0.0	<5
(Friendship) 'Lowfat'	8 oz	210	11.0	35.0	170	0	3.0	14
(Knudsen) 'Cal 70'	6 oz	70	6.0	11.0	90	0	0.0	0
(Knudsen) 'Lowfat'	8 oz	240	11.0	43.0	135	0	4.0	15
(New Country) 'Lowfat' French	6 oz	150	5.0	31.0	90	0	2.0	(mq)
(Weight Watchers) 'Ultimate 90'	1 cup	90	10.0	13.0	120	na	0.0	5
(Yoplait)	6 oz	180	9.0	29.0	120	0	3.0	15
(Yoplait) 'Crunch 'N Yogurt' w/granola, nonfat	7 oz	220	8.0	43.0	125	na	2.0	5
(Yoplait) 'Custard Style'	6 oz	180	7.0	30.0	110	0	4.0	20
(Yoplait) 'Custard Style'	4 oz	130	5.0	20.0	70	0	3.0	15
(Yoplait) 'Fat-free'	6 oz	150	8.0	28.0	110	0	0.0	5
(Yoplait) 'Light Custard Style' fat-free	6 oz	90	6.0	17.0	85	na	0.0	5

Food Name	Serv. Size	Total Cal.	Prot. GMS	Carbs GMS	Sod. MGS	Fiber GMS	Fat GMS	Chol. MGS
(Yoplait) 'Nonfat'	8 oz	180	11.0	35.0	140	0	0.0	5
WILD BERRY *(Light n' Lively)* lowfat,								
1% milkfat, cultured	4.4 oz	140	5.0	28.0	70	na	1.0	5
YOGURT, FROZEN								
(Alta•Dena) apricot mango, nonfat	4 oz	90	3.0	20.0	210	na	0.0	0
(Baskin Robbins) See Part III.								
(Ben & Jerry's)								
apple pie	1/2 cup	170	4.0	32.0	90	0	3.0	10
banana strawberry	1/2 cup	160	4.0	32.0	60	1.0	2.0	5
blueberry	1/2 cup	160	4.0	32.0	60	1.0	2.0	5
cherry Garcia	1/2 cup	170	4.0	31.0	70	0	3.0	10
chocolate fudge brownie	1/2 cup	190	6.0	35.0	130	2.0	4.0	10
chocolate raspberry swirl	1/2 cup	200	5.0	40.0	72	1.0	2.5	5
coffee almond fudge	1/2 cup	200	6.0	30.0	82	1.0	7.0	15
English toffee crunch	1/2 cup	190	4.0	32.0	110	0	6.0	10
(Bison) chocolate	3.5 oz	94	3.0	18.0	50	(tr)	2.0	5
(Breyers)								
black cherry	1/2 cup	120	3.0	24.0	50	(tr)	1.0	10
chocolate	1/2 cup	120	3.0	24.0	65	(tr)	1.0	10
peach	1/2 cup	110	3.0	22.0	50	(tr)	1.0	10
red raspberry	1/2 cup	120	3.0	23.0	50	(tr)	1.0	10
strawberry	1/2 cup	110	3.0	22.0	45	(tr)	1.0	10
strawberry-banana	1/2 cup	110	3.0	22.0	45	(tr)	1.0	10
vanilla	1/2 cup	120	3.0	23.0	55	0	1.0	15
(Colombo)								
banana split, lowfat, 'Sundae Style'	3 oz	100	2.0	20.0	50	na	1.0	5
Bavarian chocolate chunk, 'Gourmet'	3 oz	120	3.0	18.0	40	(tr)	4.0	10
caramel fudge sundae, lowfat,								
'Sundae Style'	3 oz	100	3.0	21.0	60	na	1.0	5
caramel-pecan chunk, 'Gourmet'	3 oz	120	4.0	19.0	150	(tr)	3.0	10
chocolate peanut butter twist,								
'Sundae Style'	3 oz	110	3.0	18.0	65	na	3.0	5
dream, 'Gourmet'	3 oz	90	3.0	16.0	45	0	2.0	10
Heath bar crunch, 'Gourmet'	3 oz	130	3.0	19.0	75	(tr)	5.0	15
mocha Swiss almond, 'Gourmet'	3 oz	120	3.0	17.0	45	(tr)	5.0	10
nonfat, lite	4 oz	95	4.0	21.0	70	na	0.0	0
peanut butter cup, 'Gourmet'	3 oz	140	4.0	16.0	90	(tr)	7.0	5
plain, lowfat	4 oz	99	3.0	18.0	35	na	2.0	10
plain, 'Nonfat Lite'	4 oz	95	4.0	21.0	70	na	0.0	0
strawberry passion, 'Gourmet'	3 oz	100	1.0	18.0	40	(tr)	2.0	5
wild raspberry cheesecake, 'Gourmet'	3 oz	100	2.0	18.0	40	(tr)	2.0	5
(Crowley)								
cherry	3 oz	80	2.0	16.0	40	(tr)	1.0	5

Food Name	Serv. Size	Total Cal.	Prot. GMS	Carbs GMS	Sod. MGS	Fiber GMS	Fat GMS	Chol. MGS
chocolate	3 oz	80	2.0	15.0	40	(tr)	2.0	10
peach	3 oz	80	2.0	16.0	40	(tr)	1.0	5
raspberry	3 oz	80	2.0	16.0	40	(tr)	1.0	5
strawberry	3 oz	80	2.0	16.0	40	(tr)	1.0	5
vanilla	3 oz	80	2.0	15.0	40	0	2.0	10
(Dannon)								
cappuccino, nonfat, 'Light'	4 oz	80	4.0	19.0	70	na	0.0	0
caramel pecan, 'Pure Indulgence'	4 oz	180	4.0	22.0	70	na	8.0	20
cherry vanilla swirl, nonfat, 'Light'	4 oz	90	4.0	21.0	65	na	0.0	0
chocolate, nonfat, 'Light'	4 oz	80	4.0	19.0	70	na	<1.0	0
chocolate, 'Pure Indulgence'	3 oz	130	5.0	24.0	75	na	3.0	10
chocolate nut, chunky, 'Pure Indulgence'	4 oz	190	5.0	24.0	60	na	9.0	20
chunky chocolate nut, 'Pure Indulgence'	4 oz	190	5.0	24.0	60	na	9.0	20
cookies and cream, 'Pure Indulgence'	4 oz	180	4.0	18.0	95	na	7.0	20
Heath bar crunch, 'Pure Indulgence'	4 oz	170	4.0	25.0	100	na	7.0	25
peach, nonfat, 'Light'	4 oz	80	4.0	19.0	70	na	0.0	0
red raspberry, nonfat, 'Light'	4 oz	90	3.0	21.0	65	(tr)	0.0	0
strawberry, nonfat, 'Light'	4 oz	80	4.0	19.0	70	na	0.0	0
vanilla, nonfat, 'Light'	4 oz	80	4.0	20.0	70	na	0.0	0
vanilla, 'Pure Indulgence'	3 oz	130	5.0	25.0	50	na	3.0	10
(Dreyer's)								
black cherry vanilla, nonfat, 'Inspirations'	4 oz	90	4.0	19.0	80	na	0.0	0
blueberry, 'Inspirations'	3 oz	80	2.0	15.0	40	(tr)	1.0	5
cherry, 'Inspirations'	3 oz	80	2.0	15.0	40	(tr)	1.0	5
chocolate, 'Inspirations'	3 oz	80	2.0	15.0	40	(tr)	1.0	5
peach, 'Inspirations Perfectly Peach'	3 oz	80	2.0	15.0	40	(tr)	1.0	5
raspberry, 'Inspirations'	3 oz	80	2.0	15.0	40	(tr)	1.0	5
strawberry, 'Inspirations'	3 oz	80	2.0	15.0	40	(tr)	1.0	5
strawberry-banana, 'Inspirations'	3 oz	80	2.0	15.0	40	(tr)	1.0	5
vanilla chocolate swirl, nonfat, 'Inspirations'	4 oz	90	4.0	19.0	85	na	0.0	0
vanilla-raspberry swirl, 'Inspirations'	3 oz	80	2.0	15.0	45	(tr)	1.0	5
(Elan) chocolate almond	1/2 cup	160	5.0	23.0	65	(tr)	7.0	(mq)
(Häagen-Dazs)								
chocolate	3 oz	130	6.0	21.0	40	(tr)	3.0	25
peach	3 oz	120	4.0	20.0	30	(tr)	3.0	31
praline pandemonium, 'Exträas'	4 oz	240	7.0	33.0	115	na	9.0	45
strawberry	3 oz	120	4.0	21.0	30	(tr)	3.0	29
strawberry cheesecake craze, 'Exträas'	4 oz	210	7.0	31.0	100	na	7.0	50
vanilla almond crunch	3 oz	150	5.0	22.0	65	(tr)	5.0	33
(Natural Nectar) chocolate, 'Fi-Bar Lite'	2.5 oz	190	4.0	29.0	140	na	6.0	5
(Sealtest)								
black cherry, nonfat, 'Free'	1/2 cup	110	2.0	24.0	50	(tr)	0.0	0
chocolate, nonfat, 'Free'	1/2 cup	110	3.0	24.0	55	(tr)	0.0	0

Food Name	Serv. Size	Total Cal.	Prot. GMS	Carbs GMS	Sod. MGS	Fiber GMS	Fat GMS	Chol. MGS
peach, nonfat, 'Free'	1/2 cup	100	2.0	23.0	35	(tr)	0.0	0
red raspberry, nonfat, 'Free'	1/2 cup	100	2.0	23.0	40	(tr)	0.0	0
strawberry, nonfat, 'Free'	1/2 cup	100	2.0	22.0	35	(tr)	0.0	0
(TCBY) See Part III.								
YOGURT, FROZEN, SOFT-SERVE								
(Bresler's)								
'Gourmet' all flavors, 1 oz	1/2 cup	29	0.9	5.5	15	(tr)	0.5	2
'Lite' all flavors, 1 oz	1/2 cup	27	1.1	6.0	11	(tr)	0.0	0
(Crowley)								
banana, 'Peaks of Perfection,' 3.5 oz	1/2 cup	100	3.0	19.0	50	(tr)	2.0	5
chocolate, 'Peaks of Perfection,' 3.5 oz	1/2 cup	100	4.0	19.0	60	(tr)	2.0	5
lemon, 'Peaks of Perfection,' 3.5 oz	1/2 cup	100	3.0	19.0	50	(tr)	2.0	5
plain, 'Peaks of Perfection,' 3.5 oz	1/2 cup	90	2.0	20.0	40	0	1.0	5
raspberry, 'Peaks of Perfection,' 3.5 oz	1/2 cup	100	3.0	19.0	50	(tr)	2.0	5
strawberry, 'Peaks of Perfection,' 3.5 oz	1/2 cup	100	3.0	19.0	50	(tr)	2.0	5
vanilla, 'Peaks of Perfection,' 3.5 oz	1/2 cup	100	3.0	19.0	50	0	2.0	5
(Dannon)								
blueberry	1/2 cup	100	3.0	18.0	50	(tr)	2.0	5
butter pecan	1/2 cup	100	3.0	18.0	55	(tr)	2.0	5
cappuccino	1/2 cup	100	3.0	18.0	55	0	2.0	5
cheesecake	1/2 cup	100	4.0	18.0	55	0	2.0	5
chocolate	1/2 cup	120	5.0	23.0	65	(tr)	2.0	5
lemon meringue	1/2 cup	100	4.0	18.0	55	(tr)	2.0	5
peach	1/2 cup	100	4.0	18.0	55	(tr)	2.0	5
piña colada	1/2 cup	100	4.0	18.0	55	(tr)	2.0	5
raspberry	1/2 cup	100	3.0	18.0	50	(tr)	2.0	5
red raspberry, 'Nonfat'	1/2 cup	90	3.0	21.0	65	(tr)	0.0	0
strawberry	1/2 cup	100	3.0	18.0	50	(tr)	2.0	5
strawberry-banana	1/2 cup	100	3.0	18.0	50	(tr)	2.0	5
(Häagen-Dazs)								
banana, nonfat	1 oz	25	1.0	5.0	15	na	0.0	0
chocolate	1 oz	30	1.0	4.0	13	(tr)	1.0	3
chocolate, nonfat	1 oz	30	1.0	6.0	20	(tr)	0.0	0
coffee	1 oz	28	1.0	4.0	13	0	1.0	3
raspberry	1 oz	30	1.0	5.0	15	na	1.0	3
strawberry, nonfat	1 oz	25	1.0	5.0	10	na	0.0	0
vanilla	1 oz	28	1.0	4.0	13	0	1.0	3
YOGURT BAR, FROZEN								
(Dole)								
cherry 'Fruit & Yogurt'	1 bar	80	2.0	17.0	22	na	<1.0	na
raspberry 'Fruit & Yogurt'	1 bar	70	1.0	17.0	18	na	<1.0	na
strawberry 'Fruit & Yogurt'	1 bar	70	1.0	17.0	16	na	<1.0	na

Food Name	Serv. Size	Total Cal.	Prot. GMS	Carbs GMS	Sod. MGS	Fiber GMS	Fat GMS	Chol. MGS
(Häagen-Dazs)								
cherry chocolate fudge	1 bar	230	5.0	28.0	50	na	12.0	35
peach	1 bar	100	2.0	18.0	20	na	1.0	15
piña colada	1 bar	100	2.0	21.0	25	na	1.0	15
raspberry and vanilla	1 bar	100	3.0	19.0	20	na	1.0	15
strawberry daiquiri	1 bar	100	2.0	20.0	20	na	1.0	20
tropical orange passion	1 bar	100	2.0	21.0	30	na	1.0	20
YOGURT DESSERT *(Sara Lee)*								
'Free & Light'	1/10 pkg	120	2.0	26.0	90	na	1.0	0
YOGURT FLAVORED DRINK								
(Dannon) all flavors	8 oz	190	6.0	32.0	110	(tr)	4.0	10
(Yogloo) fruit basket	10 oz	170	3.0	40.0	80	na	0.0	na
(Yogloo) original	10 oz	170	3.0	40.0	80	na	0.0	na
(Yogloo) peach	10 oz	170	3.0	40.0	80	na	0.0	na
(Yogloo) strawberry	10 oz	170	3.0	40.0	80	na	0.0	na

Z

Food Name	Serv. Size	Total Cal.	Prot. GMS	Carbs GMS	Sod. MGS	Fiber GMS	Fat GMS	Chol. MGS
ZITI ENTREE, FROZEN								
(Budget Gourmet) 'Side Dish' in marinara								
sauce	6.25 oz	220	9.0	25.0	380	(mq)	9.0	15
ZUCCHINI. See also SQUASH, SUMMER.								
baby, raw	1 large	3	0.4	0.5	0	na	0.1	0
baby, raw	1 med	2	0.3	0.3	0	na	0.0	0
boiled, drained	4 oz	18	0.7	4.5	3	>.6 c	0.1	0
raw	1 lb	62	5.0	12.5	11	2.2	0.6	0
raw, trimmed	1 oz	4	0.3	0.8	1	.1	<.1	0
w/skin, boiled, drained, mashed	1/2 cup	19	0.8	4.7	4	1.7	0.1	0
w/skin, boiled, drained, sliced	1/2 cup	14	0.6	3.5	3	1.3	0.0	0
w/skin, raw, sliced	1/2 cup	9	0.8	1.9	2	.8	0.1	0
Canned								
in tomato juice	1/2 cup	33	1.2	7.8	424	>.6 c	0.1	0
Italian style	1/2 cup	33	1.2	7.8	426	>.6 c	0.1	0
(Del Monte) in tomato sauce	1/2 cup	30	1.0	8.0	485	(mq)	0.0	0
(Progresso) Italian style	1/2 cup	50	1.0	8.0	540	2.0	2.0	<1
Frozen								
w/skin, unprepared	10-oz pkg	48	3.3	10.2	6	3.4	0.4	0
(Seabrook)	3.3 oz	16	1.0	3.0	2	>1.0 c	0.0	0
(Southern)	3.5 oz	18	1.2	3.6	20	(mq)	0.1	0
(Stilwell) 'Quick Krisp' breaded	3.3 oz	200	4.0	24.0	410	(mq)	10.0	15